LIBRARY
NSCC WATERD
60 MAYO FLA...
DARTMOUTH, NS B2Y 0A5 CANADA

W9-AEX-804

BERKOWITZ'S
Pediatrics
A PRIMARY CARE APPROACH

5th Edition

Carol D. Berkowitz, MD, FAAP

Distinguished Professor of Clinical Pediatrics
David Geffen School of Medicine at
University of California Los Angeles
Executive Vice Chair
Department of Pediatrics
Harbor-UCLA Medical Center
Torrance, CA

American Academy of Pediatrics
141 Northwest Point Blvd
Elk Grove Village, IL 60007-1019

American Academy of Pediatrics Department of Marketing and Publications Staff

Maureen DeRosa, MPA
Director, Department of Marketing and Publications

Mark Grimes
Director, Division of Product Development

Alain Park
Senior Product Development Editor

Carrie Peters
Editorial Assistant

Sandi King, MS
Director, Division of Publishing and Production Services

Theresa Wiener
Manager, Publications Production and Manufacturing

Jason Crase
Manager, Editorial Services

Houston Adams
Digital Content and Production Specialist

Julia Lee
Director, Division of Marketing and Sales

Linda Smessaert
Brand Manager, Clinical and Professional Publications

Library of Congress Control Number: 2013949728

ISBN: 978-1-58110-846-0

eISBN: 978-1-58110-851-4

MA0699

The recommendations in this publication do not indicate an exclusive course of treatment or serve as a standard of care. Variations, taking into account individual circumstances, may be appropriate.

Brand names are furnished for identification purposes only. No endorsement of the manufacturers or products mentioned is implied.

Every effort has been made to ensure that the drug selection and dosages set forth in this text are in accordance with the current recommendations and practice at the time of publication. It is the responsibility of the health care professional to check the package insert of each drug for any change in indications and dosages and for added warnings and precautions.

The publishers have made every effort to trace the copyright holders for borrowed material. If they have inadvertently overlooked any, they will be pleased to make the necessary arrangements at the first opportunity.

Berkowitz's Pediatrics: A Primary Care Approach, 5th Edition

Copyright © 2014 American Academy of Pediatrics. All Rights Reserved. No part of this publication may be reproduced or transmitted in any form or by any means, electronic or mechanical, including photocopying, recording, or any information retrieval system, without written permission from the Publisher (e-mail permissions editor at marketing@aap.org).

Copyright © 2000, 1996 W.B. Saunders Company

Printed in the United States of America.

9-347/0614

1 2 3 4 5 6 7 8 9 10

Preface

The expansion of immunizations has reduced or eliminated many of the infectious diseases that confronted the children and adolescents for whom pediatric clinicians cared. New and more challenging morbidities, including obesity, violence, and mental health concerns, confront pediatric patients, their families, and their health care professionals. This fifth edition of *Berkowitz's Pediatrics: A Primary Care Approach* examines a series of emerging entities that pediatricians are expected to be knowledgeable about and able to address. The edition also updates information about the ever-changing health care scene. Because we interface with other disciplines and are increasingly working as members of health care teams, we must be equipped to understand the principles of their practices and communicate effectively with them. And lastly, our multicultural society includes children from all parts of the world and from all kinds of families, and we need to be prepared to address their needs.

My thanks to all the contributors and to the staff of the American Academy of Pediatrics, especially Alain Park, Jason Crase, Carrie Peters, Linda Smessaert, and Theresa Wiener, and my assistant, Claudette Hoskins, for all their help.

Carol D. Berkowitz

Contributors

Sudhir K. Anand, MD
Emeritus Professor of Clinical Pediatrics
David Geffen School of Medicine at University of California Los Angeles
Chief, Division of Pediatric Nephrology
Harbor-UCLA Medical Center
Torrance, CA

David Atkinson, MD
Associate Professor of Clinical Pediatrics
David Geffen School of Medicine at University of California Los Angeles
Division of Pediatric Cardiology
Harbor-UCLA Medical Center
Torrance, CA

Sarah J. Atunah-Jay, MD, MPH
T32 Research Fellow, Division of Medicine
The Warren Alpert School of Medicine
Brown University
Providence, RI

Justine Bacchetta, MD, PhD
Department of Pediatrics
David Geffen School of Medicine at University of California Los Angeles
Los Angeles, CA

Andrew J. Barnes, MD, MPH
Assistant Professor of Developmental-Behavioral Pediatrics
Division of Academic General Pediatrics
University of Minnesota
Minneapolis, MN

Lindsay S. Baron, MD
Attending Physician, Pediatric and General Radiology
Lowell General Hospital
Lowell, MA

Maneesh Batra, MD, MPH
Associate Professor of Pediatrics
University of Washington School of Medicine
Seattle, WA

Andrew K. Battenberg, MD
Resident, Department of Orthopaedic Surgery
Harbor-UCLA Medical Center
Torrance, CA

Carol D. Berkowitz, MD
Distinguished Professor of Clinical Pediatrics
David Geffen School of Medicine at University of California Los Angeles
Executive Vice Chair, Department of Pediatrics
Harbor-UCLA Medical Center
Torrance, CA

Karen C. Bodnar, MD, IBCLC
Assistant Clinical Professor of Pediatrics
Harbor-UCLA Medical Center
Torrance, CA

Emily Borman-Shoap, MD
Assistant Professor of Pediatrics
Pediatric Residency Program Director
University of Minnesota
Minneapolis, MN

Iris Wagman Borowsky, MD, PhD
Associate Professor and Director
Division of General Pediatrics and Adolescent Health
Department of Pediatrics
University of Minnesota
Minneapolis, MN

Calla R. Brown, MD
Resident, Departments of Internal Medicine and Pediatrics
University of Minnesota
Minneapolis, MN

Casey Buitenhuys, MD
Clinical Instructor of Medicine
David Geffen School of Medicine at University of California Los Angeles
Fellow, Pediatric Emergency Medicine
Harbor-UCLA Medical Center
Torrance, CA

David B. Burbulys, MD
Professor of Medicine
David Geffen School of Medicine at University of California Los Angeles
Associate Director, Emergency Medicine Residency Program
Harbor-UCLA Medical Center
Torrance, CA

Jonnie Burton-Mota, MD
Assistant Clinical Professor of Pediatrics
Division of Pediatric Hospital Medicine
Harbor-UCLA Medical Center
Torrance, CA

Kelly Callahan, MD, MPT
Assistant Professor of Pediatrics
David Geffen School of Medicine at University of California Los Angeles
Harbor-UCLA Medical Center
Torrance, CA

Gangadarshni Chandramohan, MD, MS
Associate Professor of Pediatrics
David Geffen School of Medicine at University of California Los Angeles
Division of Pediatric Nephrology
Harbor-UCLA Medical Center
Torrance, CA

Grant P. Christman, MD
Assistant Professor of Clinical Pediatrics
Keck School of Medicine of the University of Southern California
Division of Hospital Medicine
Children's Hospital Los Angeles
Los Angeles, CA

Noah Craft, MD, PhD
Los Angeles Biomedical Research Institute
Torrance, CA
Medicine-Pediatrics Resident
University of Minnesota
Minneapolis, MN

Catherine A. DeRidder, MD
Assistant Professor of Clinical Pediatrics
Keck School of Medicine of the University of Southern California
Los Angeles County & University of Southern California Medical Center
Los Angeles, CA

Alejandro Diaz, MD
La Maestra Community Health Centers
San Diego, CA

Sabrina D. Diaz, MA, MMFT
Los Angeles Biomedical Research Institute
Harbor-UCLA Medical Center
Torrance, CA

Steven Donohoe, BS
David Geffen School of Medicine at University of California Los Angeles
Los Angeles, CA

Robin Winkler Doroshow, MD, MMS, MEd
Associate Professor of Pediatrics
The George Washington University School of Medicine and Health Sciences
Pediatric Cardiologist
Children's National Medical Center
Associate Professor of Pediatrics
Georgetown University School of Medicine
Director, Division of Pediatric Cardiology
Georgetown University Hospital
Washington, DC

Nima Eftekhary, MD
Resident Physician, Department of Orthopaedic Surgery
New York University Hospital for Joint Diseases
New York, NY

Melissa K. Egge, MD
Santa Clara Valley Medical Center
San Jose, CA

W. Suzanne Eidson-Ton, MD, MS
Health Sciences Associate Clinical Professor of Family and Community Medicine
University of California Davis School of Medicine
Sacramento, CA

Nwando Eze, MD
Department of Pediatrics
Orange, CA

Andrea Fang, MD
Pediatric Emergency Medicine Fellow and Health Sciences Clinical Instructor
Harbor-UCLA Medical Center
Torrance, CA

Marianne Gausche-Hill, MD
Professor of Clinical Medicine
David Geffen School of Medicine at University of California Los Angeles
Vice Chair and Chief, Division of Pediatric Emergency Medicine
Director, Pediatric Emergency Medicine and EMS Fellowships
Harbor-UCLA Medical Center
Torrance, CA

George Gershman, MD
Professor of Pediatrics
David Geffen School of Medicine at University of California Los Angeles
Chief, Division of Pediatric Gastroenterology and Nutrition, Department of Pediatrics
Harbor-UCLA Medical Center
Torrance, CA

Rick Goldstein, MD
Attending Physician in Pediatric Palliative Care
Dana-Farber Cancer Institute
Boston Children's Hospital
Harvard Medical School
Boston, MA

Geeta Grover, MD
Developmental and Behavioral Pediatrician
The Center for Autism and Neurodevelopmental Disorders
Santa Ana, CA
Children's Hospital of Orange County, Orange, CA
Associate Clinical Professor of Pediatrics
Irvine College of Medicine
University of California, Irvine
Irvine, CA

H. Mollie Greves Grow, MD, MPH
Assistant Professor of Pediatrics
University of Washington
Research Faculty
Seattle Children's Research Institute

Mark Hanudel, MD
Pediatric Nephrology
UCLA Medical Center
Los Angeles, CA

Thomas R. Hawn, MD, PhD
Professor, Department of Medicine
Division of Allergy and Infectious Diseases
University of Washington School of Medicine
Seattle, WA

Kenneth R. Huff, MD
Professor of Pediatrics and Neurology
David Geffen School of Medicine at University of California Los Angeles
Chief, Division of Neurology, Department of Pediatrics
Harbor-UCLA Medical Center
Torrance, CA

Lynn Hunt, MD
Clinical Professor of Pediatrics
University of California, Irvine
Santa Ana, CA

Stanley H. Inkelis, MD
Professor of Pediatrics
David Geffen School of Medicine at University of California Los Angeles
Director, Pediatric Emergency Medicine
Harbor-UCLA Medical Center
Torrance, CA

Walter Jimenez, MD
Institute for Cancer Care
Mercy Medical Center
Baltimore, MD

Jesse Joad, MD, MS
Professor of Pediatrics
Associate Dean Diversity and Faculty Life Emerita
University of California, Davis
Davis, CA

Doron D. Kahana, MD
Assistant Clinical Professor of Pediatrics
David Geffen School of Medicine at University of California Los Angeles
Division of Pediatric Gastroenterology, Hepatology & Nutrition
Harbor-UCLA Medical Center
Torrance, CA

Tom Kallay, MD
Associate Professor of Pediatrics
David Geffen School of Medicine at University of California Los Angeles
Director, Simulation and Skills Center, Division of Pediatric Critical Care
Harbor-UCLA Medical Center
Torrance, CA

Elaine S. Kamil, MD
Health Sciences Professor of Pediatrics
David Geffen School of Medicine at University of California Los Angeles
Director, Pediatric Nephrology
Cedars-Sinai Medical Center
Los Angeles, CA

Khalid M. Khan, MD
Department of Pediatrics
Georgetown University Medical Center
Washington, DC

Jane S. Kim, MD
Assistant Professor, Pediatric Radiology
Department of Diagnostic Radiology & Nuclear Medicine
University of Maryland Medical Center
Baltimore, MD

Kenny Yat-Choi Kwong, MD
Chief, Division of Allergy-Immunology
Associate Clinical Professor of Pediatrics
Department of Pediatrics
Harbor-UCLA Medical Center
Torrance, CA

Kathy K. Langevin, MD, MPH
Assistant Clinical Professor, Dermatology
David Geffen School of Medicine at University of California Los Angeles
Los Angeles, CA

Joseph L. Lasky III, MD
Clinical Associate Professor, Pediatrics and Neurosurgery
David Geffen School of Medicine at University of California Los Angeles
Chief, Pediatric Hematology/Oncology
Harbor-UCLA Medical Center/Los Angeles Biomedical Research Institute
Torrance, CA

Steve L. Lee, MD
Associate Professor of Surgery and Pediatrics
David Geffen School of Medicine at University of California Los Angeles
Chief of Pediatric Surgery
Harbor-UCLA Medical Center
Torrance, CA

Charlotte W. Lewis, MD, MPH
Associate Professor, Department of Pediatrics
Divisions of General Pediatrics and Craniofacial Medicine
Adjunct Associate Professor, Pediatric Dentistry
University of Washington School of Medicine
Seattle, WA

Catherine S. Mao, MD
Associate Professor of Clinical Pediatrics
David Geffen School of Medicine at University of California Los Angeles
Division of Pediatric Endocrinology
Harbor-UCLA Medical Center/Los Angeles Biomedical Research Institute
Torrance, CA

Kevin Madden, MD
Fellow, Harvard Palliative Medicine Fellowship Program
Dana-Farber Cancer Institute
Boston Children's Hospital
Harvard Medical School
Boston, MA

Deborah McCurdy, MD
Professor, Department of Pediatrics
Division of Allergy, Immunology, Rheumatology
David Geffen School of Medicine at University of California Los Angeles
Los Angeles, CA

ChrisAnna M. Mink, MD
Clinical Professor of Pediatrics
David Geffen School of Medicine at University of California Los Angeles
Department of Pediatrics
Harbor-UCLA Medical Center
Torrance, CA

Julie E. Noble, MD
Clinical Professor of Pediatrics
David Geffen School of Medicine at University of California Los Angeles
Director, Pediatric Managed Care
Director, Low Risk Nursery
Harbor-UCLA Medical Center
Torrance, CA

Suzinne Pak-Gorstein, MD, PhD, MPH
Assistant Professor, Department of Pediatrics
University of Washington School of Medicine
Codirector, Global Health Pathways
Seattle Children's Hospital
Seattle, WA

Eduard H. Panosyan, MD
Assistant Clinical Professor of Pediatrics
David Geffen School of Medicine at University of California Los Angeles
Division of Pediatric Hematology/Oncology
Harbor-UCLA Medical Center
Los Angeles Biomedical Research Institute
Torrance, CA

Miriam F. Parsa, MD, MPH
Assistant Clinical Professor, Department of Pediatrics, Division of Rheumatology
David Geffen School of Medicine at University of California Los Angeles
Los Angeles, CA

Bonnie R. Rachman, MD
Professor of Pediatrics
David Geffen School of Medicine at University of California Los Angeles
Division of Pediatric Critical Care
Harbor-UCLA Medical Center
Torrance, CA

Christian B. Ramers, MD, MPH
Assistant Medical Director, Research /Special Populations
Family Health Centers of San Diego
San Diego, CA

Joseph Ravera, MD
Fellow in Pediatric Emergency Medicine
Harbor-UCLA Medical Center
Torrance, CA

Nasser Redjal, MD
Professor of Clinical Pediatrics and Allergy/Immunology
David Geffen School of Medicine at University of California Los Angeles
Director, Allergy/Immunology Managed Care
Harbor-UCLA Medical Center
Torrance, CA

Katherine E. Remick, MD
Clinical Instructor of Pediatrics
David Geffen School of Medicine at University of California Los Angeles
Fellow, Pediatric Emergency Medicine
Harbor-UCLA Medical Center
Torrance, CA

Teresa Rosales, MD
Clinical Professor of Ophthalmology
David Geffen School of Medicine at University of California Los Angeles
Jules Stein Eye Institute
Pediatric Ophthalmologist, Private Practice
Long Beach, CA

Timothy K. Ruttan, MD
Dell Children's Medical Center of Central Texas
Pediatric Emergency Medicine
University of Texas Southwestern at Austin
Austin, TX

Isidro B. Salusky, MD
Professor of Pediatrics
David Geffen School of Medicine at University of California Los Angeles
Director, Pediatric Dialysis Program
Program Director, General Clinical Research Center
University of California Los Angeles
Los Angeles, CA

Nefthi Sandeep, MD
Fellow, Division of Pediatric Cardiology, Department of Pediatrics
Children's National Medical Center
Washington, DC
Research Fellow
National Heart, Lung, and Blood Institute
National Institutes of Health
Bethesda, MD

Lucinda S. Santos, MHA
Los Angeles Biomedical Research Institute at Harbor-UCLA
Torrance, CA

Eric R. Schmitt, MD, MPH
Assistant Clinical Professor of Emergency Medicine
University of California, San Francisco, Fresno Medical
Education Program
Attending Physician, Department of Emergency Medicine
Community Regional Medical Center
Fresno, CA
Attending Physician, Department of Emergency Medicine
Children's Hospital of Central California
Madera, CA

Erica Sibinga, MD, MHS
Assistant Professor of Pediatrics
Johns Hopkins School of Medicine
Baltimore, MD

Monica Sifuentes, MD
Professor of Clinical Pediatrics
David Geffen School of Medicine at University of California Los Angeles
Associate Program Director, Vice Chair of Education, Department
of Pediatrics
Harbor-UCLA Medical Center
Torrance, CA

Lynne M. Smith, MD
Professor of Clinical Pediatrics
David Geffen School of Medicine at University of California Los Angeles
Vice Chair for Academy Affairs, Department of Pediatrics, Division
of Neonatology
Harbor-UCLA Medical Center
Torrance, CA

Blanca Solis, MD
Associate Physician
Primary Care Network
University of California, Davis
Davis, CA

Robin Steinberg-Epstein, MD
Director of Developmental and Behavioral Pediatrics and Clinical
Professor of Pediatrics
University of California, Irvine School of Medicine and Children's Hospital
of Orange County
Developmental Behavioral Pediatrician
For OC Kids Neurodevelopmental Center

Kenneth W. Steinhoff, MD
Associate Clinical Professor, Department of Pediatrics
Child Psychiatrist
Child Development Center, Department of Pediatrics
University of California, Irvine
Irvine, CA

Miriam T. Stewart, BA
Johns Hopkins School of Medicine
Baltimore, MD

Sara T. Stewart, MD
Associate Professor of Pediatrics
David Geffen School of Medicine at University of California Los Angeles
Harbor-UCLA Medical Center
Torrance, CA

Benjamin H. Taragin, MD
Associate Professor of Radiology and Pediatrics
Director, Pediatric Radiology
Division of Radiology
Children's Hospital at Montefiore
Montefiore Medical Center of The Albert Einstein College of Medicine
Bronx, NY

Alan Tomines, MD
Associate Clinical Professor of Pediatrics and Health Services
David Geffen School of Medicine at University of California Los Angeles
and UCLA Fielding School of Public Health
Harbor-UCLA Medical Center
Torrance, CA

Hendry Ton, MD, MS
Health Sciences Associate Clinical Professor of Psychiatry and
Behavioral Sciences
University of California Davis School of Medicine
Davis, CA

Derek Wong, MD
Assistant Professor of Clinical Pediatrics
David Geffen School of Medicine at University of California Los Angeles
Division of Medical Genetics
Harbor-UCLA Medical Center
Torrance, CA

Jennifer K. Yee, MD
Assistant Professor of Pediatrics
David Geffen School of Medicine at University of California Los Angeles
Division of Pediatric Endocrinology
Harbor-UCLA Medical Center
Torrance, CA

Ki-Young Yoo, MD
Assistant Clinical Professor, Division of Dermatology, Department
of Medicine
David Geffen School of Medicine at University of California Los Angeles
Los Angeles, CA

Kelly D. Young, MD, MS
Health Sciences Clinical Professor of Pediatrics
David Geffen School of Medicine at University of California Los Angeles
Department of Emergency Medicine
Harbor-UCLA Medical Center
Torrance, CA

David P. Zamorano, MD
Assistant Professor, Department of Orthopaedic Surgery
California School of Medicine, Irvine
Irvine, CA

Contents

SECTION II

Health Maintenance and Anticipatory Guidance

SECTION III

Acute and Emergent Problems

SECTION IV

Head, Neck, and Respiratory System

SECTION V

Hematologic Disorders

SECTION VI

Cardiovascular System

SECTION VII

Genitourinary Disorders

SECTION VIII

Orthopedic Disorders

SECTION IX

Gastrointestinal Disorders

SECTION X

Neurologic Disorders

SECTION XI

Dermatologic Disorders

SECTION XII

The New Morbidity

SECTION XIII

Chronic Diseases of Childhood and Adolescence

Primary Care: Skills and Concepts

CHAPTER 1

Primary Care: Introduction

Julie E. Noble, MD

Primary care is defined as the comprehensive health care that patients receive from the same health care professional over a longitudinal period. The term was first used in the 1960s to designate the role of the primary care physician in response to the abundance of subspecialists and lack of generalists among practicing physicians. It is generally accepted that primary care physicians include pediatricians, family physicians, and internists. In 1966, *The Graduate Education of Physicians: The Report of the Citizens Commission on Graduate Medical Education* (the Millis Committee Report) to the American Medical Association recognized the importance of primary care and recommended a national commitment to educating primary care physicians. Primary care was further defined in 1974 by Charney and Alpert, who separated it into component parts: first contact, longitudinal care, family orientation, and integration of comprehensive care. To understand the depth of primary care, the component parts should be explored.

First contact occurs when a patient arrives for medical care at the office of a primary care physician. The visit includes an intake history, complete physical examination, screening tests appropriate for age, and an assessment of problems with treatment (if indicated). Of great importance is the establishment of the physician-patient relationship. Physicians become the primary medical resource and counselors to these patients and their families and the first contacts when successive medical problems arise.

Longitudinal care, the second component of primary care, implies continuity of care over time. Physicians assume responsibility for issues concerning health and illness. In pediatrics, such care involves monitoring growth and development, following school progress, screening for commonly found disorders, making psychosocial assessments, promoting health, preventing illness with immunizations, and safety counseling programs.

Family orientation is the third component of primary care. Patients must be viewed in the context of their environment and family. Otherwise, practitioners cannot adequately care for patients. In pediatrics, a child's problems become the family's, and the family's problems become the child's. This has become increasingly apparent with the recognition that problems of poverty, drug use, HIV exposure, obesity, teenage pregnancy, and gang involvement directly affect a child's health and quality of life. The psychosocial forces in a particular child's life are intricately interwoven into his or her health care, and the assessment of these forces is an essential component of the primary care of that child. Environmental exposures have a direct effect on a child's health, and a primary care physician must have a knowledge of those environmental threats.

As pediatric medical problems become more complex, many health and educational resources in the community may be used to supplement care. Primary care physicians integrate and coordinate these services in the best interest of patients, thus providing **integration of comprehensive care,** the fourth component of primary care. Working with social service agencies, home care providers, educational agencies, and government agencies, physicians can use multiple resources for the benefit of patients. Understanding the resources of the community is an important part of a primary care physician's education.

Medical Home

When patients select a primary care physician, they have identified a medical home. That home incorporates the physical, psychologic, and social aspects of individual patients into comprehensive health care services, thus meeting the needs of the whole person. This concept of the medical home was first documented by the American Academy of Pediatrics (AAP) in 1967 in the book *Standards of Child Health Care,* which noted that a medical home should be a central source of all the child's medical records. The idea of a medical home developed into a method of providing comprehensive primary care and was successfully implemented in the 1980s by Calvin Sia, MD, FAAP, in Hawaii. He is considered to be the "father" of the medical home. In policy statements published in 1992 and 2002, the AAP defined the characteristics of a medical home to be "accessible, continuous, comprehensive, family-centered, coordinated, compassionate, and culturally effective." To make that home work for patients, geographic and financial accessibility are key elements. The most important aspect of a home is that it is a place where patients feel cared for.

Since its implementation in pediatrics in 2004, the medical home model was adopted by the American Academy of Family Physicians and American College of Physicians. Its definition was expanded to include use of electronic information services, population-based management of chronic illness, and continuous quality improvement. The concept has been accepted as a form of high-quality health care. Cost and quality benefits have been well documented. Recognizing these benefits, large corporations with practitioners formed the Patient-Centered Primary Care Collaborative to promote the idea of designated medical homes. As part of that collaborative, the National Committee for Quality Assurance adopted eligibility criteria for a practice to define itself as a medical home. Requirements for the designation include the adoption of health information technology and decision-support systems, modification of clinical practice patterns, and ensuring continuity of care. With the advent of health care reform in the United States, as part of the effort to control the rising cost of health care, the federal government has endorsed the concept of the medical home model. The Academic Pediatric Association has defined the *family-centered* medial home to delineate the dependency of the child to the family and community in the medical home model.

Role of the Primary Care Pediatrician

As a primary care physician, the role of the pediatrician has not only included the care of acute illnesses and injuries but also the preventive aspects of well-child care with its focus on immunizations, tracking growth and development, and anticipatory guidance. Now there is a renewed emphasis on the importance of the role of the pediatric primary care physician in assessing the psychosocial aspects of pediatric patients. Termed the *new morbidity* by Robert Haggerty, MD, in the 1970s, recognizing these social issues, including family dysfunction; developmental problems, including learning disabilities; and behavioral problems, including emotional disorders, has become a significant part of the role of the physician. In 1993, the AAP stated that pediatricians are obliged to have knowledge of physical and environmental factors and behaviors affecting health, normal variations of behavior and emotional development, risk factors and behaviors affecting physical health, and behavior problems. The focus of the pediatrician should be detection, evaluation, and management, with referrals if needed. Newer morbidities secondary to the increasing complexity of our society were outlined in 2001 by the AAP. These include school problems, mood and anxiety disorders, adolescent suicide and homicide, firearms, school violence, drug and alcohol abuse, HIV, obesity, and the effects of the media on children. Other psychosocial factors such as poverty, homelessness, single-parent families, divorce, working parents, and child care necessitate that pediatricians work with social service agencies to deliver appropriate care to their patients. The role of the primary care physician is continually expanding in an effort to deliver comprehensive care to each patient in a medical home. Often this care is rendered by physician-led teams that include other health care professionals.

Subspecialist Care

Medical knowledge and technology have made amazing advancements in the past several decades. Total knowledge of all fields is impossible for individual physicians. As a result, the role of the subspecialist physician has developed as an adjunct to that of the primary care physician. New fields of subspecialties, such as child abuse pediatrics, have arisen as a response to increased knowledge. Primary care physicians should seek subspecialist consultation when the suspected or known disease process is unusual or complicated, when it demands specialized technology, or when they have little experience with the disease. Generally, subspecialists evaluate patients and concentrate on the organ system or disease process in their area of expertise.

Primary care physicians can use a subspecialist for a consultation or referral. When initiating a consultation, primary care physicians seek advice from the consultant on workup or management of the patient. Consulting physicians assess the patients with a history and physical examination, focusing on their specialty. They then recommend possible additional laboratory tests, offer a diagnosis and treatment plan, and send the patients back to their primary care physicians for coordination of further care.

Use of the subspecialist is termed **secondary care.** For example, an 8-year-old girl with weight loss and persistent abdominal pain has an upper gastrointestinal radiograph series that reveals a duodenal ulcer. She is sent by her primary care physician to a pediatric gastroenterologist for **consultation,** with a request for an endoscopy to allow definitive diagnosis and up-to-date management guidelines. The girl then returns to the primary care physician with recommendations for treatment and further care. Electronic, abbreviated consultations can now be done through an e-consultation system. These consultations give the primary care physician a treatment plan from the subspecialist to implement without a need for the subspecialist to see the patient.

Primary care physicians can also generate a referral to a subspecialist, which differs from a consultation. A **referral** requests that the subspecialist assume complete care of the patient. This transfer of a patient to a tertiary care site establishes a subspecialist as the coordinator of further health care for the patient. For example, a 4-year-old boy with recurrent fevers, hepatosplenomegaly, and blasts on peripheral blood smear is referred to a pediatric oncologist for diagnosis, the latest treatment, and ongoing medical care.

When requesting advice from subspecialists, whether on a consultative or referral basis, primary care physicians should outline specific questions with a probable diagnosis to be addressed by the subspecialist. For example, a consultation requesting evaluation of a child with hematuria is inappropriate. The primary care physician should perform a basic diagnostic evaluation and suggest the most likely diagnosis. The child can then be referred appropriately. For example, a child diagnosed with nephritis should be sent to a pediatric nephrologist, whereas a child diagnosed with Wilms tumor should be sent to a pediatric oncologist.

When primary care physicians and subspecialists function cooperatively and offer 3 levels of care (primary, referral, and consultative), patients receive the highest quality medical care. In general, care provided by subspecialists is characterized as being more expensive and procedure driven. Laboratory studies are ordered with increased frequency by subspecialists, further inflating the cost of medical care. If patients have no longitudinal health care and see multiple practitioners, repeat laboratory studies are often ordered. Primary care is believed to deliver more cost-effective, improved medical care. With the spiraling cost of medical care, there continues to be a nationwide movement to produce more primary care physicians. However, it should be remembered that the role of the subspecialist is an essential supplement to the primary care physician when managing complicated disease. A balance between generalists and subspecialists needs to be maintained in the education process.

Laboratory Tests

For most conditions, the diagnosis is revealed by the history and physical examination in more than 95% of cases. Thus, good communication skills are a basic tenet of primary care. Patients frequently complain about unnecessary laboratory tests, which increase the cost of medical care, and the prescription of unnecessary medications. To lessen these problems, the primary care physician should use laboratory tests and medications discriminatingly, recognizing their value as well as their potential iatrogenic effects.

In primary care, laboratory tests should be used to help confirm a condition suspected on the basis of the history or physical examination or diagnose a condition that may not be apparent after a thorough history and physical assessment. In pediatrics especially, the value of each test result should be weighed against the inconvenience, discomfort, and possible side effects in children. Tests in at-risk children can also be used as screening tools to prevent disease or to identify a disease early so that treatment can begin and symptoms can be minimized. Laboratory studies can provide a variety of other information, including data to establish a diagnosis, knowledge necessary to select therapy or to monitor a disease, and information about the risk of future disease. Organ function, metabolic activity, and nutritional status can also be assessed, and evidence of neoplastic or infectious disease can be provided. In addition, laboratory studies can be used to identify infectious and therapeutic agents or poisons.

Screening laboratory tests are used when the incidence of an unsuspected condition is high enough in a general population to justify the expense of the test (see Chapter 11). Subclinical conditions, such as anemia, lead poisoning, and hypercholesterolemia, are part of some health maintenance assessments.

Physicians must remember that there is variability in test results and that laboratory error can occur. Laboratory results should always be viewed in the context of the patient. The sensitivity of a test, the ability of the test to detect low levels, and the specificity of a test for the substance being measured must also be considered by the physician when evaluating a test result.

Challenges for the Future

As this edition of *Berkowitz's Pediatrics: A Primary Care Approach* was being written, health care reform was being implemented in the United States. It remains apparent that the role of the primary care physician has increased in importance in health care delivery. Two of the basic tenets of primary care, accessibility and an ongoing relationship with the primary care physician (both of which are reported by patients to be very important), are now recognized as essential components of the medical home. The challenge continues to ensure continuity in health care funding to preserve the continuity of the medical home. Payment reform promises to improve payment to primary care practices and rewards high performance.

Through accountable care organizations, as proposed in health care reform, primary care physicians would be the foundation of the organization whose mission is management of the continuum of care and cost as well as to ensure quality of care.

Access to same-day care, which is part of the obligation of the medical home and essential to pediatric patients, can be difficult in the busy schedule of primary care physicians. Practices need to accommodate these visits. Community health centers can provide excellent medical homes for children in families with low income, but these centers can have challenges with accessibility and adequate referral sources. Walk-in immediate medical care clinics and retail clinics have arisen, but episodic visits in a variety of settings do not deliver comprehensive care for the patient, and these short visits may not take into account the entirety of the patient's medical history. This creates a challenge for the primary care physician and medical home to develop a system to integrate the information from these encounters into the comprehensive medical record.

With the advent of hospitalists providing inpatient care, primary care physicians may not be included in in-patient management. They then face a challenge in retrieving important information about the care of their patients.

Medical care reform incorporates accountability, demonstration of quality of care, and standards of medical practice into the medical home model. These have increased the oversight and bureaucracy of medical care exponentially. This business of medicine with redundant oversight of medical care has put a tremendous burden of administrative activities in the lap of the primary care physician. There is a significant challenge to physicians to provide care while answering to administrative structures.

The biggest challenge to pediatric primary care physicians has always been to ensure the future of health care funding to provide access and availability in a medical home of health care to all children. The Patient Protection and Affordable Care Act will provide health coverage for nearly all children, but in a multi-payer, market-driven health care system, there will remain significant challenges. There continue to be a multitude of programs, varying in each state, to pay for children's health care. Families will move among payers, disrupting continuity of care. Universal health care for children is being advocated. Without a national plan for financing, children's health care will continue to be variable, leading to disparities in children's health.

Selected References

American Academy of Pediatrics Committee on Psychosocial Aspects of Child and Family Health. The new morbidity revisited: a renewed commitment to the psychosocial aspects of pediatric care. *Pediatrics.* 2001;108(5):1227–1230

American Academy of Pediatrics Medical Home Initiatives for Children With Special Needs Project Advisory Committee. The medical home. *Pediatrics.* 2002;110(1):184–186

American Academy of Pediatrics Retail-Based Clinic Policy Work Group. AAP principles concerning retail-based clinics. *Pediatrics.* 2006;118(6):2561–2562

American Association of Medical Colleges. AAMC policy on the generalist physician. *Acad Med.* 1993;68(1):1–6

Carrier E, Gourevitch MN, Shah NR. Medical homes: challenges in translating theory into practice. *Med Care.* 2009;47(7):714–722

Cheng TL. Primary care pediatrics: 2004 and beyond. *Pediatrics.* 2004;113(6):1802–1809

Hoilette LK, Blumkin AK, Baldwin CD, Fiscella K, Szilagyi PG. Community health centers; medical homes for children? *Acad Pediatr.* 2013;13(5):436–442

Rittenhouse DR, Shortell SM, Fisher ES. Primary care and accountable care—two essential elements of delivery-system reform. *N Engl J Med.* 2009;361(24):2301–2303

Rosenbaum S. The Patient Protection and Affordable Care Act and the future of child health policy. *Acad Pediatr.* 2012;12(5):363–364

Starfield B. *Primary Care: Concept, Evaluation, and Policy.* New York, NY: Oxford University Press; 1992

Stille C, Turchi RM, Antonelli R, et al. The family-centered medical home: specific considerations for child health research and policy. *Acad Pediatr.* 2010;10(4):211–217

Tonniges TF, Palfrey JS, Mitchell M, eds. The medical home. *Pediatrics.* 2004;113(5 suppl):1471–1548

CHAPTER 2

Child Advocacy

Grant P. Christman, MD, and Julie E. Noble, MD

CASE STUDY

A 15-year-old boy is brought to the emergency department with a gunshot wound to his left leg. He says he was hanging out at the park with his friends when a random car drove by and shots were fired. Though he denies being in a gang, his mother expresses concerns in a conversation with the social worker. His physical examination reveals a gunshot wound to his left lower leg, with intact sensation, movement, and pulses in the left foot, and no other signs of injury. A radiograph shows a fractured left tibia, and he is admitted for orthopedic surgical treatment.

Questions

1. What does it mean to be a child advocate?
2. Aside from caring for individual patients, how can pediatricians promote the well-being of their communities?
3. What is the role of pediatricians in child advocacy?
4. What are the levels of advocacy?
5. How do pediatricians implement advocacy?

An advocate is someone who speaks on behalf of a person or cause. No group in our society has a greater need for advocates than children. Children are ill equipped to face the many threats to their health; they cannot obtain their own health insurance, access available social services, or even take themselves to the doctor when sick. Children also have no voice in our society. They cannot vote, donate money to political campaigns, or speak publicly to advance their interests. The word *advocate* is derived from a Latin root meaning "one who has been called to another's aid." From the beginnings of pediatrics as an independent branch of medicine, pediatricians have answered this call to advocate for the health and well-being of children.

The father of American pediatrics, Abraham Jacobi, MD, spent his career in the late 1800s and early 1900s advocating for children through legislation in New York and Washington, DC. He was a great teacher of pediatrics, introducing the discipline into academic medicine, but truly believed that physicians needed to be involved in public policy. Another founder of American pediatrics, Job Lewis Smith, MD, recognized the need for a clean water supply and decent housing to decrease the high infant mortality rate of his time. He worked through public advocacy to improve conditions not only for his patients but for children in general. The American Academy of Pediatrics (AAP) was founded on federal advocacy principles. In June 1921, the Sheppard-Towner Act on maternal and child health legislation was introduced into Congress. It was the first involvement of the federal government on behalf of children and provided federal matching funds to states for services for pregnant women and new mothers. The American Medical Association (AMA), worried that the legislation would lead to socialized medicine, condemned the act, while the AMA Section on Diseases of Children supported the legislation. When the act was up for reauthorization in 1930 and the AMA still opposed it, the pediatric group left the AMA and founded the AAP. This organization has been advocating for children ever since.

The New Morbidity

Advocacy has become increasingly important because the new morbidities in pediatric medicine are related to community forces. As our society has become more complicated, major health concerns have become even more intertwined with the environments in which children are involved. Child health outcomes improved dramatically in the 1900s with the development of vaccines, antibiotics, and new and improved surgical care to treat the classic morbidities of infectious disease, infant mortality, poor nutrition, epidemics, overcrowding, and chronic disease. But there emerged new morbidities that were negatively affecting child health outcomes. These morbidities of the 1960s to 1980s, as described by Robert Haggerty, MD, included family dysfunction, learning disabilities, emotional disorders, and educational problems. In the 1980s to 2000s, Judith Palfrey, MD, documented new challenges for pediatricians: social disarray, political ennui, the sequelae of high-tech care, and new epidemics of violence, AIDS, cocaine, and homelessness. The newest morbidities of the 21st century include the increased prevalence of childhood obesity, the rise in certain mental health issues, and significant health disparities among cultural and socioeconomic groups.

Though there has been improvement in recent years, many children in America continue to face challenges in obtaining access to quality health care. Over the past several decades, government programs like Medicaid and the Children's Health Insurance Program have expanded the availability of health care to children of limited financial means. As of 2012, there were still 6.6 million children younger than 18 years with no health insurance coverage, representing 8.9% of that population. Among children in poverty the uninsured rate was 12.9%, versus 7.7% for children not in poverty. Racial and ethnic minorities were also more likely to be uninsured, with Hispanic children having the highest rate at 14.1%. Roughly one-third of all children were receiving coverage from public insurance programs.

It is clear that these significant issues affecting child health cannot be adequately dealt with on an individual basis but require advocacy on a community or national scale to improve child health outcomes and life for children.

Community Pediatrics

Community pediatrics has developed as the vehicle to implement advocacy. Robert Haggerty, MD, first originated the concept in 1968 in an article published in the *New England Journal of Medicine*. In his work as department chair of pediatrics at the University of Rochester, NY, he developed an extensive advocacy agenda for the children of the community of Rochester. Subsequently, the AAP published a policy statement from its Committee on Community Health Services, "The Pediatrician's Role in Community Pediatrics." The policy delineates 5 components of community pediatrics: a *perspective* from the individual patient to all the children in the community; a *recognition* that family, education, society, culture, spirituality, economy, environment, and politics all affect the health of children; a *synthesis* of clinical practice and public health principles directed to providing health care to a child and promoting the health of all children; a *commitment* to collaborate with the community to optimize health care for all children, especially disadvantaged children; and an *integral part* of the role of the pediatrician. All of these components are recommended as a part of pediatric practice, and training in advocacy has been instituted in pediatric training programs. Examples of potential involvement in the community include serving as a board member, developing health agendas, working with an existing organization to design and fund a community service project, and being a source of information for the community on child health issues.

Levels of Advocacy

Every pediatrician functions as a child advocate on a daily basis. With every patient encounter, the pediatrician advocates for care in the best interest of the patient. This first level of advocacy includes treating the *individual's* immediate medical needs, performing screening tests, giving anticipatory guidance, and coordinating referrals as needed. The pediatrician may step beyond direct medical care to advance the welfare of the child, for example, by writing letters to help a patient obtain social services or visiting a patient's school for an Individual Education Plan meeting. The second level of advocacy is *community* advocacy. Pediatricians are an integral part of the community, and the community directly affects the health of their patients. Thus, pediatricians have a responsibility to improve conditions in their community to benefit children. To do this, they must be familiar with the services that are available for children. They can develop relationships with child care centers, schools, community coalitions, city governments, and local organizations to advocate for

the best interests of children. On a *state* level, pediatricians can work to improve health care resources or develop policies to help and protect children. Opportunities for involvement include working on legislation, budgets, regulations, and initiatives or working with the executive branch of local and state government. The next level of advocacy would be the *federal* level, at which pediatricians can be involved with their senators and representatives lobbying for child health issues. Pediatricians may also be involved in testifying before a congressional subcommittee. The final level of advocacy is the *international* level. For example, pediatricians may decide to work with the World Health Organization to improve immunizations for all children worldwide. Global child health is now a focus of many advocacy training programs.

Becoming a Child Advocate

To become an effective child advocate, pediatricians must first identify an issue that they want to change or set a goal to improve the lives of children. The more specific the issue or goal, the easier it is to develop a solution. Ideas often come from clinical practice, where repeatedly engaging in individual advocacy efforts on behalf of patients with the same problems suggests the need for a larger solution. The first step is to obtain background information about the problem and to collect objective data that supports the need for change, then to define the nature of the problem and the affected population in clear and precise terms.

Community Projects

Pediatricians may find that the issue would be best addressed through a community advocacy project. In developing such a project, relationship with the community is of the utmost importance, and pediatricians should endeavor to become familiar with the community as a whole. Community exploration, potentially as simple as walking or driving through the community and looking around, can reveal areas of need, such as dilapidated housing or unsafe streets. Equally important is the discovery of the community's assets, institutions such as churches, schools, and banks, which give the community strength and could provide support and counsel for the project. Pediatricians should view themselves as members of the community, acting from within and in collaboration with the community, rather than as outsiders bringing about change externally.

The next step is to develop an intervention. After the possible solutions are considered, pediatricians should collaborate with community stakeholders to develop and implement the solution that is the most practical. Having credibility in the community makes the task of collaboration much easier. Everyone is more effective working with others, but collaboration necessitates the ability to compromise and be flexible in implementation plans. Larger projects may require funding, and grants may be sought from advocacy organizations, the government, or even local businesses. Data should be collected during the intervention to monitor the success of the project. If the project is successful, its methods may be adopted by child advocates in other communities.

Legislative Advocacy

Though initially daunting for physicians without political expertise, involvement in the legislative process is often the only way to effect a desired change for children's health. Information about the content and progress of existing bills is readily available online, and legislators can be contacted by letter, e-mail, or phone to offer a position. It is helpful to become familiar with the process by which a bill becomes a law at the state and federal levels; the identities of the important players change as a bill progresses through various subcommittees and committees and ultimately to a floor vote.

Pediatricians may also arrange to meet with a legislator or staff member at a district or capital office to discuss their position personally. In the dual role of scientist and healer, pediatricians are in a unique position to inspire the heart and the mind. It is important to state the problem clearly and explain why a new law is the solution, to present well-researched facts that support the position, and to stick to layman's terms, avoiding medical jargon whenever possible. Pediatricians should minimize the appearance of self-interest by focusing on how the proposal will help children, rather than how it will benefit the profession. It may also help to connect with the legislator by sharing a story about a patient encountered in practice who has been affected by the problem, especially if the patient is a constituent of the legislator (though the patient's identity must never be discussed without his or her consent). Leaving behind a concise fact sheet summarizing the position and pertinent background information will help ensure that the position is not forgotten when the legislator is considering the issue at a later date.

Pediatricians should be prepared to encounter opposition from some legislators and avoid responding with angry statements that would alienate a legislator. Effective advocacy requires building relationships with legislators over the long term, and a legislator who opposes a position one year may be a potential supporter the next year, when the political climate changes, or may be a potential ally on another important issue. There are a number of other pitfalls to avoid, such as making or agreeing with partisan statements or claiming to represent an organization like the AAP or an institution like a university without authorization. When asked a question they do not know the answer to, pediatricians should avoid guessing and should instead offer to do further research and contact the legislator with the requested information.

When developing a new legislative proposal from scratch, the challenge is to remember that although the factors contributing to child health may be numerous and complex, legislative proposals must by nature be concrete and limited. It may be best to start small and work for incremental change. The first step is to identify a clear and, if possible, measurable objective and define the target population. Other important information to know when drafting a proposal includes what the potential funding sources would be (if applicable) and which government agencies might be involved in implementation or enforcement. Pediatricians should partner with one or more legislators early on, as some of the finer points of the legislative process will be outside the experience of the average pediatrician, and because a bill must be sponsored by a legislator to be considered for passage. Building a coalition of support within the community, involving important stakeholders such as politicians, businesspeople, other health care professionals, educators, and parents, will help the bill gain political support.

Opposition should be expected, and potential sources of opposition should be identified in advance. If opposition from a powerful interest group is anticipated, it may help to meet with a representative of that group to explain the proposal. Potential arguments might include ways in which the proposal is really in the group's self-interest, the moral imperative to help children, or that opposing an initiative to benefit children might generate negative publicity. Compromising on aspects of the proposal should be considered, when doing so might turn an enemy into an ally. When facing intractable opposition from powerful interests, pediatricians and supporters should recruit even stronger allies into their coalition.

The process of turning a policy idea into real legislation may be lengthy. A bill may have to be reintroduced repeatedly over several years before achieving passage. Once a bill becomes a law, advocates must continue working to ensure that the bill is reauthorized when applicable and that regulatory processes develop favorably. Physicians who are recognized as experts in child health policy will be called on to testify before committees in Congress or the state legislature on policy issues affecting children.

Media Advocacy

The media, including newspapers, magazines, radio, television, and the Internet, are extremely influential in our society. News stories about child health and welfare may not always be written from a child-friendly point of view. Pediatricians play an important role in providing the media with better information and a different angle on a story. For instance, a pediatrician reading a newspaper story about a child who exhibited signs of autism spectrum disorder (ASD) shortly after his 1-year physical might write a letter to the editor discussing the lack of scientific evidence for a connection between vaccinations and ASD. Over time pediatricians can develop relationships with local journalists, who can then turn to them for information when covering child health stories.

A directed media campaign may also be a key element in an advocacy project. At the community level, the media can help spread ideas, notify the public of events, and bring out potential allies and coalition members. When advocating for legislation, pediatricians can use the media to reach legislators directly and, equally important, to reach thousands of the legislators' constituents all at once, who may in turn help pressure their legislators for change. In such situations, it is essential to plan a media strategy ahead of time by determining the most important target audience, selecting the appropriate types of media to approach, crafting a message appropriate to those media, and preparing thoughtfully for encounters with journalists.

Getting Connected

The AAP is a vital resource for pediatricians interested in child advocacy, with its Federal Advocacy Action Network, as well as the various state chapters advocating at the state level. Other national organizations that pediatricians may become involved with include Docs for Tots, Children's Defense Fund, and the Child Welfare League of America. Toolkits for advocacy are available through these organizations.

Improving the health of all children through advocacy is considered to be the responsibility of pediatricians and can be a tremendously rewarding part of pediatric practice.

CASE RESOLUTION

In the case scenario, treating this teen for his orthopedic injury is only the first part of thorough pediatric care. His social history and the environment in which he lives are essential information for the pediatrician to obtain to be an advocate for this patient and prevent a second admission for a subsequent and potentially worse injury. A social work evaluation is performed and reveals that he lives in poverty in the inner city and does indeed belong to a gang. The patient and his family are counseled on his high-risk behavior, and he is referred to the police department for its Gang Alternative Program. His pediatrician becomes concerned about the high prevalence of gang activity in the community and explores coalitions in the area that recognize similar concerns. A potential solution is identified: establishing high-quality after-school programs that involve teens in productive activities. The Boys & Girls Clubs of America organization is contacted, and it has an interest in establishing a center in this community. The pediatrician volunteers to be on the board and help develop after-school programs.

Selected References

American Academy of Pediatrics. *AAP Advocacy Guide.* Elk Grove Village, IL: American Academy of Pediatrics; 2009. http://www.aap.org/moc/loadsecure.cfm/advocacyguide/pdf_version/AdvocacyGuide.pdf. Accessed January 23, 2014

American Academy of Pediatrics Committee on Community Health Services. The pediatrician's role in community pediatrics. *Pediatrics.* 2005;115(4):1092–1094

American Academy of Pediatrics Community Pediatrics Training Initiative. *Community-based Resident Projects Toolkit: A Guide to Partnering with Communities to Improve Child Health.* Elk Grove Village, IL: American Academy of Pediatrics; 2011. http://www.aap.org/commpeds/CPTI/Toolkit-Bod-2005.pdf. Accessed January 23, 2014

American Public Health Association. *APHA Media Advocacy Manual.* Washington, DC: American Public Health Association; 2011. http://www.apha.org/about/news/mediaadvocacy.htm. Accessed January 23, 2014

Bar-on ME. The use of public education in practice. *Pediatr Rev.* 2001;22(3):75–81

Berman S. Training pediatricians to become child advocates. *Pediatrics.* 1998;102(3 Pt 1):632–636

DeNavas-Walt C, Proctor BD, Smith JC. *Income, Poverty, and Health Insurance Coverage in the United States: 2012.* US Census Bureau Current Population Reports P60-245. Washington, DC: US Government Printing Office; 2013. http://www.google.com/url?sa=t&rct=j&q=&esrc=s&source=web&cd=1&ved=0CCYQFjAA&url=http%3A%2F%2Fwww.census.gov%2Fprod%2F2013pubs%2Fp60-245.pdf&ei=FF_hUoCrA4OvsQSNooD4Cw&usg=AFQjCNFVVpYExyol6OVXGkf2ux_QopMSIA&bvm=bv.59568121,d.cWc&cad=rja. Accessed January 23, 2014

Kaczorowski J, ed. Community pediatrics: making child health at the community level an integral part of pediatric training and practice. *Pediatrics.* 2005;115(suppl 3):1119–1212

Palfrey JS. *Child Health in America: Making a Difference through Advocacy.* Baltimore, MD: Johns Hopkins University Press; 2006

Palfrey JS, Hametz P, Grason H, McCaskill QE, Scott G, Chi GW. Educating the next generation of pediatricians in urban health care: the Anne E. Dyson Community Pediatrics Training Initiative. *Acad Med.* 2004;79(12):1184–1191

Paulson JA. Pediatric advocacy. *Pediatr Clin North Am.* 2001;48(5):1307–1318

Rudolf MC, Bundle A, Damman A, et al. Exploring the scope for advocacy by paediatricians. *Arch Dis Child.* 1999;81(6):515–518

Sheehan K, ed. Pediatric advocacy. *Pediatr Ann.* 2007;36(10):624–625

Sia CC. Abraham Jacobi Award address, April 14, 1992. The medical home: pediatric practice and child advocacy in the 1990s. *Pediatrics.* 1992;90(3):419–423

Taylor D, Raman R. Look how far we've come as advocates for children—but consider where we still need to go! *Contemp Pediatr.* 2005;22:54–64

CHAPTER 3

Global Child Health

Suzinne Pak-Gorstein, MD, PhD, MPH, and Maneesh Batra, MD, MPH

CASE STUDY

You are watching television when the programming is interrupted by breaking news that a severe earthquake has struck a developing country that you have recently visited. You wonder if and how you could become involved in efforts to help the country respond to the disaster, prevent diseases, and rebuild its health structure.

Questions

1. What are the global trends in childhood disease and mortality?
   How does this compare with the United States?
2. What is global health (GH)?
3. What is the role of a pediatrician in GH?
4. What are the key organizations in GH that pediatricians work in?
5. How can pediatricians carry out international work in an ethical and effective manner?

Background

Worldwide, an estimated 7.6 million children younger than 5 years died in 2010, which translates into more than 21,000 children dying each day. This figure actually represents a one-third reduction from the 11.9 million child deaths estimated in 1990. Still, significant disparities in child mortality persist and have become increasingly concentrated in specific regions of the world that bear a disproportionate burden. Africa and Asia combined account for 83% of all child deaths, with one-third of these deaths occurring in south Asia and half in sub-Saharan Africa. Less than 1% of deaths occur in high-income countries.

Three diseases—pneumonia, diarrhea, and malaria—accounted for 41% of all child deaths worldwide in 2010. Most of these lives could be saved through increased coverage of low-cost prevention and treatment measures, including antibiotics for acute respiratory infections, oral rehydration therapy for diarrhea, immunizations to protect against pneumococcal pneumonia and rotaviral diarrhea, and the use of insecticide-treated mosquito nets and appropriate drugs for malaria.

Undernutrition is an underlying cause of at least one-third of all deaths in children younger than 5 years. Reducing chronic and acute undernutrition will have a substantial effect on reducing child mortality. Furthermore, improved coverage of specific nutritional interventions, such as early and exclusive breastfeeding, are cost-effective and reduce the prevalence of pneumonia and diarrhea.

An estimated 40% of deaths in children younger than 5 years occur in the first month of life, and most of these deaths occur at home in the first postnatal week. Hence, improving newborn care is essential to the goal of improving child health. Increased access to basic, inexpensive interventions is needed to reduce neonatal mortality rates globally, including delivery by skilled birth attendants,

hygienic umbilical cord care, and training community health workers to assess and begin early treatment for neonatal infections.

In September 2000 world leaders from 190 nations came together to adopt the United Nations Millennium Declaration, committing to reduce extreme poverty through a series of time-bound targets. The 8 Millennium Development Goals (MDGs) range from halving extreme poverty to providing universal primary education and reducing child mortality by two-thirds—all by the target date of 2015 (Box 3-1). The MDGs form a blueprint ratified by more than 190 nations and have galvanized unprecedented efforts to meet the needs of the world's poorest people.

Though progress has been made toward achieving MDG 4, the pace has been modest and insufficient to meet the goal of two-thirds reduction in childhood mortality by 2015. Enormous gaps in child mortality rates exist between high- and low-income countries, with

---

Box 3-1. Millennium Development Goals

The **Millennium Development Goals (MDGs)** were developed and signed by all United Nations member countries in September 2000. There are 8 goals with 21 targets and a series of measurable indicators for each target.

Goal 1: **Eradicate extreme poverty and hunger.**

Goal 2: **Achieve universal primary education.**

Goal 3: **Promote gender equality and empower women.**

Goal 4: **Reduce the child mortality rate.**
   Target: Reduce the under-5 mortality rate by two-thirds between 1990 and 2015.

Goal 5: **Improve maternal health.**

Goal 6: **Combat HIV/AIDS, malaria, and other diseases.**

Goal 7: **Ensure environmental sustainability.**

Goal 8: **Develop a global partnership for development.**

a rate of 3 child deaths per 1,000 live births in Singapore compared with 185 in Sierra Leone in 2011.

Large inequities in child health also exist within countries. For example, in Bolivia and Peru, the richest fifth have almost universal access to a skilled attendant at birth, compared with only 10% to 15% among the poorest fifth. Women in poor rural households accounted for two-thirds of unattended births.

How does the United States compare to the rest of the world with respect to child mortality rates and health inequities? While the United States has one of the world's highest expenditures on health ($8,402 per capita in 2010, United Nations Development Programme), it ranks among the poorest among highly developed nations with respect to its under-5 mortality rate (8 deaths per 1,000 live births), which is higher than rates in most of Europe, including countries with far fewer resources such as Estonia, Croatia, and Hungary. Although the under-5 mortality rate in the United States has improved in recent decades, it is still higher than many other wealthy nations—2.3 times that of Iceland and more than 75% higher than the rate of the Czech Republic, Finland, Italy, Japan, Norway, Slovenia, and Sweden. Great health inequities are also apparent within the United States. Native American children ages 1 to 4 years have the highest death rates (49 per 100,000), followed by African American children (46 per 100,000), while non-Hispanic white children have the lowest death rates (28 per 100,000).

It has been projected that policy interventions aimed at country-level inequities would have a major effect on the under-5 mortality rate for the country as a whole, even in low-inequality regions. Worldwide, about 40% of all under-5 deaths could be prevented by bringing rates in the poorest 80% of the population down to those of the richest 20%.

While the Institute of Medicine has defined *global health* (GH) to encompass "health problems, issues, and concerns that transcend national boundaries, and may best be addressed by cooperative actions…", the World Health Organization has emphasized GH to signify health problems that affect global politics and economies and arise from disparities in sociopolitical and economic status. Inequalities in health within and between countries arise from inequalities within and between societies. These disparities in social and economic conditions impact children's risk of illness as well as the actions that families take to prevent or treat illness when it occurs. Consequently, the emerging field of GH intersects medical and social science disciplines such as demographics, economics, epidemiology, political economy, and sociology.

Integrating Global Health Into Pediatrician Careers

The most vulnerable groups in a society are children, and the strongest medical advocate for the health of children is the pediatrician. Consequently, pediatricians have been leaders in addressing global and local health disparities, and their collective voice has been powerful. Global health work varies widely in scope and extent. The duration of GH activities ranges from singular short-term medical missions to long-term postings in resource-limited settings. Involvement in GH

encompasses the direct provision of clinical services, technical assistance for program development, research, education and training of health care workers, and governmental advocacy for policy changes. The goals of GH activities range from forging novel directions in areas of basic sciences and epidemiologic, clinical, and operations research to addressing the needs of the world's poorest communities. Ideally, GH experiences should be transformative for the poor communities of the world as well as the clinicians who engage in these experiences.

By committing to a single international site (eg, hospital, rural clinic, community) and working with a partner based at that site, the pediatrician can engage in a longitudinal supportive relationship that is sustainable and effective. Pediatricians can also make a sustainable impression by empowering in-country partners through training of trainers, such as community health workers, supervisors, and clinicians responsible for health professional trainees.

Pediatricians have also played an important role in responding to humanitarian emergencies in the United States as well as in other countries, such as the aftermath of the Haiti earthquake. In addition, pediatricians with skills in research and evaluation may contribute to GH through clinical research and program evaluations.

Many GH opportunities do not require an overseas trip. While vulnerable populations and inequities to health certainly exist in low-income countries, significant inequities abound in the United States. Among developed countries, those with the highest health status have the lowest levels of health inequality. The United States ranks at the bottom of this list, with one of the poorest health rankings and the highest inequalities in health. Opportunities to carry out *local* GH work are plentiful and include supporting the care and resettlement of local refugee and immigrant families, supporting international adoptees, serving migrant farmworkers, and supporting Native American health issues.

The pediatrician may also work locally for GH by advocating for equity of health care at all levels domestically and globally, working in the home office of a US-based GH organization, and providing expertise to support international organizations dedicated to vulnerable children. Finally, pediatricians can make a significant impact in GH by lobbying the US government for more international relief funding or supporting corporations with ethical international trade practices.

Beyond the Hospitals: Global Public and Community Health and Advocacy

As a growing number of US medical students and residents seek training opportunities in developing country settings, most of these trips are spent in a foreign hospital on a pediatric ward providing direct clinical care. In addition to observing and managing tropical diseases and more severe forms of commonly encountered pediatric conditions, visiting physicians and students learn and experience common themes in these low-resource settings: underpaid and under-trained health workers, hospital administration untrained in health management, dilapidated facilities, basic medicine shortage, lack of tools in testing and imaging, and higher mortality rates.

Because the needs at such hospitals and clinics are glaring, the physician instinctively seeks to fill the gaps with what defines quality health care in the United States—more medicines, equipment, clinical staffing (through visiting physicians), and perhaps training. However, the long-term effect of a brief visit, even repeated visits, may be further improved through efforts to prevent disease using public health approaches and focusing on communities.

With further training in areas such as public and community health or health service management, the pediatrician may act as an "agent of change" by undertaking systems-based quality improvement approaches, public health measures, and community-based strategies to have lasting positive effects on child health.

Box 3-2 lists some key categories of GH organizations. In collaboration with community groups, the clinician or student can effectively empower community health workers and work within local community-based nongovernmental organizations (NGOs) to contribute to lasting and contextually appropriate change.

"Experiencing" how most of the world lives is a tremendous gift, honor, and burden that accompanies these experiences. Continuing to advocate for children living in poverty in the world after returning from a short-term medical experience is a fantastic way to enact one's ongoing responsibility. Additionally, though perhaps less glamorous than traveling overseas, working within the US health care and political system to promote awareness for change has the potential to catalyze lasting and significant improvements in child health. Similarly, through work to empower local refugee communities in the United States or to advocate for more equitable access to health care for vulnerable immigrant children, pediatricians can make a significant and lasting difference in the efforts to close the gap in health disparities.

Ethical Issues in Global Health

The traditional model for medical experiences for US-based physicians presumes that in the United States we possess the knowledge, skills, and resources to improve the conditions of people living in developing countries. However, most students and physicians who have participated in such an experience report that the greatest benefit from such experiences is for themselves.

Though the desire to improve the conditions of children by providing clinical care is well-intentioned and altruistic, there is potential for short- and long-term harm. In the short term, caring for children in such settings with conditions that are unfamiliar to visiting students or physicians and out of the scope of their training can lead to errors in diagnosis and management. For students, often there is less supervision of their clinical work in these settings, which can result in harm to patients and students' growth as physicians. In the long term, provision of clinical care by visiting students or physicians can undermine the existing health system infrastructure.

As the number of US medical students, trainees, and physicians who visit developing countries for short-term training experiences continues to grow, concern for medical tourism and the long-term effect of these training experiences on the under-resourced hosts is rising. Key factors for ensuring effective, sustainable, and ethical

---

Box 3-2. Global Health Organizations: Some Examples

International Health or Multilateral Organizations

World Health Organization (WHO)
United Nations Children's Fund (UNICEF)

Bilateral Government Organizations

US Agency for International Development (USAID)
Centers for Disease Control and Prevention (CDC)
Peace Corps

International Donor Foundations

Bill & Melinda Gates Foundation
Wellcome Trust
Children's Investment Fund Foundation (CIFF)

US-Based Nongovernmental Organizations (NGOs)

Partners In Health
Global Health Council
Save the Children

International NGOs

Specialized services or training
Short-term service/training trips (eg, cleft palate repairs)
Emergency relief and rehabilitation
Doctors Without Borders (Médecins Sans Frontières)
International Committee of the Red Cross
CARE International
International Rescue Committee (IRC)

Consultant Organizations: For-profit and Not-for-profit

Seed Global Health (formerly known as Global Health Service Partnership)
FHI 360 (formerly known as Family Health International)
John Snow, Inc. (JSI)
• Global health (GH) consultant organizations may take government contracts to provide international support.

Faith-Based Organizations

World Vision
Aga Khan Foundation
American Friends Service Committee

Academic Institutions

An increasing number of academic institutions are developing GH programs in partnership with international groups, overseas academic institutions, or ministries of health.
Consortium of Universities for Global Health (CUGH)

Local and Domestic

Global health advocacy organizations
Refugee resettlement agencies
Indian health services

Resources

American Academy of Pediatrics Section on International Child Health (AAP SOICH)
Academic Pediatrics Association Global Health Special Interest Group (SIG)
Physicians for Social Responsibility (PSR)

international collaborations include forethought, planning, and long-term partnership.

Proper *predeparture preparation and education* for any overseas medical experience is a critical first step. Proper education entails orientation regarding the country and its sociopolitical context and public health priorities. Knowledge of the key medical problems facing the communities as well as international and local treatment guidelines and strategies to deliver care within the confines of existing local resources are also important.

Suchdev et al and others have outlined fundamentals for the creation of a meaningful international partnership with a community. The first step is the development of a **mission** or an identified shared purpose with partners prior to visiting a new international site. Also, it is critical to establish a **collaboration** with a local agency, such as an NGO or governmental agency, to promote sustainability and enhance effectiveness of the care delivered. Another important component for long-term impact and partnership is to ensure that the **education** of community members, other physicians, and trainees is a part of the mission and that appropriate educational experiences are structured into the trip and planning. Closely related to this is the appreciation of the reciprocal nature of any education: The visiting physician is in a position to be learning just as much if not more than the local providers about working in the local setting.

A fourth fundamental for meaningful partnerships involves ensuring that **service** is truly being provided to the community by *learning about the health priorities* of the community from the NGO or other local agency. Also, it is important to encourage **teamwork** by working with appropriate supervision, including physicians from the host country. Effective international collaboration also requires sensitivity to the *costs and burden* that a visitor will have on the host. Finally, assurance of partnership effectiveness requires building an **evaluation** process early on that incorporates the perspectives of all the players, including local officials, health professionals, and community members. This would include assessment of whether educational objectives are being met for all stakeholders, including the host site.

CASE RESOLUTION

You learn about a US-based nongovernmental organization (NGO) with a long history of partnership and work in the earthquake-stricken country. You research that NGO further and find that it is a reputable group with long-term interests in the country. You speak to friends who have recently visited the country and learn more about what skills and resources are needed. You make arrangements to join a team of experienced health workers from the NGO by taking time from work and garnering support from your family to manage with your absence. You undergo an in-depth orientation of the site, people, sociopolitical situation, team roles, and expected activities through a series of discussions with all participants.

Selected References

Liu L, Johnson HL, Cousens S, et al. Global, regional, and national causes of child mortality: an updated systematic analysis for 2010 with time trends since 2000. *Lancet.* 2012;379(9832):2151–2161

Rajaratnam JK, Marcus JR, Flaxman AD, et al. Neonatal, postneonatal, childhood, and under-5 mortality for 187 countries, 1970–2010: a systematic analysis of progress towards Millennium Development Goal 4. *Lancet.* 2010;375(9730):1988–2008

Suchdev P, Ahrens K, Click E, Macklin L, Evangelista D, Graham E. A model for sustainable short-term international medical trips. *Ambul Pediatr.* 2007;7(4):317–320

United Nations Development Programme. *Human Development Report 2010. The Real Wealth of Nations: Pathways to Human Development.* Geneva, Switzerland: United Nations Development Programme; 2010. http://hdr.undp.org/en/reports/global/hdr2010. Accessed October 16, 2013

Victora CG, Wagstaff A, Schellenberg JA, Gwatkin D, Claeson M, Habicht JP. Applying an equity lens to child health and mortality: more of the same is not enough. *Lancet.* 2003;362(9379):233–241

CHAPTER 4

Talking With Children

Geeta Grover, MD

CASE STUDY

The moment you walk into the examination room, the 2-year-old girl begins to cry and scream uncontrollably. She clings to her mother and turns her face away. The mother appears embarrassed and states that her daughter reacts to all physicians this way. After reassuring the mother that you have received such welcomes before, you sit down at a comfortable distance from the girl and her mother. You smile at the girl and compliment her on her dress, but she does not seem to be interested in interacting with you at this point. You place an age-appropriate book on the examination table, indicating to the child that the book is for her. You begin your interview with the mother and try not to look at the girl. Out of the corner of your eye, you see that her crying is easing a bit and she has begun to examine the book you had placed on the table.

Questions

1. How does children's age influence their understanding of health and illness?
2. Should physicians speak directly with children about their illnesses?
3. At what age can children begin to communicate with physicians about their illnesses?
4. At what age are children able to begin making decisions that affect their health?
5. How can positioning and placement of children in the examination room affect the overall tone and quality of the visit?

Effective doctor-patient communication, which is difficult enough when patients are adults, becomes even more challenging when patients are children. In pediatrics, interviewing involves balancing the needs of parents and children. Whereas parents may be more focused on issues pertaining to disease, treatment, or aspects of parenting, children look to physicians with different needs and concerns, depending on their age. To have a meaningful and satisfying exchange with children, pediatricians must take into account children's age, intelligence, and developmental maturity because all of these factors affect their concepts of health and illness. As children grow and develop, their understanding of health and illness matures and develops as well.

Developmental Approach to Communicating With Children

Childhood is a time of not only great physical growth but also of tremendous social, emotional, and cognitive maturation. An appreciation of the cognitive stages of development helps pediatricians develop a healthy relationship with their patients by allowing them to communicate with children in an age-appropriate manner. Piaget defined 4 stages of cognitive development, which occur in the same sequence but not at the same rate in all children (Table 4-1). Children in the sensorimotor stage (birth–2 years of age) experience the world and act through sensations and motor acts. They are developing the concepts of object permanence, causality, and spatial relationships. Children in the preoperational stage (2–6 years) understand reality only from their own viewpoint. As egocentric thinkers, they are unable to separate internal from external reality,

Table 4-1. Piaget's Stages of Cognitive Development		
Age[a]	*Stage*	*Characteristics*
Birth–2 y	Sensorimotor	Experiences world through sensations and motor acts
2–6 y	Preoperational	Egocentric thinking; imitation and fantasy play
6–11 y	Concrete operational	Mental processes only as they relate to real objects
>11 y	Formal operations	Capacity for abstract thought

[a]Approximate ages.

and fantasy play is important. School-aged children (6–11 years) are capable of concrete operational thinking. These children can reason through problems that relate to real objects. Older children (>11 years) have the capacity for abstract thought, which defines the stage of formal operations.

An appreciation of how children's cognitive development affects their understanding of illness and pain aids physicians in developing therapeutic relationships. Bibace and Walsh have outlined a developmental approach to children's understanding of illness: Children's explanations of illness are classified into 6 categories consistent with Piaget's cognitive developmental stages. Children 2 to 6 years of age view illness as caused by external factors near the body (phenomenalism and contagion). Young children engage in so-called magical thinking; proximity alone provides the link between cause and illness. Children 7 to 10 years of age should be able to differentiate between self and nonself. At this stage they begin to understand that although illness may be caused by some factor outside the body, illness itself is located inside the body (contamination and internalization). Children older than 11 years understand physiological and psychophysiological explanations for illness (Table 4-2).

A similar developmental sequence applies to children's understanding of pain. Gaffney and Dunne have outlined a developmental approach to this understanding. Younger children may attribute pain to punishment for some transgression or wrongdoing on their part. They may not understand the relationship between pain and illness (eg, "Pain is something in my tummy."). Children with concrete operational thought can appreciate that pain and illness are related, but they may have no clear understanding of the causation of pain (eg, "Pain is a feeling you get when you are sick."). Older children and adolescents begin to understand the complex physical and psychologic components of pain. For example, they realize that although the bone in the arm is broken, pain is ultimately felt in the head (eg, "Pain goes up some nerves from the broken bone in my arm to my head.").

Guidelines for Doctor-Child Communication

A developmental framework that takes into account children's language skills and causal reasoning abilities is essential in providing appropriate health care to children. Successful communication with children depends not only on spoken words but also nonverbal cues and the environment itself. A pleasant, child-friendly environment with bright colors, wall decorations, and toys helps make children feel more comfortable. Health care practitioners should be sincere because children are extremely sensitive to nonverbal cues. Pediatricians should take a few minutes to enjoy children; this not only gives children a chance to evaluate their physicians but also allows clinicians to begin assessing areas of development. A general principle of the pediatric examination is to begin with the least invasive portions of the examination (eg, heart, lungs, abdomen) and save the most invasive for last (eg, oropharynx, ears). Pediatricians should maintain their self-control in difficult situations. If they approach their limit, they should step outside for a few minutes or ask someone for assistance. Overall guidelines for communicating with children are provided in Box 4-1. Age-specific guidelines follow.

Birth to 6 Months

Examination of newborns and infants of this age is usually pleasant. Although verbal interaction is limited, it is important to play with newborns and infants, hold them, and talk to them. By watching physicians interact with their infants, new parents have an opportunity to learn how to behave with their infants. Newborns and infants have not yet developed a fear of strangers and can usually be easily examined in parents' arms or on the examination table.

7 Months to 3 Years

This is perhaps the most challenging age group with regard to developing rapport and performing examinations. After entering the

| \multicolumn{3}{c}{**Table 4-2. Children's Concepts of Illness**} |
Age	Concept of Illness	Example
	Preoperational	*How do people get colds?*
2–6 y	Phenomenalism	"From the sun."
	Contagion	"When someone else gets near them."
	Concrete Operational	*How do people get colds?*
7–10 y	Contamination	"You're outside without a hat and you start sneezing. Your head would get cold—the cold would touch it—and then it would go all over your body."
	Internalization	"In winter, people breathe in too much air into their nose and it blocks up the nose."
	Formal Operations	*How do people get colds?*
>11 y	Physiological/ psychophysiological	"They come from viruses, I guess."
		How do people get a heart attack?
		"It can come from being all nerve-racked. You worry too much, and the tension can affect your heart."

Modified and reproduced with permission from Bibace R, Walsh ME. Development of children's concepts of illness. *Pediatrics.* 1980;66(6):912–917

| \multicolumn{2}{c}{**Box 4-1. Physician-Child Communication**} |
Dos	Don'ts
Provide a pleasant environment.	Limit the child's participation.
Pay attention to nonverbal cues.	Threaten the child.
Be sincere and honest.	Compare the child to others.
Enjoy the child.	Get into power struggles.
Speak age appropriately.	
Get down to the child's eye level.	
Examine from least to most invasive.	
Respect the child's privacy.	
Maintain self-control.	
Have a sense of humor.	

examination room, pediatricians should take a few moments to converse or play with these infants and children. Such actions help put children at ease and allow them to get to know their doctors. Children who are 1 to 2 years of age will probably busy themselves, exploring the room during the history taking. By acknowledging them periodically, physicians build rapport that will help later during the examination. Two- to 3-year-olds are usually very apprehensive of the examination. Physicians should get down to children's eye level when speaking to them. Reassurances such as, "You're not going to get any shots today," can help alleviate their fears. Because stranger anxiety has developed, physicians should try to do as much of the examination as possible with children in parents' laps. Distractions such as stethoscope toys, flashing penlights, or keys may be helpful.

3 to 6 Years

Children's expressive capabilities are growing at tremendous rates during this period. Children can usually be engaged in conversation. They should be given repeated opportunities for participation, but they should not feel pressured to take part. Children may doubt physicians' true intentions and will probably only speak once their comfort level has been achieved. Children should be involved; they can be asked simple questions about their illness (eg, "Where does it hurt?"). In addition, children should be given some control during the examination (eg, "Should I look in your mouth next or your ears?"), and they should be allowed to handle physicians' equipment. Knowing what to expect next and having some control over the examination can help to decrease fear and increase cooperation.

7 to 11 Years

Examination of children in this age group can be rewarding. Physicians should make a point to speak directly with children and not just with parents concerning the chief complaint and history. Children can usually provide a good history of their illness, although their concept of time may be misleading. For example, a "long, long time" may mean hours, days, or months, and parents need to clarify this. Children should be asked about school, friends, and favorite activities. Answers to such questions give physicians an idea of children's social and emotional well-being, which may be affecting their physical health. Physicians sometimes overlook children's need for privacy at this age. Drapes should be used appropriately during the examination, and physicians should be sensitive to the presence of other children or adults in the room.

Physicians should begin to involve older children in the management of their illness. Children's understanding of their illness and its management should be assessed (eg, children with asthma could be asked, "What is this inhaler for? When are you going to use it? Show me how."). Children should be given an opportunity to express their fears and anxieties, and these concerns should be discussed (eg, "Asthma can be scary, especially when you can't catch your breath. Have you ever felt like that? Tell me about it."). Children should be involved in the management of their illness, which allows them to develop a sense of responsibility for their own health and medical care. Active participation in their health care visits leads to greater visit satisfaction, knowledge, and competence of prescribed medical therapies.

Older Than 12 Years

Communication with adolescents is discussed in detail in Chapter 6.

Children and Health Literacy

Health literacy (see Chapter 31) is a person's ability to receive, understand, and use information to make appropriate health decisions. At what age does an individual become responsible for his or her own health? Although in the medical setting, children often have limited involvement in medical decision-making about their own health, in the community, children are routinely making decisions that affect their well-being: A 4-year-old chooses water instead of a soda at a friend's birthday; a 6-year-old runs home to put on her helmet before she rides her neighbor's new bike; an 8-year-old recognizes that her cough is the first sign of an impending asthmatic attack and goes to the school nurse to use her inhaler; a 12-year-old refuses the cigarette she is being offered. Health attitudes and behaviors learned during childhood affect adult lifestyle choices and thereby health. Health literacy skills should be encouraged from a young age. If information is presented in an age-appropriate manner, children between the ages of 3 and 18 years are capable of understanding and using health information. In today's world of patient-centered care and ever-increasing accessibility to health information through new technologies, it is imperative that we encourage our patients to be knowledgeable consumers beginning at a young age.

Barriers to Effective Communication With Children

The manner in which adults speak to children is influenced by what they think children can understand. Physicians tend to overestimate the understanding capabilities of younger children and underestimate those of older children. Lack of appreciation for the cognitive sophistication of children may lead to frustration for all involved. Younger children are presented with information they may not be able to comprehend, and older children may feel frustrated because they are being spoken to in a childlike manner.

Overestimating children's receptivity to medical information can be particularly problematic in the case of children with chronic illness. It is easy to assume that children with chronic medical conditions or those with more hospitalizations would have more sophisticated understanding of illness causation. Although these children may seem more savvy and knowledgeable about medical procedures, there is little research to support the assumption that they have more sophisticated understanding of illness causation than would be expected based on their age or developmental level, or that they are better able to understand and retain medical information than their peers without chronic medical concerns.

Another potential barrier in communicating with children is limiting their participation. Physicians tend to elicit information from children but exclude them from diagnostic and management information. Older children want to know about their illness and are capable of learning about management.

All physicians have been frustrated or pushed to the limit at one time or another when working with children. In such situations, physicians should remember that children are probably not trying to irritate them on purpose. Crying or lack of cooperation generally stems from fear or a sense of lack of control over the situation. Pediatricians should avoid taking part in a battle over power or control with children. Threatening remarks (eg, "If you're not good, I'll have to give you a shot.") or comparisons between children (eg, "Your brother is younger than you and he didn't cry.") not only are ineffective but may make the situation worse. A clear perspective, empathy, and a sense of humor are much more useful.

CASE RESOLUTION

You learn from the mother that her daughter has been in good health. The mother has brought in the child for a routine health maintenance visit. You assess that the child's development is normal and her immunizations are up-to-date. As you and the mother talk, the child appears more relaxed and less frightened. You use the book to engage and distract the child during the examination. She begins to respond to your questions and cooperate with the examination, but she chooses to remain on her mother's lap. Praising a child who is cooperative helps reinforce preferred behavior.

Selected References

Bibace R, Walsh ME. Development of children's concepts of illness. *Pediatrics.* 1980;66(6):912–917

Borzekowski DL. Considering children and health literacy: a theoretical approach. *Pediatrics.* 2009;124(Suppl 3):S282–S288

Erickson SJ, Gerstle M, Feldstein SW. Brief interventions and motivational interviewing with children, adolescents, and their parents in pediatric health care settings: a review. *Arch Pediatr Adolesc Med.* 2005;159(12):1173–1180

Gaffney A, Dunne EA. Developmental aspects of children's definitions of pain. *Pain.* 1986;26(1):105–117

Ginsburg HP, Opper S. *Piaget's Theory of Intellectual Development.* 3rd ed. Englewood Cliffs, NJ: Prentice-Hall; 1988

Myant KA, Williams JM. Children's concepts of health and illness: understanding of contagious illnesses, non-contagious illnesses and injuries. *J Health Psychol.* 2005;10(6):805–819

Nobile C, Drotar D. Research on the quality of parent-provider communication in pediatric care: implications and recommendations. *J Dev Behav Pediatr.* 2003;24(4):279–290

Perrin EC, Perrin JM. Clinicians' assessments of children's understanding of illness. *Am J Dis Child.* 1983;137(9):874–878

van Dulmen AM. Children's contributions to pediatric outpatient encounters. *Pediatrics.* 1998;102(3 Pt 1):563–568

Vatne TM, Slaugther L, Ruland CM. How children with cancer communicate and think about symptoms. *J Pediatr Oncol Nurs.* 2010;27(1):24–32

CHAPTER 5

Talking With Parents

Geeta Grover, MD

CASE STUDY

An 8-month-old boy with a 1-week history of cough and runny nose, a 2-day history of vomiting, diarrhea, and fever, and a temperature of 101°F (38.3°C) is evaluated in the emergency department (ED). The mother is very concerned because her son's appetite has decreased and he has been waking up several times at night for the last 2 days.

A nurse interrupts and says that paramedics are bringing a 5-year-old trauma victim to the ED. The appearance of the 8-month-old child is quickly assessed; he seems active and alert. Bilateral otitis media is diagnosed. Before leaving the examination room the physician says to the mother, "Your son has a viral syndrome and infection in his ears. I am going to prescribe an antibiotic that you can begin giving him today. Give him Tylenol as needed for the fever. Don't worry about his vomiting and diarrhea; just make sure that he drinks plenty of liquids and don't give him milk or milk products for a few days. Bring him back here or to his regular doctor if his fever persists, he doesn't eat, he has too much vomiting or diarrhea, he looks lethargic, or if he isn't better in 2 days."

Questions

1. How much information can most parents absorb at one time? Did this mother receive more information than she can be reasonably expected to remember?
2. How do you assess parental concerns? Did the physician address the mother's worries sufficiently?
3. How do you know whether a parent has understood all the information? Was this mother given a chance to clarify any questions she had?
4. What are some barriers to effective doctor-patient communication?
5. How does the setting itself influence communication?

Communication is the foundation of the therapeutic relationship between physicians, patients, and their families. Effective communication in the pediatric setting involves the exchange of information among physicians, parents, and children. In addition, observing the interaction between parents and children gives physicians an opportunity to assess parenting skills and the dynamics of the parent-child relationship. The communication needs of parents and children are quite different; this makes the exchange of information challenging. Parental concerns should be addressed in a sensitive, empathetic, and nonjudgmental manner. A nonthreatening, pleasant demeanor and age-appropriate language help facilitate communication with children (see Chapter 4).

Pediatrics encompasses not only the traditional medical model of diagnosis and treatment of disease but also maintenance of the health and well-being of children through longitudinal care and the establishment of ongoing relationships between physicians and families. Personal relationships between physicians and families create an atmosphere in which information can be exchanged openly. The pediatrician's role in such relationships is to not only diagnose and treat but also to listen, advise, guide, and teach.

The doctor-patient relationship is truly a privilege. Patients entrust physicians with their innermost thoughts and feelings, allow them to touch private parts of their bodies, and trust them to perform invasive procedures or administer medications. Mutual respect is essential for the development of a healthy relationship between physicians, parents, and children. Through practice and continued awareness of interpersonal abilities, physicians can develop good communication skills. All physicians eventually develop their own personal interviewing and examination style. What seems awkward and difficult at first soon becomes routine and even enjoyable as physicians become more comfortable with patients.

Parental Concerns

Parents' preconceived ideas and concerns about their children's illnesses can greatly influence the exchange of information between physicians and patients. At health maintenance or well-child visits, it is important for pediatricians to address nonmedical and psychosocial concerns of parents, such as their children's development, nutrition, and growth. Often these questions stem from discussions with other parents or increasingly from information received through various Internet and media resources (see Chapter 9). Although such concerns may seem trivial to pediatricians, they may be extremely important to parents. In addition to addressing the needs of the child, the health maintenance visit also gives the pediatrician an opportunity to assess and address parental needs. Parental depression, substance abuse, family violence, or marital discord can all have profound effects on children's health and development. When evaluating children brought in for illness, it is important to ask parents what concerns them the most. Parental fears may be much different than medical concerns. Failure to give parents the opportunity to ask questions or to address these concerns in a sensitive manner may lead to dissatisfaction and poor communication.

The Pediatric Interview

Pediatric interviews are conducted in a variety of settings for many different reasons. The first interaction between the physician and parents may be during the prenatal interview before the birth of the child, in the hospital following the delivery, or in the doctor's office during the well-baby visit. Later, the physician may see children in the office for regular health maintenance visits or in the office, emergency department (ED), or hospital for an acute illness.

The specific clinical situation dictates the information that needs to be gathered and appropriate interviewing techniques. During the prenatal visit, physicians should discuss common concerns and anxieties about the new baby with prospective parents. In addition, parents have an opportunity to interview physicians and evaluate their offices and staff.

In the emergency setting, physicians must elicit pertinent information needed to make decisions about management within a short period. Absence of long-term relationships can make communication in the ED particularly challenging. Focused, closed-ended questions should be used primarily. The periodic health maintenance visit is at the opposite end of this spectrum. Here the use of broad, open-ended questions is more appropriate; closed-ended questions should be used as needed for clarification.

Communication Guidelines

Overall principles, applicable regardless of the setting, include interacting with the child and family in a professional yet sensitive and nonjudgmental manner. Common courtesies, such as knocking before entering the room, dressing and behaving in a professional manner, introducing oneself, and addressing parents and children by their preferred names, are always appreciated and welcomed. Taking a few moments to socialize with families develops a more personal relationship that may allow more open conversation about sensitive and emotional issues.

Family-centered care is an approach to health care in which the physician realizes the vital role that families play in ensuring the health and well-being of children. Family-centered–care physicians convey respect for parents' insight into and understanding of their children's behavior and needs and actively seek out their observations and incorporate their family preferences into the care plan as much as possible. Benefits of family-centered care include a stronger alliance between the physician and family; increased patient, family, and professional satisfaction; and decreased health care costs.

The medical visit may be divided into 3 parts: the interview, physical examination, and concluding remarks. Examples of doctor-parent and doctor-child communications for each of these components are given in Table 5-1.

Interview

The goal of the interview is to ascertain the chief complaint, determine appropriate medical history, and gain an understanding of the family's perspective of the illness or its specific concerns. It is important to address cognitive (informational) and affective (emotional) needs of the family during the interview. The interview usually begins with open-ended questions to give parents and children an opportunity to discuss their concerns and outline their agenda for the visit. Not uncommonly, the real reason for the visit may not be disclosed until the family believes the physician is trustworthy and honest. *Generous listening* is a technique of receiving and respecting information without judgment or any agenda to analyze it and figure out what to do next. Generous listening creates a space of safety that allows parents and children to say what they perceive to be true. Once issues have been laid out, closed-ended questions can be used to clarify and further define the information presented. It often becomes necessary to guide the interview, especially when parents have several broad issues on their agenda for that visit and time does not permit their discussion.

Physicians should gently acknowledge parental concerns and define time limitations. These actions allow physicians to focus on the most salient issues of that visit. Physicians should limit their use of medical jargon (scientific terms) and be aware of nonverbal communication. A sincere, empathic, and compassionate communication style helps parents feel that their situation is truly understood even if physicians can do very little to help them. Pauses and silent periods should be used, especially when discussing emotionally difficult issues, to convey to parents and children that their physician cares enough to listen. Physicians should not underrate their own knowledge, but at the same time they should recognize their limitations and use consultants appropriately. Finally, physicians' understanding of the chief complaint and history should be summarized so parents have an opportunity to clarify points of disagreement.

Today there are increasing demands for primary care physicians to address not only the physical but also the psychosocial health needs of their patients. Patient-centered care is a comprehensive approach to medical care that encourages communication between physicians, patients, and their families. Clinicians address the immediate pressing medical concerns in the context of each patient's unique environmental circumstances and underlying psychosocial concerns, both of which may directly or indirectly affect health-related outcomes. Empathy, unconditional positive regard, and genuineness are essential physician characteristics in this collaborative approach. Motivational interviewing (MI) is one such patient-centered, collaborative, and directive interaction style that offers an effective means of addressing these developmental, behavioral, and social concerns within the context of a primary care setting. Motivational interviewing addresses the ambivalence and discrepancies between a person's current values and behaviors and their future goals. In contrast to more traditional medical approaches that rely primarily on authority and education, MI is a collaborative approach that relies on elicitation of the patient's ideas about change.

| Table 5-1. Communication Guidelines and Techniques ||
Techniques	Examples
Interview	
Open-ended questions.	"How is Susie?"
Closed-ended questions.	"Does she have a cough?"
Repetition of important phrases.	"She has had a high fever for 4 days now?"
Clarification.	"What do you mean by 'Susie was acting funny'?"
Pauses and silent periods.	
Limit medical jargon.	"Susie has an ear infection" vs "Susie has otitis media."
Guide the interview.	"Right now I am most interested in hearing about the symptoms of this illness."
Be aware of nonverbal communication.	Use eye contact and phrases such as "I see."
Acknowledge parental concerns.	"Worrying about hearing loss is understandable."
Empathize.	"A temperature of 104°F can be very frightening."
Remember common courtesies.	Knock before entering.
Recognize personal limitations.	"I am not an expert in this area. I would like to consult with a colleague."
Summarize.	"So she has had fever for 4 days but the rash and cough began 1 week ago?"
Physical Examination	
Show consideration for the child.	"It's OK to be afraid."
Inform.	"That took me some time, but her heart sounds normal."
Explain procedures.	"You may feel a little uncomfortable during the rectal examination."
Avoid exclamations.	"Wow! I have never seen anything like this!"
Concluding Remarks	
Provide closure.	"Our time is over today. May we discuss this at the next visit?"
Minimize discharge instructions.	
Be specific.	"I am going to treat her with amoxicillin" vs "I'll prescribe an antibiotic."
Praise.	"You're doing a great job."
Confirm parental understanding.	"Please repeat for me Susie's diagnosis and treatment instructions so I'm sure I've been clear in explaining them to you."

Motivational-interviewing physicians understand that trying to move beyond a patient's readiness to change is likely to increase that patient's resistance to treatment (eg, lecturing to an adolescent who is not yet ready to quit smoking about the dangers of smoking is unlikely to be effective and may even produce more resistance). Motivational interviewing requires that the physician follow 4 principles (Table 5-2). Operationally, open-ended questions (eg, "How do you feel about smoking?"), affirmations (eg, "You are tired of having to monitor your blood sugar every day and stick to your diet."), and reflective listening (eg, "You are worried about your daughter's behavior and are concerned that if it persists, she may be expelled from school.") are important tools of MI. In addition, MI physicians ask permission before giving advice (eg, "Would it be OK if I shared some information with you?"), or the physician may state the facts but let the parent interpret the information (eg, "What does this mean to you?"). Motivational interviewing is not only effective with adults, but research with adolescents has shown MI to be an effective tool to increase self-efficacy to enact change (eg, adolescent smoking cessation).

| Table 5-2. Principles of Motivational Interviewing ||
Principle	Example
Express empathy.	Use reflective listening.
Develop discrepancy between patient's current behavior and treatment goal.	Patient, not physician, presents arguments for change.
Roll with the patient's resistance.	Avoid arguing for change.
Support the patient's self-efficacy.	Patient's own belief in the possibility of change is an important motivator.

Adapted from Miller WR, Rollnick S. *Motivational Interviewing: Helping People Change.* 3rd ed. New York, NY: Guilford Press; 2012

Physical Examination

Parents keenly observe physicians' interactions with their children during the examination. It is an important time for physicians to build a therapeutic relationship with children (see Chapter 4). The transition between the history and physical examination can be made by briefly telling children and parents what to expect during the examination. Physicians should show consideration for children's fears. Physicians often find it helpful to speak with families at periodic intervals during the examination about their observations. Prolonged periods of silence as the physician listens or palpates may be anxiety provoking for families. Physicians should be sure to explain any procedures that they or their staff are going to perform at a level that is appropriate for parents and children. In addition, physicians should try to avoid exclamations or comments to themselves during the examination (eg, "Wow, that's some murmur!"), which may be alarming to families.

Concluding Remarks

This portion of the visit, which is all too easy to rush through, is extremely important. Closure can be provided by summarizing the diagnosis or outlining plans for the following visit. Parents should be asked to participate by acknowledging closure and helping to develop a management plan. Shared decision-making and consumerism are replacing the traditional paternalistic medical model in which physicians decided what should be done and patients accepted the recommendations without question. In this shared decision-making model, it is important to assess parental readiness for knowledge (especially in emotionally difficult situations) and keep family resources and limitations in mind. Discharge instructions should be minimized, physicians should be specific, and the number of diagnoses, medications, and "as needed" instructions (indications for seeking medical advice such as "return as needed for high fever") should be limited. When complicated discharge instructions are given, additional physician time may be required to ensure parental understanding. Praising parents on care of their children can boost their self-esteem and confidence and may minimize calls and questions. Parental understanding should be confirmed; parents should be asked to repeat the diagnosis and treatment plan. Simply asking parents if they have understood is not enough because parents often say "yes" out of respect for the physician's time or embarrassment that they have not understood what has been said. For example, the physician could say, "I want to be sure that I've spoken clearly enough. Please repeat for me [child's name] diagnosis and treatment instructions."

Barriers to Effective Communication

Barriers to effective communication may be divided into systems barriers and interpersonal barriers (Table 5-3). The primary systems barriers are the setting itself and lack of continuity of care. Because of access problems within the health care system (ie, lack of health insurance coverage), many children receive only episodic care from different physicians in acute care clinics or EDs. Without the benefit of long-term relationships, doctor-patient communication may suffer.

Interpersonal barriers include physician time constraints, frequent interruptions, and cultural insensitivity. Frequent interruptions or

Table 5-3. Barriers to Effective Communication

Barriers	Examples
Systems	
Lack of continuity of care	Episodic care that is primarily illness driven
The setting itself	Emergency departments and acute care clinics
Interpersonal	
Physician time constraints	Appearing impatient or preoccupied
Frequent interruptions	Pager goes off or asked to come to the phone
Cultural insensitivity	Suggesting treatments that are not acceptable within the family's belief systems

apparent impatience on the part of physicians conveys to parents and children that they do not care or they are too busy for them. Language differences may pose a significant barrier depending on the region in which physicians practice. Ideally, physicians themselves should be able to speak with parents and children. If translators are needed, children must not play this role because this places them in an awkward situation. Parents of other patients must not be used because this violates patients' privacy. Only professional translators are recommended. Physicians should be sensitive to cultural differences (eg, gender issues, views on illness, folk remedies, beliefs). Suggesting treatments that are not culturally acceptable or are contrary to folk wisdom simply decreases compliance with prescribed treatment plans. For example, many Eastern cultures believe in the concept of "hot" and "cold" foods and illnesses. Suggesting to a mother that she feed primarily "hot" foods to a child she believes to have an illness that is also "hot" may not be acceptable to her. Such information is rarely volunteered and must be elicited through sensitive patient interviewing.

Effective communication is not only essential for accurate diagnosis but also correlates with improved patient recall of instructions and adherence to prescribed courses of treatment. Poor communication can have negative consequences for the patient (eg, compromised care) and physician (eg, medicolegal consequences). Effective communication enhances medical outcomes and patient satisfaction.

CASE RESOLUTION

The doctor-patient interaction presented in the case history illustrates several of the "not to" points discussed herein. The physician did not acknowledge parental concerns or make sure that the mother had understood the diagnosis and treatment plan. The mother was presented with more information than she could have reasonably been asked to remember. This interaction could have been improved if the physician conveyed to the mother that her concerns were appreciated and then reassured her that her child was going to be all right. Furthermore, the physician should have told the mother the name and dosage schedule of the antibiotic to be prescribed and limited the number of "as needed" instructions.

Selected References

American Academy of Pediatrics Committee on Hospital Care and Institute for Patient- and Family-Centered Care. Patient- and family-centered care and the pediatrician's role. *Pediatrics.* 2012;129(2):394–404

Dixon SD, Stein MT. *Encounters with Children: Pediatric Behavior and Development.* 4th ed. Chicago, IL: Mosby-Year Book; 2006

Erickson SJ, Gerstle M, Feldstein SW. Brief interventions and motivational interviewing with children, adolescents, and their parents in pediatric health care settings: a review. *Arch Pediatr Adolesc Med.* 2005;159(12):1173–1180

Grover G, Berkowitz CD, Lewis RJ. Parental recall after a visit to the emergency department. *Clin Pediatr (Phila).* 1994;33(4):194–201

Hagan JF, Shaw JS, Duncan PM, eds. *Bright Futures: Guidelines for Health Supervision of Infants, Children, and Adolescents.* 3rd ed. Elk Grove Village, IL: American Academy of Pediatrics; 2008

Korsch BM, Freemon B, Negrete VF. Practical implications of doctor-patient interaction analysis for pediatric practice. *Am J Dis Child.* 1971;121(2):110–114

Levetown M; American Academy of Pediatrics Committee on Bioethics. Communication with children and families: from everyday interactions to skill in conveying distressing information. *Pediatrics.* 2008;121(5):e1441–e1460

Miller WR, Rollnick S. *Motivational Interviewing: Helping People Change.* 3rd ed. New York, NY: Guilford Press; 2012

Remen RN. Generous listening. http://www.rachelremen.com/generous-listening. Accessed October 16, 2013

Tates K, Meeuwesen L. Doctor-parent-child communication: a (re)view of the literature. *Soc Sci Med.* 2001;52(6):839–851

Teutsch C. Patient-doctor communication. *Med Clin North Am.* 2003;87(5):1115–1145

Young KT, Davis K, Schoen C, Parker S. Listening to parents. A national survey of parents with young children. *Arch Pediatr Adolesc Med.* 1998;152(3):255–262

CHAPTER 6

Talking With Adolescents

Monica Sifuentes, MD

CASE STUDY

This is a first-time visit for a 15-year-old girl who is accompanied by her mother. The mother is concerned because her daughter's grades have been dropping since beginning high school, and she appears fatigued and irritable. The mother reports no new activities or recent changes in the home situation and no new stressors in the family. Both parents are employed, the girl has the same friends she has always had, and her siblings currently are doing well academically. The girl is healthy and has never been hospitalized. After the mother leaves the room, the girl is interviewed alone.

Questions

1. When interviewing adolescents, what is the significance of identifying their stage of development?
2. What are important areas to cover in the adolescent interview?
3. What issues of confidentiality and competence need to be discussed with adolescents before conducting the interview?
4. When should information be disclosed to others, despite issues of confidentiality?

Adolescence is a time of unique change. Unlike other periods in life when individuals have at least some knowledge or experience to guide them, adolescence can be characterized by feelings of physical awkwardness, emotional turmoil, and social isolation. In addition, the teenage years are dreaded by most parents, who often feel ill equipped to handle the unpredictability of their children's responses to puberty. So instead of "taking the bull by the horns," some parents choose the route of quiet observation. They fully intend to "be there" for their children but wait to be approached. Hence, many adolescents do not have the active guidance or timely advice of parents during the teenage years and prefer to spend their time alone or in the company of friends or acquaintances. Fortunately, most adolescents pass through this period uneventfully. In fact, many individuals go through this period gladly, finally being permitted to drive a car or go out on a date.

Physicians must use a different approach when interviewing adolescents because information comes directly from the teenager, rather than the parents. Unlike an interview with a younger pediatric patient, the adolescent interview should focus on several psychosocial issues that may be uncomfortable to discuss with the parent present. Each teenager should therefore be interviewed alone. The goal of the interview is to help the adolescent become more comfortable discussing health-related issues with the physician, give the adolescent the opportunity to become more responsible for his or her health care, and discover any psychosocial problems that might interfere with a relatively smooth passage through adolescence.

Stages of Adolescence

Adolescents are stereotypically labeled as difficult, complex, time-consuming patients with complicated problems or complaints that lead to nonmedical diagnoses. In addition, they are often accompanied by overbearing, demanding parents, or sometimes no parents at all.

The quality and quantity of information obtained during the medical and psychosocial interview can be greatly enhanced by taking developmental milestones into consideration. Adolescence can be divided into 3 developmental stages: early, middle, and late (Table 6-1). For example, interest in discussing long-term educational goals varies depending on the age of the adolescent. Most 18-year-olds are prepared to discuss college plans, specific vocational interests, and employment opportunities. In contrast, 12-year-olds are still anchored in the concreteness of early adolescence and often are ill prepared to discuss plans for higher education. Current middle school experiences are much more important to this age group and should therefore be the focus of discussion. Peer pressure is most prominent during middle adolescence; therefore, 14-year-olds with friends who smoke cigarettes and drink beer probably use the same illicit substances.

Table 6-1. Developmental Milestones During Adolescence			
	Early Adolescence (11–13 y)	*Middle Adolescence (14–16 y)*	*Late Adolescence (17–21 y)*
Thought processes	Concrete	±Abstract	Abstract
Parental supervision	+	±	−
Risk-taking behavior	+	±	−
Peer pressure	±	+ +	+

Modified from March CA, Jay MS. Adolescents in the emergency department: an overview. *Adolesc Med.* 1993;4(1):1–10.

Knowledge of these developmental differences allows the interviewer to more effectively explain instructions and diagnoses to teenagers. For example, 19-year-olds can better understand the effects of untreated or recurrent chlamydia cervicitis on long-term fertility than 13-year-olds. This is not to say that physicians should not discuss these possible consequences with a sexually active 13-year-old with chlamydia, but they should use more concrete wording and repeat the information at future visits. Age guidelines are not rigid, however, and each interview should be individually tailored to the particular adolescent and the circumstances surrounding the visit.

Issues of Confidentiality and Competence

A discussion about **confidentiality is essential** and can be approached in 2 ways. Each method has distinct advantages as well as disadvantages. Interviewers should use the approach that they find most comfortable; this allows conversation to flow more naturally.

The first approach involves informing adolescents at the beginning of the interview that most issues discussed are held in strict confidence and will not be repeated to anyone. Exceptions are suicidal or homicidal behavior and a history of or ongoing sexual or physical abuse. In any of these instances, other professionals are told of the disclosed information, and parents or guardians ultimately are informed of the disclosure. The advantages to this approach are that discussion of these "logistics" at the beginning of the interview is less awkward, making the ground rules clear from the start. This contributes to an atmosphere of trust and honesty. The disadvantage is possible inhibition by adolescents who are unsure about disclosing particular incidents (eg, those concerning sexual abuse); some teenagers are now almost certain not to share this information for fear of involving other professionals or family members. Interviewers should be nonjudgmental, reassuring, and empathetic to reduce the possibility of such an occurrence.

The second, less popular approach to the discussion of confidentiality involves informing adolescents at the end of the interview or when and if one of the exceptions to maintaining confidentiality arises. Proponents of this approach argue that adolescents tend to respond more honestly to questions when they do not believe physicians will inform others, including their parents or legal guardians. Physicians have a legal responsibility, however, to report sexual and physical abuse; in cases of suicidal or homicidal behavior, it is in the patient's best interest to inform other professionals of this disclosure. The disadvantage to this method is that these issues often arise at very emotional times during the interview, and it is difficult to interrupt the patient to discuss mandated reporting. If physicians wait until the end of the interview to inform adolescents about mandated reporting, however, patients may leave the office feeling deceived and probably will not return for future visits. For this reason, most health care professionals prefer to inform adolescents at the onset of the interview about confidentiality with the hope that it contributes to the development of a trusting relationship.

An assessment of the adolescent's ability to make health-related decisions is another important aspect of the interview. **Competence** is the ability to understand the significance of information and assess alternatives and consequences sufficiently to identify a preference. Various factors besides age must be considered, such as level of maturity, intelligence, degree of independence, and presence of any chronic illness. This last factor is included because adolescents with chronic conditions may have already participated in decisions about their health care. Regardless, it can be difficult to assess competence from just one visit. It may not even be necessary to make an assessment emergently, except in certain cases, such as with an unplanned pregnancy.

Although it is imperative to interview adolescents alone, every attempt should be made to involve parents in all health-related decisions. Although specific state laws allow physicians to treat minors in emergent situations and in cases of suspected sexually transmitted infections (STIs) without parents' consent, physicians should urge adolescents to inform their parents of any ongoing problems disclosed during the interview. The ultimate decision, however, rests with the adolescent. Physicians can assist adolescents in discussing delicate issues with their parents by role-playing with teenagers or by sitting in on the conversation between the adolescents and their parents.

Psychosocial Review of Systems

A major part of the adolescent interview involves taking an adequate psychosocial history, which can be completed in 20 to 30 minutes in most cases. The approach, known by the acronym **HEADDSSS** (*h*ome environment, *e*mployment and *e*ducation, *a*ctivities, *d*iet, *d*rugs, *s*afety, *s*exual activity/*s*exuality, *s*uicide/depression), allows interviewers to evaluate the critical areas in adolescents' lives that may contribute to a less than optimal environment for normal growth and development (Questions Box). Questions about sexuality, sexual orientation, and gender identification must be asked in a nondirected, nonjudgmental fashion, giving adolescents time to respond. This information is imperative to adequately assess risks for conditions such as social isolation, unintended pregnancy, and STIs, including HIV. In addition, an inquiry about sexual and physical abuse is indicated during this part of the interview.

Because many adolescents now have access to the Internet 24/7 via their cellular telephone, home computer, or other electronic device, it is important to discuss screen time with them and their parents. In addition to reviewing the amount of time actually spent on an electronic device each day, physicians also should inquire about texting, sexting, and whether the patient is a victim of cyberbullying.

Issues That Need Immediate Attention

Many issues discussed during the psychosocial interview can be a source of anxiety for adolescents. Certain problems must be taken more seriously than others and may demand immediate attention. Suicidal ideation, with or without a previous attempt, definitely requires a more in-depth analysis of the gravity of the problem. The physician or other health care practitioner should make sure that

Talking With Adolescents: HEADDSSS

H: Home environment
- With whom does the adolescent live?
- Have there been any recent changes in the living situation?
- How are things between parents/other adults living in the home?
- Are the parents employed?
- How does the adolescent get along with the parents and siblings?

E: Employment and education
- Is the adolescent currently in school?
- What does the adolescent enjoy about school? Dislike?
- How is the adolescent performing academically?
- Has the adolescent ever been truant or expelled from school?
- Are the adolescent's friends attending school?
- Is the adolescent currently employed? How many hours does he or she work each week?
- What are the adolescent's future education/employment/vocational goals?

A: Activities
- What does the adolescent do in his or her spare time?
- How much time is spent on technology (the computer, cell phone, other electronic devices)?
- What does the adolescent do for fun? Is the adolescent ever bored?
- With whom does the adolescent spend most of his or her time?

D: Diet
- What is a typical meal for the adolescent?
- Does the adolescent have any food restrictions?
- What does the adolescent think about his or her current weight and body shape?
- Is there a recent history of changes in his or her weight?
- Has the adolescent dieted in the last year?

D: Drugs
- Do any of the adolescent's friends smoke tobacco, use drugs or alcohol?
- Is the adolescent currently using, or has he or she ever used, tobacco?
- Is the adolescent currently using, or has he or she ever used, any illicit drugs? What about steroids? Alcohol?
- Does the adolescent ever feel pressured by friends to use drugs or alcohol?

S: Safety
- Does the adolescent use a seat belt and bicycle helmet?
- Does the adolescent participate in high-risk situations, such as riding in the car with someone who has been drinking?
- Does the adolescent feel safe at home? At school? In his or her neighborhood? At work?
- Is there a firearm in the adolescent's home? If so, what does the adolescent know about firearm safety?

S: Sexual activity/sexuality
- What is the adolescent's gender identity and sexual orientation?
- Is the adolescent currently in a relationship?
- Is the adolescent sexually active?
- If so, what was the age of the adolescent's first sexual experience?
- What types of sexual experiences has he or she had?
- How many sexual partners has the adolescent had in his or her lifetime?
- Does the adolescent have a history of sexually transmitted infections?
- Does the adolescent (or the partner) use condoms, or another method of protection?
- Does the adolescent (or the partner) use any methods of contraception?
- Does the adolescent have a history of sexual or physical abuse?

S: Suicide/depression
- Is the adolescent bored all the time? Ever sad or tearful? Tired and unmotivated?
- Has the adolescent ever felt that life is not worth living or ever thought of or tried to hurt himself or herself? More importantly, does the adolescent have a suicide plan or access to a firearm?

For more detailed information, see the Goldenring entries under Selected References.

Reprinted with permission from Goldenring JM, Rosen DS. Getting into adolescent heads: an essential update. *Contemp Pediatr.* 2004;21:64. Copyright © Advanstar Communications.

---

adolescents feel they can tell or make verbal contact and call someone if they feel like hurting themselves. Mental health professionals should be involved in the clinical assessment of these precarious situations. Other issues that require immediate attention include possible danger to others, possible or confirmed unplanned pregnancy, and a history of or ongoing sexual or physical abuse.

Concluding the Interview

The adolescent interview should be conducted at a time when the adolescent is relatively healthy and the interviewer has set aside ample time for a thorough, uninterrupted discussion. However, all topics need not be addressed during the initial interview if time does not permit. Issues that are not covered at this visit can be addressed at the next one. The number of appointments needed to discuss or work through a particular problem is unlimited.

At the end of each visit, the interview should be summarized, any difficult topics should be identified, and the issue of confidentiality should be reviewed. Adolescents should then be asked to identify a person whom they can trust or confide in should any problems arise before the next visit. In some instances, this issue may already have been discussed during the interview. Adolescents also should be given the opportunity to express any other concerns not covered in the interview and ask additional questions.

Physicians should clearly point out to the adolescent any significant risk factors or risk-taking behaviors that have been identified during the interview and assess the teenager's readiness to change this behavior. For those adolescents who are not engaging in high-risk behaviors, physicians should acknowledge that things seem to be going well, praise them with positive feedback, and review their individual strengths and accomplishments. Available resources, such as teen hotlines and popular Web sites, should be given to the adolescent prior to inviting the parents or guardians back into the examination room. General concerns should then be reviewed with the parents while maintaining the adolescent's confidentiality. Parents also should be given appropriate written or electronic resources to review, particularly if a sensitive subject has been discussed, and invited to call you if they have any questions or concerns. The follow-up appointment should be arranged with the adolescent prior to the conclusion of the visit.

CASE RESOLUTION

The adolescent in the case history initially should be informed about confidentiality and the specific exceptions to maintaining it. Nonthreatening topics, such as home life, school, employment, and other outside activities, should be explored first, followed by questions about sexuality, sexual orientation, sexual activity, and illicit drug use. Suicidal behavior or depression and safety issues should also be reviewed with the teenager alone and again with the parent if there is a need for a more formal or immediate mental health evaluation. In addition, computer and cell phone use as well as sleep hygiene should be evaluated. Identified high-risk behaviors and their consequences should be discussed with the adolescent at the end of the interview, and a plan for future visits should be arranged. The mother should then be invited back into the examination room prior to the conclusion of the visit.

Selected References

Akinbami LJ, Gandhi H, Cheng TL. Availability of adolescent health services and confidentiality in primary care practices. *Pediatrics.* 2003;111(2):394–401

Bravender T, Price CN, English A. Primary care providers' willingness to see unaccompanied adolescents. *J Adolesc Health.* 2004;34(1):30–36

Breuner CC, Moreno MA. Approaches to the difficult patient/parent encounter. *Pediatrics.* 2011;127(1):163–169

Cavanaugh RM. Managing the transitions of early adolescents. *Adolesc Health Update.* 2008;20:1–10

English A, Kenney KE. *State Minor Consent Laws: A Summary.* 3rd ed. Chapel Hill, NC: Center for Adolescent Health and the Law; 2010

Ford C, English A, Sigman G. Confidential health care for adolescents: position paper for the Society for Adolescent Medicine. *J Adolesc Health.* 2004;35(2):160–167

Ginsburg KR. Viewing our adolescent patients through a positive lens. *Contemp Pediatr.* 2007;24:65–76

Goldenring JM, Cohen E. Getting into adolescent heads. *Contemp Pediatr.* 1988;5:75–90

Goldenring JM, Rosen DS. Getting into adolescent heads: an essential update. *Contemp Pediatr.* 2004;21:64–90

Gutgesell ME, Payne N. Issues of adolescent psychological development in the 21st century. *Pediatr Rev.* 2004;25(3):79–85

Guttmacher Institute. State policies in brief. An overview of minors' consent law. http://www.guttmacher.org/statecenter/spibs/spib_OMCL.pdf. Created March 1, 2014. Accessed March 17, 2014

Hawkins JD, Smith BH, Catalano RF. Delinquent behavior. *Pediatr Rev.* 2002;23(11):387–392

Klein DA, Goldenring JM, Adelman WP. Probing the scars. How to ask the essential questions. *Contemp Pediatr.* 2014;31:16–28

Knight JR, Sherritt L, Shrier LA, Harris SK, Chang G. Validity of the CRAFFT substance abuse screening test among adolescent clinic patients. *Arch Pediatr Adolesc Med.* 2002;156(6):607–614

Kokotailo PK, Gold MA. Motivational interviewing with adolescents. *Adolesc Med.* 2008;19:54–68

Kreipe RE. Introduction to interviewing: the art of communicating with adolescents. *Adolesc Med.* 2008;19:1–17

Ott MA, Labbett RL, Gold MA. Counseling adolescents about abstinence in the office setting. *J Pediatr Adolesc Gynecol.* 2007;20(1):39–44

Van Hook S, Harris SK, Brooks T, et al. The "Six T's": barriers to screening teens for substance abuse in primary care. *J Adolesc Health.* 2007;40(5):456–461

CHAPTER 7

Telephone Management and E-medicine

Emily Borman-Shoap, MD, and Iris Wagman Borowsky, MD, PhD

CASE STUDY

The mother of an otherwise healthy 10-month-old girl calls and tells you that her daughter has a fever. The girl's rectal temperature has been 103°F to 104°F (39.4°C–40.0°C) for the past 2 days. Although she is cranky with the fever, she plays normally after receiving acetaminophen. The girl is eating well and has no runny nose, cough, vomiting, diarrhea, or rash.

Mother also mentions 2 other concerns that she has been meaning to bring up with you. The first is questions about feeding and how to introduce solid foods; the other is sleep problems. Her daughter has been waking up several times a night for the past month, and mom is feeling exhausted.

Questions

1. How do telephone and face-to-face encounters between physicians and patients differ?
2. What are some general guidelines for effective doctor-patient communication over the telephone?
3. What historical information is necessary for appropriate telephone management?
4. What points are important to cover in home treatment advice?
5. For nonurgent issues, how can telephone encounters or e-medicine play a role in patient care?

Parents are increasingly accessing their pediatrician through avenues other than a typical office visit. Telephone management and electronic communications make up a substantial portion of a pediatrician's time. It is estimated that pediatricians spend more than 25% of their total practice time engaged in telephone medicine. Telephone management includes triage of acute illness complaints as well as ongoing preventive care and chronic condition management. Electronic communication may also play a role in acute, chronic, and preventive care.

Telephone Management for Acute Illness

The key components of a telephone management encounter for acute illness mirror an office visit: establish rapport, gather a complete history, formulate an assessment and plan, ensure adequate follow-up, and document the encounter. The key difference is that there is no opportunity for physical examination in a telephone encounter. Thus, gathering a thorough history becomes even more critical.

Telephone Communication Skills: Establishing Rapport

Parents commonly call their pediatricians because they are worried about their child. The friendly voice of a health care worker who is ready to lend an ear goes a long way toward reassuring an anxious parent. Calls should begin with a *verbal handshake.* Staff should identify themselves and the place where the call is received and offer to help. They should learn the caller's name, his or her relationship to the child, and the child's name and gender; these names, as well as the child's gender, should be used in the conversation, thereby creating a more personal atmosphere.

Telephone calls for medical advice are often received in busy environments, such as emergency departments (EDs) or clinics, where other patients are waiting to be seen. It is easy to be abrupt under these circumstances and not give complete attention to callers. If calls are not emergencies, practitioners can take the caller's telephone number and return the call as soon as possible. If callers do not feel that their concerns have been fully acknowledged, they are likely to feel dissatisfied, even if they are given sound advice. Furthermore, research on doctor-patient relationships suggests that lack of friendliness or warmth in the doctor-patient relationship and patient dissatisfaction are associated with noncompliance with medical advice. Studies show that the length of a patient visit does not correlate with patient satisfaction. Telephone encounters do not necessarily have to be lengthy; the average length of a call is reported to be 3 to 5 minutes, depending on the setting. Calls must be pleasant, however, and they must address callers' concerns. Open-ended questions such as, "Tell me about your child's illness," or "Are there any other symptoms?" are useful at the beginning of a call because they give callers an opportunity to explain the situation without interruptions.

Establishing rapport over the telephone is more difficult than in person because the practitioner is limited to verbal communication. In face-to-face encounters, physicians can use words as well as means of nonverbal communication, such as facial expressions, eye contact, gesturing, and touch, to convey warmth and empathy. Practitioners should use various aspects of **verbal communication** to convey sincere interest in callers' concerns, and they should pay attention to these verbal cues in callers. Many components of verbal communication (in addition to words themselves), including vocal expression, pace, articulation, tone, volume, and pauses, affect telephone interactions. Health care professionals should speak clearly and use vocabulary that callers understand; **medical jargon should be avoided.** A friendly yet respectful tone and a calm, professional manner should be maintained.

Careful listening is crucial to obtaining the information necessary to make medical decisions over the telephone. One of the major goals of health care professionals is to recognize and respond to callers' main concerns and expectations. Researchers have found the following questions useful in the identification of parents' chief concerns: "What worries you the most about [use child's name] illness?" and "Why does that worry you?"

For callers who ramble, health care professionals may need to focus the conversation. Asking the question, "What can I do to help?" should clarify the reason for the call. If information needs to be verified, practitioners can summarize what they have heard and ask if they have understood correctly.

Angry callers may elicit defensive or confrontational behavior from health care professionals. Responding to anger with arguments, however, is time-consuming, stressful, and pointless. Practitioners should be warm and understanding so that callers who want to discuss their feelings are comfortable. Acknowledging anger may encourage open discussion and problem-solving (eg, "You sound upset. Is there anything I can do to help?"). Empathizing with callers (eg, "I don't blame you for being upset"; "That must have been very frustrating.") may also help.

Practitioners can build confidence in callers by complimenting them on the way they have handled things so far (eg, "You did the right thing by giving your child acetaminophen for the fever. That is exactly what I would have done"; "I'm glad that you called about this."). The practitioner may even be able to offer reassurance to parents who are not managing their child's illness correctly by commenting that many parents try the same treatment. A different treatment approach can then be suggested.

Before the end of the conversation, callers should be given an opportunity to ask questions and encouraged to call again if additional problems occur.

Telephone History Taking

Most calls for triage of an acute problem concern upper respiratory symptoms, fever, rash, trauma, or gastrointestinal complaints—the same problems most commonly seen in the office. Many patients with these chief complaints can be safely managed at home through standardized history taking and home care advice. Several excellent published telephone management protocols can aid the health care team in advising patients efficiently and appropriately. Many practices use nurses as the first point of contact for telephone triage, with the pediatrician serving as second-tier triage for more complex or worrisome complaints.

How much history should be obtained over the telephone? Enough information should be gathered to make an appropriate decision. Questions should be directed at **determining whether an emergency exists** and **making a diagnosis.** Practitioners should follow the same organized approach they would use in the office setting (Questions Box). Key features, such as age of the patient and past medical history, should guide questioning. For example, if the mother of a 20-day-old girl reports that her daughter has a temperature of 102°F (38.9°C), the newborn must be seen immediately. An older child with the same chief complaint of fever may be safely managed at home, depending on the answers to other questions about additional symptoms. Similarly, knowing that a child who has been exposed to chickenpox has a compromised immune system is crucial in providing appropriate telephone advice.

Additional specific questions should then be asked to clarify the child's condition and obtain all the information necessary to make a good decision. Many practitioners have the option to access electronic medical records (EMRs) remotely to review the child's record. This can greatly aid in obtaining a thorough history. If review of the medical record is possible, it is reassuring to tell the child's caregiver that you can access this information, by stating, for example, "I am reviewing your child's medical record in the computer so that I can be sure I have all of the information I need to give you good advice."

The physician should focus on the critical features that will affect disposition of the patient (emergency department vs office visit vs home care). For example, with a child who is vomiting or has diarrhea, the state of hydration is critical; with a cough, the occurrence of breathing difficulty; and with head trauma, loss of consciousness. Methods of teaching telephone management skills include role-playing, listening to mock calls by simulated parents, and reviewing tapes of actual calls.

Telephone Advice: Communicating Your Assessment and Management Plan

If the situation is an emergency, this should be explained to the caller, and appropriate follow-up plans should be made (ie, sending an ambulance for life-threatening conditions such as respiratory depression or uncontrollable bleeding, or advising the caller to bring the child by car to the ED or physician's office within a specified amount of time for potentially dangerous complaints, such as right lower quadrant pain or possible fracture). If the call is not an emergency, health care professionals must decide if and when the child should be seen by a physician and the appropriate course of home treatment.

Because most childhood illnesses are mild and self-limited, evaluation of the safety of medical advice obtained over the telephone

Telephone Management: Acute Illness

Questions

- How old is the child?
- What is the child's chief problem? What are the child's symptoms?
- How long has the child had these symptoms?
- How is the child acting?
- Does the child have any chronic illnesses?
- Is the child taking any medications?
- What is the caller most worried about?

requires large samples to detect poor outcomes associated with mismanagement. Research has described a "wellness bias" in which practitioners, who primarily see patients with mild, self-limited illnesses, may downplay the severity of reported symptoms and choose the most benign diagnostic possibility. This bias may be more pronounced in a telephone encounter, for which the physician cannot see the child. One study reported telephone encounters in which physicians seemed to make a decision early in the conversation and then "shut out" additional information that should have led to the consideration of more serious diagnoses. The safest approach is to always have a high index of suspicion for a serious condition. Questions can then be asked to confirm or dispel those suspicions.

Research shows that parents need and expect to receive an explanation of their child's illness. Practitioners should clearly state what the child's illness seems to be, what probably caused it, and what the parents can expect (eg, length of time that the child is likely to be sick, additional symptoms that may appear).

Before giving any treatment advice, health care professionals should ask callers the following questions: "What have you done so far?"; "Have you given the child any medications?"; and "How is this treatment working?" If the therapy seems appropriate, callers should be complimented and encouraged to continue the treatment. The regimen should be modified as indicated. Instructions for home treatment should be clear and as easy to implement as possible. If the instructions are complicated or lengthy, callers may want to write them down. When prescribing medication, ask if the child has any known drug allergies, and give the dose, frequency of administration, and information about possible side effects. Practitioners should verify that the caller can follow the telephone advice (eg, a parent has a thermometer and knows how to use it).

Closing the Encounter: Ensuring Appropriate Follow-up

Practitioners should confirm that callers understand the information and instructions and agree with the plan. Asking questions such as, "What questions do you have?" encourages callers to raise uncertainties and ask for needed clarification. Most importantly, if the decision is to manage at home, callers should always receive specific instructions about when to call back. Caregivers should call if the child's symptoms change, persist, worsen, or cause anxiety. Also, symptoms specific to the child's condition should be followed (eg, child has fever for more than 2 days, irritability, decreased urination). If physicians plan to check up on children by telephone, they should confirm and record the appropriate callback number(s). Parents who seem unduly anxious or uncomfortable with home treatment should be given the opportunity to have their child seen by a physician.

Documentation

All calls for medical advice should be documented in the child's medical record for medical reasons (eg, better follow-up, improved continuity of care) and legal purposes. The form used for documentation should include the date and time of the call; the name, identity, and telephone number of the caller; the name and age of the child; the chief complaint; other symptoms; possible diagnoses; advice given; and the name of the person who took the call.

Privacy and Technology Considerations

Practitioners should be aware that many calls take place over cellular phones. The caller may be able to see the phone number that you are calling from. Callers should be given clear instructions as to the appropriate avenue for calling the physician back (eg, "Please call back to the nurse triage line if you need to talk to me again."). Some practitioners may choose to block their numbers so they are not visible by caller identification. Others may feel comfortable having a parent call directly to their cell phone but should give the parent clear guidelines about doing so.

Many cell phones are capable of taking and sending pictures. This can be a valuable additional piece of information when evaluating symptoms such as rash. However, the physician should discuss with the caller that data sent by cell phone may not be secure.

Telephone Management: Preventive Care and Care Coordination

Telephone encounters can provide an excellent opportunity for preventive care and anticipatory guidance. Issues such as sleep problems or behavioral issues may be difficult to discuss during an office visit while the child is present. Telephone follow-up provides an opportunity to minimize distraction during conversation between parent and practitioner. Some pediatric offices develop protocols to charge a fee for prolonged telephone consultation.

Telephone follow-up can also help to facilitate care coordination for children with chronic health care conditions. For example, a clinic practitioner who recommends medication changes for a child presenting with poorly controlled asthma can have a follow-up call with the parents one month later to assess asthma symptoms. Using telephone follow-up when appropriate allows practitioners to adapt their care to the patient's needs (patient-centered care) and minimize missed work and school for patients and families.

E-medicine

An increasing avenue for communicating with patients is virtual medicine. Studies suggest that up to 75% of patients would like to communicate with their physician through e-mail. Patients who do choose electronic communication as a means of interacting with their physician report high rates of satisfaction. Patients and parents who choose electronic message as a form of communication with their physician tend to have higher degrees of education.

E-mail communication can be convenient for patients and families and may increase patient-centered care. Specific American Academy of Pediatrics, American Medical Association, and American Medical Informatics Association (AMIA) guidelines exist for the use of e-mail with patients. However, it should be noted that traditional e-mail poses a variety of data security concerns. Therefore, many EMRs have now incorporated the ability for patients and their parents to interact directly with the EMR. This includes the ability to view laboratory test results, immunization records, growth charts, and patient problem lists. Parents may also have the ability to send a secure message to the health care team with a health care question. Clinics should create guidelines for patients and parents about appropriate issues to be addressed through electronic messaging, expected response time, and who will provide a response (ie, nurse or physician).

Communication through the EMR should be kept professional, concise, and to the point. Written communication has the benefit that it can eliminate the telephone tag phenomenon when trying to connect with a parent for a phone call. However, physicians should remember that written communication will be interpreted through the lens of the reader. Delicate or complex conversations should be first broached on the phone or in person. Similar guiding principles apply with telephone and e-mail communications: establish rapport, give clear advice, and provide guidance for follow-up. Attention should be paid to correct grammar and spelling in e-mails because errors may decrease confidence in the physician. Electronic communication can also be a useful method to provide patient education materials, such as a link to a helpful Web site.

Conclusions

Telephone management and e-medicine represent the changing face of medical practice. Physicians should be prepared to deliver care that meets the needs of the patient, and this may necessitate being creative with how and where care is delivered. The approach needs to be tailored to each patient scenario, and physicians should continually strive to adapt their approach so that they can provide effective and appropriate patient-centered care in and out of the office.

CASE RESOLUTION

In the case history at the beginning of this chapter, the pediatrician learns several facts that lead to the recommendation that the child be seen that day (the next day if the call is made at night). These facts include the child's age, the height and duration of the fever, and lack of any symptoms of localized infection.

The other concerns of feeding questions and sleep issues present excellent opportunities for management through a follow-up phone call, electronic communication, or office visit, depending on parent preference and clinic resources.

Selected References

American Academy of Pediatrics. Section on Telehealth Care Web site. http://www.aap.org/sections/telecare. Accessed November 19, 2013

American Academy of Pediatrics Section on Telephone Care and Committee on Child Health Financing. Payment for telephone care. *Pediatrics.* 2006;118(4):1768–1773

Brown JL, Swiontkowski MF. *Pediatric Telephone Medicine: Principles, Triage, and Advice.* 3rd ed. Philadelphia, PA: J. B. Lippincott; 2003

Bunik M, Glazner JE, Chandramouli V, Emsermann CB, Hegarty T, Kempe A. Pediatric telephone call centers: how do they affect health care use and costs? *Pediatrics.* 2007;119(2):e305–e313

Gerstle RS; American Academy of Pediatrics Task Force on Medical Informatics. E-mail communication between pediatricians and their patients. *Pediatrics.* 2004;114(1):317–321

Kempe A, Bunik M, Ellis J, et al. How safe is triage by an after-hours telephone call center? *Pediatrics.* 2006;118(2):457–463

Kempe A, Luberti A, Belman S, et al. Outcomes associated with pediatric after-hours care by call centers: a multicenter study. *Ambul Pediatr.* 2003;3(4):211–217

Lee TJ, Baraff LJ, Guzy J, Johnson D, Woo H. Does telephone triage delay significant medical treatment? Advice nurse service vs on-call pediatricians. *Arch Pediatr Adolesc Med.* 2003;157(7):635–641

Lee TJ, Guzy J, Johnson D, Woo H, Baraff LJ. Caller satisfaction with after-hours telephone advice: nurse advice service versus on-call pediatricians. *Pediatrics.* 2002;110(5):865–872

Poole SR. *The Complete Guide: Developing a Telephone Triage and Advice System for a Pediatric Office Practice During Office Hours and/or After Hours.* Elk Grove Village, IL. American Academy of Pediatrics; 2003

Reisman AB, Brown KE. Preventing communication errors in telephone medicine. *J Gen Intern Med.* 2005;20(10):959–963

Schiller JH, Christner JG, Stansfield RB, Watnick CS, Mullan PB. What parents want from emails with their pediatrician: implications for teaching communication skills. *Patient Educ Couns.* 2013;92(1):61–66

Schmitt BD. *Pediatric Telephone Protocols: Office Version.* 14th ed. Elk Grove Village, IL: American Academy of Pediatrics; 2013

Ye J, Rust G, Fry-Johnson Y, Strothers H. E-mail in patient-provider communication: a systematic review. *Patient Educ Couns.* 2010;80(2):266–273

CHAPTER 8

Informatics

Alan Tomines, MD

CASE STUDY

You are a physician in a small pediatric practice. Your hospital is planning to acquire an electronic health record, which will be made available within the hospital and to the offices of its affiliated practices. The hospital chief of staff asks you to sit on the hospital's informatics committee to participate in the vendor selection process and assist with the implementation of the selected system. You have previously used the hospital's computer to check patients' laboratory results, and your practice uses computers for billing and scheduling. However, you don't consider yourself a technology expert and express your trepidation to the chief of staff, who asks you to speak with the head of the informatics committee.

Questions

1. What are the important informatics concepts to understand?
2. What are the important drivers of health care information technology?
3. What are the challenges to implementing successful health information systems?
4. What are the special pediatric considerations in health information systems?

To make the best possible clinical decisions, physicians must have information about their patients' health that is current, accurate, complete, and reliable. This information should be available wherever and whenever it is needed. Where possible, the physician should be presented with information that will encourage an evidence-based approach to decision-making, and the decisions made should be communicated to other health care professionals in a manner that is clear and error-free. The physician should also be able to receive feedback on the quality of care provided. Health care information technology (HIT) holds the promise of increasing access to patient health information, improving patient safety, reporting and measuring desired health outcomes, and making health care more efficient; at the same time, it holds the promise of decreasing health care expenditures. However, the implementation of HIT is not without challenges.

Basic Concepts

Although the terms *data, information,* and *knowledge* are sometimes used interchangeably, these concepts are distinct. Data are mere observations or facts (eg, hemoglobin equal to 9 g/dL). Information is data placed in meaningful context (eg, hemoglobin equal to 9 g/dL in a breastfed 3-month-old). Knowledge is the understanding of information, including an assessment of its completeness (eg, hemoglobin equal to 9 g/dL in a breastfed 3-month-old may represent a physiological nadir but may also represent blood loss, increased destruction of red blood cells, or decreased production of red blood cells). Any structured collection of data may be referred to as a *database.*

Information technology refers to any hardware or software that supports the acquisition, storage, retrieval, transformation, interpretation, and dissemination of data and information. An *information system* is the sum of the people and work processes that are supported by information technology. Depending on the degree to which technology is applied, the processes of an information system may be automated, manual, or a combination of both.

What Is Informatics?

Medical informatics is the science that deals with the appropriate application of information technology to health care work processes. To apply information technology appropriately, specialists in informatics (referred to as *informaticians* or *informaticists*) focus first on improving the quality of data and the efficiency of work flow in the patient care setting; it is in this optimized environment that technology may be applied most effectively. Medical informatics places great emphasis on non-technologic considerations that can influence the successful implementation of health information systems, including information science, cognitive psychology, project management, organizational and change management, health care policy, and ethics.

As a field, medical informatics can itself be subdivided into specific clinical domains, such as nursing, pharmacy, veterinary medicine, dentistry, and imaging. *Biomedical informatics* is a term of broader scope that encompasses medical informatics, bioinformatics (having the primary domain of genomics and bioengineering), and public health informatics. Outside of the United States, *health informatics* is the term more frequently used to convey the same breadth.

Electronic Health Information Systems

Although all electronic health information systems ultimately deal with managing some aspect of patient care, they are divided here into 4 coarse groupings: electronic records of patient care, administrative systems, ancillary clinical systems, and telemedicine. Box 8-1 lists several common abbreviations used in electronic health information systems.

Electronic Records of Patient Care

An electronic medical record (EMR) represents the clinical documentation and legal record of care provided to a patient by a health care professional or organization. An EMR can usually create and store traditional clinical documentation, such as progress notes and consultations. However, a full-fledged EMR represents more than an electronic version of the traditional paper-based record. Important components of an EMR include a clinical data repository (CDR), a clinical decision-support system (CDSS), and computerized physician order entry (CPOE). A CDR is a real-time database containing all of the clinically relevant patient data in an institution. A CDSS is a special computer program that applies medical knowledge to data from a CDR to produce patient-specific care recommendations. A CPOE is a special computer program that allows providers to write electronic orders that are directed to the appropriate clinical staff or ancillary department. A CPOE can decrease errors due to illegible handwriting, decrease delays in the receipt and execution of orders, and allow for orders to be entered away from the care setting. In addition, a CPOE (when paired with a CDSS) can prevent harm due to drug-drug interactions, drug-allergy interactions, or errors in age- or weight-based dosing.

An EMR generally operates within the functional boundary of a hospital or practice. However, information about a patient's health is not limited to traditional health care settings. A personal health record (PHR) is a summary of an individual's health history, usually self-maintained, that contains information collected from encounters with different health care professionals, medicolegal documents (eg, living wills, advance directives), and other health information that may be relevant to patients (eg, regimens for nontraditional remedies, results of home testing for blood pressure). The concept of a PHR is not new; patients with multiple medical problems have long maintained paper-based PHRs out of necessity—to have at least one reliable and portable source containing a complete medical history. The electronic PHR is an evolving entity, ranging from scanned paper documents stored on portable devices (eg, CD-ROM or other removable media) to Web-based applications that interface with EMRs and capture data from medical devices. The PHR is not considered a legal record of care.

The electronic health record (EHR) represents the next stage in the evolution of the EMR. An EHR will have all of the desired functionality of a full-fledged EMR but will exchange data among multiple different EMRs to provide the entire longitudinal history of the patient. In addition, an EHR will support functionality related to research and public health, such as identification of

Box 8-1. Abbreviations Used in Informatics	
ARRA	American Recovery and Reinvestment Act of 2009
CDR	clinical data repository
CDSS	clinical decision-support system
CPOE	computerized physician order entry
EHR	electronic health record
EMR	electronic medical record
eRx	electronic prescribing
HIE	health information exchange
HIPAA	Health Insurance Portability and Accountability Act of 1996
HIS	hospital information system
HIT	health care information technology
HITECH	Health Information Technology for Economic and Clinical Health Act
IIS	immunization information system or registry
LIS	laboratory information system
P4P	pay for performance
PACS	picture archiving and communication system
PHI	protected health information
PHR	personal health record
RIS	radiology information system

patient-appropriate clinical trials, mandatory reporting of notifiable disease, and provision of anonymized clinical data to support clinical and public health research.

A health information exchange (HIE) is an enabling technology that acts as a hub for the secure exchange of data between EMRs. An EMR that is connected to an HIE has the ability to exchange health information with other EMRs that are connected to that HIE, precluding physicians and hospitals from having to establish an interface between their EMR and every other EMR in which a patient might have data. While an HIE generally serves a specific geographic region, the interconnection of HIEs provides the capability for an EMR in one region to share data with an EMR in another region, reducing the barriers to accessing a patient's entire history of episodic care.

Ancillary Clinical Systems

Ancillary clinical systems provide information management and automation for specific domains, including pharmacy, laboratory, imaging, and immunizations.

A pharmacy information system tracks patients' prescription and payment information and can improve patient safety by checking for medication interactions and appropriate dosing. A related concept is electronic prescribing (e-prescribing or eRx), which is a specialized form of CPOE that allows clinicians to prepare and transmit prescriptions electronically to a pharmacy information system. When connected to an EMR/EHR, a pharmacy information system can help to support the medication management cycle of prescription writing and transmission (via CPOE), dispensing (pharmacy information system), and medication administration and monitoring (as documented in an EMR/EHR).

A laboratory information system (LIS) manages the receipt of laboratory orders (eg, from CPOE), tracking of specimens, capture of data from automated analyzers, and presentation of laboratory results to the ordering health care professional via direct access to the LIS or an interface that transfers the results to an EMR/EHR. Electronic laboratory results can support patient safety through timelier access as well as automated decision support.

A picture archiving and communication system (PACS) manages the storage and distribution of patients' electronic medical images, which are often captured directly from computerized or digital radiography devices, as well as other imaging modalities (eg, computed tomography, magnetic resonance imaging, ultrasound). A radiology information system (RIS) incorporates the functionality of a PACS while managing other imaging service activities, such as reporting, scheduling, and billing.

An immunization information system (IIS or immunization registry) is used to document and track patient vaccinations. An IIS can send reminder or recall notices, as appropriate, to physicians and parents when vaccinations are due or delinquent or when administered vaccines are determined to be ineffective or unsafe. As an IIS is usually maintained regionally by public health entities, it also collects reports on adverse vaccine events and provide summaries of regional vaccination prevalence. These systems are usually able to exchange data with capable EMRs/EHRs.

Administrative Systems

A hospital information system (HIS) comprises all of the clinical and nonclinical information systems of an institution. An HIS may be a single integrated information system or may represent multiple interconnected information systems. Hospitals and large practices often have separate information systems to manage individual administrative functions, such as appointment scheduling, insurance eligibility, and billing and payment. A practice management system is an information system designed to manage administrative tasks for small- and medium-sized clinical practices.

Telemedicine

Telemedicine is not an information system but a related concept of interest in informatics. Telemedicine is the use of information and communication technologies to deliver health care over a distance, often to support patient care in rural or underserved areas. There are many specialties within telemedicine, roughly corresponding to distinct medical specialties, such as teleradiology (the transmission of radiologic images electronically for interpretation) and telesurgery (the use of video and robotic technology to perform surgery). The use of e-mail and Web sites to consult with patients is also a form of telemedicine.

Drivers

The key health care drivers for the adoption of HIT are the improvement of patient safety, measurement of health care outcomes, increased efficiency of work flow in the patient care setting, and reduction of health care expenditures.

Patient safety, through the reduction of preventable errors, is the primary driver of information technology adoption in many health care organizations. In its report *To Err Is Human: Building a Safer Health System,* the Institute of Medicine (IOM) estimated that up to 98,000 US deaths annually are attributable to medical errors. Most errors were noted to be preventable and caused by systems and processes that increase, or fail to prevent, human errors. Computerized physician order entry is an example of information technology that has the potential to improve patient safety by alerting the physician to errors before an order is submitted.

Changes in the health care marketplace are driving the measurement of health care outcomes. Pay for performance (relating payment to measures of quality of care provided), medical "report cards" that permit comparison of health care plans and professionals, and Accountable Care Organizations are examples of market drivers. Information technology is critical to collecting and analyzing data to calculate these measures. In addition, a CDSS may improve health care outcomes through guideline adherence by reminding physicians and patients about necessary care services that may have been overlooked.

Improvements in efficiency are another driver in the adoption of information technology. The automation of highly repetitive, data-intensive activities, such as billing or scheduling, is an example of where efficiency can be improved. However, introduction of information technology into a clinical setting without thorough consideration of work flow may actually decrease efficiency.

Health care spending is approaching 20% of the gross domestic product of the United States and is increasing at a rate nearly twice that of inflation. Information technology is considered to be a potential source of cost savings by reducing duplication of diagnostic studies and decreasing the time spent on administrative tasks. In addition, in the IOM report *Crossing the Quality Chasm: A New Health System for the 21st Century,* the use of e-mail was touted as a method for meeting the needs of patients more quickly and at lower cost than a traditional visit.

Challenges

Despite the significant health care drivers for adopting HIT, there are a number of challenges that prevent the easy implementation of systems.

The ease with which information systems can exchange electronic patient data should not belie the care that must be taken to protect patient data. Protected health information (PHI) is any information about a patient (eg, name, medical record number) that may be used to identify a patient. Privacy is the patient's right to keep this information a secret. Confidentiality is the assurance made by health care professionals that private information will not be revealed. Security involves the policies and technologies that support the assurance of confidentiality. The Health Insurance Portability and Accountability Act of 1996 defines the measures that must be taken to ensure that PHI is secure and made available only to authorized individuals or organizations. Appropriate concerns exist about breaches of patient privacy when data are stored electronically. Although health information systems often employ sophisticated technical barriers to protect patient data, it is often the case that data breaches are the result of people failing to adhere to policy safeguards. Educating health care professionals is critical to ensuring the confidentiality of patient data.

The cost of implementing health information systems can be prohibitive for health care delivery organizations, particularly small practices. To address this barrier, the Health Information Technology for Economic and Clinical Health (HITECH) Act was included in the American Recovery and Reinvestment Act of 2009. The HITECH Act authorizes Medicare and Medicaid incentives to be provided to clinicians and hospitals that adopt EHRs and demonstrate their *meaningful use* by meeting specific objectives toward improved health care delivery and outcomes. These objectives include using EHRs for fundamental activities, such as recording patient demographics and vital signs; maintaining active problem, medication, and allergy lists; providing patients with summaries of outpatient visits and inpatient discharge instructions; eRx and ordering; and providing drug-drug and drug-allergy checks. The objectives also include more esoteric or complex functions, such as providing data to public health agencies for disease surveillance and immunization and cancer registries; generating lists of patients with specific conditions for quality improvement and research, identifying and providing patient-specific education resources; and supporting medication reconciliation and care summaries across health care settings. To assure physicians and hospitals that they are adopting EHRs that allow them to meet meaningful use regulations, the US Department of Health and Human Services has developed a process and criteria for certifying EHRs. In the first 18 months of the meaningful use program, more than 75% of eligible hospitals qualified for financial incentives, although smaller hospitals and critical access hospitals have lower participation than larger hospitals.

The management of organizational change is an important part of successful information system implementations. Introduction of technology inevitably results in changes in the work flow of physicians and nurses and may lead to repurposing of administrative staff. Resistance to change should be anticipated; strategies to mitigate resistance should be employed, including involvement of health care professionals in the selection and deployment of HIT.

Human-computer interaction is the study of the interactions between people and information technology. It is important for users to perceive that the technology is useful (supports the work being done) and that the technology is usable (readily learned, efficient, and helps them to avoid and correct errors). The topic of usability of HIT is an emerging area of research in the field of informatics.

The effect of technology on patient-physician interaction must also be considered. Time constraints or computers located in examination rooms may compel some physicians to do electronic documentation during patient visits. While some patients look favorably on the use of HIT, physicians should be sensitive to patients who feel that technology is intrusive; where appropriate, physicians should acknowledge the intrusion and identify potential benefits to the patient (including efficiency of access to information and more efficient communication of prescriptions to pharmacies or orders to ancillary services).

Pediatric Considerations

Although pediatric patients represent approximately one quarter of the US population, pediatric functionality is often underdeveloped in electronic health information systems. When considering these systems for pediatric settings, particular attention should be focused on the highly specific data, task, and policy needs of pediatric practice.

The presence of functionality to support clinical tasks that are generally, if not uniquely, pediatric should always be examined. Immunization management, including the ability to assess a patient's status or exchange data with an IIS, is highly desirable. Weight-based dosing and the tracking of growth parameters are other functions that are often overlooked. Age-specific documentation and educational materials can be well-managed electronically.

The data and terminology of an information system should suit the highly specific needs of pediatric practice. Units of measure should reflect the requisite data precision. For example, the age of a patient in hours (rather than years, months, or even days) and weight in grams is critical to appropriate care in the neonatal period. Laboratory values should be accompanied by age-appropriate normal ranges. Patient identification must account for the frequent changes in names and numerical identifiers that may occur in infancy or during change of custody. Pediatric terminology, such as developmental milestones, type of cry, or characterization of stool, are often overlooked in information systems designed for adults.

Pediatric policy issues should also be reflected in the design of an information system. Authorization for the child (or the child's parents, guardians, or other legal authority) to view all, none, or parts of a child's medical record should be enforced electronically as it would be for the paper medical record. Likewise, secondary use of patient data for public health, research, or commercial purposes should be allowed or restricted as appropriate.

At this time, there is no electronic medical home for the care of children. The electronic history of care may be distributed across EMRs, IISs, school health information systems, and specialty registries for rare conditions, trauma, or foster care. With the emergence of HIEs as a conduit for data exchange, it may be possible to create a virtual medical home. It is important that pediatricians work toward reducing the legislative, technologic, and cultural barriers to linking child health information systems without compromising the security or confidentiality of PHI.

Pediatricians should be actively involved in the acquisition and development of information technology to ensure that child-specific data and policy needs are addressed. Pediatricians should also be involved in national policy initiatives to ensure that health information systems are certified for pediatric use and integrated to support care that is child-centered.

CASE RESOLUTION

In the case history at the beginning of this chapter, the pediatrician speaks with the head of the informatics committee. The pediatrician learns that she has been asked to participate because of her understanding of physician work flow in the office setting and to advocate for the highly specific data needs and policies associated with the pediatric population. Her expertise will help to identify issues that, if addressed, may contribute to successful acceptance of the information system by pediatricians and other physicians and improved outcomes for patients.

Selected References

Adler-Milstein J, Furukawa MF, King J, Jha AK. Early results from the hospital Electronic Health Record Incentive Programs. *Am J Manag Care.* 2013;19(7):e273–e284

Blumenthal D, Tavenner M. The "meaningful use" regulation for electronic health records. *N Engl J Med.* 2010;363(6):501–504

De Leon SF, Silfen SL, Wang JJ, Kamara TS, Wu WY, Shih SC. Patient experiences at primary care practices using electronic health records. *J Med Pract Manage.* 2012;28(3):169–176

Gerstle RS; American Academy of Pediatrics Task Force on Medical Informatics. E-mail communication between pediatricians and their patients. *Pediatrics.* 2004;114(1):317–321

Hinman AR, Davidson AJ. Linking children's health information systems: clinical care, public health, emergency medical systems, and schools. *Pediatrics.* 2009;123(Suppl 2):S67–S73

Institute of Medicine Committee on Quality of Health Care in America. *To Err Is Human: Building a Safer Health System.* Kohn LT, Corrigan JM, Donaldson MS, eds. Washington, DC: National Academies Press; 2000

Kaushal R, Barker KN, Bates DW. How can information technology improve patient safety and reduce medication errors in children's health care? *Arch Pediatr Adolesc Med.* 2001;155(9):1002–1007

Kemper AR, Uren RL, Clark SJ. Adoption of electronic health records in primary care pediatric practices. *Pediatrics.* 2006;118(1):e20–e24

Middleton B, Bloomrosen M, Dente MA, et al. Enhancing patient safety and quality of care by improving the usability of electronic health record systems: recommendations from AMIA. *J Am Med Inform Assoc.* 2013;20(e1):e2–e8

Shiffman RN, Spooner SA, Kwiatkowski K, Brennan PF. Information technology for children's health and health care: report on the Information Technology in Children's Health Care Expert Meeting, September 21-22, 2000. *J Am Med Inform Assoc.* 2001;8(6):546–551

Sittig DF, Singh H. Legal, ethical, and financial dilemmas in electronic health record adoption and use. *Pediatrics.* 2011;127(4):e1042–e1047

Spooner SA; American Academy of Pediatrics Council on Clinical Information Technology. Special requirements of electronic health record systems in pediatrics. *Pediatrics.* 2007;119(3):631–637

CHAPTER 9

Counseling Families About Internet Use

Alan Tomines, MD

CASE STUDY

A 16-year-old girl is accompanied by her mother for a routine visit. The girl is doing well in school, is active in team sports, and has a small circle of friends that are well-known to her mother. The mother describes no new problems at home, nor any changes in behavior, except that she is concerned that her daughter "spends too much time on the computer."

Questions
1. What are the commonly used Internet services?
2. What are the benefits and risks of the Internet?
3. What strategies may be used to make the Internet safer to use?
4. What signs may indicate that an adolescent is engaging in risky behaviors on the Internet?

The Internet is a worldwide system of interconnected computer networks. At its inception, it was the exclusive domain of the military and academia; today, the Internet is a public gateway to electronic information, communication, and commercial services. The Internet has profoundly changed the way that we learn, work, play, and interact with others. Its influence is so pervasive that it has become an integral part of the education and socialization of children, making it a subject of interest for parents, physicians, and researchers. Physicians can provide pragmatic counsel to families that focuses on the benefits and risks of the Internet, strategies for safer use, and assessment of online behavior in adolescents. Physicians should also be prepared to discuss health information that families find on the Internet.

A Brief History of the Internet

The Internet began in the 1960s as ARPANET (Advanced Research Projects Agency Network), a US Department of Defense project to share government-funded, university-based computer resources across a reliable communications network. Through the 1970s, ARPANET found acceptance with academics and researchers as a conduit for scientific information exchange, due in large part to **e-mail** (electronic mail), a technology for sending and receiving messages.

Recognizing the potential of the ARPANET, the National Science Foundation (NSF) began a separate effort to connect the computer science departments at non-ARPANET universities; initially dubbed CSNET (Computer Science Network) and later renamed NSFNET (NSF Network), this new network further expanded electronic information exchange. In 1990 the ARPANET was retired, with many of its networks being absorbed into NSFNET. The resulting network,

renamed the *Internet,* extended its reach into the business sector and to international researchers but remained relatively inaccessible to the general public.

During the early 1990s, the European Organization for Nuclear Research (CERN) developed protocols to facilitate the sharing of physics research data over the Internet. These protocols allowed computer files, on different computers and having different formats (eg, text and images), to be shared as single documents that could be viewed using a special computer program (browser). This system of linked documents was collectively dubbed the *World Wide Web (WWW,* or simply *the Web),* with collections of documents referred to as *Web pages* or *Web sites.* In 1993 CERN made its work freely available, leading to the rapid proliferation of commercial and individual Web sites.

Internet Services and Concepts

Today the most commonly used Internet services are e-mail and the Web. A person actively using an Internet service is said to be **online.** Use of the Web is sometimes referred to as *surfing the Web* or *surfing the 'Net* and is facilitated by **search engines** (programs that use keywords or topics to find related documents, images, Web sites, or other services on the Internet) such as Google and Yahoo! Internet services may be accessed by a wide range of computing devices, from traditional personal computers to more mobile platforms (eg, laptop computers, tablets, smartphones [mobile phones that provide access to Internet services]). Regardless of the computing device used, Internet access is usually provided by an **Internet service provider** (ISP), a company that has an Internet connection that it shares with consumers on a subscription basis.

Because of their popularity in the pediatric age group, there are a few specialized Internet services of which physicians should take special note. Web logs (or **blogs**) are Web-based journals. Like a traditional paper-based diary, a blog can be used to express activities, thoughts, or feelings. Blogs may be public (available for anyone to read) or private (having restricted access); the owner of a blog may allow readers to add comments to the blog. **Social networking** Web sites, such as Twitter, Facebook, and Tumblr, are similar in content to blogs, with the added dimension that users are encouraged to create a network of online friends by establishing links to other users' Web pages. Blogs and social networking Web sites are examples of **asynchronous** services (in which communication between users does not have to take place in real time) whose content may be moderated by the owner of the service to ensure that content is appropriate. In contrast, **chat rooms** are Internet venues that permit the real-time exchange of text messages between multiple simultaneous participants. **Instant messaging** is similar to a chat room, although it is generally limited to one-on-one exchanges of real-time messages. Although sometimes referred to as *text messaging,* instant messaging is a more inclusive term that better reflects the immediacy of interaction and expansion of content to include images and multimedia (eg, streaming audio and video files). Instant messaging is a popular premium service with mobile phone subscriptions, making it possible to have a continuous online presence. Adolescents have shown an increasing preference for instant messaging—estimated to be used by one-third of all teens.

Internet Benefits and Access

Physicians should be able to identify the benefits of Internet use. The Internet provides access to a wealth of educational resources and cultural experiences through the use of text, images, and multimedia. Access to these resources allows children to exercise their reading, writing, information-seeking, and technology skills. The Internet also provides the opportunity to exchange messages frequently with family and friends. In addition, children with common interests can use e-mail, chat, blogs, or social networking to communicate, commiserate, and encourage; PatientsLikeMe (www.patientslikeme.com) is an example of a social networking Web site that allows children (and their families) with common medical conditions to share their collective experiences.

Physicians may also take a role in reducing disparities to Internet access. Internet use and access is correlated with socioeconomic status. While nearly 95% of adolescents in the United States are regularly online, millions do not have access. Pediatricians may help families gain access to the Internet by identifying institutions that provide safe online environments, such as libraries, community centers, and schools. In addition, patient-centered Internet-based health interventions are increasingly being studied as a supplement to traditional health care delivery; addressing disparities to Internet access may increase opportunities for these interventions, particularly in underserved communities.

Physicians should also be aware that children with disabilities might have a difficult time using the Internet without **assistive technology** (hardware or software designed to improve the accessibility of computers). Children who are visually impaired or blind may be aided by the use of special software, including screen magnifiers, braille embossers, or screen readers (software that uses a computer-generated voice to read e-mail and Web pages); however, it is important to note that many Web sites are not developed to be compatible with screen readers. Children who are hearing impaired or deaf may be aided by ensuring that their computers are set to provide visual cues rather than audio prompts; this functionality is usually built into the operating system of a computer. Children with mobility or dexterity challenges might find it difficult to use a traditional keyboard and mouse; alternative keyboards and pointing devices, computer touch screens, and tablet devices can be suggested as supporting technologies. Pointing devices that employ sound or infrared beams, as well as software that responds to the spoken word, may be viable alternatives where manual control is not possible.

Internet Threats

While the Internet has many benefits, being online does entail some risks. To understand these risks, it is helpful to understand many of the Internet's neutral properties. The Internet is interactive: Unlike traditional media (eg, newspapers, radio, television), the Internet user may have real-time interactions with a person or a sophisticated computer program. The Internet has few restrictions: Anyone can put almost anything on the Internet, without regard to credibility or appropriateness. The Internet is public and permanent: Although information on a Web site may be removed, it is possible for anyone that visits a Web site to make an electronic copy of what is there, and many Web sites are archived historically (www.archive.org) and remain publicly retrievable long after they seem to be gone. The Internet is anonymous: People are not necessarily who they represent themselves to be. These properties do not encourage, but do enable, the most common Internet threats: strangers/predators; interpersonal victimization; and pornography, gaming, gambling, and shopping.

Internet predators are the greatest concern of parents. More than 90% of teens have shared personal information about themselves online, including name, birth date, interests, or contact information (eg, e-mail address, phone number). More than one-third of adolescents online have "friends" that they have never met in person. Approximately three-fifths of online adolescents have received an instant message or e-mail from a stranger, and 17% have been contacted by someone who made them feel scared or uncomfortable.

Online interpersonal victimization is the receipt of unwanted harassment or sexual attention over the Internet. One-fifth of children have reported being victimized, and a high risk factor was talking about sex with someone online. Cyberbullying is a specific type of online interpersonal victimization involving repetitive contact with electronic messages or images that are harmful or threatening. Cyberbullying may be as prevalent online as "traditional" bullying, with nearly one-fifth of middle school–aged children reporting that they had been cyberbullied at least once in the last 12 months. Approximately 88% of teens had witnessed other people being mean or cruel online, with 21% saying that they have joined in.

While children may be individually targeted by strangers or cyberbullies, they may also passively encounter undesired Internet content. More than 40% of children reported having been exposed to pornography online, and nearly two-thirds of them described this exposure as unwanted. In adolescents between the ages 15 and 17 years, more than 70% reported accidentally being exposed to online pornography. A high risk factor for exposure to pornography was the downloading of images.

Sexting is the exchange of sexually explicit text, images, or multimedia, generally via instant messaging. Sexting sits at the convergence of pornography and cyberbullying, with the added danger that some adolescents may not perceive sexting as harmful or threatening. In some jurisdictions, minors that have participated in sexting have been charged with possessing child pornography.

Strategies for Safer Internet Use

The American Academy of Pediatrics (AAP) has provided age-specific guidance for a safer Internet experience: For children through age 14 years, parents should be actively involved with all online activities, establish rules for safe online behavior, and use Internet safety tools; by age 15, parents may permit Internet access without restriction but should continue to reinforce rules.

Parents may be actively involved by educating themselves about the Internet and their children's Internet access, sharing time with their children online, and advocating for a safer Internet environment. Some parents may not be technically savvy and may require basic instruction on Internet technology. Classes may be available through libraries, community centers, local parent-teacher association, or online primers such as TeachParentsTech.org (www.teachparentstech.org). Parental education on Internet safety can begin with Web-based resources, such as the Federal Trade Commission (FTC) OnGuardOnline.gov (www.onguardonline.gov), National Center for Missing & Exploited Children NetSmartz Workshop (www.netsmartz.org), iKeepSafe (www.ikeepsafe.org), and INOBTR ("I Know Better") (www.inobtr.org). Parents should be aware of other venues where their children may access the Internet, such as schools, libraries, and friends' homes, and they should find out what Internet safety policies and technologies have been instituted in these environments.

By sharing time online, parents can promote and model responsible Internet behaviors. Parents should talk about what they see together on the Internet and encourage children to share what they have experienced when online alone, whether good or bad. Placing the computer in a public location in the home will encourage the idea that the Internet is a shared experience; however, parents should be aware that mobile devices allow children to access the Internet covertly. Children should be provided with a separate account to access the Internet, which their parents can also access. Having a separate account will allow parents to directly restrict the software and content that children can access and to periodically review Web sites visited and e-mails or messages sent and received. Parents should understand that some children are savvy enough to erase their Web browsing history; consequently, the absence of a Web browsing history may be a cause for suspicion. Parents should also monitor instant messaging activity regularly on smartphones.

Parents should act as advocates to safeguard the Internet for children. When a child encounters inappropriate Internet content or messages that are hurtful or distressing, parents should alert their ISP, as well as the owner of the Web site where the content or messages were discovered. Where appropriate, parents should also contact the appropriate legal authorities and the National Center for Missing & Exploited Children (www.missingkids.com). Commercial Web sites that collect personal information from children younger than 13 years are required to follow the Children's Online Privacy Protection Act of 1998, which is enforced by the FTC. According to this law, Internet Web site operators must post their policy indicating what personal information is collected, how that information will be used, and if that information will be shared with a third party. Parents must consent to the collection and use of personal information and may revoke this consent at any time.

Parents should set and enforce house rules for Internet use. Children should not communicate with or plan to meet strangers known only to them through the Internet; nor should they respond to messages that are unsolicited or that make them feel uncomfortable. Children should not share personal information or pictures with others on the Internet; nor should they download files from the Internet. Children should be encouraged to be good citizens, including not doing anything that may be hurtful to others or plagiarizing information that they find freely on the Internet. For older children, safety pledges can be used as formal agreements of acceptable use. Time limits should be set and strictly enforced. The AAP recommends no more than 2 hours of total screen time (computer and television) for children older than 2 years. Any activities that are not allowed should be specifically identified.

Even with house rules in place, physicians should recommend the use of Internet safety tools to protect against inappropriate use and external threats. Although not directly targeted at children, parents should be aware of software to protect against malware. Malware generally includes viruses and worms (software programs that can corrupt the information saved on a computer), spyware (software that tracks Internet activity and sends this information to another person), and pop-ups (a new browser window that may contain marketing or other undesired content). Viruses and worms are generally downloaded as attachments in e-mail, whereas spyware and pop-ups are introduced by surfing the Web. Parents should also protect against spam (unsolicited e-mail), which may contain undesired content or solicitations.

Filters are special computer programs that allow acceptable Internet content to be presented and block content deemed to be inappropriate. Filtering may use one or more of the following methods: "blacklists" of Web sites that are specifically blocked; "white lists" of Web sites that are specifically permitted; the blocking of specific words or terms; and the maturing technology of blocking suspicious image content. Filters are neither perfectly specific nor perfectly sensitive and may require parental adjustment to achieve an acceptable level of filtering. Parents may contact their ISP to enable filtering of content before it enters the home (**server-side filtering**). If server-side filtering is too restrictive for some members in the household or not restrictive enough for others, parents may acquire filtering software that is installed directly on computers in the home (**client-side filtering**). Client-side filters work with standard Web browsers, although special child-oriented Web browsers may be acquired that have client-side filtering built in.

Monitoring software automates parental tracking of Internet usage by creating a reviewable record of Web sites and images viewed, messages sent and received, and even individual keystrokes entered. The potential benefits of monitoring software should be weighed against the invasiveness to the privacy of the child. Monitoring software often includes time-limiting capability, which can be set to allow Internet access only during certain hours of the day and to disable access to the Internet after a specified amount of time has elapsed.

Adolescents on the Internet

As with other aspects of their lives, adolescents should feel that they can discuss what they see on the Internet with their parents without imperiling their access to the Internet. Most adolescents have access to the Internet from home, and nearly all have access to the Internet at school or at a friend's house. Parents should be aware that adolescents who have restrictive Internet rules at home are more likely to attempt Internet access outside the home, where their activity may be more difficult to monitor.

Adolescents may engage in risky online behaviors, including communicating with and planning to meet in person strangers met online. From a review of past cases, the Federal Bureau of Investigation has identified specific behaviors that may indicate a child is engaging in risky online behaviors, including spending several hours online, especially at night; having pornographic images on the computer; turning the monitor off or quickly changing the screen when a parent enters the room; and using unrecognized user names or accounts. Other non-Internet behaviors that should arouse suspicion include phone calls from unknown adults, outgoing calls to unrecognized phone numbers, gifts or packages received, or unexplained credit card activity.

The physician should consider addressing online activities in the adolescent psychosocial review of systems. Asking adolescents about online activities may unveil risky online behaviors or provide an opportunity to discuss concerns about their health and well-being. Nearly one-third of adolescents have searched the Internet for health information, most often related to sex and sexually transmitted infections, nutrition, and exercise and fitness. Additionally, adolescent girls also search for information on physical abuse, sexual abuse, and dating violence. Online activities worthy of inquiry include health topics searched for on the Internet, maintenance of a social networking page, sharing personal information on the Internet, communicating with strangers, meeting people known only via the Internet, and engaging in (or being a victim of) cyberbullying or sexting. Adolescents should also be reminded that the Internet is not private and that colleges and employers may discover information about the adolescent on what seem to be "private" social networking pages.

Health Information on the Internet

Patients regard physicians as the preferred and most trusted source for health information; however, patients do seek out health information on the Internet prior to, or sometimes in lieu of, consulting with their physician. It is important to remind families that health information on the Internet may be outdated, incomplete, incorrect, intentionally misleading, or easily misinterpreted. When patients have questions about information that they find on the Internet, physicians should take care not to disregard the information outright. Inquiries should be viewed as opportunities to address points of concern. Most often, patients simply want their physician's opinion of the information, as opposed to a specific treatment.

Providing patients with Web sites that provide reliable information can improve the quality of information seen and reduce the overwhelming quantity of information that parents must sort through. Physicians may help support patients by identifying evidence-based health information resources on the Internet, such as HealthyChildren.org, the official AAP Web site for parents (www.HealthyChildren.org); the National Library of Medicine MedlinePlus (www.medlineplus.gov); the Centers for Disease Control and Prevention (www.cdc.gov); and the US Department of Health and Human Services healthfinder.gov (www.healthfinder.gov). Specialists should be prepared to identify online information sources and support groups, particularly for rare, chronic, or debilitating conditions. Physicians should caution families caring for children with special medical conditions about the characteristics of less reliable online resources or support groups, which may include novel or alternative treatment regimens, advice to stop treatment, or charging of fees for participation or treatment.

CASE RESOLUTION

In the case history at the beginning of this chapter, the pediatrician finds out that the girl uses the computer for 1 to 2 hours every afternoon to complete her homework assignments and is on the Internet for 2 to 3 hours every evening surfing the Web, checking her Facebook and Tumblr pages, or posting tweets to her Twitter account. The pediatrician advises the girl that, for safety reasons, personal information should never be shared over the Internet, adding that colleges and employers often research prospective candidates using the Internet. The pediatrician also asks whether she has received, witnessed, or participated in hurtful or distressing communications online. With the mother and daughter, the pediatrician discusses the option to have a parent-child contract that clearly establishes the rules for acceptable Internet use in and out of the home, including appropriate time limits. The pediatrician also directs the mother to Internet-based resources for safeguarding the home environment and to a workshop for new Internet users at the local library.

Selected References

Ahmad F, Hudak PL, Bercovitz K, Hollenberg E, Levinson W. Are physicians ready for patients with Internet-based health information? *J Med Internet Res.* 2006;8(3):e22

Chung JE. Patient-provider discussion of online health information: results from the 2007 Health Information National Trends Survey (HINTS). *J Health Commun.* 2013;18(6):627–648

Demartini TL, Beck AF, Klein MD, Kahn RS. Access to digital technology among families coming to urban pediatric primary care clinics. *Pediatrics*. 2013;132(1): e142–e148

Glowniak J. History, structure, and function of the Internet. *Semin Nucl Med*. 1998;28(2):135–144

Jimison H, Gorman P, Woods S, et al. *Barriers and Drivers of Health Information Technology Use for the Elderly, Chronically Ill, and Underserved. Evidence Report/ Technology Assessment No. 175*. Rockville, MD: Agency for Healthcare Research and Quality; 2008. AHRQ Publication No. 09-E004. http://www.ncbi.nlm.nih. gov/books/NBK38653. Accessed December 6, 2013

Kowalski RM, Limber SP. Electronic bullying among middle school students. *J Adolesc Health*. 2007;41(6 Suppl 1):S22–S30

Lenhart A, Madden M, Smith S, Purcell K, Zickuhr K, Rainie L. Teens, kindness and cruelty on social network sites. Pew Research Center's Internet & American Life Project. http://pewinternet.org/Reports/2011/Teens-and-social-media.aspx. Published November 9, 2011. Accessed December 6, 2013

Madden M, Lenhart A, Duggan M, Cortesi S, Gasser U. Teens and technology 2013. Pew Research Center's Internet & American Life Project. http://www. pewinternet.org/Reports/2013/Teens-and-Tech.aspx. Published March 13, 2013. Accessed December 6, 2013

Moreno MA, Egan KG, Bare K, Young HN, Cox ED. Internet safety education for youth: stakeholder perspectives. *BMC Public Health*. 2013;13:543

Sim NZ, Kitteringham L, Spitz L, et al. Information on the World Wide Web— how useful is it for parents? *J Pediatr Surg*. 2007;42(2):305–312

Smith PK, Mahdavi J, Carvalho M, Fisher S, Russell S, Tippett N. Cyberbullying: its nature and impact in secondary school pupils. *J Child Psychol Psychiatry*. 2008;49(4):376–385

Stopbullying.gov. Cyberbullying. http://www.stopbullying.gov/cyberbullying/ index.html. Accessed December 6, 2013

Wolak J, Mitchell K, Finkelhor D. Unwanted and wanted exposure to online pornography in a national sample of youth Internet users. *Pediatrics*. 2007;119(2): 247–257

CHAPTER 10

Cultural Competency Issues in Pediatrics

W. Suzanne Eidson-Ton, MD, MS; Hendry Ton, MD, MS; Blanca Solis, MD; and Jesse Joad, MD, MS

CASE STUDY

You are seeing A.J., a 12-year-old Mexican American boy for a well-child visit. His mother speaks Spanish and "a little" English, is single, and works full time in motel custodial services. After school and during summers, A.J. is cared for by his older brother (17 years old) and his maternal grandmother, who lives a block away. His weight and body mass index are well above the 95th percentile for his age. When discussing his diet, you learn that his mother buys packaged foods that he can make for himself when she is away. She is concerned that he will not eat if she does not buy the processed, fatty foods that he likes.

Further, these types of foods are more plentiful than healthier options at the local market where she shops. A.J. sometimes eats at his grandmother's home, but she is elderly and not cooking much anymore. When discussing physical activity, he states that he wants to play soccer. His mother is concerned about this, however, because he often complains of headaches and stomachaches when it is time for practice, and she does not want to buy the equipment if he will quit after a few weeks, as has happened in the past.

This case study illustrates many important issues faced by those who provide health care to children. In this chapter, we intend to address the cultural competencies important for the practice of pediatrics, as well as some health and health care disparities faced by certain populations of children.

Definition of Culture

Culture is defined as a set of meanings, norms, beliefs, and values shared by a group of people. It is dynamic and evolves over time and with each generation. Culture encompasses a body of learned behaviors and perspectives that serve as a template to shape and orient future behaviors and perspectives from generation to generation and as novel situations emerge. It shapes how and what symptoms are expressed and influences the meaning that one attributes to symptoms, including one's beliefs about the causes, effects, and potential remedies for these symptoms. Culture is considered to be broad, encompassing not only race and ethnicity but also sexual orientation, gender roles, gender identity, socioeconomic status, nationality, and other group affiliations. The interaction between the culture of the patient and family and that of the physician is often significant and can lead to bias in assessment and treatment. These biases, in turn, can contribute to health and health care disparities.

Health Disparities

Health disparities are defined as differences in health outcomes across different groups. Health *care* disparities, as defined by the Institute of Medicine in the document *Unequal Treatment: Confronting Racial*

and Ethnic Disparities in Health Care, are "racial or ethnic differences in the quality of health care that are not due to access-related factors or clinical needs, preferences, and appropriateness of intervention." Health disparities and health care disparities exist within the United States and particularly affect minority populations. While health disparities may be due to many social determinants of health, such as class and access to safe neighborhoods, healthy food, and health care, health care disparities are directly related to what happens to certain patients in the health care system once they have accessed care.

Hispanic children in the United States face significant health and health care disparities. In particular, related to this chapter's case study, the highest prevalence of overweight children is in the Hispanic population. Hispanic children also have a lower fitness level and watch more television that white children in the United States. The reasons behind these disparities are complex and multifactorial, some of which will be discussed as follows. Hispanic children also face disparities in the health care they receive. For example, the duration of their routine well-child visits is shorter and they are less likely to receive counseling at these visits compared with white children.

In addition to these examples of lack of access to quality health care, there are many social, political, and cultural elements that contribute to health care disparities observed in certain ethnic groups. Individual physicians may have limited effects on the economic, environmental, and political issues that contribute to poor outcomes. It is nevertheless important to understand these issues and how they may contribute to patients' health outcomes. For example, lack of access to quality, low-cost foods in one's neighborhood, lack of transportation, advertising practices that target low-income communities, and lack of access to safe playgrounds are examples of social determinants that contribute to obesity. It is also essential to understand the influence of culture on patients' health beliefs, health behavior, and health status. We will discuss cultural issues further later in this chapter.

Finally, acculturation is likely to have an effect on health, health beliefs, and health behaviors as well. Second-generation Hispanic adolescents are twice as likely as first-generation Hispanic adolescents to be obese or overweight. Acculturation across generations in Hispanics has been associated with decreased fruit and vegetable consumption, increased soda consumption, and decreased physical activity. However, acculturation is a complex variable in relationship to pediatric obesity. For example, in one study, Mexican American mothers who were less acculturated had children with higher body mass indexes.

Cultural Competence

Physicians who strive for cultural competence try to minimize their bias and seek to incorporate cultural assets into their work with patients. Cross and colleagues describe cultural competence as a continuum. While this continuum was used to characterize organizations, it is also relevant for physicians. At the most negative pole, *cultural destructiveness* comprises attitudes and practices that are meant to be harmful to cultures and individuals within the particular culture. Clinicians at this level may overtly discriminate against individuals based on their culture (eg, intentionally making homophobic, racist, or sexist remarks to colleagues). Clinicians who have *cultural incapacity* do not overtly discriminate but lack the ability and willingness to recognize and intervene when discrimination happens. As a result, they ultimately reinforce culturally oppressive behaviors and policies. In the *cultural blindness* phase, one believes that culture makes no difference and that all people are the same. This viewpoint ignores cultural strengths, encourages assimilation, and often leads to blaming of the victims of racial injustices for their problems. Clinicians at this stage may have difficulty believing in the validity of health disparities, despite the enormous body of evidence supporting this. While they strive to give quality care to everyone, they fail to recognize culture-specific experiences that affect patients' health (eg, poverty or violence based on race, sexual orientation, or gender) and miss opportunities to incorporate culturally relevant strengths into treatment (eg, collaboration with traditional healers, extended family, or faith-based organizations). *Cultural precompetence* is characterized by a willingness to deliver quality services and a commitment to civil rights but a lack of knowledge and experience to implement culturally relevant services. Clinicians here often struggle with knowledge that disparities exist and perhaps they continue to contribute to them, yet they are at a loss as to what to do about it. A physician at the stage of *cultural competence,* in contrast, seeks to expand his or her cultural knowledge and resources, often in consultation with culturally diverse communities. He or she also continuously self-assesses and adapts traditional service models to enhance care for culturally diverse patients. Finally, a physician with

cultural proficiency holds cultural diversity in highest esteem and continuously advocates for increased cultural competence throughout the system of care. It is important to recognize that physicians move back and forth along this continuum dynamically, influenced by their own experiences. For example, a physician who identifies with being in the culturally competent phase when working with Hispanic patients may find himself or herself having cultural incapacity when working with gay or lesbian patients.

Communication

Initially, when addressing the patient in the case study in this chapter, it is very important to maximize communication with the patient and his mother. Effective communication results in an improved physician-patient relationship, treatment adherence, and health outcomes. Poor communication may have negative consequences. Patients with limited English proficiency (LEP), in particular, have greater barriers to health care, poorer quality of health, and poorer health status. In a Joint Commission on the Accreditation of Health Care Organizations (JCAHO) study involving 6 hospitals, researchers found that patients with LEP were at greater risk for iatrogenic harm. In contrast, use of interpreters is associated with greater follow-up with preventive and primary care services. Ideally, one would have a trained medical interpreter to communicate with the patient's mother. It would be inappropriate for the patient to communicate for his mother, although this happens often in clinical practice. It is clearly a difficult position for this boy to interpret health information for his mother. There is no guarantee that he understands what the physician is communicating or that he is interpreting correctly for his mother. It also disturbs the appropriate power balance between the mother and her son. Here are strategies for using interpreters.

1. Meet with the interpreter briefly prior to the interview to discuss overall goals for the interview and ground rules (eg, use word-for-word interpretation).
2. Use nonverbal behaviors such as eye contact, nodding, or facial expressions to let the patient know that the physician understands what is being communicated.
3. Speak directly to the patient and address the patient in the first person.
4. Use short, simple statements and stick to one topic at a time.
5. Avoid medical jargon and ambiguous statements.
6. Meet briefly with the interpreter after the interview to confirm pertinent information, ask about cultural information, and discuss feedback.
7. Remember that interpreters are not medical professionals. Therefore, consider information volunteered by interpreters as reliable as collateral information provided by other non–health professionals.

Unconscious Bias

In addition to ensuring effective communication, it is important to address unconscious biases that one may have as the physician for this patient. While few health care professionals intentionally discriminate based on culture, studies suggest that physicians are likely to have unconscious biases that can significantly affect their care of patients.

Physicians can take steps to decrease unconscious bias. It is essential to first acknowledge that bias really does exist in the health care system and within the lived experience of patients as well as physicians. It is good practice for health care professionals to explore the Project Implicit Web site (https://implicit.harvard.edu/implicit) and take the online tests designed to detect bias across various cultural dimensions, including race, gender, and sexual orientation. Most people who take these tests realize rather quickly that they carry biases which they had no idea existed within themselves. For many, acknowledging one's own biases may be the most difficult step. The next step is to work toward replacing one's biases with positive and realistic associations about other groups. For example, seeking out dialogue and companionship with people culturally different from oneself can help to replace one's negative assumptions with more positive associations. Finally, it is important to be mindful of the potential influence of unconscious bias on medical decision-making, whether treating a patient of similar background to the physician or a patient of a very different background. While it is essential to consider cultural context, it is also important to keep in mind that each patient is a unique individual. In situations in which bias may be present, physicians should speak less and listen more, striving to avoid assumptions.

Eliciting Patients' Perspectives

A patient's and physician's understanding of a health issue is an important part of overall clinical collaboration. Typically, the patient's history is obtained with limited consideration to the patient's beliefs about the health problem. Difficulties may arise if the patient or a family members disagree with the physician's explanations of the illness. Openly disagreeing with a physician's assessment and treatment recommendations is considered disrespectful in many cultures. The patient and family may instead acknowledge the physician's status by expressing agreement but maintain their own ideas about how to address the issue. A.J.'s mother, for example, may report her intention to follow through with his physician's recommendation to change to a healthier diet, but may in fact continue with the ready-made foods because she feels there are difficulties getting healthier foods given her long work hours and the availability of healthy food in her neighborhood. The physician may characterize obesity as a primarily biological problem, whereas A.J.'s mother might see it as primarily a problem of access and time.

Further, A.J.'s mother may not see his overweight status as a problem at all. The relationship of pediatric obesity to cultural ideals and norms around food, eating, and parenting is complex. There is some evidence in ethnographic studies that, in some Hispanic cultures, feeding children and especially giving "treats" is a way of showing love. Parents who have children who are "healthy eaters" may not want to limit their children's enjoyment of food. In addition, body size ideals vary across communities, and there is some evidence that

in some Hispanic communities, children meeting criteria for being overweight are considered more attractive and healthier than thinner children, who may be consider frail. In addition, poverty and the experience of food scarcity can further exacerbate overeating when food is more accessible. Finally, particularly when other friends or family members offer food to children, it may be considered socially unacceptable for the parent to refuse or criticize the type of food being offered (Kaufman and Karpati, 2007). Understanding these types of cultural norms can be helpful in treating individual patients. However, it is important to remember that particular individuals and families have their own cultural norms that may or may not be consistent with others in their ethnic group.

Conflicts in health beliefs between the physician and patient/family may result in treatment non-adherence and dropout. It is important that the physician and patient/family discuss their respective health perspectives. The more that the physician understands the patient's and family's health beliefs, the more effective the physician will be at addressing differences and building on common ground. Likewise, patients and families may feel a greater level of comfort with a physician's recommendations if their questions and concerns about the physician's perspectives are addressed. The following questions can help a physician further understand patients' health beliefs. These questions can also be used to facilitate discussion about health issues identified by the physician.

1. About which problem are you most concerned?
2. What do you think about my concerns (ie, the physician's identified problems [in this example, obesity])?
3. What do you think has caused the problem?
4. What are your concerns about this problem? How does it affect you?
5. What treatments do you think might work for it?
6. What are your goals for treatment?
7. What is your understanding of the treatment offered? What are your concerns about it? What are the barriers for completing or carrying out the treatment?

Decision-making

It is also important to understand how a patient or family makes medical decisions. Many physicians look to a child's parents as the primary decision-makers. This process may be culturally influenced. Parents from strongly collectivistic cultures, in which the needs and priorities of the group supersede those of the individual, may wish to have others, such as senior family members, spiritual leaders, or clan leaders, be involved in health care decision-making. Failure on the part of the physician to allow the inclusion of these people in decision-making may result in parents feeling forced into a decision, precipitate conflict within the family, and lead to the family or community blaming the parents if a bad outcome occurs. Here are suggested questions for facilitating a discussion around decision-making.

1. How do you usually make decisions about health care?
2. Do you involve anyone else in that process? Who? What are their roles?

3. Who usually makes the final decision?
4. How comfortable are you with using that process to make decisions about your current situation?

CASE STUDY, continued

At a follow-up visit for A.J., you ask to speak with him alone. During your assessment, you learn that he is attracted to boys but has not shared this with anyone. He is certain that his brothers will not approve and his mother will be heartbroken. He is sometimes teased at school because he is "not tough enough," and he fears some of the bigger bullies might try to jump him if he hangs around after school to participate in any after-school sports activities.

At this visit, it is extremely important to remain nonjudgmental and supportive of the patient's early sexual identity development. See chapters 43 and 141 for suggestions on addressing the sexual identity and bullying issues presented by this patient. Another resource is the Fenway Institute National LGBT Health Education Center (www.lgbthealtheducation.org/training/learning-modules).

There are several other factors to consider with respect to health disparities in this case. In the National Longitudinal Study of Adolescent Health, in which 20,000 adolescents were surveyed in 1995, male and female Hispanic adolescents were more likely to report same-sex romantic attraction than their peers of other ethnic groups, significantly more so than their white and Asian peers. In addition, male and female Hispanic adolescents were more likely than their peers to be victims of violence. Therefore, the issues of sexual minorities and bullying are important to consider in addressing adolescent health disparities in culturally diverse communities in the United States. It is also important to understand A.J.'s sexual orientation in the context of his family and ethnic community. While there are certainly challenges for lesbian, gay, bisexual, transgender, and questioning (LGBTQ) youth in Hispanic families, particularly when there is the strong influence of antigay religious views, there are also strengths for LGBTQ individuals with strong cultural identities. For example, in one study, young urban Hispanic men who have sex with other men were less likely to engage in risky sexual behavior if they were connected to their ethnic community.

These are some examples of the complicated intersection of sexual identity and ethnic identity in cultural issues in pediatrics. There is more information about youth sexual identity formation, as well as bullying, in other chapters.

CASE RESOLUTION

You are supportive of your patient in his early sexual identity development, discuss safe adults in A.J.'s life with whom he can explore his feelings and concerns, and identify lesbian, gay, bisexual, transgender, and questioning community resources. You also discuss A.J.'s and his mother's perspectives about food, his weight, and his activity level, using a medically trained interpreter for his mother. You identify some of this family's strengths: A.J.'s mother's desire to help him be healthier; A.J.'s relationship with his grandmother, who cooks healthy traditional foods; and A.J.'s supportive relationship with his older brother. After discussion, the patient decides that he would like to learn to cook from his grandmother and will commit to cooking dinner for a family meal once a week, which delights his mother. His brother has also agreed to take him to soccer practice and games for a neighborhood soccer team. The patient likes this idea, as he feels safe from bullies around his brother and feels that soccer will help him be stronger and more confident. You arrange for a follow-up visit in several months to check in with A.J. and his mother about their progress and to brainstorm about further interventions.

Selected References

Caprio S, Daniels SR, Drewnowski A, et al. Influence of race, ethnicity, and culture on childhood obesity: implications for prevention and treatment: a consensus statement of Shaping America's Health and the Obesity Society. *Diabetes Care.* 2008;31(11):2211–2221

Cross T. Services to minority populations. Cultural competence continuum. *Focal Point.* 1988;3:1-9

Flores G, Abreu M, Tomany-Korman SC. Limited English proficiency, primary language at home, and disparities in children's health care: how language barriers are measured matters. *Public Health Rep.* 2005;120(4):418–430

Flores G; American Academy of Pediatrics Committee on Pediatric Research. Racial and ethnic disparities in the health and health care of children. *Pediatrics.* 2010;125(4):e979–e1020

Gaw AC. *Concise Guide to Cross-Cultural Psychiatry.* Washington, DC: American Psychiatric Publishing; 2001

Green AR, Carney DR, Pallin DJ, et al. Implicit bias among physicians and its prediction of thrombolysis decisions for black and white patients. *J Gen Intern Med.* 2007;22(9):1231–1238

Institute of Medicine. *The Health of Lesbian, Gay, Bisexual, and Transgender People: Building a Foundation for Better Understanding.* Washington, DC: National Academies Press; 2011

Institute of Medicine. *Unequal Treatment: Confronting Racial and Ethnic Disparities in Health Care.* Smedley BD, Stith AY, Nelson AR, eds. Washington, DC: National Academies Press; 2003. http://www.nap.edu/openbook.php?record_id=10260&page=R1. Accessed February 19, 2014

Jacobs EA, Shepard DS, Suaya JA, Stone EL. Overcoming language barriers in health care: costs and benefits of interpreter services. *Am J Public Health.* 2004;94(5):866–869

Kaufman L, Karpati A. Understanding the sociocultural roots of childhood obesity: food practices among Latino families of Bushwick, Brooklyn. *Soc Sci Med.* 2007;64(11):2177–2188

Kumanyika SK. Environmental influences on childhood obesity: ethnic and cultural influences in context. *Physiol Behav.* 2008;94(1):61–70

Matsumoto D. *Culture and Psychology.* San Francisco, CA: Brooks/Cole Publishing Co; 1996

O'Donnell L, Agronick G, San Doval A, Duran R, Myint-U A, Stueve A. Ethnic and gay community attachments and sexual risk behaviors among urban Latino young men who have sex with men. *AIDS Educ Prev.* 2002;14(6):457–471

Popkin BM, Udry JR. Adolescent obesity increases significantly in second and third generation U.S. immigrants: the National Longitudinal Study of Adolescent Health. *J Nutr.* 1998;128(4):701–706

Russell ST, Truong, NL. Adolescent sexual orientation, race, and ethnicity, and school environments: a national study of sexual minority youth of color. In: Kumashiro KK. *Troubling Intersections of Race and Sexuality: Queer Students of Color and Anti-Oppressive Education.* Lanhan, MD: Rowman & Littlefield Publishers, Inc; 2001

Schulman KA, Berlin JA, Harless W, et al. The effect of race and sex on physicians' recommendations for cardiac catheterization. *N Engl J Med.* 1999;340(8): 618–626

Schyve PM. Language differences as a barrier to quality and safety in health care: The Joint Commission perspective. *J Gen Intern Med.* 2007;22(Suppl 2):360–361

Stewart MA. Effective physician-patient communication and health outcomes: a review. *CMAJ.* 1995;152(9):1423–1433

Sussner KM, Lindsay AC, Peterson KE. The influence of maternal acculturation on child body mass index at age 24 months. *J Am Diet Assoc.* 2009;109(2):218–225

Timmins CL. The impact of language barriers on the health care of Latinos in the United States: a review of the literature and guidelines for practice. *J Midwifery Womens Health.* 2002;47(2):80–96

CHAPTER 11

Principles of Pediatric Therapeutics

Bonnie R. Rachman, MD

CASE STUDY

An 18-month-old girl who has had a cough, runny nose, and fever for 2 days is brought to your office for evaluation. The previous night she awoke from sleep crying and pulling at her ear. The patient has no other symptoms. Her mother states she has had previous ear infections, the most recent occurred 2 months ago. The last time she took amoxicillin she broke out in hives. Otherwise the patient has no significant medical history.

On physical examination, the patient is febrile to 102°F (38.9°C) and has yellow rhinorrhea. The ear examination reveals a red, bulging, nonmobile tympanic membrane in one ear, while the other ear appears normal. The remainder of the examination is benign.

Questions

1. What are the current practice guidelines for antibiotic treatment of otitis media? How does treatment change with the age and symptoms of the patient?
2. How does the previous reaction to a medication influence the antibiotic choice?
3. How do factors such as child care, work, and family plans affect the choice of medication?
4. What role do over-the-counter medications have in the management of the patient's symptoms?

A drug or therapeutic can be defined as any substance that is ingested, absorbed, or injected that alters the body's function. Examples include prescription medications, over-the-counter (OTC) medications, homeopathic preparations, herbal remedies and teas, vitamin supplements, and illicit substances. Different drug categories have differing safety profiles and regulation levels. Prescription drugs are the most regulated. Homeopathic preparations, some vitamin formulations, and most herbal remedies may have little, if any, standardization, safety testing, or regulation. Illicit drugs have no quality testing.

The use of prescription and OTC medications is very common in pediatrics. The Slone Survey, a random digit-dial survey of medication use, found that families with children reported more than 55% of children younger than 12 years had taken some medication preparation within the last 7 days. Of those taking a medication, 22% were taking at least one prescription medication. In a given month, more than 50% of preschool-aged children had received some OTC medication. The number of children aged 12 years and younger being administered an OTC medication in a given period is more than twice that of a prescription medication. The most commonly used OTC medications are acetaminophen and ibuprofen. In the adolescent age group, aged 12 to 17 years, more OTC products are used for acne and less for allergies or pain relief. Given that the use of OTC medications is so prevalent and that many OTC medications contain multiple active ingredients, concerns about their safety profile for children is an issue that needs to be addressed by pediatricians with families at routinely scheduled office visits as well as by regulatory agencies.

Another concern is the use of prescription or OTC medications as drugs of abuse. Of particular concerns are adolescents who abuse alcohol, illicit drugs, and medications, including OTC cough medications containing dextromethorphan. In the 2011 Monitoring the Future survey of eighth, 10th, and 12th graders nationwide, approximately 5% of the survey participants reported using OTC cough medicine to "get high" in the past year. Also, in the past year, 49% reported abuse of alcohol, 25% reported abuse of marijuana, 6% reported abuse of Vicodin, and 4% reported abuse of OxyContin.

Furthermore, according to Centers for Disease Control and Prevention data from 2004 to 2005, more than 70,000 children annually were brought to the emergency department (ED) for medication overdoses (in more than 26,000 visits, OTC medications were implicated). Eighty-two percent of ED visits for medication overdoses resulted from unsupervised ingestions of prescription and OTC drugs, with peak incidence in 2-year-olds.

Most drugs prescribed for children have not been tested in children. Before the US Food and Drug Administration (FDA) initiated a pediatric program (Best Pharmaceuticals for Children Act of 2007), only about 20% of drugs approved by the FDA were labeled for pediatric use. Currently, about one-third of drugs prescribed to children have been studied for safety and efficacy in pediatric populations. The practice of prescribing drugs for off-label conditions is found in approximately 50% of all physician prescriptions. By necessity, doctors have routinely given drugs to children off label, which means the drug has not been approved for used in children based on the demonstration of safety and efficacy in adequate, well-controlled clinical trials. It does not imply that the drugs are unsafe. The Pediatric Research Equity Act of 2007 (PREA) requires pediatric studies and covers drugs and biologics. Under the PREA, the FDA can require pediatric studies of a drug submitted in a new drug application if it determines the product is likely to be used in a substantial number of pediatric patients or if the product would provide a meaningful benefit in the pediatric population over existing treatment. In a systematic review of the frequency of off-label use of antibiotics in clinical pediatric practice, the percentage of off-label antibiotic prescriptions varied from 1% to 94%. Some of the wide variation observed in pediatric patients might be attributed to the heterogeneity among the study populations' ages of children.

Differences in pharmacokinetics among infants, children, and adolescents can result in differences in drug efficacy and toxicity. To choose the most important therapeutic, health care professionals must consider a number of factors, including patient characteristics, disease epidemiology, safety profile, patient compliance, and cost-effectiveness (Box 11-1).

Patient Characteristics

Infants and children have differing physiological characteristics than adults, including immaturity of metabolic and organ function. Body weight and surface area are considerations in drug dosing for pediatrics. In addition, the therapeutic window for many drugs is smaller for children than adults. Pharmacologic factors, including age-based variability in absorption, metabolism, and excretion of drugs in children compared with adults, as well as age-specific contraindications of certain medications, pose special vulnerabilities to the adverse effects of overdosing. Conversions of doses from ingredient amounts to volumes for liquids labeled for home use are also problematic.

The patient's medical history plays an important part in the choice of an appropriate therapeutic. Depending on the patient's condition and medical and surgical history, the absorption, metabolism, or usual effectiveness of a therapeutic may be altered. Children with short bowel syndrome can potentially have difficulty absorbing oral medications depending on which portion of the bowel was removed. Children with mental retardation who are given central nervous system–altering medications can be difficult to monitor for changes in mental status seen with systemic infection. In addition, children with glucose-6-phosphate dehydrogenase deficiency can suffer from drug-induced hemolytic anemia when given certain drugs, such as sulfonamides. Malnourished children are at greater risk for drug toxicity because low serum albumin levels decrease the amount of bound drug and result in increased levels of unbound drug in circulation.

Box 11-1. Factors in Choosing Appropriate Therapeutics	
Patient Characteristics	*Patient Compliance*
Age	Taste
Medical history	Purpose of treatment
Allergies	Storage
Use of other medications	Side effects
Diagnosis	*Cost-effectiveness*
Epidemiology	Drug availability
Age-specific factors	Formulary restrictions
Safety Profile	
Therapeutic index	
Black box warning	

Allergies to medications and reactions to prior drugs are important pieces of information to glean from the patient and family. Specific information about symptoms or problems while taking a drug are of great significance because side effects can be mislabeled as drug allergies. Drug allergies are reactions that have an immunologic basis. Of the 4 types of immune mechanisms associated with drug allergies, IgE mediated reactions are of the greatest concern because they can result in anaphylaxis. Adverse reactions, such as vomiting, can be idiosyncratic or nonimmune mediated. A side effect is an expected but undeniable consequence of taking a medication. Families often attribute any symptoms a patient experienced while taking a medication to a drug allergy. It is therefore important to know which side effects are associated with a medication to determine whether an allergy is present. Any medication that has been associated with an allergic reaction (eg, skin eruptions, swelling, urticaria, respiratory difficulty) should not be used without consulting a specialist.

Also important is to consider what other medications the patient is taking. This may influence the drug of choice. Metabolism of one drug may influence the metabolism of another. Drug metabolism is divided into 2 types.
1. Phase 1 reactions include oxidation, reduction, and hydrolysis.
2. Phase 2 reactions involve adding subgroups to a drug.

Other drugs can affect reactions during either phase. For example, the enzyme activity of the P 450 system involved in oxidation can be induced or inhibited depending on other medications being taken, resulting in an altered rate of metabolism. A common drug used in pediatrics that inhibits the P 450 system is erythromycin, while phenobarbital and phenytoin induce the system. Drug interactions are not a contraindication to the use of a therapeutic, but the dose or serum level may need to be closely monitored.

Diagnosis

Etiologies for many common diseases may differ depending on the patient's age group. Some drugs to which the patient's condition may be susceptible are contraindicated in certain patient populations.

Treatment duration may also vary depending on the patient's age group (eg, an adult with an uncomplicated urinary tract infection may receive only a 1- to 3-day course of treatment, while a child may receive 7 to 10 days of treatment because of the high recurrence of infection that has been observed with a shorter treatment duration).

Safety Profile

Medications have benefits and risks; these constitute a safety profile. When choosing a medication, the safety profile (ie, risks vs benefits) must be evaluated. Some risks may be caused by the duration of treatment, dose, or interactions with other medications. Therapeutic index, which is one way to quantify the risk associated with a specific dose, may be a consideration in medication choice. The therapeutic index is the difference between the dose that provides a desired effect and the dose that provides an undesired effect. For example, a medication with a wide therapeutic index is one in which a desired effect is achieved with a dose much lower than that required to produce a toxic effect. In general, a medication with a wide therapeutic index, such as ibuprofen, is considered safer than a medication with a narrow therapeutic index. The higher the morbidity and mortality associated with a condition, the more narrow the accepted therapeutic index can be. Food-drug interactions and drug-drug interactions are other risks that can be anticipated. There are also risks that are independent of the dose of the therapeutic, which are called idiosyncratic effects. These are unexpected and usually unavoidable risks associated with the medication.

In the United States, a black box warning, also known as a black label warning, is a type of warning that appears on prescription drugs that may cause serious side effects. The name came about from the black border that usually surrounds the text of the warning. Black box warnings mean that medical studies indicate that a drug carries a significant risk of serious or even life-threatening adverse effects. Examples of a medication used in pediatrics that has black box warnings are antidepressants. This warning does not prevent the use of the medication but requires the physician and family to evaluate the risks and benefits of its use.

Patient Compliance

Medications and therapeutics are only useful if the patient takes the medication as prescribed. Factors that contribute to patient adherence include, but are not limited to, administration convenience and ease of taking the medication, the patient's and family's understanding of the benefits and risks of the medication, and side effect profile.

Because children are dependent on their caregivers to administer medications properly, the caregiver must understand why the drug was prescribed, how it should be dispensed, and why it must be taken for a specific length of time. For a medication to achieve its maximal therapeutic usefulness, accurate dosing is important. A staff member should demonstrate how to measure and dispense the medication. The caregiver should then be asked to demonstrate the process. This will make an important difference in adherence to the medication regimen.

In pediatrics, palatability is a major factor in patient adherence. If children do not like the taste or texture of a medication, they will refuse to take it. Physicians who prescribe medications for children should be familiar with the taste and texture and be prepared to find alternatives. Prednisone is a common example of this; it is available as a pill and a suspension. The suspension may taste differently depending on the preparation prescribed. Children often vomit the less-palatable version. Knowing in advance what children will take may prevent future problems associated with noncompliance.

Cost-effectiveness

Cost-effectiveness is defined as outcome per unit cost. Outcome is the treatment of the condition or alleviation of the symptoms for which the medication was prescribed. Cost includes the price of the medication or treatment as well as the physician's and family's time. Therefore, if a patient is prescribed a medication that is less effective for the child's condition because of cost, it many end up costing more because of the need for additional doctor visits and more medications. In many practice settings, the pharmacy has a set formulary of medication limiting the selection of medications for specific conditions. From the patient side, many families have limited or no health insurance and may have to pay the full cost of a medication. The cost of treating a common condition such as otitis media can differ as much as 10-fold depending on the medication prescribed. Thus, an appropriate drug of choice is influenced by the out-of-pocket cost to the family. The perceived cost-effectiveness of a therapeutic is different for each situation and depends on external factors affecting the physician and family.

Drug Dosing

Compared with the adult population, in which drug doses are based on a standard dose for an individual regardless of age, size, or weight, pediatric medications are usually dosed based on weight or body surface area. For medication dosing determined by weight, when a child reaches 40 to 50 kg, the dosing is often changed to a standard adult dose. With the increasing prevalence of childhood obesity, many school-aged children weigh more than 50 kg, thereby making it important to know the maximum daily dose because calculating milligrams per kilogram can easily exceed this amount. For drugs with narrow therapeutic indexes, such as chemotherapy or immunosuppressive medications, body surface area is used to determine appropriate dosing. Once a therapeutic agent is chosen, an appropriate dosing schedule must be determined. Dosing guidelines can be presented as total dose per 24 hours or an amount per dose. An example for dosing acetaminophen for a 1-year-old is given in Box 11-2.

Box 11-2. Dosing Example: Acetaminophen

A 1-year-old has a fever, and the family wants to know how much acetaminophen to give her. She weighs 11.2 kg. The recommended dose of acetaminophen is 10 to 15 mg/kg every 4 to 6 hours. Acetaminophen is sold as a suspension with the concentration of 160 mg/5 mL.

1. Determine the amount of medication needed by multiplying the weight of the child by the recommended dose.

$$11.2 \text{ kg} \times 10 \text{ mg/kg} = 112\text{-mg acetaminophen}$$

2. Determine the volume of medication based on the concentration of acetaminophen to be used.

Dosing volume =

(amount of medication) ÷ (concentration of medication)

Suspension

$$\text{Dosing volume} = 112 \text{ mg} \div 160 \text{ mg/5 mL}$$
$$= (112 \times 5)/160$$
$$= 3.5 \text{ mL}$$

This family can be instructed to give the 1-year-old 3.5 mL of the suspension of acetaminophen orally every 4 to 6 hours as needed for fever.

Mediation Errors and Adverse Drug Events

Pediatric patients are at greatest risk for medication errors because of the need to calculate dose based on weight. The risk for errors with the potential for harm are 3 times higher in children than adults. The incidence of adverse drug events in pediatrics is about 2.3%. More than half of these errors occur during the prescribing phase when the medication dose is calculated. Dosing error checking is complicated by the fact that children's weights vary from as little as 500 g to much more than 100 kg. Therefore, a dose range for a medication may be very large. The second most common causes of error in pediatric prescriptions is missing information and illegibility.

The American Recovery and Reinvestment Act of 2009 provided much needed momentum toward widespread EHRs, which include e-prescribing. Systems that have computerized physician order entry or e-prescribing can reduce medication errors by having alerts for inappropriate dosing, improved legibility, warnings for drug interactions, and just-in-time information on the most appropriate drug choice. Not all errors will be rectified by e-prescribing; examples of errors that elude decision-support programs include inappropriate selection of medication for the condition being treated and failure to recognize a change in patient status.

CASE RESOLUTION

After obtaining the history and performing a physical examination, the pediatrician determines that the patient has acute otitis media. Depending on the age of the child and the severity of symptoms, American Academy of Pediatrics clinical practice guidelines suggest a stratified approach to therapeutics. For children younger than 2 years, pediatricians can treat with antibiotics if the diagnosis is certain or observe the patient without antibiotics if the patient is otherwise healthy. In this case, the pediatrician discusses the options with the family and, because of the severity of pain and previous ear infections, chooses to treat the infection. The antibiotic of choice for treatment of otitis media is amoxicillin at a dose of 80 to 90 mg/kg/d. The mother states that her daughter had hives with amoxicillin, a type 1 hypersensitivity. Other antibiotic choices would include cefdinir 14 mg/kg/d in 1 to 2 doses per day. Treatment of pain is essential with otitis media. The patient can take oral acetaminophen or ibuprofen.

The mother raises concern about her daughter's cough and runny nose and would like to use an over-the-counter cough medication. The US Food and Drug Administration does not recommend use of cough preparations in this age group. Educating the mother about conservative therapies, including nasal suctioning, humidification, and nasal saline, to treat her respiratory symptoms is more appropriate.

If the patient were not allergic to amoxicillin, it would have been the drug of choice. It is inexpensive, has a narrow microbiological spectrum, and is palatable. Amoxicillin does require refrigeration, which would be of concern if the family were traveling. While this case illustrates several obvious constraints, it is important to emphasize that choosing the appropriate medication is dependent on the intrinsic needs of the patient and extrinsic factors that can affect adherence and ultimately the effectiveness of treatment.

Selected References

American Academy of Pediatrics Council on Clinical Information Technology. Electronic prescribing systems in pediatrics: the rationale and functionality requirements. *Pediatrics.* 2007;119(6):1229–1231

American Academy of Pediatrics Steering Committee on Quality Improvement and Management and Committee on Hospital Care. Principles of pediatric patient safety: reducing harm due to medical care. *Pediatrics.* 2011;127(6):1199–1210

Bell EA, Tunkel DE. Over-the-counter cough and cold medications in children: are they helpful? *Otolaryngol Head Neck Surg.* 2010;142(5):647–650

Gerstle RS, Lehmann CU; American Academy of Pediatrics Council on Clinical Information Technology. Electronic prescribing systems in pediatrics: the rationale and functionality requirements. *Pediatrics.* 2007;119(6):e1413–e1422

Hersh AL, Shapiro DJ, Pavia AT, Shah SS. Antibiotic prescribing in ambulatory pediatrics in the United States. *Pediatrics.* 2011;128(6):1053–1061

Hughes RG, Edgerton EA. Reducing pediatric medication errors: children are especially at risk for medication errors. *Am J Nurs.* 2005;105(5):79–80

Lieberthal AS, Carroll AE, Chonmaitree T, et al. The diagnosis and management of acute otitis media. *Pediatrics.* 2013;131(3):e964–e999

Pollock M, Bazaldua OV, Dobbie AE. Appropriate prescribing of medications: an eight-step approach. *Am Fam Physician.* 2007;75(2):231–236

Shaddy RE, Denne SC; American Academy of Pediatrics Committee on Drugs and Committee on Pediatric Research. Guidelines for the ethical conduct of studies to evaluate drugs in pediatric populations. *Pediatrics.* 2010;125(4):850–860

US Food and Drug Administration. Science & research. Pediatrics. http://www.fda.gov/ScienceResearch/SpecialTopics/PediatricTherapeuticsResearch/default.htm. Updated November 25, 2013. Accessed January 27, 2014

Vernacchio L, Kelly JP, Kaufman DW, Mitchell AA. Medication use among children <12 years of age in the United States: results from the Slone Survey. *Pediatrics.* 2009;124(2):446–454

Young SS, Blandino DA, Engle JP, et al. *Appropriate Use of Common OTC Analgesics and Cough and Cold Medications.* Leawood, KS: American Academy of Family Physicians; 2008

CHAPTER 12

Pediatric Pain and Symptom Management

Rick Goldstein, MD

CASE STUDY

You are caring for a 5-year-old girl with stage 4 neuroblastoma who is at home receiving palliative care. Her tumor is refractory. She receives oral chemotherapy and transfusions as an outpatient to offset the bone marrow depletion caused by her tumor. Pain from her metastases is becoming increasing problematic, most especially in her chest wall and right femur. Her spine is also involved, but she does not experience weakness. Though fatigued, she derives great pleasure from attending school and being surrounded by friends and family members, playing as she is able. She hates the hospital and her parents have chosen to avoid it, intending to keep her comfortable at home until she dies. You have remained closely involved throughout her illness and would like to help with the management of her symptoms.

Questions

1. What is the approach to pain management in children?
2. How does one assess the level of pain in children?
3. What is meant by *adjuvant therapy*?
4. What is the role of distraction in pain management?
5. What are non-pain symptoms that can cause distress?
6. What is the management of non-pain symptoms?

Ill or injured children experience distressing physical symptoms. This is particularly true when their illness or injuries are chronic or life-limiting. The appropriate management of such symptoms is fundamental to minimizing their suffering and optimizing their quality of life. Pain can not only diminish a child's physical well-being but also affect her psychological, social, and spiritual health. A child experiencing poorly controlled pain will withdraw interpersonally and be unable to engage in the activities that make life, however limited, meaningful. Similarly, a child troubled by nausea will experience distress from the symptom while also losing the simple pleasure of eating and other satisfying comforts. Symptom management improves the lives of children who are medically fragile.

Research on parents of children who are seriously ill has found that their greatest concerns are about their children's symptoms not being satisfactorily controlled. Studies of dying children have noted that distressing symptoms often go untreated. Wolfe et al, in landmark research investigating the symptoms and suffering of children dying from cancer, found that most of the children experienced fatigue, pain, dyspnea, anorexia, nausea and vomiting, and constipation in the last month of their lives (Figure 12-1). Similar findings have since been noted in other populations. Children who are neurologically impaired are particularly at risk because of their limited verbal abilities and atypical responses to pain. Symptom management of seriously ill children has been improved significantly since early studies. As more children with chronic and serious illnesses are cared for and sometimes die at home, the management of their illnesses will increasingly involve their primary care pediatrician.

This chapter will review the basic medical approaches to pain and symptom management in children, particularly those with serious illnesses. In addition to pain, approaches to nausea, anorexia, fatigue, and secretions will be presented. The focus will be on the medical management issues a primary care pediatrician may attempt to manage in the community setting. When the primary care pediatrician is insufficiently familiar with such treatment, consultation with pain or palliative care specialists is appropriate.

Pain

Pain is an integrated biophysical and "existential" construct. It involves complex mechanisms of nociception modulated by biochemical factors, neuroplasticity, genetic and familial factors, and one's past experience with painful events. Each child experiences pain in a unique way and quickly develops learned behaviors related to it. As such, there is no simple correlation between the objective degree of injury and the experience of pain. More accurately, physical, psychological, interpersonal, and existential factors all contribute in important ways to the experience of pain. A comprehensive approach to pain will address all of these elements.

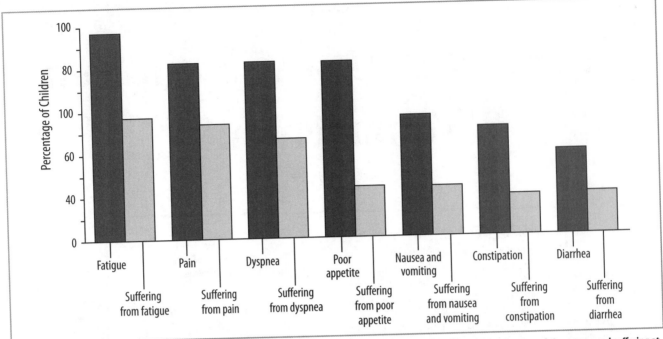

Figure 12-1. The presence and degree of suffering from specific symptoms in the last month of life. (From Wolfe J, Grier HE, Klar N, et al. Symptoms and suffering at the end of life in children with cancer. *N Engl J Med.* **2000;342[5]:326–333. Reprinted with permission.)**

Assessment

Pain can be divided into 2 basic types: nociceptive and neuropathic. An understanding of their presentations can help differentiate the source of pain in children. Nociceptive pain is the activation of peripheral nerve receptors by noxious stimuli causing tissue damage, and its intensity is related in part to the location and the amount of damage. Somatic pain refers to nociceptive pain from musculoskeletal, bony, or superficial sources (eg, skin, mucosa). Deep somatic pain tends to be localized and concentrated and described as stabbing, aching, or throbbing, eg, bone pain is deep and aching. Superficial somatic pain is sharper and can be burning or pricking. The source of nociceptive pain can also be visceral. Visceral pain is usually poorly localizable; can be described as cramping, gnawing, or pressure; and may follow daily patterns of varying intensity.

Neuropathic pain is caused by injury or dysfunction of the central nervous system (CNS) or peripheral nerves. It can be described as burning, tingling, shooting, or scalding. Its presence points to neuropathies, CNS insult, or evolving damage to the nervous system. Understanding whether the source of pain is somatic, visceral, or neuropathic helps guide treatment choices.

Pain has been referred to as the "fifth vital sign" and should be a part of the medical evaluation of every child. Pain is phenomenological and thus, while its existence is "real" and "objective," it can only be experienced by the affected person. Though it is not a completely subjective experience, it can only be truly articulated by the person in pain and, fundamentally, the patient's report of the presence or severity of pain is the key to the assessment. In children, and especially children with developmental issues, objective assessment tools may be useful to identify the presence of pain and quantify its severity. In most patients these scales are also helpful in understanding the symptom of pain over time.

Pain scales assess the intensity of pain. Analog pain scales (Figure 12-2), generally scoring intensity on a scale of 1 to 10, have some reliability when used in the same patient over time. Younger children may have difficulty with the concept of quantity or the meaning of greater intensity. An important modification of the analog scale for children with impaired communication skills or cognition is an individualized numeric rating scale, where parents' observations of their child's facial expression, body movements, activity and interaction, cry, and ability to be consoled as they experience worsening pain are used to label the points of the scale.

For children older than 3 years, the Wong-Baker FACES Pain Rating Scale (Figure 12-3) is often used. After showing children the faces, they are instructed that each face is for a person who has no pain (hurt), some pain, or a lot of pain. The child is then asked to choose the face that best describes how he is feeling. More comprehensive pain assessment tools are available that also assess function and mood, but they are not widely used. The perspective of parents and others familiar with the child is crucial to any assessment of a child's pain.

Obviously, the child in pain must be relieved of it. However, it is advantageous to make a strong effort to understand the source of the pain and treat conditions amenable to non-pain medication. For example, chest pain may be caused by candidal esophagitis or abdominal pain due to constipation. Thinking clearly about the source of pain and not simply providing analgesic agents in a reflexive manner has the benefits of preserving alertness, sparing side effects, and sustaining the least impaired quality of life. It also can permanently eliminate the pain by eliminating the underlying condition responsible for it.

Figure 12-2. Visual analog pain scale. (From McCaffery M, Pasero C. *Pain: Clinical Manual.* St Louis, MO: Mosby; 1999. Reprinted with permission.)

Figure 12-3. Wong-Baker FACES Pain Rating Scale. (From Wong-Baker FACES Foundation [2014]. Retrieved January 1, 2014, with permission from www.WongBakerFACES.org.)

Medical Management

Opioids are the mainstay of pain management. Familiarity with the basic principles of treatment with these agents is fundamental to care for children with serious acute and life-limiting illness. In cases of complex pain or those involving daunting polypharmacy, it may be best to seek guidance from pain or palliative care specialists. Certain medications (ie, methadone or selective norepinephrine reuptake inhibitors) or invasive approaches (ie, intrathecal pumps, regional blocks, and surgical or radiotherapeutic approaches to pain control), as well as the management of chronic pain, particularly in adolescents, should involve consultation with or referral to pain and palliative care specialists. The optimal management of pain includes addressing psychosocial and spiritual distress and making efforts at enhancing a child's function.

Opioids have no ceiling doses. Dose escalation should proceed until the pain is controlled, provided that side effects are tolerable. Children on long-term opioid treatment often receive surprisingly high doses yet, provided the treatment is successful in controlling pain, are comfortable and functional. As a general rule, infants younger than 6 months should be started at one-third the general pediatric dose. Intolerable pain is more easily prevented than relieved, and efforts should be directed at "staying ahead of the pain." Anticipated side effects of opioids include constipation, pruritus, and nausea and vomiting. The pruritus and nausea and vomiting are usually short-lived, disappearing in a week, but constipation persists. All patients on scheduled opioids should also receive scheduled doses of stool softeners and stimulant laxatives.

Barriers exist in patients and physicians that may prevent the optimal use of opioids. Foremost is the concern about respiratory depression. In opioid-naïve patients, this risk is minimized by appropriate dosing. Even in patients requiring dose escalation, the risk is low and respiratory depression is preceded by sedation rather than an abrupt event. When needed, naloxone can be used to reverse a worrisome respiratory effect, though at the cost of the return of pain. Physicians may also be unfamiliar with appropriate dosing, may not view pain control as a priority of care, or may be worried about difficulties ensuring follow-up and ongoing assessment. Families, for their part, may believe that pain is an inevitable part of the child's disease, may worry about the "symbolism" of starting a morphine drip as a hastening of death, or may worry about addiction or the stigma of having their child on such medications. Cultural and religious factors may also elicit reluctance. When these concerns arise, they should be addressed directly. In truth, the greatest concern should be to minimize any suffering caused by inadequately treated pain.

Parents and some physicians may overestimate the benefit of distraction in pain management. Distraction is best thought of as an assessment tool and may be an adjunct, but not a treatment, for pain. If a child can be substantially distracted from her pain for a significant period, the pain need not be managed with medication. But if the child's distress is apparent despite the distraction, the pain needs pharmacologic intervention. What must be avoided is a distressed child engaging in the distraction to please adults while her pain goes unabated. Similarly, there is no place for the use of placebos in the treatment of pain.

The World Health Organization 2-step approach to pharmacologic management of pain, revised in 2012 from the Pain Relief Ladder, is the most important guide to pain management in children. It presents a stepwise and additive approach to "capture" a child's pain as well as to augment the pharmacologic treatment of pain. The model is premised on using a 2-step strategy, dosing at regular intervals, using the appropriate route of administration, and adapting treatment to the individual child.

Children with mild pain who have not been on any analgesic medication are managed with oral analgesics, ie, acetaminophen and ibuprofen (step 1). In certain cases, intravenous (IV) acetaminophen or ketorolac may be used. Adjuvants may be added if appropriate. Acetaminophen can be given orally or rectally. Compounded ibuprofen can be given rectally, though its efficacy is still under study. The topical application of these agents in ketoprofen cream or aspirin cream may also be of benefit. Rarely, there may be a role for a COX-2 inhibitor. All nonsteroidal anti-inflammatory drugs (NSAIDs) have ceiling doses and gastrointestinal toxicities. Except for acetaminophen, all affect platelet function.

Adjuvants are non-analgesic medications that are helpful in the management of a child's pain. For example, anxiety experienced by a child who is medically fragile may potentiate the child's pain and distress, even at step 1. A benzodiazepine may be helpful in such cases. A lidocaine patch can help with some somatic pain. Certain forms of mild to moderate pain (ie, neuropathic pain) may be adequately addressed with gabapentin or pregabalin and can spare opioids in part or completely.

Step 2 addresses children with moderate to severe pain and involves the addition of opioids to the treatment plan (Table 12-1). "Weak opioids" are no longer recommended (eg, codeine, tramadol). Research has shown that codeine may be a weaker analgesic than a standard dose of many NSAIDs, and it has a ceiling effect. Its oral bioavailability is widely unpredictable at 15% to 80%. Most importantly, codeine is a prodrug that must be metabolized by the liver into morphine. This is problematic because it is estimated that 35% of children do not metabolize codeine in the anticipated way, leading to great uncertainties in a calculated effect. The use of tramadol is only weakly recommended because of concerns about risks for seizures and hyper-serotonergic symptoms with its use. The initiation of opioids in smaller children in step 2 typically involves the use of oral oxycodone at the appropriate dose. Where dose escalation is likely, morphine has advantages due to its multiple formulations.

When pain persists or worsens, morphine, hydromorphone, or oxycodone are recommended initial choices. Doses are escalated until pain is controlled, using the least invasive form of administration necessary. This step may involve the addition of controlled-release preparations of opioid or methadone, while using shorter-acting agents for breakthrough pain. To calculate the as-needed (prn) dose for breakthrough pain, a rule of thumb is that the prn dose is 10% to 15% of the 24-hour total opioid dose or its equivalent, given every 1 to 2 hours.

An in-depth discussion of methadone and fentanyl exceeds the scope of this chapter, but it is worth making several points about them. Neither have active metabolites, making them important options for patients with renal failure where accumulated metabolites from other opioid agents can cause myoclonus, confusion, or hyperalgesia. Fentanyl, a potent analgesic, is available in a transdermal patch, which is an important non-IV, non-oral option for children having difficulty swallowing. They must have adequate body fat because the drug is deposited across the rate-limiting membrane into fat reservoirs and is absorbed from that reservoir into the child's bloodstream. Methadone has some distinct analgesic advantages. It is inexpensive, its half-life allows for more convenient twice-a-day or 3-times-a-day dosing, and it is especially helpful in treating neuropathic pain. It is complicated to dose, however, and its long and variable half-life make it a more complicated choice for those not familiar with its use.

The management of moderate and severe pain over time can lead to the development of difficult unintended effects, including sedation, nausea and vomiting, pruritus, or urinary retention. At high doses or when metabolites accumulate, patients may develop delirium, myoclonus, or hyperesthesia. Opioid rotation can be very helpful in these situations. This method involves converting one form of opioid to an equivalently analgesic dose of another. Doses can be calculated using equianalgesic dosing charts (Table 12-2). A critical concept of opioid rotation in the conversion is allowing for incomplete cross-tolerance.

Rotation of the opioid agent (ie, using a different opioid) holds the promise of maintaining analgesia with lesser amounts of the newly introduced drug and eliminating side effects. *Tolerance* is the term used to describe the need over time for greater amounts of a specific opioid to achieve the desired analgesic effect. While there is no ceiling dose for opioids, with higher doses there may be an accompanying increase in adverse effects (ie, the emergence of the intolerable side effects noted previously, the accumulation of toxic metabolites, or high costs due to the required amounts of the drug). Because of differences in receptor binding between opioids, the cross-tolerance from one opioid to another is not complete. An equianalgesic dose of another opioid will require less of the medication and achieve a more favorable balance between analgesia and side effects.

The reduction in equianalgesic dosing for cross-tolerance is between 25% and 50%. In cases of poorly controlled pain, a lesser reduction is appropriate. The steps in a rotation are (1) calculating the daily dose of current opioid in oral morphine equivalents, (2) determining the equianalgesic dose of the agent to be introduced, (3) reducing the calculated amount by one-third to allow for cross-tolerance, and (4) dividing the total daily dose into the units of bolus dosing or continuous infusion.

Table 12-1. Dosing of Selected Step 2 Analgesic Medications

Drug Name	Initial Oral Dosing	Initial IV Dosing	Preparations	Comments
Oxycodone	0.1–0.2 mg/kg q 4–6 h	NA	1-mg/mL and 20-mg/mL solutions; 5-, 10-, 15-, 20-, or 30-mg tablets	Available in controlled-release tablets (OxyContin) May be administered PO, sublingual, or PR
Morphine	0.15–0.3 mg/kg q 4 h	50–100 µg/kg q 2–4 h Continuous infusion 10–30 µg/kg/h	2-mg/mL, 4-mg/mL and 20-mg/mL solution 10-, 15-, 30-mg tablets 5-, 10-, 20-, 30-mg suppository	May be administered PO, IV, sublingual, or PR Available in controlled-release tablets (MS Contin)
Hydromorphone	60 µg/kg q 3–4 h	15–20 µg/kg q 4 h Continuous infusion 5 µg/kg/h	1-mg/mL oral solution 2-, 4-, 8-mg tablets 3-mg suppository	May be administered PO, IV, sublingual, or PR Controlled-release tablets not available in United States

Abbreviations: IV, intravenous; NA, not applicable; PO, orally; PR, far point of accommodation; q, every.

Drug	Oral/Rectal Route	Parenteral Route	Conversion Ratio to Oral Morphine	Equianalgesic Dose of Oral Morphine
Morphine sulfate	30 mg of oral morphine	10 mg of parenteral morphine	Parenteral morphine is **3 times** as potent as oral morphine.	30 mg
Oxycodone	20 mg of oral oxycodone	NA	Oral oxycodone is **roughly 1.5 times** more potent than oral morphine.	30 mg
Hydrocodone	20 mg of oral hydrocodone	NA	Oral hydrocodone is **roughly 1.5 times** more potent than oral morphine.	30 mg
Hydromorphone	7 mg of oral hydromorphone	1.5 mg of parenteral hydromorphone	Oral hydromorphone is about **4–7 times** as potent as oral morphine. Parenteral hydromorphone is **20 times** as potent as oral morphine.	30 mg
Fentanyl	NA	15 µg/h	Transdermal fentanyl is **approximately 80 times** as potent as morphine (This is based on studies converting from morphine to fentanyl. Currently, there are no empirical studies converting fentanyl to morphine.)	30 mg

Abbreviation: NA, not applicable.

Adapted with permission from VS Periyakoil, MD; Opiods and pain management module; Stanford eCampus Palliative Care Curriculum. http://palliative.stanford.edu. Accessed May 1, 2014.

For example, a child is receiving 120 mg oxycodone and 80 mg total prn morphine orally each day. He vacillates between barely adequate pain control and over-sedation. He is no longer able to walk. The decision is made to rotate his opioid to IV hydromorphone. A dosage of 120 mg oxycodone is equivalent to 180 mg oral morphine (oxycodone is 1.5 times more potent than oral morphine) and, when added to the 80-mg oral morphine being used prn, the equivalent daily dose of oral morphine is 260 mg. Parenteral hydromorphone is 20 times as potent than oral morphine, so the equianalgesic amount of parenteral hydromorphone is 13 mg. Reducing by one-third for cross-tolerance but rounding up given the barely adequate pain control, the total daily equianalgesic dose of parenteral hydromorphone is 9 mg. That can be divided by 24 to determine the hourly infusion rate of a continuous IV infusion (375 µg/hour) or divided by 6 to determine the bolus dose to be given every 4 hours (1.5 mg). Finally, to determine a prn dose, 10% to 15% of the daily hydromorphone dose is 1 mg, offered every 1 to 2 hours.

Physicians lacking experience in pain management often worry about the difficulty of addressing uncontrolled pain. In addition to feeling distress about their patients' discomfort, physicians are concerned that an escalation in medication will make the child apneic and unnecessarily hasten death. Because expert and effective management is a critical skill in the care of seriously ill children, especially those facing the end of life, the primary care physician may choose to consult with palliative care or pain treatment specialists to ensure that the child's needs are adequately addressed. Alternatively, hospice medical directors can provide palliative care consultations if hospital-based teams are not available.

The risk of respiratory depression while using an accepted escalation rationale is actually quite small. Patients may fall asleep when their pain is "captured," but this is generally due to exhaustion related to the previously unrelieved pain. Even in mild to moderate pain, patients do not notice a change in dose increases when they are less than 25% above baseline. In cases of moderate to severe pain, a dose escalation of 50% to 100% is appropriate. Research has shown that pain relief during a pain crisis can be achieved quickly with a rapid medication escalation under close supervision. The recommended approach is to provide doses every 10 minutes, increasing by 50% every third dose, until the symptom is relieved. For instance, using the previous example, 1 mg hydromorphone would be given, then repeated 10 minutes later, then followed 10 minutes later by 1.5 mg hydromorphone, then repeated 10 minutes later, etc, until the pain is adequately controlled. The pain is generally "captured" within 30 to 40 minutes. The manner in which the urgency is addressed will depend on the expressed goals of care in each case.

The management of neuropathic pain presents a considerable challenge. The source of neuropathic pain is the insult or dysfunction of the central, peripheral, or autonomic nervous system. Pediatric patients may experience this pain due to degenerative CNS processes or injury, as well as treatment-related injuries to the nervous system from drug toxicities, radiation therapy, or surgery. Infection may also cause neuralgia. Children describe neuropathic pain as jolts of burning, stabbing, or shooting. It also causes allodynia, dysesthesia, and hyperalgesia. The results of various approaches to the treatment of neuropathic pain are mixed, and a multimodal approach, including an emphasis on physical therapy and more than one therapeutic agent, is recommended. Adjuvant medications are offered as a first line in children, with gabapentin beginning at 10 mg/kg/day divided 3 times a day and titrating upward to doses as high as 60 mg/kg/day. Strong opioids may be included in an appropriate regimen. Tricyclic antidepressants tend to be used less for children in the management of neuropathic pain because of concerns of arrhythmia risk.

Dystonia and neuro-irritability, while not properly neuropathic pain, present similar challenges in children with neurodegenerative conditions. Generalized dystonia is a condition in which there are sustained, erratic, painful muscle contractions that cause twisting and repetitive movements or abnormal postures. *Neuro-irritability* is a term used to describe the difficulty in settling and persistent crying seen in some chilldren who are cognitively impaired with metabolic and neurodegenerative conditions. These symptoms are distressing and often occur in children whose impairments make an assessment of their experience difficult. Benzodiazepines, typically diazepam, are the first line for dystonia (Table 12-3). Trihexyphenidyl is also commonly considered, as is valproate, baclofen, carbamazepine, or tetrabenazine. In severe, intractable cases, the implantation of deep brain stimulators is being increasingly considered, although the empiric basis for that decision remains under study. Anticonvulsants are the mainstay in the treatment of neuro-irritability. Phenobarbital is often the first medication tried. The treatment of these conditions is generally determined in consultation with a child neurologist.

Management of Non-pain Symptoms (Table 12-3)

Dyspnea

There are many similarities between the treatment of severe dyspnea and severe pain. Dyspnea is caused by increased work of breathing, hypoxia, and hypercapnia and the driving desire of the brain to relieve them. Experientially, it may cause a feeling similar to being underwater too long and needing to surface. Like pain, it has a physical basis, but the distress is potentiated by psychological, interpersonal, and existential aspects. After oxygen, opioids are the treatment of choice, and they are dosed at one-third of the dose for pain treatment. While this is another situation in which inexperienced physicians are typically worried about worsening the patient's condition by causing respiratory depression, there is strong evidence for the effectiveness of low-dose opioids in alleviating dyspnea. Opioids reduce breathlessness and provide benefit to patients with limited risk of respiratory depression at appropriate doses. Due to the anxious state dyspnea often causes and the fact that anxiety worsens dyspnea, an appropriate dose of a benzodiazepine is also helpful, although never as the principal medication. Simple environmental measures, such as the breeze from an electric fan on the patient's face or uncluttering the room, also bring relief.

Nausea and Vomiting

Nausea and vomiting are common symptoms in children with complex illnesses or facing the end of life and significant sources of distress and discomfort. They can have different etiologies, principally

gastrointestinal, CNS, or treatment-related. Children with neurologic impairments can suffer from retching, and many of their medications have nausea among their side effects. Children are especially vulnerable to anticipatory nausea, a conditioned behavioral response in anticipation of a medication or procedure that has caused nausea and vomiting in the past. Anorexia can be a symptom of low-grade nausea. An approach to nausea and vomiting based on an understanding of the cause of the symptom exacerbation and understanding the symptom mechanism can prove valuable. A careful history and physical examination, with special attention to medications and procedures, is crucial.

While a patient's presentation may be complex, there are 4 pathways to nausea and vomiting. The vomiting center, which lies in the brain stem, receives input from the chemoreceptor trigger zone (CTZ), the cerebral cortex, peripheral pathways in the gastrointestinal tract, and the vestibular system. The CTZ responds to toxins (and medications) in blood and spinal fluid; the cerebral cortex responds to sensory input, anxiety, meningeal irritation, and elevated intracranial pressure; peripheral pathways are stimulated by mechanical stretch in intestinal obstruction and by mucosal injury; and the vestibular system is affected by motion and labyrinth disorders. Each pathway involves different neuro-receptors for mechanism-based therapy to target.

The CTZ can be suppressed by the blockage of dopamine type 2 receptors with haloperidol, prochlorperazine, chlorpromazine, or metoclopramide. Peripheral pathways can be addressed by identifying the underlying cause and with the blockage of 5-HT_3 receptors by ondansetron. The cortex can be addressed with anxiolytics, attention to sensory stimuli (eg, smells, tastes), and in cases of elevated intracranial pressure, high-dose steroids. Dronabinol may also be helpful. The vestibular system is managed by blocking muscarinic acetylcholine and histamine receptors with scopolamine, hyoscyamine, and diphenhydramine. (Promethazine is useful in adults but is to be avoided because of its implication in sudden death in some children.)

The causes of nausea and vomiting are often not pure but involve multiple pathways. For instance, opioid-induced nausea and vomiting may be due to constipation or gastroparesis, stimulation of the CTZ, or sensitization of the labyrinth. Choices must be made about how to approach the possible causes in a stepwise manner. The literature suggests that mechanism-based therapy is more effective, employs a systematic approach that identifies all possible contributors, and encourages the treatment of underlying causes. It uses medication in a targeted manner, lessening the risk of untoward effects and oversedation. Finally, it is worth pointing out that the risk of extrapyramidal side effects is greater in children, and when using high doses of metoclopramide or the phenothiazines, premedication with diphenhydramine is recommended.

Anorexia

Anorexia is an anticipated symptom at the end of life. Some parents have great difficulty with this symptom and can feel overwhelmed by the loss of a concrete expression of their nurturing. They want

	Table 12-3. Medications Used for Common Symptoms in Pediatric Palliative Care		
Symptom	*Medication*	*Starting Dose*	*Comments*
Dystonia	Diazepam	0.5 mg/kg/dose IV/PO q 6 h prn; initial dose for children <5 y is 5 mg/dose; for children ≥5 y, dose is 10 mg/dose	May be irritating if given by peripheral IV
	Trihexyphenidyl	0.1 mg/kg/d PO	Would initiate in consultation with child neurologist; not for children <3 y; 2-mg/5-mL liquid available
	Phenobarbital	3 mg/kg/d PO	Helpful with neuro-irritability; many liquid concentrations
	Baclofen	5 mg PO tid, increase by 5 mg/dose prn	Helpful with neuropathic pain and spasticity; abrupt withdrawal may result in hallucinations and seizures; not for children <10 y.
Nausea	Metoclopramide	0.1–0.2 mg/kg/dose q 6 h, up to 10 mg/dose (prokinetic and mild nausea dosing) For chemotherapy-associated nausea 0.5–1 mg/kg q 6 h prn PO/IV/SC; give with diphenhydramine	Helpful when dysmotility an issue; may cause extrapyramidal reactions, particularly in children following IV administration of high doses; contraindicated in complete bowel obstruction or pheochromocytoma
	Ondansetron	0.15 mg/kg/dose q 8 h to max of 8 mg/dose Some institutions also use daily dosing for chemotherapy.	Significant experience in pediatrics; good empiric therapy for nausea in palliative care population; higher doses used with chemotherapy; oral dissolving tablet contains phenylalanine.
	Lorazepam	0.025 mg/kg up to 2 mg IV/PO q 6 h	May be given sublingually; particularly helpful with anticipatory nausea; avoid use in neonates.
	Scopolamine patch	1.5-mg patch, change q 72 h	Good for motion-induced nausea/vomiting; handling patch and contacting eye may cause anisocoria and blurry vision; may fold patches but do not cut them.
	Prochlorperazine	0.4 mg/kg/d PO/PR divided q 8 h	Available in suppositories and 1-mg/mL syrup; not for children <2 y
Anorexia	Megestrol acetate	10 mg/kg/d in 1–4 divided doses, up to 15 mg/kg/d or 800 mg/d.	For children >10 years; acute adrenal insufficiency may occur with abrupt withdrawal after long-term use; use with caution in patients with diabetes mellitus or history of thromboembolism; may cause photosensitivity.
	Cyproheptadine	0.25–0.5 mg/kg/d PO divided q 6 h	
Respiratory secretions	Glycopyrrolate	0.04–0.1 mg/kg po q 4–8 h	Excessive drying of secretions can cause mucus plugging of airways; anticholinergic side effects possible.
	Scopolamine patch	1.5-mg patch, change q 72 h	Excessive drying of secretions can cause mucus plugging of airways; handling patch and contacting eye may cause anisocoria and blurry vision; may fold patches but do not cut them.
	Atropine 1% ophthalmic drops	One drop sublingual, titrate to effect	
Fatigue	Methylphenidate	Norms not established Begin with a fraction of a 0.3 mg/kg/d.	Daytrana patch can be helpful.

Abbreviations: IV, intravenous; PO, orally; PR, far point of accommodation; prn, as needed; q, every; SC, subcutaneous; tid, 3 times a day.

Modified from Wolfe J, Ullrich C. Pain and symptom control in pediatrics. In: Walsh D, ed. *Palliative Medicine*. Philadelphia, PA: Saunders Elsevier; 2009, with permission.

their child to eat to be better able to fight his illness. Food preparation and feeding him is something concrete they can do for their child. A child who is dying wants to please his parents as much as healthy children, maybe more so. It is important to acknowledge the feelings behind the desire of parents for their child to eat. Small portions of the child's favorite foods or new favorites he asks for may be comforting to all.

There are times earlier in an illness when it may be appropriate to improve appetite. Cyproheptadine has a long history of safe use in children and has been shown to be helpful in some cases. Megestrol acetate has been shown effective in increasing weight but not muscle mass and may be considered in children older than 10 years. Cannabinoids, while stimulating appetite, have not been demonstrated to increase weight. Steroids, while likely to improve appetite, often come at an unacceptable cost of irritability and immunosuppression.

One other consideration related to feeding is whether children are starving when they no longer have the desire to eat. Research comparing the "anorexia-cachexia syndrome" with starvation shows 2 very different metabolic states. Differences in energy expenditure, protein synthesis and proteolysis, glucose metabolism, and hormonal levels reinforce the view that anorexia-cachexia is a hypermetabolic state, while starvation in healthy individuals is an effort by the body to conserve itself. An understanding of this difference enables physicians to explain to parents how the disease is robbing the child's energy and that it is not the fault of their efforts or the lack of food. In fact, research on adults dying of advanced cancer found that even the patients who ate the most lost weight.

Respiratory Secretions

Respiratory secretions are a common symptom in children who are seriously ill. Children with neuromuscular diseases and neurologic impairment can have problems managing secretions. The presence of a tracheostomy can further complicate matters. The use of suction- and cough-assist machines is important, particularly in the setting of acute respiratory illnesses that cause increased secretions. In children at this stage of illness, drying agents (eg, glycopyrrolate, atropine, scopolamine, hyoscyamine) are sometimes helpful, but they may increase the risk of acute obstruction by thickening secretions and causing mucus plugging.

Terminal secretions (the "death rattle") are understandably very distressing to parents. The child does not typically notice them. They are not relieved by suctioning but sometimes respond to repositioning. Drying agents are usually prescribed in this setting. There is not much advantage to switching between agents if the effect is not substantial, though more than one agent should be tried. Glycopyrrolate stands alone among these agents as the only one that does not cross the blood–brain barrier and thus is the least likely to cause CNS effects.

Fatigue

Fatigue is a highly prevalent symptom at the end of life. In one study of children with terminal cancer, 96% were found to have experienced fatigue in their last month. This symptom is especially disheartening because fatigued children may have the desire to do things that provide a quality of life but not be up to the task. Fatigue may be caused by illness, treatments, stress, isolation, poor sleep hygiene and circadian disorientation, mood, or the lack of pleasure or activity. The sedative effects of some medications certainly contribute. Sleep, exercise, nutrition, anemia treatment, increased interactions, and activity all have been shown to have a beneficial effect in decreasing fatigue. Medical therapy with methylphenidate or modafinil may be helpful, dosed at lower amounts than typically prescribed for attention-deficit/hyperactivity disorder.

CASE RESOLUTION

The patient lived for 4 more months, was never again admitted to the hospital, and until her last days, remained engaged and as playful as her fatigue allowed. Her primary care pediatrician teamed with the pediatric palliative care team at the closest children's hospital and was assisted with many of the symptom management decisions. In her last days, she was on methadone, morphine boluses, lorazepam, citalopram, gabapentin, ondansetron, MiraLax, senna, and as-needed methylphenidate. Her pediatrician made home visits and remained available for evolving symptoms. The pediatrician was in the child's home at the time of her death, ensuring comfort, declaring the death, and affirming the value of her life.

Selected References

Breau LM, Camfield CS, McGrath PJ, Finley GA. The incidence of pain in children with severe cognitive impairments. *Arch Pediatr Adolesc Med.* 2003;157(12):1219–1226

Pritchard M, Burghen EA, Gattuso JS, et al. Factors that distinguish symptoms of most concern to parents from other symptoms of dying children. *J Pain Symptom Manage.* 2010;39(4):627–636

Solodiuk J, Curley MA. Pain assessment in nonverbal children with severe cognitive impairments: the Individualized Numeric Rating Scale (INRS). *J Pediatr Nurs.* 2003;18(4):295–299

Ullrich CK, Dussel V, Hilden JM, et al. Fatigue in children with cancer at the end of life. *J Pain Symptom Manage.* 2010;40(4):483–494

Wee B, Hillier R. Interventions for noisy breathing in patients near to death. *Cochrane Database Syst Rev.* 2008;(1):CD005177

Williams DG, Hatch DJ, Howard RF. Codeine phosphate in paediatric medicine. *Br J Anaesth.* 2001;86(3):413–421

Wolfe J, Grier HE, Klar N, et al. Symptoms and suffering at the end of life in children with cancer. *N Engl J Med.* 2000;342(5):326–333

Wood GJ, Shega JW, Lynch B, Von Roenn JH. Management of intractable nausea and vomiting in patients at the end of life: "I was feeling nauseous all of the time…nothing was working." *JAMA.* 2007;298(10):1196–1207

World Health Organization. *WHO Guidelines on the Pharmacological Treatment of Persisting Pain in Children with Medical Illnesses.* Geneva, Switzerland: World Health Organization; 2012. http://www.who.int/medicines/areas/quality_safety/guide_perspainchild/en/index.html. Accessed November 19, 2013

CHAPTER 13

Complementary and Alternative Medicine in Pediatric Primary Care

Miriam T. Stewart, BA, and Erica Sibinga, MD, MHS

CASE STUDY

A 14-year-old girl is brought to your office to follow up on her migraine headaches. She has no other significant medical history but has experienced intermittent migraine headaches over the past few years. The headaches occur approximately weekly in the evenings, do not wake her from sleep, and improve with ibuprofen (400 mg), as had been previously prescribed at your office. At this visit, the girl states that she wishes she didn't have to take medicine for her headaches. Her mother reports that a family friend has suggested acupuncture or herbs for the headaches and asks whether there are other complementary and alternative medicine (CAM) approaches that they could try.

Questions

1. What are CAM therapies?
2. How does a provider explore if there are any CAM approaches that are appropriate for the treatment of chronic or recurrent conditions such as headaches in a child or an adolescent?
3. What is the best way to determine if a family is using CAM?
4. What is the best way to communicate with a family about CAM therapies?
5. What is the best way to monitor the safety of CAM approaches?

Complementary and Alternative Medicine (CAM)

Complementary and alternative medicine (CAM) refers to a wide variety of therapies that are not typically part of "conventional" medical approaches. Conventional medicine (also called allopathic or Western medicine) is the general approach of medical doctors (MDs), doctors of osteopathy (DOs), and allied health professionals. The specific therapies thought of as CAM versus allopathic may change over time, as CAM practices may be incorporated into allopathic medicine.

Complementary and alternative medicine therapies may be used in a number of different ways. When CAM therapies are used in addition to allopathic care, they are termed *complementary*; this is by far the most common way CAM therapies are used. *Alternative* medicine refers to therapies used instead of allopathic care. A small but growing number of practitioners as well as academic centers are using allopathic and non-allopathic approaches, a practice referred to as *integrative medicine*.

Epidemiology

The use of CAM has risen steadily over the past several decades and now comprises a significant subset of health-related visits and expenditures. In 2007, more than one-third (38.3%) of American adults surveyed reported having used some form of CAM in the previous 12 months. As of 1997 the number of visits to CAM providers exceeded those to primary care physicians, and out-of-pocket expenditures for CAM were estimated at $27 billion per year. These statistics demonstrate the importance of physician awareness of CAM and support the routine inclusion of questions about CAM in the medical history.

A growing body of evidence reveals that the pediatric population is also using CAM. A large-scale survey of caregivers found that 1 in 9 children use CAM (11.8%). Higher prevalence, up to 60%, has been found in certain populations, such as children with cancer, epilepsy, sickle cell disease, and other chronic diseases. Adolescents are more likely to use CAM than younger children, and CAM is more often used in the western United States than in other regions of the country. Other factors associated with CAM use in children include parental education beyond high school, higher household income, coverage by private health insurance, use of prescription medications, and number of health conditions, doctor visits, or school days missed for illness in the past year. Non-Hispanic whites are more likely to use CAM than Hispanics or blacks, though the strength of this association diminishes when data are adjusted for confounding factors. When worry about cost delays or prevents the receipt of conventional medical care, children are more likely to use CAM. The strongest predictor of CAM use in children is CAM use by a parent; children whose parents use CAM are 5 times more likely to use CAM. When discussing CAM with families who are using it for their children, pediatricians need to be aware that parents may also be using CAM.

Motivations for Using CAM

Complementary and alternative medicine can be used for health maintenance, for symptomatic relief, as an adjunct to curative conventional medical care, for relief from side effects of conventional medical care, or in place of conventional medical care. Families choose to use CAM for many reasons. Word of mouth and belief in the efficacy of the treatment can be strong motivators. Some parents express a desire for more options and feel a sense of empowerment in their parental role as a result of CAM use. Complementary and alternative medicine may also be more congruous with a family's values, philosophies about health, and understanding of the basis of disease. Parents may fear the side effects of conventional medicines or be dissatisfied with the care their child receives in conventional medical settings. Families may seek the additional personal attention afforded by CAM providers. For some families, CAM offers additional hope when conventional medical care fails. Underlying all these motivations is the desire for the child's health and well-being and the quest for safe and effective treatments for disease. Physicians and families can find common ground in this most basic of motivations, which can inform conversations about CAM and conventional medical care.

CAM Categories

Complementary and alternative medicine therapies can be thought of as falling into 1 of 5 categories: whole medical systems, mind-body therapies, biomechanical therapies, bioenergetic therapies, and biochemical therapies (Table 13-1). Besides whole medical systems, these categories are chosen to reflect purported similarities in underlying mechanism of effect. A particular therapy may be used as part of a whole medical system approach or on its own. For example, acupuncture may be part of an individualized, comprehensive traditional Chinese medicine (TCM) treatment approach, also consisting of herbs and lifestyle recommendations, or a standardized acupuncture treatment may be used without evaluation and treatment by a TCM provider, in which case it can be thought of as a bioenergetic therapy. Additionally, a particular therapy may belong to more than one category; for example, herbal preparations may have a biochemical and placebo (mind-body) effect.

Whole Medical Systems

Whole medical systems, including allopathic medicine, are whole-system approaches to treatment, consisting of an underlying theory of healing, standardized training, and diagnostic and treatment approaches reflective of the underlying theory. For instance, TCM is based on the theory that illness and symptoms result from yin-yang energy imbalances. These energy imbalances are diagnosed through history and physical examination and treated by altering the energy balance using acupuncture (or other mechanical or thermal stimuli), herbs, and lifestyle changes (eg, diet, sleep, physical activity).

Mind-Body Therapies

These therapies are intended to enhance the mind's ability to benefit health. A number of mind-body therapies are integrated into allopathic treatment, such as psychotherapy, group therapy, imagery, and biofeedback. Others are still considered CAM, such as meditation and hypnotherapy.

Biomechanical Therapies

Biomechanical therapies aim to improve health through physical manipulation of the body. This may involve working with muscles, as with massage, or spinal alignment, as with chiropractic and osteopathic approaches. Massage therapies range from relatively light muscle work to deep tissue massage, as well as physical therapy to work with muscles and joints. Spinal manipulation therapies are used commonly in the United States and are most often practiced by chiropractors or DOs.

Bioenergetic Therapies

Bioenergetic therapies are directed at improving health through altering the body's energy as it runs through, on, or around the body. Because allopathic training does not include the concept of energy in this way, bioenergetic therapies tend to draw skepticism from allopaths. With increasing scientific evidence of its beneficial effects, acupuncture is purported to affect the body's vital energy (chi) as it courses through energy channels called meridians. In 1997 a National Institutes of Health consensus panel declared the evidence sufficient for integration of acupuncture into a number of allopathic treatments, including treatment of chemotherapy-associated nausea and emesis, anesthesia-associated nausea and emesis, and pain syndromes. Homeopathic remedies are theoretically bioenergetic therapies, as the "ingredients" are successively diluted beyond the point of significant molecular presence; therefore, it is the resulting change in the energy of the diluents (sometimes called the "memory of the molecule") that is responsible for the therapeutic effect. Additionally, a number of therapies aim to affect energy at or near the surface of the body, including therapeutic touch and Reiki, which involve a trained practitioner identifying the energy imbalance and directing his or her own energy to improve the patient's energy balance and promote healing.

Table 13-1. Selected Examples of Complementary and Alternative Medicine Therapies by Categories

	Modality	Description: At a Glance	Licensure and Regulation
Whole Medical Systems	Ayurveda	• Originated in India several thousand years ago and is still used by 80% of the population exclusively or in combination with Western medicine. • Health and disease are thought to relate to a person's constitution (prakriti), which is composed of a unique combination of the 3 life forces (doshas). Imbalances between the doshas can lead to disease. • Treatments are tailored to the individual's unique constitution and are aimed at eliminating impurities, reducing symptoms, increasing resistance to disease, reducing worry, and increasing harmony in the patient's life. • Treatments include herbs, vitamins and minerals, massage, yoga (see page 68), enemas, and specialized diet and lifestyle recommendations.	• Ayurvedic medicine is not accredited in the United States, although several states have accredited ayurvedic schools. • In India, ayurvedic medicine can be studied at the bachelor's and doctorate level.
	Native American healing	• Broad term that encompasses the healing traditions of hundreds of indigenous tribes. Has been practiced in North America for more than 40,000 years. • Can combine religion, spirituality, herbal medicine, shamanic healers, purification activities, and symbolic rituals in the treatment of medical and emotional problems. Treatments may be individual or involve the entire community. • Treatment is often a slow process that is spread over days and weeks. There is a strong belief in the therapeutic value of the relationship with the healer.	• There is no government oversight of education of or licensure for Native American healers.
	Naturopathy	Developed in Germany and the United States in the late 19th to early 20th centuries. • Central belief is that nature has healing power; practitioners view their role as supporting the body's inherent ability to restore health. • Naturopathic practitioners strive to use the most natural, least invasive approach to restore and maintain health. • Treatment modalities used by naturopaths include nutrition, vitamins and minerals, herbal medicines, homeopathy (see page 70), therapeutic massage and joint manipulation, hydrotherapy, exercise, and lifestyle counseling.	• Naturopathic physicians (ND or NMD degree) complete a 4-year graduate-level program at a naturopathic medical school accredited by the Council on Naturopathic Medical Education, which is recognized by the US Department of Education. States vary in their licensing of naturopathic physicians and the scope of naturopathic practice, including the ability to prescribe drugs, perform minor surgery, and assist in childbirth. • The American Association of Naturopathic Physicians (www.naturopathic.org) is the national professional society of naturopathic physicians.
	Traditional Chinese medicine (TCM)	• Originated in China more than 5,000 years ago; rooted in the Taoist philosophy. • Views the human body and mind as an integrated whole in which tissues, organs, and parts function interdependently. • Yin-yang theory—the concept of 2 opposing but interdependent forces that shape the world—is a core principle. Health and disease relate to balance between yin and yang in the body. • Treatments to restore balance include herbs, massage, acupuncture (see page 70), diet, and exercises such as tai chi (see page 70) and qigong.	• Most states license acupuncture but vary in their inclusion of other TCM treatments in licensure. • Acupuncture and TCM schools are accredited by the federally recognized Accreditation Commission for Acupuncture and Oriental Medicine.

Table 13-1. Selected Examples of Complementary and Alternative Medicine Therapies by Categories, continued

Modality	Description: At a Glance	Licensure and Regulation
Mind-Body Therapies		
Biofeedback	• Technique that trains people to improve their health by controlling certain bodily processes that normally happen involuntarily, including heart rate, blood pressure, muscle tension, and skin temperature. • Biofeedback practice involves attaching the patient to electrodes (or other monitoring devices) that monitor the desired process (eg, muscle tension, skin temperature). The therapist leads the patient in exercises designed to assist in controlling the desired variable, while the electrodes provide real-time feedback on the patient's success. • Biofeedback is used in a variety of conditions, including high blood pressure, headaches, chronic pain, and urinary incontinence.	• The Biofeedback Certification International Alliance certifies individuals who have met their educational and training standards, which include didactic training, supervision hours, patient sessions, and case presentations. • Pelvic floor muscle dysfunction is a subspecialty within biofeedback that provides specialized training. Only licensed health care providers may apply for certification in this specialty.
Hypnotherapy	• Hypnotherapists use exercises that bring about deep relaxation and an altered state of consciousness, also known as a trance. • Through hypnosis, people learn how to master their own states of awareness. By doing so they can affect their own bodily functions and psychologic responses. • Hypnotherapy has been studied for a number of conditions, including state anxiety (eg, before medical procedures or surgeries), headaches, smoking cessation, pain control, hot flashes in breast cancer survivors, and irritable bowel syndrome. It is also used in managing pain during childbirth.	• Most hypnotherapists are licensed medical doctors, registered nurses, social workers, or family counselors who have received additional training in hypnotherapy. Several national bodies provide training certificates. • The American Society of Clinical Hypnosis (www.asch.net) is the largest organization of health professionals using clinical hypnosis and provides hypnotherapy training.
Meditation/ mindfulness	• There are many types of meditation, most of which originated in ancient religious and spiritual traditions. Some of these include mindfulness meditation, transcendental meditation, and Zen Buddhist meditation. • In meditation, a person learns to focus attention. Some forms of meditation instruct the practitioner to become mindful of thoughts, feelings, and sensations and to observe them in a nonjudgmental way. • Meditation is believed to result in a state of greater calmness, physical relaxation, and psychologic balance and can change how a person relates to the flow of emotions and thoughts. • Meditation has been studied in a variety of populations and is used for general wellness and various health problems, including anxiety, pain, depression, stress, insomnia, and physical or emotional symptoms that may be associated with chronic illnesses such as AIDS and cancer.	• There is a broad diversity of meditation practices, each of which may have its own training programs and certification policies. • There is no national or state-based accreditation for meditation practitioner education or licensing. However, meditation programs may be eligible for continuing education credits toward licensing for health professionals. • The University of Massachusetts Medical School Center for Mindfulness in Medicine, Health Care, and Society (www.umassmed.edu/cfm) is a long-standing mindfulness program associated with an academic institution and is a source for training and research on mindfulness and mind-body medicine.
Yoga	• Yoga practice was developed in ancient India, with fully developed practice appearing around 500 BC. There are numerous branches or paths of yoga. • Derived from the Sanskrit word meaning "union," yoga strives to connect the body, breath, and mind with the goal of energizing and balancing the whole person. • Yoga practice can be individual or class-based and consists of physical postures (asanas), breathing exercises, and meditation. • Yoga is used for maintaining health and has also been studied in a wide variety of conditions, including anxiety, arthritis, asthma, cancer, back pain, diabetes, heart disease, pregnancy (when modified for pregnancy), and chronic headaches.	• There is no government oversight of yoga training or practice. • There are numerous organizations and training programs in the United States and worldwide that offer training. • The Yoga Alliance is the most widely recognized educational and professional organization for yoga in the United States. It accredits yoga training programs based on a minimum training standard. Teachers who complete Yoga Alliance–accredited training are eligible to become Registered Yoga Teachers.

Table 13-1. Selected Examples of Complementary and Alternative Medicine Therapies by Categories, continued

Biomechanical Therapies

Modality	Description: At a Glance	Licensure and Regulation
Alexander technique	• Educational method whose emphasis is on changing faulty postural habits to improve mobility and performance. • Treatment has 2 components: table work (hands-on manipulation) and guided activity, in which the practitioner observes the person in action and gives verbal, visual, and physical cues to help the person perform the activity with greater ease. • People use the Alexander technique for improved performance in performing arts and sports as well as in treatment of musculoskeletal problems, repetitive stress injuries, and chronic pain.	• To be certified by the American Society for the Alexander Technique (www.amsatonline.com), practitioners must complete 1,600 hours of training over 3 years. • There is no government oversight of training or licensure.
Chiropractic	• Developed in the United States at the end of the 19th century. • Based on the notion that the relationship between the body's structure—most notably the alignment of the spine—and its coordination by the nervous system affects health. • People most often seek chiropractic care for musculoskeletal complaints (back, neck, and shoulder pain), headaches, and extremity problems. • Hands-on spinal adjustment and manipulation is a core treatment in chiropractic care, but treatment can also include heat and ice, electrical stimulation, exercise, and counseling about diet, exercise, and lifestyle.	• Chiropractic practitioners must meet the licensing and continuing education requirements of the states where they practice. • All states require chiropractors to complete a doctor of chiropractic (DC) degree at an accredited college. • The American Chiropractic Association (www.acatoday.org) is the largest professional organization representing chiropractic doctors.
The Feldenkrais Method	• A method of somatic education that uses gentle movement and directed attention to movement patterns to expand movement options and improve functioning. • Treatment can be carried out via verbal guidance in a class setting or with hands-on gentle manipulation. • People use the Feldenkrais Method to maintain well-being and enhance performance in performing arts and athletics, as well as in the treatment of a variety of conditions including multiple sclerosis, stroke, cerebral palsy, and repetitive stress injuries.	• Feldenkrais practitioners must complete 700 to 800 hours of training over 3 to 4 years to apply for certification. Certification and training is governed by the Feldenkrais Guild of North America (www.feldenkrais.com). • There is no government oversight of training or licensure.
Massage therapy	• Massage therapy has been in use for thousands of years in diverse cultures, including China, Japan, India, Egypt, and Europe. • The term *massage therapy* encompasses more than 100 distinct techniques, but the core practice is manipulation of the muscles and soft tissues of the body using the hands and fingers. • People use massage for general wellness, as well as in a wide range of conditions including sports injuries, stress, pain, musculoskeletal complaints, anxiety, and depression.	• Most states have laws regulating massage therapy and typically require a minimum number of training hours and passage of a national examination. Massage training can be accredited by state boards or an independent agency. • The National Certification Board for Therapeutic Massage & Bodywork certifies massage practitioners who pass a national examination. • The American Massage Therapy Association (www.amtamassage.org) is the nation's largest professional organization for massage practitioners.
Osteopathy	• Developed in the United States at the end of the 19th century. • Core principle is that disease and illness begin with structural problems in the spine and resulting abnormalities in the function of the nervous system. • Doctors of osteopathy receive conventional medical training but are also trained in osteopathic manipulation techniques and craniosacral therapy, both of which involve hands-on manipulation of bones and tissues. • People seek care from osteopathic doctors for conventional medical care and specifically for musculoskeletal conditions.	• Doctors of osteopathy (DOs) complete a 4-year training program in conventional medicine and osteopathy and also complete medical residencies in their specialty of choice. • Doctors of osteopathy are recognized for full practice rights in all 50 states once they are licensed. • The American Osteopathic Association (www.osteopathic.org) is the primary professional organization and accreditation agency for osteopathy in the United States.

Table 13-1. Selected Examples of Complementary and Alternative Medicine Therapies by Categories, continued

Modality	Description: At a Glance	Licensure and Regulation
Bioenergetic Therapies		
Acupuncture	• Acupuncture is a modality of TCM (see page 67). The earliest recorded use of acupuncture dates from 200 BCE. • The core principle of acupuncture is the belief that a particular type of life force or energy (chi) circulates through the energy pathways (meridians) in the body. Chi maintains the dynamic balance of yin and yang. An imbalance of chi can cause symptoms and disease. • Acupuncture treatment involves stimulation of specific points along the meridians using pressure (acupressure), thermal energy (moxibustion), or very fine acupuncture needles. • Acupuncture has been studied in a variety of conditions, including chronic pain, postsurgical recovery, chemotherapy-related nausea, musculoskeletal problems, headaches, addiction, asthma, and menstrual problems.	• Most states require a license to practice acupuncture, although licensing and education standards vary from state to state. Licensure confers the title of LAc. • In 1997, the National Institutes of Health recognized acupuncture as a mainstream medicine healing option with a statement documenting the procedure's safety and efficacy for treating a range of health conditions. • The American Academy of Medical Acupuncture (www.medicalacupuncture.org) maintains a database of licensed physicians who are also trained to perform acupuncture.
Homeopathic remedies	• Developed by a German physician at the end of the 18th century. • Based on 2 core principles: the principle of similars ("like cures like") states that a disease can be cured by a substance that produces similar symptoms in a healthy person, and the principle of dilutions ("law of minimum dose") states that the lower the dose of the medication, the greater its effectiveness. Homeopathic remedies are so dilute that few or no molecules of the healing substance remain in the diluent. It is believed that the substance has left its imprint, which stimulates the body to heal itself. • Homeopathic remedies are derived from natural substances that come from plants, minerals, or animals.	• Homeopathic remedies are prepared according to the guidelines of the *Homoeopathic Pharmacopoeia of the United States*, which was written into federal law in 1938. • The US Food and Drug Administration requires that homeopathic remedies meet legal standards for strength, purity, and packaging, but because they contain little or no active ingredient, they do not have to undergo the same safety and efficacy testing as other over-the-counter medications. • If a homeopathic remedy claims to cure a serious disease such as cancer, it needs to be sold by prescription.
Reiki	• Developed in Japan in the early 20th century. • Based on the idea that there is a universal energy that supports the body's innate healing abilities. Practitioners seek to access this energy, allowing it to flow to the body and facilitate healing. • During treatment, the practitioner's hands are placed lightly on or just above the client's body, palms down, using a series of 12 to 15 hand positions to promote the flow of energy. Each position is held for 2 to 5 minutes. • People use Reiki for relaxation, stress reduction, symptom relief, and general well-being. It can also be used to help promote peace at the end of life.	• No licensing or government accreditation exists for the training or practice of Reiki. • Multiple organizations offer training programs and certifications.
Tai chi	• Originated in ancient China as a component of TCM. • Rooted in the principles of yin-yang balance and the balanced flow of a vital life force or energy (chi). • There are many different styles, but all involve slow, deliberate movements that flow into each other. Meditation, deep breathing, and maintenance of good posture during continuous movement are foci of the practice. • People use tai chi to improve overall fitness, balance, coordination, and agility. It is also used for chronic pain, gout, heart disease, high blood pressure, arthritis, osteoporosis, diabetes, headaches, and sleep disorders.	• No licensing or government accreditation exists for the training or practice of tai chi. • There are a variety of organizations that offer training programs and certification for tai chi.
Therapeutic touch	• Developed in the 1970s in the United States. • Based on the belief that problems in the patient's energy field that cause illness and pain can be identified and rebalanced by a healer. • The technique consists of using the hands to release harmful energy and direct healthy energy for healing purposes. During a session, the hands are held 2 to 6 inches away from the body and there is no direct physical contact between practitioner and patient.	• No licensing or government accreditation exists for the training or practice of therapeutic touch. • Multiple organizations offer training programs, including some hospitals. • Many therapeutic touch practitioners are nurses or other licensed health professionals.

Table 13-1. Selected Examples of Complementary and Alternative Medicine Therapies by Categories, continued

	Modality	Description: At a Glance	Licensure and Regulation
Biochemical Therapies	Dietary supplements	• Dietary supplements contain one or more dietary ingredients, including vitamins, minerals, herbs, or amino acids, or their constituents. Herbal medicines are considered a subset of dietary supplements in the United States. • Some dietary supplements have been proven to prevent or treat disease (eg, folic acid in the prevention of neural tube defects, calcium and vitamin D in the prevention of osteoporosis), while other claims about dietary supplements are unproven. • The most commonly used dietary supplements are fish oil, *Echinacea*, flaxseed, ginseng, multivitamins, vitamins E and C, calcium, and B-complex vitamins.	• In the United States, dietary supplements can be sold without being tested to prove they are safe and effective. They must be made according to good manufacturing practices. • In the United States, no organization regulates the manufacture or certifies the labeling of dietary supplements.
	Herbal medicine	• Herbal medicine refers to using a plant's seeds, berries, roots, leaves, bark, or flowers for medicinal purposes. • Plants have been used for medicinal purposes since long before recorded history in a wide range of human cultures. • According to the World Health Organization, 80% of the world's population relies on herbal medicines for some part of their primary care. Nearly one-third of Americans use herbs. • The most commonly used herbal supplements in the United States include *Echinacea*, St John's wort, gingko, garlic, saw palmetto, ginseng, goldenseal, chamomile, feverfew, ginger, valerian, evening primrose, and milk thistle. • Herbal remedies are used in conventional medicine as well as a variety of complementary and alternative medicine practices, including naturopathy, TCM, ayurveda, and Native American healing. Many people also use herbal remedies on their own, without the advice of a health care professional.	• In the United States, herbal supplements are classified as dietary supplements and thus can be sold without being tested to prove they are safe and effective. They must be made according to good manufacturing practices. • In the United States, no organization regulates the manufacture or certifies the labeling of herbal preparations.

Information in this table is adapted from the Health Topics pages at the National Center for Complementary and Alternative Medicine Web site (http://nccam.nih.gov/health/atoz.htm), the University of Maryland Medical Center Complementary and Alternative Medicine Guide (http://umm.edu/health/medical/altmed), and the American Cancer Society Complementary and Alternative Medicine page (www.cancer.org/Treatment/TreatmentsandSideEffects/ComplementaryandAlternativeMedicine/index).

Biochemical Therapies

These therapies are intended to improve health through their biochemical effects. Conceptually related to the biochemical mechanism of effect of allopathic medications, herbal remedies and dietary supplements have a few important differences. First, herbal remedies are by nature complex mixtures of chemicals, so their effects are likely caused by multiple biochemical reactions. Second, there is currently no federal regulation or oversight of the production of herbs or supplements in the United States, as there is with pharmaceuticals, so quality control is extremely variable. Third, safety concerns are not addressed before they are available commercially to consumers, as with pharmaceuticals, but only after products are on the market and adverse events are reported to the US Food and Drug Administration (FDA). Because of the lack of oversight of production and pre-market safety, it is important for practitioners to research not only the evidence for an herb's effect and potential adverse effects but also the particular formulation's production and quality control.

Approaching CAM Use From an Allopathic Perspective

As with any treatment option, the safety (risks) and efficacy (benefits) of a CAM modality must form the basis for therapeutic decision-making about its use. Table 13-2 can be a helpful guide in directing physician responses to a particular CAM therapy.

Assessing Efficacy

Data on the efficacy of CAM treatments are increasingly available as CAM becomes a greater focus of research effort and funding in the United States and worldwide. When searching the medical literature for CAM evidence, international and foreign-language articles can be useful, as certain CAM modalities may have been studied in greater depth or over a longer period in other countries. As with any research data, it is important to consider study design, outcome measures, sources of bias, methods of data analysis, and applicability of results for a given indication, patient, or patient population. With herbal remedies and supplements, it is also important to acknowledge that formulations differ, so efficacy as reported in a clinical trial may be altered if a different formulation is used.

Table 13-2. Guide to Complementary and Alternative Medicine Treatment Recommendations

		Is the therapy effective?	
		Yes	No
Is the therapy safe?	Yes	**Recommend**	**Tolerate**
	No	**Monitor closely or discourage**	**Discourage**
If there is insufficient evidence to assess safety or efficacy			
• Establish a plan with the family for monitoring response to treatment.			
• Discourage if adverse reactions develop.			
• Tolerate if no adverse reactions develop.			

Assessing Safety

The huge diversity of CAM makes it difficult to discuss safety in general terms. Each CAM modality has its own unique risk profile. However, awareness of broad categories of risk can help physicians prevent bad outcomes.

- *Delay of allopathic care:* In studies of CAM risks in the pediatric population, the risk associated with the highest morbidity and mortality is delay of allopathic care. This delay can come about for a number of reasons, including a family's perception that care from a CAM provider obviates the need for allopathic care, a family's inability to afford allopathic care, or a family's belief that allopathic care will be harmful. It may be helpful to contract with families that they will seek allopathic care prior to or in conjunction with CAM care for a new symptom or acute illness to rule out disease processes that require allopathic treatment.

- *Drug-drug interactions:* Certain supplements and herbal remedies may interfere with or alter the effects of conventional medicines. Particular attention has been given to substances that are inhibitors or inducers of hepatic drug metabolism by the cytochrome P-450 enzyme, with St John's wort (used for depression) and grapefruit juice being the most well-known examples. See "Resources" on page 73 for online resources for checking drug-drug interactions with herbal remedies and supplements.

- *Adverse reactions:* Allergic reactions, side effects, and idiosyncratic reactions are possible with CAM therapies as well as conventional therapies. Close follow-up is helpful in monitoring response to therapy.

Regulation and Licensure

Licensure and accreditation for CAM providers varies from state to state. Chiropractic care, massage therapy, acupuncture, naturopathy, and homeopathy have licensing bodies in some states. In states where licensing exists for a CAM modality, it is incumbent on the physician to ensure that any referrals are made to licensed practitioners. None of these licenses authorizes the practitioner to practice medicine. Other CAM modalities may have a national organization that supervises training and certifies practitioners. Though these are not subject to government oversight, there still may be value in preferentially seeking out providers who are approved by their national organization, as these providers have had to meet a standard established by their colleagues.

Regulation of herbal remedies and supplements is the subject of ongoing scrutiny and debate. Currently, the FDA does not regulate production or marketing of these products, so it is often difficult to verify their composition, safety, or efficacy unless they have been independently studied. The burden of researching products and manufacturers falls to the consumer.

Communication About CAM Use

Most caregivers of children who use CAM do not disclose this use to their pediatrician despite the fact that most report a desire to discuss it. The high rate of nondisclosure is alarming, as it places patients at risk for drug-drug interactions with conventional medications, robs physicians of the opportunity to monitor for adverse reactions, and interferes with the development of trust in the doctor-patient relationship. Reasons cited by patients and caregivers for nondisclosure include

- Negative experiences with past disclosures to physicians.
- Fear of disapproval or judgment on the part of physicians.
- Belief that physicians do not need to know.
- Lack of time with physicians.
- Physicians do not ask.

Many of these barriers can be improved by the physician.

Physicians may be reticent to discuss CAM, as evidenced by the fact that CAM discussions are patient-initiated in most cases. Physicians may worry about legal liability if there is a bad outcome. They may fear conflict with families over use of CAM. They may be afraid to reveal their lack of knowledge about CAM and may worry that this lack of knowledge will threaten a family's trust in their abilities. They may feel pressured by time constraints and overwhelmed by the need to acquire new knowledge. There is often a disconnect between the meaning that patients and families attribute to CAM use—more options and a greater sense of empowerment—and the meaning that physicians may attribute to it—irrationality given lack of evidence and the threat of interference with conventional medical care. This disconnect can influence patients and physicians to avoid the subject of CAM.

Communication Tips

- Make questions about CAM use a routine part of the medical encounter.
- Pose questions about CAM use in an open and nonjudgmental way.
  —Suggested opening: "For me to take the best possible care of your child, it is helpful for me to know about all the ways your family manages health and illness. Are there any treatments, medications, herbs, or supplements that your child uses that we have not talked about yet? Does your child see any other providers for health-related care or treatments?"
- Explore details of CAM use. Ask families not only what CAM modalities they are using but also why they chose the treatment, how it works, whether they have noticed a difference, and if there have been any downsides to the treatment.
- Validate the family's desire for health and well-being for their child.
- Do not be afraid to acknowledge the limits of your knowledge. If asked to provide a recommendation about an unfamiliar CAM modality, offer to do further research and revisit the question at a follow-up visit.
- Seek out information about CAM, including literature on safety or efficacy.
- Involve families in the thinking process of risks versus benefits of a CAM intervention or modality. Provide evidence-based advice when possible. If there is little or no evidence to support or discourage use of a CAM modality, share this information with families.
- Make a plan with families to monitor the child's response to treatment, including measurable outcomes (eg, symptom relief, increased quality of life) and any adverse effects.
- Encourage families to share information about CAM use on an ongoing basis, even if they choose to continue a treatment about which you have raised concerns.
- Document CAM-related discussions in the medical record.

Effective communication about CAM use is a wonderful opportunity to improve rapport and better understand a patient and his or her family. Communication can be a powerful tool for ensuring safety and reducing harm, as well as for broadening physician knowledge and building trust with families. Even if they do not initiate or recommend a CAM treatment, pediatricians can play an important role by monitoring a child's response to the treatment over time and engaging the family in a discussion about risks and benefits if adverse reactions arise. Discussion about CAM may also bring about a greater understanding of families' explanatory models of illness as well as their expectations of health care professionals and their beliefs about conventional medicines. Deeper insight into a family's health beliefs and values can facilitate more successful patient-physician partnership and better patient care.

Resources

CAM on PubMed
http://nccam.nih.gov/research/camonpubmed
The National Center for Complementary and Alternative Medicine provides a link to a PubMed search box that is limited to the CAM subset of PubMed.

Cochrane Reviews
www.cochrane.org/cochrane-reviews
Link to more than 700 Cochrane Reviews on CAM interventions. The Cochrane Collaboration is an independent, international network of leaders in the health care field who are committed to helping health care professionals make evidence-based decisions. Subgroups devoted to specific topic areas produce systematic reviews of available evidence for health-related interventions. The CAM-related subgroup is coordinated through the University of Maryland School of Medicine Center for Integrative Medicine.

ConsumerLab.com
www.consumerlab.com
This for-profit organization carries out independent testing of dietary supplements and herbal remedies by request of manufacturers and for the benefit of the public. In either case, samples for testing are not obtained directly from the manufacturer but from the consumer marketplace. The ConsumerLab.com seal that appears on vitamin bottles can be purchased by manufacturers once their product has been tested by ConsumerLab.com.

Georgia Regents University Augusta Robert B. Greenblatt M.D. Library Complementary and Alternative Medicine Resources
www.gru.edu/library/greenblatt/resources/links/cam.html
A list of helpful links to governmental, university-based, and nonprofit sources for information on research, training, policy, regulation, and integration of CAM.

Longwood Herbal Task Force
www.longwoodherbal.org
Detailed, evidence-based monographs on individual herbal remedies including a review of available evidence, contraindications/cautions, and safety information. Administered by a group of faculty from the Boston Children's Hospital, MCPHS University, and Dana-Farber Cancer Institute.

National Center for Complementary and Alternative Medicine at the National Institutes of Health

http://nccam.nih.gov

The National Center for Complementary and Alternative Medicine (NCCAM) is the federal government's lead agency for scientific research on CAM. The Web site provides information about CAM modalities for providers and patients, results of clinical trials supported by NCCAM, lists of ongoing trials, and information about training and funding opportunities in the field of CAM.

Natural Standard

http://naturalstandard.com

Subscription-based site that includes evidence-based information on CAM modalities as well as online tools to check for drug-drug interactions.

University of Maryland Medical Center Complementary and Alternative Medicine Guide

http://umm.edu/health/medical/altmed

Provides information on CAM therapies that is searchable by modality name and by symptom/disease. Also provides information on drug-drug interactions and side effects of herbal remedies.

CASE RESOLUTION

Explaining that this is not your area of expertise, you ask the family to return in one week to discuss this further. After consulting the National Center for Complementary and Alternative Medicine Web site and a brief review of the medical literature, you find that there are data on efficacy and safety of CAM therapies for migraine headache prevention, including acupuncture and self-hypnosis. At the follow-up visit, you discuss these options with the family. The girl is interested in both modalities but decides to try acupuncture first. You offer her support for this choice and ask that she keep close track of her headaches and return in one month to let you know how she's doing with the acupuncture treatments and her headaches.

Selected References

Barnes PM, Bloom B, Nahin RL. Complementary and alternative medicine use among adults and children: United States, 2007. *Natl Health Stat Report.* 2008;(12):1–23

Eisenberg DM, Kessler RC, Foster C, Norlock FE, Calkins DR, Delbanco TL. Unconventional medicine in the United States. Prevalence, costs, and patterns of use. *N Engl J Med.* 1993;328(4):246–252

Kabat-Zinn J. *Full Catastrophe Living: Using the Wisdom of Your Body and Mind to Face Stress, Pain, and Illness.* Rev ed. New York, NY: Bantam Books; 2013

Kemper KJ. *The Holistic Pediatrician: A Pediatrician's Comprehensive Guide to Safe and Effective Therapies for the 25 Most Common Ailments of Infants, Children, and Adolescents.* 2nd ed. New York, NY: HarperCollins; 2002

Kemper KJ, Vohra S, Walls R; American Academy of Pediatrics Task Force on Complementary and Alternative Medicine and Provisional Section on Complementary, Holistic, and Integrative Medicine. The use of complementary and alternative medicine in pediatrics. *Pediatrics.* 2008;122(6):1374–1386

Kligler B, Lee R. *Integrative Medicine: Principles for Practice.* New York, NY: McGraw-Hill; 2004

Rakel D. *Integrative Medicine.* 3rd ed. Philadelphia, PA: Elsevier Saunders; 2012

CHAPTER 14

Principles of Pediatric Surgery

Steve L. Lee, MD

CASE STUDY

A 4-month-old boy is evaluated by his pediatrician for swelling in the groin and is diagnosed with a right inguinal hernia. His parents are told that their child will be referred to a pediatric surgeon. The parents are concerned about surgery in such a young infant and ask their pediatrician multiple questions. Is he big enough to have surgery? Will he be able to eat before the surgery? Will he be in pain? Will he need to have blood drawn? Will he need to be hospitalized? Will he be put to sleep for the procedure?

Questions

1. What are the typical questions parents ask if their child is undergoing surgery?
2. What is the role of the primary care physician in advising patients and parents about surgical procedures?
3. What is the role of the operating surgeon in advising patients and parents about the surgery?
4. What are general guidelines for feeding infants and children prior to surgery?
5. What are the risks of general anesthesia in infants and children?
6. How long is the hospitalization following surgery?
7. What should parents do before meeting with the surgeon?
8. How do you prepare children who are about to undergo surgery?
9. What laboratory studies are needed prior to surgery?

No matter what the age of the patient, the prospect of surgery is generally anxiety-provoking for the patient and the patient's parents. As with any stressful patient encounter, communication is the key to educating, calming, and reassuring patients and their parents. This is particularly true when patients are being referred, even initially, for surgical consultation. Pediatricians can have a significant effect by providing basic information to parents about surgical care. It is also important for primary care physicians and surgeons to communicate with each other to provide the highest level of care.

Preoperative Care

Initial Consultation

The first task of the primary care physician is to initiate a referral to a pediatric or general surgeon. The initial surgical visit will be to confirm the diagnosis and discuss surgical and nonsurgical options for treatment. Typically, no surgical procedures are performed during this consultation. This point must be clarified, as many children and parents mistakenly think that surgery will occur at the time of the first encounter and are therefore unduly anxious. Some parents will even schedule time off unnecessarily, expecting to have to care for their postoperative child. They become disappointed and even angry when the surgery is not performed. Sometimes the diagnosis of the primary care physician is incorrect; the surgeon can reassure parents about the correct diagnosis obviating the need for any surgery.

A significant amount of information is given to parents and children during the surgical consultation. The diagnosis is confirmed and a decision is made whether the patient will require an operation. The operation is described in detail to parents and to the patient when age-appropriate to do so. In addition, a thorough review of the risks of the operation is performed. The surgeon also gives an estimate of how long the procedure will take. There is a general discussion on the expected recovery, such as whether the procedure will be as an outpatient versus inpatient, where hospitalization occurs, how long the child will miss school, and whether there are any activity restrictions.

To avoid confusion, parents are encouraged to make a list of questions prior to this first encounter and make sure each question is answered. Parents should also write down the answers to refer to them at a later time. Once parents agree to proceed with surgery, the surgeon starts the process and paperwork. Often, this will be the only visit required before the date of the operation. However, some hospitals require patients to be seen by the surgeon within 30 days of a procedure; thus, a return visit may be required if the date of surgery is beyond that time frame. Also, some centers require patients to have a preoperative evaluation with the anesthesia team prior to surgery.

Anesthetic Preparation in Infants and Children

Anesthesia is extremely safe in infants and children. The risk of a poor outcome from general anesthesia is less than 1%. In most institutions, pediatric anesthesiologists provide anesthetic care for infants and young children. If pediatric anesthesiologists are not available, anesthetic care for infants and children is often limited to a set of experienced general anesthesiologists.

There are many types of anesthetics that can be used, including moderate sedation (also known as conscious sedation), regional anesthesia, and general anesthesia. Typically, the type of anesthesia will be determined by the surgeon and anesthesiologist; however, the anesthesiologist makes the final decision. Although the least amount of anesthesia is desired, all patients must be treated as if they may need to undergo general anesthesia in case moderate sedation or regional anesthetic is inadequate.

To minimize the risk of aspiration with general anesthesia, the stomach must be empty of food and liquids. Although each hospital has its own policies, Box 14-1 lists frequently recommended guidelines for the interval between meals and surgery. In general, most infants and children will have to miss one meal prior to surgery. Often this meal can be replaced with clear liquids.

All medications should be continued unless otherwise directed by the surgeon or anesthesia staff. Medications can be taken with a small sip of water on the morning of surgery. It is also recommended to bring a list of medications on the date of the operation. All medications will be reviewed by surgical staff prior to the operation.

Laboratory Studies

Laboratory studies should be performed if indicated by the patient's underlying comorbidities or current disease process. Blood products may be needed during or after surgery if there is blood loss. If blood loss is anticipated, parents or other family members will be given the option of directly donating blood prior to the procedure. However, directly donating blood takes time (days to weeks depending on the specific blood bank) and may not be an option for urgent and emergency operations. In addition, the cost of directly donating blood is often the responsibility of the patient. If primary care physicians need laboratory tests to be drawn for other reasons, often this blood work can be obtained while the patient is under anesthesia.

Box 14-1. Guidelines for Interval Between Eating/ Drinking and Surgery in Infants and Children

<6 mo
4 h human milk/formula
2 h clear liquids[a]

6–36 mo
8 h solids
6 h human milk/formula
2 h clear liquids[a]

>36 mo
8 h solids/milk
2 h clear liquids[a]

[a]Formula, milk, orange juice, and colas are *NOT* considered clear liquids. Clear liquids include any liquid that can be seen through (eg, water, sugar water, apple juice, Jell-O, broth).

Imaging Studies

Any imaging studies obtained by the primary care physician should be brought to the surgical consultation by the parents. Hard copies or electronic files of the study itself and final report by the radiologist are highly recommended. If imaging studies are needed for further workup or preoperative planning, these studies can be ordered by the surgeon. If studies are to be ordered preoperatively by the primary care physician, it is recommended to contact the surgeon to confirm which specific studies to order. This communication will avoid obtaining unnecessary studies or the need to repeat studies (if studies were not done appropriately).

Patients Requiring Urgent/Emergency Surgery

Patients with acute conditions will often present to their pediatrician or primary care physician. Common conditions include abdominal pain consistent with appendicitis, abscess requiring drainage, incarcerated hernia, or vomiting due to pyloric stenosis. Such patients will need to be directed to the emergency department (ED) for further management, and the pediatric surgeon should be notified. Any time a patient is sent to the ED, it is essential to remind the parents to not give the patient anything to eat or drink (nil per os, or NPO). If parents feed patients en route to the ED, this will delay treatment due to anesthetic concerns. The NPO guidelines (Box 14-1) will still be enforced even in urgent conditions; only in life-threatening emergencies will NPO guidelines typically be disregarded. In most acute situations, patients are often dehydrated from vomiting, poor oral intake, or third spacing. Thus, prior to surgery, it is essential that patients are adequately resuscitated. Standard intravenous (IV) fluid resuscitation of 20 mL/kg of lactated Ringer injection or normal saline should be administered followed by continuous administration of maintenance (or higher) fluids. Appropriate antibiotics should also be administered as indicated. Patients with acute appendicitis should be started on single-, double-, or triple-agent broad-spectrum antibiotics depending on their symptoms and preference of the surgical team. Patients with abscesses should be administered antibiotics with excellent gram-positive coverage, with special attention to methicillin-resistant *Staphylococcus aureus*, given its high prevalence. Pain medication should be given as needed, even if the surgeon has not evaluated the patient. It is rare that a true surgical condition will be masked by an appropriate dose of pain medication. Finally, basic laboratory studies, such as a complete blood cell count and electrolyte panel, should be obtained.

Perioperative Care

The final operating room schedule for elective cases is made the day before surgery. Thus, the specific time of an elective procedure is not known until one day prior to surgery. Often the surgeon can give parents an estimated start time. Families will be called the day before surgery to confirm the time of the procedure and when and where to arrive. Often, patients are asked to arrive 1½ to 2 hours before the scheduled start time. This extra time is to ensure patient safety by completing all necessary steps before the actual operation.

In general, patients are put under anesthesia in the operating room. For infants and young children, an IV line is placed after the patient is asleep. To minimize anxiety, preanesthetic sedation is administered orally before proceeding to the operating room. Once in the operating room, patients are often administered an inhalational anesthetic, followed by placement of the IV line, then intubation. Some institutions allow parents to accompany their child to the operating room and see the child put to sleep with the inhalational anesthetic.

Once the operation is complete, patients are brought to the recovery room. Parents typically are allowed in the recovery room until the time of discharge. Criteria for discharge from the recovery room are listed in Box 14-2. For children who have undergone surgery as outpatients, careful written instructions are provided to parents along with follow-up appointments and telephone numbers in case problems should arise. Children who are inpatients are discharged from the recovery room to the pediatric inpatient service, along with appropriate orders for nursing personnel.

There continues to be controversy over postoperative management of former premature infants following general anesthesia. Former premature infants are at higher risk of postoperative apnea. Reasonable recommendations for typical outpatient operations include overnight admission with apnea monitoring for former premature infants who are less than or equal to 50 weeks' postconception. However, each institution has its own specific policy, and the exact age for required admission varies. The decision for admission is also based on the patient's current health and comorbidities and should be made by the surgeon, anesthesia team, primary care physician, and the patient's parents. Table 14-1 lists the most common elective and urgent/emergency operations and anticipated postoperative hospitalization stays.

Postoperative Care

Parents will often call their pediatrician with questions postoperatively; thus, the pediatrician should be knowledgeable about routine postoperative care. Most children recover from anesthesia and surgery faster than adults. Unless otherwise specified, such as following an appendectomy for perforated appendicitis, a normal diet can be resumed as soon as the patient desires. If patients are not tolerating a normal diet, a bland diet and plenty of fluids are recommended. Furthermore, patients should resume taking all of their preoperative medications the evening or next morning after surgery.

Nearly all surgical wounds are closed with absorbable sutures and covered with thin adhesive strips. Additional dressings can be removed in 1 to 2 days or as needed. Again, unless otherwise specified, most wounds can get wet (shower or quick bath) 48 hours after surgery. Dressings, except for thin adhesive strips, should be removed prior to bathing. Wounds do not need to be covered unless they are open or there is drainage.

The surgeon will provide details about activity limitations and returning to school. Often heavy physical activity, such as physical education in school or with organized sports, should be avoided until the surgeon sees the patient following discharge. While heavy physical activity is to be avoided after surgery, patients should be

Box 14-2. Criteria for Discharge After Outpatient Surgery

Stable and vital signs appropriate for age

Age-appropriate ambulation

Ability to tolerate oral fluids

No bleeding

No respiratory distress

No pain that cannot be controlled by oral medication

Age-appropriate alertness

Table 14-1. Common Elective and Urgent/Emergency Operations and Anticipated Postoperative Hospitalization

Procedure	Length of Hospitalization
Elective	
Inguinal hernia repair	Outpatient
Umbilical hernia repair	Outpatient
Cyst excision	Outpatient
Central venous catheter insertion/removal	Outpatient
Orchiopexy	Outpatient
Laparoscopic cholecystectomy	Outpatient
Lymph node biopsy	Outpatient
Ostomy takedown	3–4 d
Lung resection	3–4 d
Imperforate anus repair	3–4 d
Pectus excavatum repair (Nuss procedure)	4–5 d
Urgent/Emergency	
Laparoscopic or open appendectomy for non-perforated appendicitis	1–2 d
Laparoscopic or open appendectomy for perforated appendicitis	5–7 d
Pyloromyotomy	1 d
Intussusception reduction	1 d
Bowel resection	5–7 d
Bowel obstruction	5–7 d
Tumor resection (Wilms or neuroblastoma)	7 d
Choledochal cyst or portoenterostomy	5–7 d
Pull through for Hirschsprung disease	5–7 d

encouraged to walk as well as to cough and breathe deeply many times a day. Patients can return to school when they are feeling up to it and have no more than minimal pain.

Main reasons to contact the surgeon after the operation are for temperature above 101.5°F (38.6°C), worsening or persistent pain, persistent emesis, and any wound drainage or redness. Additional instructions specific to the operation are also provided.

CASE RESOLUTION

In this case, the pediatrician reassured the parents that many patients have been referred to this surgeon. The parents were assisted by the pediatrician in crafting their questions for the surgeon. The surgeon subsequently confirmed the diagnosis of an inguinal hernia and recommended surgery. All details were provided and the parents had their questions answered. The patient was scheduled for outpatient surgery and everything went smoothly. Postoperatively, there were no concerns, and the patient saw the surgeon and pediatrician in follow-up.

Selected References

Landsman IS, Hays SR, Karsanac CJ, Franklin A. *Pediatric Anesthesia.* In: Coran A, Adzick D, Krummel T, Laberge JM, Shamberger R, Caldmone A, eds. *Pediatric Surgery.* 7th ed. Philadelphia, PA: Mosby; 2007:201–226

Malviya S, Swartz J, Lerman J. Are all preterm infants younger than 60 weeks postconceptual age a risk for postanesthetic apnea? *Anesthesiology.* 1993;78(6): 1076–1081

CHAPTER 15

Image Gently:
Approach to Pediatric Imaging

Lindsay S. Baron, MD; Jane S. Kim, MD; and Benjamin H. Taragin, MD

CASE STUDY 1

A 15-year-old boy comes to your office complaining of 1 week of back pain after exertion. He reports no significant recent trauma. He does play varsity basketball but has not had any recent falls during games. He is otherwise healthy with no significant medical history.

The pain does not prevent him from playing sports or going to school. He has no history of prior episodes of back pain. He says the pain is relieved by nonsteroidal anti-inflammatory drugs. On physical examination, he has left-sided paraspinal focal tenderness in the L3-L4 region. He has limited range of motion twisting to that side.

CASE STUDY 2

A 10-year-old girl is brought to your office with runny nose, congestion, cough, and headache. You saw this patient 4 months ago as well as 6 weeks ago, when she had similar complaints. Her mother reports full compliance with the antibiotic regimen you prescribed but states that her daughter's symptoms have never fully resolved. On physical examination, the child is afebrile with purulent nasal discharge. There is tenderness to palpation over the cheeks and forehead.

Questions
1. What, if any, is the appropriate imaging for each patient?
2. How does one decide the appropriate imaging studies to obtain on a patient?
3. What is the ALARA principle?
4. What information is available for counseling patients about the risks of diagnostic radiation?
5. Where can one find appropriate imaging recommendations for pediatric patients?
6. Does the history influence the choice of imaging studies?
   a. What imaging would be appropriate for the patient in case study 1 if there was recent significant trauma?
   b. What imaging would be appropriate for the patient in case study 2 if her symptoms were new and started last week?

Overuse of medical imaging is a growing problem in the United States that has financial and medical repercussions. The primary care physician must often decide what, if any, is the proper imaging for patients with common complaints. In many situations, clinical assessment and physical examination are adequate for diagnosis. In some instances, however, imaging provides vital information that cannot be adequately obtained from other sources. Often, patients and their families insist on diagnostic imaging and can be under the impression that the more technologically advanced the evaluation, the better the care.

Currently, approximately 370 million studies that use diagnostic radiation are performed yearly in the United States (Figure 15-1). The most dramatic increase has been in the use of computed tomography (CT) scans. In 1982 there were 1 million CT scans performed in the United States. In 2006 there were 67 million CT scans performed, and of this number it is estimated that 4 to 7 million of these were performed in children. In response to this, many concerned health care professionals and radiologists gathered to create the national *Image Gently* campaign, focusing on minimizing the use of diagnostic radiation and using appropriate pediatric imaging for children in the United States.

Basic Concepts

Diagnostic radiology examinations that use ionizing radiation include plain radiography, fluoroscopy, CT, and nuclear medicine. Ionizing radiation causes damage to DNA molecules and may lead to cell death or a mutation. The induction of cancer takes several years, and the effects are hereditary (may be passed down to the next generation).

One of the most common ways to measure radiation dose is by the effective dose (unit: sieverts), which takes into account all of the exposed tissues and each organ's relative radiosensitivity. Certain organs are more radiosensitive than others, and children in particular are at an increased risk for breast cancer, thyroid cancer, and leukemia. It is important to note that children are more radiosensitive than adults, secondary to their growth of rapidly proliferating cells. The effective dose also provides a way to compare radiation dose across different imaging modalities. For example, a single CT

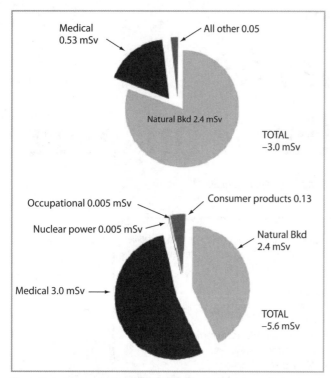

Figure 15-1. US annual per capita effective radiation dose from various sources. Upper: Chart for 1980. Lower: Chart for 2006. Bkd, background. (From Mettler FA Jr, Bhargavan M, Faulkner K, et al. Radiologic and nuclear medicine studies in the United States and worldwide: frequency, radiation dose, and comparison with other radiation sources—1950–2007. *Radiology.* **2009;253[2]:520–531, with permission.)**

Table 15-1. Average Effective Dose in Millisieverts of Different Imaging Studies

Diagnostic Procedure	Typical Effective Dose (mSv)[a]	Number of Chest X-rays (PA film) for Equivalent Effective Dose[b]	Time for Equivalent Effective Dose From Natural Background Radiation[c]
Chest x-ray	0.02	1	2.4 d
Skull x-ray	0.1	5	12 d
Lumbar spine	1.5	75	182 d
IV urogram	3	150	1.0 y
Upper GI examination	6	300	2.0 y
Barium enema	8	400	2.7 y
CT of head	2	100	243 d
CT of abdomen	8	400	2.7 y

Abbreviations: CT, computed tomography; GI, gastrointestinal; IV, intravenous; PA, posteroanterior.

[a]Average effective dose in millisieverts (mSv) as compiled by Mettler FA Jr, Huda W, Yoshizumi TT, Mahesh M. Effective doses in radiology and diagnostic nuclear medicine: a catalog. *Radiology.* 2008;248(1):254–263.

[b]Based on the assumption of an average "effective dose" from chest x-ray (PA film) of 0.02 mSv.

[c]Based on the assumption of an average effective dose from the natural background radiation of 3 mSv per year in the United States.

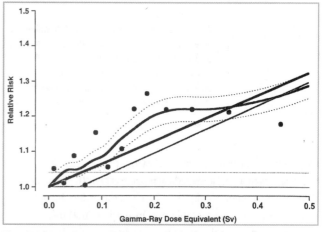

Figure 15-2. Relative risk of contracting cancer in atomic bomb survivors. (Reprinted with permission from Pierce DA, Preston DL. Radiation-related cancer risks at low doses among atomic bomb survivors. *Radiat Res.* **2000;154[2]:178–186.)**

scan imparts an effective dose that is equivalent to 100 to 250 chest radiographs in children (Table 15-1).

ALARA Principle (As Low as Reasonably Achievable)

In recent years, there has been increasing attention and research into the radiation imparted to patients from diagnostic imaging. Much of this concern stems from data derived from the atomic bomb survivors of World War II. Based on the distance of survivors from ground zero, the radiation dose to each individual was calculated. More than 50,000 of these patients were followed for more than 50 years. The data showed an increased cancer risk for many of the survivors. Based on this observation, a mathematical model was created, indicating that the risk of cancer proceeds in a linear fashion without threshold (Figure 15-2). According to this model, even a small amount of radiation increases the risk of cancer. Current estimates vary regarding diagnostic radiation and cancer. Based on research by multiple radiation biologists, the American College of Radiology (ACR) estimates that for adults, one fatal cancer will be induced for every 1,000 CT scans performed. That risk is increased in children, with one fatal cancer occurring for 500 to 1,000 CT scans performed. This is superimposed on the national cancer incidence of 42%.

On the basis of this research, the *Image Gently* campaign was founded, which stresses a multifaceted approach intended to minimize radiation exposure to children. The campaign has brought together 60 medical and professional organizations representing more than 700,000 imaging specialists from the fields of pediatrics, radiology, physics, and radiology technology. The As Low as Reasonably Achievable (ALARA) principle is based on the notion that any amount of radiation exposure, no matter how small, can increase the chance of negative biological effects. The aim of the ALARA principle is to balance the goals of minimizing the amount of radiation and obtaining sufficient imaging quality, leading to accurate diagnostic information.

Role of the Radiologist

Another guiding principle requires communication and coordination between medical specialties. When in doubt, a call to the local radiologist, whether he or she is a dedicated pediatric radiologist or not, will often be helpful in determining which test is reasonable for a specific patient. All practicing radiologists have been made aware of the *Image Gently* campaign and are trying to effectively care for pediatric patients while minimizing diagnostic ionizing radiation. There are many ways that the radiologist can tailor examinations to minimize radiation. The first step often involves asking whether nonionizing diagnostic examinations, such as ultrasound or magnetic resonance imaging (MRI), can be performed to answer the same diagnostic question. In particular, ultrasound can often be used as a screening examination to evaluate conditions that can be clarified with other studies if needed. Radiologists are also focusing on monitoring equipment and protocols for studies. All US commercial CT scanners include multiple methods to adjust the imparted radiation dose. A low-dose technique should be used whenever it is appropriate. Breast and gonadal shielding offer additional protection to children.

Available Resources

The ACR has established appropriateness criteria for imaging of specific medical conditions and presentations, coauthored by clinicians and radiologists. They are available free online and can be downloaded and incorporated into computerized ordering and electronic health record systems (www.acr.org/Quality-Safety/Appropriateness-Criteria).

Lastly, the *Image Gently* Web site (www.imagegently.org) offers educational materials for parents to help them understand the risks and benefits of diagnostic imaging and the associated radiation. The site also has printable child imaging history cards so parents can keep track of all the diagnostic radiation examinations performed on their child (Figure 15-3).

Determining the Appropriate Imaging Study

Case Study 1: The Importance of the History

Back pain is a common complaint in active adolescent patients. Many studies have evaluated the use of imaging in patients with nontraumatic back pain. In the absence of significant trauma, most studies have found that there is little value in imaging otherwise healthy adolescents complaining of musculoskeletal pain. If this patient had significant trauma or focal neurologic findings suspicious for significant cord or disc injury, MRI would be the most appropriate examination. Plain films of the spine are not helpful in assessing disc disease or intra–central nervous system injury. Plain films are helpful in older patients to evaluate the extent of multilevel disc disease. Obtaining a comprehensive history and performing a complete physical examination will help define the differential diagnosis and assist in the determination of the appropriate imaging study. See Resources at the end of the chapter for a link to the ACR Appropriateness Criteria for suspected spine trauma.

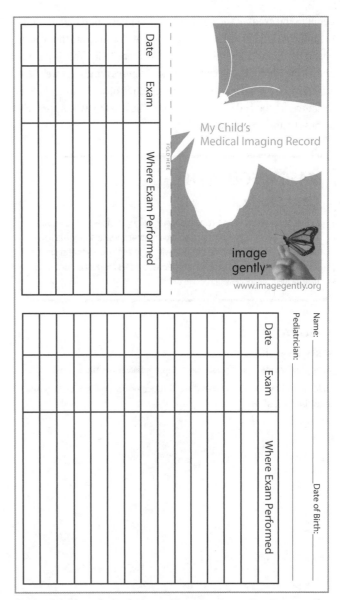

Figure 15-3. **Log to record a child's exposure to imaging studies. (Courtesy of Image Gently.)**

> ### *CASE RESOLUTION*
> #### *Case Study 1*
> The physician should recommend rest, nonsteroidal anti-inflammatory drugs, and stretching exercises for 4 to 6 weeks. If the pain still persists, magnetic resonance imaging of the lumbar spine without contrast would be a reasonable next step in the workup of this patient.

Case Study 2: Symptom Duration and Response to Treatment

Imaging should be obtained in cases of chronic sinusitis that do not respond to treatment and persist without resolution for months. Computed tomography of the sinuses is useful in evaluation of the soft tissues, extent of disease, and any potential intracranial complications. Computed tomography also provides important anatomic detail in the event of the need for surgical intervention. Plain radiography has limited utility in evaluation of sinusitis due to the lack of soft tissue and anatomic detail and low sensitivity. This is particularly true in very young children whose sinuses are not yet well aerated. Imaging is not appropriate in the setting of acute sinusitis. See Resources at the end of the chapter for a link to the ACR Appropriateness Criteria for child sinusitis.

CASE RESOLUTION
Case Study 2

The physician should order a computed tomography scan of the sinuses because the patient has signs and symptoms of chronic sinusitis despite treatment. If the patient was presenting for the first time with signs and symptoms of sinusitis, medical treatment would be indicated. If the patient does not respond to medical management, imaging should be considered.

Resources

ACR Appropriateness Criteria

Main page: www.acr.org/Quality-Safety/Appropriateness-Criteria

Child sinusitis: www.acr.org/~/media/ACR/Documents/AppCriteria/Diagnostic/SinusitisChild.pdf

Suspected spine trauma: www.acr.org/~/media/ACR/Documents/AppCriteria/Diagnostic/SuspectedSpineTrauma.pdf

Radiation dose assessment: www.acr.org/~/media/ACR/Documents/AppCriteria/Radiation%20Dose%20Assessment%20IntroductionApr%202013.pdf

Image Gently Web Site

www.imagegently.org

Selected References

Bulas D, Goske M, Applegate K, Wood B. Image Gently: improving health literacy for parents about CT scans for children. *Pediatr Radiol.* 2009;39(2):112–116

Frush DP. Radiation safety. *Pediatr Radiol.* 2009;39(suppl 3):385–390

Goske MJ, Applegate KE, Boylan J, et al. The Image Gently campaign: working together to change practice. *AJR Am J Roentgenol.* 2008;190(2):273–274

Miglioretti DL, Johnson E, Williams A, et al. The use of computed tomography in pediatrics and the associated radiation exposure and estimated cancer risk. *JAMA Pediatr.* 2013;167(8):700–707

Pearce MS, Salotti JA, Little MP, et al. Radiation exposure from CT scans in childhood and subsequent risk of leukaemia and brain tumours: a retrospective cohort study. *Lancet.* 2012;380(9840):499–505

CHAPTER 16

Simulation in Pediatric Health Care

Tom Kallay, MD

CASE STUDY

A 1-year-old boy is in your office for a routine visit and vaccinations. Upon receiving his vaccinations, he experiences an anaphylactic episode. The emergency equipment and medications are difficult to find. The child receives epinephrine and nebulized albuterol with minimal improvement. You are worried he will need airway support, but it is not clear if the equipment is serviceable. Your staff calls 911; the paramedics arrive and eventually take the child to the nearest emergency department. You and your staff feel that you could have been better prepared. You decide to take measures to optimize the function of your staff and office environment for the rare emergency.

Questions
1. What is simulation?
2. How does simulation apply to health care?
3. What modalities of simulation are available for medical training?
4. How does one create and deliver simulation training?
5. Why should a primary care physician use simulation?

Simulation is a powerful tool for learning. In broad terms, it is a learning technique using people or technology to mimic real-life encounters. These encounters are practiced in simulated conditions, and typically the learner receives performance feedback as if he or she were in the real situation.

Simulation has a long legacy of use for education and evaluation in many high-risk industries. Examples include flight simulators for pilots and astronauts, war games for the military, or technical operations for nuclear power personnel. It allows users from novice to expert to practice and develop knowledge and skills without the threat of causing harm to people. Today, these industries employ robust simulation programs that are embedded into the culture of training and skill maintenance, and there is a growing body of evidence that simulation is a safe and effective way to educate and evaluate professionals in these fields. Because health care is a high-risk industry as well, it seems intuitive that simulation would have a place in medical training with the purpose of improving patient safety and outcomes. Despite this premise, simulation has not played a large role in medical education until relatively recently.

Simulation in Medicine

History

Simulation in medicine began in 1960 with Resusci Anne, a mannequin designed for mouth-to-mouth resuscitation training. This was a new resuscitation technique conceived by Peter Safar and James Elam in 1957, which influenced Norwegian toymaker Asmund Laerdal to create the mannequin for practicing the principles of airway, breathing, and circulation (ABCs). The airway could be obstructed, and it was necessary to hyperextend the neck and thrust the chin forward to insufflate the lungs. An internal spring placed in the chest permitted the practice of cardiac compressions, and subsequently cardiopulmonary resuscitation (CPR) training was born.

The advent of computer-controlled mannequins took place in 1967 at the University of Southern California. Medical educator Stephen Abrahamson, along with anesthesiologist Dr J. Samuel Denson, collaborated with a group of engineers from the Sierra Engineering Company to create Sim One. This prototype device was a computerized adult-sized mannequin that featured breathing, heart sounds, functional pupils, and an anatomically correct airway. It was used for airway management training for anesthesia residents from the late 1960s to the 1970s, with a noted benefit of training without placing patients at risk. However, ultimately, Sim One did not gain acceptance and the program was terminated. For the next 3 decades, simulation in medical education remained relatively dormant.

The Growth of Simulation in Medicine

"…no industry in which human lives depend on the skilled performance of responsible operators has waited for unequivocal proof of the benefits of simulation before embracing it."—David M. Gaba, MD

The 1999 Institute of Medicine (IOM) report *To Err Is Human: Building a Safer Health System* drew attention to the perils of the health care system, highlighting the human and financial costs of medical errors. This period witnessed a resurgence of simulation in medicine as a response to the reinvigorated emphasis on patient safety. Government and medical institutions began to embrace simulation as a way to improve health practitioner and team performance to improve outcomes. In 2001, the Agency for Healthcare Research and Quality (AHRQ) published an analysis of patient safety practices and dedicated a chapter to the potential benefits of simulation.

As more evidence came that simulation could be applied to patient safety, it began to find its way into the language of accreditation and certification. The Accreditation Council for Graduate Medical Education has embraced simulation as an effective way to train and now mandates that simulation resources be available for programs such as anesthesia and surgery—and more programs are likely to follow. For recertification in anesthesiology, the American Board of Anesthesiology has now incorporated simulation activities into the process of obtaining board certification.

In the realm of pediatrics, there is a body of literature demonstrating the benefits of simulation. It has been used to improve skills ranging from complex resuscitations to lumbar puncture (LP) and has demonstrated applicability to inpatient and outpatient settings.

For example, the literature on pediatric outpatient emergencies shows that offices are frequently ill-equipped to handle an emergency. In 2000, the American Academy of Pediatrics Committee on Pediatric Emergency Medicine published *Childhood Emergencies in the Office, Hospital, and Community: Organizing Systems of Care*. It highlighted how preparation of the staff, office environment, and community are crucial for delivering high-quality emergency care and made the argument that simulated mock scenarios or codes are an essential part of an office emergency preparedness plan. Currently, there are many resources that provide the tools necessary for providing simulation education for pediatrics.

Simulation in the health care field continued to grow. In 2004, the Society for Simulation in Healthcare was established by professionals using simulation for education, testing, and research in health care. Members now include physicians, nurses, allied health and paramedical professionals, researchers, and educators from around the globe, and there is an annual meeting. In 2006, the AHRQ awarded $5 million to fund 19 projects through its Advances in Patient Safety Through Simulation Research portfolio (R18). In response to demand, the medical simulation equipment industry has blossomed, and currently there are products that can simulate virtually any situation encountered in medicine. With the development of not only the technology but the technique of simulation, it has become apparent that for health care, as in other high-stakes industries, simulation has found its place.

This chapter will provide a broad overview of simulation in health care—the associated terminology, available resources for health care education, and technique for providing this mode of training.

Terminology

The term *simulator* is used to describe the equipment, eg, a simulated arm for venipuncture, a computerized mannequin that replicates human physiology, or a virtual reality computer with programming designed to practice laparoscopic surgery. *Simulation* is used to describe a technique, as described by the Institute of Medicine.

> *The act of imitating a situation or a process through something analogous. Examples include using an actor to play a patient, a computerized mannequin to imitate the behavior of a patient, a computer program to imitate a case scenario, and an animation to mimic the spread of an infectious disease in a population* (Institute of Medicine, 2010)

Simulation-based medical training is used to describe a systematically designed program that provides information, demonstration, and practiced-based learning activities which are supported by the concept of deliberate practice (discussed later in the chapter).

A *simulation center* is an area designed to provide some or all the modes of simulation described previously. It can range in size from a 200-square-foot room to a 10,000-square-foot building replicating a hospital with fully equipped patient rooms, clinics, and operating rooms. There are opportunities to practice all facets of medicine, depending on the learning goals. Spaces can be fashioned to appear like an emergency department or clinic office and may be wired with cameras and microphones so learner actions and statements can be recorded and reviewed for evaluation and feedback. Some centers may use a control room adjacent to the simulation area, separated by one-way mirrors, that allows the facilitator to observe and control the scenario without being in the room with the learner. If high-fidelity mannequins are used, they are controlled from this room via computer, and facilitators communicate with role players in the scenario by two-way radio. There may be conference areas for viewing live simulations and debriefing, as well as storage areas for equipment. Multidisciplinary centers provide the best opportunity for cross-training among health care practitioners and building camaraderie.

In situ simulation describes simulation activities embedded in an actual clinical environment. The advantage is that medical scenarios can be practiced in the working environment, which provides the closest approximation of reality. It is excellent for team training because all members of the medical staff can participate. Another advantage to in situ simulation is that it affords the ability to test the working environment for conditions that can predispose one to make an error.

For example, a recent study involving prehospital practitioners used in situ simulation to identify causes of errors during a standardized, simulated out-of-hospital pediatric emergency. The study was designed to determine the most common, underlying causes of clinically significant errors committed by teams of prehospital practitioners and associated error-producing conditions. Forty-five 2-person emergency medical service crews from various locations in Michigan participated in a validated simulation of a 6-month-old with altered mental status, seizures, and respiratory arrest from intracranial hemorrhage using their own equipment and medications. The simulations were performed out of hospital using a mobile simulation vehicle—a 24-foot trailer with a control area and a simulated child's room. Practitioners were evaluated using a validated performance checklist concordant with the 2005 Pediatric Advanced Life Support guidelines and then participated in a facilitated debriefing designed to identify root causes of errors.

The findings revealed errors in oxygen delivery, equipment organization and use, glucose measurement, drug administration, and inappropriate CPR. Delay in delivery of oxygen resulted from broken or missing equipment; only half of the teams measured blood glucose while some teams did not have a glucometer in their pediatric bags. Medication errors were common, such as wrong dosing due to calculation errors, a failure to cross-check doses with partners, or improper administration. Errors in CPR included failure to check for a pulse or initiating compressions when they were not necessary. These findings demonstrated how in situ simulation can be an effective tool for identifying the cognitive, procedural, teamwork, and environmental sources of errors.

While an effective tool, in situ simulation does have shortcomings. In a busy hospital or clinic environment, staff may feel overburdened by performing extra tasks during work that may be perceived as unnecessary. It is the responsibility of the individual organizing a simulation practice session to ensure that patient care is not compromised during the activity; also of importance is to build a culture of patient safety in which staff feel a responsibility to provide excellent individual and team function in a well-prepared environment.

Medical Simulation Resources

Resources available for simulation in health care can be categorized into 5 areas: mannequin based, screen based, virtual reality, task trainers, and standardized patients (SPs) (Box 16-1). How these tools are used depends on the educational needs.

Mannequins are lifelike representations of human beings and range in size from a premature neonate to a full-sized adult. The spectrum of functionality spans from a simple form, like Resusci Anne, to a high-fidelity mannequin. *High fidelity* implies that the mannequin is computer driven and has features that represent human physiology, such as breathing, heart sounds, or blood pressure. These are technology dependent and often expensive and require expertise in maintenance and operation. Mannequins are typically used for mock codes, which can be applied to virtually any health care setting, such as an office, inpatient ward, or operating room.

Box 16-1. Resources for Medical Simulation Training

- Mannequin: simple or computer driven
- Screen-based simulation programs
- Virtual reality programs
- Task trainers
- Standardized patients

Screen-based simulated programs are more affordable and logistically easier. Unlike a mock code, which often requires the coordination of more than one person, they can be performed by an individual at any location with a computer. Software programs are available that contain libraries of clinical scenarios in which history, examination findings, images, and laboratory tests can be represented graphically. Users can select diagnostic and therapeutic options as they work through the case and generate a record of performance. Feedback can be provided by preprogrammed software or an instructor at a later time.

There are many commercially available programs for pediatrics, and there is some evidence as to their effectiveness. A 2009 study examined the ability of screen-based simulation to improve emergency and pediatric resident knowledge, confidence, and skills in a critical pediatric resuscitation. Improvement was demonstrated in knowledge and confidence but less in the skill area. These findings suggest that screen-based simulation may be an effective way to supplement resuscitation training.

Task trainers are 3-dimensional representations of body parts that allow the user to improve technique or develop psychomotor skill in many areas, such as intravenous line insertion, LP, or bag-valve mask. There are task trainers for virtually every procedure and discipline, with options ranging from premature neonates to adults. Some provide feedback to the learner based on the quality of the performance; this may be visual, auditory, or printed. For example, when practicing bag-valve-mask on a baby head, there is an airway connected to inflatable lungs which allow learners to visualize the effectiveness of their technique. Task trainers are especially useful for practitioners to gain familiarity with the equipment being used, whether it is for the first time or after a period of disuse.

Virtual reality and haptic systems employ the most sophisticated computer programming for procedural practice. *Virtual reality* refers to the recreation of environments or objects as a complex, computer-generated image; haptic systems provide the capability of tactile learning, and programs have the ability to provide detailed feedback on procedural skill based on the kinetic actions of the user. Typically, virtual reality and haptic systems are used with a task trainer; most of the products available are for vascular access, surgical procedures, bronchoscopy, or endoscopy. There is evidence demonstrating that virtual reality is superior to traditional training; it is a likely that simulation-based medical education will further incorporate virtual reality in the future. Currently, virtual reality programs are fairly cost-prohibitive and limited in scope; this may change as programming and options continue to develop.

Standardized patients have been used in graduate medical education for years. An SP is an actor playing a role and provides trainees an opportunity to practice communication, physical examination skills, or history taking. While typically playing the role of a patient, SPs can also play the role of a family member or a fellow health care practitioner.

Standardized patients offer the opportunity of providing a multifaceted learning experience when incorporated into mock scenarios. In creating a scenario for a child in diabetic ketoacidosis (DKA), for example, a script is written for an individual playing the role of an upset mother having difficulty on learning her child has diabetes. Learners would have to apply their knowledge in assessing and treating DKA, in addition to using their skills in conveying difficult information to the mother. Afterward, feedback can be provided to the learners as to their medical knowledge, decision-making, and communication. The term *confederate* is sometimes applied to role players in scenarios, as they are working together with the instructor.

Technique

The Culture of Simulation

This section will describe the elements that are needed when designing and delivering education using simulation. But before these steps are illustrated, it is important to discuss the culture of simulation learning and how it fits with our current culture of medicine.

Traditional medical education emphasizes the importance of error-free practice, with intense pressure to achieve perfection during diagnosis and treatment. Furthermore, when mistakes are made, the psychologic toll for the practitioner cannot be underestimated. It is often said that there are 2 victims in the case of a medical error: the patient and the health care practitioner. Reports of provider depression, substance abuse, and suicide highlight the need for engendering a productive rather than destructive response to medical errors, which is one of the central aims of simulation. The technique of practicing skills or decision-making in an environment absent of the "shame and blame" response can assist in developing healthy reactions to mistakes, in which the factors leading to the error are objectively reviewed and analyzed and improvements instituted. When a mistake is made, the goal is to change the thinking from what the repercussions will be to how we can better ourselves to improve care for our patients. As the practice of medicine is an art, so is the practice of making oneself a better health care practitioner.

The learning environment for simulation education activities must connote a safe learning environment in which mistakes can be made without reproach. In fact, simulation is an area where it is *desirable* for health care practitioners to make mistakes, so the practice of improvement can occur. It is the responsibility of the facilitators to explicitly state this to help create an atmosphere conducive to constructive discussion.

Simulation activities also provide an opportunity for health care professionals to train together and build effective communication skills and team camaraderie. The training of health care professionals—nurses, physicians, medical or physician assistants—generally occurs in parallel, which can have the unintended consequences of poor communication between team members. This potentially can create an environment that may not always be conducive to fair, open discussions of mistakes, which are needed if optimal learning and improvement is to occur. When delivered with creativity and enthusiasm in a nonthreatening environment, simulation can provide a venue for building effective relationships between practitioners while importing educational benefits.

Steps for Delivering Simulation Learning

Developing simulation activities requires multiple steps and careful planning to achieve learning goals (Box 16-2). Health care professionals are often busy with little extra time, so in addition to making simulations accessible, the educational product must be sound and worth the time spent. Learning events that are not well planned or delivered can have an adverse effect on an individual's perception of simulation education, which can have a negative effect on their learning.

The first step in delivering simulation learning is the creation of a mock code or scenario, followed by deliberate practice, a concept of instruction applicable to scenario or procedural training.

Mock Scenario Development

The first step to take in creating a scenario is to identify what needs to be improved; this may be related to medical knowledge, technical skill, communication, team function, or a combination of these. Adverse as well as routine events in the office or hospital setting often provide opportunities for learning and improvement and can set the educational framework.

The case study provided in the beginning of the chapter, for example, highlights a situation in which a mock code could be helpful in improving performance. Practicing a mock scenario of anaphylaxis can address multiple needs: teamwork, communication, locating and operating equipment, performing proper advanced life support techniques, and disposition. Once a scenario is developed, it could be practiced by the office staff until performance standards are met.

When writing a mock code or scenario, the first task is to create succinct learning objectives. Writing clear objectives is an underappreciated skill and is a crucial part of any educational program. Good objectives are important because they focus teaching and enable the

---

Box 16-2. Steps for Providing Simulation-Based Medical Education

1. Determine learning needs.
2. Create learning objectives.
3. Create learning lesson.
   a. Script, if performing mock scenario
   b. Simulated patient history and physical examination, laboratory data, images, and case progression
   c. Consequences of anticipated interventions and disposition
   d. Identification of required equipment and space
   e. Identification of role-players
4. Session delivery.
   a. Create a safe learning environment.
   b. Deliberate practice.
5. Feedback/debriefing.
   a. Advocacy inquiry
   b. Plan for improvement

evaluation of the effectiveness of the activity. A helpful way to start thinking about objectives is to begin with the phrase, "By the end of this session, the learner will be able to…" followed by the learning objective. Objectives should be specific and measurable and use words that are open to few interpretations. An example of how word choice can affect instruction and learner expectations follows:

| Open to many interpretations: | "By the end of the session, the learner will understand the complications of bag-mask ventilation." |
| Open to fewer interpretations: | "By the end of the session, the learner will be able to list the complications of bag-mask ventilation." |

The learning objective in the first example is vague; it may be answered in multiple ways. Also, the instructor does not have a clear standard for how to measure what has been learned. The second objective not only focuses the teacher and learner but provides a concrete way to measure knowledge by asking for a finite list. Depending on educational needs, typically 2 to 4 objectives are sufficient for a session. If there are too many objectives, it can be overwhelming and have a dilutional effect on the knowledge being imparted. Box 16-3 provides examples of words open to fewer or more interpretations.

Once the learning objectives are established, a script is written that describes the flow of events and consequences of anticipated interventions. Also included would be a list of required equipment or props, role-players needed with instructions on how to act, a history and physical examination of the simulated patient, and laboratory tests or images. It is helpful to write the scenario such that an individual other than the writer can use it for future sessions. Eventually, if multiple scenarios are written, a catalog of cases with various clinical scenarios can be developed which can serve as a sustainable learning resource. There are many templates available that can help in writing a scenario, with varying degrees of complexity. The important thing is to find a method that fits your time and needs.

Box 16-3. Words or Phrases Open to More or Fewer Interpretations

Open to More Interpretation
Know
Understand
Be able
Know how
Appreciate
Grasp the significance of
Learn
Open to Fewer Interpretations
List
Recite
Demonstrate
Perform
Rank (ie, rank as important)
Describe

Once preparation is complete, the session can be delivered. How well the instructor introduces the simulation learning experience can set the tone for all that follows. Before any simulation begins, the facilitator helps participants be clear about what is expected of them and helps them understand the benefits and limits of the simulated clinical setting. Learners must understand whether and how the case, event, or procedure will later be debriefed (discussed and analyzed) and whether the simulation will be video recorded. It must be explicit that the focus is on learning, not on catching people in a mistake. This helps create an environment where participants feel safe in sharing thoughts and feelings about the upcoming simulation and debriefing without fear of being shamed or humiliated.

Participants often worry that simulations are designed to expose their weaknesses or humiliate them. To counter these thoughts, facilitators should convey that they assume learners have good intentions and are trying to do their best but will likely make mistakes along the way. As previously stated, mistakes are actually desirable in the simulation environment because they provide focus on areas in need of improvement—and this subsequently can help improve care for patients.

After the scenario is complete, the next step is to debrief the case. This is the time to review the stated objectives; however, the overall goal of debriefing is to allow trainees to explain, analyze, and synthesize information and emotional states to improve performance in similar situations in the future. This can be challenging, as voicing critical thoughts can lead to hurt feelings or defensiveness on the part of the learner. It is the responsibility of the instructor to lead a discussion that encourages objective reflection of practice without being confrontational. There are published techniques, such as advocacy-inquiry, that can help in guiding debriefing sessions.

Advocacy-inquiry is founded in the theory of reflective practice, which is a way of analyzing one's own work practices and examining the foundation of their existence. When incorrect actions are performed, the goal of debriefing is to elicit the framework of the participants' thought processes, which have been formed by their knowledge and experience. There may have been a previous situation in which an instructor provided incorrect information or there was miscommunication, yet it had a significant formative effect on the learner's understanding and subsequent behavior.

An advocacy is an observation, whereas an inquiry is a question. When the 2 are paired together, the instructor is stating in the advocacy his or her hypothesis and testing the hypothesis with an inquiry in a nonthreatening manner. For example, during a mock code drill for a patient with asystole, you notice that cardiac compressions were not started immediately. During the debriefing, you might state, "So, I noticed that you were working on providing oxygen to the patient after you noticed the lack of a heart rate. I was thinking there was possibly an additional maneuver to be done . I'm curious—how were you seeing the situation at that time [inquiry]?" Rather than a judgmental comment ("Do you realize that it took you 2 minutes before you started compressions?"), the instructor is using advocacy-inquiry to elicit the learner's framework of thinking that guided his or her actions. The participant might state, "I was once admonished during my training for not adhering strictly to the ABCs, so I was working on providing the airway and breathing first," which provides the instructor an opportunity to refine the thought process of the learner for a patient with asystole.

Just as the delivery of simulated scenarios requires practice, so does the facilitation of a productive debriefing process. Included in the references is a good resource available for learning the technique of debriefing.

While simulated clinical scenarios or mock codes are complex processes, the task of teaching procedures is generally more straightforward. The concept of deliberate practice applies well to simulation-based procedural training.

Deliberate Practice

Education research has demonstrated that acquisition of expertise in medicine or other fields (eg, professional sports, musical performance, chess) is based on a set of principles governed by the concept of deliberate practice. Deliberate practice is one of the cornerstones of simulation-based medical education. To summarize, it dictates that the learner will engage in repetitive performance of cognitive or psychomotor skills with direct assessment, which provides the learner with feedback geared to improve performance. The elements of deliberate practice are listed in Box 16-4.

Coupled with simulation, deliberate practice has been shown to improve performance in many medical and surgical specialties. Studies ranging from general pediatrics to vascular surgery have demonstrated improvements in skills, knowledge, and team function when simulation with deliberate practice is used.

A randomized, controlled trial evaluated the effectiveness of deliberate practice simulation-based training to improve infant LP skills among pediatric residents, compared with a control group receiving audiovisual training only. After a baseline assessment of LP skill and knowledge, all participants viewed an educational audiovideo presentation. The intervention group went on to

participate in a simulation-based deliberate practice session on an infant LP simulator. The primary outcome was self-reported clinical success on the first infant LP after training.

Fifty-one residents reported on 32 LP encounters; 94% of the intervention group reported success, compared with 47% in the control group, a significant difference. However, when evaluated on an observed clinical examination at 6 months, there was no difference between groups. These findings suggest that while simulation training with DP is effective, there is a temporal decline in skills demonstrating the need for continual practice and retraining.

In adult medicine, a randomized trial with wait-list controls evaluated the acquisition of advanced cardiovascular life support skills among internal medicine residents using a mannequin simulator. Residents who received the simulation-based medical education with deliberate practice scored 38% higher on a reliable skills evaluation than residents in the wait-list control group. After crossover and a deliberate practice session with the control group, the scores surpassed the performance outcomes of the first intervention group. The authors concluded that deliberate practice, in addition to time and experience, is helpful in achieving competence.

The concept of close observation by experts with provision of constant real-time feedback can be applied to virtually any procedure. However, deliberate practice is only one tool in achieving procedural excellence; continual practice is a key component to maintaining a high level of performance.

Benefits of Simulation

Despite all the points demonstrating that simulation is a valid teaching tool for medical training, there are concerns about its role. The time taken away from real patient experience, significant effort and time required to create and deliver simulation training, cost of equipment, and potential for humiliation are all points that cause trepidation. Furthermore, is it effective?

Simulation is still an evolving science, and there is a growing body of evidence that it can be effective in improving medical knowledge and skills, team function and communication, and patient safety and outcomes and also save hospital costs when analyzed by return on investment. Health care payers and liability insurers have noticed simulation as the potential effects on patient safety are now being realized. For the development of the health care professional, it does not and should not replace the benefits of real patient experience but can serve as an important component in his or her education. Once one grasps the technique, there are ways to provide simulation education without elaborate and expensive simulators but with some creativity using lower-cost materials. The future of simulation in medicine depends on the dedication and ingenuity of the health care simulation community to see that improved patient safety and educational outcomes can be realized using this method. Potential benefits and applications of simulation are outlined in Box 16-5.

Box 16-4. Features of Deliberate Practice

1. Highly motivated learners with good concentration
2. Engagement with a well-defined learning objective or task
3. Appropriate level of difficulty
4. Focused, repetitive practice
5. Rigorous, precise measurements
6. Informative feedback from educational sources (eg, simulators, instructors)
7. Monitoring, correction of errors, and more deliberate practice
8. Evaluation to reach a mastery standard
9. Advancement to another task or unit

From McGaghie WC, Siddall VJ, Mazmanian PE, Myers J; American College of Chest Physicians Health and Science Policy Committee. Lessons for continuing medical education from simulation research in undergraduate and graduate medical education: effectiveness of continuing medical education: American College of Chest Physicians Evidence-Based Educational Guidelines. *Chest.* 2009;135(3 Suppl):62S–68S, with permission.

Box 16-5. Benefits and Applications of Simulation

- Avoidance of risks to patients and learners
- Tailoring of procedural training or scenarios to educational need and attributes of learner
- Practicing of skills and scenarios as many times as necessary
- Enhancing of transfer of skills from classroom to clinical arena
- Determination of educational needs
- Training for optimal team or organizational function
- Practicing communication skills
- Providing opportunity to practice rare critical events
- Assisting in the testing of new equipment or facilities
- Refresher training for staff at all levels
- Serving as formative or summative assessment tool at all levels

Conclusion

Health care simulation is a technique to augment real experiences with guided, interactive encounters that approximate reality. The last 20 years have witnessed tremendous growth in the health care training industry, with applications in medical education and patient safety practices. It provides a way to train without placing patients at risk and can be tailored to meet the needs of learners at any level. When delivering simulation education, it is important to highlight to participants the goal of improvement and acceptance of errors to connote a safe learning environment. Future work must be done to continue advancing this technique to assist in improving the health care system for our patients.

CASE RESOLUTION

You review what occurred in your office with the child in anaphylaxis and identify what the educational and environmental needs are. You determine that your educational objectives are related to finding and operating the emergency equipment. You obtain an inexpensive mannequin to serve as a model for the child and write the script of the case. You discuss with your office staff what your plans are and that the goal is to improve office function in emergent situations. You schedule an appropriate time and deliver the mock scenario with the entire office staff. It is discovered that some of the equipment is not operational, and some staff members do not know how to operate the defibrillator. Afterward, you lead a discussion with the group, review the points that are in need of improvement, and make a plan to rectify the equipment issues and knowledge gaps. The mock code intervention was universally well received by the staff, and they felt that the program helped improve the office's ability to handle emergency situations.

Resources for Physicians

American Academy of Pediatrics Life Support Programs: www.aap.org/en-us/aap-store/life-support-programs/Pages/life-support-programs.aspx

Anesoft Simulator professional health care simulation software for the computer, tablet, and smartphone: http://anesoft.com

Selected References

American Academy of Pediatrics Committee on Pediatric Emergency Medicine. *Childhood Emergencies in the Office, Hospital, and Community: Organizing Systems of Care.* Seidel JS, Knapp JF, eds. Elk Grove Village, IL: American Academy of Pediatrics; 2000

Biese KJ, Moro-Sutherland D, Furberg RD, et al. Using screen-based simulation to improve performance during pediatric resuscitation. *Acad Emerg Med.* 2009;16(Suppl 2):S71–S75

Cohen ER, Feinglass J, Barsuk JH, et al. Cost savings from reduced catheter-related bloodstream infection after simulation-based education for residents in a medical intensive care unit. *Simul Healthc.* 2010;5(2):98–102

Greenberg LW, Ochsenschlager D, O'Donnell R, Mastruserio J, Cohen GJ. Communicating bad news: a pediatric department's evaluation of a simulated intervention. *Pediatrics.* 1999;103(6 Pt 1):1210–1217

Issenberg SB, McGaghie WC, Petrusa ER, Lee Gordon D, Scalese RJ. Features and uses of high-fidelity medical simulations that lead to effective learning: a BEME systematic review. *Med Teach.* 2005;27(1):10–28

Kessler DO, Auerbach M, Pusic M, Tunik MG, Foltin JC. A randomized trial of simulation-based deliberate practice for infant lumbar puncture skills. *Simul Healthc.* 2011;6(4):197–203

Lammers R, Byrwa M, Fales W. Root causes of errors in a simulated prehospital pediatric emergency. *Acad Emerg Med.* 2012;19(1):37–47

McGaghie WC, Siddall VJ, Mazmanian PE, Myers J; American College of Chest Physicians Health and Science Policy Committee. Lessons for continuing medical education from simulation research in undergraduate and graduate medical education: effectiveness of continuing medical education: American College of Chest Physicians Evidence-Based Educational Guidelines. *Chest.* 2009;135(3 Suppl):62S–68S

Rudolph JW, Simon R, Rivard P, Dufresne RL, Raemer DB. Debriefing with good judgment: combining rigorous feedback with genuine inquiry. *Anesthesiol Clin.* 2007;25(2):361–376

Scott DJ, Pugh CM, Ritter EM, Jacobs LM, Pellegrini CA, Sachdeva AK. New directions in simulation-based surgical education and training: validation and transfer of surgical skills, use of nonsurgeons as faculty, use of simulation to screen and select surgery residents, and long-term follow-up of learners. *Surgery.* 2011;149(6):735–744

Toback SL, Fiedor M, Kilpela B, Reis EC. Impact of a pediatric primary care office-based mock code program on physician and staff confidence to perform life-saving skills. *Pediatr Emerg Care.* 2006;22(6):415–422

Wayne DB, Butter J, Siddall VJ, et al. Mastery learning of advanced cardiac life support skills by internal medicine residents using simulation technology and deliberate practice. *J Gen Intern Med.* 2006;21(3):251–256

CHAPTER 17

Pediatric Hospital Medicine

Grant P. Christman, MD

CASE STUDY

A 15-month-old girl presents to a community hospital emergency department with fever, cough, and rhinorrhea. On initial evaluation, she is found to be in moderate respiratory distress, with decreased air movement and patchy bilateral wheezes and crackles on lung examination. Her oxygen saturation is 87% on room air and rises to 96% with the application of 1 L per minute of supplemental oxygen by nasal cannula. The physician diagnoses the patient with bronchiolitis and gives a treatment of nebulized albuterol and an oral dose of prednisone. The hospital has no inpatient pediatric service, so the emergency physician calls the local children's hospital to arrange a transfer. The emergency physician signs the patient out to a hospitalist, who accepts her onto the inpatient pediatric service and arranges for transport.

Questions

1. What is the role of hospitalists in inpatient pediatric care?
2. How can pediatricians implement principles of family-centered care and evidence-based medicine into the clinical care of hospitalized children?
3. How can physicians promote quality improvement and patient safety in the hospital setting?
4. What communication strategies can hospitalists use to ensure safe transitions of care within the hospital and back to the outpatient medical home after discharge?

Every primary care physician (PCP) must periodically make the decision to hospitalize a patient who can no longer be cared for effectively in an outpatient setting. In 2010, there were 3 million total hospitalizations of children and young adults 0 to 21 years of age, or 3.5 per 100 persons in this age group. Common reasons for hospitalization include the need for close monitoring due to existing or expected clinical deterioration, initiation of an intensive diagnostic workup, expected need for surgical procedures, and administration of complex, technology-intensive, or risky treatments.

In the traditional model of providing hospital care, the PCP admits the patient to the hospital and then continues to personally direct the patient's care: rounding on the patient in the hospital daily; writing all orders for diagnostic studies, medications, and other care; and consulting directly with subspecialists as needed. Because of economic and structural pressures from a changing health care system, a second model has emerged in which, once the PCP admits the patient to the hospital, further care is coordinated by a pediatrician specializing in inpatient medicine: a hospitalist.

The term **hospitalist** was first coined by Wachter and Goldman in 1996. Though hospitalists existed prior to that time, the prevalence of hospitalists has increased significantly in the decades since. The Society of Hospital Medicine defines the scope of the hospitalist's work to include the clinical care of acutely ill, hospitalized patients; education, research, and leadership in the field of hospital medicine; and working to enhance the performance of hospitals and health care systems.

While hospitalists are unable to provide the uninterrupted continuity of care that PCPs provide in the traditional model, hospitalist systems offer a different advantage: the extended physical presence of a physician in the hospital who is responsible for the patient's care—as much as 24 hours a day, 7 days a week in some systems—which is impossible to sustain for a PCP with a busy outpatient practice.

Inpatient Pediatric Care

Every patient presenting for admission to the hospital requires a thorough initial evaluation (history and physical examination) following a direct verbal handoff from the health care professional requesting admission. If admission is requested by someone other than the PCP (eg, emergency physician, surgeon following a surgical procedure), the hospitalist should consider contacting the PCP to establish a relationship, gather more information about the presenting complaint, and learn more about the patient's established medical problems and routine care. Primary care physicians may not always be available; as such, it is helpful if patients have been thoroughly educated on their medical conditions and carry a list of their medications and allergies with them.

Inpatient pediatric care should be **patient- and family-centered care**, which has been defined by the American Academy of Pediatrics as "health care that is grounded in a mutually beneficial partnership among patients, families, and providers that recognizes the importance of the family in the patient's life." In the hospital setting, this may take the form of **multidisciplinary family-centered**

rounds, a system in which doctors, nurses, and other allied health professionals round together on hospitalized patients with their families at the bedside. During rounds, health professionals educate patients and families, hear their preferences, and include them in the medical decision-making process. Some families may prefer not to participate in rounds, and this preference should be respected as well. If there is a language barrier, in-person or telephonic interpreters should be used to facilitate the rounding process, in accordance with the principle of equitability of care. A **child life specialist** may be consulted to help the patient cope with the hospitalization, including daily rounds and anxiety-provoking or painful procedures, by clarifying what is discussed in terms the child can understand and helping the child process or be distracted from these events through various types of creative play.

Patient- and family-centered care is complemented by the application of **evidence-based medicine** principles to medical decision-making. Questions of diagnosis, prognosis, treatment, or avoidance of harm should be clearly defined to facilitate an effective review of the medical literature. One way of developing a focused clinical question is through the **PICO** process, wherein the physician identifies the applicable *p*atient population, *i*ntervention (eg, treatment, diagnostic test, prognostic factor), *c*omparison (control or placebo group), and *o*utcome (eg, diagnosis, prognosis, harm to the patient). For example, in formulating a diagnostic workup for a 5-year-old patient presenting with an asthma exacerbation, the physician might ask whether school-aged children with asthma (P) who receive a chest radiograph (I), as compared with children who receive no imaging (C), have a shorter length of hospital stay (O).

Advances in technology have made it possible to consult medical evidence at the point of care, even in the patient's room during bedside rounds, with the use of laptops, tablets, and in-room computers. When searching through primary research studies, such as randomized controlled trials, to answer a clinical question, the physician must determine whether the results are valid and generalizable to the patient under consideration. It may be more efficient and just as legitimate to use a summary of the evidence, such as a systematic review, which may be available through an established medical journal or a Web-based service.

Hospitalists should also make use of **clinical practice guidelines** as a way of providing standardized and evidence-based care. The Institute of Medicine (IOM) defines clinical practice guidelines as "statements that include recommendations intended to optimize patient care that are informed by a systematic review of evidence and an assessment of the benefits and harms of alternative care options." In applying clinical practice guidelines, hospitalists should consider factors specific to the individual patient, such as comorbid conditions, limited availability of services in specific hospital settings, and patient values and preferences, that may warrant deviating from aspects of care recommended by the guideline.

In addition to providing routine inpatient care, some hospitalists also provide certain types of specialized care, such as procedural sedation, palliative care consultations (for patients with terminal or complex conditions), and surgical comanagement. Hospitalists often play a role in accepting patients for admission to the inpatient service, facilitating hospital-to-hospital transfers, and providing physician-assisted transport. Because of medical and technologic advances leading to improved survival, hospitalists are increasingly caring for the growing population of **children with medical complexity**. Providing quality care to these children is challenging due to their dependence on medical technologies and multiple medications, the paucity of applicable clinical evidence to support management strategies, and the need for time-intensive and complex care coordination. Depending on the resources available to the family and the PCP's familiarity with the patient (which may be limited if the patient has had frequent or prolonged hospital stays), transitioning the patient to the outpatient medical home may be particularly challenging.

Patient Safety and Quality Improvement

While it is important for individual physicians to engage in clinical practice that is family centered and evidence based, the next step is to ensure that quality care is being systematically delivered at the hospital level, and where it is not, that **quality improvement (QI)** programs are initiated. In its 2001 report, *Crossing the Quality Chasm: A New Health System for the 21st Century,* the IOM defined *quality health care* as being safe, effective, efficient, patient centered, timely, and equitable. Opportunities to improve the quality of care delivered by the hospital may be suggested by issues faced in individual patient encounters, quality metrics tracked by hospital administration (eg, length of stay, readmissions), or feedback from patients, their families, and their PCPs.

One model for the creation of QI projects is the **Plan-Do-Study-Act (PDSA) cycle.** In the *plan* phase, the hospitalist identifies a problem or aim, defines a change that could be made to address the problem, and determines how the effectiveness of the change will be measured. It is usually necessary to form a team of like-minded physicians, administrators, and nurses and other allied health professionals early in the planning process. In the *do* phase, the change is implemented and data are collected about its effectiveness. These data may include **process measures** (how consistently the change is implemented) and **outcome measures** (the effect of the change on, eg, the patient population, hospital system, costs). In the *study* phase, data are analyzed and successes and failures of the program identified. Finally, in the *act* phase, the team determines whether the change should be continued and adopted more widely in the hospital, modified in some way, or discarded altogether. Depending on the project, additional PDSA cycles may be needed to maximize the breadth and depth of the effect. Successes should be shared publicly with the hospital community to promote support for further QI efforts.

Physicians should also promote a **culture of safety** in the hospital, meaning that the hospital's processes and workforce are dedicated to the promotion of **patient safety**. **Adverse events**, a term encompassing all injuries caused by medical management, are common and often caused by preventable medical errors, especially medication errors (eg, incorrect dosing, administering medications to the wrong patients). Common initiatives to improve patient safety include use of electronic health records and computerized order entry, review of orders by multiple health professionals, promotion of sterile technique and hand washing, work-hour limitations to prevent fatigue, and having time-outs before procedures to verify the patient's identity and site of the procedure. Hospitals should hold regular morbidity and mortality conferences to review cases in which adverse events occur. These conferences should be confidential and focus not on blaming individual practitioners but rather identifying systemic failures that may be corrected to prevent future adverse events. When adverse events occur, patients and their families should be informed in a timely fashion according to procedures established by the hospital.

Transitions of Care

Inpatient systems in which hospitalists work in shifts typically have physician-to-physician handoffs of patient care responsibility at least once every 24 hours. Resident work hours in teaching hospitals have been limited to promote patient safety, but this also results in more frequent patient handoffs. If there is inadequate communication, handoffs may increase risk for medical errors and adverse events. Safe handoffs may be promoted by written handoff notes and strategies for effective verbal handoffs. One such strategy uses the **I-PASS** mnemonic, with the letters standing for a 5-step process in verbal handoffs: *i*llness severity (stable or unstable), *p*atient summary (summary statement, events leading up to admission, hospital course, ongoing assessment, plan), *a*ction list (to-do list, time line, and ownership), *s*ituation awareness and contingency planning (know what's going on, plan for what might happen), and *s*ynthesis by receiver (receiver summarizes what was heard, asks questions, and restates key action items).

The discharge process should begin as soon as the patient is hospitalized. Goals of the hospitalization, discharge criteria, potential barriers to discharge, and an anticipated date of discharge should be identified in concert with the patient and family and reviewed on daily rounds. The hospitalist should formulate the discharge plan together with the other practitioners and allied health professionals involved in the care of the patient, including subspecialists, nurses, social workers, and discharge planners. For patients with complex needs, issues to address may include procurement of durable medical equipment, insurance coverage for medications, scheduling of follow-up appointments, and provision of other services such as in-home nursing. The use of written or computerized discharge checklists may help ensure that no element is delayed long enough to prolong the hospital stay or forgotten altogether.

The final result of the discharge process is the transition of care from the hospitalist back to the PCP and medical home. If communication is poor, this transition carries with it the potential for significant information loss (about, eg, the hospital course, new diagnoses, future outpatient care needs such as subspecialty referrals and laboratory testing) and resulting adverse events for the patient. Ideally, the hospitalist should strive to communicate periodically with the PCP throughout the hospitalization, especially at the time of any important events. Most essential is communication at the time of discharge, which may take the form of verbal updates by telephone, e-mailed updates, or faxing or e-mailing discharge summaries.

Conclusion

The use of hospitalists to provide inpatient pediatric care has been on the rise in the past 2 decades since the term was first introduced. Studies of hospitalist systems suggest that the quality of care provided by hospitalists is equivalent to, and in some ways may improve on, care delivered via the traditional model. When attention is paid to maintaining communication, hospitalists have the potential to be partners in care with PCPs and the outpatient medical home.

CASE RESOLUTION

The patient is admitted to a monitored bed and, after the initial assessment, the hospitalist concurs with the diagnosis of bronchiolitis. Based on current clinical practice guidelines, the hospitalist discontinues the use of systemic steroids and bronchodilators. The hospitalist obtains the primary care physician's number from the family and places a call on the day of admission, learning that the patient has a penicillin allergy that was not reported by the parents during the history and physical examination. The hospitalist also begins to explore the possibility of initiating a quality improvement project in the management of bronchiolitis that would use clinical practice guidelines to create a set protocol for admissions with an order template in the electronic health record. The patient improves over the subsequent 3 days and is transitioned off oxygen. The hospitalist, together with a discharge planner, reconnects with the primary care physician, faxes a discharge summary, and arranges a follow-up appointment 3 days after discharge.

Selected References

American Academy of Pediatrics Committee on Hospital Care, Institute for Patient- and Family-Centered Care. Patient- and family-centered care and the pediatrician's role. *Pediatrics.* 2012;129(2):394–404

Eichner J, Cooley WC. Coordinating the medical home with hospitalist care. *Hosp Pediatr.* 2012;2(2):105–108

Guyatt G, Rennie D, Meade M, Cook D, eds. *Users' Guide to the Medical Literature: A Manual for Evidence-Based Clinical Practice.* 2nd ed. New York, NY: McGraw Hill; 2008

Institute of Medicine. *Clinical Practice Guidelines We Can Trust.* Washington, DC: National Academy Press; 2011

Institute of Medicine. *Crossing the Quality Chasm: A New Health System for the 21st Century.* Washington, DC: National Academy Press; 2001

Institute of Medicine. *To Err is Human: Building a Safer Health System.* Washington, DC: National Academy Press; 2000

Leonard MS. Patient safety and quality improvement: medical errors and adverse events. *Pediatr Rev.* 2010;31(4):151–158

Rosen P, Stenger E, Bochkoris M, Hannon MJ, Kwoh CK. Family-centered multidisciplinary rounds enhance the team approach in pediatrics. *Pediatrics.* 2009;123(4):e603–e608

Schriefer J, Leonard MS. Patient safety and quality improvement: an overview of QI. *Pediatr Rev*. 2012;33(8):353–360

Society of Hospital Medicine. Definition of a hospitalist and hospital medicine. http://www.hospitalmedicine.org/AM/Template.cfm?Section=Hospitalist_Definition&Template=/CM/HTMLDisplay.cfm&ContentID=24835. Approved November 4, 2009. Accessed March 10, 2014

Starmer AJ, Spector ND, Srivastava R, et al. I-PASS, a mnemonic to standardize verbal handoffs. *Pediatrics*. 2012;129(2):201–204

US Department of Health and Human Services, Health Resources and Services Administration, Maternal and Child Health Bureau. *Child Health USA 2012*. Rockville, MD: US Department of Health and Human Services; 2013

Wachter RM, Goldman L. The emerging role of "hospitalists" in the American health care system. *N Engl J Med*. 1996;335(7):514–517

Zaoutis L, Chang V, eds. *Comprehensive Pediatric Hospital Medicine*. Philadelphia, PA: Mosby Elsevier; 2007

CHAPTER 18

Pediatric Genomic Medicine

Derek Wong, MD

CASE STUDY

A 4-year-old boy with moderate global developmental delay is brought to his pediatrician's office for evaluation. The patient has an unremarkable family history and a normal physical examination. Previous evaluation included a normal karyotype and fragile X DNA test. The patient's parents would like to know if there is anything else that can be done to determine the etiology of the delay. In addition, his mother has recently read about companies that offer multiple genetic tests to consumers and wonders if these tests will be useful as well.

Questions

1. How is microarray technology useful in pediatric practice?
2. How is next-generation sequencing technology affecting current practice?
3. What are the limitations of these new technologies?
4. What is direct-to-consumer genetic testing?

As a result of the Human Genome Project (HGP), the first essentially complete human sequence was published in 2003. Very rapid progress in DNA sequencing technology has decreased the cost of sequencing an individual from $750 billion in the HGP to less than $10,000 per person in 2013. Currently, microarray analysis has resulted in dramatically increased yields for patients with developmental delay, autism spectrum disorders (ASDs), and multiple congenital anomalies. Genetic panels for a variety of conditions, such as familial cardiomyopathy and X-linked intellectual disability, offer testing for 20 to 1,000 genes at the same price as sequencing 2 to 4 genes cost a few years ago. Several companies offer direct-to-consumer genetic testing, designed to provide information without physician input. Pharmacogenomics, which promises individualized drug therapy based on genomic data, is moving from specialized disease therapeutics to common diseases. The promise of a $1,000 genome has been hailed as the beginning of a new era of personalized medicine, in which each patient will have a tailor-made set of interventions to optimize his or her health. As with most breakthrough technologies, these advances will be balanced by significant limitations.

Epidemiology: Human Genome Anatomy

Human cells have 2 haploid genomes, each containing 3 billion base pairs with an estimated 20,000 to 25,000 protein encoding genes, plus a variable number of copies of the mitochondrial genome. On average, 2 humans share 99.9% of their DNA. There are at least 10 million single nucleotide polymorphisms (SNPs), which are single base changes that are present in a substantial percentage of the population ($>$1%). A small percentage of SNPs fall within the coding or regulatory regions of genes and directly influence gene function. The remaining SNPs have no known effect on protein production but may be inherited in recognizable patterns (haplotypes) with other SNPs.

Recently, it has become evident that most human genetic variation is not because of SNPs. Instead, copy number variants (CNVs), in which DNA segments containing up to several million base pairs are duplicated or deleted, account for a substantial portion of variation between individuals. Although studies have found that 12% of the genome is subject to CNV (Redon et al), the effect of this variation on an individual's phenotype is unknown.

Although most autosomal-recessive disorders are rare, most humans are carriers of several disease alleles. In a recent study (Bell et al), there was an average of 2.8 recessive mutations per person in 448 genes involved in severe autosomal-recessive conditions.

Pathophysiology: The Genotype/Phenotype Correlation and Environment

There are numerous examples of genetic background affecting the presentation of rare genetic disorders. Although most patients with untreated classic phenylketonuria develop intellectual disability, some patients with high blood levels have normal IQ on a regular diet. Patients with thalassemia are affected by the alpha to beta globin gene ratio. Therefore, β-thalassemia "carriers" with one mutation may become symptomatic if they have duplicated alpha chains. Understanding susceptibility to common genetic disorders will require an understanding of a complex network of interacting genes.

Genomic data provide information about only one predisposing factor to a disease state. Many diseases are caused by a combination of genetic susceptibility and environmental forces. The first examples of this interaction that were discovered were monogenic conditions such as complement deficiency, which predisposed patients to bacterial meningitis, or cancer susceptibility genes that caused extreme radiation sensitivity. However, the gene-environment connection is known to be much deeper, with certain environmental conditions causing methylation of the genetic code, silencing multiple genes without changing DNA sequence. These epigenetic changes may persist across generations, causing, for example, mothers exposed to wartime famine to produce children who are born to conserve energy. If these children are fed a typical American diet, they are prone to obesity and diabetes. Fetal cells that persist in maternal circulation (fetal microchimerism) may play a role in tumor prevention and susceptibility to autoimmune disease. Finally, our bodies contain more bacteria than human cells. The interaction of the bacterial and human genomes plays an important role in some disease states.

Clinical Presentation/ History and Physical Examination

A thorough history and physical examination will continue to be a critical component of patient assessment in the genomic age of medicine. Large databases will need to be created to correlate human genotypes to corresponding phenotypes, which are defined by the patient's clinical presentation. Even when genetic and epigenetic sequencing is commonplace, the only way to measure the effect of the disease on the individual is by clinical assessment.

Laboratory Testing

Microarray testing has had a dramatic effect on common pediatric conditions such as developmental delay and ASD. Comparative genomic hybridization (CGH) microarray testing uses closely spaced DNA probes to detect chromosomal deletions or duplications at 100 to 10,000 times the resolution of a standard karyotype. The diagnostic yield for developmental delay and multiple congenital anomalies has increased from 3% to 4% to 15% to 20% using this technology. For example, patients with ASDs with normal karyotypes may have microdeletions or microduplications of 16p11.2. Several relatively common genetic conditions, such as 1p36 deletion syndrome, have been delineated through the use of microarray testing.

Single nucleotide polymorphism microarray testing is a newer technology that has largely replaced CGH microarray. Single nucleotide polymorphism microarrays detect the same chromosomal imbalances as CGH microarrays, but in addition the SNP microarray can pinpoint regions of homozygosity that represent identical sequences on both alleles. This information is useful in a consanguineous couple because it highlights areas where mutated autosomal-recessive disease genes are likely to be found. In addition, SNP microarrays can detect some patients with uniparental isodisomy (inheritance of 2 identical alleles from one parent) and may suggest the presence of an imprinting disorder such as Prader-Willi syndrome.

There are several limitations of microarray testing. Although microarray testing has largely replaced the standard karyotype, microarrays cannot detect balanced translocation carriers or mosaic patients with a percentage of abnormal cells of less than 25% to 30%.

Some microarray deletions or duplications are known normal variants. Some patient samples show an abnormal result, but the lack of parental samples may hinder interpretation of the significance of the finding.

Next-generation sequencing is a phrase used to describe new methods that allow parallel sequencing of billions of base pairs at relatively low cost. Whole exome sequencing concentrates on the 1% of the genome that is the protein coding region and has become available on a clinical basis in the last several years. A recent report shows a diagnostic yield of 25% of this technology on 250 samples (Yang et al). Within the next several years, whole genome sequencing is expected to become available, allowing discovery of variation in regulatory elements located outside the coding regions. These technologies will create a major paradigm shift by averting many costly and invasive procedures, such as muscle biopsy, and decreasing the time to diagnosis.

Next-generation sequencing technology has significant drawbacks that must be addressed in the near future. Some genes, particularly those with high guanine-cytosine content, are not well captured or sequenced with current high-volume technologies. Thus, whole exome sequencing may miss 10% or more of the genome, and in some cases a next-generation disease panel supplemented by traditional sequencing may be more appropriate. Exome sequencing cannot capture triplet repeat genes such as fragile X. Microduplications and microdeletions are not normally detected with current technologies and must be captured using a microarray.

A patient's next-generation sequencing results will have thousands of differences from reference sequences. Until huge databases of genomes from millions of patients are available, bioinformatic algorithms must be used to sift through the data and determine which changes are potentially relevant. Parental testing is often essential for these studies and may not be available. In general, results may be divided into 3 categories: known mutations, SNPs or other alterations that do not cause disease, and variants of unknown significance. The last category may contain tens or hundreds of altered genes, and matching potential mutations to a given phenotype is very difficult. Technology will drive down the price of sequencing over time, but the cost of bioinformatics will dominate the price of these new technologies as the amount of data increases.

Direct-to-Consumer Genetic Testing

Several companies market genetic tests that report disease risk by analyzing multiple SNPs along with common disease mutations. The companies argue that consumers have the right to know their genetic information, and some offer genetic counseling services. However, the tests may lack sensitivity and specificity because the analysis is based on limited genetic markers without family history or phenotypic information. Many consumers (and their physicians) are ill-equipped to understand the nature of the results, and patients of nonwhite ethnicity may have many indeterminate results. In 2010, the US Food and Drug Administration decided to develop regulations for the sale of direct-to-consumer genetic tests.

Treatment: Pharmacogenomics

Individualized pharmacologic treatment is one of the ultimate goals of the HGP. Although pharmacogenomics is a very young field, several tests are available that reduce the risk of an adverse drug reaction. Patients with variant thiopurine methyltransferase alleles may have severe toxicity to drugs, such as azathioprine and 6-mercaptopurine, that are used in multiple disorders. Children with a 1555A>G mutation in the mitochondrial genome are susceptible to aminoglycoside-induced hearing loss, even after the first dose. Pharmacogenomics for common diseases such as asthma is currently under investigation and may allow a more rational choice of multidrug regimens.

Future Developments

Despite huge potential, the effect of the HGP has yet to be felt in most areas of medicine, including pediatrics. However, during the next decade, genomics will revolutionize the diagnosis of mendelian disorder. The effect of the HGP on common diseases and therapy is less obvious. It is unclear whether consumers will use genomic information to alter their lifestyles, whether the information comes from their physicians or direct-to-consumer testing. In addition, whole exome and whole genome sequencing create a variety of ethical issues. If a patient presents with heart disease, and testing shows an increased risk for Alzheimer disease, should this information be disclosed to the patient? It is certain that pediatricians will need to familiarize themselves with genomic medicine because the number of tests will overwhelm the available medical genetics specialists and genetics counselors.

CASE RESOLUTION

The patient's microarray testing shows a small microdeletion in chromosome 6. Parental testing indicates that the microdeletion is present in the patient's father, who has had normal development. Further testing includes whole exome sequencing, which shows a potential missense mutation in *CASK,* a gene on the X chromosome that may cause developmental delay. This alteration is not found in the patient's mother, implying that it is most likely deleterious. The parents receive genetic counseling about future pregnancies.

Resource

National Human Genome Research Institute, All About the Human Genome Project (HGP)
www.genome.gov/10001772

Selected References

Bell CJ, Dinwiddie DL, Miller NA, et al. Carrier testing for severe childhood recessive diseases by next-generation sequencing. *Sci Transl Med.* 2011;3(65):65ra4

Bloss CS, Schork NJ, Topol EJ. Effect of direct-to-consumer genomewide profiling to assess disease risk. *N Engl J Med.* 2011;364(6):524–534

Clancy S. Copy number variation. *Nature Education.* 2008;1(1):95

Feero WG, Guttmacher AE, Collins FS. Genomic medicine—an updated primer. *N Engl J Med.* 2010;362(21):2001–2011

Hines RN, McCarver DG. Pharmacogenomics and the future of drug therapy. *Pediatr Clin North Am.* 2006;53(4):591–619

Gonzaga-Jauregui C, Lupski JR, Gibbs RA. Human genome sequencing in health and disease. *Annu Rev Med.* 2012;63:35–61

Kuehn BM. Inconsistent results, inaccurate claims plague direct-to-consumer gene tests. *JAMA.* 2010;304(12):1313–1315

Li MM, Andersson HC. Clinical application of microarray-based molecular cytogenetics: an emerging new era of genomic medicine. *J Pediatr.* 2009;155(3):311–317

Redon R, Ishikawa S, Fitch KR, et al. Global variation in copy number in the human genome. *Nature.* 2006;444(7118):444–454

Solomon BD, Hadley DW, Pineda-Alvarez DE, et al. Incidental medical information in whole-exome sequencing. *Pediatrics.* 2012;129(6):e1605–e1611

Yang Y, Muzny DM, Reid JG, et al. Clinical whole-exome sequencing for the diagnosis of mendelian disorders. *N Engl J Med.* 2013;369(16):1502–1511

CHAPTER 19

Principles of Quality Improvement: Improving Health Care for Pediatric Patients

Bonnie R. Rachman, MD

CASE STUDY

During a routine staff meeting at your group pediatric practice, it was noted that many of the patients followed by your practice are behind in their immunizations. The reasons for this are unclear, as you and your colleagues are strong proponents of the timely administration of preventive immunizations. You want to develop a mechanism to determine what factors are leading to a delay in vaccine administration.

Questions

1. What is quality improvement?
2. How does assessing the delivery of recommended health maintenance relate to quality?
3. How is the prevention of medical errors related to quality improvement?
4. What is the difference between harm and error?
5. What factors are associated with medical errors?
6. What is meant by organizational culture?

History

The origin of medical quality improvement lies not in medicine but in industry and dates back to the 1920s. Dr Walter A. Shewhart was an American physicist, engineer, and statistician. In 1924 Dr Shewhart presented a memo in which he showed a schematic control chart. The diagram and text set forth all the essential principles and considerations involved in quality control. Dr Shewhart pointed out the importance of reducing variation in a manufacturing process and noted that continual process adjustment in reaction to nonconformance actually increased variation and degraded quality. He went on to develop **data presentation rules** that continue to be important today: Data have no meaning apart from their context, and data contain signal and noise. To be able to extract information, one must separate the signal from the noise within the data.

In the 1950s Dr Shewhart's colleague, W. Edwards Deming, while working in Japan, taught top management how to improve design and, subsequently, service, product quality, testing, and sales. Deming, applying Dr Shewhart's concepts, described the Plan-Do-Study-Act cycle as an approach to quality improvement. He opined, "The key is to practice continual improvement and think of manufacturing as a system, not as bits and pieces."

In the 1970s Avedis Donabedian, a physician, proposed a model for assessing health care quality by describing 7 pillars of quality (Box 19-1). He posited that structure is the environment in which health care is provided, process is the method by which health care is provided, and outcome is the result of the care provided. He emphasized the importance of measurement and evaluation of health care quality, ensuring completeness and accuracy of medical records, observer bias, patient satisfaction, and cultural preferences for health care.

Box 19-1. 7 Pillars of Quality
Efficacy
Efficiency
Optimality
Acceptability
Legitimacy
Equity
Cost

In 1991 Drs Paul Batalden and Don Berwick helped form the Institute for Healthcare Improvement (IHI), which has led to the application of quality improvement science to health care in the United States and internationally. The IHI promotes the adoption of measurement and feedback to improve the quality of health care. It is an easily accessible resource for education and information related to quality improvement in health care.

Historically, efforts for improving quality focused on "quality assurance." The goal was to minimize "defects" as measured by audits. Now the emphasis is on quality improvement, which focuses on moving the entire performance curve toward a greater level of performance by adopting best practices instead of simply focusing on low performers. Ongoing measurement is vital to sustaining any improvement. The process of quality improvement requires careful planning, thorough documentation, consistent analysis, and open-mindedness to results.

Quality Improvement in Pediatrics

Pediatrics is a specialty that emphasizes health maintenance and disease prevention. Studies have shown that recommended targets are not being consistently realized. Mangione-Smith and colleagues reported that children received only 46.5% of recommended care for preventive services, acute illness management, and ongoing care of chronic conditions. Shaughnessy and Nickel reported that 21% of outpatient prescriptions in a family medicine practice had at least one error. Other investigators found that medication samples were dispensed with inadequate documentation. In a pediatric emergency department in Canada, 100 prescribing errors and 39 medication administration errors occurred per 1,000 patients. In a sample of new prescriptions for 22 common medications in outpatient pediatric clinics, approximately 15% were dispensed with potential dosing errors.

The Learning from Errors in Ambulatory Pediatrics study aimed to learn the scope of, range of, potential causes of, and possible solutions to medical errors in pediatric ambulatory care. The study found that among 14 pediatric practice sites, there were 147 medical errors reported during the 4-month study period. The largest group of errors was related to medical treatment (37%). Of the medical treatment errors, 85% were medication errors. There were also errors associated with patient identification (22%); preventive care, including immunizations (15%); diagnostic testing (13%); and patient communication (8%).

There are many examples of errors in the inpatient arena as well. A study looking at inpatient medication errors found that among 1,000 children in 12 independent children's hospitals, 1 in 15 children was exposed to wrong medications, side effects, or drug interactions. Takata and Currier reported a rate of 11.1 adverse events per 100 pediatric inpatients; 22% of these errors were deemed preventable. In a 2005 Joint Commission on Accreditation of Healthcare Organizations report, the root cause of more than 70% of 2,400 sentinel events was communication failure between health care professionals or between families and health care professionals. In those events, 75% of patients died because of this type of failure.

Kurtin and Stucky describe 5 barriers or challenges to high-quality care in the pediatric and adult arenas (Table 19-1). The first is widespread unnecessary variation in care. To prevent medical error, one needs to understand how, when, and where it occurs; look at the system that allowed the error to happen; and keep the system open and blame-free (Box 19-2).

Factors associated with risk of error are not the individuals who work in the system but rather the system in which the individuals work. To decrease the risk of error, the language of patient safety must be understood, and a deeper understanding of the principles of systems analysis work models and other solutions must be developed.

Definitions

To understand quality improvement and improve patient safety, one must be familiar with the terminology. The National Patient Safety Foundation defines *patient safety* as the avoidance, prevention, and amelioration of adverse outcomes or injuries stemming from the processes of health care. The Institute of Medicine (IOM) defines *patient safety* as freedom from accidental injury.

Table 19-1. Barriers to High-Quality Care

Barrier	Explanation
Unnecessary variation in care	Diagnostic or therapeutic interventions performed at the discretion of the ordering physician and not required by the patient's condition
Gap between knowledge and practice	May be many years; time it takes a proven new practice to go from medical literature to routine clinical care
Failure of physicians to understand and work in the hospital's complex systems of care	Challenges to accessing information/data/personnel/materials to facilitate patient care
Need to improve patient safety	No consistent mechanism in place
Slow adoption and routine use of practices that can improve clinical outcomes and patient safety	Use of clinical pathways may mitigate.

Box 19-2. Factors Associated With Errors

Communication failures
Frequent distractions and interruptions
Inadequate supervision
Drug ordering issues
Limited access to patient information
Noisy work environment
Lack of 24-hour pediatric pharmacy
Emergency situations

An *adverse event* is defined as injury caused by medical management rather than underlying condition. Some are not preventable. One example of a non-preventable adverse event is the patient who receives the appropriate antibiotic at the appropriate time in an appropriate dose who has an allergic reaction to the medication. This differs from *medical error*, which is the failure of a planned action to be completed as intended (error in execution) or the use of a wrong plan to achieve an aim (error of planning). *Outcomes* summarize the effectiveness of care, including adverse events.

James Reason, who did extensive work on organization models of accidents, further delineates the terminology. A *slip* is an error in execution; the observable action deviates from what was planned. A *lapse* is an error in execution due to a memory failure. A *mistake* is a knowledge-based failure; the plan is carried out correctly but the planned action was wrong for the situation. An *active error* (sharp-end error) typically occurs in a patient care area by a frontline practitioner; the effects may be felt immediately. A *latent error* (blunt error) is caused by a system-based problem and may relate to poor design, incorrect installation, look-alike packaging, soundalike names, faulty maintenance, or bad management decisions. These are more difficult to identify and hard to recognize. Health care workers frequently develop work-arounds to bypass the problem. This often leads to the belief that the work-around is normal.

A *system* is a set of interdependent human and nonhuman elements interacting to achieve a common aim. In a hospital, it may be a unit or a department. *Processes* are how care is delivered. (Are policies routinely followed? Are evidence-based medicine guidelines implemented? Does the transfer of patients occur in an organized manner?) *Work models* provide a conceptual framework for investigating events and processes so all contributing factors are evaluated. Plan-Do-Study-Act is an example of a conceptual framework. The premise of all work models is that an organized, systematic approach to event investigation results in reliable data that may be used to develop a new *system*.

Continuous quality improvement (CQI) is the continued process of reviewing and improving processes and procedures associated with providing goods or services. It may evaluate structure, process, or outcome as independent components of the CQI process or all simultaneously, as considerable overlap exists between the components and quality of care.

When evaluating the quality of health by comparing outcomes, it is important to understand the concept of *risk adjustment*. *Risk adjustment* allows statistical adjustment of patient differences, such as severity of illness, to make comparisons of outcomes clinically meaningful. This enables the translation of statistically significant tests into clinically meaningful results.

Errors and How They Occur

The pervasiveness of the medical error problem is enormous. In 1999, the IOM published *To Err Is Human: Building a Safer Health System*. This report stated that medical error accounted for approximately 44,000 to 98,000 deaths annually in US hospitals. This is more deaths than from AIDS, motor vehicle crashes, or breast cancer. The types of events included adverse drug events, improper transfusions, surgical injuries, wrong-site surgeries, suicides, and mistaken patient identity. Most errors occurred in intensive care units, operating rooms, and emergency departments. The annual total cost was estimated to be between $17 billion to $29 billion. The cost of additional care was $8 billion. This figure does not account for lost income and productivity. The IOM made many recommendations in this report, including a balanced approach between regulatory and market-based initiatives as well as the establishment of a national focus to create leadership, research, tools, and protocols to enhance the knowledge base about safety. It recommended raising performance standards and expectations for improvements in safety through the actions of oversight organizations, professional groups, and group purchasers of health care. An additional recommendation was to implement safety systems in health care organizations to ensure safe practices at the delivery level. In 2001, the IOM published a follow-up report, *Crossing the Quality Chasm: A New Health System for the 21st Century*. Safety was deemed the key dimension of quality. Only a systems approach would work to improve quality in health care; trying harder was inadequate. A stepwise correction of problems in the system is the key to success. The culture of blame must be overcome; human error was to be expected. Table 19-2 lists types of errors and their definitions.

Medical errors are not usually an isolated event or done by a single person. Normally there are numerous safe points and double checks built into the process, but each layer of safety has gaps or holes. When these holes line up, the error reaches the patient. Standardized approaches can reduce variability and improve system efficiency. The goal is to make the holes as small as possible or even make them disappear. There are many factors associated with medical error, including human factors triggered by interruptions, fatigue, time pressures, anger, anxiety, fear, and boredom. Mistakes can result from a wrong plan of action. Mistakes involve misinterpretation of a problem, lack of knowledge, and habitual patterns of thought. A violation is a purposeful rule violation whether reasoned or reckless. The factors associated with risk are not the individuals who work in the system but rather the system in which the individuals work.

Table 19-2. Types of Errors in Health Care	
Error	**Definition**
Diagnosis	Error of delay in diagnosis; failure to employ indicated tests, the use of outmoded tests or therapy, or the failure to act on results of monitoring or tests
Treatment	Error in the performance of an operation, procedure, or test; an avoidable delay in treatment or responding to an abnormal test or inappropriate/not indicated care
Medication	Most frequent type of error; includes an error in the dose or method of using a drug
Prevention	Failure to provide prophylactic treatment or inadequate monitoring or follow-up of treatment

Harm Versus Error

The ultimate goal is to reduce patient harm. Early quality improvement efforts targeted the elimination of error. It had been believed that reducing error would decrease harm. This is not true; most medical errors never harm patients and may be clinically insignificant. One example would be the acetaminophen dose that is given 1 hour late. Why does one differentiate? Focusing on harm puts the microscope on the system, not the individual.

Quality Improvement and Organizational Culture

"This is the way we do things around here."

Patients expect to receive quality health care without experiencing preventable harm. The IOM has defined *quality* in health care as "the degree to which health services for individuals and populations increase the likelihood of desired health outcomes and are consistent with current professional knowledge." One of the things that influence quality in health care is organizational culture.

Many pediatricians are never taught about organizational culture. It is the invisible powerful dictator of how things are done in an organization. It is a latent and often unconscious set of forces that determine individual and collective behavior, ways of perceiving, thought patterns, and values. Hospitals have their own cultures. Subcultures exist among physicians and nurses as well as within departments, such as critical care. It may be challenging to understand all of a hospital's different subcultures.

Promoting change is rarely easy. Some people may adapt and change appropriately, while others resist and become dysfunctional. To make changes, there must be an environment in which teamwork can grow. Groupthink must be avoided. *Groupthink* is a term coined by Yale psychologist Irving Janis. It is "a way of thinking that people may adopt when they are members of a cohesive or homogeneous group; in particular, a group whose members seek unanimity of thought to the point that they cannot consider alternative ideas." It can prevent critical thinking and debate. Without disagreement, creativity can be lost. Negative effects of groupthink include an illusion of invulnerability, insulated leaders who may be protected from contradictory evidence, and members who accept confirming data and reject data that fail to fit their views. Alternatives are not considered and individuals with conflicting views are discounted or demonized. Talented leaders welcome diversity of thoughts and ideas. Leaders must empower team members to have open discussions and offer ideas.

Communication is a key component of organizational culture. Communication involves 2 parts: message and meaning. Message is stated; meaning is interpreted and may be interpreted differently among people. Strategies to improve communication are legion. Included in these strategies are methods for remaining calm in high-workload, stressful situations. Other strategies include more verbalization, verbalizations that relate to problem-solving, speaking in first-person plural, and coordinating tasks to the right person's experience level. Good communication encourages input from team members. Offering positive feedback builds confidence, reduces

stress, and clarifies ambiguities. Team evaluations provide input on how well team members are communicating with each other and the progression toward achieving team goals. Benchmarking against a similar team may provide valuable information. An outside consultant may be used to observe the team and provide feedback. Internally, the use of informal, regular meetings to discuss the team's progress and provide debriefing sessions to discuss the team process may be constructive in moving the team forward toward its goals and ensuring effective communication. Team conflict is experienced by all teams at one time or another. It happens when people come together to resolve a problem, dialogue about care improvement, or discuss changing processes to improve care. It needs to be managed effectively so issues at hand can be resolved while still providing the best-quality patient care.

Teamwork has been defined by numerous organizations. The IOM in 2003 used this definition: "All health professionals should be educated to deliver patient-centered care as members of an interdisciplinary team, emphasizing evidence-based practice, quality improvement approaches, and informatics." The IOM defines a *multidisciplinary team* as one in which members cooperate, communicate, and integrate care to ensure that patient care is continuous and reliable.

Measuring Quality

Ideally, measurements should evolve from the IOM quality aims (Box 19-3). Improvement measures may not be sufficiently valid and reliable for public dissemination yet may still be useful for benchmarking, to identify best practice, or as part of quality improvement initiatives.

Adult measures may not be appropriate for pediatrics. Pediatrics is unique due to heterogeneity, including age, size, diagnoses, and treatment modalities including medication dosing.

Measures must be reliable. The definition of *reliability* is the ability of the measure to perform similarly under stated conditions over time. In health care, reliability is often used interchangeably with the concept of precision. *Precision* is the ability of a measurement process to reproduce its own outcome. To achieve precision, a reliable system requires clear and concise definitions of the data fields to be collected. An effective approach is to train data collectors. There must also be a robust method for data coding and entry. Reliability needs to be intermittently assessed within and between observers over time to ensure consistency.

Measures must also be valid. A measure is *valid* if it adequately represents the attribute of interest. Internal validity is the soundness of the developed indicator. External validity is the ability of the indicator to be applied to a broader population.

Box 19-3. Institute of Medicine Quality Aims	
Timeliness	Safety
Efficiency	Equity
Effectiveness	Patient-centeredness

Measures must be feasible and usable. *Feasibility* is the actual ability to gather measures. For a measure to be usable, the intended audience must be able to understand the findings and use them in an appropriate fashion. It is *usable* if it is able to uncover meaningful differences between groups.

Three types of measures are essential to quality improvement.

1. *Outcomes measures:* Address how the health care services provided to patients affect their health, functional status, and satisfaction.
2. *Process measures:* Address the health care services provided to patients.
3. *Balancing measures:* Evaluate unintended consequences or the stability of the system being changed in the project.

A balanced set of measures for a quality improvement effort should include at least one outcome, one process, and one balancing measure.

Error Metrics

How does one measure harm? How does one measure safety?

Measuring harm is often done with occurrence reports. This identifies 2% to 8% of all adverse events in an inpatient setting. It may be done with retrospective, concurrent, or trigger-based chart review. There are no standardized methods for reporting, investigating, or disseminating information related to preventable adverse events. In the past, the qualitative concept of patient safety has been translated in quantitative metrics. Three frameworks that have been used include measuring error, measuring patient injuries, and measuring risk.

Error-based patient safety metrics are premised on the idea that the goal of medicine is to successfully implement the correct plan of care. It is an attractive measure of assessing safety because many errors occur and are somewhat easy to find. There are many problems with error metrics, as very few measures of error represent the true rate.

$$\text{Error rate} = (\text{identified errors})/(\text{potential opportunities for that error to occur})$$

The numerator (identified errors) may be hard to obtain because with reported events, one only knows the errors reported, not the actual number of occurrences. Therefore, it is nothing more than a rate of reporting.

Some other modalities proposed to get the true numerator include chart review. The difficulty with chart review includes the number of steps in the process—error occurs, each error is recognized by a practitioner, the error is documented by a practitioner, the chart is reviewed, the reviewer recognizes the event during the chart review, and the error is attributed correctly. Ethnographic study, the direct observation of people, has the same pitfalls.

Other confounders include hindsight bias. For problems to be effectively rectified, the correct understanding and attribution of events that created the error must occur. The retrospective analysis of error creates the potential for incorrect or simplistic identification of causes for events. Subsystem failures are difficult to identify as a contributing cause to an adverse event. The incorrect or inadequate attribution of causality creates the potential for misguided actions to "solve" the wrong problem.

Focusing solely on active errors leaves latent failures and, consequently, the whole system more vulnerable to adverse events. Identifying errors is important, but solely focusing on errors may lead to the blame game. Trends may be a barometer for the organization's culture as it relates to patient safety. Identified errors provide learning opportunities, preventing harm to other patients.

Injury-based patient safety metrics focus on unintended outcomes, such as catheter-related bloodstream infections, ventilator-associated pneumonia, in-hospital cardiac arrest, and deaths. Improvement efforts are more likely to focus on system vulnerabilities with a high potential for adverse events.

Risk-based patient safety metrics are a measurement of hazards or risks. Using a systems view, errors and injuries are the result of hazards or risks within the system of care. The focus is on hazardous conditions that increase the likelihood of downstream errors. Efforts are centered on 3 core areas: systematic risk identification, risk assessment, and risk reduction/elimination. It is proactive and saves counting errors and injuries (makes it less important). The elimination of risk includes the substitution of less risky alternatives, the development of administrative controls, and individual protection. It incorporates information gathered from the frontline bedside practitioner. The focus on risk reduction may decrease the need to quantify error rates or injury prevalence. This requires a shift in thinking from counting errors and injuries to proactively identifying risk. The intent is to identify systems-level problems that may be amenable to quality improvement efforts.

Patient Safety/Error Prevention

The Institute for Safe Medication Practices has developed a rank order of error-reduction strategies. They range from most effective (forcing functions and constraints) to least effective (education/information). In between are strategies such as (from most to least effective) automation and computerization, standardization and protocols, checklists and double-check systems, and rules and policies.

Education and information dissemination are important and helpful; they increase awareness. However, lectures are quickly forgotten and signs are often ignored. It is the least effective means to prevent the occurrence of error. Rules and policies are required by several agencies. They are a good resource but not an effective means of preventing a specific event.

Checklists, double-check systems, and bundles are very effective when they are a routine part of practice, but they are not foolproof. The best example of a double-check system is the surgical sponge and instrument counts done at the end of a surgical case. Checklists and bundles are also being used for other procedures like central line placement. Standardization minimizes the risk of error, and protocols bring a standard approach to a clinical issue. They are designed to eliminate variation from practitioner to practitioner and patient to patient. Weak points may still exist and be prone to error. Automation and computerization are 2 of the best means to prevent medical error from occurring. They are only as safe and good as the person entering the data. Forcing functions and constraints is the best way to prevent error through safeguards. In this manner, systems and products are engineered to be safer from the ground up.

Plan-Do-Study-Act cycles are one way of developing and implementing change leading to improved patient safety and quality of care. Plan-Do-Study-Act cycles force small-scale, stepwise thinking; allow for making predictions; force thoughtful deliberation on the increased knowledge; and subsequently facilitate change. The use of small-scale change can cause rapid adaptation and implementation of change in various health care settings.

Conclusions

The key elements to a system change are the will to do whatever it takes to make a change to a system, the ideas on which to base the design of the new system, and the execution of the changes to the system. Change is difficult, but sustaining change is even more complex. Hardwired sustainability in a new system is imperative. The "old way" has to be more difficult or inconvenient to perform. In health care, spreading improvements depends on key individuals; one critical success factor is the role of leadership. Leaders must inspire and communicate a shared vision, model the way, challenge the current process, no longer accept the status quo, and enable others with resources, training, and time. The successes must be celebrated.

CASE RESOLUTION

During your staff meeting, you decide to use a Plan-Do-Study-Act cycle to examine the practice's vaccine administration practice, identify barriers to timely vaccine administration, and develop a plan to ensure that vaccines are administered in a timely fashion.

Plan: The charts of all patients seen for routine care in the past 3 months are pulled. They are audited using a premade check sheet to identify vaccines given, vaccines missed, and barriers to administration. After analyzing the data, it becomes clear that many opportunities for immunization were missed because of inability to get parental consent. This seemed to coincide with a television program that discussed increasing rates of autism spectrum disorders (ASDs) associated with vaccination.

Do: At your next routine staff meeting, you present the data to your colleagues. You recommend rebutting the television show with a fact sheet and a discussion with parents by the physician. Your colleagues agree to implement this change because it is low cost and easy to put into practice.

Study: Three months after implementation, you re-collect data and find there are fewer missed opportunities for immunization and that your program has had some success. Some parents are still resistant to immunizing their children for fear of ASDs.

Act: You present the follow-up data to your colleagues and they agree to implement the current strategy. Data will be reexamined in 3 months to see if the program continues to be effective.

Selected References

Agency for Healthcare Research and Quality. Improving health care quality. http://www.AHRQ.gov/news/qualfact.htm. Accessed January 27, 2014

Aguayo R. *Dr. Deming: The American Who Taught the Japanese About Quality.* New York, NY: Fireside; 1991:40–41

Association of Public Health Observatories. *The Good Indicators Guide: Understanding How to Use and Choose Indicators.* Coventry, United Kingdom: NHS Institute for Innovation and Improvement; 2008. http://www.apho.org.uk/resource/item.aspx?RID=44584. Accessed January 27, 2014

Best M, Neuhauser D. Walter A. Shewhart, 1924, and the Hawthorne factory. *Qual Saf Health Care.* 2006;15(2):142–143

Carey RG, Lloyd RC. *Measuring Quality Improvement in Healthcare: A Guide to Statistical Process Control Applications.* Milwaukee, WI: American Society for Quality; 2001

Counte MA, Meurer S. Issues in the assessment of continuous quality improvement implementation in health care organizations. *Int J Qual Health Care.* 2001;13(3):197–207

Dharma Haven. Dr. Deming's management training. http://www.dharma-haven.org/five-havens/deming.htm. Revised April 27, 1998. Accessed January 27, 2014

Dill JL, Generali JA. Medication sample labeling practices. *Am J Health Syst Pharm.* 2000;57(22):2087–2090

Dodek P, Cahill NE, Heyland DK. The relationship between organizational culture and implementation of clinical practice guidelines: a narrative review. *JPEN J Parenter Enteral Nutr.* 2010;34(6):669–674

Donabedian A. *An Introduction to Quality Assurance in Health Care.* New York, NY: Oxford University Press; 2003

Griffin E. *A First Look at Communication Theory.* 8th ed. McGraw-Hill; 2011.

Institute of Medicine. Committee to design a strategy for quality review and assurance in Medicare. In: Lohr KN, ed. *Medicare: A Strategy for Quality Assurance.* Vol 1. Washington, DC: National Academies Press; 1990

Institute of Medicine. *Crossing the Quality Chasm: A New Health System for the 21st Century.* Washington, DC: National Academy Press; 2001

Institute of Medicine. *Health Professions Education: A Bridge to Quality.* Washington, DC: National Academy Press; 2003

Institute of Medicine Committee on Quality of Health Care in America. *To Err is Human: Building a Safer Health System.* Kohn LT, Corrigan JM, Donaldson MS, eds. Washington, DC: National Academy Press; 2000

The Joint Commission. Sentinel event. http://www.jointcommission.org/sentinel_event.aspx. Accessed January 27, 2014

Kenney C. *The Best Practice: How the New Quality Movement Is Transforming Medicine.* New York, NY: Public Affairs; 2008

Kotter JP. *Leading Change.* Boston, MA: Harvard Business Review Press; 2012

Kozer E, Scolnik D, Macpherson A, et al. Variables associated with medication errors in pediatric emergency medicine. *Pediatrics.* 2002;110(4):737–742

Langley GJ, Moen RD, Nolan KM, Nolan TW, Norman CL, Provost LP. *The Improvement Guide: A Practical Approach to Enhancing Organizational Performance.* 2nd ed. San Francisco, CA: Jossey-Bass; 2009

Leape LL, Lawthers AG, Brennan TA, Johnson WG. Preventing medical injury. *QRB Qual Rev Bull.* 1993;19(5):144–149

Magnetti S, Behal R. Organizational factors and human factors related to harmful medical event outcomes in 23 academic medical centers using electronic medical error-event reporting systems for targeting patient safety programs. Boston, MA: Academy Health Annual Research Meeting; 2005. Abstract 4205

Mangione-Smith R, DeCristofaro AH, Setodji CM, et al. The quality of ambulatory care delivered to children in the United States. *N Engl J Med.* 2007;357(15): 1515–1523

McPhillips HA, Stille CJ, Smith D, et al. Potential medication dosing errors in outpatient pediatrics. *J Pediatr.* 2005;147(6):761–767

Measure Type Definition. http://www.health.state.mn.us/healthreform/baskets/measurement090609_definition.pdf. Accessed February 18, 2014

Miles P. Health information systems and physician quality: role of the American Board of Pediatrics maintenance of certification in improving children's health care. *Pediatrics.* 2009;123(Suppl 2):S108–S110

Mohr JJ, Lannon CM, Thoma KA, et al. Learning from errors in ambulatory pediatrics. In: Henriksen K, Battles JB, Marks ES, et al, eds. *Advances in Patient Safety: From Research to Implementation. Vol 1. Research Findings.* Rockville, MD: Agency for Healthcare Research and Quality; 2005. http://www.ncbi.nlm.nih.gov/books/NBK20472. Accessed January 27, 2014

National Patient Safety Foundation. Definitions and hot topics. http://www.npsf.org/for-healthcare-professionals/resource-center/definitions-and-hot-topics. Accessed January 27, 2014

Reason J. *Human Error.* Cambridge, United Kingdom: Cambridge University Press, 1990

Reason J. Human error: models and management. *BMJ.* 2000;320(7237):768–770

Shaughnessy AF, Nickel RO. Prescription-writing patterns and errors in a family medicine residency program. *J Fam Pract.* 1989;29(3):290–295

Smith D, Bell GD, Kilgo J. *The Carolina Way: Leadership Lessons From a Life in Coaching.* New York, NY: Penguin Press; 2004

Takata G, Currier K. Enhancing patient safety through improved detection of adverse drug events. Presented at: 13th Annual Forum on Quality Improvement in Health Care (Institute for Healthcare Improvement); December 2001; Orlando, FL

Takata GS, Mason W, Taketomo C, Logsdon T, Sharek PJ. Development, testing, and findings of a pediatric-focused trigger tool to identify medication-related harm in US children's hospitals. *Pediatrics.* 2008;121(4):e9927–e9935

Western Electric. Western Electric—a brief history. *Western Electric News.* 1913;2(2). http://www.beatriceco.com/bti/porticus/bell/westernelectric_history.html#Western%20Electric%20-%20A%20Brief%20History. Accessed January 27, 2014

Health Maintenance and Anticipatory Guidance

CHAPTER 20

Neonatal Examination and Nursery Visit

Julie E. Noble, MD

CASE STUDY

You are performing an examination on a 16-hour-old newborn who was born at 39 weeks' gestation to a 28-year-old healthy primigravida via normal spontaneous vaginal delivery. There were no complications at delivery and Apgar scores were 8 at 1 minute and 9 at 5 minutes. The newborn weighed 7 lb, 1 oz (3,200 g) and was 19.7 inches (50 cm) long at birth with a head circumference of 34 cm. The mother received prenatal care beginning at 10 weeks' gestation; had no prenatal problems, including infections; and used no drugs, alcohol, or tobacco during the pregnancy. Her blood type is O Rh-positive. She is negative for hepatitis B surface antigen, HIV, and group B streptococcus and nonreactive for syphilis. The father is also healthy.

On physical examination, the newborn is appropriate size for gestational age with a length and head circumference in the 50th percentile. Aside from small bilateral subconjunctival hemorrhages, the rest of the physical examination is entirely normal.

Questions

1. What parts of the maternal history are important to review before performing a newborn's physical examination?
2. What further history is important for a complete newborn assessment?
3. What aspects of the physical examination of newborns are essential to explain to parents?
4. What physical findings mandate a more extensive workup prior to discharge?
5. What is the routine hospital course for a normal newborn?
6. What are important points to cover with parents at the time of discharge for a normal term newborn?
7. What laboratory studies, if any, should be performed prior to discharge?

The initial newborn physical examination is an important first encounter with the pediatrician, the newborn, and the newborn's mother and, if available, father, all establishing relationships with each other. The key purpose of this examination is to assess the status of the newborn and detect any underlying medical problems. Relaying this information to parents is essential and answers the question foremost in a parent's mind: "Is my baby 'normal'?" By performing a physical examination in the parents' presence during the newborn's first 24 hours of life, pediatricians can play a major role in allaying parental anxiety. More than 90% of newborns are normal, but the pediatrician's role includes identifying medical problems or high-risk conditions in the prenatal screening (including ultrasound), neonatal examination, and history. Evaluation and treatment, if necessary, can be initiated before discharge from the nursery.

Pediatric Prenatal Visit

Ideally, the pediatrician has spoken with the parents at a prenatal visit before meeting them in the hospital. The prenatal meeting provides an opportunity for parents to interview the physician, as well as the rest of the office staff, about general policies and procedures for well-child appointments, sick visits, and contacting the physician after hours. It also is a time to discuss what will take place at the hospital and explain the role of allied health care professionals (eg, lactation specialists) in the overall care of the mother and newborn. For pediatricians and other health care practitioners, the prenatal visit is a time to gather vital medical information about the current pregnancy, identifying any high-risk conditions, and to inquire about any problems with previous deliveries. The pediatrician should also review any pertinent family history. In addition, the pediatrician needs to note specific needs of the parents, which may include cultural rituals or ceremonies surrounding the birth of a newborn, such as circumcision. Whether the newborn will be born at home, in a birthing center, or in the more traditional hospital setting, arrangements should be made to accommodate the wishes of the family. The prenatal visit allows physicians to assess any psychosocial issues that may negatively influence initial mother-newborn bonding, such as maternal drug use, no paternal involvement, absence of a supportive social network, or lack of housing. Any of these issues may necessitate social service intervention. The social environment that will surround the newborn at home will have a great effect on her future.

This appointment is the ideal time to establish the medical home and emphasize the importance of breastfeeding and educate the mother on its many benefits. Anticipatory guidance issues, including positioning the newborn on her back to sleep, safe bedding, and child passenger safety, can also be discussed.

Neonatal Nursery Visit

At the time of birth, the newborn will receive a screening examination and risk assessment by the nursery personnel when he is stable after any needed resuscitation. If there are no noted abnormalities, the pediatrician is notified of the birth, and the recommendation from the American Academy of Pediatrics (AAP) and American College of Obstetricians and Gynecologists *Guidelines for Perinatal Care* notes that the pediatrician should evaluate the newborn within 24 hours. Meanwhile, in the delivery room, the newborn is dried, Apgar scores are assigned, and the newborn is placed skin to skin on the mother's chest, with a blanket placed over the mother and newborn, to facilitate bonding and early breastfeeding.

If there are perinatal or delivery complications, such as maternal fever, maternal medication during labor and delivery, meconium aspiration, asphyxia, prematurity, obvious newborn malformations, or distress, the newborn should be supported as necessary and kept on a radiant warmer for assessment. The physician should promptly be notified to perform the neonatal physical examination, evaluating any problem and initiating treatment.

Evaluation

Perinatal History

The perinatal history is the beginning of the newborn's medical history and is very significant to the newborn evaluation. To obtain all of the pertinent history, it may be necessary to review the maternal medical record. Results of maternal laboratory tests, such as blood type; rapid plasma reagin status; purified protein derivative; HIV and hepatitis B status; and chlamydial, gonococcal, and group B streptococcus cultures, should be noted (Questions Box). The pediatrician should also obtain triple screen, prenatal ultrasound, and amniocentesis results, if performed. Delivery room events and Apgar scores should be reviewed before performing the neonatal physical examination. This review helps the physician focus the examination on findings suggested by previous medical history. The occurrence of any unusual circumstances surrounding the delivery should be explained to parents at the time of the examination. They may not have understood the need for a vacuum-assisted or emergent cesarean delivery. It is important to be prepared to discuss the medical implications of such events.

Physical Examination

Every attempt should be made to perform the neonatal physical examination at the mother's bedside. This gives the physician the opportunity to meet with parents and gives parents a chance to have

Questions

Neonatal Examination

- Did the mother receive prenatal care? If so, since what month of gestation?
- Were all prenatal studies normal?
- Does either parent have a history of sexually transmitted infections, such as syphilis, gonorrhea, or herpes?
- Does either parent have a history of alcohol, tobacco, or illicit drug use?
- Did the mother take any prescribed or over-the-counter medications routinely during pregnancy?
- Did the mother have any complications, such as bleeding or decreased fetal movement, during pregnancy?
- Were there any indications of a complicated delivery, including administration of maternal medications?
- Is there a family history of congenital anomalies or diseases?
- Is the mother planning to breastfeed?
- Does the neonate have any siblings? If so, what are their ages?
- Is anyone available to help with the new baby or siblings?

all of their initial questions answered immediately. In certain circumstances, such as when the newborn is premature or when the mother is being treated for a medical complication, an initial bedside examination may be impossible to perform. In any event, the physician or other health care practitioner should speak to parents about the results once the examination has been completed.

The neonatal examination should be performed with the newborn completely unclothed and the newborn's body temperature maintained. The newborn should be assessed for evidence of birth trauma and congenital malformations, and an assessment of normal physiology of organ systems should be done. The newborn's birth weight, length, and head circumference should be plotted; physicians should keep in mind that these measurements are often made in the delivery room and may be subject to error. The diagnosis of small for gestational age (SGA) (weight less than 10th percentile) or large for gestational age (LGA) (weight greater than 90th percentile) can predispose a newborn to several medical problems. Temperature, respiratory rate, and heart rate should be reviewed via the nursery record. Feeding, voiding, and stooling patterns are also available in the nursery record.

The newborn evaluation should include an expanded Ballard score, which includes parameters for neuromuscular and physical maturity to accurately estimate gestational age. A late preterm or near-term newborn, from 35 to 37 weeks of gestation, frequently does not have the physiological maturity to feed vigorously and maintain body weight, glucose, or body temperature. These newborns are at high risk for readmission for treatment of jaundice, dehydration, and hypoglycemia. They should be followed very closely.

The newborn's overall appearance should be noted, particularly for the presence of any dysmorphic features. Physicians should determine whether the newborn looks normal or has any abnormal facial features, such as low-set ears and widely spaced eyes (see Chapter 72).

Skin

In the newborn, a thick layer of white vernix caseosa composed of sebaceous secretions and epidermal cells can frequently be seen. The presence and location of any rashes or birthmarks should be carefully described and pointed out to the parents. The particular location of the lesion as well as the pathology of the epidermal lesion may aid in its specific diagnosis. Skin lesions from birth trauma must be documented and treated as necessary. Bruising should be differentiated from the benign dermal melanosis often located in the sacral area. Skin color should also be noted: Cyanosis may be indicative of congenital heart disease, the presence of jaundice suggests hyperbilirubinemia, or plethora may be a sign of polycythemia.

Head

Head size and shape, including the size of the fontanels and position of the sutures, should be evaluated. The head may be significantly molded into a cone deformity secondary to pelvic pressure at the time of delivery. This resolves within days after birth, and with its resolution there may be a significant change in the head circumference. A cephalhematoma, which is a subperiosteal bleed that does not cross the suture line, appears as a unilateral or bilateral discrete lump on the side of the head. This finding may predispose the newborn to hyperbilirubinemia, and resolution may take up to 2 months. A cephalhematoma should be differentiated from a caput succedaneum, which is scalp edema that crosses the midline, and may be ballotable. Edema usually resolves rapidly. Skull fractures may occur with birth trauma and may present as a step-off or crepitus on palpation of the skull. They are associated with cephalhematoma but rarely need treatment. All head findings may be a source of concern to parents.

Eyes

The eyes should be evaluated for subconjunctival hemorrhages, colobomas, extraocular movements, and presence of red reflexes. If it is not possible to elicit a red reflex, an ophthalmologic evaluation is essential. Its absence suggests conditions such as congenital cataracts or retinoblastomas.

Ears

The placement, size, and shape of the ear pinnae should be noted as well, along with any preauricular or postauricular pits or appendages. The presence of a significant auricular abnormality may correlate with hearing loss or suggest a genetic syndrome.

Nose

The nose should be checked carefully for patency of the nares. This can be easily accomplished by occluding airflow from one nostril and observing airflow from the other. Choanal atresia is an important condition to rule out because newborns are obligate nose breathers until 3 months of age, and choanal atresia may lead to respiratory distress. A nasal fracture can also occur during the delivery process. This presents as an asymmetric nose. If the physician presses on the nasal tip and the nares are symmetric, the diagnosis is a deformity that will resolve. If the nose falls to one side, there is a probable nasal septum fracture that should be evaluated promptly by an otolaryngologist.

Mouth

The oropharynx should be examined closely for any defects in the hard or soft palate. A bifid uvula may indicate a submucosal defect of the soft palate that may be difficult to appreciate without palpation (see Chapter 73). Common normal findings in the oropharynx, including Epstein pearls located at the midline on the hard palate and epithelial cysts along the gum line, should also be noted. Loose natal teeth should be removed to prevent the possibility of aspiration (see Chapter 74). The tongue should be evaluated for macroglossia or a tight lingual frenulum (ankyloglossia), which may interfere with effective breastfeeding.

Chest

The neck should be palpated for sternocleidomastoid hematomas and the clavicles for fractures, which are more common in newborns who are LGA or a delivery complicated by shoulder dystocia. The chest should be inspected for respiratory effort and lungs auscultated to ensure normal breath sounds throughout. The quality of the newborn's cry should be assessed. Laryngeal webs or a paralyzed vocal cord may present in the newborn. Chest wall deformities, such as pectus excavatum, should be noted. If an absent rib is suspected, a radiograph is needed. The presence of breast buds is normal, but supernumerary nipples are minor malformations, although no treatment is indicated. Widely spaced nipples are a common minor malformation in patients with Turner syndrome.

Heart

The heart should be auscultated to ensure that it is in the proper position on the left side of the chest. Cardiac murmurs should be appreciated and documented. The presence of a murmur does not always indicate complex congenital heart disease. In the first 24 hours, a murmur may be a closing ductus, and newborns can also have functional murmurs. Peripheral pulmonic stenosis is a common benign heart murmur in the newborn that is characterized by transmission to the back. Every murmur should be evaluated on an individual basis. If assessment is indicated, 4 extremity blood pressures, a pulse oximetry reading, an electrocardiogram (ECG), and a chest radiograph should be obtained. If there are abnormal findings or the murmur is associated with cyanosis, tachypnea, poor feeding, or congenital anomalies, there is high suspicion of a pathologic cause. A consultation from specialists in pediatric cardiology should be sought and an echocardiogram obtained.

Abdomen

The abdomen is easiest to palpate prior to feeds. It should be assessed for any masses or organomegaly (eg, polycystic kidneys, hepatosplenomegaly, adrenal hemorrhage) that warrant further investigation. Bimanual palpation may be helpful to identify masses. The umbilicus should be examined to identify 3 vessels as well as the quality of the cord. A small, atretic cord can explain a low weight in the newborn. Erythema and swelling of the skin around the cord may indicate omphalitis, a serious infection.

Genitalia

In female neonates, the labia majora may be swollen, but the urethra and vaginal opening should be visualized to ensure patency. It is common to see hymenal tags. Clitoral size should be noted. Parents should be told that a physiological vaginal discharge and the presence later of a pink or blood-tinged discharge are a normal neonatal response to maternal estrogen withdrawal. In male newborns, the penis should be examined for size and length. The foreskin should be retracted sufficiently to reveal the location of the urethral meatus to assess for hypospadias. A testicular examination can rule out hydroceles, inguinal hernias, and cryptorchidism.

Skeleton

The newborn skeleton should be assessed for evidence of a skeletal dysplasia. All long bones should be examined for a potential fracture secondary to birth trauma. The neonatal hip examination is important to detect developmental dysplasia of the hip, seen more commonly after a breech position in utero. The Ortolani maneuver is performed to detect a dislocated hip. The "clunk" felt when performing the examination is the relocation of the femoral head of the affected hip in the joint capsule. In contrast, a "click" may indicate normal perinatal ligament laxity. The Barlow maneuver detects an unstable hip with the possibility of dislocation. If either test result is positive, it is diagnostic for a hip that is or could be dislocated and warrants an orthopedic consultation. Treatment with a Pavlik harness is initiated until confirmatory testing by an ultrasound is reliable at 6 weeks of age. The spine should be palpated completely to the sacrum. Sacral defects, deep sacral pits, or sacral tufts of hair warrant an investigation for such conditions as spina bifida occulta. Fingers and toes should be counted and assessed for syndactyly. The feet may be turned inward, outward, or up and should be gently moved to a normal position to ensure flexibility. Deformities secondary to intrauterine pressure are common. Clubfoot or equinovarus deformations should receive orthopedic evaluation.

Neurologic Examination

A newborn's resting position should be assessed to evaluate tone. All extremities should be flexed. The newborn then can be held prone under the shoulder girdle for further evaluation of tone, and extremities should continue flexed. Newborns should be observed for motor activity, moving arms and legs symmetrically. Response to sensory stimulation and deep tendon reflexes should be elicited. Facial movements should be closely observed for symmetry. Primitive reflexes, such as suck, rooting, grasp, stepping, and especially Moro, are an important part of the newborn neurologic examination. The behavior of the newborn can also yield information about an intact neurologic system. He should respond to sound, fixate on a face, and be capable of attempts at self-consolation.

Normal findings of the nursery physical examination are summarized in Box 20-1. Significant findings must be addressed immediately when noted at the initial nursery examination, including evidence of hydrocephalus, a ductal-dependent cardiac lesion, cyanotic congenital heart disease, a diaphragmatic hernia, an abdominal mass, or a

possible chromosomal abnormality such as trisomy 13 or trisomy 18, which can all be life-threatening. The physical conditions associated with trisomy 21 are rarely life-threatening, although suspicion of the diagnosis does warrant a genetics consultation and evaluation for cardiac and abdominal anomalies (see Chapter 39).

Laboratory Tests

Few laboratory tests are needed for the normal newborn. The only test that all US newborns receive is the state-mandated newborn screening test prior to discharge from the nursery (see Chapter 22). Heel-stick blood usually is evaluated for inheritable conditions, such as phenylketonuria, galactosemia, hypothyroidism, hemoglobinopathies, cystic fibrosis, congenital adrenal hyperplasia, and a panel assessing inborn errors of metabolism. The newborn screen varies by state and depends on the prevalence of a particular disease in a given region (see Chapter 22), but there is a federal effort to standardize testing. In all states, hearing screening is also part of the mandated newborn screening. Screening methods may be by automated auditory brain stem response, otoacoustic emission testing, or conventional auditory brain stem response. The newest screening test has

---

Box 20-1. Common Benign Physical Findings in Newborns

Skin
Milia, erythema toxicum, salmon patch, nevus flammeus, hemangiomas, dermal melanosis, lanugo (body hair), vernix

Head
Cephalhematoma, caput succedaneum, molding

Face
Swollen overall appearance, minor malformations

Eyes
Swollen eyelids, subconjunctival hemorrhages

Ears
Preauricular appendages/pits, folded pinnae

Nose
Flattened nose, milia over bridge

Mouth and Throat
Epstein pearls, epithelial pearls, natal teeth, shortened frenulum

Chest
Supernumerary nipples, breast buds, galactorrhea, pectus excavatum or carinatum

Genitalia
Females: swollen labia, hymenal tags, vaginal discharge
Males: hydrocele, undescended testicle (palpated in inguinal canal)

Hips
Click

Extremities
Feet turned up, in, or out, but malleable

Neurologic Examination
Primitive reflexes: Moro, grasp, rooting, stepping

been the addition of pulse oximetry at 24 hours of life to rule out transposition of the great vessels, tetralogy of Fallot, and hypoplasia of the left heart.

Another laboratory test that is often performed when indicated in a newborn is a serum glucose in newborns at high risk for hypoglycemia (which includes newborns who are SGA or LGA, newborns of diabetic mothers, and newborns who are symptomatic). A hematocrit is necessary in jaundiced, pale, or ruddy-appearing newborns; SGA and LGA newborns; and twins and multiples. In cases of ABO or Rh incompatibility, serum bilirubin and antiglobulin (Coombs) tests are important to obtain. Screening for hyperbilirubinemia to prevent kernicterus is recommended for all newborns. Bilirubin screening can be done easily by a transcutaneous reading followed by a serum level if the transcutaneous reading is elevated (see Chapter 117).

Imaging Studies

Routine radiographs are not indicated in neonates whose examination is normal and should be ordered only if indicated by the examination. Some minor malformations, such as pectus excavatum, do not need radiographs. Vertebral radiographs, ultrasound of the lumbosacral spine, or magnetic resonance imaging is appropriate in the neonate with a deep sacral pit or sacral tuft of hair for the diagnosis of spina bifida occulta. Clavicular radiographs are indicated if swelling or pain is located in the clavicular area or if an asymmetric Moro reflex is elicited. A chest radiograph, ECG, and echocardiogram are warranted for a significant murmur. If a prenatal ultrasound indicates that the newborn has hydronephrosis, a follow-up renal ultrasound should be obtained. If multiple anomalies are found, a renal ultrasound looking for malformations of the kidneys should be performed, and skeletal survey might also be helpful. More extensive studies are indicated if an emergent physical finding is discovered.

Management

After stabilization in the delivery room, the newborn should be thoroughly dried and given to the mother for breastfeeding and bonding. If mother and baby are healthy, the newborn should stay with the mother. An initial bath is only necessary to remove blood or meconium after the newborn's temperature is stable. The administration of intramuscular vitamin K to prevent hemorrhagic disease of the newborn and the application of ophthalmic ointment or silver nitrate in the newborn's eyes to prevent gonorrheal infection is universal. Hepatitis B vaccine is recommended for all newborns at birth regardless of mother's serology. Every hospital should encourage rooming-in of the newborn with the mother. The newborn should feed in the delivery room if breastfeeding or within 2 hours of birth and continue to feed every 2 to 3 hours to prevent hypoglycemia. The preferred feeding method is breastfeeding, and the mother should receive sufficient postpartum support to ensure success (see Chapter 26). Vital signs should be monitored every 30 minutes until stable during the transition to extrauterine life, which can last 4 to 8 hours, then every 4 hours. Daily weights as well as strict documentation of voiding and stooling are necessary to monitor the newborn for adequacy of intake and dehydration. Weight loss is

expected, but more than 7% requires physician assessment. Umbilical cord care remains an area of controversy, and it appears that leaving the cord to dry is sufficient treatment.

If desired, circumcision is usually performed on the day of discharge (see Chapter 24). The newest guidelines from the AAP note that the benefits of circumcision outweigh the risks. Local anesthesia is universally recommended for the procedure. Following the procedure, parents are instructed to leave the gauze or Plastibell in place. It will fall off spontaneously. Petroleum ointment may also be placed on the corona of the penis to prevent its sticking to the diaper. The physician should be notified if excessive bleeding or oozing occurs (eg, soaking of the diaper with blood) after discharge from the nursery.

Discharge Planning and Counseling

In most cases, mother and newborn should be discharged home together. The recommended hospital stay is 48 hours for a vaginal delivery and 96 hours for a cesarean delivery. The physician should reexamine the newborn at the day of discharge to identify problems that might have developed as well as counsel the mother. A bilirubin assessment is required. Again, this examination is best performed at bedside. The newborn's physical findings and hospital course should be reviewed with the mother and father. If studies other than routine neonatal screening were performed, parents should also be informed of the results.

Discharge is the best time to review anticipatory guidance issues. Topics that should be covered at the bedside include feeding patterns and what to expect, sleeping and elimination patterns in the newborn, umbilical cord care, bathing the newborn, and safety issues such as car safety seats, sleeping position, and safe sleep environments. Guidelines on symptoms of illness and when to call the office or emergency department should also be addressed. These include a rectal temperature of 100.4°F (38.0°C) or above, respiratory distress, irritability, lethargy, decreased feeding, and evidence of dehydration. If parents have any concerns about their newborn, they should be encouraged to call the physician's office. A follow-up visit should be arranged at day 3 to 5 of life for any newborn being breastfed to give breastfeeding support as well as to assess the newborn for evidence of jaundice or dehydration. An early follow-up appointment may also be indicated in a newborn with social risk factors and near-term newborns who are at higher risk for complications. If the newborn is born via cesarean delivery or is formula feeding, a follow-up visit at one week after discharge may be appropriate.

Early newborn discharge is an option if desired by the mother. There are published recommendations from the AAP for guidance on discharge at younger than 48 hours. Generally, the history, including social risk factors, physical examination, and hospital course, should all be low risk and the newborn should have been observed for at least 12 hours. If the newborn is stable and sent home at less than 48 hours, a mandatory follow-up appointment should be scheduled in 2 days. If a newborn has had a home birth, that newborn needs a medical evaluation within 24 hours of birth and subsequently 48 hours later. Hospitalists have been assuming more of the hospital care for newborns in many communities. It is necessary that the complete hospital record and results of screening tests accompany the newborn to the medical home. This coordination of transfer of care can be a challenge, but is essential for optimal care.

CASE RESOLUTION

In the case study presented at the beginning of the chapter, the parents should be told that the newborn's weight, length, and head circumference are all normal. The examination is reviewed at bedside and the subconjunctival hemorrhages should be shown to the parents and their benign self-limited nature explained. Parents should be reassured about all other normal aspects of the physical examination. The newborn's blood type from cord blood should be obtained because the mother is O Rh-positive. Routine neonatal screening, feeding, sleeping, elimination, bathing, and safety should be reviewed. Prior to discharge, the newborn should receive the hepatitis B vaccine, newborn screening tests, and bilirubin assessment. A follow-up appointment should be made in 48 hours after discharge to follow breastfeeding progress. Results of all newborn screening tests should be reviewed when available.

Selected References

American Academy of Pediatrics, American College of Obstetricians and Gynecologists. *Guidelines for Perinatal Care*. 7th ed. Elk Grove Village, IL: American Academy of Pediatrics; 2012

American Academy of Pediatrics Committee on Fetus and Newborn. Hospital stay for healthy term newborns. *Pediatrics*. 2010;125(2):405–409

American Academy of Pediatrics Committee on Fetus and Newborn. Planned home birth. *Pediatrics*. 2013;131(5):1016–1020

American Academy of Pediatrics Section on Cardiology and Cardiac Surgery Executive Committee. Endorsement of Health and Human Services recommendations for pulse oximetry screening for critical congenital heart disease. *Pediatrics*. 2012;129(1):190–192

American Academy of Pediatrics Task Force on Circumcision. Circumcision policy statement. *Pediatrics*. 2012;130(3):585–586

Cohen GJ; American Academy of Pediatrics Committee on Psychosocial Aspects of Child and Family Health. The prenatal visit. *Pediatrics*. 2009;124(4):1227–1232

Coloherty J, Eichenwald E, Stark A, eds. *Manual of Neonatal Care*. 6th ed. Philadelphia, PA: Lippincott Williams & Wilkins; 2008

Fernhoff PM. Newborn screening for genetic disorders. *Pediatr Clin North Am*. 2009;56(3):505–513

Lauer BJ, Spector ND. Hyperbilirubinemia in the newborn. *Pediatr Rev*. 2011;32(8):341–349

Maisels MJ, Bhutani VK, Bogen D, Newman TB, Stark AR, Watchko JF. Hyperbilirubinemia in the newborn infant ≥35 weeks' gestation: an update with clarifications. *Pediatrics*. 2009;124(4):1193–1198

Ramachandrappa A, Jain L. Health issues of the late preterm infant. *Pediatr Clin North Am*. 2009;56(3):565–577

Sayers SM. Indigenous newborn care. *Pediatr Clin North Am*. 2009;56(6):1243–1261

US Preventive Services Task Force. Screening of infants for hyperbilirubinemia to prevent chronic bilirubin encephalopathy: US Preventive Services Task Force recommendation statement. *Pediatrics*. 2009;124(4):1172–1177

Warren JB, Phillipi CA. Care of the well newborn. *Pediatr Rev*. 2012;33(1):4–18

CHAPTER 21

Perinatal Maternal Mood and Anxiety Disorders: The Role of the Pediatrician

Carol D. Berkowitz, MD

CASE STUDY

You are evaluating a 3-week-old newborn who is the product of a 39-week gestation to a 30-year-old gravida 1, para 1 mother who has been breastfeeding the newborn. Birth weight was 3,650 g, and the baby now weighs 3,380 g. The mother expresses concern about her ability to breastfeed. She also admits to being exhausted and feeling detached from the baby and overwhelmed by being a mom, something she had looked forward to since she was a little girl. She has difficulty concentrating and has no appetite. She asks you if it is normal to feel this way.

Questions

1. What is the spectrum of perinatal mood and anxiety disorders?
2. What are the signs and symptoms of peripartum depression?
3. What are the risks to newborns of mothers who experience peripartum depression and other mood disorders?
4. What is the role of the pediatrician in assessing mothers for perinatal mood and anxiety disorder?
5. What screening instruments are available to assist in assessing mothers for perinatal mood and anxiety disorders?
6. What are the risks and benefits of the use of psychopharmacology during pregnancy and postpartum?
7. What resources are available to offer to mothers who may be experiencing perinatal mood disorders?

The term *perinatal maternal mood and anxiety disorders* is the preferred nomenclature used to denote the set of mental health issues facing mothers (and fathers) related to the pregnancy and birth of a neonate. Peripartum depression had been used to encompass a cadre of mental health problems that new mothers may experience, but now there is recognition that mental health issues can be present preconception, through pregnancy, and through the infant's first year of life, and these issues include not only depression but other disorders. Despite public disclosures and open discussions by celebrities such as Brooke Shields and Gwyneth Paltrow, the condition is underrecognized, and many mothers go undiagnosed and untreated. The pediatrician is in an ideal position to assess a mother for the presence of these symptoms following the birth of a baby because the pediatrician usually sees the mother-baby dyad prior to the obstetric postpartum visit at 6 weeks following the baby's birth. The recommended time points for screening for postpartum depression coincide with well-baby checks: 2 weeks, 2 months, and 6 months. In addition, women are likely to follow up with their baby's pediatric appointments more than their own. While fatigue is a common complaint of new mothers as well as new fathers, other symptoms, particularly those of impaired functioning and diminished ability to care for the baby, may suggest a more significant disturbance.

Epidemiology

Maternal depression is the number one complication of pregnancy, exceeding diabetes and hypertension. The incidence of peripartum depression varies with the population studied, with the estimated range being from 5% to 25%. Between 14% and 23% of pregnant women experience depressive symptoms while pregnant, and approximately 13% of women take an antidepressant at some time during their pregnancy. The prevalence is felt to be much higher at 40% to 60% in certain groups, including low-income women, certain ethnic minorities (including Hispanic and African American), pregnant and parenting teenagers, mothers of multiple births, and women who served in the military in Iraq and Afghanistan. The World Health Organization notes that depression is the fourth leading cause of disease burden in the world. In spite of the high prevalence across all groups, fewer than 50% of cases of maternal depression are identified.

Often, there is reluctance on the part of obstetricians or psychiatrists to treat pregnant women with antidepressants because of concerns about the potential effects of the medications on the developing fetus. These effects include fetal malformations, cardiac defects, pulmonary hypertension, and reduced birth weight. However, untreated depression and anxiety in pregnancy also increase the risk of preterm delivery, low birth weight, and newborns' own ability to regulate emotions and stress. The American College of Obstetricians and Gynecologists and the American Psychiatric Association have issued joint guidelines on the management of pregnant women with depression, which discuss the indications for psychotherapy as well as psychopharmacology in the pregnant woman. Pediatricians are usually not involved in this part of the decision-making process but should be knowledgeable about the possible complications that the newborn may experience following birth from exposure to antidepressants or untreated maternal mental illness. Approximately 6% to 10% of fathers experience peripartum depression, with the highest rates seen between 3 and 6 months following the birth of the baby. Paternal rates of depression are higher when there is maternal depression, and the effect on the infant is greater than if the father is not affected. Depressed fathers have a higher rate of substance abuse.

There is a wide range of symptomatology that can be categorized under peripartum mood disorders (Box 21-1). **Baby blues** or **maternity blues** are used to describe the very common experience of new mothers, said to affect 50% to 80% of postpartum women in the first few days after delivery. There is no *Diagnostic and Statistical Manual of Mental Disorders, Fifth Edition, Text Revision (DSM-5-TR)* categorization of baby blues. Generally, symptoms improve over 1 to 2 weeks and functioning is not impaired, although baby blues may herald later depression. Mothers experience sadness, crying, mood swings, anxiety, and worrying.

A diagnosis of **postpartum depression** meets the criteria of depression according to *DSM-5,* which include a depressed mood, diminished pleasure (anhedonia), changes in appetite and sleep, psychomotor agitation or retardation, fatigue, feelings of worthlessness or inappropriate guilt, decreased ability to concentrate, and recurrent thoughts of death or suicide. Suicide is the leading cause of death in mothers during the first year postpartum. Technically, symptoms of depression must begin within 4 weeks of delivery and may persist for 1 year, though the onset is often insidious and doesn't come to attention until much later than 1 month postpartum.

Postpartum psychosis is less frequent, occurring in 1 to 3 per 1,000 deliveries within the first 4 weeks after delivery. There is severe impairment, with paranoia, mood shifts, hallucinations, delusions, and suicidal and homicidal ideation. Sometimes there is a history of a preexisting bipolar disorder. Affected mothers require hospitalization, in part because the infanticide rate is 4% to 5%.

Other disorders that have been recognized as being pregnancy and birth related or exacerbated include anxiety disorders, panic disorder, postpartum post-traumatic stress disorder, postpartum

---

Box 21-1. Peripartum Mood Disorders Symptomatology

Baby Blues
- Sadness
- Crying
- Mood swings
- Anxiety
- Worrying
- First few days after delivery
- Resolves in 1 to 2 weeks

Postpartum Depression
- Meets *Diagnostic and Statistical Manual of Mental Disorders, Fifth Edition, Text Revision,* criteria for depression
- Depressed mood
- Diminished pleasure
- Change in appetite
- Change in sleep
- Fatigue
- Feelings of worthlessness or guilt
- Inability to concentrate
- Recurrent thoughts of death or suicide

Postpartum Psychosis
- Severe impairment
- Paranoia
- Mood shifts
- Hallucinations
- Delusions
- Suicidal/homicidal ideation
- Usually requires hospitalization

---

bipolar disorder, and postpartum obsessive-compulsive disorder; 5% of mothers report intrusive thoughts of harming their baby.

It is estimated that 400,000 neonates are born to mothers who are depressed. These neonates are at risk for a host of adverse physical and developmental consequences.

Pathophysiology

The precise pathophysiology of maternal depression has not been elucidated, but sleep deprivation related to the demands of caring for a newborn, genetic factors, other biological or inflammatory processes (cytokines), and hormonal changes are felt to be contributing factors. While there are rapid decreases in the levels of estrogen, progesterone, and cortisol, the hormonal levels noted in mothers who experience postpartum depression do not differ from women who do not experience postpartum depression. Perhaps more significantly, there are a number of risk factors that have been associated with its development, including prior history of depression in general but especially during a previous pregnancy; mood disorders, including premenstrual dysphoric disorder; substance abuse; alcohol dependence; low socioeconomic status; a history of infertility; prior perinatal loss (eg, miscarriage, sudden infant death syndrome, bed-sharing death); lack of social support or community network; unintended or unwanted pregnancy; or a family history of depression. Other social/familial factors include marital discord, divorce, and intimate partner violence. Homicide is the leading cause of death among pregnant women. It is important to recognize that depression can affect adoptive mothers, who experience stress and anxiety during the adoptive process and remain concerned that the birth mother may reclaim her baby.

Perinatal depression is less easy to recognize in fathers. The depression is often covert or masked. Men are less likely to seek help or have ongoing access to health care professionals. They may feel excluded from the mother-baby relationship. Often they become workaholics as a means of dealing with the depression

Evaluation

Mother

Screening for perinatal mood disorders is felt to be within the scope of the pediatric practice. Studies have shown that mothers are comfortable being queried by pediatricians about how they are doing. Some pediatricians express concern about the appropriate strategies for screening and what to do if they determine that a mother has symptoms of depression.

It is important to couch any depression screening in language that makes a new mother feel comfortable and not judged in any way. Postpartum Support International has developed the "universal message" to share with depressed new mothers: (1) You are not crazy; (2) you are not alone; and (3) with the right help, you will get better.

There are several instruments that help screen for postpartum depression. A simple tool, called the Patient Health Questionnaire-2 (PHQ-2), begins with a background statement related to depression as a common and treatable condition that often goes unrecognized. There follows justification citing the recommendation of the US Preventive Services Task Force that all adults be checked for depression. The question, "Over the past 2 weeks, how often have you been bothered by any of the following problems?" is asked, with the following 2 categories: "Little interest or pleasure in doing things," and "Feeling down, depressed, or hopeless." For both categories, the following responses are possible: 0, not at all; 1, several days; 2, more than half the days; 3, nearly every day. A score of 3 or more has a sensitivity of 83% and a specificity of 92% for major depressive episode, and indicates a more extensive assessment is necessary to make the diagnosis of depression.

A second instrument is the Edinburgh Postnatal Depression Scale (EPDS). A sample question from the scale is given in Box 21-2. The scale was developed in 1987 and consists of 10 questions completed by the mother. The mother is asked to check the response that comes the closest to how she has been feeling in the previous 7 days, with there being 4 choices ranging from often to never. All items must be completed, and the mother must respond by herself unless she has limited English skills. The maximum score is 30. A score greater than 10 indicates risk for depression. A positive response to question 10,

---

Box 21-2. Sample Question From Edinburgh Postnatal Depression Scale

As you are pregnant or have recently had a baby, we would like to know how you are feeling. Please check the answer that comes closest to how you have felt IN THE PAST 7 DAYS, not just how you feel today.

Here is an example, already completed.

I have felt happy:

☐ Yes, all of the time.

☒ Yes, most of the time.

☐ No, not very often.

☐ No, not at all.

This would mean: "I have felt happy most of the time" during the past week. Please complete the other questions in the same way.

Modified with permission from Cox JL, Holden JM, Sagovsky R. Detection of postnatal depression. Development of the 10-item Edinburgh Postnatal Depression Scale. *Br J Psychiatry.* 1987;150: 782–786.

---

which asks about suicidality by itself, is considered a positive screen. The instrument is available in more than 40 languages. A third instrument is the Patient Health Questionnaire-9. Like the EPDS, the questionnaire includes 10 questions (9 questions and a follow-up question if any of the first 9 indicated any problems) related to the signs and symptoms of depression. The respondent notes whether the symptoms are present "not at all," "several days," "more than half the days," or "nearly every day." A score is then generated based on the mother's answers to assess her degree of depression. Mothers may be asked to complete these questions while in the waiting area.

Infants and Children

Infants and children may experience a number of problems as a consequence of maternal depression. These children may develop disorders of attachment, particularly insecure attachment, and they are at risk for the subsequent development of conduct or other behavior disorders. Language development may be adversely affected because depressed mothers speak fewer words and have fewer social interactions with their children. Maternal depression has also been associated with the decision not to breastfeed or the early cessation of breastfeeding. Classic environmental failure to thrive can be related to maternal depression and reduced mother-baby interactions. The effects of maternal depression can be detected in 2-month-old infants who regard depressed mothers less frequently, have poorer state regulation, interact with objects less frequently, and have lower levels of overall activity than infants of nondepressed mothers. These symptoms are attributed to the notions of the need for reciprocity between the mother and infant: mirror neurons, skill beget skill, and serve and return. The persistent absence of responsive care disrupts brain development. Long-term effects of maternal depression on child development have been demonstrated in magnetic resonance imaging of the brains of such children and increased cortisol levels at the time of school entry. Children are characterized as anxious, wary, and withdrawn. Social skills are noted to be poor. Early diagnosis and intervention may prevent the development of these problems.

Management

The major role of the pediatrician is to assist in the early identification of mothers who are experiencing perinatal mood and anxiety disorders and to make the appropriate referral for more definitive management. Support for this recommendation comes from a number of sources, including the 1999 and 2001 reports of the Surgeon General; *Bright Futures: Guidelines for Health Supervision of Infants, Children, and Adolescents;* the American Academy of Pediatrics (AAP) National Center for Medical Home Implementation; and AAP policies on family-centered care. Practices that include the presence of social workers or mental health specialists can avail themselves of these individuals to assess, counsel, and refer these mothers as appropriate. The mother may be referred back to her obstetrician for a visit prior to the 6-week checkup. Alternatively, mothers may be referred to local mental health specialists when such resources are known and available.

The pediatrician should also be familiar with the possible effects of psychotropic medications on the fetus and newborn and recommendations about these medications in relation to breastfeeding. The decision to initiate psychotropic medication during pregnancy is made by the obstetrician or psychiatrist caring for the mother. There is no antidepressant specifically FDA approved for use during pregnancy. All antidepressants cross the placenta and are never Category A (no risk). Animal studies reveal no teratogenic effects of these medications, and the treating physician has to balance the risks of untreated depression versus selected serotonin reuptake inhibitors (SSRIs). Paroxetine (Paxil) has been associated with abnormalities of the right ventricular outflow tract. There is an increased risk of a septal defect with the use of any SSRI. It is noted that the risk of preterm labor increases from 6% to 22% when SSRIs are used, but the risk of preterm labor with untreated maternal depression is 20%. Newborns who have been exposed to SSRIs may exhibit poor neonatal adaption or neonatal abstinence syndrome. Symptoms include respiratory distress, irritability, jitteriness, hypotonicity, poor latching and feeding, and, rarely, seizures. The incidence of persistent pulmonary hypertension increases from 1 to 6 in 1,000. Even if the mother is on an SSRI, she should be encouraged to breastfeed. There is the most experience with sertraline (Zoloft) and paroxetine (Paxil). Low levels of drug are detected in human milk but not in the newborn's blood.

There are a number of Internet sites that are very helpful in providing information about community resources. Postpartum Support International (www.postpartum.net; 800/944-4PPD [4773]) provides geographically specific information. The site can be accessed even while the mother is in the pediatrician's office. To get the needed information, go to the site, click on "get help," click on the map for the specific location, and click on an e-mail for the region, and a reply will arrive within 24 hours. It is also important to have an emergency protocol in place, such as calling 911 or a psychiatric emergency team, should a woman endorse suicidality while in the pediatrician's office. Having such resources and protocols in place

can go a long way toward reducing pediatricians' anxiety about screening for depression and suicidality.

Some perinatal programs offer home visitation or the use of doulas (women who support other women through labor, delivery, and after the birth of a baby in a nonmedical capacity), which assist mothers-to-be as well as recent mothers with the demands of birth and parenting. Such programs may offer a preventive and early intervention approach to peripartum depression by offering help and emotional support to new mothers.

When older children have been affected by maternal depression, there are other treatment modalities that focus on the mother and the child to help address attachment disorders. Research on these dyadic interventions has demonstrated they are associated with decreased psychiatric symptoms and significant improvement in functioning of the mother and the child. Internalizing and externalizing child behaviors are reduced when maternal depression, anxiety, or other conditions are addressed. Some programs include parent-child interactive therapy and parent-child psychotherapy. A program called Circle of Security involves video-based intervention that focuses on strengthening caregiver giving.

Prognosis

The prognosis for perinatal mood and anxiety disorders and their effects on newborns, infants, and children are contingent on early recognition and appropriate intervention. Promoting screening is critical to ensuring a positive outcome. Unfortunately, pediatricians still face barriers, which include the need to screen for a number of other conditions (eg, parental smoking, interpersonal violence), insufficient time, inadequate training, lack of appropriate resources, and lack of payment for services. A number of models have demonstrated that screening for perinatal mood and anxiety disorders can be successfully undertaken in a pediatric practice. The Assuring Better Child Health & Development project has been implemented in 28 states and involves the AAP chapters in those states. Pediatricians in Illinois can be paid through Medicaid if they administer the EPDS. *Bright Futures,* the health maintenance guidelines developed by the AAP and Health Resources and Services Administration, endorse assessing parental social and emotional well-being. Incorporating questioning into the well-child visits at 1, 2, 4, and 6 months is recommended and can be billed using *Current Procedural Terminology* code **99420**. Additional information about individual state initiatives can be found at www.nashp.org/abcd-resources (National Academy for State Health Policy).

CASE RESOLUTION

While many of this mother's symptoms are common, her self-assessment that she is unable to function suggests that she is experiencing postpartum depression rather than baby blues. You ask her if it is all right to contact her obstetrician to see if she could be seen sooner. She agrees. When you reach her obstetrician, she schedules the mom to come in the following morning. The obstetrician tells you she has a therapist in her office who will be able to meet with the mother at that time.

Selected References

Choi Y, Bishai D, Minkovitz CS. Multiple births are a risk factor for postpartum maternal depressive symptoms. *Pediatrics.* 2009;123(4):1147–1154

Earls MF; American Academy of Pediatrics Committee on Psychosocial Aspects of Child and Family Health. Incorporating recognition and management of perinatal and postpartum depression into pediatric practice. *Pediatrics.* 2010;126(5):1032–1039

Hanley GE, Oberlander TF. The effect of perinatal exposures on the infant: antidepressants and depression. *Best Pract Res Clin Obstet Gynaecol.* 2014;28(1):37–48

Mattocks KM, Skanderson M, Goulet JL, et al. Pregnancy and mental health among women veterans returning from Iraq and Afghanistan. *J Womens Health (Larchmt).* 2010;19(12):2159–2166

Olson AL, Dietrich AJ, Prazar G, Hurley J. Brief maternal depression screening at well-child visits. *Pediatrics.* 2006;118(1):207–216

Yonkers KA, Wisner KL, Stewart DE, et al. The management of depression during pregnancy: a report from the American Psychiatric Association and the American College of Obstetricians and Gynecologists. *Obstet Gynecol.* 2009;114(3):703–713

CHAPTER 22

Newborn Screening

Derek Wong, MD

CASE STUDY

A 1-week-old boy is brought to his pediatrician's office for a positive newborn screening test result for congenital adrenal hyperplasia. The baby was a product of a 38-week gestation and was born by normal spontaneous vaginal delivery to a 30-year-old gravida 2, para 2 woman with an unremarkable pregnancy. Birth weight was 3,300 g, and the baby is feeding and acting appropriately. Family history is unremarkable, and the physical examination is normal.

Questions

1. What are the proposed benefits of newborn screening?
2. Which newborn screening tests are most commonly performed?
3. How are the results of newborn screening tests reported to physicians?
4. How should a patient with an abnormal newborn screening result be managed?
5. What are the most common causes of false-positive and false-negative results?
6. What are the ethical issues and future challenges surrounding newborn screening?

Newborn screening programs are designed to identify neonates at risk for catastrophic outcomes from treatable illnesses. During the past 40 years, technologic advances such as tandem mass spectrometry have made it possible to test for more than 50 metabolic disorders from a single blood spot. New techniques in molecular biology allow for rapid diagnostic testing of conditions such as cystic fibrosis.

From the inception of newborn screening in the 1960s until 2005, each state chose a different set of conditions for its newborn screening program based on disease prevalence, cost, availability of treatment, and false-positive rate. In 2005, an expert panel from the American College of Medical Genetics and Genomics recommended 29 core disorders for which newborn screening was most effective (Table 22-1), as well as 25 secondary disorders that are in the differential diagnosis of a core disorder. In 2010, severe combined immunodeficiency (SCID) was added to the list of core disorders. By the end of 2013, all states offered testing for the 29 original core disorders, although screening for secondary disorders and SCID was variable. The full Recommended Uniform Screening Panel includes those disorders, hearing screening (covered in Chapter 76), and critical congenital heart disease, the testing of which by pulse oximetry was endorsed by the American Academy of Pediatrics (AAP) in 2011, and pilot projects have begun in several states. The availability of enzyme replacement therapy for lysosomal storage disorders has led to their inclusion in several state panels (Table 22-2).

Primary care physicians have 3 crucial roles in the newborn screening process. First, they provide education to parents about the newborn screening process. Second, they ensure that specimens are drawn under proper circumstances and that the results are promptly followed up. Finally, they provide medical follow-up and referral in positive cases. Physicians need to have contact information for state newborn screening programs and local pediatric subspecialists. The following Web sites link to contact information for these groups:

- State newborn screening programs: National Newborn Screening & Global Resource Center (http://genes-r-us.uthscsa.edu)
- Geneticists, metabolic and clinical: Society for Inherited Metabolic Disorders (www.simd.org) and American College of Medical Genetics and Genomics (www.acmg.net)
- Pediatric endocrinologists: Pediatric Endocrine Society (https://www.pedsendo.org)
- Pediatric hematologists: American Society of Pediatric Hematology/Oncology (www.aspho.org)
- Pediatric pulmonologists: Cystic Fibrosis Foundation (www.cff.org) (under Care Center Network)

Epidemiology

More than 4 million newborns are screened each year in the United States. The National Newborn Screening 2006 Incidence Report shows that as a result of newborn screening, 1 in 3,200 newborns were diagnosed with a metabolic disorder, 1 in 2,200 were diagnosed with congenital hypothyroidism, 1 in 2,200 were diagnosed with sickle cell disease or a related hemoglobinopathy, and 1 in 29,000 were diagnosed with congenital adrenal hyperplasia. Several disorders are more common in particular ethnic groups. For example, cystic fibrosis has an incidence of 1 in 2,500 in whites, and sickle cell disease has an incidence of 1 in 400 in African Americans.

Table 22-1. Core Newborn Screening Disorders[a]	
Disorder	*Possible Signs and Symptoms in Neonates[b]*
Organic Acid Disorders	
Glutaric aciduria type 1	Macrocephaly
Biotinidase deficiency	
Multiple carboxylase deficiency	
HMG-CoA lyase deficiency	Vomiting, lethargy, tachypnea
Cobalamin A, B deficiency	Seizures, coma, anion gap acidosis
Isovaleric aciduria	Hyperammonemia
Methylmalonic acidemia	Anemia, neutropenia, thrombocytopenia
Propionic acidemia	
3-methylcrotonyl-CoA carboxylase deficiency	
β-ketothiolase deficiency	Asymptomatic[c]
Fatty Acid Oxidation Disorders	
Medium-chain acyl-CoA dehydrogenase deficiency	Lethargy, coma, sudden death, hypo-ketotic hypoglycemia
	Reye-like syndrome
Very long-chain acyl-CoA dehydrogenase deficiency	Lethargy, coma, sudden death, hypo-ketotic hypoglycemia
Long-chain L-3-OH acyl-CoA dehydrogenase deficiency	Cardiomyopathy, arrhythmias
Trifunctional protein deficiency	Cholestasis, Reye-like syndrome
Carnitine uptake defect	Asymptomatic[c]
Amino Acid Disorders	
Maple syrup urine disease	Poor feeding, vomiting, lethargy, seizures, coma, maple syrup odor
Citrullinemia	Hyperammonemia, vomiting, seizures, lethargy, coma
Argininosuccinic aciduria	
Tyrosinemia type 1	Hepatomegaly, increased PT/PTT, liver failure, boiled cabbage odor
Homocystinuria	Asymptomatic[c]
Phenylketonuria	Asymptomatic
Hemoglobinopathies	
Sickle cell disease (HbS)	Dactylitis
Sickle β-thalassemia	Asymptomatic[c]
Hemoglobin C sickle cell disease	
Other	
Congenital hypothyroidism	Umbilical hernia, enlarged fontanelle, macroglossia, jaundice
Congenital adrenal hypertrophy	Virilization in females; salt-wasting crisis
Galactosemia	Cataracts, jaundice, poor feeding, sepsis
Cystic fibrosis	Meconium ileus, intestinal obstruction
Severe combined immunodeficiency	Recurrent infections

Abbreviations: HMG, 3-hydroxy-3-methylglutaryl; CoA, coenzyme A; PT, prothrombin time; PTT, partial thromboplastin time.

[a]Most of these conditions may not be asymptomatic outside of the neonatal period.

[b]Many neonates with these disorders are completely asymptomatic.

[c]*Asymptomatic* covers the first month of life and does not exclude very rare case reports of neonatal presentation.

Clinical Presentation

Most neonates with disorders detected by newborn screening are clinically asymptomatic in the first 2 weeks of life, but the remainder may have significant signs and symptoms (see Table 22-1). The presence of such features may lead to a more urgent workup or hospitalization. Unfortunately, severe forms of some metabolic disorders may cause coma and encephalopathy by 48 hours of age. In these cases, newborn screening results are critical, for they will suggest a probable diagnosis and allow early optimization of therapy.

Table 22-2. Additional Disorders Screened in Individual States[a]
Amino Acid Disorders, Organic Acid Disorders
5-oxoprolinuria (pyroglutamic aciduria)
Carbamoyl phosphate synthetase deficiency
Ethylmalonic encephalopathy
Hyperornithinemia-hyperammonemia-homocitrullinuria syndrome (HHH syndrome)
Hyperprolinemia
Methylene-tetrahydrofolate reductase deficiency
Nonketotic hyperglycinemia
Ornithine carbamoyltransferase deficiency
Lysosomal Storage Diseases
Fabry disease
Gaucher disease
Glycogen storage disease type 2 (Pompe disease)
Hunter syndrome (MPS 2)
Hurler syndrome (MPS 1H)
Krabbe disease
Niemann disease types A and B
Hemoglobinopathies
Glucose-6-phosphate-dehydrogenase deficiency
Infectious Diseases
HIV
Toxoplasmosis

Abbreviation: MPS, mucopolysaccharidosis.

[a]This list may not reflect current practice. Some of the testing is in a pilot phase and may not be accurate or specific.

Differential Diagnosis

While newborn screening techniques are continually improved, false-positive and false-negative errors occur. Mislabeled specimens, technical errors, and reporting errors can occur in any laboratory. Any specimen collected before 12 hours of age is at risk for a false-negative metabolic result or a false-positive hypothyroidism result. Premature newborns have a reduced metabolic capacity and therefore exhibit higher metabolite levels and increased false-positive results compared with term newborns. Anemia or polycythemia can affect the amount of serum per blood spot and increase false-negative results, and transfusion may alter galactosemia and hemoglobinopathy testing. Neonates on hyperalimentation may have increased amino acid and lipid levels, especially if the newborn screen is drawn from a central line. To ensure accurate and uniform testing, it is imperative to communicate relevant clinical information to the state newborn screening office.

Newborn Screening Practices

Parental Education and Consent

All parents should be informed of the state screening program at the prenatal visit or during the initial newborn examination. Written materials that explain the screening program are available from the state screening office, and online materials explaining abnormal results are available on fact sheets at Web sites such as http://pediatrics.aappublications.org/cgi/content/full/118/3/e934. Health care practitioners are responsible for educating parents on the method for obtaining the blood specimen, risks and benefits of screening tests, conditions to be screened, and implications of positive results.

It is important to tell parents that positive results do not necessarily mean that their newborn has a particular disorder; the results must be confirmed by more specific tests. In addition, parents should know that disorders in some children are missed because of sampling errors, faulty testing, or inadequate accumulation of the abnormal metabolite at the time of testing.

Newborn screening is mandatory in all states, although many states allow exemptions for religious beliefs or other reasons. In most states, parents have given informed consent if practitioners have discussed the state-mandated program with them and they have agreed to participate. A few states require signed consent to opt into the newborn screening program, and several more require consent to disclose identifiable information. Physicians should document parental refusal regardless of state laws.

Specimen Collection and Handling

Proper specimen collection and handling are essential components of a successful screening program. All newborns should be screened before discharge from the hospital, ideally between 48 to 96 hours of age. Early screening increases the chance of a false-negative metabolic result or a false-positive hypothyroidism result. For this reason, some states have a mandatory second screen between 1 and 6 weeks of age, while others require a second screen only if the first screen is obtained before a specified time (12–48 hours depending on the state). Late screening increases the sensitivity of metabolic testing but also increases the chances for a delay in diagnosis of life-threatening conditions such as galactosemia. If possible, blood samples should be obtained prior to any transfusions or dialysis. Otherwise, screening tests should still be performed as outlined previously, and arrangements should be made to have them repeated at an appropriate time. It is likely that guidelines that recommend screening premature or sick newborns at birth, 48 to 72 hours, and 28 days/discharge will be considered for implementation into state newborn screening programs in the near future.

Only a few drops of blood are needed for each disk on the filter paper, but the sample must saturate the paper evenly. The use of needles and glass capillary tubes for blood collection is discouraged because they may cause hemolysis or micro-tears in the filter paper. Specimens must be individually air-dried in a horizontal position, thus avoiding contamination and excessive exposure to heat. They should be mailed to the laboratory within 24 hours of collection. Inadequate specimen collection and handling can lead to test inaccuracies, delays in reporting results to physicians, and unnecessary repetition of screening tests. Therefore, all individuals who are involved in the newborn screening process should adhere strictly to the procedures set forth by their state program.

Reporting of Results

In most states, all results of neonatal screening tests, whether normal or abnormal, are reported to the physician of record. Normal results are mailed to the physician for placement in the patient's medical record. Abnormal results are usually reported by telephone or letter, depending on the severity of the potential condition. Results are also sent to the hospital where the neonate was born for inclusion in the medical record. The physician of record is responsible for contacting parents about the need for confirmatory testing and, if necessary, referral to an appropriate subspecialist. If a newborn is no longer under the care of this physician or if the family cannot be located, state and local public health departments can be called on to assist in the search for the newborn and family.

Diagnostic and Therapeutic Considerations

A health care team consisting of a primary care physician and staff, state newborn screening office personnel, state newborn screening laboratory, local laboratories, and subspecialty physician is responsible for care and follow-up of patients with positive newborn screening results. All newborns with abnormal results, whether borderline or clearly significant, should be evaluated by their primary care physician. A complete history and physical examination as well as a family history should be obtained. Abnormal results for some newborn screening tests, such as very long-chain acyl–coenzyme A (CoA) dehydrogenase deficiency, may normalize with a second screen. Therefore, most follow-up evaluation centers on targeted diagnostic tests. Depending on the nature of the suspected disorder, initiation of treatment before confirmatory laboratory results are known may be appropriate. For example, prophylactic antibiotics should be administered if sickle cell anemia is suspected. After confirmatory results have been received, the treatment can be modified or halted.

Potentially life-threatening conditions in the newborn period, such as galactosemia, maple syrup urine disease, and congenital adrenal hyperplasia, are particularly important to evaluate and treat emergently. Depending on the clinical picture, suspected disorder, and experience of the physician, telephone consultation with a specialist or immediate referral to a regional medical center may be necessary.

Nearly all of the diseases in the current newborn screening panel are inherited in an autosomal recessive manner. Families of affected newborns should be offered genetic counseling for future pregnancies, in addition to written information about the newly diagnosed condition. Depending on the condition, older siblings may need to be evaluated. In some conditions, such as 3-methylcrotonyl-CoA carboxylase deficiency, a positive newborn screen result may reflect an affected asymptomatic mother whose metabolites have passed to her newborn.

Current Issues and Future Challenges

Protecting patient privacy is of the utmost importance, and nearly all programs have laws to protect a patient's personal information, blood spots, and genetic information. There is great concern among parents and physicians that insurance companies will use newborn screening information to discriminate against children and their families.

There is no dispute that newborn screening saves lives. Additionally, the cost of newborn screening programs is outweighed by the reduction in morbidity and mortality from a purely economic standpoint. However, some diseases under consideration for newborn screening, such as lysosomal storage disorders, have extremely costly treatments that may total several million dollars over the lifetime of the patient and produce significant morbidity. Cost-benefit analysis will be crucial to shaping future newborn screening panels. Pediatricians and other health care professionals need to advocate for insurance coverage for newborn screening panels because patients may be charged more than $100 for testing.

Currently, a large percentage of false-positive results occur in premature neonates, in part due to the lack of age-specific laboratory values for all metabolites. In several states, a lack of appropriate cutoff values led to a large number of false-positive results among babies in neonatal intensive care units that strained the state programs. In the future, careful pilot testing of new tests in newborns of all gestational ages will be needed to improve the screening process.

There is debate about the benefit of early detection of disorders such as cystic fibrosis. While recent studies have suggested that patients benefit from early therapy, it is unclear how much early detection improves the long-term pulmonary or nutritional status of affected children. Some disorders, such as short-chain acyl-CoA dehydrogenase deficiency, are asymptomatic in most individuals and have a high rate of false-positive tests because of the presence of common polymorphisms in the population. The lifelong treatment of patients who would otherwise remain asymptomatic, the added burden of a genetic diagnosis, and family stress caused by a false- or true-positive result have led several countries to remove this disorder from their newborn screening panels. Fortunately, there has been a large amount of progress made in reducing false-positive results using new algorithms for second-tier testing.

Several newborn screening tests detect asymptomatic carrier status in newborns. While the knowledge of a patient's carrier status may be of some advantage for childbearing, it has no immediate benefit for the newborn and may lead to discrimination and stigmatization. Parents of affected newborns (who are usually asymptomatic carriers) face the same dilemma and should be given the option to refuse testing for carrier status.

New challenges will emerge as genetic technology advances toward the ultimate goal of sequencing a patient's entire genome. Practitioners will have to weigh the decision of whether to inform parents about non-treatable or late-onset conditions. The AAP Committee on Bioethics advises against screening for such conditions, but the debate has been reopened as testing for spinal muscular atrophy has been developed. Finally, some conditions that are caused by a complex interaction between genetics and environment, such as celiac disease, may require screening at school age. Pediatricians should be involved in decisions concerning the addition of new disorders to existing newborn screening programs because they are key players in the implementation of these programs.

CASE RESOLUTION

The patient in the case study at the beginning of the chapter should have a full evaluation, including an electrolyte panel, due to the possibility of salt-wasting congenital adrenal hyperplasia. Confirmatory testing, including measurement of precursor hormones such as 17-hydroxyprogesterone and subsequent molecular testing, and glucocorticoid therapy should be considered in consultation with a pediatric endocrinologist.

Selected References

American Academy of Pediatrics Committee on Bioethics. Ethical issues with genetic testing in pediatrics. *Pediatrics*. 2001;107(6):1451–1455

American Academy of Pediatrics Section on Cardiology and Cardiac Surgery Executive Committee. Endorsement of Health and Human Services recommendation for pulse oximetry screening for critical congenital heart disease. *Pediatrics*. 2012;129(1):190–192

American College of Medical Genetics and Genomics. ACMG *ACT Sheets* and confirmatory algorithms. https://www.acmg.net/ACMG/Resources/ACT_Sheets_and_Confirmatory_Algorithms/ACMG/Resources/ACT_Sheets_and_Confirmatory_Algorithms/ACT_sheets_Homepage.aspx?hkey=1654e248-53f2-41a9-8d93-f3d96de05e0a. Accessed February 20, 2014

Hewlett J, Waisbren SE. A review of the psychosocial effects of false-positive results on parents and current communication practices in newborn screening. *J Inherit Metab Dis*. 2006;29(5):677–682

Kaye CI; American Academy of Pediatrics Committee on Genetics. Introduction to the newborn screening fact sheets. *Pediatrics*. 2006;118(3):1304–1312

Kaye CI; American Academy of Pediatrics Committee on Genetics. Newborn screening fact sheets. *Pediatrics*. 2006;118(3):e934–e963. http://www.pediatrics.aappublications.org/cgi/content/full/118/3/e934. Accessed February 20, 2014

Matern D, Oglesbee D, Tortorelli S. Newborn screening for lysosomal storage disorders and other neuronopathic conditions. *Dev Disabil Res Rev*. 2013;17(3):247–253

Sun A, Lam C, Wong DA. Expanded newborn screening for inborn errors of metabolism: overview and outcomes. *Adv Pediatr*. 2012;59(1):209–245

CHAPTER 23

Caring for Twins and Higher-Order Multiples

Sabrina D. Diaz, MA, MMFT, and Lynne M. Smith, MD

CASE STUDY

An expectant mother visits you. She has been advised by her obstetrician that an ultrasound shows she is pregnant with twins. She asks about care of twins and what special considerations she should keep in mind as she looks forward to the delivery. In particular, she is concerned about the feeding schedule and whether she will be able to breastfeed.

Questions

1. What is the incidence of multiple births?
2. What is the difference between fraternal and identical twins?
3. What major medical problems may affect twins and higher-order multiples?
4. What developmental and behavioral problems are associated with raising multiples?

With the advent of artificial reproductive therapy, the incidence of twins and higher-order multiples is increasing. Counseling the parents of multiples provides a unique opportunity for pediatricians. Much of what is known about caring for multiples comes from work with twins. Many societies have been fascinated with twins, and many myths and superstitions surround their birth. Some people believe that a mother of twins must have been unfaithful to her husband because a father cannot sire 2 children. Native Americans of the Iroquois nation believed that one twin was good and the other was evil. To prevent the recurrence of twins, the Khoikhoi removed one of the father's testicles.

Parents of multiples often have many questions about the care of their children, but they rarely pose them to health care professionals. In one study in which 18 out of 29 mothers breastfed their twins, only 3 received information about breastfeeding from their physicians. One mother had been told by her obstetrician that she could not breastfeed her twins. Physicians should become knowledgeable about caring for multiples and the unique challenges they present to parents related to feeding, sleeping, and behavior.

Epidemiology

Since 1980, there has been a 101% increase in twin deliveries in the United States, and the number of higher-order multiples has increased 5-fold. Twin rates have also increased in Finland, Norway, Austria, Sweden, Australia, Hong Kong, Japan, Canada, Singapore, and Israel. A major contributor to the increase in multiple births is that women are starting their families later than in previous generations. Between 1980 and 2006, twin birth rates increased 190% for mothers who were 40 years or older. Because of the increased risk of infertility with advanced maternal age, more couples are choosing to conceive with assisted reproductive technologies, including ovulation-stimulating drugs, in vitro fertilization (IVF), and intracytoplasmic sperm injection. As of 2009, assisted reproductive technology resulted in multiple gestations in approximately 50% of pregnancies and accounted for 20% of all multiple births nationwide. Forty-seven percent of newborns conceived from assisted reproductive technology are multiple-gestation births, compared with only 3% of newborns nationwide. Single embryo transfer has lower success rates than multiple embryo transfer, increasing the likelihood of multiple births. In addition, advanced maternal age is associated with increased follicle-stimulating hormone levels and the release of multiple eggs by the ovary, increasing the chance of multiple births.

The overall natural incidence of twin births is about 32 in 1,000. Twins account for just slightly more than 1% of all births, and 20% of neonates born at fewer than 30 weeks' gestation are twins. The average incidence of monozygotic or identical twins, which is the same for all women regardless of race and age, is about 1 in 300 births. The incidence of dizygotic or fraternal twins varies among different groups and method of conception. In the United States, African Americans and whites have comparable incidences of liveborn twin deliveries, and both have significantly higher rates than Hispanic women. A maternal family history of dizygotic twins correlates most strongly with an increased incidence of twins. A family history of monozygotic twins or a paternal family history of dizygotic twins does not increase the risk of twins.

Pathophysiology

Higher-order multiples, conceived naturally or via artificial reproductive technology, may be fraternal or a combination of monozygotic twins and fraternal siblings. Monozygotic twins result from the splitting of a single egg. They may share a placenta (monochorionic, figures 23-1A and 1B) and, in rare cases, may also share an amniotic sac (monoamnionic). When splitting occurs early (after several cell divisions of the zygote), each fetus develops its own chorion and amnion, leading to dichorionic and diamnionic placentas. Dizygotic twins result from 2 eggs, with each egg fertilized by a different sperm. Dizygotic twins have 2 placentas (Figure 23-1C). Although these placentas may fuse together like 2 pancakes, they are almost always dichorionic and diamnionic (Figure 23-1D). Ultrasound at 14 weeks or sooner has been found to be 96% predictive of monochorionic twins and can also predict monoamnionic twins, anomalies, and syndromes.

Following birth, many parents want to determine whether twins are monozygotic or dizygotic. Different-sex twins are almost always dizygotic, although monozygotic twins of different sexes have been reported in the literature. This occurs when one twin loses a Y chromosome and becomes a phenotypic female with Turner syndrome (XO). Occasionally the male twin may be XXY and have Klinefelter syndrome.

To determine whether twins are monozygotic or dizygotic after birth, a number of procedures can be undertaken. Visual or pathologic examination of the placenta is helpful. About two-thirds of monozygotic twins have a common chorion and share one placenta. Finding a single chorion usually means the twins are monozygotic, unless the placentas of dizygotic twins have fused together. DNA testing is the preferred method for determining zygosity. Most commercially available testing, often referred to as zygosity testing, involves examining DNA obtained from buccal swabs from each child. Identification of short tandem repeats via polymerase chain reaction is typically accurate 99% of the time and is similar to techniques used in forensic medicine. Commercial laboratory charges range from $100 to $200, though prices vary significantly depending on the company and whether zygosity is being tested for twins or higher-order multiples.

Recent research on monozygotic twins has also focused on the effect of epigenetics, or how the environment affects genetics. By analyzing the DNA of monozygotic twins, researchers are hoping to identify epigenetic tags that mark a change in gene expression. Although DNA cannot be altered, DNA methylation, which affects the strength of gene expression, may be a process that in the future can be manipulated to reverse some complex disorders, such as autism spectrum disorder.

Differential Diagnosis

Diagnosing multiples is not difficult, but physicians should be aware of the problems these newborns may experience.

Perinatal Complications

Multiple births are associated with a significantly higher risk for perinatal complications relative to singleton births. The maternal complication most commonly reported with multiples is pregnancy-induced hypertension. Maternal preeclampsia rates are higher in twins and increase nearly 5-fold with triplets. In addition, mothers of twins who conceived via IVF have a higher rate of preeclampsia than mothers of twins who conceived naturally. Other maternal complications include placenta previa, antepartum hemorrhage, gestational diabetes mellitus, anemia, uterine atony, and maternal death.

Neonatal mortality is 4-fold higher in twins and 15-fold higher in higher-order multiples. Neonatal morbidity is much higher in multiple births because of the increased incidence of prematurity and growth restriction. The risk for these complications increases with the number of fetuses. The perinatal mortality of monozygotic twins is 8 times that of singletons and 4 times that of dizygotic twins. Twins and higher-order multiples are also at increased risk for cerebral palsy.

Monozygotic twins are at greater risk for death and cerebral palsy because of complications such as severe birth weight discordance and twin transfusion syndrome (TTS). Twin transfusion syndrome is seen in 10% to 15% of monochorionic pregnancies and results from unbalanced blood flow due to vascular anastomoses within the shared placenta. The diagnosis is suspected by ultrasound when one fetus is growth restricted with oligohydramnios and the other fetus has evidence of volume overload with polyhydramnios. Both twins are ultimately at risk to become hydropic or die. Without treatment, TTS-induced death of at least one twin is as high as 80% to 100%. Of additional concern, the death of one twin is associated with neurologic damage or subsequent death of the surviving twin, with 1 in 10 surviving twins developing cerebral palsy.

Until recently, treatment was drainage of amniotic fluid in the twin with polyhydramnios to reduce the risk of preterm delivery. Endoscopic laser ablation of placental anastomoses has emerged as the treatment of choice for severe TTS pregnancies diagnosed and treated prior to 26 weeks' gestation. Laser ablation addresses the primary pathology and results in an average gestation at delivery of 33 weeks, which is a significant improvement from the average

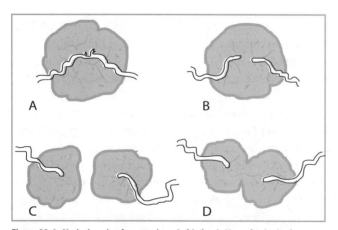

Figure 23-1. Variations in placentas in twin births. A, Monochorionic placenta, cords close together. B, Monochorionic placenta, cords farther apart. C, Dichorionic placentas, separate. D, Dichorionic placentas, fused.

29 weeks with serial amniotic fluid reductions. Laser ablation is not without risks, however; reported complications include premature rupture of membranes, amniotic fluid leakage into the maternal peritoneal cavity, vaginal bleeding, and chorioamnionitis.

One percent of monozygotic twins are monochorionic–monoamnionic. Although monoamnionic twins have a lower risk of TTS, they are at very high risk for cord accidents. Monoamnionic pregnancies are monitored closely, and once the fetuses reach viability, emergent delivery is indicated if fetal distress is noted to avoid fetal death. Because fetal death significantly increases the risk of cerebral palsy and other neurologic disorders in the surviving twin, it is no longer recommended to allow fetal death in one monoamnionic twin to lengthen the gestation of the non-distressed twin.

Congenital Malformations

Twins and higher-order multiples have an increased risk of anomalies. Monochorionic twins have a higher risk of cardiac anomalies than dichorionic twins, increasing their need for fetal echocardiograms. Multiples conceived via IVF or intracytoplasmic sperm injection have increased risk for anomalies and aneuploidy. Disorders of genetic imprinting (eg, Beckwith syndrome, Angelman syndrome) are also increased with intracytoplasmic sperm injection. These genetic complications are thought to be secondary to the underlying cause of infertility instead of artificial reproductive technologies. Because the costs associated with infertility treatments are substantial, many couples choose not to obtain a comprehensive chromosomal analysis looking for deletions or translocations on themselves prior to using reproductive technologies. Nuchal translucency and chorionic villus sampling can be used to detect and confirm suspected aneuploidy as early as the first trimester. Chorionic villus sampling is not widely available and ranges from $1,000 to $2,000; however, many insurance companies will cover the procedure in women older than 35 years or with risk factors that may increase the baby's likelihood of having a serious health problem.

In addition to increased risks for malformations, multiples are at risk for deformations secondary to crowding, including torticollis, hip dislocation, plagiocephaly, and foot deformities. Monochorionic twins are also at risk for becoming conjoined twins, estimated to occur in 1 in 50,000 to 200,000 gestations, with more than 50% dying in utero or stillborn and 35% dying within the first 24 hours. Although monochorionic twins are more common in males, conjoined twins are often female. Conjoining occurs because of incomplete splitting of the embryo or after a secondary fusion between 2 previously separate embryos. Prenatal ultrasound is commonly used to diagnose this condition; more recently, prenatal magnetic resonance imaging has been used to evaluate specific anomalies. Due to surgical advances, some parents continue the pregnancy with hopes the live-born neonates can be separated.

Postnatal Complications

Approximately 60% of twins and 90% of triplets are born prematurely, increasing the risk of morbidity and mortality. Though growth in twins tends to be normal until 30 to 34 weeks' gestation, growth restriction is commonly associated with multiple births. Twins conceived by IVF are more likely to be born at a low birth weight than spontaneously conceived twins. Smaller twins have an increased incidence of hypoglycemia in the newborn period and have higher rates of targeted learning deficits and school failures during childhood. In addition, children born with growth restrictions have an increased risk for obesity and diabetes in later life. Selective intrauterine growth restriction (IUGR), when only one twin is affected by IUGR, occurs in 10% of monochorionic twins. This occurs when the twin with IUGR has reversed flow or persistent absent flow in the umbilical artery.

Evaluation

History

A general medical history should be obtained, including a history of the pregnancy. Any specific medical complaints should also be addressed (Questions Box).

Physical Examination

The initial evaluation of newly born twins involves assessment of gestational age and determination of the presence of any medical problems or anomalies (see Chapter 20). Older twins may undergo health maintenance visits at which routine as well as specific complaints are addressed.

Laboratory Tests

Newborns should be assessed for the presence of anemia or polycythemia with a hemoglobin determination. Hypoglycemia may occur in the newborn period and should be assessed frequently until glucose levels are stable. If the twins are premature, they may have many of the problems seen in preterm newborns, such as neonatal respiratory distress syndrome and necrotizing enterocolitis.

Older children should receive an appropriate evaluation for age, with a specific focus on any behavioral concerns.

Management

The focus of the management of multiples involves counseling parents about issues related to routine care and anticipated stress of caring for more than one newborn simultaneously. Parents often care for 2 or more children at the same time, but multiples present unique issues related to multiple children who are developmentally and chronologically at the same point. Many parents experience anxiety

Questions

Caring for Twins

- Did the mother have any problems during the pregnancy?
- How long did the pregnancy last?
- Did the mother take any medications, including fertility drugs?
- Did the children have any problem after the delivery or in the newborn nursery?

about the upcoming challenges they will face. Baby care books that specifically deal with birthing and raising multiples are available. Support groups and Web sites also provide information for families of multiples.

Feeding multiple newborns is often an exhausting challenge for parents, and consultation with a lactation expert is recommended. The physical demands of feeding multiple newborns are often compounded by women recovering from prenatal complications such as preeclampsia. Because prematurity is common, newborns may have an immature suck reflex, making feeding more challenging. Few multiples are still exclusively breastfed by 4 months of age, and common reasons cited for unsuccessful breastfeeding of multiples include maternal stress, depression, fatigue, perceiving they were producing insufficient milk, and time burden. Despite these obstacles, parents should know that breastfeeding is possible even for triplets and understand the benefits of breastfeeding to the newborns' health. It is recommended that mothers begin breastfeeding as soon as possible to establish their milk supply. If supplemental nutrition is needed, utilizing a medicine dropper, syringe, spoon, cup, or finger feeding instead of a bottle will reduce the risk for newborns developing a preference for an artificial nipple.

Some options for breastfeeding twins are as follows:

1. Feed both babies at the same time, with one on each breast. This method is recommended only after adequate breastfeeding has been established in each twin, typically not until after 1 week of age. It is advised that the baby having fewer problems latching be placed on the breast first so that the milk ejection reflex is already established for the poorer-feeding baby. Because the babies may not drink the same amount, it is important that they feed on the opposite breast for the next feeding to maximize milk production.

   Babies may be put in a number of positions. The mother can be sitting and cradling (across the chest) one baby while holding the other like a football. Alternatively, the mother may cradle both babies so that they are cross-positioned over one another with their legs make an X across the mother's lap, or she may have both under her arms in a football position. Breastfeeding pillows designed for feeding multiples are helpful, and electric breastfeeding pumps are essential.

2. Feed the babies at different times. The mother breastfeeds one and then the other, starting with the more vigorous feeder. This approach may pose a problem; both babies may be hungry at the same time and maternal fatigue may inhibit success because the chance for sleep is diminished with this method. Some mothers prefer this method because it provides individualized attention and opportunities for attachment with each baby.

3. Breastfeed one baby and bottle-feed the other, which gives the mother a free hand. Most parents use a combination of breastfeeding and bottle-feeding. A mother can let the first baby feed on demand but wake up the second one when the first one is done. Eighty percent of parents of twins acknowledge that they prop the bottle instead of holding it, and they should be counseled against this. There are several effective feeding positions

that do not require bottle propping, and parents should be encouraged to adopt one of these positions.

Breastfeeding triplets and higher-order multiples is even more challenging than breastfeeding twins. Mothers of triplets exclusively breastfeeding report they feed 2 babies, one on each breast, and the third follows on both breasts. Because the hind milk has higher fat content, it is important to rotate the feeding order of the babies. Another popular option is to breastfeed 2 and have the third bottle-feed simultaneously.

Feeding twins or higher-order multiples may decrease the amount of sleep a mother gets. Because sleep deprivation is associated with maternal depression and exclusively breastfeeding mothers of multiples report more sleep problems compared with mothers who do not breastfeed or who formula-feed and breastfeed, these factors should be discussed when offering feeding options to parents. Encouraging paternal involvement with feeding may alleviate some maternal stress and sleep deprivation.

Sleeping in the same crib is no longer recommended because of concerns about co-sleeping. It is important to counsel parents about **car safety seats.** Parents who cannot afford the cost of multiple car safety seats may resort to placing one baby in the car safety seat and the others on the seat of the car, a dangerous practice that is illegal throughout the United States. Parents should be advised about the need for car safety seats for all babies.

Bathing should be done separately in the interest of safety until babies can sit up.

Toilet training is reportedly easier with some twins because one twin learns from the other via modeling or peer pressure.

Maintenance of individuality for multiples may be challenging. Researchers suggest that mothers can bond to only one newborn at a time, a concept called monotropy. In addition, mothers bond more strongly with the twin who leaves the hospital first. Twins are often dressed alike and given similar names because this may facilitate the bonding process. To help with individual development, physicians are encouraged to obtain history and examine each child individually. Physicians should attempt to distinguish the children from one another independent of parental reminders. Twins should not be referred to as "the twins" but by their respective names. As multiples get older, issues related to classrooms and birthday parties frequently arise, and they should be consulted concerning their preferences. Individual birthday parties and gifts should be considered. (Some multiples comment on their disappointment at receiving the same present for birthdays and holidays. There is no surprise in opening gifts if the other twin opened a gift first.)

Whether multiples should be placed in the same or different classrooms is unclear. Placement in different classrooms is advocated to support each child's individual development. However, there are no data to support separate classroom placement with regard to social development or decreasing problem behaviors. Researchers have investigated the effect of separate classes in a longitudinal study and also found no difference in educational achievement between twins who share classrooms and those in separate classrooms. It is currently recommended that school districts have a flexible policy addressing school placement of twins. A checklist has been created to assist families and schools in determining the best school placement for twins (www.twinsandmultiples.org/dloads/school_checklist.pdf). Families with higher-order multiples are more likely to have children in separate schools because of the higher risk that some of the children will have developmental delays.

Sibling rivalry is common among co-multiples as well as other siblings within a family. Older siblings may resent the attention paid to the new babies, so family and friends should be reminded to shower attention on the older siblings. Because twins often exclude siblings and peers socially, parents are encouraged to schedule times when one twin and sibling are with one parent and the other twin is alone with another family member. Isolating twins (or 2 triplets from a third) fosters more sibling interaction and less dependency between the twins. These separations are encouraged to begin early in development because the later in development isolation is introduced, the less agreeable multiples are to the separations.

Developmental differences among multiples may also contribute to sibling rivalry. The smaller or more delayed child may become jealous of their co-multiple. Conversely, typically developing children may become frustrated when the sibling with special needs receives more attention than they receive.

Until age 3 years, **language development** is delayed in twins relative to singletons. A contributing factor to language delay is less time for individual facilitated play, which is helpful for language development. If twins communicate with a private language, they have an increased risk of language and cognitive delays. Language delays usually become much less pronounced by mid-childhood.

The risk for **cerebral palsy** is increased with higher multiples because of the increased rates of prematurity and IUGR. Fetal death of a co-multiple and monochorionic placentas are the biggest risk factors for developing cerebral palsy.

Attention-deficit/hyperactivity disorder is more common in twins. The temper tantrums multiples display can be severe and are understandable given the heightened need to gain parental attention from their sibling. Having twins in the home is a risk factor for **child abuse,** either to a twin or to their siblings.

Prior to delivery, parents should be made aware that **maternal depression** is frequently reported after the birth of multiples. The physical stress of caring for multiple newborns can be overwhelming, and parents often feel isolated at home. The incidence of depression is higher in mothers of twins than of singletons, with sleep deprivation being a cited contributing factor. It is important to suggest that parents of multiples obtain outside aid, including help from high school students after school and family members, to decrease fatigue and increase their ability to experience respite even for short periods.

In addition to exhaustion and isolation, the increased financial demands that accompany multiple newborns can strain the parents' relationship. Mothers often have to leave work earlier in the pregnancy than women with singleton pregnancies, adding financial burden. The medical costs associated with prematurely delivered newborns can be substantial. To cover for the loss of income at a time of increasing family expenses, the father is often required to work more hours. This increased occupational stress comes at a time when child care demands at home have increased significantly. Financial burdens are especially difficult with multiples conceived artificially because of the cost associated prior to birth. This may be a contributing factor to why parents of twins conceived artificially reported less satisfaction than parents of twins conceived naturally.

Grief is another significant contributor to parental depression. Approximately 15% of children from multiple births grow up as a singleton survivor. Birthday celebrations serve as reminders to the parents of the death of the other child. Parents grieving the loss of one of their twins have comparable grief to those grieving the loss of a singleton pregnancy. It is imperative that physicians caring for the family acknowledge the parents' grief because family and friends often do not acknowledge the parents' pain if there is a surviving newborn.

Surviving children born prematurely or small for gestational age are at increased risk for developmental delays. The stress of raising a child with special needs is also a source of grief because parents mourn the loss of their dreams of having a normal child.

Prevention

Regardless if conceived naturally or via artificial reproductive technology, it is impossible to guarantee singletons or higher-order multiples. Nonetheless, a maternal family history of dizygotic births increases the likelihood of high-order multiples. Artificial reproductive technology often results in higher-order multiples. However, the number of embryos implanted via artificial reproductive technology has decreased following high-profile births of grand multiples that highlighted the financial difficulties placed on families, as well as the increased risk for developmental delays in the children.

Prognosis

Although multiples have a higher incidence of perinatal problems, appropriate anticipatory guidance and routine health maintenance can help families optimize their children's outcome.

Resources for Parents

Baby Center: www.babycenter.com

Center for Loss in Multiple Birth: www.climb-support.org

Luke B, Eberlein T. *When You're Expecting Twins, Triplets, or Quads: Proven Guidelines for a Healthy Multiple Pregnancy.* 3rd ed. New York, NY: HarperCollins Publishers; 2011

MOST (Mothers of Supertwins): http://MOSTonline.org

Multiples of America: www.nomotc.org

Neifert M. *Dr. Mom's Guide to Breastfeeding.* New York, NY: Penguin Group; 1998

CASE RESOLUTION

The mother in the case scenario is advised that breastfeeding is not only possible but recommended. She is told about the options for timing and positioning of the newborns. The issues of family history and child passenger safety are also discussed, and anticipatory guidance on the potential stress of raising multiples is given.

Selected References

Chauhan SP, Scardo JA, Hayes E, Abuhamad AZ, Berghella V. Twins: prevalence, problems, and preterm birth. *Am J Obstet Gynecol*. 2010;203(4):305–315

Cowan JM, Demmer LA. Assisted reproductive technology and preimplantation genetic diagnosis: impact on the fetus and newborn. *NeoReviews*. 2007;8(3):e127–e132

Flidel-Rimon O, Shinwell ES. Breast feeding twins and high multiples. *Arch Dis Child Fetal Neonatal Ed*. 2006;91(5):F377–F380

Hansen M, Kurinczuk JJ, Bower C, Webb S. The risk of major birth defects after intracytoplasmic sperm injection and in vitro fertilization. *N Engl J Med*. 2002;346(10):725–730

Hay DA, Preedy P. Meeting the educational needs of multiple birth children. *Early Hum Dev*. 2006;82(6):397–403

Klock SC. Psychological adjustment to twins after infertility. *Best Pract Res Clin Obstet Gynaecol*. 2004;18(4):645–656

Martin JA, Hamilton BE, Ventura SJ, Osterman MJK, Wilson EC, Matthews TJ. Births: final data for 2010. *National Vital Statistics Reports*. 2012;61:1–71

Martino D, Loke YJ, Gordon L, et al. Longitudinal, genome-scale analysis of DNA methylation in twins from birth to 18 months of age reveals rapid epigenetic change in early life and pair-specific effects of discordance. *Genome Biol*. 2013;14(5):R42

Miller P. A thing or two about twins. *National Geographic*. 2012;1:1–6

Moore JE. Q&A's about multiple births. *Contemp Pediatr*. 2007;24:39–55

Pharoah PO, Dundar Y. Monozygotic twinning, cerebral palsy and congenital anomalies. *Hum Reprod Update*. 2009;15(6):639–648

Polderman TJ, Bartels M, Verhulst FC, Huizink AC, Van Beijsterveldt CE, Boomsma DI. No effect of classroom sharing on educational achievement in twins: a prospective, longitudinal cohort study. *J Epidemiol Community Health*. 2010;64(1):36–40

Shinwell ES, Haklai T, Eventov-Friedman S. Outcomes of multiplets. *Neonatology*. 2009;95(1):6–14

Siegel SJ, Siegel MM. Practical aspects of pediatric management of families with twins. *Pediatr Rev*. 1982;4:8–12

Sutcliffe AG, Derom C. Follow-up of twins: health, behaviour, speech, language outcomes and implications for parents. *Early Hum Dev*. 2006;82(6):379–386

Thorpe K. Twin children's language development. *Early Hum Dev*. 2006;82(6):387–395

CHAPTER 24

Circumcision

Nwando Eze, MD, and Lynne M. Smith, MD

CASE STUDY

An expectant mother visits you prenatally. She talks about circumcision in addition to issues relating to breast-feeding and car passenger safety. Her husband is circumcised. She is unclear about the medical indications for circumcision and asks your opinion about circumcision in the newborn period.

Questions

1. What are the benefits of circumcision?
2. What are the indications for circumcision in older children?
3. What are the techniques used to perform circumcision?
4. What are the complications of circumcision?

Male circumcision, a procedure in which the foreskin of the penis is removed, has been performed for more than 4,000 years. It is routinely performed in certain groups, most notably among Jewish and Muslim people. In many other cultures (eg, Abyssinian, Australian [aborigine], Polynesian), circumcision is presumably performed to facilitate intercourse. Circumcision can be viewed as a ritual procedure, but its role as a medical one has long been an area of controversy.

The benefits of male circumcision have been debated for years. Over the past 20 years, even the American Academy of Pediatrics (AAP) has changed its official position on the medical indication for circumcision. The AAP stated in 1999 and reaffirmed in 2005 that there were potential benefits to circumcision, though the procedure was not medically indicated. However, in 2012, the AAP released an updated policy stating that the health benefits of circumcision outweigh the risks of the procedure. This statement was based on a systematic evaluation of peer-reviewed literature that demonstrated preventive health benefits of elective male circumcision, including reductions in the risk of urinary tract infections (UTIs) in the first year of life, decreased risks of heterosexual acquisition of HIV and other sexually transmitted infections (STIs), and a decreased incidence of penile cancer. Additionally, the statement noted that male circumcision does not adversely affect penile sexual function/sensitivity or sexual satisfaction and that complications related to circumcision are infrequent and rarely severe.

Disadvantages of routine circumcision in newborns include cost-effectiveness and the risk of complications. The procedure is sometimes criticized as an archaic and maiming ritual. Female circumcision, which may involve clitoridectomy or resection and closure of the labia minora or majora, is infrequently practiced in Western culture and is not discussed here. *There are no medical benefits attributable to female circumcision.*

Circumcision in newborns has been performed in a routine and preventive manner, much the same way immunizations are administered. Primary care physicians should be aware of the risks and benefits of the procedure to be able to counsel parents and make referrals to consultants when certain medical conditions arise.

Epidemiology

The prevalence of neonatal circumcision, a procedure that became increasingly popular in the United States in the 1950s and 1960s, once ranged from 69% to 97% depending on cultural mores. In the United States, the procedure is commonly performed during the newborn period. Changing cultural patterns have resulted in a lower frequency of circumcision—down to 57% in 2008—which reflects, in part, state Medicaid programs no longer covering circumcision. Rates also vary by race, religion, and geographic region. In 2008, the circumcision rate in the western United States was 30%, compared with 74% in the Midwest, 67% in the Northeast, and 61% in the South. The higher Hispanic birth rate in the West contributes to these regional differences because Hispanic neonates are less likely to receive a circumcision. The estimated prevalence of circumcision for Australian-born men is 59% (newborn rate estimated 10%–20%); in Canada, 32%; and in the United Kingdom, 15%. Circumcision is the second most common surgical procedure after vasectomy in adult males. It is the most commonly performed operation in male children.

A reported 10% of uncircumcised males ultimately require circumcision as adults because of complications of phimosis and balanitis. Uncircumcised males with diabetes are particularly prone to these complications.

Clinical Presentation

Most often, parents will query their child's pediatrician about the advisability of a circumcision, and the newborn will not have any clinical symptoms. Older infants and children in need of a circumcision can present with symptoms of phimosis, in which the foreskin balloons out on urination; paraphimosis, in which a retracted foreskin cannot be returned to its normal position; or recurrent problems of infection or inflammation of the foreskin (posthitis), glans (balanitis), or both (balanoposthitis).

Pathophysiology

In uncircumcised males, the foreskin adheres to the glans until about age 6 years. A gradual, normal lysing of the adhesive bands connecting the foreskin to the under-portion of the glans then occurs. Nonphysiological phimosis occurs as a result of scarring of the preputial wing. Lysing of adhesions in an effort to treat the phimosis usually leads to further adhesions. If the foreskin is retracted and remains in that position, paraphimosis develops.

Differential Diagnosis

The differential diagnosis relates to conditions that may be managed with a circumcision, including phimosis, paraphimosis, and infection and inflammation of the penis. Conditions such as hypospadias may be mistaken for a partially circumcised penis because the condition is associated with absence of the ventral foreskin. A careful history will differentiate hypospadias from a circumcision.

Evaluation

History

In cases involving newborns, history should include the presence of any coagulopathies involving family members, which would preclude the performance of a circumcision. In older infants and children, history should include problems relating to voiding, such as ballooning of the foreskin or difficulty initiating the urinary stream.

Physical Examination

The physical examination should assess the genitalia, particularly to determine if there is evidence of hypospadias, in which the urethral orifice is not located at the tip of the glans. In such a situation, circumcision should be delayed because the foreskin is used to reconstruct the urethra. In cases of phimosis, the degree of phimosis should also be assessed.

Laboratory Tests

Routine laboratory tests are not indicated, although a urinalysis may be obtained in children with a history of prior UTI. Coagulation studies would be appropriate if there is a family history of a bleeding disorder.

Imaging Studies

Imaging studies are not indicated in most children undergoing circumcision. Such studies would be relevant if there was concern that the urogenital anatomy was abnormal.

Prognosis

The prognosis is excellent with complications being exceedingly rare.

Benefits

It has been stated that circumcision facilitates penile hygiene by removing the foreskin, which may serve as a repository for bacteria, smegma, and dirt. Ability to retract the foreskin increases with age (Table 24-1); thus, penile hygiene is easier to achieve in older children. The term **phimosis** refers to inability to retract the foreskin. In male infants beyond the newborn period, phimosis is the major indication for circumcision. Phimosis is normal in children up to about 6 years of age but is non-physiological if urination results in ballooning of the foreskin, regardless of age. When the retracted foreskin acts as a tourniquet in the mid-shaft of the penis, **paraphimosis** occurs, preventing the return of lymphatic flow. Paraphimosis is commonly related to traumatic retraction of the foreskin, typically during cleaning or by medical personnel during bladder catheterization. Because of this, parents are no longer advised to retract the foreskin in an effort to lyse adhesions. The incidence of paraphimosis is increasing in adults secondary to body piercing. Newly placed penile rings can cause enough pain to prevent foreskin retraction.

Balanitis, or inflammation of the glans, is not uncommon in infants. It is frequently associated with *Candida* infection, and the glans is swollen and erythematous. Posthitis, or inflammation of the foreskin, is also often secondary to *Candida* infection. Other organisms, including gram-negative microbes, may be associated with balanitis. The presence of recurrent balanitis is an indication for circumcision. In older males, indications for circumcision include phimosis, paraphimosis, balanitis, posthitis, and balanoposthitis.

Urinary tract infections reportedly occur 10 times more often in uncircumcised (1:100) than circumcised infants (1:1,000). In young uncircumcised boys, UTIs are directly related to colonization of the foreskin with urotoxic organisms. Pyro-nephritogenic, fimbriated *Escherichia coli* bind to the inner lining of the foreskin within the first few days of life. Other bacteria preferentially bind to this mucosal surface, including fimbriated strains of *Proteus mirabilis* and non-fimbriated *Pseudomonas, Klebsiella,* and *Serratia* species. Multiple studies have demonstrated an increased incidence of UTIs as the rate of circumcision has decreased. A 2012 meta-analysis of 22 studies examining the incidence of UTIs in males found a 23% lifetime risk of UTI in uncircumcised males versus 8.8% in circumcised males. Thus, the lifetime risk of UTI

Table 24-1. Ability to Retract the Foreskin in Boys (by Age)	
Age	*Percentage With Retractable Foreskin*
Birth	4%
6 mo	15%
1 y	50%
3 y	80%
6 y	90%

significantly exceeded the 1.5% circumcision complication rate, the majority of these complications being minor. Complications associated with UTIs, particularly bacteremia, meningitis, and subsequent death, have occurred.

In Western countries, penile cancer is reported in 0.7 to 0.9 per 100,000 men but is as great as 4.2 per 100,00 men in Paraguay. These regional differences are thought to be related to lack of circumcision of the penis. Only a few isolated cases of cancer of the penis occur in circumcised men. The estimated lifetime risk of penile cancer is 1 in 600 in uncircumcised males compared with 1 in 50,000 to 1 in 12 million in circumcised males. From 1930 through 1990, 10,000 men died from penile cancer; there were 1,280 new cases found in 2007 with 290 deaths. The reported mortality of invasive penile cancer is 25%. Phimosis is strongly associated with invasive penile cancer, with other cofactors such as human papillomavirus (HPV) infection and poor hygiene possibly contributing. Smoking is consistently associated with penile cancer and is further reason to strongly advocate for smoking cessation programs.

Cervical carcinoma among the partners of uncircumcised men has been reported with increased incidence. In addition, current partners of circumcised men with a history of multiple sexual partners have a decreased risk of cervical cancer compared with partners of uncircumcised men. Circumcision in adolescent boys and men in Uganda found a significantly decreased incidence of HPV and human herpesvirus 2 infection. Circumcision has also been associated with a lower risk of HIV infections. Three randomized, controlled trials conducted in South Africa, Kenya, and Uganda confirmed findings in observational studies that circumcision is protective against HIV infection. In addition, circumcision was not associated with increased HIV risk behavior. Based on these findings, in 2007 the World Health Organization stated that male circumcision should be part of a comprehensive strategy for HIV prevention. It remains critical, however, to promote the practice of safe sex, as circumcision confers only partial protection from HPV, human herpesvirus 2, and HIV.

Risks

Risks related to circumcision are related to complications from the procedure (Box 24-1) and discussed under "Management" on page 136. It should be noted that elective circumcision should be performed only if the newborn is stable and healthy.

Box 24-1. Complications Associated With Circumcision	
Bleeding	Inclusion cysts
Infection	Penile lymphedema
Repeat circumcision	Urethrocutaneous fistulae
Phimosis	Penile cyanosis
Skin bridges	Penile necrosis
Urinary retention	Wound dehiscence
Meatitis	

Parent Counseling

Parents of Newborns

In the newborn period, proper counseling of parents, including a discussion of the risks and benefits of circumcision, is important. Opponents to neonatal circumcision cite psychologic trauma to neonates from so painful a procedure. Local anesthesia minimizes this effect. Parents should be informed about the benefits of circumcision, including a reduction in occurrence of UTIs, STIs, and cancer of the penis and cervix. Problems related to the foreskin itself, such as phimosis, paraphimosis, posthitis, and balanitis, should also be discussed.

It is appropriate to tell parents that boys who are not circumcised in the neonatal period may need to be circumcised later in life. Parents should be informed about the risks associated with circumcision in newborns, which are discussed in greater detail on page 136. In older individuals, risks include hemorrhage, infection, and injuries to the penis and urethra. In addition, parents should be told that approximately 2% of circumcised neonates require a second circumcision due to inadequate foreskin removal.

Research has shown that parents are more influenced by the circumcision status of the father, religion, and race than by physician attitude concerning their ultimate decision about circumcision. The 2012 AAP policy statement emphasizes that parents should consider health benefits and risks in light of their own religious, cultural, and personal preferences, as the medical benefits alone may not outweigh these other considerations for individual families. Counseling during the second trimester of pregnancy results in no change in parents' decision about circumcision. Parents of newborn boys should be instructed in care of the penis at the time of discharge from the newborn hospital stay, whether or not the newborn is circumcised.

Parents of Infants and Older Children

The need for circumcision in male infants who present with UTIs is problematic. Evaluation usually tries to determine the existence of other predisposing conditions that could lead to the UTI. Investigators disagree on the need for circumcision following an initial UTI in uncircumcised boys. No clear-cut evidence indicates that circumcision at this time decreases the incidence of future UTIs, so the decision is parental rather than medical. In children who present with significant phimosis or paraphimosis, circumcision is usually recommended to prevent recurrences of these problems. Medical management, including the use of topical steroids for phimosis, may obviate the need for surgery in some children. Such treatment involves the daily external application of betamethasone cream from the foreskin tip to the corona glandis for 4 to 6 weeks. History, including the duration of symptoms and whether the child has had similar episodes in the past, helps formulate appropriate management.

Management

The medical attitude toward circumcision has changed over the last 40 years, with an initial inclination toward circumcision, followed by a move away from circumcision. The present position on circumcision as described by the AAP Task Force on Circumcision suggests that newborn circumcision has potential medical benefits and advantages as well as disadvantages and risks. When circumcision is considered, benefits and risks should be explained to parents, and informed consent should be obtained. Parents should be advised that the frequency with which third-party payers pay for circumcisions, particularly for routine circumcisions in the newborn period, has decreased. However, Kacker and colleagues have recently published an economic model justifying Medicaid coverage of circumcision in the United States that may lead to changes in payment for circumcision.

Contraindications

Circumcisions should only be performed in completely healthy neonates. Contraindications to circumcision are well defined. Any abnormalities of the penis, such as hypospadias, absence of any portion of the foreskin, or chordee, preclude circumcision. Ambiguous genitalia and prematurity are contraindications. Circumcision should be delayed in premature and ill term newborns until they are ready for discharge. Patients with a personal or family history of bleeding diathesis should not be circumcised. Newborns from such families should be assessed for evidence of coagulation problems. If these are present, circumcision should not be carried out.

Circumcision Procedure

Numerous techniques are used to perform circumcisions. These procedures may involve clamp techniques with Gomco, Mogen, or Plastibell clamps. Any of these techniques is believed to give comparable results in the hands of trained, experienced operators. Formal surgical excision may also be carried out, usually in older children and adults. Three guidelines should be followed to decrease the incidence of complications: marking of the coronal sulcus in ink, dilation of the preputial wing, and retraction of the foreskin so that the urethral meatus is visualized. This prevents cutting the meatus. Electrocautery should never be used in conjunction with metal clamps because of the danger of extensive injury.

Appropriate anesthesia in newborns undergoing circumcision is the standard of care. The pain and stress of circumcision is evidenced by changes in neonate state and behavior. Non-pharmacologic techniques such as positioning and sucrose pacifiers are insufficient to prevent procedural pain but may be used in conjunction with other forms of analgesia. Local anesthesia is the preferred method of pain management. Dorsal penile nerve block, the subcutaneous injections of local anesthetic at the base of the penis, is effective at reducing pain responses during circumcision. Ring block, the subcutaneous circumferential injections of a local anesthetic around the mid-shaft of the penis, has also been shown to be effective and avoids the potential complication of injecting local anesthesia toward the dorsal vessels. Topical application of lidocaine/prilocaine cream (eg, EMLA) or oral sucrose solution on a pacifier also reduces pain and its associated stress but to a lesser extent than local anesthesia. For older, prepubertal children requiring formal surgical excision, suture-less circumcision using tissue glues has been associated with reduced operative time and an improved cosmetic result.

Complications

A number of complications are associated with circumcision in newborns (Box 24-1). The most common complication is **bleeding**, which may occur in 0.2% to 8% of cases. Bleeding can usually be controlled using local pressure. More significant bleeding may require local pressure with 1:1,000 adrenaline-soaked gauze or with the use of other topical agents such as Surgicel. The second most frequently seen complication is **infection**, reported in up to 8% of circumcised newborns. Plastibell clamps are associated with a higher incidence of infection than Gomco clamps. Most infections usually respond to local treatment, although intravenous antibiotics should be considered because neonatal sepsis and necrotizing fasciitis may occur secondary to infections following circumcision.

Poor cosmetic outcome is also a complication of circumcision. **Phimosis** may occur if removal of the foreskin is insufficient. If the foreskin is inadequately freed up from the inner preputial epithelium, a concealed penis, with the shaft retracted backward into the abdominal wall, may develop. **Skin bridges** may form between the glans and shaft, leading to accumulation of smegma or tethering of the erect penis. Most post-circumcision adhesions are reported to resolve at the time of puberty with the onset of masturbation or sexual activity.

In the immediate postsurgical period, urinary retention may occur secondary to tight surgical bandages. This complication can be prevented by applying local pressure rather than tight bandages to obtain hemostasis. Meatitis and meatal ulcers possibly caused by irritation from ammonia or damage to the frenulum artery at the time of circumcision have been reported in circumcised males. Inclusion cysts that represent implantation of smegma are also seen. Additional injuries following circumcision may include penile lymphedema, urethrocutaneous fistulae secondary to misplaced sutures, penile cyanosis, and necrosis secondary to tight Plastibell clamps. Wound dehiscence, which involves separation of the penile skin from the mucous membrane, and denudation of the penile shaft may occur more frequently with Gomco clamps than Plastibell.

> ### *CASE RESOLUTION*
>
> The risks and benefits of circumcision should be discussed with the mother. The father should be encouraged to participate in the decision-making process.
>
> If the parents elect not to have their son circumcised, they should be instructed on the appropriate care of the uncircumcised penis, which involves gentle external washing without retraction of the foreskin.

Selected References

Alanis MC, Lucidi RS. Neonatal circumcision: a review of the world's oldest and most controversial operation. *Obstet Gynecol Surv.* 2004;59(5):379–395

American Academy of Pediatrics Task Force on Circumcision. Circumcision policy statement. *Pediatrics.* 2012;130(3):585–586

American Academy of Pediatrics Task Force on Circumcision. Male circumcision. *Pediatrics.* 2012;130(3):e756–e785

Anderson JE, Anderson KA. What to tell parents about circumcision. *Contemp Pediatr.* 1999;16:87–103

Binner SL, Mastrobattista JM, Day MC, Swaim LS, Monga M. Effect of parental education on decision-making about neonatal circumcision. *South Med J.* 2002;95(4):457–461

Brady-Fryer B, Wiebe N, Lander JA. Pain relief for neonatal circumcision. *Cochrane Database Syst Rev.* 2004;(4):CD004217

Castellsagué X, Bosch FX, Muñoz N, et al. Male circumcision, penile human papillomavirus infection, and cervical cancer in female partners. *N Engl J Med.* 2002;346(15):1105–1112

Dubrovsky AS, Foster BJ, Jednak R, Mok E, McGillivray D. Visibility of the urethral meatus and risk of urinary tract infections in uncircumcised boys. *CMAJ.* 2012;184(15):E796–E803

Fergusson DM, Boden JM, Horwood LJ. Circumcision status and risk of sexually transmitted infection in young adult males: an analysis of a longitudinal birth cohort. *Pediatrics.* 2006;118(5):1971–1977

Gee WF, Ansell JS. Neonatal circumcision: a ten-year overview: with comparison of the Gomco clamp and the Plastibell device. *Pediatrics.* 1976;58(6):824–827

Kacker S, Frick KD, Gaydos CA, Tobian AA. Costs and effectiveness of neonatal male circumcision. *Arch Pediatr Adolesc Med.* 2012;166(10):910–918

Kim HH, Li PS, Goldstein M. Male circumcision: Africa and beyond? *Curr Opin Urol.* 2010;20(6):515–519

Lane V, Vajda P, Subramaniam R. Paediatric sutureless circumcision: a systematic literature review. *Pediatr Surg Int.* 2010;26(2):141–144

Merrill CT, Nagamine M, Steiner C. *Circumcisions Performed in U.S. Community Hospitals, 2005.* Rockville, MD: Agency for Healthcare Research and Quality; 2008. HCUP Statistical Brief #45. http://www.hcup-us.ahrq.gov/reports/statbriefs/sb45.pdf. Accessed October 16, 2013

Minhas S, Manseck A, Watya S, Hegarty PK. Penile cancer—prevention and premalignant conditions. *Urology.* 2010;76(2 Suppl 1):S24–S35

Morris BJ, Wiswell TE. Circumcision and lifetime risk of urinary tract infection: a systematic review and meta-analysis. *J Urol.* 2013;189(6): 2118–2124

Schoen EJ. Ignoring evidence of circumcision benefits. *Pediatrics.* 2006;118(1):385–387

Tobian AA, Serwadda D, Quinn TC, et al. Male circumcision for the prevention of HSV-2 and HPV infections and syphilis. *New Engl J Med.* 2009;360(13):1298–1309

Van Howe RS. Is neonatal circumcision clinically beneficial? Argument against. *Nat Clin Pract Urol.* 2009;6(2):74–75

Warner L, Cox S, Kuklina E, et al. Updated trends in the incidence of circumcision among male newborn delivery hospitalizations in the United States, 2000-2008. Paper presented at: National HIV Prevention Conference; August 26, 2011; Atlanta, GA

CHAPTER 25

Nutritional Needs

Jonnie Burton-Mota, MD

CASE STUDY

At a routine health maintenance visit, a mother asks if she may begin giving her 4-month-old daughter solid foods. The infant is taking about 4 to 5 oz of formula every 3 to 4 hours during the day (about 32 oz per day) and sleeps from 12:00 am to 5:00 am without awaking for a feeding. Her birth weight was 7 lb (3,182 g), and her present weight and length (13 lb [5,909 g] and 25" [63.5 cm], respectively) are at the 50th percentile for age. The physical examination, including developmental assessment, is within normal limits.

Questions

1. What are some of the parameters that may be used to decide when infants are ready to begin taking solid foods?
2. Up to what age is human milk or infant formula alone considered adequate intake for infants?
3. At what age do infants double their birth weight? At what age do they triple their birth weight?
4. What problems are associated with the early introduction of solid foods?

Good nutrition is essential for normal growth and development. The physician plays an important role not only in assessing the growth of children but also in counseling parents about the nutritional needs of maturing children. The primary care physician should be knowledgeable about key nutritional concepts for children, including normal growth patterns and assessment of the child's nutritional status, changing nutritional requirements and feeding patterns from infancy through adolescence, and common feeding and nutritional disorders.

Growth Patterns and Nutritional Requirements of Normal Children

Monitoring the growth and nutritional status of infants and children is an integral component of well-child care. The average normal expected increases in weight, height, and head circumference for the first several years of life are listed in Table 25-1.

The energy and nutritional requirements of children vary with age. Postnatal growth is most rapid during the first 6 to 12 months of life; hence, caloric and protein needs are very high at this time. The average daily energy and protein needs of children from birth to 18 years of age are presented in Table 25-2.

On average, newborns weigh 7.7 lb (3.5 kg), are about 20 inches (50 cm) long, and have a head circumference of 14 inches (35 cm). They lose about 5% to 10% of their birth weight during the first several days of life and usually regain this weight by the age of 10 to 14 days. During the first several months of life, weight gain serves as an important indicator of infants' general well-being. Failure to gain weight during this time may be a clue to a wide variety of problems, ranging from underfeeding to malabsorption. Newborns and infants gain about 30 g/day (roughly 1% of their birth weight per day) for

the first 3 months of life and about 10 to 20 g/day for the rest of the first year. Infants double their birth weight by 6 months of age and triple their birth weight by 12 months of age. Children aged 2 years to puberty gain ~2 kg/year (4.4 lb/year). On average, children weigh

Table 25-1. Normal Expected Increase in Weight, Height, and Head Circumference of Newborns, Infants, and Children

Normal Weight Gain	
Age	Expected Weight Increase
0–3 mo	25–35 g/d
3–6 mo	12–21 g/d
6–12 mo	10–13 g/d
1–6 y	5–8 g/d
7–10 y	5–11 g/d
Normal Height Increase	
Age	Expected Height Increase
0–12 mo	10"/y (25 cm/y)
13–24 mo	5"/y (12.5 cm/y)
2 y–puberty	2.5"/y (6.25 cm/y)
Normal Increase in Head Circumference	
Age	Expected Increase in Head Circumference
0–3 mo	2 cm/mo
4–6 mo	1 cm/mo
7–12 mo	0.05 cm/mo
Total increase	12 cm in first y

Table 25-2. Energy and Protein Needs of Children

Age (y)	Calories (kcal/kg/d)	Protein (g/kg/d)
0–1	90–120	2.5–3.0
1–7	75–90	1.5–2.5
7–12	60–75	1.5–2.5
12–18	30–60	1.0–1.5

about 10 kg at 1 year of age, 20 kg at 5 years of age, and 30 kg at 10 years of age. A rough rule of thumb that can be used to estimate the expected weight of a child based on age is $2 \times$ age (years) $+ 10 =$ weight (kg). A prepubertal child who does not gain at least 1 kg/year should be monitored for nutritional deficits.

Infants and young children grow about 10 inches (25 cm) during the first year of life, 4 inches (10 cm) during the second year, and 3 inches (7.5 cm) during the third and fourth years. School-aged through preadolescent children grow approximately 2.5 inches/year. This is followed by another growth spurt, the prepubertal-pubertal growth spurt. Girls grow 3 to 4 cm every 6 months and boys grow 5 to 6 cm every 6 months during this period.

Feeding Patterns of Infants and Children

Liquid Foods

Human breast milk is generally recommended as the exclusive nutrient for newborns and infants during the first 6 months of life and then could continue with complementary foods through 12 months of age. However, there are situations in which breastfeeding is not possible for the mother or is contraindicated because of a disease or medication. Therefore, although breastfeeding is the most advantageous for mother and baby and should be encouraged, mothers should never be made to feel inadequate or guilty if they are unable to breastfeed. Human milk or an iron-fortified infant formula provides complete nutrition for infants during the first 4 to 6 months of life. During the first month or 2 of life, newborns and infants take about 2 to 3 oz of formula (approximately 10 minutes on each breast) every 2 to 3 hours.

Because human milk is more easily digested than formula, it passes out of the stomach in 1½ hours; formula may take up to 4 hours. Therefore, during the first 4 to 6 weeks of life, breastfed newborns want to feed more frequently (8–12 times in 24 hours) than formula-fed newborns (6–8 times in 24 hours), with an increased number of nighttime feedings as well. By about 3 to 5 months of age, breastfed and bottle-fed infants do not differ in the number of nighttime feedings, although some breastfed infants continue to wake out of habit.

Most infants 6 months or younger consume about 4 to 5 oz per feeding every 4 to 5 hours. Under routine circumstances, human milk is preferred to infant formulas because it has emotional, nutritional, and immunologic advantages. Breastfeeding allows infants and mothers to develop a unique relationship that can be emotionally satisfying (see Chapter 26).

The composition of human milk varies over time. Colostrum, the first milk produced after delivery, is high in protein, immunoglobulin (Ig), and secretory IgA. Colostrum gradually changes to mature milk 7 to 10 days after delivery. The nutrient content of human milk of mothers who deliver preterm compared with those who deliver at term may vary considerably. Individual assessment may be necessary to determine the appropriateness of human milk for preterm newborns.

Nutritionally, human milk is uniquely tailored to meet the specific needs of babies. Human milk provides approximately 20 kcal/oz, the same as routine infant formulas. Table 25-3 compares the composition of human milk and several infant formulas. Human milk has relatively low amounts of protein compared with cow's milk (1% vs 3%), yet the levels are sufficient to provide for satisfactory

Table 25-3. Composition of Human Milk and Select Infant Formulas (Calories: 20 kcal/oz)

Formula	Protein	Carbohydrate	Fat
Human milk (mature)	40% casein and 60% whey	Lactose	Human milk fat
Cow's milk	80% casein and 20% whey	Lactose	Butterfat
Enfamil with LIPIL	Nonfat cow's milk and whey	Lactose	Palm olein, soy, coconut, and high-oleic sunflower oils; DHA, ARA
Similac Advance	Nonfat cow's milk and whey	Lactose	High-oleic safflower oil, coconut and soy oils, DHA, ARA
Enfamil ProSobee	Soy protein and methionine	Corn syrup solids	Palm olein, soy, coconut, and high-oleic sunflower oils
Similac Soy Isomil	Soy protein and methionine	Corn syrup solids and sucrose	High-oleic safflower oil, soy and coconut oils; DHA, ARA
Nutramigen with LIPIL	Casein hydrolysate, cystine, tyrosine, tryptophan	Corn syrup solids and cornstarch	Palm olein, soy, coconut, and high-oleic sunflower oils; DHA, ARA
Pregestimil with LIPIL	Casein hydrolysate, cystine, tyrosine, tryptophan	Corn syrup solids, modified cornstarch, and dextrose	MCT, high-oleic safflower and soy oils, DHA, ARA
Similac Expert Care Alimentum	Casein hydrolysate, cystine, tyrosine, tryptophan	Sucrose modified tapioca starch	Safflower oil, MCT, soy oil, DHA, ARA

Abbreviations: ARA, arachidonic acid; DHA, docosahexaenoic acid; MCT, medium-chain triglycerides.

growth of babies. Protein content is highest at birth at 2.3 g/dL, then declines over the first month to 1.8 g/dL, yet it ensures adequate protein status throughout the first year of life.

Qualitative differences also make human milk more desirable. Casein-whey ratio in human milk is about 30:70, making it easier to digest than most infant formulas, which tend to have higher casein-whey ratios at 82:18. Whey is more easily digested and associated with faster gastric emptying compared with casein. Newborns and infants that breastfeed tend to digest their milk more easily, have softer stools, and be less satiated overnight, requiring more feeds, than those fed formula. Other whey proteins such as IgA, lysozyme, and lactoferrin all contribute and help host defenses.

Lactose is the major carbohydrate of human and cow's milk, but it is present in higher concentrations in human milk. Lactose in human milk also contributes to softer stool consistency with non-pathologic fecal flora and improved absorption of minerals. Oligosaccharides in human milk found in the carbohydrate polymers and glycoproteins have been structurally shown to mimic bacterial antigen receptors and may have a role in host defense. Fat is the primary source (50%) of calories in human milk. The fat in cow's milk, which contains primarily saturated fatty acids, is not as well digested by newborns and infants as human milk fat, which is predominantly composed of polyunsaturated fats. Within the last decade, the long-chain polyunsaturated fatty acids docosahexaenoic acid (DHA) and arachidonic acid (ARA) have been added to most infant formulas to simulate the higher levels found in human milk. Although research suggests that DHA and ARA supplementation may enhance vision and improve growth and cognitive development in formula-fed infants, the exact degree of effect remains unclear.

Human milk from well-nourished women should provide adequate amounts of all vitamins and other micronutrients. However, vitamin K, vitamin D, iron, and fluoride are not present in sufficient quantities to satisfy all nutritional needs over a prolonged period, and supplementation should be considered. The American Academy of Pediatrics recommends that all newborns receive a prophylactic dose of 0.5 to 1 mg of parenteral vitamin K in the immediate newborn period to help prevent bleeding disorders. Even though the vitamin D content of human milk is low compared with cow's milk, newborns and infants of healthy mothers have generally not been observed to develop rickets if there is sufficient exposure to sunlight. Newborns require about 1 minute of exposure to sunlight on the face to produce enough vitamin D. However, adequate sun exposure is difficult to assess, and there are increasing concerns about the harmful effects of sunlight. Compared with the previous recommendation of an average intake of 200 IU of vitamin D per day, the 2010 Institute of Medicine recommendation calls for an average intake of 400 IU of vitamin D per day to meet the needs of most infants younger than 12 months. Although human milk contains less iron than iron-fortified formulas (fortified to about 12 mg/L of iron), the bioavailability of the iron in human milk is greater. Breastfed infants do not need iron supplementation until 6 months of age. Exclusively breastfed infants and infants who are fed ready-to-eat formulas or formulas prepared with bottled water may need supplementation with 0.25 mg of fluoride per day if they develop dental caries and parents are not first using fluorinated tap water. Giving all infants older than 6 months fluoride is no longer recommended because of increased fluorosis (see Chapter 28).

Human milk has several immunologic advantages, which are allergy and infection protective, over standard cow's milk–based formulas. Its allergy-protective characteristics are attributed, in part, to the decreased intestinal permeability associated with human milk compared with standard formulas. The host defense factors present in human milk include Ig, complement, and cellular components (eg, macrophages, neutrophils, lymphocytes). Studies have shown that the incidences of viral and bacterial illnesses are lower in exclusively breastfed infants compared with their formula-fed peers.

Breastfeeding is the recommended method of infant feeding during the first 6 months of life, but it is not always possible and is occasionally contraindicated. Although maternal infection is usually not a contraindication to breastfeeding, maternal HIV infection is one exception to this recommendation in the United States. This is not necessarily true, however, in many developing countries, where the risk of death during the first year of life without breastfeeding is greater than the risk of HIV infection. Antibiotics are generally safe during breastfeeding, but certain other drugs are contraindicated.

Solid Foods

Supplemental foods may be added to infants' diets between the ages of 4 to 6 months. Solid foods should be introduced as soon as infants require the additional calories and are developmentally mature (eg, infant can sit and support his or her head). Early introduction of solid foods has been associated with an increased incidence of food allergy and may contribute to overeating and obesity. Factors that indicate infants may be ready for solid foods include current weight twice that of birth weight, or about 13 lbs; consumption of more than 32 oz of formula per day (if on a formula only diet); frequent feeding (regularly more than 8–10 times per day or more often than every 3 hours); and persistent dissatisfaction due to hunger.

The quantity of formula should be limited to no more than 32 oz to allow for the introduction of solid foods. An iron-fortified infant cereal, most commonly rice cereal because it does not contain gluten, is usually the first solid food offered to infants. Other single-grained cereals, such as barley cereal or oatmeal, are also appropriate early supplemental foods. It is not unusual for infants to reject their first several spoonfuls of cereal because the tastes and textures are new. If they refuse the feeding, it should be stopped. Solid foods should be reintroduced in 1 week. Fruits and vegetables may be introduced within a few weeks. The order is not as important as the need to add only one new food at a time and no more than 1 to 2 new foods per week. Meats may be introduced after 6 months of age.

Although commercially prepared infant juices are an important source of vitamin C and may provide a smooth transition to solid foods, excessive juice intake may be associated with dental caries, diarrhea, growth failure, and increased sugar with little to no nutritious value. About 2 oz of water or apple juice can be given at 4 to 6 months of age as needed to loosen stools in those infants who are constipated. This can be gradually increased to about 4 oz/day. Once infants have accepted the juice, juice can be mixed with a small quantity of cereal and offered to infants with a spoon. Solid foods should not be mixed in the bottle; caregivers should wait until the infant can accept spoon feedings. The vitamin C in juice increases the bioavailability of the iron in the cereal.

Precooked infant cereals, such as rice cereal, can be mixed with a variety of liquids, including human milk, formula, water, or infant fruit juices. Initially, the cereal should be mixed to a thinner consistency (eg, about 1 tablespoon of cereal to 2 oz of liquid); once infants have accepted the new taste and texture, the mixture should gradually be worked to a thicker consistency. By about 7 to 8 months of age, infants should be taking 4 to 6 tablespoons of cereal mixed with enough liquid to give the mixture the consistency of mustard. Mixed cereal grains may be given to older infants.

A wide variety of commercially prepared baby foods designed to be developmentally appropriate and labeled by stage (ie, first, second, third) are available. The jars of different stages contain the amount of food that an infant at a given age should be able to eat at one sitting. This is not always the case, however, and opened jars of baby food may safely be stored in the refrigerator for 2 to 3 days. Infants should not be fed directly from the jar because saliva on the spoon mixes with the remaining food and digests it, causing it to liquefy. Vegetables and meats may be offered at room temperature but should be warmed slightly for greater palatability. Fruits and desserts may be at room or refrigerator temperature. Home-cooked fruits and vegetables should be thoroughly washed, pureed, and strained before giving to infants. Home-prepared foods tend to have a shorter shelf life than commercially bought baby foods because of lack of preservatives, but some may find that they are more palatable to the infant.

First-stage foods, for infants 4 to 6 months of age, include strained infant juices, single-grain cereals, and pureed strained fruits and vegetables such as bananas, carrots, and peas. These foods contain no egg, milk, wheat, or citrus, to which some infants may be sensitive. Second-stage foods, for infants about 6 to 9 months of age, are smooth, mixed-ingredient foods, such as mixed vegetables, or meat dinners, such as chicken noodle. Third-stage foods, or junior foods, are for infants about 9 to 10 months of age who can sit well without support, have some teeth, and have begun self-feeding. These more coarsely textured foods contain a wider variety of nutrients, such as vegetable and meat dinner combinations. Finger foods, such as crackers, cheese wedges, or cookies, can also be introduced by 9 to 10 months of age, once infants have developed a pincer grasp. Most infants are eating the same meals as the rest of the family (table foods) by about 1 year of age. Foods that can easily be aspirated, such as raw carrots, nuts, and hard candies, should be avoided until children are older than 4 years.

Baby foods can be prepared at home as long as they are finely pureed or strained and contain enough liquid to make them easy for infants to swallow. One danger of preparing foods at home is that sugar, salt, or spices can be easily added to make foods palatable to adults. These ingredients are not necessary for infants. In addition, homegrown, home-prepared vegetables may be contaminated with high levels of nitrates (eg, because of contaminated well water) and nitrites (eg, in vegetables such as carrots, beets, and spinach). Nitrates and nitrites have been implicated in the development of methemoglobinemia, especially in infants younger than 6 months. Methemoglobinemia decreases the oxygen-carrying capacity of the blood, leading to anoxic injury and death. This is more of a concern in rural areas that primarily use well water.

Weaning from the breast or bottle to a cup usually occurs at 6 to 12 months of age but may be delayed up to 18 months of age in some children. Homogenized, vitamin D–fortified cow's milk may be given at 12 months of age. Fat-free (skim) and low-fat (1%) milk should not be given before 2 years of age.

Diet of Children and Adolescents

The caloric and protein needs of children decrease in the second year of life, paralleling the decrease in growth rate during this time. Milk intake also decreases and may drop to 16 oz/day by 24 to 36 months of age. Except for increased caloric requirements, the diet of school-aged children and adolescents should be similar to that of normal adults. Evidence that foods eaten during childhood may have long-lasting effects on adult health is increasing, and it is important that children develop healthy eating habits early in life. Atherosclerosis, osteoporosis, and obesity are some of the diseases that may have their beginnings during childhood.

The US departments of Agriculture (USDA) and Health and Human Services (HHS) have replaced the food pyramid with a new visual aid—a circular plate on a square mat. Half of the plate consists entirely of vegetables and fruits, whereas the other half of the plate is divided into one-quarter protein and one-quarter grains, with a small side of dairy. It's a much more visually descriptive tool that guides how to divide daily meals. The Web site www.choosemyplate.gov provides individual dietary guidance according to a child's age, sex, and activity level based on the USDA/HHS dietary guideline for Americans older than 2 years.

To promote lifelong heart healthy habits, the American Heart Association (AHA) released a statement of dietary recommendations for children and adolescents. It recognizes that children are often offered nutrient-poor foods that are high in fat and sugar and overly processed. The AHA recommendations support USDA guidelines and include eating fruits and vegetables daily while limiting fruit juice intake, using vegetable oils, using butter instead of soft margarines, eating whole grain rather than refined grain breads and cereals, using nonfat or low-fat milk and dairy products, eating more fish, and reducing salt intake. Specific AHA guidelines are

1. Limit total fats to less than 25% to 35% of total daily calories.
2. Limit saturated fat to less than 7% of total daily calories.
3. Limit trans fat to less than 1% of daily calories.
4. Remaining fat should come from natural sources of monounsaturated and polyunsaturated fats, such as unsalted nuts and seeds, fish (especially oily fish such as salmon, trout, and herring at least 2 times a week), and vegetable oils such as canola oil.
5. Limit cholesterol intake to less than 300 mg a day or, if you have coronary artery disease, less than 200 mg a day.

The AHA also encourages behaviors for parents and caregivers that promote healthy habits for the whole family. These recommendations ask parents and caregivers to choose mealtimes, provide a social context for eating by having regular family meals, lead by example in their own eating habits, and allow children to self-regulate food intake and not to force them to finish meals if not hungry.

Children who consume a varied diet do not need routine vitamin supplementation. However, children and teens who are considered picky eaters, as well as children at nutritional risk, may benefit from supplementation. This includes children and teens who are anorexic or those who follow fad diets, those with chronic diseases, those who consume a vegetarian diet, and those with failure to thrive. A standard pediatric vitamin-mineral supplement should contain no more than the dietary reference intakes of its components. Parents should be counseled to teach their children that supplements are not candy and to keep them out of reach. Serious overdoses can occur, especially with iron-containing formulations.

Bone health is determined by calcium and vitamin D intake as well as weight-bearing physical activity. Recent data suggest the possibility of other important health benefits throughout life of these key nutrients and behavior, in addition to bone growth and development. The 2010 Institute of Medicine guidelines call for a recommended daily allowance of 600 IU per day of vitamin D for children older than 1 year and 1,300 mg of calcium per day for children 9 to 18 years of age. Unfortunately, calcium intake for most US children, particularly adolescents, is generally below the recommended levels. Barriers to adequate calcium intake may be due to the preference of sweetened juice and soft drinks over milk as well as lactose intolerance in certain populations. Nondairy calcium sources include salmon, white beans, broccoli, and calcium-fortified foods such as orange juice, breakfast cereals, and soy milk. Adequate calcium intake can be achieved by eating 3 (or 4 for adolescents) age-appropriate servings of dairy products or other calcium-rich food per day. In children and adolescents who do not consume adequate amounts of calcium from dietary sources, a calcium supplement is recommended. This can be in the form of a multivitamin in the younger child or calcium carbonate tablets with or without vitamin D for the adolescent.

Adolescence is a period of tremendous physical and emotional growth, both of which greatly affect nutritional needs and habits. Although their rapid physical growth requires increased energy and nutrients, the common eating habits of teens do not always support their needs. Teens tend to skip meals, eat outside the home, consume fast food and snacks, and experiment with different restrictive fad diets or various forms of vegetarianism.

Teen athletes also have their own unique nutritional concerns. They want to maximize performance while maintaining the desired physique for their particular sport or weight class. While there are many nutritional supplements, such as creatinine, carnitine, various amino acids, and dehydroepiandrosterone, that claim to enhance athletic performance, none has thus far been fully evaluated scientifically. Instead, teen athletes should be counseled on the importance of a basic nutrient: water. Proper hydration does enhance performance and prevents heat injury. Approximately 4 to 8 oz of fluid for every 15 minutes of exercise is recommended regardless of actual thirst. Carbohydrate loading before competition is believed to enhance performance; however, this practice has no effects on non-endurance events and may confer only a modest effect for endurance events by prolonging time to exhaustion. In counseling a teen athlete, specific questions should also be directed to elicit any unhealthy practices to maintain or lose weight.

Vegetarianism is gaining popularity among adolescents. Reasons for choosing vegetarianism are varied, including health benefits, means for weight loss, animal cruelty concerns, and religious beliefs. It is important to ask vegetarians about their specific restrictions, as these relate to their nutritional risks. Semi-vegetarians are those who avoid red meat but eat fish and chicken in moderation. Lacto-ovo vegetarians consume animal products, such as dairy and eggs, but avoid animal flesh. Vegans do not eat any animal products, such as dairy, eggs, honey, or gelatin. Those who follow a macrobiotic diet restrict not only animal products but also refined and processed foods, foods with preservatives, and foods that contain caffeine or other stimulants.

A well-planned vegetarian diet can provide all necessary nutrients; however, many teens experiment with vegetarianism in a non-vegetarian household and require guidance. The nutrients that may be deficient in a vegetarian diet are protein, calcium, vitamin D, vitamin B_{12}, iron, and zinc. Protein intake is usually not a concern for lacto-ovo vegetarians because eggs and dairy have high-quality proteins. Vegans and macrobiotic followers have a variety of plant-based protein sources from which to choose, such as legumes, cereals, nuts, seeds, and fruits. Because vitamin B_{12} is only found in animal-based foods, vegans and macrobiotic followers must ensure adequate intake via supplements or by consuming vitamin B_{12}-fortified foods, such as soy and nut beverages and cereals.

Lastly, familiarity with the latest fad diets is an asset for any primary care practitioner. These diets are usually restrictive in certain nutrients and recommend unusual dietary patterns that are inconsistent with current USDA guidelines. Although there are some suggestions that these diets work for some adults, there are almost no scientific data for children and adolescents. Popular plans include Atkins and other high-fat/low-carbohydrate diets; the Zone diet, which emphasizes a very specific ratio of protein and carbohydrates; the Ornish diet, which is extremely low in fat; the South Beach Diet, which alters the types of carbohydrates for an optimal glycemic index; and the more exotic liquid or detoxification plans. To keep abreast of the latest fads, refer to the Academy of Nutrition and Dietetics (www.eatright.org), which maintains an annual review of such popular fad diets.

Evaluation

History

Nutritional assessment begins with a complete dietary history. The dietary assessment should emphasize the quantity, quality, and variety of foods in the diet. Any special or restricted dietary habits should be noted (eg, vegetarian diet, vegan diet, occasional vegetable juicing/fasting). A 3-day food record listing the types and quantities of food eaten throughout the day can be very helpful in evaluating dietary history.

In addition, the child's routine medical, family, and social history all may influence nutritional status. For example, the economic status of families may affect the variety and type of foods they may be able to purchase, and the level of education of parents influences their ability to understand the concepts of a healthy diet. Poverty and ignorance of nutritional needs are among the most common reasons for malnutrition in children. But it can never be assumed that a family cannot comprehend the importance of eating a healthy nutritious diet as well as the significance of daily physical activity. Therefore, it is of vital importance that the pediatrician stress to families the value of healthy food choices at each physical examination. Family access to food can be estimated by asking parents about how often the family skips meals during the average month. Such information assesses food insecurity within a household. Specific cultural food preferences and feeding practices should also be included in the history.

Physical Examination

Weight, length or height, head circumference, weight for length, and body mass index (BMI) should be measured or calculated routinely and plotted on a longitudinal basis on appropriate growth curves. In addition to the charts provided by the Centers for Disease Control and Prevention and World Health Organization, additional charts are available for special populations for which growth is altered, such as infants and children with low birth weight and prematurity, Down syndrome, Turner syndrome, Williams syndrome, and several other chromosomal and genetic disorders. Changes in the rate of growth over time are more useful than a single measurement in the assessment of nutritional problems. Calculation of the height age (age for which the child's height is at the 50th percentile), weight age (age for which the child's weight is at the 50th percentile), and ideal weight for actual height may be useful when deviations from normal are noted.

In addition to the overall impression about nutritional status, certain findings on physical examination may be characteristic of particular nutritional disorders. The evaluation of the hair, skin, eyes, lips and oral mucosa, dentition, and musculoskeletal system should be emphasized because the examination of these areas is most likely to show the effects of malnutrition. Muscle wasting; hepatosplenomegaly; skeletal deformities; decayed teeth; rough, dry skin; hair that is easily plucked; and irritability may all be signs of inadequate nutrition.

Laboratory Tests

Suspected malnutrition or nutrition-related disorders, based on history and physical examination, can be further investigated with laboratory studies. Tests that may be used in the evaluation of anemia, one of the most common nutrition-related disorders seen in children, include a complete blood cell count, reticulocyte count, serum iron, ferritin, and total iron-binding capacity. Investigation of suspected malnutrition begins with an assessment of protein status, with measures of indicators such as serum albumin, total protein, and transthyretin. Liver function tests and a lipid profile may also be useful in the evaluation of suspected malnutrition. Screening tests that may be used in the evaluation of failure to thrive (FTT) include thyroid function studies, urinalysis, and bone age (see Chapter 133). More specific tests, such as serum vitamin levels (eg, folate or vitamin B_{12} levels in suspected malabsorption) or hormone assays (eg, growth hormone levels in the evaluation of short stature), may be obtained in certain instances.

Common Feeding and Nutritional Problems of Childhood

Several gastrointestinal (GI) problems have been attributed to diet. A small amount of spitting up is seen in most children, especially during the first 6 months of life. However, vomiting can be a sign of several disorders, ranging from viral GI tract infections to more severe illnesses, such as pyloric stenosis, urinary tract infection, GI obstruction, or inborn error of metabolism (see Chapter 111). Constipation, which is seen more commonly in formula-fed than breastfed infants, may be due to insufficient fluid intake (see Chapter 115). The simple addition of 4 to 6 oz of water to an infant's diet or temporary use of apple or prune juice may solve the problem. Enemas and suppositories should not be recommended routinely.

Chronic nonspecific diarrhea of childhood, or "toddler's diarrhea," may be seen in infants and children 6 months to 5 years of age with low dietary fat intake and excessive fruit juice consumption (see Chapter 114). Failure to absorb sugars, especially sorbitol and fructose, can lead to an osmotic diarrhea.

Underfeeding or a diet that is not nutritionally balanced may result in FTT (see Chapter 133). The opposite problem, obesity, is one of the most common nutritional problems of children in the United States (see Chapter 135). The prevalence of this condition in children 6 to 11 years of age is estimated to be about 20% to 25%. Finally, the eating disorders anorexia nervosa and bulimia nervosa are estimated to affect about 1 in 100 adolescent females 16 to 18 years of age (see Chapter 137).

The picky eater is a common parental concern in the primary care setting. For practitioners who work with the Hispanic population, the child who "no come nada," literally translated as the child who "does not eat anything," is a similar common parental concern. Parents can be reassured by their child's normal weight for height or BMI and growth velocity. They should be counseled that it is normal for preschoolers to exert their individuality by limiting food preferences, the fact that it may take up to 10 exposures for a child to accept a new food, the difference between child and adult portion sizes, and the concept that children can self-regulate food intake to sustain normal growth and health.

Nutritional disorders include malnutrition and deficiencies of vitamins and minerals. Iron deficiency anemia is one of the most common nutrition-related problems seen in children and adolescents. Malnutrition is one of the leading causes of childhood morbidity and mortality worldwide. Although primary protein-calorie malnutrition (PCM) is rare in most parts of the United States, surveys conducted on pediatric wards have demonstrated that about one-third of pediatric inpatients with chronic disease have evidence of some degree of PCM. The most common deficits were weight for height below 90% of standard (ie, evidence of acute malnutrition) and height for age below 95% of standard (ie, evidence of chronic malnutrition). The 2 forms of PCM are marasmus (severe caloric depletion) and kwashiorkor (inadequate protein intake). Untreated PCM can result in impaired growth, poor intellectual development, and impaired immune functioning.

Resources

ChooseMyPlate.gov: www.choosemyplate.gov

US Department of Agriculture Food and Nutrition Information Center: https://fnic.nal.usda.gov

---

CASE RESOLUTION

The infant described in the case history is probably ready to begin some solid foods because she is consuming 32 oz of formula per day and continues to be hungry. In addition, she has reached a weight of 13 lb and has almost doubled her birth weight. The mother is counseled to begin feeding her daughter a single-grain infant cereal mixed with formula. (The cereal should be fed by spoon, not given in a bottle.) Within a few weeks, once the infant is taking the cereal well, other first foods, such as fruits and vegetables, may be introduced.

Selected References

Abrams SA. Dietary guidelines for calcium and vitamin D: a new era. *Pediatrics.* 2011;127(3):566–568

Academy of Nutrition and Dietetics. Eat right. http://www.eatright.org. Accessed February 27, 2014

American Academy of Pediatrics. *Pediatric Nutrition.* Kleinman RE, ed. 7th ed. Elk Grove Village, IL: American Academy of Pediatrics; 2014

Cahill JB, Wagner CL. Challenges in breastfeeding. *Contemp Pediatr.* 2002;19: 94–138

Centers for Disease Control and Prevention. Growth chart training: introduction. http://www.cdc.gov/nccdphp/dnpao/growthcharts. Accessed February 27, 2014

Chandran L. Is there a role for long-chain polyunsaturated fatty acids in infant nutrition? *Contemp Pediatr.* 2003;20:107–124

Chandran L, Gelfer P. Breastfeeding: the essential principles. *Pediatr Rev.* 2006;27(11):409–417

Fiocchi A, Assa'ad A, Bahna S; Adverse Reactions to Foods Committee; American College of Allergy, Asthma and Immunology. Food allergy and the introduction of solid foods to infants: a consensus document. *Ann Allergy Asthma Immunol.* 2006;97(1):10–21

Fiorino KN, Cox JM. Nutrition and growth. In: Robertson J, Shilkofski N, eds. *The Harriet Lane Handbook: A Manual for Pediatric House Officers.* 17th ed. St Louis, MO: Mosby; 2005:525–608

Garcia RS. No come nada. *Health Aff (Millwood).* 2004;23(2):215–219

Gidding SS, Dennison BA, Birch LL, et al. Dietary recommendations for children and adolescents: a guide for practitioners: consensus statement from the American Heart Association. *Circulation.* 2005;112(13):2061–2075

Greer FR, Krebs NF; American Academy of Pediatrics Committee on Nutrition. Optimizing bone health and calcium intake of infants, children, and adolescents. *Pediatrics.* 2006;117(2):578–585

Heird WC. Progress in promoting breast-feeding, combating malnutrition, and composition and use of infant formula, 1981-2006. *J Nutr.* 2007;137(2):499S–502S

Kleinman RE. Chronic nonspecific diarrhea of childhood. *Nestle Nutr Workshop Ser Pediatr Program.* 2005;56:73–84

Larson N, Neumark-Sztainer D. Adolescent nutrition. *Pediatr Rev.* 2009;30(12): 494–496

Moilanen BC. Vegan diets in infants, children and adolescents. *Pediatr Rev.* 2004;25(5):174–176

Ogden CL, Kuczmarski RJ, Flegal KM, et al. Centers for Disease Control and Prevention 2000 growth charts for the United States: improvements to the 1977 National Center for Health Statistics version. *Pediatrics.* 2002;109(1):45–60

US Department of Agriculture. ChooseMyPlate.gov. http://www.choosemyplate.gov. Accessed February 27, 2014

Wagner CL, Greer FR; American Academy of Pediatrics Section on Breastfeeding and Committee on Nutrition. Prevention of rickets and vitamin D deficiency in infants, children, and adolescents. *Pediatrics.* 2008;122(5):1142–1152

CHAPTER 26

Breastfeeding

Julie E. Noble, MD, and Karen C. Bodnar, MD, IBCLC

CASE STUDY

A 25-year-old woman, pregnant with her first child, comes into your office with her husband for a prenatal visit. She would like to know what advice you can give her about breastfeeding. She expects a normal delivery, has had no breast surgery, and is not on any medications, but does smoke cigarettes occasionally. She plans to return to work when the baby is 4 months old.

Questions

1. What is the normal physiology of lactation?
2. What are the benefits of breastfeeding?
3. What are the contraindications to breastfeeding?
4. What management maximizes a mother's success at breastfeeding?
5. How do you manage some of the common problems that may arise during breastfeeding?

Human milk is the natural food source for human newborns and infants. It is a complete nutritional product made specifically for human newborns and infants, and all **formulas** are incomplete attempts at replication. **Human milk** is made of water, fat, lactose-containing carbohydrates, and protein, as well as vitamins, **immunoglobulins,** enzymes, hormones, and even phagocytes and lymphocytes. It is a dynamic fluid that changes in composition as newborns and infants grow. Early **colostrum** is high in lactose and protein, composed of casein and whey, and very immunologically active. Through lactogenesis, it becomes mature milk with much greater quantity, lower protein and higher fat content, but still immunologically active.

Epidemiology

In previous generations, newborns and infants were totally dependent on breastfeeding by their mother or a wet nurse for their survival. When formula feeding was attempted at foundling hospitals in Europe and the United States in the 1800s, the mortality rate in exposed newborns and infants was as high as 85%. Thus, the advantages of breastfeeding were recognized and still promoted in the early 1900s. Following the advent of pasteurization, cow's milk formula became much safer. Formula development allowed more mothers to enter the workforce, which became a necessity during World Wars I and II. With poorer urban mothers working outside the home and upper-class mothers choosing not to breastfeed, preferring the freedom that formula feeding allowed, breastfeeding rates declined over the course of the 20th century. **Formula** feeding became the norm as formula companies successfully marketed formulas. In 1972, at the nadir, only 22% of babies were ever breastfed. However, current scientific understanding of the many benefits of breastfeeding for baby and mother has been the impetus to again promote breastfeeding as the preferred food source for newborns and infants.

In the United States today, following the Centers for Disease Control and Prevention **Healthy People initiative,** which included a national agenda calling for an increase in the rate of breastfeeding, 76.5% of mothers are initiating breastfeeding. But the rate of mothers sustaining breastfeeding to 1 year of age is only 27%. Rates are lower in low socioeconomic groups and among women with lower levels of education. Ethnic disparities also exist, with the African American population having the lowest rates in the United States.

Multiple health professional organizations have endorsed breastfeeding. In 1991, the World Health Organization and United Nations Children's Fund developed the Baby-Friendly Hospital Initiative, delineating 10 steps to undertake in the hospital to promote successful breastfeeding. This initiative is used worldwide to improve breastfeeding rates. The American Academy of Pediatrics published its policy statement, "Breastfeeding and the Use of Human Milk," in 2005 and a revised version in 2012. This policy endorses breastfeeding and delineates the physician responsibility to promote and support it. In 2011, the US Department of Health and Human Services issued *The Surgeon General's Call to Action to Support Breastfeeding.* There is now a national imperative to promote breastfeeding.

Anatomy and Physiology of Lactation

The breasts consist of lobules and alveoli where milk is produced, as well as the **ductile system,** leading to 10 to 15 milk duct openings in the nipple. During pregnancy, the breast responds to **estrogen, placental lactogen, prolactin,** and **progesterone.** The breasts enlarge as the lobules further mature and differentiate. The nipples darken and the surrounding areolas enlarge. In the first 24 hours of a baby's life, only a small volume of colostrum, around 40 to 50 mL total, is produced because prolactin, from the anterior pituitary, is inhibited by progesterone. With the drop in progesterone after delivery, **prolactin** begins to stimulate increased milk production. This increased production, termed *lactogenesis stage 2,* occurs on average on day 3 or 4 after the delivery. With the stimulus of suckling, **oxytocin** is released from the posterior pituitary and causes contraction of myoepithelial cells, which squeeze milk from the alveoli. While initial production of **milk** is not dependent on newborn suckling, the more the neonate feeds and the more often the breast is effectively emptied, the more milk will be produced. If milk is not removed, an autocrine hormone called feedback inhibitor of lactation (FIL) acts locally within each breast to inhibit milk production.

Benefits of Breastfeeding

For the baby, the benefits to being breastfed are myriad. Studies have demonstrated that breastfed infants have a decreased incidence and severity of **infectious illnesses,** including diarrhea, respiratory infections, otitis media, bacterial meningitis, and urinary tract infections. The incidence of otitis media is 100% higher in formula-fed infants than exclusively breastfed infants. There have also been studies demonstrating better performance on **cognitive testing** among children who were breastfed as infants. Among preterm infants fed human milk, the incidence of necrotizing enterocolitis is also significantly reduced. Breastfeeding in infancy also reduces the later incidence of **atopy, allergies, asthma, childhood obesity, type 2 diabetes,** and even childhood **cancer.** Decreased rates of **sudden infant death syndrome** (see Chapter 61) have also been documented. All of these benefits are increased by increasing the length and exclusivity of breastfeeding.

For the mother, an immediate benefit to breastfeeding is oxytocin-induced decreased postpartum blood loss and enhanced newborn and infant bonding. Lactation amenorrhea may serve subsequently as birth control. Breastfeeding has also been associated with quicker return to prepregnancy weight as well as decreased risk of breast cancer, ovarian cancer, diabetes, and osteoporosis in the mother. There is also some evidence to suggest that breastfeeding decreases the risk of postpartum depression.

Societal benefits from breastfeeding include markedly decreased annual health care costs. An estimated savings of $10.5 billion yearly could be generated if 80% of American families breastfed exclusively for the first 6 months of babies' lives. A decreased incidence of illness among newborns and infants would also enable mothers to miss fewer workdays, increasing their productivity and benefiting the workplace. In addition, with an increased breastfeeding rate there would be a reduction in environmental waste from bottles and **formula** containers.

Barriers to Breastfeeding

There have been many studies evaluating barriers in the United States to breastfeeding. Understanding these barriers is essential to devising strategies for effective interventions to improve breastfeeding rates. With effective physician, nursing, and peer support, most mothers should be able to breastfeed successfully. One of the most important barriers is the lack of knowledge in pregnant women about the benefits of breastfeeding. Education beginning at the first prenatal visit is vitally important. Campaigns encouraging breastfeeding as the social norm through public health venues can help with education of the general populace.

Some mothers report feeling uncomfortable breastfeeding in public. Identifying this issue and helping these mothers to feel more supported or find privacy when they need it can help them to succeed with breastfeeding. Currently there are laws in 45 states that protect a mother's right to breastfeed in public.

Many new mothers have poor family support for breastfeeding, and the whole family needs to be included in breastfeeding counseling. The mother will not be successful if her family is encouraging her to use formula.

Some mothers find that their place of employment does not make accommodations for a breastfeeding mother. It may be that the workplace needs to be reminded of laws promoting breastfeeding in the workplace. The Patient Protection and Affordable Care Act includes a provision that the workplace must provide adequate break time and a private place for nursing mothers to pump for up to 1 year. Some states offer additional protections.

Hospitals may have practices or policies that interfere with successful breastfeeding, including high cesarean delivery rates or no rooming-in policy. Physicians should work with their hospitals to minimize these potential barriers. Some medical professionals become barriers to exclusive breastfeeding because they lack the knowledge to properly manage problems as they arise.

Contraindications

Absolute contraindications to breastfeeding are few but need to be addressed. If a neonate has **galactosemia type 1** as detected by newborn screening and is therefore unable to metabolize lactose or galactose, he may not breastfeed. Newborns can also inherit defects in protein metabolism that may call for a special diet, precluding breastfeeding. In most states, newborn screening now includes testing for most of these metabolic disorders.

Maternal infections prohibiting breastfeeding include active, untreated tuberculosis; HIV; and human T-cell lymphotropic virus types 1 and 2. In addition, if herpetic vesicles are present on the breast, the mother should not breastfeed.

Most medications are safe for a mother to use while breastfeeding, and the risk to the newborn or infant of not breastfeeding often outweighs the risk of exposure to subclinical doses of the medication in human milk. Each medicine should be reviewed for potential contraindications or possible negative effects on milk supply. Chemotherapeutic agents, antimetabolites, radioactive isotopes, and drugs of abuse are all contraindicated for breastfeeding. However, a mother with a history of drug use may benefit from breastfeeding as long as her toxicology results are closely monitored and are negative.

Breastfeeding Management

The management of breastfeeding should begin in the prenatal period. The US Preventive Services Task Force endorses promotion and support for breastfeeding at all health care encounters.

The pregnant woman should be educated by her pediatrician and obstetrician on the benefits of breastfeeding. Her history should be reviewed for potential contraindications. If none exists, she should be encouraged to breastfeed. If she commits to breastfeeding before the baby is born, she is more likely to be successful. Involving her partner in these discussions has also been shown to improve breastfeeding success rates.

At the time of delivery, if there are no complications, the neonate should be dried, assigned initial Apgar scores, and placed skin to skin on the mother's abdomen or chest for warmth and contact. The newborn will find his way to the breast and latch on. This early breastfeeding experience will greatly facilitate further breastfeeding. The neonate should not be separated from the mother except for medical reasons. A hospital policy for rooming-in will greatly facilitate breastfeeding. A healthy full-term newborn has no medical need for formula supplements.

During the hospital stay, the newborn should breastfeed on demand on both breasts for as long as he wants. Generally he should nurse at least 8 times a day. Without pacifiers or supplemental feeds, the neonate will learn to breastfeed more quickly. The mother should be counseled on appropriate latch-on, positioning of the newborn, and manual expression of milk. Breastfeeding support should be available from all involved hospital staff, and a certified lactation consultant can be very helpful.

Urine and stool output can be a reliable indicator of the success of breastfeeding. A successful breastfeeding neonate should urinate 3 times per day and stool 3 to 4 times per day by 3 to 5 days of age. By day 5 to 7 of life, he should urinate 4 to 6 times per day and pass 3 to 6 stools per day. Weight loss should be monitored and should not exceed 7% to 10% of his birth weight. Mothers whose newborns are taken to the neonatal intensive care unit must be helped with pumping or hand expressing their breasts within the first hours after delivery. By encouraging initial and frequent expression of milk, a mother's milk supply can be established even when her newborn is not able to directly nurse.

Vitamin K (1.0 mg intramuscularly) is indicated within the first 6 hours of life to prevent hemorrhagic disease of the newborn. During the first 6 months of life, the only supplement to breastfeeding that is needed is vitamin D 400 IU daily started in the first few days of life to prevent rickets.

After hospital discharge, the breastfeeding newborn should be seen by his physician at day 3 to 5 of life and again at 2 weeks of age to support breastfeeding. Early assessment may prevent many breastfeeding problems and will allow the physician to intervene early if problems arise, preventing discontinuation of breastfeeding. New mothers need encouragement and reassurance. At each visit, the neonate should be assessed for weight, feeding schedules, voiding and stooling patterns, and jaundice. The mother's breasts should be examined and a feeding observed. Mothers who are giving formula supplementation in the first weeks need help to improve milk transfer and wean formula supplements. Referral to a lactation specialist and follow-up in days is appropriate.

The infant should exclusively breastfeed until 6 months of age. At that time an iron source is needed, and iron-fortified cereal can be given with a gradual introduction of other pureed foods. The recommendation is that breastfeeding continue until at least 1 year of age or as long as the mother and infant are content.

If a mother plans on returning to work, she should be counseled to initiate exclusive breastfeeding and wait until the infant is 1 to 2 months of age prior to introducing a bottle of expressed milk. When separated from the infant, she should pump her breasts at regular intervals. The milk can be saved in the refrigerator for up to 5 days or in the freezer for up to 6 months (ideal) or even 12 months (acceptable) for later use. Milk should be used within 4 to 6 hours if at room temperature. In general, milk should be stored in 2- to 4-ounce bags or containers, which are labeled with the date. When she is back with the infant, she should put the infant to breast at the usual interval. Many mothers can work and breastfeed well past a child's first birthday.

Sometimes pediatricians will be consulted about weaning the breastfed infant. There is no age at which weaning must occur, and in many cultures toddlers nurse until the age of 3 to 4 years. While some infants readily give up the breast, others are more reluctant to do so. There are no easy solutions to dealing with a reluctant toddler, and some suggestions include the adage, "Don't offer, but don't refuse." Lactation consultants may be a valuable resource at this time.

Potential Problems

Attachment

Latching-on is the first step that is essential for successful breastfeeding. A neonate with a correct latch will have the nipple and significant portion of the areola under the nipple in his mouth with her lips flanged outward. If a newborn is not latching effectively, the mother will experience pain and the newborn should be removed from the nipple and attached again. If pain persists, a medical professional should evaluate the mother-baby dyad for problems. Causes can include poor latch, inverted nipples, flat nipples, ankyloglossia (tongue-tie), small mandible, or nipple confusion. Treatment may consist of help with positioning, nipple shields, frenotomy, or syringe feeding until the newborn learns to latch.

Sore Nipples

Breastfeeding should not be painful. If the mother is experiencing pain, the neonate is probably not latching correctly and may be chewing on the nipple. This may cause cracked and even bleeding nipples. The newborn should be positioned on the breast to get as much of the areola in the mouth as possible. Cracked nipples can be treated with lanolin or hydrogel pads and repositioning. Expressed milk left to dry on cracked or bleeding nipples has healing properties. If there is significant injury, the mother may need to pump that breast for 24 hours while the nipple heals. The newborn can be syringe fed if necessary to avoid exposure to artificial nipples. Nipple pain that is not resolved with improved positioning requires further evaluation.

Occasionally sore nipples are secondary to a candidal infection, and mother and baby should be treated with an antifungal medication, such as nystatin. Bacterial infection and Raynaud phenomenon are also uncommon causes of nipple pain.

Engorgement/Mastitis

When there is milk stasis for any reason, a mother may become **engorged.** The breast will appear full, firm, lumpy, and tender. Treatment is to empty the breast, and the newborn or infant is the most effective breast pump. Warm packs or a hot shower before feeding can be helpful. Sometimes an electric breast pump expedites emptying, softens the breast, and facilitates baby latching. If it is not possible to empty an area of the breast, such as in cases of a prior surgery that has severed some ducts, FIL will decrease and stop milk production in this area.

If engorgement is left untreated, it may lead to mastitis. **Mastitis** is defined as breast inflammation with signs of systemic infection frequently including fever and body aches. If a mother develops mastitis, she should continue to breastfeed. Emptying the breast is important, but treatment also consists of oral antibiotics and rest. There are isolated reports of breastfed babies acquiring a bacterial infection if the mother has mastitis. Mastitis involves a cellulitis of the breast, and the organisms are usually not in the ducts or **milk.** Babies may refuse to breastfeed on an affected breast if the taste of the milk is affected. The mother may then elect to breastfeed the baby on the unaffected side and pump the affected breast. Ineffective treatment of mastitis may cause it to progress into a breast abscess requiring more invasive treatments, such as surgical drainage. Incisions should be made parallel to ducts to avoid severing them and away from the areola so the baby can continue to latch. If there is frank pus coming from the nipple, the baby should not breastfeed until the discharge has resolved. The mother should pump the affected breast to empty the milk and support her supply.

Low Supply

The most common reason for early cessation of breastfeeding is perceived low milk supply. While 95% of Western women are physiologically able to produce sufficient milk, many supplement with formula when it is not medically necessary. Supplementation may be due to difficulty with latch or unrealistic expectations of newborn behavior causing a lack of confidence. Formula supplementation leads to decreased breastfeeding, and in time, milk supply will decrease if the breasts are not emptied by the baby, a pump, or hand expression.

To encourage exclusive breastfeeding, medical professionals must be able to support a mother's confidence and ability to breastfeed. They must be able to assess milk transfer as well as baby hydration and weight gain. When supplementation is necessary, medical professionals must enable mothers to express their breasts, and often this milk is the only supplement needed. Any formula supplements given in the first few days should be stopped when mothers experience lactogenesis stage 2. At office visits, if babies have been given formula unnecessarily, physicians must help families by addressing breastfeeding problems and closely following the baby's weight as supplements are decreased and eliminated. In later months, mothers may express concern that they have less milk when, in fact, infants have become more efficient eaters.

When babies have poor weight gain, a thorough investigation must be undertaken to see if the difficulty stems from a problem with the baby, mother's milk supply, milk transfer, or some combination of these. It is critical to provide the baby with sufficient calories and to protect the mother's supply with pumping during this time. For mothers who do lack sufficient milk, more frequent and effective emptying of the breast may solve the problem, but if this fails, galactagogues (human milk stimulants) may be useful in some cases.

Hyperbilirubinemia/Dehydration

If neonates lose more than 7% to 10% of their birth weight, they are at risk for becoming dehydrated and have a higher likelihood of significant jaundice. Increased intake is necessary, and the frequency of feeds should be increased. If newborns are not latching on well, expressed **milk** can be given by syringe. Neonates should be closely monitored, and **formula** can be offered after human milk if milk supply is insufficient. If insufficient supply is the problem, the mother should be assisted in increasing her milk supply. Using a breast pump will increase supply because increased demand increases supply. If the newborn appears significantly jaundiced, blood levels of bilirubin should be obtained. Physiologic jaundice is related to hepatic immaturity with decreased conjugation of bilirubin as well as decreased excretion. Breastfeeding babies tend to have higher levels of unconjugated bilirubin. Increased feeding will frequently resolve the problem as hydration status improves and frequency of stooling increases. Occasionally, especially in late preterm neonates, treatment with phototherapy is needed. The baby should be evaluated for any other causes of jaundice and should be followed closely (see Chapter 117) and treated as indicated.

Resources for the Breastfeeding Mother

Many hospitals and health care organizations have lactation specialists who can assist nursing mothers and answer questions related to lactation. Health facilities may loan or rent **electric breast pumps** to new mothers to help establish a good supply of milk. Some mothers may choose to purchase such pumps, especially if they are planning to continue to breastfeed after returning to work. Recent legislation has designated breast pumps as medical devices that are covered by health insurance.

Access to information can also be obtained through community agencies or national organizations such as **La Leche League International** (www.lalecheleague.org) or the Special Supplemental Nutrition Program for Women, Infants, and Children (WIC) program. Such agencies provide a resource to the clinician in assisting mothers with breastfeeding.

CASE RESOLUTION

In the case presented, the mother should be informed of the many benefits of breastfeeding to the baby, herself, and society. She should be encouraged to breastfeed because she has no contraindications. You recommend she stop cigarette smoking completely for her own health as well as the baby's; however, if she is unable, breastfeeding is still superior to formula. In the hospital she should request that her newborn be placed skin to skin with her in the delivery room and continue rooming-in to breastfeed on demand. Reassure her that the hospital and your office will give her support and guidance with breastfeeding. Even though she is anticipating going back to work, she should initially nurse exclusively. She can begin to introduce the bottle with pumped milk at 1 to 2 months of age. Her workplace should provide an area for nursing mothers to pump and refrigerate the milk. You encourage her to explore the lactation policies at her place of work and to seek out new mom support groups.

Selected References

American Academy of Pediatrics, American College of Obstetricians and Gynecologists. *Breastfeeding Handbook for Physicians.* Schanler RJ, Krebs NF, Mass SB, eds. 2nd ed. Elk Grove Village, IL: American Academy of Pediatrics; 2014

American Academy of Pediatrics, American College of Obstetricians and Gynecologists. *Guidelines for Perinatal Care.* Riley LE, Stark AR, eds. 7th ed. Elk Grove Village, IL: American Academy of Pediatrics; 2012

American Academy of Pediatrics Section on Breastfeeding. Breastfeeding and the use of human milk. *Pediatrics.* 2012;129(3):e827–e841

Brenner M. You can provide efficient, effective, and reimbursable breastfeeding support—here's how. *Contemp Pediatr.* 2005;22:66–76

Chandran L, Gelfer P. Breastfeeding: the essential principles. *Pediatr Rev.* 2006;27(11):409–417

Chung M, Raman G, Trikalinos T, Lau J, Ip S. Interventions in primary care to promote breastfeeding: an evidence review for the US Preventive Services Task Force. *Ann Intern Med.* 2008;149(8):565–582

Feldman-Winter LB, Schanler RJ, O'Connor KG, Lawrence RA. Pediatricians and the promotion and support of breastfeeding. *Arch Pediatr Adolesc Med.* 2008;162(12):1142–1149

Lawrence RA, Lawrence RM. *Breastfeeding: A Guide for the Medical Profession.* 7th ed. Maryland Heights, MO: Elsevier Mosby; 2011

Sachs HC; American Academy of Pediatrics Committee on Drugs. The transfer of drugs and therapeutics into human breast milk: an update on selected topics. *Pediatrics.* 2013;132(3):e796–e809

US Department of Health and Human Services. *The Surgeon General's Call to Action to Support Breastfeeding.* Washington, DC: US Department of Health and Human Services, Office of Surgeon General; 2011. http://www.surgeongeneral.gov/library/calls/breastfeeding/calltoactiontosupportbreastfeeding.pdf. Accessed November 19, 2013

US Preventive Services Task Force. Primary care interventions to promote breastfeeding: US Preventive Services Task Force recommendation statement. *Ann Intern Med.* 2008;149(8):560–564

Wellstart International. *Lactation Management Self-Study Modules Level I.* Naylor AJ, Wester RA, eds. 4th ed. Shelburne, VT: Wellstart International; 2013

CHAPTER 27

Sleep: Normal Patterns and Common Disorders

Geeta Grover, MD

CASE STUDY

During a routine 6-month health maintenance visit, a mother states that although her 6-month-old son falls asleep very easily at about 10:00 pm every night while breastfeeding, he wakes every 2 to 3 hours and cries until she nurses him back to sleep. A review of the dietary history reveals that the infant is breastfed about every 3 hours and was begun on rice cereal 2 weeks ago. His immunizations are current. The boy has no medical problems, and his physical examination is normal.

Questions

1. How old are most infants when they can begin to sleep through the night (at least 5 hours at a stretch) without a feeding?
2. What factors contribute to frequent nighttime awaking during infancy?
3. What advice can be given to parents to facilitate an infant's sleeping through the night?
4. What are sleep disturbances experienced by older children and adolescents?

Sleep disorders are common during infancy and childhood. Getting children to go to bed, fall asleep, stay asleep, and stay in bed can be no small challenge. Parents frequently ask pediatricians about sleep-related problems at routine health maintenance visits. Age-appropriate suggestions on how to help children sleep well are usually welcomed by parents.

Epidemiology

A broad range of physical, emotional, and social consequences have been associated with inadequate sleep in children. Impaired motor skills, an increased risk for obesity, mood disorders, and impaired concentration and academic performance are some of the consequences associated with insufficient sleep. Achieving adequate sleep at every age is an important pediatric health issue.

Sleep problems are one of the most common concerns seen in pediatric practice. Bedtime struggles and frequent night awaking occur in 20% to 25% of children younger than 3 years. In preschool-aged children, nighttime fears (eg, of noises, of the dark) or separation anxiety often contributes to these problems. Estimates of parent-reported sleep problems in school-aged children range between 11% and 40%. As children get older, nightmares and night terrors may contribute to night awaking. About 5% of individuals experience nightmares, which usually begin before the age of 10 years and are seen more often in girls than in boys. Night terrors are a specific form of partial night awaking from deep sleep that may begin during the preschool years. The incidence in children is reported to be between 1% and 4%, with the greatest frequency

between 5 and 7 years of age. Such terrors are more common in boys than in girls, and a familial tendency has been reported. Febrile illness and obstructive sleep apnea may be predisposing factors.

In most Western countries, children are expected to sleep in their own beds. However, in many cultures, it is not uncommon for newborns, infants, and young children to sleep in their parents' bed (the "family bed"). Bed sharing in newborns and infants younger than 10 to 12 weeks is associated with a higher incidence of sudden infant death syndrome, especially if the mother smokes. Accidental asphyxia from overlaying or the presence of soft bedding or overheating may contribute to bed sharing–related deaths. Parents should always be advised about safe sleeping practices (see Chapter 61). In older infants and children, co-sleeping is not a problem in and of itself, and the decision to co-sleep, like the decision to breast-feed or bottle-feed, is an entirely personal one. Most newborns and infants who share a bed with their parents have sleep-onset associations to facilitate falling asleep. Therefore, parents who share a bed with their young children commonly have to lie down with them for 20 to 30 minutes to get them to fall asleep. Several studies have shown that co-sleeping infants are 2 to 3 times more likely to have night awaking than those who sleep alone. Furthermore, newborns and infants who are breastfeeding and bed sharing sleep the shortest periods prior to awaking. Parents who only plan on co-sleeping with their newborns and infants for a limited period will need a clear transition plan, such as ending this practice by 5 to 6 months of age, before infants are old enough to object excessively. For children with sleep problems, bed sharing is not a good solution. However, in the absence of any preexisting sleep problems or psychological concerns, co-sleeping, as a lifestyle choice, has not been associated with any long-term developmental, behavioral, or psychological problems in the co-sleeping children.

Clinical Presentation

Parents may raise concerns about their child's sleep pattern during a routine health maintenance visit. Because some parents may be reluctant to "bother" their physician with such seemingly minor concerns, the physician should routinely question parents about their child's sleep patterns and offer anticipatory guidance as appropriate.

Pathophysiology

To understand disturbances associated with sleep, the physiology of normal sleep and the development of normal sleep behavior in children must be understood.

Sleep States

Normal sleep has 2 distinct states, **rapid eye movement (REM)** and **non–rapid eye movement (NREM)** sleep. Rapid eye movement sleep develops at about 29 weeks' gestation and persists throughout life. It is an active, lighter stage of sleep that occurs in association with rapid eye movements. Other features of REM sleep include suppression of muscle tone; rapid, irregular pulse and respiratory rate; and body twitches. Dreams occur during REM sleep. The electroencephalogram (EEG) pattern of REM sleep is very similar to stage 1 NREM sleep.

Non–rapid eye movement sleep begins at about 32 to 35 weeks' gestation. During NREM sleep, pulse and respiratory rates are slower and more regular and body movements are minimal. Most of the restorative functions of sleep occur during this state. After the first several months of life, NREM sleep may be divided into 4 stages ranging from drowsiness to very deep sleep. Each stage represents a progressively deeper state of sleep and has a characteristic EEG tracing: stage 1 has low-voltage, fast activity; stage 2 is notable for the presence of sleep spindles and K complexes against a low-voltage background; and stages 3 and 4 are identified by varying amounts of high-amplitude, slow waves known as delta waves.

The Sleep Cycle

Rapid eye movement and NREM sleep together make up the sleep cycle. Typically, the deepest sleep takes place during the first several hours of the night, with lighter stages of NREM and REM sleep occurring during most of the rest of the night. Although sleep stages are the same in infants and adults, several differences between the onset and duration of REM and NREM sleep in infants and adults exist. First, the sleep cycle is shorter in infants (50–60 minutes) than in adults (90–100 minutes), which means that infants have more periods of active REM sleep compared with adults. Second, the total amount of time spent in REM sleep decreases with increasing age. Term newborns spend about 50% of their total sleep time in REM sleep (up to 80% in premature newborns); this decreases to about 30% by 3 years of age and to 20% by adulthood. Third, infants may have very little REM latency, entering their first REM cycle very shortly after falling asleep. Adults, in comparison, generally enter their first REM period about 90 minutes after the onset of sleep.

Sleep/Wake Patterns

Sleep patterns follow a normal developmental sequence in children; the amount of sleep children need changes with maturation (Figure 27-1). Healthy term newborns sleep 16 to 17 hours per day. Because they are unable to sleep for more than a few hours at a time, sleeping and waking periods are fairly evenly distributed throughout the day and night. Many infants are able to sleep through the night (at least 5 hours uninterrupted) by the age of 3 months; most infants are capable of this by 4 months. Brief arousals are a normal part of the sleep cycle at all ages, but children should be able to return to

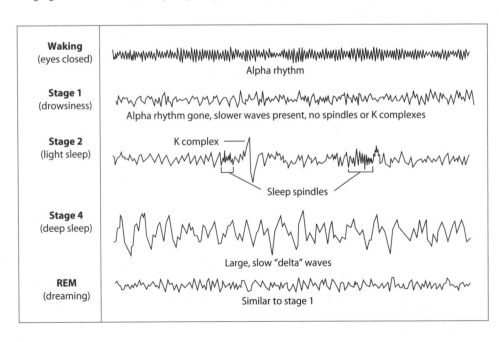

Figure 27-1. Typical sleep patterns in childhood. (Reprinted with permission of Scribner Publishing Group, a division of Simon & Schuster, Inc. from the Touchstone edition of *Solve Your Child's Sleep Problems,* New, Expanded and Revised by Richard Ferber, MD. Copyright © 1985, 2006 by Richard Ferber, MD. All rights reserved.)

sleep on their own without requiring parents' attention. Children should definitely be able to fall asleep on their own by the age of 4 to 6 months. Otherwise, parental participation to fall asleep becomes required at every awaking throughout the night.

By 12 months of age, infants sleep about 14 hours per day, divided into 2 naps during the day and a period of about 10 hours at night. During the second year of life, most children stop napping in the morning. By 2 years of age, they require about 13 hours of sleep per day (1–2 hours in an afternoon nap and 11–12 hours at night). Most children take an afternoon nap until 3 years of age, and some children continue this until 5 years of age. The amount of nighttime sleep children need gradually continues to decline, decreasing from about 12 hours during the preschool years to about 8 to 9 hours during adolescence.

Sleep Abnormalities

The etiology of sleep disorders can be complex, involving the interaction of children's temperamental characteristics, psychosocial stressors in the home, parental child-rearing philosophies, and the developmental nature of normal sleep states and sleep cycles.

Differential Diagnosis

The differential diagnosis of sleep disorders may be distinguished by problems associated with falling asleep or frequent night awaking (Box 27-1). Falling asleep may present 2 types of difficulties: problems associated with settling children to sleep and bedtime refusal.

In infants, **inappropriate sleep-onset associations** are the most common reason for difficulty settling to sleep. These infants require parental participation (eg, holding, rocking, feeding) to fall asleep. They have not learned the critical skills of self-calming and initiating sleep on their own. Because these infants do not have the self-soothing behaviors necessary to fall back asleep after normal nighttime arousals, they may also have nighttime awaking. Brief arousals are a normal component of sleep. Nighttime awaking is different because parents' participation is needed to resettle the infant. The difficulty that infants experience falling back to sleep on their own, not the awaking itself, is the problem.

An example of an inappropriate sleep-onset association is the infant or child who needs to be breastfed or bottle-fed to fall asleep. The term **trained night feeder** has been coined to describe children who need to be fed before going back to sleep after normal nighttime awaking. Although they are developmentally old enough to receive all nutrition during the day, they have become conditioned to require nighttime feedings. These children are often breastfed or bottle-fed until they fall asleep and only then placed in the crib. They are conditioned to require feeding to initiate sleep, and when they experience normal nighttime arousals, they require the breast or bottle to go back to sleep.

The term **trained night crier** refers to infants or children who, like trained night feeders, lack the self-comforting and self-initiating skills necessary to fall asleep on their own. Trained night criers awake, cry, and want to be held, comforted, or entertained before they can go back to sleep.

Box 27-1. Practical Approach to the Differential Diagnosis of Sleep Disorders in Children

Difficulty Falling Asleep

Circadian and sleep schedule disturbances
- Irregular sleep/wake patterns
- Advanced sleep phase
- Delayed sleep phase
- Regular but inappropriate sleep schedules without phase shifts (eg, late evening naps)

Habits, associations, and expectations
- Inappropriate sleep-onset associations
- Bedtime refusal/struggles
- Poor or inconsistent limit setting

Overstimulation

Psychosocial
- Separation anxiety
- Nighttime fears (eg, of the dark, of monsters)
- Family and social stresses

Medical
- Acute illness
- Underlying medical problems
- Medications (eg, antihistamines, stimulants, codeine, anticonvulsants)

Nighttime Awaking

Normal variation (eg, breastfed infant)

Habits, associations, and expectations
- Inappropriate sleep-onset associations (eg, age-inappropriate night awaking for feeding)

Psychosocial
- Nighttime fears
- Family and social stresses

Medical
- Acute illness
- Underlying medical problem
- Medications

Nightmares

Arousal disorders (eg, night terrors, sleepwalking, sleep talking)

Miscellaneous Sleep Disorders

Intrinsic sleep disorders
- Narcolepsy
- Sleep apnea (obstructive or central)
- Restless legs syndrome
- Periodic leg movements

Sleep/wake transition disorders (eg, head banging, rocking)

Acute illness may also be a cause of sleep disturbances. Children with otitis media may awake at night because of pain. They may continue to experience awaking after the infection has resolved, however, and require comforting or some sort of attention to fall asleep again.

In infants and children between the ages of 9 and 18 months, **separation** and **separation anxiety** may also affect sleep patterns. Children may cry when parents leave the room and have difficulty settling to sleep. Ability to climb out of the crib or bed can be associated with nighttime awaking in older toddlers. The transition from a crib to a bed is usually made between 2 and 3 years of age. Children who can climb out of their cribs or beds may come out of their rooms repeatedly for drinks of water, trips to the bathroom, or to sleep in the parents' bed. Such factors as nighttime fears of the dark influence sleep behaviors during the preschool years (3–5 years of age). Children's growing needs for autonomy and control over their environment may lead to bedtime refusals during the toddler and preschool years.

Disorders of the sleep/wake cycle may contribute to sleep schedule irregularities. Circadian rhythms govern the regularity and degree of wakefulness and sleepiness. The circadian clock inherent in humans is not an exact 24-hour pattern but can be modified or entrained onto one by environmental cues. Regular and consistent structure needs to be provided by parents because development of children's sleep/wake rhythms depends on an interaction of the child's inherent biological rhythms with the environment. Entrainment requires predictable occurrence of time cues such as light and dark, mealtime, and bedtime. A consistent awaking time in the morning is one of the most important of these cues.

Irregular sleep/wake cycles may be seen in children living in chaotic environments with irregular mealtimes and sleep/wake schedules. A delayed sleep phase and regular but inappropriate sleep/wake schedule are the most common forms of sleep rhythm disturbance. Children with **delayed sleep phase** have a resetting of their circadian rhythm; they are not sleepy at bedtime and have excessive morning sleepiness. This is a common problem because the inherent circadian clock has a cycle closer to 25, not 24, hours. This clock has not been entrained to a 24-hour schedule in these children.

Examples of **regular but inappropriate sleep/wake schedules** include children who nap at the "wrong" time (eg, a child who regularly naps at 7:00 pm for 1 hour and then has trouble going to bed at 9:00 pm) and infants who seem to have day and night confused. These children sleep most of the day and stay up most of the night.

Night terrors (pavor nocturnus), **sleepwalking** (somnambulism), and **sleep talking** (somniloquism) are all forms of partial awaking that occur during deep or stage 4 NREM sleep, most often during the transition from stage 4 NREM sleep to the first REM sleep period. Sleepwalking and sleep talking usually occur during the school-aged years, whereas night terrors begin during the preschool years.

Nightmares and night terrors may begin during the preschool years and may continue throughout childhood. Night terrors are different from nightmares and occur during a different stage of the sleep cycle (Table 27-1). With night terrors, children usually sit up in bed and cry or scream inconsolably for up to 15 minutes. They may appear dazed and have signs of autonomic arousal, such as tachycardia, tachypnea, and sweating. These children cannot be consoled. When they finally go back to sleep, they do not remember the event in the morning. Because parents are often frightened by the

Table 27-1. Nightmares Versus Night Terrors

Characteristic	*Nightmare*	*Night Terror*
Time of night	Late	Early, usually within 4 hours of bedtime
Sleep stage	Rapid eye movement sleep	Partial arousal from deep non–rapid eye movement sleep
State of child	Scared but consolable	Disoriented, confused, and inconsolable
Memory of event	Clear recall of dream	Usually none
Return to sleep	Reluctant because of fear	Easily, unless fully awake
Management	Reassure child	Reassure parents

experience, they may think the child is having a seizure or is suffering from an emotional disturbance and may seek medical advice. Although attacks may be precipitated by stressful events or fatiguing daytime activities, night terrors do not indicate excessive stress or emotional disturbance in children's lives unless they recur.

Nightmares usually occur during the last third of the night during REM sleep, whereas night terrors more often take place during the early part of the night. Nightmares are scary dreams that may awake children, who can often remember them. Children can usually be consoled by parents but are reluctant to go back to sleep because of their fears.

Excessive daytime sleepiness can be a symptom of medical problems such as depression, sleep apnea, narcolepsy, or illness. Viral illness is perhaps the most common medical cause of such sleepiness in children. Inadequate sleep at night may also be a potential cause of sleepiness during the day. Screening for daytime impairments (eg, decline in academic performance, inattention) is important in children suspected of having sleep disorders. Primary sleep disorders, such as obstructive sleep apnea, have been shown to be associated not only with excessive daytime sleepiness but also with cognitive deficits and impaired attentional capacity.

Narcolepsy, a disorder of excessive sleepiness, is characterized by an overwhelming desire to sleep during the daytime despite adequate sleep at night. Its symptoms include excessive daytime sleepiness, cataplexy, sleep paralysis, and hypnagogic hallucinations. Cataplexy is an abrupt loss of muscle tone that is usually precipitated by an emotional reaction, such as laughter or anger. Sleep paralysis is an inability to move or speak that occurs as patients fall asleep or awaken. Hypnagogic hallucinations, which can be visual or auditory, occur while falling asleep. Narcolepsy affects about 0.05% to 0.1% of the general population. The prevalence increases to 50% of family members when the family history is positive. The exact genetic basis of inheritance is unknown. The age of onset is usually between 10 and 20 years. Diagnosis is often delayed or missed for months to years in some cases because not all symptoms may be present initially. Diagnosis is important because pharmacologic therapy with central nervous system (CNS) stimulants may provide some symptomatic relief.

Sleep-related breathing disorders (SRBDs) occur across a spectrum with habitual snoring as the least severe form and **obstructive sleep apnea syndrome (OSAS)** as the most severe form. Risk factors associated with the development of SRBDs include obesity, presence of chronic sinus problems, recurrent wheezing, nasal allergies, family history of obstructive sleep apnea, and certain disorders that present with craniofacial abnormalities (eg, Down syndrome, Prader-Willi syndrome). Obstructive sleep apnea syndrome in children is a disorder of breathing during sleep. It is characterized by prolonged partial upper airway obstruction or intermittent complete obstruction (obstructive apnea) that disrupts normal gas exchange and sleep patterns. Risk factors for OSAS include adenotonsillar hypertrophy, obesity, craniofacial anomalies, and neuromuscular disorders. Obstructive sleep apnea syndrome is thought to be secondary to a combination of adenotonsillar hypertrophy and reduced neuromuscular tone of the upper airway during sleep. Large tonsils and adenoid alone do not necessarily indicate that the child has OSAS. Symptoms include nightly snoring (often with intermittent pauses or gasps), disturbed sleep, and daytime neurobehavioral problems. Obstructive sleep apnea syndrome should be distinguished from **primary snoring,** which is defined as snoring without obstructive apnea, arousals from sleep, or abnormalities in gas exchange. Obstructive sleep apnea syndrome can not only disturb the quality of sleep but can also cause potentially serious complications, such as failure to thrive and, in severe cases, cor pulmonale.

Restless legs syndrome, or periodic leg movements, is a recently described condition characterized by uncomfortable creeping or crawling feelings, mainly occurring in the lower extremities, when the child is resting or inactive and relieved by movement. The condition may be attributed to growing pains in younger children (see Chapter 107) and can be associated with delayed sleep onset.

Evaluation

History

Evaluation of children with sleep difficulties begins with a thorough, detailed sleep history taken from parents and children, if old enough (Questions Box). The use of a specific screening questionnaire, such as the Children's Sleep Habits Questionnaire by Judith Owens, MD, MPH, may facilitate the evaluation. It is designed to screen for the most common sleep problems in children aged 4 to 12 years. It is not intended to be used to diagnose specific sleep disorders but rather to identify children possibly needing further evaluation. Dr Owens has also developed a simple screening acronym, BEARS (bedtime resistance/sleep-onset delay; excessive daytime sleepiness; awaking at night; regularity, patterns, and duration of sleep; and snoring and other symptoms), which can be useful as an initial screen to determine if further assessment may be necessary.

Evaluation should also include an assessment of children's temperament and psychological well-being. Children's developmental status and level of function should be evaluated as well. Children with developmental, neurologic, and psychological concerns have higher rates of sleep disturbances. For example, it is estimated that

Questions

Sleep

- Does the child have regular nap times and bedtimes, or do these depend on changing parental schedules?
- What time does the child go to bed?
- What does the child do in the hour before bedtime? Is there a consistent bedtime routine?
- Does the child watch television, play video games, or use the Internet or mobile telephone in the hour before bed?
- Where does the child sleep (eg, ask about co-sleeping, noise, temperature)?
- Is the child able to fall asleep on his or her own, or does he or she require a parent's participation?
- Does the child require feeding or fluids at night?
- When does the problem occur relative to bedtime and what does the child do (detailed explanation)?
- How often does the problem occur?
- How long has the child been having sleep problems?
- How does the parent respond?
- Does the child snore?
- When does the child wake up in the morning? Is the child difficult to awake?
- Is the child sleepy during the day?
- How much caffeine does the child consume (eg, in coffee, tea, soda, chocolate)?
- Is the child taking any medications?
- Is there a family history of sleep disturbances?
- Is there any stress within the home due to marital or financial difficulties that may affect the home environment and cause the child to be anxious or stressed?

25% to 50% of children with attention-deficit/hyperactivity disorder seen in clinical practice will have sleep problems, especially difficulties in initiating and maintaining sleep.

Physical Examination

Physical examination is important to rule out organic causes of sleep difficulties. Special attention should be paid to the airway and nervous system. Acute illness (eg, otitis media), obstructive sleep apnea resulting from adenoidal or tonsillar hypertrophy (most commonly), colic, gastroesophageal reflux, and any CNS disease or abnormality may all alter the sleep/wake cycle.

Laboratory Tests

In most cases, a detailed history and physical examination should be sufficient to establish the reason for sleep disturbance; laboratory assessment is usually not necessary. Further evaluation, when warranted, should be tailored to the child's clinical presentation. An EEG may be useful if a central abnormality, such as a seizure disorder, is suspected. Polysomnography, the simultaneous monitoring of EEG, electrocardiogram, chin muscle tone, eye movements, and respirations during a night of sleep in a sleep laboratory, may be very useful in certain children when significant sleep disturbances, such as nocturnal seizures, narcolepsy, or OSAS, are suspected. Any child suspected of a sleep-related breathing disorder (eg, history of snoring or abnormal breathing during sleep) should be evaluated for OSAS.

Management

The goal of management is to help children develop a healthy pattern of sleeping, not simply eliminate the immediate problem. Healthy sleep associations include providing a consistent schedule of naps and bedtime, along with a pleasant bedtime routine. It is important to put newborns and infants in their cribs while they are relaxed and drowsy but not already asleep. This gives them the opportunity to develop skills to put themselves to sleep. If they become accustomed to being fed or rocked until they fall asleep, they will seek the same means of falling asleep every time they normally wake up during the night. In addition, overstimulation in the evening may make settling to sleep difficult for toddlers or young children. Instead, a routine such as a bath followed by a story in the child's bedroom with a clearly defined end point when the parent leaves the child in the crib or bed sleepy but awake may help facilitate sleep. Children must learn to fall asleep on their own.

Trained night feeders and trained night criers are newborns and infants who have not learned to fall asleep on their own. The basic treatment for these infants is to put them in their cribs when they are sleepy but awake and ignore subsequent crying. Their last memory before falling asleep should not be of their parents holding or feeding them. If the crying persists, contact with the newborns and infants should be brief and boring. Scheduled awaking is a technique in which infants are slightly aroused by the parent 15 to 60 minutes before an expected spontaneous awaking in an effort to prevent spontaneous awaking. Scheduled awaking may be an effective treatment alternative for some trained night criers. If infants awake for a feeding, parents should try to stretch the interval between waking and feeding so that infants have an opportunity to practice self-calming techniques. Specific sleep disorders can be addressed individually. Older toddlers and preschoolers who delay going to bed or refuse to stay in their rooms at night need clear, firm limits. It is important that these children have consistent bedtime routines and nighttime interventions for when they awake. A gate may need to be installed in the bedroom doorway to prevent children who refuse to stay in their rooms at night from moving about the house and potentially hurting themselves or disturbing others. Parents of children who have night terrors may require reassurance that their children are not suffering from significant emotional problems or stressors. A night-light may help alleviate the anxieties of preschoolers who are unable to sleep at night because of their fears of darkness. Disturbances of the sleep/wake schedule can be corrected over time by gradually shifting children's schedules in the desired direction. For example, children with a delayed sleep phase who go to bed very late can have their morning wake-up time progressively advanced about 15 minutes per day; this is followed by a progressive advancement in their bedtime until the desired schedule is reached.

The fast-moving pace and stresses of modern life, including 24/7 access to technologies, subject children and adolescents to increased stimulation, which can affect their sleep patterns. Whereas at the turn of the century, artificial lighting and radio were considered to be the causes of delayed bedtimes, today, television viewing, video games, the Internet, and mobile telephones lead to overstimulation. This overstimulation may result in many children and adolescents not getting the sleep they need. Implementation of good sleep hygiene practices is an important first step for school-aged children and adolescents who are experiencing sleep problems, especially sleep-onset problems. *Sleep hygiene* refers to the establishment and maintenance of schedules and conditions conducive to healthy, restorative sleep. Good sleep hygiene practices are outlined in Box 27-2. It is important to remember that adolescents require at least as much sleep as they did as preadolescents—about 9 hours of sleep per night. Referral to a sleep specialist may be necessary for some children, especially when significant sleep disturbances, such as narcolepsy, nocturnal seizures, or OSAS, are suspected.

Prognosis

Unfortunately, newborns and infants with sleep problems tend to grow into children with sleep problems. Researchers have found that about 40% of infants with sleep problems at the age of 8 months still had a problem at 3 years. It is to the parents' advantage to help their children develop healthy sleep habits rather than ignore the problems and hope that children outgrow them.

Box 27-2. Good Sleep Hygiene

Environment
- Dark
- Quiet
- Comfortably cool

Schedule
- Regular bedtime
- Regular awaking time
- Naps, if needed, should be early in the day with consistent time and duration

General
- No frightening/stimulating television, video games, or stories and no vigorous physical activities in the hour before bedtime.
- Unplug and charge technology devices outside children's bedrooms to avoid surreptitious access during sleep hours.
- Limit caffeine, especially after lunchtime.
- Consistent and calming bedtime routine.
- Consistent soothing methods.
- Children put to bed drowsy but awake.

CASE RESOLUTION

The 6-month-old described in the case history has disordered sleep associations. He has been conditioned to nighttime feedings, although he is old enough not to require them for nutrition. The physician suggests several things the mother can do to try to solve her son's sleep problem. She can begin by gradually lengthening the interval between daytime feedings to 4 to 5 hours. When he cries at night, she can wait progressively longer before feeding him and can then eventually eliminate the feedings altogether. He will learn to fall asleep on his own without requiring feeding.

Selected References

American Academy of Pediatrics Task Force on Sudden Infant Death Syndrome. SIDS and other sleep-related infant deaths: expansion of recommendations for a safe infant sleeping environment. *Pediatrics.* 2011;128(5):e1341–e1367

Bhargava S. Diagnosis and management of common sleep problems in children. *Pediatr Rev.* 2011;32(3):91–99

Burnham M, Lawler J. *The Complete Idiot's Guide to Sleep Training for Your Child.* New York, NY: Alpha Books; 2006

Byars KC, Yolton K, Rausch J, Lanphear B, Beebe DW. Prevalence, patterns, and persistence of sleep problems in the first 3 years of life. *Pediatrics.* 2012;129(2): e276–e284

Ferber R. *Solve Your Child's Sleep Problems: New, Revised, and Expanded Edition.* New York, NY: Fireside; 2006

Iglowstein I, Jenni OG, Molinari L, Largo RH. Sleep duration from infancy to adolescence: reference values and generational trends. *Pediatrics.* 2003;111(2): 302–307

Matricciani LA, Olds TS, Blunden S, Rigney G, Williams MT. Never enough sleep: a brief history of sleep recommendations for children. *Pediatrics.* 2012;129(3): 548–556

Michael L, Morton K. Sleep disorders in children explained. What's keeping your child from a full night's rest? http://www.end-your-sleep-deprivation.com/sleep-disorders-in-children.html. Accessed November 20, 2013

Moon RY, Fu L. Sudden infant death syndrome: an update. *Pediatr Rev.* 2012;33(7):314–320

Moturi S, Avis K. Assessment and treatment of common pediatric sleep disorders. *Psychiatry.* 2010;7(6):24–37

Okami P, Weisner T, Olmstead R. Outcome correlates of parent-child bedsharing: an eighteen-year longitudinal study. *J Dev Behav Pediatr.* 2002;23(4): 244–253

Owens JA. The ADHD and sleep conundrum: a review. *J Dev Behav Pediatr.* 2005;26(4):312–322

Owens JA, Dalzell V. Use of the 'BEARS' sleep screening tool in a pediatric residents' continuity clinic: a pilot study. *Sleep Med.* 2005;6(1):63–69

Owens JA, Moturi S. Pharmacologic treatment of pediatric insomnia. *Child Adolesc Psychiatr Clin N Am.* 2009;18(4):1001–1016

Owens JA, Spirito A, McGuinn M. The Children's Sleep Habits Questionnaire (CSHQ): psychometric properties of a survey instrument for school-aged children. *Sleep.* 2000;23(8):1043–1051

Shamseer L, Vohra S. Complementary, holistic, and integrative medicine: melatonin. *Pediatr Rev.* 2009;30(6):223–228

CHAPTER 28

Oral Health and Dental Disorders

Charlotte W. Lewis, MD, MPH

CASE STUDY

The parents of a 9-month-old girl bring her to the office because they are concerned that their daughter has no teeth yet. Growth and development have proceeded normally, and the physical examination is unremarkable.

Questions

1. What is the mean age and range for the eruption of the first tooth?
2. What is meant by *mixed dentition?*
3. When should oral hygiene using a toothbrush begin?
4. What are risk factors for dental caries?
5. What are the indications for the application of fluoride varnish?

Dental caries comprises the most common chronic disease of childhood. Pediatricians and other health care professionals often see young children multiple times before children have their first dental visit. Primary care physicians are thus in a prime position to counsel families on preventive oral health and identify early signs of dental decay so that timely treatment can occur. In 2003, the American Academy of Pediatrics issued a recommendation that pediatricians and other pediatric health care professionals begin regular oral health anticipatory guidance and risk assessment before patients are 6 months old. This recommendation affirms the essential need for clinicians to educate themselves on normal and abnormal patterns of dental eruption and occlusion, early and advanced signs of dental caries and its complications, and appropriate preventive oral health practices. Establishing collaborative partnerships with community dentists is helpful in promoting ongoing clinician and family education and appropriate patient referrals.

Epidemiology

Caries begins in childhood and eventually affects 90% of adults. Even so, the effect of dental decay on low-income individuals is disproportionate, leading to earlier onset, more affected teeth, complications, and ultimately tooth loss during adulthood because of caries. Results of the third National Health and Nutrition Examination Survey (NHANES III) released from 1999 to 2004 indicated that 24% of 2- to 4-year-olds and 51% of 6- to 8-year-olds had caries in primary teeth. Among 12- to 19-year-olds, 59% had caries in permanent teeth. Children living below 200% of the federal poverty level (FPL) had more caries relative to children at or above 200% FPL (Figure 28-1). Poverty is the most important risk factor for caries. Children

Figure 28-1. Percent of US children with dental caries by federal poverty level category. (From US Department of Health and Human Services, National Center for Health Statistics. *National Health and Nutrition Examination Survey, NHANES III- 1999–2004.* **Hyattsville, MD: National Center for Health Statistics; 2004.)**

living below 200% FPL should be considered at high risk for caries and started on an intensive caries primary prevention program during infancy. Components of standard caries primary prevention for all children and intensive caries primary prevention for children with a high risk of caries are described in Box 28-1. Other population and individual risk factors are listed in Box 28-2.

Toothache, a complication of dental caries, afflicts millions of US children; in 2007, 14% of 6- to 12-year-olds had experienced a toothache within the previous 6 months. Toothache disproportionately affects children who are poor or minorities and those with special health care needs. Occlusal abnormalities are also common in children. At least 30% of children are estimated to have moderate to severe orthodontic needs.

Box 28-1. Caries Prevention

Standard Caries Primary Prevention for All Children

1. Encourage consumption of optimally fluoridated water (0.7 ppm of fluoride).
2. Initiate fluoride toothpaste at first tooth eruption (alternatively, children with low risk of caries can start fluoride toothpaste at age 2 years). Use a rice-grain–sized amount of toothpaste before age 2 years and a pea-sized amount after 2 years. Brush twice daily and do not rinse afterward.
3. Primary care physician should examine teeth and oral structures at every well-child care visit.
4. Regular dental visits
5. Anticipatory guidance should include the following information
   a. Frequently consuming sugar-sweetened foods and drinks (including 100% juice) increases caries.
   b. Taking a bottle/sippy cup with any kind of juice or sugar-sweetened beverage to bed increases caries.
   c. Regularly drinking optimally fluoridated water reduces caries.
   d. Using fluoride toothpaste of at least 1,000 ppm twice daily reduces caries.

Intensive Caries Primary Prevention for Children With a High Risk of Caries

Includes all of the standard recommendations as well as the following:

1. Twice-yearly fluoride varnish application beginning at first tooth eruption
2. Twice-daily toothbrushing with rice-grain–sized amount of toothpaste at first tooth eruption
3. Initiation of regular professional dental care before 12 months of age

---

Box 28-2. Population and Individual Risk Factors for Dental Decay

Population Risk Factors

- **Low socioeconomic status**
- Recent immigrant
- Latino, Native American, and other nonwhite race/ethnicity
- No dental insurance or limited access to professional dental care

Individual Risk Factors

- Currently active decay or history of decay in patient
- Maternal tooth loss from caries
- Frequent and/or prolonged intake of foods containing fermentable carbohydrates (or frequent/ongoing use of liquid medications prepared with sucrose)
- Presence of visible plaque on the teeth
- Exposed root surfaces
- Having a special health care need that increases risk for caries (eg, cleft lip) or its complications (eg, some congenital heart disease), interferes with home oral hygiene (eg, oral aversiveness), or affects ability to obtain regular professional dental care (eg, behavioral difficulties associated with autism spectrum disorder)
- Inadequate exposure to fluoride
- Reduced salivary flow
- History of radiation therapy to head or neck
- Wearing of orthodontic appliances or prostheses

Clinical Presentation

Dental development begins in utero. Subsequently, the teeth erupt into the upper or **maxillary** jaw and into the lower or **mandibular** portion of the jaw. Teeth have a crown and root section (Figure 28-2). The **crown** is the visible portion of the tooth. The **root** is that part contained within the socket of the alveolar bone. The outer, hard coating of the crown is the **enamel.** Beneath the enamel is the **dentin,** composed of microtubules for transport of nutrients from the pulp to the outer portions of the tooth. The **pulp** contains nerves and vascular structures critical for the health and viability of the tooth. Teeth are anchored to the jaw through **periodontal ligaments.**

There are 20 **primary or deciduous teeth,** which erupt between approximately 6 and 36 months of age (Figure 28-3A). The first primary teeth to erupt typically are the lower **central incisors.** These teeth erupt on average at 6 to 10 months of age. A simple but not always precise rule of thumb is that the first tooth erupts at 6 months of age and then one tooth per month erupts until all primary teeth have erupted by about 24 to 30 months of age. In the normal pattern of primary tooth eruption, the incisors erupt, followed by eruption of the first molars, then canines (cuspids), and finally the second molars (hence the helpful mnemonic for the order of primary tooth eruption in each quadrant of the mouth: forward-forward-back-forward-back for incisor-incisor-first molar-cuspid-second molar).

Figure 28-2. Tooth anatomy.

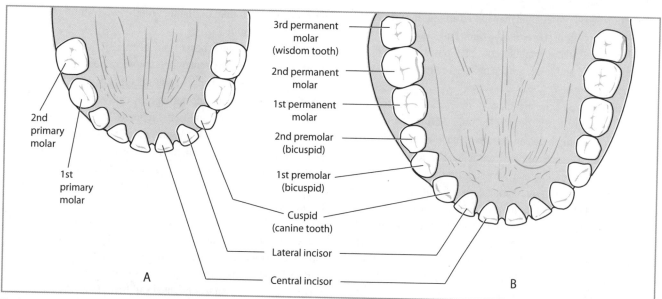

Figure 28-3. A, Primary dentition. B, Permanent dentition.

There is variation in the timing of tooth eruption in the population, and normal tooth eruption can vary by 6 to 12 months from the average. The eruption process may occasionally be preceded by a bluish discoloration to the gum, called an **eruption hematoma,** a benign process. More often, eruption of the primary teeth is associated with more generalized symptoms, such as fussiness and drooling. These symptoms are commonly referred to as teething. **Teething** does not cause diarrhea, respiratory infections, or true fever, although these entities may be present coincidentally with tooth eruption in infants.

The primary teeth are replaced by the **permanent teeth** (Figure 28-3B), which begin eruption at approximately 6 years of age. Permanent and primary teeth are present during the **mixed dentition phase,** which occurs between 6 and 13 years of age. Early mixed dentition is sometimes referred to as the "ugly duckling" stage because the permanent dentition looks large and awkward relative to the remaining primary teeth and because there may be transient malpositioning of the teeth. There are normally 32 permanent teeth; the last to erupt are the **third molars,** commonly known as **wisdom teeth,** at about 17 to 21 years of age.

Variations from the normal in number of teeth are not uncommon. **Hypodontia** refers to the presence of fewer than normal teeth. The most common teeth to be congenitally absent are the third molars, second premolars, or maxillary lateral incisors. Congenital absence of a central incisor is distinctly uncommon and should raise concern for the presence of other midline defects. Several teeth may be missing in disorders such as **Down syndrome** or **ectodermal dysplasia. Anodontia** is the congenital absence of teeth. Extra teeth are called **supernumerary teeth.** Children may be born with teeth already erupted, known as **natal teeth.** Teeth that erupt shortly after birth are referred to as **neonatal teeth** if their eruption occurs in the first month of life. These teeth are usually incisors, and at least 90% represent normal dentition rather than supernumerary teeth. The presence of natal or neonatal teeth may be familial and, on rare occasion, may suggest an underlying syndrome. In addition to variations in number, teeth may also demonstrate variations in color and structure due to abnormalities in tooth development, trauma, or extrinsic factors.

Caries may occur any time after eruption of the teeth. **Early childhood caries** (ECC), a more general term referring to what in the past was called *baby bottle tooth decay* or *nursing bottle caries,* affects a substantial portion of children. The pattern of decay seen in ECC is different from that seen in the teeth of older children and adults. Typically ECC first affects the maxillary incisors and spares the lower incisors. This pattern of decay is hypothesized to result from prolonged and frequent exposure of the teeth to sweet liquids, eg, falling asleep with a juice bottle in the mouth, whereby the beverage pools around the upper incisors but the lower teeth are protected by the overlying tongue. The **pit and fissure surfaces** of the molars are more likely sites of decay in older children. Fermentable carbohydrates, particularly those of a sticky nature, become embedded in these surfaces and are not easily reached by the bristles of a toothbrush. This allows for prolonged action of acid-producing bacteria and subsequent caries formation.

In its earliest stages, caries appears on physical examination as white, opaque areas at the gum line **(white spot lesions).** At this early stage, the lesion is potentially reversible if remineralization can occur, eg, by applying fluoride varnish to the white spots. However, once the decay has eroded the enamel, irreversible damage has occurred. Symptoms differentiate the degree and depth of caries involvement; however, young children often have difficulty localizing dental pain. A cavity into the dentin may produce intermittent pain, especially on exposure to temperature change or pressure on the affected tooth. Once cavitation has extended into the pulp, the resulting pulpitis may cause severe, persistent, often throbbing pain in the affected tooth, possibly awaking the child from sleep. Eventually the pulp undergoes necrosis and pain may disappear. However, the infection is still present and may spread around the tooth apex, forming a periapical abscess or fistula. Dental infection can progress to involve the maxilla or mandible and then move into the fascial planes of the head and neck, producing facial cellulitis, abscess, or airway obstruction.

The relationship of the maxillary to the mandibular dentition has functional and aesthetic implications. **Malocclusion** is an abnormal relationship between the upper and lower teeth and may be developmental, genetic, or environmental in etiology. Children with craniofacial disorders often have significant occlusal problems and facial asymmetries necessitating early referral for craniofacial team care. Other children may have milder malocclusion that needs orthodontic care. Normal occlusion occurs when the maxillary incisors are slightly in front of the mandibular incisors and the posterior molars interdigitate (Figure 28-4). This is called **class 1 occlusion. Class 2 occlusion** occurs when the maxillary teeth project too far anteriorly from the mandibular teeth. This may be associated with an **overjet,** commonly known as *buckteeth,* which can predispose to dental injury when children fall. **Class 3 occlusion** occurs when the mandibular teeth are anterior to the maxillary. This is also commonly referred to as an *underbite.* Other common forms of malocclusion include an **anterior open bite,** whereby the posterior teeth come together but there is an opening between the top and bottom anterior teeth, and a **crossbite,** which occurs when some of the upper teeth are located inside of the lower teeth during occlusion.

Pathophysiology

Hypodontia may be familial or occur secondary to an underlying syndrome. However, failure of one tooth to erupt is also commonly caused by another tooth in the path of eruption or insufficient space in the dental arch. Defects of tooth structure have a variety of causes. Medications, infection, jaundice, metabolic disorders, and irradiation may adversely affect normal tooth formation or mineralization. The permanent teeth begin to develop in utero and mineralize after birth, making them susceptible to prenatal and postnatal exposures. **Intrauterine infection** with rubella, cytomegalovirus, or syphilis may adversely affect tooth structure. Local oral infection (eg, a periapical abscess involving a primary tooth in early childhood) can damage the developing permanent tooth bud, resulting in a malformed permanent tooth.

Discolored teeth may be the result of intrinsic or extrinsic factors. Tetracycline given to pregnant or lactating women or children younger than 8 years can cause intrinsic staining of the permanent teeth. Exposure to high levels of fluoride during early childhood can cause **fluorosis** of the permanent dentition. Fluorosis, when it occurs in the United States, is usually mild, characterized by white striations on the permanent teeth. Children with mild fluorosis have teeth that are more resistant to dental decay. Teeth more severely affected by fluorosis may display hypoplastic enamel that is prone to staining; however, moderate and severe dental fluorosis is rare in the United States.

Inherited enamel or dentin defects may cause abnormal color of the teeth. These conditions may be isolated to the teeth, as in the case of **dentinogenesis imperfecta,** or as part of a systemic disorder, such as porphyria or osteogenesis imperfecta. A single dark tooth is usually non-vital or has bled within the tooth structure after dental trauma. Extrinsic staining is superficial and is usually due to poor oral hygiene; smoking; chewing tobacco or betel nuts; certain beverages such as coffee, tea, or wine; or medications such as liquid iron supplements.

Malocclusion can be caused by tooth crowding, an underlying craniofacial condition, abnormal jaw growth relationship, or malpositioning of the teeth, most commonly as the result of digit (usually thumb) sucking. The most common types of malocclusion associated with digit sucking are **anterior open bite,** overjet, or posterior crossbite.

Dental decay is a transmissible infectious disease in which cariogenic bacteria are passed from mother (usually) to child. *Streptococcus mutans* and *Lactobacillus* species, among other bacteria, produce acids as end products of carbohydrate metabolism. These acids dissolve the calcium-phosphate mineral of a tooth's enamel during a process called demineralization. If not reversed through remineralization, the tooth structure erodes until the demineralized area collapses, resulting in a cavity. A balance of caries-promoting and caries-inhibiting factors is constantly in play. Intraoral factors that inhibit caries include normal salivary production and regular fluoride exposure; those that promote caries are frequent intake of carbohydrates, particularly simple sugars, and xerostomia.

Differential Diagnosis

It can be difficult to differentiate tooth staining from a carious lesion, particularly when there are small areas of discoloration on the pit and fissure surfaces. If the lesion disappears with cleaning, staining is the etiology; however, staining is not always readily removed, and examination by a dentist and radiographs can help evaluate such lesions. White spots on the teeth also can have multiple etiologies. When the white spot is chalky in appearance and located along the gingival margin, demineralization that could progress to frank decay should be considered. On the other hand, small intrinsic defects of the enamel may also appear as white spots; however, these are usually located throughout the crown and not just along the gingival margin, and they also reflect light like the rest of the tooth (ie, not chalky).

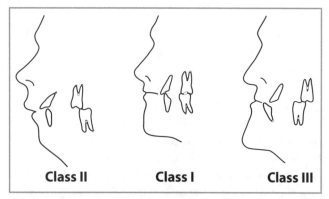

Figure 28-4. Classes of occlusion. Class I (middle) is considered most desirable from a functional and aesthetic perspective.

Class II   Class I   Class III

Evaluation

History

Dental pathology is diagnosed primarily through history and physical examination. Many physicians have not traditionally included the teeth and supporting structures as part of their routine physical examination. However, pediatricians and other health care professionals caring for children are generally the first, and often the only, health care professionals to examine a child during the early years of life and therefore play a key role in identification of dental pathology. This is particularly true in settings where access to professional dental care is limited. Early diagnosis facilitates timely referral to dental specialists who provide definitive management.

Physical Examination

During each well-child visit, the medical professional should closely assess the mouth and its structures for the pattern of eruption and dental development; the presence of caries, plaque, gingivitis, and other oral lesions (see Chapter 74); and malocclusion. Physicians should examine the gingiva of children, particularly those with dental decay or toothache, to assess for evidence of periapical abscess, which may need antibiotic therapy or incision and drainage.

The oral cavity of a young child can be examined most easily with the caregiver and examiner in a **knee-to-knee position,** with the child's head in the examiner's lap and the legs wrapped around the caregiver's waist. Older children can be examined on the examination table or while seated in a chair. It is useful to have a disposable mouth mirror and a good light source. A toothbrush can be used to prop the mouth open to allow for examination of the teeth and oral cavity. The toothbrush can later be used to demonstrate good toothbrushing techniques.

A child's occlusion is best examined by looking at the child's face from the anterior and lateral perspectives and watching the child's front and back teeth as the child opens and then bites down. Having the child bite down on a tongue depressor placed horizontally between the child's upper and lower teeth will demonstrate if there is a cant or asymmetry of the occlusion. The lateral profile of a child's face can be particularly revealing. Constructing an imaginary line between the bridge of the nose, the base of the nose, and the tip of the chin defines the shape of the lateral profile. In preschool-aged and older children, a slightly convex profile is preferable from functional and aesthetic perspectives. A concave profile is never normal and may be caused by midface underdevelopment or protrusion of the mandible. These children usually have a class 3 malocclusion. An overly convex profile may be due to an overjet or mandibular retrusion. These children usually have a class 2 malocclusion.

Laboratory Tests

An ill-appearing child with a dental abscess or facial cellulitis of odontogenic etiology should have a complete blood cell count and a blood culture obtained.

Imaging Studies

Dental radiographs are useful in evaluating for the presence and extent of dental decay. They can also aid in determining whether a tooth that has not erupted as expected is absent or prevented in some way from erupting. Finally, when there is concern for pathology, imaging, particularly a panoramic radiograph or computed tomography scan, can be useful in evaluating the facial skeleton.

Management

Much of the definitive management of dental disorders falls to dental professionals. However, physicians play an important role in educating families about prevention, identifying pathology, and facilitating dental referrals. Some dental conditions commonly fall into the realm of the primary care practitioner. For example, teething symptoms can be alleviated by giving the child a cold teething toy to suck on or with acetaminophen or ibuprofen given orally. Over-the-counter topical anesthetic agents often contain alcohol and are not recommended.

The American Academy of Pediatric Dentistry recommends the first professional dental care visit by 12 months of age. This is particularly important for children at high risk for dental caries. Occasionally, very young infants require a dental consultation. For example, if the natal or neonatal teeth interfere with feeding or are so loose as to pose an aspiration risk, they should be extracted; otherwise they require no intervention. When no teeth have erupted by 18 months of age, a dentist may choose to take radiographs to determine the status of the child's future dentition. If few developing teeth are seen, this can point to other diagnoses in which hypodontia or anodontia occur. Most superficial extrinsic tooth stains can be removed during professional cleaning. Intrinsic stains can be treated by a dentist with abrasion and bleach techniques or application of a composite veneer. Malocclusion, when not reversible or self-limited, often is treated with orthodontics. More severe cases may require orthognathic surgery.

In some communities it may be difficult to find a dental professional who will care for a child younger than 3 years, and this further emphasizes the importance of medical professionals in monitoring children's teeth and surrounding structures. Publicly insured children may also encounter difficulty accessing professional dental care. Clinicians should be aware of the closest source of specialized pediatric dental care if it is not within their own community. Dental schools or pediatric dental residency training programs generally offer specialized dental care for children, including sedation or anesthesia that may be needed to provide appropriate care.

Particularly in settings of limited access to dental care, physicians play an important role in educating families about the prevention of caries through advice about cariogenic food and beverages, regular tooth cleaning, and appropriate use of fluoride. Although physicians commonly advise parents not to allow their child to take a bottle to bed, it is particularly important that the child not take a bottle with **juice** or other sweetened beverages to bed. The evidence that human milk, formula, or cow's milk causes caries is equivocal.

Physicians can also actively intervene if early caries lesions or white spots are identified. Application of **fluoride varnish** to the teeth can help to remineralize and reverse early caries lesions. When a child has more advanced caries, prompt referral to a dental professional is indicated. Pulpal involvement and abscess formation may result if a carious lesion is ignored. If dental care is not immediately available, antibiotics (penicillin V or clindamycin) and analgesics (eg, ibuprofen) may alleviate symptoms temporarily; however, more definitive treatment (**root canal** or extraction) is necessary to remove the source of infection and prevent resurgence of symptoms and further complications. When an abscess has spread to involve the cheek, face, or neck, admission to the hospital for intravenous antibiotics and surgical drainage is usually indicated.

Prevention

Prevention of dental disorders and promotion of good oral health are the combined responsibility of the primary physician, child, family, and dentist. Important preventive practices include regular home oral hygiene; access to routine dental care; sound dietary practices, including avoiding frequent or prolonged exposure to fermentable carbohydrates, especially sucrose; sealant application; and, importantly, regular use of **fluorides.** Increasing availability of fluoridated water and fluoride-containing toothpaste has dramatically decreased the prevalence of decay in the United States and other developed countries over the last 50 years. Nevertheless, for many in the lay public, fluoride evokes controversy and undue concerns about adverse health effects. Pediatricians have an important role to play in countering misinformation and educating families about the safety, effectiveness, and appropriate use of fluoride. Fluoride can reverse or arrest early carious lesions through enhancement of tooth mineralization and reversal of tooth demineralization. The composition of the fluoride-containing enamel, fluoride apatite, is harder and less acid soluble than the original enamel that it replaces. Fluoride works best at remineralizing teeth when it is provided in a topical rather than systemic form (eg, fluoride drops are a systemic form of fluoride). Topical exposure to fluoride occurs through drinking fluoridated water, using fluoride toothpaste, and with professional applications.

There have been 2 recent changes to fluoride policies in the United States. First, the optimal fluoride level in drinking water to prevent tooth decay has been decreased to 0.7 ppm, which replaces the previous recommended range of 0.7 to 1.2 ppm. This change has been enacted because of expanded availability of fluoride from sources other than community water fluoridation and concerns for increasing incidence of dental fluorosis. Second, the American Dental Association now recommends fluoride supplements only for children who have a high risk of caries who live in fluoride-deficient communities. In a number of other countries, including Canada, England, and Australia, fluoride drops are no longer recommended in favor of early initiation of fluoride toothpaste. Relative to drops, fluoride toothpaste offers important advantages of lower cost, topical mode of action, no need for prescription, and a strong body of research evidence supporting its caries-preventive effects, particularly when used twice daily and when toothbrushing is supervised by parents or takes place in a classroom setting. Commercially available fluoride toothpaste in the United States contains 1,000 or 1,100 ppm of fluoride.

Tooth cleaning should begin with first tooth eruption, though when to add fluoride toothpaste has been confusing to parents and health care professionals. Parents worry that their child will swallow too much fluoride toothpaste before the child learns to spit out the residue. In fact, young children will swallow some toothpaste in the process of brushing, but if the appropriate amount of paste is used, the swallowed amount will be minimal. Children with high risk of caries should have their teeth brushed twice daily with a rice-grain–sized amount of fluoride toothpaste beginning at first tooth eruption. At 2 years of age, the amount of fluoride toothpaste per brushing can be increased to the size of a pea. It may also be beneficial for children who have a low risk of caries to initiate toothbrushing with fluoride toothpaste at first tooth eruption, particularly if they do not regularly consume fluoridated water (eg, children who are exclusively breastfed, children who live in fluoride-deficient communities). Some parents of children with low caries risk may choose to wait until after 2 years of age before starting use of fluoride toothpaste to avoid the risk of excessive fluoride intake that could contribute to fluorosis. There is no research evidence that "training" (ie, fluoride-free) toothpaste has any caries-preventive properties. By the age of about 7 years, most children have developed sufficient fine motor skills to begin flossing and brushing their teeth independently. Until then, parents should help their children brush and floss. It is not necessary to floss while there are still spaces between a child's teeth, as is the usual case in young children with only primary teeth. As additional teeth erupt and teeth become closely approximated, flossing is important to remove plaque between the teeth that can contribute to caries, gingivitis, and later to periodontal disease. **Sealants** placed on the pit and fissure surfaces of permanent molars can also be an important defense against caries in these surfaces. Children should be seen by a dentist for evaluation for sealant placement within 6 to 12 months of eruption of their first and second permanent molars.

Certain types of malocclusion are preventable. Because caries and trauma can lead to premature tooth loss and subsequent loss of spacing and overcrowding, prevention of these entities will minimize the need for later orthodontic treatment. Prolonged digit sucking contributes to malocclusion. If children can discontinue these practices before age 4 years, digit-associated malocclusion is usually reversible. Dentists can employ specific devices and treatment to help stop digit sucking if other methods, including behavior modification, are unsuccessful (see Chapter 53).

Prognosis

Many dental disorders are preventable. Early identification and prompt referral can prevent complications. In the past, edentulism in adulthood resulting from dental decay and periodontitis was common. Fluoride use and increased attention to preventive oral hygiene have reduced this condition as well as the incidence of permanent teeth caries; however, substantial disparities continue to adversely affect the oral health of US children and adults with low income, who are minorities, and who have special needs.

CASE RESOLUTION

The parents of the infant in the case history should be reassured that the absence of teeth in their 9-month-old daughter is normal. Her first tooth may not appear until she is 12 months old. As long as she is growing and developing normally, there is no cause for concern.

Selected References

American Academy of Pediatrics Oral Health Initiative. Protecting All Children's Teeth (PACT): A Pediatric Oral Health Training Program. www2.aap.org/ORALHEALTH/pact/index-cme.cfm. Accessed November 20, 2013

British Fluoridation Society. *One in a Million: The Facts About Water Fluoridation*. 3rd ed. The Ashton-Under-Lyne, United Kingdom: British Fluoridation Society; 2012. http://www.bfsweb.org/onemillion/onemillion.htm. Accessed November 20, 2013

Department of Health and the British Association for the Study of Community Dentistry. *Delivering Better Oral Health: An Evidence-Based Toolkit for Prevention*. 2nd ed. London, United Kingdom: Department of Health; 2009. http://webarchive.nationalarchives.gov.uk/20130107105354/http://www.dh.gov.uk/en/Publicationsandstatistics/Publications/PublicationsPolicyAndGuidance/DH_102331. Accessed November 20, 2013

Ismail AI, Hasson H. Fluoride supplements, dental caries and fluorosis: a systematic review. *J Am Dent Assoc*. 2008;139(11):1457–1468

Lewis C, Stout J. Toothache in US children. *Arch Pediatr Adolesc Med*. 2010;164(11):1059–1063

Lewis CW, Johnston BD, Linsenmeyar KA, Williams A, Mouradian W. Preventive dental care for children in the United States: a national perspective. *Pediatrics*. 2007;119(3):e544–e553

Marinho VC, Higgins JP, Sheiham A, Logan S. Fluoride toothpastes for preventing dental caries in children and adolescents. *Cochrane Database Syst Rev*. 2003;(1):CD002278

Milgrom P, Chi DL. Prevention-centered caries management strategies during critical periods in early childhood. *J Calif Dent Assoc*. 2011;39(10):735–741

Mouradian WE, Slayton RL, eds. Special issue on children's oral health. *Acad Pediatr*. 2009;9(6):371–482

US Government Accountability Office. *Report to Congressional Requesters. Medicaid. Extent of Dental Disease in Children Has Not Decreased, and Millions Are Estimated to Have Untreated Tooth Decay*. Washington, DC: US General Accounting Office; 2008. http://www.gao.gov/new.items/d081121.pdf. Accessed November 20, 2013

US Maternal and Child Health Bureau. *Topical Fluoride Recommendations for High-Risk Children. Development of Decision Support Matrix. Recommendations from MCHB Expert Panel*. Washington, DC: October 22–23, 2007. http://www.mchoralhealth.org/PDFs/TopicalFluorideRpt.pdf. Accessed November 20, 2013

CHAPTER 29

Normal Development and Developmental Surveillance, Screening, and Evaluation

Geeta Grover, MD

CASE STUDY

The parents of a 12-month-old are concerned that she is not walking yet. They report that she sat independently at 7 months and began crawling at 8 months. She can pull herself up to stand while holding on to furniture but is not cruising. Her birth and medical history are unremarkable. The physical examination is within normal limits, and review of your records reveals no concerns on a developmental screening test administered at 9 months of age.

Questions

1. What are the major areas in which development is assessed?
2. What are the gross motor, fine motor, and personal/social milestones for a 12-month-old?
3. What developmental screening tests could you administer to further assess her development?
4. How is developmental delay in children defined?

Development refers to the acquisition of functional skills during childhood. Monitoring the growth and development of children is an integral part of the assessment of pediatric patients. Recording the acquisition of developmental milestones provides a systematic approach by which to observe the progress of children over time. For ease of monitoring, these developmental milestones may be divided into 5 major domains or areas: gross motor, fine motor/adaptive, language, personal/social, and cognitive. This chapter discusses these major areas of development and the principles that govern them.

Four principles apply to all aspects of development. First, motor development is a continuous process that proceeds in the cephalocaudal direction and parallels neuronal myelination; therefore, developmental milestones reflect the maturation of the nervous system. Second, the sequence of development is the same in all children, but the rate of development may vary from child to child (eg, all children must walk before they run, but the age at which children walk or run varies from child to child). Third, the rate of attainment of milestones in one area may not parallel that in another. Fourth, certain primitive reflexes must be lost before corresponding voluntary movements can be attained (eg, the asymmetric tonic neck reflex must disappear before children can roll over).

Pathophysiology

Development is influenced by biological and environmental factors. Biological factors such as prematurity, exposure to drugs in utero, or the presence of chronic disease may place children at increased risk for developmental problems and delays. Environmental factors influencing development include parental attitudes and actions, socio-demographic factors, and cultural and societal influences. The quality of parental stimulation may influence the rate of acquisition of certain skills, especially cognitive and language abilities in preschool-aged children. Poverty and other socioeconomic factors may make it difficult for parents to provide their child with an optimal environment for growth and development.

Development in Newborns and Infants

Normal, full-term newborns enter the world capable of responding to visual, auditory, olfactory, oral, and tactile stimuli. They can be quieted and can even soothe themselves. Newborns can signal needs (eg, crying when hungry or wet), but they have a limited ability to respond to caregivers, primarily exhibiting disorganized and seemingly purposeless movements when stimulated. The newborn's reflexive generalized symmetric movements (eg, arm waving and kicking) in response to environmental stimuli are eventually replaced by cortically mediated voluntary actions in older infants and children. Additionally, in newborns, certain primitive reflexes can be elicited by appropriate peripheral stimuli. Eventually, primitive reflexes are replaced by reactions that allow children to maintain postural stability in response to a variety of sensory inputs (proprioceptive, visual, and vestibular).

Primitive reflexes are mediated by the brain stem; they are involuntary motor responses that are elicited by appropriate peripheral stimuli and are present at birth but disappear during the first 6 months of life. Normal motor development seems to be related to the suppression of these reflexes (Figure 29-1). Persistence or reappearance of these reflexes may indicate the presence of brain damage. **Postural reactions,** which are ultimately smoothly integrated into adult motor function (Figure 29-1), appear between 2 and 9 months of age. These reactions help maintain the orientation of the body in space and the interrelationship of one body part to another. The 3 major categories of postural reactions are righting, protection, and equilibrium.

The profile generated by combining primitive reflexes and postural reactions can be used to monitor the course of normal development and identify cases of problematic development. Persistence of primitive reflexes or failure of development of postural reactions can signal developmental problems. Authorities estimate that there are more than 70 primitive reflexes and postural reactions. Researchers do not agree on which of these reflexes or reactions are the most useful in the monitoring of development. The 7 most commonly used primitive reflexes are described in Box 29-1, and selected postural reactions are presented in Box 29-2.

Normal Development

A developmental assessment should include an evaluation of milestones in each of the 5 major areas. **Gross motor skills** are overall movements of large muscles (eg, sitting, walking, running). **Fine motor/adaptive skills** involve use of the small muscles of the hands, the ability to manipulate small objects, problem-solving skills, and eye-hand coordination. **Language skills** include hearing, understanding, and use of language. **Personal/social skills** involve socialization and ability to care for personal needs. **Cognitive skills** involve the ability to use higher mental processes, including comprehension, memory, and logical reasoning.

Table 29-1 outlines the normal pattern of development for each of these skills. The Table lists the average age of attainment of these skills as well as the normal ranges where available. Development is

an orderly and sequential process, and children must proceed through several stages before any given milestone is attained. Therefore, the physician should document not only *what* children can do but *how* they do it. For example, to sit without support, children first achieve head control. Several stages later they are able to sit in a

---

Box 29-1. Selected Primitive Reflexes
Moro Reflex
Allowing the baby's head to drop back suddenly results in abduction and upward movement of the arms followed by adduction and flexion. This reflex disappears by 4 months of age.
Rooting Reflex
Touching the corner of the baby's mouth results in lowering of the lower lip on the same side and movement of the tongue toward the stimulus.
Sucking Reflex
Placing an object in a baby's mouth causes vigorous sucking.
Grasp Reflex
Placing a finger in a baby's palm causes the baby to grasp it; the baby reinforces the grip as the finger is drawn upward. A similar response is seen in the foot grasp. Both of these reflexes disappear by 2 to 3 months of age.
Placing Reflex
Stroking the anterior aspect of the tibia against the edge of a table results in the lifting of the baby's leg to step onto the table.
Stepping Reflex
Holding the baby upright and slightly leaning forward produces alternating flexion and extension movements of the legs that simulate walking. This reflex disappears by 5 to 6 weeks of age.
Asymmetric Tonic Neck Reflex
With the baby lying supine, turning the head to one side results in extension of the extremities on that side and flexion of the opposite extremities (fencer position). This reflex disappears by 3 to 4 months of age.

Box 29-2. Selected Postural Reactions
Righting Reactions
These allow the body to maintain normal postural relationships of the head, trunk, and extremities during all activities. The different reactions appear at different ages, beginning shortly after birth and ranging up to 12 months of age.
Protection and Equilibrium Reactions
Protective Equilibrium Response
When gently pushed toward one side while in a sitting position, infants increase trunk flexor tone toward that side to regain their center of gravity and extend the arm on the same side to protect against falling. This response usually emerges at about 4 to 6 months of age.
Parachute Reactions
When held in ventral suspension and suddenly lowered (downward parachute), infants extend their arms as if to protect themselves from a fall; similar reactions are seen with forward and backward stimulation. These reactions appear at 8 to 9 months of age.

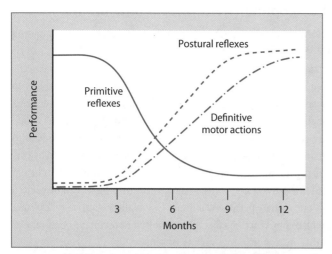

Figure 29-1. Primitive reflex profile. (Reproduced with permission from Capute AJ, Accardo PJ, Vining EP, Rubenstein JE, Harryman S. *Primitive Reflex Profile.* Baltimore, MD: University Park Press; 1978:10.)

"tripod" position with arms extended in front for support, and finally they sit with the head steady and back straight without support (Figure 29-2).

Gross Motor Skills

During the first year of life, the ultimate goal of gross motor development is walking. The first step toward this goal is head control. By 6 months of age, children are able to sit without support for a few seconds. At 9 to 10 months of age, children are able to pull themselves to a standing position, and by 12 to 17 months of age, they are able to walk. Children then learn to run, negotiate stairs, hop on one foot, and skip—in that order.

Fine Motor/Adaptive Skills

Development of the 2-finger pincer grasp is the major goal of fine motor development during the first year (Figure 29-3). The hands primarily remain in a fisted position until 3 months of age. Infants also discover the midline at this age, and shortly thereafter they may play with the hands in the midline. Four-month-olds begin reaching for desired objects; by 6 months of age, they are able to transfer objects from one hand to the other. By 7 months, they have a 3-finger pincer grasp, and by 9 to 10 months, they have developed the 2-finger grasp, which allows them to manipulate small objects such as raisins and pencils. By 14 months, they begin to scribble, and by 3 to 5 years, they are able to copy geometric shapes. Children with early preference for the use of one hand over another, especially prior to about 18 months of age, should be assessed for the presence of paresis or other neuromuscular problems. Handedness may develop by 3 years but often is not firmly established until the age of 4 to 5 years.

Language Skills

The development of normal speech and language skills is discussed in Chapter 30.

Figure 29-2. Stages in the development of sitting. A, Head control. B, "Tripod sitting." C, Head steady and back straight without support.

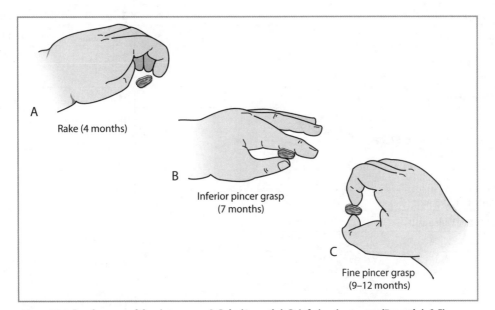

Figure 29-3. Development of the pincer grasp. A, Rake (4 months). B, Inferior pincer grasp (7 months). C, Fine pincer grasp (9–12 months).

Table 29-1. Normal Pattern of Development[a]		
Skill	*Mean Age*	*Normal Range*
Gross Motor Skills		
Reflex head turn; moves head side to side	Newborn	0–3 mo
Lifts head when prone	1 mo	1–4 mo
Lifts shoulders up when prone	2 mo	1–4 mo
Lifts up on elbows; head steady when upright	3 mo	2–5 mo
Lifts up on extended hands; rolls front to back; no head lag when pulled to sitting from supine position	4 mo	3–6 mo
Rolls back to front	5 mo	4–7 mo
Sits independently (≥30 s)	6 mo	5–9 mo
Crawls on hands and knees	8 mo	6–11 mo
Pulls to stand	9 mo	6–12 mo
Cruises	11 mo	9–14 mo
Walks	12 mo	9–17 mo
Walks backward	15 mo	13–17 mo
Runs	15 mo	13–20 mo
Kicks a ball	24 mo	18–30 mo
Walks up and down stairs (taking one step at a time and holding on)	24 mo	
Stands on one foot	30 mo	
Walks up stairs alternating steps	30 mo	28–36 mo
Peddles a tricycle	3 y	30–48 mo
Walks down stairs alternating steps/hops on one foot	4 y	
Skips	5 y	
Fine Motor/Adaptive Skills		
Tracks horizontally to midline	1 mo	
Tracks past midline/tracks vertically	2 mo	1–3 mo
Not fisted for >50% of the time; tracks 180 degrees; visual threat; discovers midline	3 mo	3–4 mo
Reaches for bright object; brings object to mouth	4 mo	
Transfers object from one hand to the other	6 mo	4–7 mo
3-finger pincer grasp	7 mo	6–10 mo
Neat pincer grasp	9 mo	7–10 mo
Bangs cubes in midline	9 mo	7–11 mo
Tower of 2 cubes; scribbles spontaneously	14 mo	14–20 mo
Tower of 4 cubes	18 mo	17–24 mo
Copies vertical and horizontal line; tower of 6 cubes	2 y	
Copies circle	3 y	
Copies cross (†)	4 y	
Copies square; draws person with 3 parts	5 y	
Copies triangle; draws person with 6 parts	6 y	
Language Skills		
Alerts to bell	Newborn	
Searches with eyes for sound	2 mo	
Cooing	3 mo	1–4 mo
Turns head to voice or bell; laughs	4 mo	3–6 mo

Table 29-1. Normal Pattern of Development[a], continued

Skill	Mean Age	Normal Range
Language Skills, continued		
Babbles	6 mo	5–9 mo
Mama/dada nonspecific	8 mo	6–10 mo
Understands the word "no"	10 mo	
Mama/dada specific	10 mo	9–14 mo
Follows 1-step command with gesture; 3–5-word vocabulary	12 mo	10–16 mo
Follows 1-step command without gesture	15 mo	12–20 mo
Can point to several body parts	18 mo	12–24 mo
50-word vocabulary	2 y	
2-word sentences; pronouns indiscriminately	2 y	20–30 mo
States first name	34 mo	30–40 mo
250-word vocabulary; 3-word sentences; speech intelligible to strangers 75% of time	3 y	
Uses pronouns appropriately	3 y	30–42 mo
Personal/Social Skills		
Regards face	Newborn	
Spontaneous social smile	6 wk	1–3 mo
Discriminates social smile; relates to parent with real joy	6 mo	
Displays stranger anxiety; plays peekaboo	7 mo	7–9 mo
Orients to name; uses gestures to get needs met	12 mo	
Drinks from a cup	15 mo	10–18 mo
Uses a spoon, spilling a little	15 mo	12–18 mo
Uses sounds, pointing, or other "showing" gestures to draw attention to object of interest	15 mo	12–15 mo
Simple pretend play (eg, feeding doll)	18 mo	
Imitates housework	18 mo	14–24 mo
Helps with undressing	2 y	22–30 mo
Washes and dries hands	2 y	
Parallel play; enjoys being next to other kids	2 y	12–30 mo
Undresses self	3 y	30–40 mo
Toilet training		24–36 mo
Imagines self as different characters	3 y	
Cooperative play	3 y	24–48 mo
Dresses without assistance	5 y	
Cognitive Skills		
Sensorimotor		Newborn–2 y
Preoperational		2–6 y
Concrete operational		6–11 y
Formal operations		>11 y
Miscellaneous Cognitive Milestones		
Concept of today	24 mo	
Concept of tomorrow	30 mo	
Concept of yesterday	36 mo	
Concept of right and left	7 y	

[a]Detailed language milestones are presented in Chapter 30, Table 30-1, page 178.

Personal/Social Skills

These skills enable children to interact and respond to the surrounding world. Deficits in the development of age-appropriate social skills/social relatedness (eg, social orienting, social referencing, joint attention, pretend play) are a defining feature of autism spectrum disorders (ASDs). For children within this spectrum, the development of social skills is characteristically "out of sync" with their overall level of functioning. Joint attention is the inclination to share enjoyment, interests, or achievement with other people, and like other developmental skills, it seems to develop in graduated stages (early skills include reciprocal smiling at the sight of a familiar person, followed by later emerging skills like the ability to isolate one's index finger and point by 12–15 months of age). Lack of joint attention seems to be a core deficit in ASDs; it also seems to be specific to ASDs. (Autism spectrum disorders are discussed fully in Chapter 128.)

Cognitive Skills

These abilities allow children to think, reason, problem-solve, and understand the surrounding environment. The concept of object permanence or object constancy, the realization that objects may exist even if they cannot be seen, develops at approximately 7 to 9 months of age. The understanding of time comes much later. Children develop the concept of "today" at 24 months of age, "tomorrow" at 30 months, and "yesterday" at 36 months. It is extremely important that health care professionals realize that children's perception and understanding of pain, disease, and illness are guided by their stage of cognitive development. The psychologist Jean Piaget generated complex generalizations by observing what children did and how they did it; his theories are the cornerstone of knowledge in this area. Piaget's 4 stages of cognitive development are presented in Box 29-3.

Developmental Delay

Children are said to be developmentally delayed if they fail to reach developmental milestones at the expected age. This age ranges widely because of the wide variation among normal children. Individual children may be delayed in one area or several areas of development.

Box 29-3. Piaget's 4 Stages of Development

Sensorimotor (Birth–2 Years)
Children approach the world through sensations and motor actions. They develop a sense of object permanence, spatial relationships, and causality.

Preoperational (2–6 Years)
Children's mental processes are linked to their own perception of reality. They do not separate internal and external reality.

Concrete Operational (6–11 Years)
Children can perform mental operations in their heads if they relate to real objects. They develop concepts of conservation of mass, volume, and number.

Formal Operations (>11 Years)
Children develop the capacity for abstract thought.

Differential Diagnosis

Three factors are involved in the differential diagnosis of children with developmental delays: determination of the area or areas of development in which delay is apparent; if motor delay is evident, determination of whether the condition is progressive or nonprogressive; and assessment to see if developmental milestones previously achieved are lost or if age-appropriate milestones were achieved at all.

Children with an early history of normal development who subsequently experience a slowing of developmental progression, often associated with cognitive delays or seizures, may have a metabolic defect. Children who attain developmental milestones and subsequently lose them may have a neurodegenerative disease (eg, multiple sclerosis, adrenoleukodystrophy) or a lesion of the spinal cord or brain. The presence of habitual rhythmic body movements (eg, body rocking, head banging) may be a sign of a pervasive developmental disorder such as ASDs.

Cerebral palsy, the classic example of nonprogressive motor abnormality, is a form of static encephalopathy characterized by abnormal movement and posture. The type of cerebral palsy depends on which area of the brain is injured. Spastic cerebral palsy, seen most commonly, is secondary to upper motor neuron injury. The ataxic form of the disease is related to lesions of the cerebellum or its pathways. Dyskinetic cerebral palsy manifests as uncontrolled and purposeless movements that often result from a basal ganglia lesion (eg, athetosis following bilirubin deposition in the basal ganglia). Onset of symptoms is in infancy or early childhood. The key factor in making the diagnosis is establishing that the motor deficits are static and not progressing.

Evaluation

When evaluating children for possible delays in development, it is important to remember that there is a great deal of variation in the age of attainment of milestones. In addition, the rate of acquisition of milestones in one area of development may not parallel that in another. Routine and ongoing assessment of a child's level of development at all periodic health maintenance visits through observation, history, physical examination, and screening tests allows the physician to form a longitudinal view of the child. The physician is thus able to identify and differentiate true deficits and delays from temporary setbacks.

History

Evaluation of children for suspected delays in development includes a complete history (Questions Box). Family history is important because other family members may have relatively delayed attainment of milestones. Perinatal factors that place children at high risk for developmental difficulties include a history of maternal drug or alcohol use during pregnancy, prematurity in the child, and congenital infections. Other historical risk factors for developmental delay include history of seizures, sepsis or meningitis, exposure to lead or other toxins, and poor feeding or growth. Environmental factors,

Questions

Normal Development

- Has anyone in the child's family had developmental problems or delays?
- Did the mother use any drugs or alcohol during pregnancy?
- Was the child premature?
- Does the child have a history of seizures?
- Has the child had meningitis or sepsis?
- Does the child have any history of not feeding well or poor growth?
- Is the child's home environment characterized by any stresses (eg, divorce, limited financial resources)?

such as stressful home conditions, history of abuse or neglect, and lack of stimulation, may also contribute to delayed development.

Physical Examination

Height and weight should be checked. Abnormal growth (ie, height or weight <fifth percentile or head circumference <fifth percentile or >90th percentile) may be a marker for developmental delay. The presence of congenital anomalies (eg, cataracts, hypertelorism, spina bifida) or neurocutaneous lesions (eg, café au lait spots) may be suggestive of chromosomal anomalies or other genetic diseases. Neuromuscular examination should emphasize age-appropriate milestones. Abnormalities in muscle tone (eg, hypotonia, hypertonia), bulk, or strength may be clues to the presence of neuromuscular disease (eg, muscular dystrophy), cerebral palsy, or Down syndrome.

Laboratory Tests

Age-appropriate assessment of the child's vision and hearing should be performed if signs of motor, cognitive, or language delays are apparent. Chromosomal studies may be conducted if dysmorphic features are noted on the physical examination. Evidence of cognitive or motor delays may warrant metabolic studies (eg, organic and amino acids).

Imaging studies of the head, such as magnetic resonance imaging scans or electroencephalograms, may be necessary if the child has a history of seizures or an abnormal neurologic examination.

Developmental Surveillance, Screening, and Evaluation

Early detection of developmental delays is a responsibility of all pediatric health care professionals. Unfortunately, current detection rates of developmental disorders are lower than their actual prevalence. About 20% of children between the ages of 3 to 17 years will have one or more developmental, learning, or emotional disorders, with 4% to 5% having developmental delays. Without the use of specific developmental screening tools, only about 30% of developmental disabilities are identified, but with the use of tools this identification rate increases to 70% to 80%.

Developmental surveillance, the ongoing process of monitoring individual children's developmental status, should be incorporated at each health maintenance visit. Surveillance involves eliciting and attending to parental concerns about their children's development and usually involves age-specific queries, such as whether the child is walking, talking, or pointing. Surveillance has been referred to as a kind of developmental growth chart. Recognition of children who may be at risk of developmental delays is the goal of developmental surveillance.

Developmental screening is the administration of a brief standardized tool to identify children at risk of a developmental disorder. Box 29-4 lists frequently used developmental screening tools. A formal developmental screening should be performed when developmental surveillance elicits a risk factor for developmental delay; in the absence of established risk factors or parental concerns, the administration of a general developmental screening tool is recommended by the American Academy of Pediatrics (AAP) at the 9-, 18-, and 24- or 30-month health maintenance visits (AAP, 2006). The AAP further recommends that in addition to a general developmental screening tool, an ASD-specific screening tool should also be administered at the 18-month visit. (See Chapter 128 for a listing of ASD-specific screening tools.) Periodic screening is necessary to detect emerging disabilities as children grow. Screening instruments should have a broad developmental focus and be brief, inexpensive, valid, and reliable. Screening tests are not diagnostic. A failed screening test should lead to a referral for further developmental evaluation.

Developmental evaluation (developmental assessment) is performed when surveillance or screening identifies a child as being at high risk of a developmental disorder. The aim is to identify the specific developmental disorder or disorders affecting the child. Developmental evaluation is performed by trained examiners. Unlike developmental screening, developmental evaluation is diagnostic.

The Bayley Scales of Infant and Toddler Development, 3rd Edition (Bayley-III), first published in 1933 by Nancy Bayley, is one of the most commonly used developmental evaluation tools. It has 5 distinct scales yielding scores for 5 developmental domains: cognitive, language, motor, social-emotional, and adaptive behavior. The Bayley-III may be used for children 1 to 42 months of age. Developmental tests like the Bayley-III (emphasizing sensorimotor-based

---

Box 29-4. Frequently Used Developmental Screening Instruments

Developmental Screening Instruments Relying on Information From Parents

- Child Development Inventory
- Child Development Review—Parent Questionnaire (CDR-PQ)
- Infant Development Inventory
- Ages & Stages Questionnaire, 3rd Edition (ASQ-3)
- Parents' Evaluation of Developmental Status (PEDS)

Screens Relying on Eliciting Skills Directly From Children

- Bayley Infant Neurodevelopmental Screener (BINS)
- Batelle Developmental Inventory, 2nd Edition (BDI-2)
- Brigance Screens III
- Denver Developmental Materials DENVER II

skills) have a poor correlation with later measures of intelligence (emphasizing language and abstract reasoning), especially before 24 to 30 months of age. As such, developmental tests are best used as measures of current developmental functioning rather than as predictors of future functioning. Intelligence tests, achievement tests, personality tests, or behavior rating scales may be used for preschool- and school-aged children having behavioral or emotional concerns, learning disabilities, or developmental disabilities.

Management

Children with identified developmental delays in one or more areas should be referred to the appropriate specialist, agency, or state program for further testing and assessment. Detailed neurologic examination may be necessary if gross motor delays are identified. Language delays may warrant formal hearing and speech assessment by an audiologist or a speech pathologist. Cognitive impairment requires formal psychometric assessment, which in some cases can be performed through the child's school.

Prognosis

Early identification of children with developmental delays is critical; it allows for early intervention, thereby making it possible for individual children to reach their maximum potential. Identification and treatment of underlying disease (eg, hypothyroidism, infection) prevents further damage. Removal of children from adverse home environments or placement of children from impoverished home environments in early intervention programs can greatly stimulate their developmental potential. The prognosis for children with mild developmental delays can sometimes be improved greatly from participation in such early intervention stimulation programs.

Selected References

American Academy of Pediatrics Council on Children With Disabilities, Section on Developmental Behavioral Pediatrics, Bright Futures Steering Committee, Medical Home Initiatives for Children With Special Needs Project Advisory Committee. Identifying infants and young children with developmental disorders in the medical home: an algorithm for developmental surveillance and screening. *Pediatrics.* 2006;118(1):405–420

Gerber RJ, Wilks T, Erdie-Lalena C. Developmental milestones: motor development. *Pediatr Rev.* 2010;31(7):267–277

Gerber RJ, Wilks T, Erdie-Lalena C. Developmental milestones 3: social-emotional development. *Pediatr Rev.* 2011;32(12):533–536

Hamilton SS, Glascoe FP. Making developmental behavioral screenings work for school-aged kids. *Contemp Pediatr.* 2010:63–87

Johnson CP, Myers SM; American Academy of Pediatrics Council on Children With Disabilities. Identification and evaluation of children with autism spectrum disorders. *Pediatrics.* 2007;120(5):1183–1215

Marks KP, LaRosa AC. Understanding developmental-behavioral screening measures. *Pediatr Rev.* 2012;33(10):448–458

Myers SM, Johnson CP; American Academy of Pediatrics Council on Children With Disabilities. Management of children with autism spectrum disorders. *Pediatrics.* 2007;120(5):1162–1182

Roberts G, Palfrey J, Bridgemohan C. A rational approach to the medical evaluation of a child with developmental delay. *Contemp Pediatr.* 2004;21:76–100

Shevell M, Ashwal S, Donley D, et al. Practice parameter: evaluation of the child with global developmental delay: report of the Quality Standards Subcommittee of the American Academy of Neurology and the Practice Committee of the Child Neurology Society. *Neurology.* 2003;60(3):367–380

Wilks T, Gerber RJ, Erdie-Lalena C. Developmental milestones: cognitive development. *Pediatr Rev.* 2010;31(9):364–367

CASE RESOLUTION

The parents of the child described in the case history may be reassured that their child is developing normally for her age. Although most children begin walking at about 12 months of age, commencement of walking anywhere up to the age of 17 months is considered to be within normal limits. The American Academy of Pediatrics recommends that standardized developmental screening should be performed when developmental surveillance identifies high risk factors and routinely at the 9-, 18-, and 24- or 30-month health maintenance visits. Administration of a formal screening tool is probably not necessary at this visit but can be considered again at the 15-month visit if there is a lack of progression in her gross motor skills or if any other risk factor is identified at that time.

CHAPTER 30

Speech and Language Development: Normal Patterns and Common Disorders

Geeta Grover, MD

CASE STUDY

The parents of a 3-year-old girl bring her to see you. They are concerned because their daughter has only an 8- to 10-word vocabulary and she does not put words together into phrases or sentences. They report that she seems to have no hearing problems; she responds to her name and follows directions well.

In general, she has been in good health. Her development, aside from delayed speech, is normal. During the physical examination, which is also normal, the girl does not speak.

Questions

1. What language skills should children have at 1, 2, and 3 years?
2. Approximately how many words should 3-year-olds have in their vocabulary?
3. By what age should children's speech be intelligible to strangers at least 75% of the time?
4. What factors may be associated with delayed speech development?
5. What tests are used to assess children's hearing, speech, and language development?

The ability to communicate through language is a uniquely human skill. Speech refers to the production of sounds, whereas language involves comprehension and expression; it is the use of words, phrases, and gestures to convey intent. **Receptive language** refers to the ability to understand others, while **expressive language** is the ability to produce communication to convey meaning to others. Normal hearing is essential for the development of speech and language.

Speech disorders include problems in the production of speech sounds. Speech disorders may affect articulation (phonologic disorders), fluency (stuttering), or voice (tone, pitch, and volume). The development of language skills in a normal sequence but at a slower pace than normal is referred to as *language delay;* language delays may affect only receptive or expressive language or both (eg, a mixed receptive-expressive language delay). An atypical sequence of language skill acquisition is referred to as a *language disorder.* Children with developmental language disorders have persistent and significant limitation in their ability to receive or express language.

The development of normal speech and language skills is an important developmental milestone that is eagerly awaited by parents. Normal patterns of language development should be as familiar to pediatricians as all other aspects of child development (see Chapter 29). It is important that children with suspected language delays be referred to specialists as early as possible. Children with delayed speech or language development should be suspected of having a hearing deficit. Diminished hearing is an important cause of delayed language development. Delays in language development can also be seen in the context of global developmental or cognitive delays or associated with autism spectrum disorders (ASDs).

Epidemiology

The prevalence of specific language impairment in school-aged children who have no hearing loss or obvious genetic or neurologic condition is about 7%. Speech and language disorders are more common in boys than girls and in children who have a family history of language, speech, or reading disorders. There is good evidence now that early language impairment is associated with later difficulties learning to read.

Clinical Presentation

Lack of response to sound at any age, failure to achieve age-appropriate expressive language skills, and parental concern about a child's hearing are the most important signs of hearing or language impairment. Deaf infants coo normally and may even babble; therefore, an infant's vocalizing does not preclude a hearing loss.

Pathophysiology

The left hemisphere of the brain is responsible for language skills in 94% of right-handed adults and approximately 75% of left-handed adults. Peripheral auditory stimuli are transmitted to the primary auditory areas in both temporal lobes. Sounds then undergo a series of analyses, primarily in 3 main areas in the left cerebral cortex: Wernicke area (or auditory association area), which is responsible for the comprehension of language; Broca motor speech (or motor encoding) area, which is responsible for the preliminary conversion of language into motor activity; and the primary and supplementary motor cortexes, which control the movements necessary for speech. This complex process is responsible for the comprehension and production of language.

Speech and language develop in a predictable, orderly sequence. Language skills can be receptive or expressive. Early receptive milestones refer to ability to hear and respond to sound, whereas later milestones reflect ability to understand spoken words. Early expressive milestones relate to speech production; later, children use language to convey their intent to others. In the first year of life, receptive skills are more advanced than expressive skills.

Children's language skills evolve primarily through parent-child interactions. Language begets language; children must first receive language before they are able to express themselves with language. Eye contact, social smiling, and ability to share attention with others, or joint attention (developed by 12–15 months of age), are children's first experiences with shared meaning, crucial for language development. Evidence exists that by the time a child is 4 years of age, the differences in word exposure between children living in higher socioeconomic environments as compared with those living in lower socioeconomic environments may be up to 30 million words. Research also suggests that expressive language vocabulary at age 3 predicts language and reading achievement up to 9 to 10 years of age. (See Chapter 31 for information about the importance of early reading exposure on children's language development.)

Knowledge of normal receptive and expressive language skills (Table 30-1) is essential to recognition and identification of developmental delays. Box 30-1 lists "danger signals" that indicate possible delays and serves as a guide for referral to specialists. It is most important to remember that by the age of 3 years, 75% of children's speech should be intelligible to strangers.

Differential Diagnosis

The various causes of delayed language development include hearing loss, disorders of central nervous system (CNS) processing, anatomic abnormalities, and environmental deprivation (Box 30-2). Although birth order (eg, the belief that younger children speak later than firstborn children because older siblings speak for them), laziness (eg, "Don't give him what he wants when he points. Make him ask for it"), and bilingualism are commonly believed to lead to speech and language delay, their contributory role has never been proved. For a complete discussion of hearing loss, refer to Chapter 76.

Table 30-1. Receptive and Expressive Language Milestones (Birth to 3 Years)

Skill	Mean Age	Normal Range
Receptive Milestones		
Alerts to sound	Newborn	
Orients to sound/turns to voice	4 mo	3–6 mo
Responds to name	4 mo	4–9 mo
Understands "no"	10 mo	9–18 mo
Follows 1-step command with gesture	12 mo	10–16 mo
Follows 1-step command without gesture	15 mo	12–20 mo
Points to several body parts	18 mo	12–24 mo
Follows 2-step command with gesture	24 mo	22–30 mo
Expressive Milestones		
Cooing (vowel sounds)	3 mo	1–4 mo
Laughs	4 mo	3–6 mo
Babbling (consonants added to vowel sounds)	6 mo	5–9 mo
Dada/Mama nonspecifically	8 mo	6–10 mo
Dada/Mama specifically	10 mo	9–14 mo
3- to 5-word vocabulary	12 mo	
Immature jargoning (gibberish with inflection)	13 mo	10–18 mo
Mature jargoning (gibberish with occasional word)	18 mo	16–24 mo
50-word vocabulary	24 mo	
2-word phrases	24 mo	20–30 mo
Uses pronouns indiscriminately	24 mo	22–30 mo
States first name	34 mo	30–40 mo
Uses pronouns appropriately	36 mo	30–42 mo
250-word vocabulary	36 mo	
75% of speech intelligible to strangers	36 mo	

Box 30-1. Danger Signals in Language Development

- Inconsistent or lack of response to auditory stimuli at any age
- No babbling by 9 months
- No intelligible speech by 18 months
- Inability to respond to simple directions or commands (eg, "sit down," "come here") by 24 months
- Speech predominantly unintelligible at 36 months
- Dysfluency (stuttering) of speech noticeable after 5 years
- Hypernasality; inappropriate vocal quality, pitch, or intensity at any age

---

Box 30-2. Causes of Delayed Language Development

- Hearing impairment
- Perinatal risk factors leading to hearing impairment
- Disorders of central nervous system processing
  —Global developmental delay
  —Intellectual disability
  —Autism spectrum disorders
- Developmental language disorders
- Disorders of language production
  —Articulation disorder
  —Dysarthria
  —Verbal apraxia
- Presence of anatomic abnormalities (eg, cleft lip, cleft palate)
- Environmental deprivation

Questions

Language Development

- Are the child's language capabilities appropriate for age?
- Do the parents feel that their child has difficulty hearing?
- Is there any family history of childhood deafness?
- Has the child been exposed to any ototoxic agents (eg, amino-glycoside antibiotics)?
- Is there a history of neonatal asphyxia, hyperbilirubinemia, or low birth weight?
- Has the child ever had bacterial meningitis?
- Did the mother have a TORCHS (toxoplasmosis, rubella, cytomegalovirus, herpes simplex, syphilis) infection during pregnancy?

Disorders of CNS processing include global developmental delay, intellectual disability, ASDs (see Chapter 128), and developmental language problems. Developmental language disorders produce speech or language delays in children in the absence of hearing loss, anatomic abnormalities of the vocal tract, intellectual disability, or global developmental delay. "Late talkers," or children who have normal comprehension but simply begin speaking late, have mild developmental language problems. Children who are completely nonverbal have more severe problems.

Anatomic abnormalities may also result in speech and language delays. Cleft palate is the abnormality most commonly associated with difficulties in speech production. Children with cleft palate characteristically have hyper-nasal speech secondary to velopharyngeal incompetence (eg, dysfunction of the soft palate). In addition, conductive hearing losses may result from chronic serous otitis media, which is common in children with cleft palate. The presence of a submucosal cleft palate, characterized by a bifid uvula, diastasis of the muscles in the midline of the soft palate with intact mucosa, and notching of the posterior border of the hard palate, should be considered in children without an overt cleft palate who have recurrent symptomatic serous otitis media and phonation difficulties.

Environmental deprivation is another cause of delayed language development, especially in families where children are not spoken or read to. Sometimes there is additional historical or physical evidence of deprivation (eg, profound failure to thrive, physical or sexual abuse) or emotional trauma (eg, domestic violence).

Evaluation

History

When evaluating children younger than 3 years, pediatricians must rely primarily on parental reports of children's language capabilities (Questions Box). Children who are 3 years and older can usually be engaged in conversation during the visit, but younger children are more likely to be uncooperative or remain silent when confronted

---

Box 30-3. High-Risk Indicators for Hearing Loss in Children (Birth to 24 months)

Neonatal Period (Birth–28 d)
- Family history of sensorineural hearing loss (SNHL)
- In utero infection associated with SNHL (eg, TORCHS [toxoplasmosis, rubella, cytomegalovirus, herpes simplex, syphilis] infections)
- Anatomic malformations of the head and neck region
- Hyperbilirubinemia at a level requiring exchange transfusion
- Low birth weight ($<$1,500 g)
- Bacterial meningitis
- Low Apgar scores
- Respiratory distress (eg, meconium aspiration)
- Mechanical ventilation for 10 days or more
- Exposure to ototoxic medications (eg, aminoglycoside antibiotics) for more than 5 days or in combination with loop diuretics
- Stigmata of syndromes known to be associated with hearing loss (eg, Down syndrome)

Infants and Children (29 d–24 mo)
- Parental concern about hearing, speech, language, or developmental delay
- Recurrent or persistent otitis media with effusion for at least 3 months
- Severe head trauma (associated with fracture of the temporal bone)
- Infections associated with SNHL (eg, bacterial meningitis, mumps, measles)
- Neurodegenerative disorders or demyelinating diseases
- Any of the newborn risk factors listed previously

Adapted with permission from American Academy of Pediatrics Joint Committee on Infant Hearing. Supplement to the JCIH 2007 position statement: principles and guidelines for early intervention after confirmation that a child is deaf or hard of hearing. *Pediatrics*. 2013;131:e1324 and American Academy of Pediatrics Committee on Practice and Ambulatory Medicine and Section on Otolaryngology—Head and Neck Surgery. Hearing assessment in infants and children: recommendations beyond neonatal screening. *Pediatrics*. 2009;124(4):1252–1263.

by strangers or new situations. Historical factors, such as a family history of childhood deafness, exposure to ototoxic agents (eg, aminoglycoside antibiotics), neonatal asphyxia or neonatal intensive care unit stay of more than 5 days, hyperbilirubinemia, maternal cocaine abuse, or low birth weight, provide valuable information in the identification of high-risk infants (see boxes 30-1 and 30-3).

Physical Examination

Examination should include a thorough assessment of the head and neck region. Microcephaly may indicate the presence of intellectual disability or structural abnormalities. Abnormalities of the external ear (eg, microtia) may be associated with sensorineural hearing loss. Otoscopic examination of the ear is essential. Presence of a middle ear effusion may be associated with a conductive hearing loss. The tympanic membrane should be examined for evidence of scarring or perforation, often secondary to recurrent otitis media. Pneumatic otoscopy provides subjective assessment of tympanic membrane mobility (compliance) when it is subjected to a pulse of air. Tympanometry (impedance audiometry) performed in the office can provide objective information about the mobility of the tympanic membrane and presence of middle ear effusions (Figure 30-1). Tympanometry is not a hearing test but rather an assessment of middle ear functioning that uses sound energy to determine the compliance of the tympanic membrane and pressure in the middle ear. Physical stigmata of any syndromes that may be associated with deafness (Box 30-4) should be noted.

Laboratory Tests

The advantages of early identification of hearing loss cannot be overemphasized. The Joint Committee on Infant Hearing "Year 2007 Position Statement: Principles and Guidelines for Early Hearing Detection and Intervention Programs" recommends that the hearing of all newborns should be evaluated at no later than 1 month of age. Newborns not able to pass the screening should have a comprehensive audiologic evaluation at no later than 3 months of age. High-risk indicators for hearing loss (see Box 30-3) serve 2 purposes. First, they help identify newborns, living in areas where universal newborn hearing screening is not yet available, who should receive an audiologic evaluation. Second, these risk indicators help identify neonates who require ongoing medical and audiologic monitoring because normal hearing at birth in these children may not preclude the development of later hearing loss (eg, delayed onset).

The evaluation of any child with delayed language development or suspected hearing loss begins with a hearing assessment. Various techniques are available, depending on the child's age and degree of sophistication required. (A detailed discussion of the various tests used to evaluate children's hearing is presented in Chapter 76.) In addition to a hearing evaluation, a full speech, language, and communication assessment (eg, assessment of pragmatic language skills) should be performed on children with suspected language delays. In the pediatric office, parent report inventories may be used to validate parental concerns, and office-based language assessment may be aided by the use of screening tests such as the Clinical Linguistic

Figure 30-1. Basic tympanometry curves. The Type A curve indicates a normally compliant tympanic membrane (TM). The Type B curve indicates little or no motion of the TM and can be seen with middle ear effusion, a scarred TM, or a cholesteatoma. The Type C curve indicates negative middle ear pressure and may be seen with a resolving middle ear effusion or eustachian tube dysfunction. Other variations can occur in these basic curves that are not illustrated here.

Box 30-4. Syndromes Commonly Associated With Hearing Impairment

Autosomal-Dominant Conditions
- Branchio-oto-renal syndrome
- Goldenhar syndrome (oculoauriculovertebral dysplasia)
- Stickler syndrome
- Treacher Collins syndrome
- Waardenburg syndrome

Autosomal-Recessive Conditions
- Alport syndrome
- Jervell and Lange-Nielsen syndrome
- Pendred syndrome
- Usher syndrome

Chromosomal Disorders
- Trisomy 13 syndrome
- Trisomy 18 syndrome

Miscellaneous Disorders
- CHARGE (coloboma, congenital heart disease, choanal atresia, growth and intellectual disability, genitourinary anomalies, ear anomalies, and genital hypoplasia) syndrome
- TORCHS (toxoplasmosis, rubella, cytomegalovirus, herpes simplex, syphilis) syndrome

---

and Auditory Milestone Scale or the Early Language Milestone Scale. These tests are used to supplement the clinical history of a child's language abilities. Children who, in addition to speech or language impairments, also have signs of possible cognitive or social skills impairments should receive a comprehensive, multidisciplinary developmental assessment.

Management

The first 3 years of life are crucial to language development. As hearing impairment is an important cause of delayed language development in young children, the Joint Committee on Infant Hearing 2007 position statement recommends that infants with confirmed hearing loss should receive appropriate interventions by 6 months of age. The history, physical examination, and initial screening can be used to suggest referral to various specialists (eg, audiologists, speech pathologists, child psychologists, otolaryngologists) for further clarification of hearing, speech, or language deficits and treatment. Early identification of hearing impairment and its degree of severity allow for early intervention in the form of amplification of sound, special education for children, and counseling and support services for the families with affected children. (See Chapter 76 for further information on management of hearing impairment.)

Language learning occurs best in interactive and responsive environments. Encourage parents of infants and young children to have fun speaking, singing, playing with toys, and reading with their children. These reciprocal parent-child interactions along with high verbal parental responsiveness stimulate children cognitively and foster language development.

Preserve the home language for bilingual children whenever possible. Bilingualism is associated with increased cognitive control in the form of improved executive function skills and mental flexibility. Evidence indicates that bilingualism does not cause language delays, although language delays can still be seen in bilingual children.

Special education is of prime importance in the management of children with language difficulties. The Education for All Handicapped Persons Act, federal legislation passed in 1975, and its subsequent comprehensive reauthorization as the Individuals with Disabilities Education Act (IDEA) in 1990 with further revision in 2004, requires that public schools provide individualized and appropriate education for all children with disabilities. Knowledge of available community resources (eg, special schools) can aid pediatricians in providing **support services** such as special community agencies and support groups for disabled children and their parents. Children with language delay in the context of global developmental or cognitive delays or ASDs require prompt referral to early intervention services.

Prognosis

Children with a history of speech and language delays should be monitored carefully for the emergence of reading difficulties. Reading is a language-based skill that requires the appreciation of subtle differences among speech sounds (eg, phonologic awareness) and the ability to link these sounds to written symbols. The emergent literacy model of reading development assumes that reading, writing, and oral language develop concurrently from interactions in social contexts.

Children with speech and language delays require long-term monitoring of academic, emotional, and behavioral functioning. Treated early, speech and language delays and disorders generally improve over time. The final prognosis is dependent on the nature and severity of the underlying cause and the interventions provided.

CASE RESOLUTION

The child described in the case history has delayed development of expressive language skills. At the age of 3 years, she should have a 250-word vocabulary and speak in 3-word sentences; in addition, her speech should be primarily intelligible to strangers. Because of the delay, she should be referred immediately for a hearing assessment and speech and language evaluation. Hearing loss is an important diagnosis to rule out. Simply because her parents report no hearing problems does not mean she does not have a deficit. She may have learned to respond to nonverbal cues, or she may hear only some things.

Selected References

American Academy of Pediatrics Committee on Practice and Ambulatory Medicine and Section on Otolaryngology–Head and Neck Surgery. Hearing assessment in infants and children: recommendations beyond neonatal screening. *Pediatrics*. 2009;124(4):1252–1263

American Academy of Pediatrics Joint Committee on Infant Hearing. Supplement to the JCIH 2007 position statement: principles and guidelines for early intervention after confirmation that a child is deaf or hard of hearing. *Pediatrics*. 2013;131:e1324

American Speech-Language-Hearing Association. The advantages of being bilingual. http://www.asha.org/about/news/tipsheets/bilingual.htm. Accessed November 20, 2013

Bialystok E, Craik FI, Luk G. Bilingualism: consequences for mind and brain. *Trends Cogn Sci*. 2012;16(4):240–250

Cates CB, Dreyer BP, Berkule SB, White LJ, Arevalo JA, Mendelsohn AL. Infant communication and subsequent language development In children from low-income families: the role of early cognitive stimulation. *J Dev Beh Pediatr*. 2012;33(7):577–585

Fierro-Cobas V, Chan E. Language development in bilingual children: a primer for pediatricians. *Contemp Pediatr*. 2001;18:79–98

Harlor AD, Bower C; American Academy of Pediatrics Committee on Practice and Ambulatory Medicine and Section on Otolaryngology–Head and Neck Surgery. Hearing assessment in infants and children: recommendations beyond neonatal screening. *Pediatrics*. 2009;124(4):1252–1263

Hart B, Risley TR. The early catastrophe. The 30 Million Word Gap by Age 3. *American Educator*. 2003;27:4–9

Joint Committee on Infant Hearing. Year 2007 position statement: principles and guidelines for early hearing detection and intervention programs. *Pediatrics*. 2007;120(4):898–921

Lee J. Size matters: early vocabulary as a predictor of language and literacy. *Applied Psycholinguistics*. 2011;32:69–92

McQuiston S, Kloczko N. Speech and language development: monitoring process and problems. *Pediatr Rev* 2011;32(6):230–239

Nelson HD, Nygren P, Walker M, Panoscha R. Screening for speech and language delay in preschool children: systematic evidence review for the US Preventive Services Task Force. *Pediatrics*. 2006;117(2):e298–e319

Tierney CD, Brown PJ, Serwint JR. Development of children who have hearing impairment. *Pediatr Rev*. 2008;29(12):e72–e73

Zebrowski PM. Developmental stuttering. *Pediatr Ann*. 2003;32(7):453–458

CHAPTER 31

Literacy Promotion in Pediatric Practice

Lynn Hunt, MD

CASE STUDY

You are seeing a 6-month-old boy for the first time for a well-child visit. The child has a completely negative history and seems to be thriving. The patient's mother works part-time as a housekeeper and his father is a seasonal worker in agriculture. The infant is up-to-date on his immunizations except for his 6-month shots. The family history is noncontributory, but his mother mentions that her 6-year-old daughter needs to repeat kindergarten. Teachers have advised the mother that her oldest daughter is cooperative, but she has not mastered letters and early reading yet. Mother says she is not concerned because the teacher said with "a little more time" her daughter will be fine.

Questions

1. How are reading and language developmentally related?
2. What are the consequences of low literacy when children get older?
3. How are literacy and health outcomes related?
4. What are the components of the Reach Out and Read model?

Early literacy promotion in the office setting is now recognized as an essential part of pediatric primary care. The American Academy of Pediatrics (AAP) and the Canadian Paediatric Society encourage health care professionals to include literacy promotion in the routine clinical care of toddlers and young children. We know from the ever-expanding evidence of early brain development that reading aloud, speaking to babies, singing, and sharing books can permanently change neuronal connections in the brain. These connections forged by reciprocal attention and spoken language are important for learning during the school years as well as the emotional health of the child.

Literacy promotion can begin even before a baby learns to speak and long before a child is ready to learn to read. Eventual mastery of reading will depend on skills such as language ability, imagination, and familiarity with books and the reading process. Children develop many of these skills in the first few years of life even before they go to preschool. In fact, a child's language ability by 3 years of age is strongly correlated with later academic performance. Parent-child interactions are crucial, and guidance for parents on literacy promotion activities at home should begin in the first year of the child's life.

Reading aloud to children on a regular basis is one of the most effective ways to promote early literacy and language development. Language skills are the foundation for later reading ability and are dependent largely on the amount and quality of language exposure. The architecture of a developing brain is physically altered by experiences during infancy. At birth a baby's brain contains 100 billion neurons, which go on to form trillions more connections. Those connections that are stimulated by frequent use will persist, while less-used synapses will be eliminated as the brain matures. Reading aloud and book sharing may help ensure the preservation of brain connections associated with skills such as memory, creativity, comprehension, and language. Reading aloud is also a positive nurturing activity which in itself will promote other important neuronal connections and healthy development. The AAP recommends avoiding television or other electronic media for children younger than 2 years because young children learn best by interacting with people; screens are not the same.

Reading aloud exposes children to vocabulary they don't hear in daily conversations (eg, 3 bears, beanstalks). Reading aloud also stimulates the imagination (eg, cows jumping over the moon). Over time, children learn that the abstract letters on the page represent words, and they become aware of different, smaller sounds making up words. All of these experiences lead to reading readiness.

Consequences of Low Literacy

There are significant consequences to low literacy as children get older. Poor academic skills are consistently linked with higher dropout rates, entrance into the juvenile justice system, and unemployment. One-third of all juvenile offenders are reported to read below the fourth-grade level, and more than 80% of adult prison inmates are high school dropouts.

Literacy level and health outcomes are also intimately related. *Health literacy* is defined as the degree to which individuals can obtain, process, and understand the basic information they need to make appropriate health decisions. Multiple studies have demonstrated that low literacy affects health and well-being negatively. Individuals with limited health literacy are more likely to engage in risky behavior and less likely to receive the care they need. Adolescents with low reading ability are more likely to smoke, use alcohol, carry a weapon, and be in a physical fight requiring medical treatment. Conversely, higher levels of literacy are associated with positive health outcomes such as appropriate use of inhaled asthma medication or choosing to breastfeed a baby.

Promoting literacy is good medicine not only for the individual but also for society. Besides the societal effect of school failure, individuals with limited literacy incur medical expenses that are up to 4 times greater than patients with adequate literacy skills. Low literacy costs the health care system billions of dollars every year in preventable visits and hospital stays.

Literacy Promotion in the Medical Office

The AAP endorses the Reach Out and Read model of early literacy promotion, and this model is incorporated in the official AAP Bright Futures guidelines for pediatric health care professionals.

The Reach Out and Read model has 3 main components.

1. *Anticipatory guidance:* During regular well-child visits, health care professionals encourage parents to read aloud to their young children at home. The advice is age-appropriate, and concrete examples are provided or modeled by the physician.

2. *Books:* A new developmentally and culturally appropriate book is given by the physician to patients and parents at each well-child visit so that parents have the tools to follow the physician's advice.

3. *Waiting rooms:* Literacy-rich waiting rooms contribute to the literacy message. Gently used books for parents to read to their child while waiting and displays or information about local libraries are encouraged. Where appropriate and feasible, community volunteers read aloud in waiting rooms, modeling for parents the pleasures and techniques of reading aloud to very young children.

Reach Out and Read had its origins in an urban clinic serving a high proportion of low-income families and has always had a special focus on children growing up in poverty. For complex reasons, poverty is a powerful predictor of children's exposure to language. Children in low-income homes are 40% less likely to be read to on a daily basis than other children. Pioneer researchers Hart and Risley estimate that by age 4 years, children living below the poverty line will hear 30 million fewer words in total than those growing up in higher-income households.

Providing advice to parents is easiest and most effective when a book is brought in at the beginning of a visit. That way, physicians can naturally weave in guidance that is appropriate to the age of the child (Box 31-1 and Table 31-1). Advice should be brief and to the point, supportive, and part of a general conversation about the child's development and behavior.

Another advantage of presenting the book early in the visit is the amount of developmental and relationship information that can be observed. The book is a tool that can speed informal developmental surveillance. If a 2-year-old exclaims, "Doggie says wow-wow!" there is no doubt she is putting 2 words together. If a 1-year-old uses an

---

Box 31-1. Anticipatory Guidance for Parents

Specific guidance can help parents with age-appropriate expectations for how their children will handle books and respond to stories.

- *Newborns and very young babies* need to hear a parent's voice as much as possible: talking, singing, and telling stories are all good.
- *6-month-olds* may put books in their mouths; this is developmentally normal and appropriate and is why we give them chewable board books. It is not in any way an indication that the child is too young for a book!
- *12-month-olds* may point with one finger to indicate interest in a picture; parents should see this as developmental progress.
- *18-month-olds* may turn board book pages and may insist on turning back again and again to a favorite picture.
- *2-year-olds* may not sit still to listen to a whole book but will still enjoy looking at individual pages or having parents read them stories bit by bit.
- *3-year-olds* may retell familiar stories and may memorize their favorite book.
- *4- and 5-year-olds* may start to recognize letters or their sounds. They can understand and follow longer stories.
- *School-aged children* will start to be able to read to you—but don't stop reading to them, and enjoy taking turns.

Adapted from Reach Out and Read. http://www.reachoutandread.org/resource-center. Used with permission.

---

index finger to point and looks to see if his mother is watching, the physician can gain information about fine motor ability and the child's social interaction in only a few moments.

Children benefit from storytelling and book time in whatever fashion is most comfortable for the parent. Ideally books should be in the family's preferred language or bilingual. It is best for parents to use the language that is easiest for them because it is more important for children to hear a language with rich vocabulary and complex sentences than to learn English first. If no book is available in the appropriate language or parents are not confident with their own reading skills, the primary care physician should encourage parents to look at books, name pictures, and talk about what is going on in the pictures with their children. Physician knowledge of local programs for adult literacy and English as a second language is often useful because parents may ask for resources when literacy is discussed in the examination room.

Primary Care Physicians Can Make a Difference

The primary care setting is the ideal venue for literacy promotion for several reasons. First, almost all parents will bring in their child for immunizations, so there is an opportunity to reach a broad group, not just those seeking learning experiences for their children. In fact, 96% of all children younger than 6 years see their physician at least once annually. Second, each child is seen for multiple visits from a very young age, providing repeat opportunities to discuss reading aloud during the critical first years. Further, suggestions supporting literacy-focused activities are a logical extension of the advice about

Table 31-1. Developmental Milestones of Early Literacy

Motor	Cognitive	What Parents Can Do
6–12 Months		
• Reaches for books • Book to mouth • Sits in lap, head steady • Turns pages with adult help	• Looks at pictures • Vocalizes, pats pictures • Prefers pictures of faces	• Hold child comfortably; face-to-face gaze. • Follow baby's cues for "more" and "stop." • Point and name pictures.
12–18 Months		
• Sits without support • May carry book • Holds book with help • Turns board pages, several at a time	• No longer mouths right away • Points at picture with one finger • May make same sound for particular picture (labels) • Points when asked, "Where's…?" • Turns book right side up • Gives book to adult to read	• Respond to child's prompting to read. • Let child control the book. • Be comfortable with toddler's short attention span. • Ask "Where's the…?" and let child point.
18–24 Months		
• Turns board pages easily, one at a time • Carries book around the house • May use book as a transitional object	• Names familiar pictures • Fills in words and familiar stories • "Reads" to dolls or stuffed animals • Recites parts of well-known stories • Attention span highly variable	• Relate books to child's experiences. • Use books in routines, bedtimes. • Ask child "What's that?" and let child answer. • Pause and let child complete the sentence.
24–36 Months		
• Learns to handle paper pages • Goes back and forth in books to find favorite pictures	• Recites whole phrases, sometimes whole stories • Coordinates text with picture • Protests when adult gets a word wrong in a familiar story • Reads familiar books to self	• Keep using books in routines. • Read at bedtime. • Be willing to read the same story over and over. • Ask "What's that?" • Relate books to child's experiences. • Provide crayons and paper.
3 Years and Older		
• Competent book handling • Turns paper pages one at a time	• Listens to longer stories • Can retell familiar story • Moves finger along text • "Writes" name • Moves toward letter recognition	• Ask "What's happening?" • Encourage writing and drawing. • Let child tell story.

Adapted from Reach Out and Read. Milestones of early literacy development. http://www.reachoutandread.org/resource-center. Used with permission.

growth and development parents are already receiving at these visits. And when parents trust and value advice from their primary care physician, early literacy messages assume greater credibility.

The effectiveness of this primary care model to promote reading aloud to young children has been demonstrated in multiple research studies. Parents who received even one book were much more likely to read aloud to their children and report reading as a favorite activity of their child. The effect was greatest for the poorest families, an important finding for children who may need this intervention the most. The outcome was similar for non–English-speaking families, and the findings held even if the book was given in English. Finally, and most encouraging, toddlers and preschoolers who had received care in clinics applying the Reach Out and Read model had higher scores on language and vocabulary assessments than children not served by the program.

Literacy promotion and the Reach Out and Read model of giving books along with advice provide benefits for all concerned. Medical professionals have a tool to assist with development surveillance and a way to build stronger bonds with families. Parents receive important information about reading aloud and advice tailored to the age of their child. And most importantly, children receive the benefits of reading aloud as well as beautiful, developmentally appropriate books.

CASE RESOLUTION

You speak to the mother about the value of reading aloud to her children. You give the 6-month-old a board book with pictures of baby faces. You demonstrate, showing how the 6-month-old is interested in the pictures and watches intently as you turn the pages. At the end of the visit you also find a gently used rhyming book that the mother can take home for her 6-year-old.

Selected References

American Academy of Pediatrics. Bright Futures. http://brightfutures.aap.org. Accessed November 20, 2013

American Academy of Pediatrics. Early Brain and Child Development: Building Brains, Forging Futures, http://www.aap.org/en-us/advocacy-and-policy/aap-health-initiatives/EBCD/Pages/About.aspx. Accessed November 20, 2013

American Medical Association. Health literacy.http://www.ama-assn.org/ama/pub/about-ama/ama-foundation/our-programs/public-health/health-literacy-program.page. Accessed November 20, 2013

Reach Out and Read. *Leyendo Juntos (Reading Together): Literacy Promotion for Pediatric Primary Care Providers.* Boston, MA: Reach Out and Read; 2011. http://www.reachoutandread.org/FileRepository/LeyendoJuntosProviderGuide.pdf. Accessed November 20, 2013

Reach Out and Read. What children like in books. http://www.reachoutandread.org/FileRepository/WhatChildrenLikeinBooks.pdf. Accessed November 20, 2013

Summary of studies of relationship between health services, outcomes, costs, or disparities and literacy. http://www.ncbi.nlm.nih.gov/books/NBK82444/table/appendixes.app10.t1/?report=objectonly. Accessed May 2, 2014

CHAPTER 32

Gifted Children

Iris Wagman Borowsky, MD, PhD, and Calla R. Brown, MD

CASE STUDY

A 3-year-old girl is brought to your office for well-child care. Her parents believe that she may be gifted because she is much more advanced than her sister was when she was the same age. The parents report that their younger daughter walked at 11 months of age and was speaking in 2-word sentences by 18 months. She is very "verbal," has a precocious vocabulary, and constantly asks difficult questions such as, "How do voices come over a radio?" The girl stays at home with her mother during the day but recently began going to a preschool program 2 mornings a week. She enjoys preschool and plays well with children her own age. She also likes to play with her sister's friends from school.

The girl is engaging and talkative. She asks questions about what you are doing during the examination and demonstrates impressive knowledge of anatomy. The physical examination is normal.

Questions

1. How are gifted children identified?
2. What characteristics are associated with giftedness?
3. What are the best approaches for dealing with the education of gifted children?
4. What is the role of the pediatrician in the management of gifted children?

Giftedness has been defined in several ways. The psychometric definition of giftedness is based on scores obtained on standardized intelligence tests. The 2 most frequently used cutoff points are 2 standard deviations above the mean (IQ = 130–135) and 3 standard deviations above the mean (IQ = 145–150). Children with these scores are in the upper 2% and 0.1% of the IQ distribution, respectively. IQ, which is considered to be fairly stable after the age of 3 or 4 years, is the best single predictor of scholastic achievement at all levels, from elementary school to college.

A second definition of giftedness is based on real-life achievements or performance of exceptional skills rather than on test scores. Children with special talents (other than general intelligence) in areas such as music, mathematics, ice skating, chess, or drama fit this description. Other definitions of giftedness recognize motivation, commitment, perseverance, high self-esteem, and creativity as personality traits that allow children with above-average ability to develop exceptional talents. This collective group of traits is often referred to as the "potential to achieve" academic or other success.

Epidemiology

The prevalence of giftedness depends on the somewhat arbitrary definitions of giftedness and the varied approaches for identification of gifted children. Traditional screening systems identify 3% to 5% of students for participation in gifted programs in schools. Some schools use an alternative system in which 10% to 15% of children are recognized as above average. In an effort to foster giftedness in these children, schools offer them enriched programs.

Intellectual giftedness in children has been associated with the social, economic, and educational background of their families.

Factors that correlate with higher IQ scores in children are more years of parental education, higher IQ scores of mothers, increased family income, smaller family size, and longer intervals between siblings. Children from low-income and minority backgrounds are less likely to be identified as gifted than other children. African American, Hispanic, and Native American students are underrepresented by 30% to 70% in gifted programs in the United States.

Larger head size at 1 year of age and greater height and weight at 4 years of age have also been reported in children with high IQs. Although researchers have found that children who are academically gifted, as a group, begin to walk, verbalize, and read earlier, this research is still in its infancy; thus, these factors are not useful for predicting giftedness in individual children.

Evaluation

One of the primary goals of child health promotion is **developmental monitoring.** The early identification of developmental delays, which allows for prompt intervention, is one of the primary purposes of such monitoring. Techniques for developmental assessment include **review of developmental milestones** with parents and discussion of parental concerns, **informal observation** of children in the office, and **formal screening with standardized tests,** such as the Denver II.

Identification of Gifted Children

Although parents' first concern is usually to confirm that their child is developing normally, it is not uncommon for parents to ask if their child is gifted. Such questions are typically motivated by parents' desire to optimally encourage their child's development. Sharing information and observations with parents during developmental monitoring may facilitate parent-child interaction and child development. In a competitive society, the pediatrician should look for signs that above-average abilities are the result of undue pressures placed on children, such as incessant teaching or over-scheduling of time.

Infancy and early childhood may not be the best time to determine whether a child is gifted. Age of attainment of developmental milestones and performance on standardized tests (eg, Bayley Scales of Infant and Toddler Development) during the first 2 years of life are unreliable predictors of intellectual giftedness. Reasons for this lack of reliability may include weaknesses in the tests and variable rates of child development that result in transient precocity or delay. Tests that focus on visual memory tasks in infants may be better predictors of later academic intelligence; this possibility requires more research. In addition, many special talents that comprise giftedness, such as creativity or artistic or musical ability, may not manifest themselves until children are older.

The determination of giftedness in older children may involve several factors (Box 32-1). The early identification of giftedness allows for the development of an appropriate educational program that is optimally matched to a particular child's ability to learn. Without early identification and intervention, children who are intellectually gifted may become disillusioned with school, lose interest in learning, fail to develop study skills because they are never challenged to think and work hard, and develop a pattern of underachievement that may be difficult to reverse by the middle grades.

Special Groups of Gifted Children

Giftedness is harder to identify in some children. In **children who are physically disabled,** giftedness is often obscured by their obvious physical disability, which demands attention. These children may participate in special programs in which their physical needs are the major concern at the expense of their academic or artistic potential. In addition, poor self-esteem associated with the disability may prevent these children from realizing their potential. To identify giftedness in children who are physically disabled, parents and teachers must make a concerted effort to search for potential and encourage its development. Strengthening a child's capacities may involve training in the use of a wheelchair or computer or taking frequent breaks to prevent fatigue.

Giftedness also commonly goes unnoticed in children who are **learning disabled.** It is quite possible for exceptional and poor abilities to coexist in a given child. In fact, an estimated 10% of gifted

---

Box 32-1. Factors Used in the Identification of Giftedness in Children
• Intelligence tests
• Standardized achievement tests
• Grades
• Classroom observations
• Parent and teacher rating scales
• Evaluation of creative work in a specific field (eg, poems, drawings, science projects)

---

children have a reading problem, reading 2 or more years below grade level. Albert Einstein, Auguste Rodin, and John D. Rockefeller are famous examples of brilliant individuals who had reading and writing problems. An extreme example of the occurrence of extraordinary and deficient abilities together in one individual is the child savant. Affected children possess amazing abilities in one area (eg, music, drawing, mathematics, memory), but they are delayed in other respects. In addition, they have behavioral problems that resemble autism, such as repetitive behavior, little use of language, and social withdrawal.

Learning disabilities may obscure children's talents, thus preventing awareness of their potential. Conversely, children's giftedness may mask their weaknesses, depriving them of needed help. Worst of all, gifted children who are learning disabled may manage to barely "get by" in the regular classroom setting and fail to receive recognition for strengths or weaknesses. Large differences on intelligence and achievement tests between scores in different areas, such as language and spatial abilities, may indicate giftedness and a learning disability. Attention should be given to weaknesses and strengths. Research suggests that programs that focus on strengths, not deficits, enhance self-esteem in gifted children who are learning disabled and can be extremely beneficial in their academic development.

The identification of giftedness is also difficult in **children who underachieve.** Parents may approach the pediatrician with the following frustrating problem: Their child is doing poorly at school, although they believe that the child is bright because of the child's abilities and participation in advanced activities at home. Underachievement may result from a learning disability, poor self-esteem, lack of motivation, or the absence of rewards, at home or at school, for succeeding in academics.

As previously stated, giftedness is less likely to be recognized in children from families of low income or who are ethnically diverse. Many of the tests used to identify giftedness have been "normed" on white, English-speaking, middle-class children. Validation of newer methods of assessment that are less fraught with cultural and socioeconomic bias is ongoing. Until there are validated tests that are sensitive to socioeconomic differences, other means for identifying giftedness, such as assessment of creative work and teacher and student nominations, should be stressed.

Management

At Home

Loving, responsive, stimulating parenting should be encouraged for all children, including those who are gifted. Parents of gifted children may feel inadequate, fearing that their child is smarter than they are. The pediatrician can provide **parental reassurance** by telling parents, "You must have been doing something right for your child to have been identified as gifted." Children's librarians, periodicals written for parents and teachers of gifted children (eg, *Gifted Child Today),* and the local chapter of the National Association for Gifted Children are good resources for parents.

Parents are often overwhelmed with complex questions from their precocious preschool-aged children about issues ranging from homelessness and world hunger to theology and the creation of the universe. The pediatrician should tell parents that they should not be afraid to admit that they do not know all the answers and should work together with their child to find the answers.

The pediatrician may need to warn parents about putting too much pressure on their gifted children. For example, enrolling children in multiple classes often leaves little free time for unstructured play. Play affords many opportunities for self-learning, interaction with peers, and development of creativity and initiative. Parents of infants, toddlers, and preschoolers should be encouraged to take cues from their children. If children have a rich environment with plenty of objects and books to explore, diverse experiences, and stimulating interactions, they will develop their own interests. Other educational materials and special instruction can then be provided in a particular area of interest.

Children who are gifted are often mistakenly considered to fit the stereotype of troubled, socially awkward "nerds." With the exception of children at the genius extreme (IQ>180), gifted children are generally more sociable, well-liked, trustworthy, and emotionally stable than their peers, with lower rates of mental illness and delinquency. Nevertheless, they have the same emotional needs as other children. Gifted children may prefer to play with older children whose interests and abilities are closer to their own. This should be allowed as long as these relationships are healthy.

Parents should be encouraged to treat children who are gifted the same way they do their other children. Siblings of gifted children may become resentful if attention is centered on their brother or sister. They may feel inferior, particularly if gifted children surpass them in school. Tensions may be magnified if gifted children become friends with their older siblings' friends. To preserve a sense of self-worth and competence in siblings, the pediatrician should recommend to parents that they set aside special time to spend with each of their children. Parents should encourage other talents (eg, musical abilities, athletic abilities) in siblings. Older siblings should receive the special privileges and responsibilities that come with age, such as staying up later or doing different chores. Any tensions within the family should be openly discussed and addressed.

At School

Parents often seek advice from their pediatrician about educational planning for children who are gifted. A learning environment with the optimal degree of challenge—hard enough to require new learning and stave off boredom, but not so hard as to be discouraging—is the goal for all children. Parents of young children should look for preschools with flexible programs and capable teachers to accommodate children with precocious skills. Parents of school-aged children must decide whether **acceleration** (starting school earlier or skipping grades) or **enrichment** (staying in the same grade but supplementing the regular curriculum) is more appropriate (Table 32-1). The choice depends on the particular child.

Parents and teachers of gifted children are usually concerned that children in accelerated programs may have problems with social adjustment if their classmates are older. Existing evidence, however, suggests that children who are gifted benefit socially from acceleration. Gifted children in accelerated programs participate in school activities (except contact sports) more often than gifted children placed with classmates of the same age. Even when children who are gifted are placed with children their own age, they tend to make friends with older children with whom they share more interests. Gifted children also make up any curricular content missed by grade skipping. Because the process may be difficult to reverse, acceleration may not be the best option when the decision is a borderline one.

Enrichment involves keeping gifted children with same-age classmates but supplementing the regular curriculum. Regular class placement with a teacher who is willing to offer extra work (eg, special projects) in addition to grade-level assignments, part-time programs to supplement regular class work (eg, field trips, foreign language classes), honors classes that group bright children together for their basic curriculum, and independent study by the family at home are all examples of enrichment programs. These programs may work well for some children who are gifted, depending in large part on the resources and funding available and the experience, creativity, and enthusiasm of the teachers involved.

Some enrichment programs may isolate gifted from non-gifted children, however, and encourage labeling of the gifted students as "elite." If children are required to make up the regular class work that they miss when they are involved in the enrichment program, they may find themselves overloaded with homework.

Table 32-1. Acceleration Versus Enrichment in Gifted Education		
	Advantages	*Disadvantages*
Acceleration	May provide suitable academic challenge	Difficult to reverse
	May have social benefits	May have to skip more than one grade to be properly challenged
	Can be offered by all schools	
	Inexpensive	
Enrichment	Classmates are same age	May be expensive and inaccessible to many families due to tuition and transportation costs
	May expose children to subjects they would not otherwise learn	Inadequate for children who are highly gifted
	Appropriate for children who are mildly gifted	May isolate gifted from non-gifted children and encourage "elite" label
		May lead to excessive homework if children have to make up work of regular class

Often a **combination of acceleration and enrichment** programs is the best option. Acceleration or enrichment alone may not be enough for the brightest children. Acceleration may not be sufficient for markedly advanced children who would have to skip 2 or 3 grades to be appropriately challenged. The pediatrician should recommend that parents work closely with teachers to achieve the best learning environment for their children. Some factors that should be considered are age, physical size, motor coordination, emotional maturity, personality, and particular areas and degrees of giftedness of the child. Acceleration may be a better option for a large, outgoing child than for a small one. Gifted children should be asked what they would like to do.

When evaluating the suitability of an educational situation for their gifted child, parents should watch for some warning signs. Excessive homework should not be expected or tolerated because it cuts into the child's time to play and develop socially. The emphasis in gifted education should be on broadening perspectives, not increasing busy work. If children who are gifted are developing a sense of elitism or peer animosity, the nature and philosophy of the program should be questioned. Boredom with schoolwork, not needing to study, signs of depression, or symptoms suggestive of school phobia, such as recurrent abdominal pain or headaches on school mornings, should prompt investigation into the suitability of the child's program.

Homeschooling, either partial to complement classroom curricula or full time, is an educational alternative. To decide if this is the best choice for the family and the child who is gifted, recommend that parents who are considering homeschooling gather as much information as possible, including talking to other parents who are homeschooling their children, reviewing sample curricular materials, and contacting school districts and state departments about requirements and specific steps.

Schools with students from low-income or minority backgrounds tend to use their limited resources to help students who are doing poorly in school, rather than gifted students. In addition, children from low-income or minority backgrounds may experience further barriers to academic achievement, including lack of informational materials about gifted programs in parents' native languages and difficulty meeting requirements because of lack of transportation and parental employment responsibilities. Research has shown that programs for gifted children from such backgrounds benefit all students by creating positive role models and promoting the school as a place for the cultivation of excellence. In addition to providing support for individual gifted children and their families, the pediatrician may choose to engage in an active advocacy role within the community by, for example, promoting diverse educational experiences for students of all backgrounds, helping policy makers to discover and remove barriers to participation, and working with community organizations to educate families from minority or low-income backgrounds about educational opportunities for their children who are gifted.

Prognosis

Children who are gifted are a diverse group, comprising children with exceptional academic, artistic, or other abilities, combined with the creativity and commitment to achieve their potential. Children may be gifted in one area and average or even below average in another area. The purpose of identifying gifted children is to provide them with an educational environment to help maximize their potential. The pediatrician is poised to help children and their families recognize that other factors in addition to cognition, including social development, concepts of self-worth, self-discipline, and resilience, are also vitally important to the overall success and well-being of the child. Pediatricians can serve as a resource for parents in raising children who are gifted and helping children and families to obtain appropriate evaluation, educational programs, and supportive resources. The prognosis for gifted children is excellent.

CASE RESOLUTION

In the case presented, the physician should reaffirm the parents' observations that their child is gifted. The parents should be encouraged to explore programs in which their daughter's talents may be fostered, but at the same time, they should understand that even gifted children need time for play and unstructured activities.

Selected References

Davidson Institute for Talent Development. http://www.davidsoninstitute.org. Accessed November 22, 2013

Liu YH, Lien J, Kafka T, Stein MT. Discovering gifted children in pediatric practice. *J Dev Behav Pediatr.* 2005;26(5):366–369

Lovett BJ, Lewandowski LJ. Gifted students with learning disabilities: who are they? *J Learn Disabil.* 2006;39(6):515–527

Morawska A, Sanders MR. Parenting gifted and talented children: what are the key child behaviour and parenting issues? *Aust N Z J Psychiatry.* 2008;42(9):819–827

National Association for Gifted Children. http://www.nagc.org. Accessed November 22, 2013

Olszewski-Kubilius P, Clarenbach, J. *Unlocking Emerging Talent: Supporting High Achievement of Low-Income, High-Ability Students.* Washington, DC: National Association for Gifted Children; 2012. http://www.nagc.org/uploadedFiles/Conventions_and_Seminars/National_Research_Summit/Unlocking%20Emergent%20Talent%20FULL%20No-Tint.pdf. Accessed November 22, 2013

Pfeiffer SI. The gifted: clinical challenges for child psychiatry. *J Am Acad Child Adolesc Psychiatry.* 2009;48(8):787–790

Plucker JA, Callahan CM, eds. *Critical Issues and Practices in Gifted Education: What the Research Says.* 2nd ed. Waco, TX: Prufrock Press Inc; 2014

Ramos E. Let us in: Latino underrepresentation in gifted and talented programs. *J Cult Divers.* 2010;17(4):151–153

Robinson NM, Olszewski-Kubilius PM. Gifted and talented children: issues for pediatricians. *Pediatr Rev.* 1996;17(12):427–434

Rosenberg MD, Robokos D, Kennedy RF. The gifted child. *Pediatr Rev.* 2010;31(1):41–43

Shaunessy E, Karnes FA, Cobb Y. Assessing potentially gifted students from lower socioeconomic status with nonverbal measures of intelligence. *Percept Mot Skills.* 2004;98(3 Pt 2):1129–1138

University of Connecticut. Neag Center for Gifted Education and Talent Development. http://www.gifted.uconn.edu. Accessed November 22, 2013

Vaivre-Douret L. Developmental and cognitive characteristics of "high-level potentialities" (highly gifted) children. *Int J Pediatr.* 2011;2011:420297

CHAPTER 33

Children and School: A Primer for the Practitioner

Geeta Grover, MD

CASE STUDY

An 8-year-old boy is brought in by his parents in early April because his third-grade teacher informed them that he is currently failing in school and may not be promoted to the fourth grade. Review of his medical, developmental, and school histories reveals that he was a very colicky infant and continued to be difficult as a toddler. His language skills were somewhat delayed, although not enough to warrant a full evaluation. His preschool teacher felt that he was easily distracted when doing seat work. In kindergarten he had some difficulty learning all of his letters, numbers, and sounds. Early reading was difficult in kindergarten and first grade but improved by the end of the year. Second grade was fairly good except for continued concerns about inattention and distractibility. By third grade he was struggling more, especially with writing, and not reaching grade level in several areas. He also continued to be inattentive and distractible in his classroom.

Examination reveals a well-developed and well-nourished boy whose growth parameters are within normal limits for his age. He appears somewhat anxious in the examination room, and when asked about school he tells you that he feels he is just not as smart as the other children in his class.

Questions

1. Should grade retention be considered when a child is failing in school?
2. What are the advantages and disadvantages of grade retention?
3. What is the differential diagnosis of school failure?
4. What steps should be taken at this time by the parents and the school for the boy in this scenario?

Because of their routine contact with young children and their families, pediatricians are often the professionals most knowledgeable about child development. Pediatricians' longitudinal perspective on their patients' lives places them in a unique position to evaluate, diagnose, and manage not only children's medical needs but also their developmental, social-emotional, behavioral, and educational ones. Traditionally, the 5-year-old health maintenance visit has been regarded as the "school readiness" visit. However, waiting until this date to address concerns about educational readiness is too late. **School readiness** must be promoted from infancy through early childhood.

During the school-aged years, pediatricians should continue to monitor children's school progression by inquiring about academic, social-emotional, and behavioral development. Parents often turn to pediatricians for advice on their children's behavioral or academic difficulties at school, which may be leading to **school failure.** The evaluation and management of school failure requires a multidisciplinary approach under the guidance, support, and advocacy provided by pediatricians. It is important that pediatricians have an understanding of the evaluation and management of children's school readiness needs and school difficulties, should such arise.

Epidemiology

School readiness is the term used to describe those qualities and traits that are considered prerequisites for a child to be ready to be successful in school. According to national surveys of kindergarten teachers, about one-third of children are not ready for school when they enter, and of these children, 25% will repeat kindergarten or first grade. Language deficiencies and problems with emotional maturity are cited most often as the factors that most restrict school readiness.

School failure is a multifaceted issue and epidemiologically complex. Overall, about 20% of children have one or more developmental, learning, behavioral, or emotional disorders. Only 10% to 15% of children in the United States are receiving special education services because of difficulties with school performance. Finally, we know that children with concerns such as these are 2 to 3 times more likely to drop out of school than children without any of these concerns.

Approximately 10% to 15% of school-aged children repeat or fail a grade in school. Children who have disabilities are nearly 3 times more likely to repeat a grade than children without disabilities. About 1 in 5 children who repeat a grade in school has some identifiable disability. Grade failure is also more common among boys, children living in poverty, minorities, and those in single-parent homes.

Given that the average child in the United States spends nearly 50% of her waking day in a school or a similar learning situation for approximately 12 or 13 years, it follows that a lack of success in these settings will lead to difficulties for much, or all, of adult life. Undetected school difficulties can create a lifelong pattern of frustration and failure. Children with **attention-deficit/ hyperactivity disorder (ADHD)** are 2 to 3 times more likely to drop out of high school than their peers without ADHD; children with ADHD who attend college are less likely to graduate than their non-ADHD peers (see Chapter 129). About 40% of all juvenile offenders have learning disabilities; many have never received any help for their disabilities. Even more alarming is that 85% of juvenile delinquents and more than 60% of adult prisoners are functionally illiterate—somehow these children slipped through the cracks of the educational system.

Clinical Presentation

Defining **school readiness** is not an easy task because the intellectual, physical, social, and emotional development among kindergarten-aged children varies tremendously. Generally, school readiness means that children are adequately prepared to participate in formal schooling (Box 33-1). Readiness implies not only adequate pre-academic skills but also adequate physical, developmental, language, social-emotional, and behavioral skills to allow children to be successful in the formal schooling environment.

With regard to **school failure,** the non-specificity of children's presenting signs and symptoms and of parental complaints make it challenging to determine a specific etiology. For instance, parental concern about a child's inability to focus could suggest an attention disorder, learning disability, mood disorder, or perhaps all 3. Parental concerns can be categorized into 3 broad areas: learning (eg, learning disability, problems with higher-order cognition including intellectual disability), attention (eg, ADHD), and emotional/ behavioral (eg, anxiety, depression, serious emotional disturbance). Signs of school difficulties are presented in Box 33-2. It is important to look not only at academic skills but also at other components of the educational experience, such as social and emotional experiences. Finally, it is important to ascertain the basis for the perception that a child is failing. Does the problem exist in the eyes of the student, parent, teachers, or everyone?

Academic achievement across subjects must be assessed, especially in the areas of reading, mathematics, and writing. In addition, it is also important to evaluate students who have good skills but fail to perform satisfactorily in the areas of writing, planning, organization, project completion, test taking, or classroom participation. Difficulty with academic performance may lead to school failure in spite of satisfactory academic skills.

In addition to academic skills and performance, the development of good social skills and peer relations is equally important. Some students have difficulties "fitting in," which leads to a disappointing educational experience in spite of academic excellence.

Box 33-1. Kindergarten Readiness Skills

Academic
- Counts to at least 10
- Recognizes some printed letters and perhaps a few words (eg, name)
- Beginning to understand connection between oral and written language (evidence of phonologic skills)
- Recognizes and matches shapes and colors that are eg, the same or different

Personal, Social, Emotional, and Developmental
- Able to separate from parents for several hours at a time
- Takes care of personal hygiene and toileting
- Verbally communicates personal needs
- Able to relate personal experiences, ideas, thoughts, and feelings with words
- Sustains attention to task for 10 to 15 minutes
- Able to understand and follow directions with 2 or 3 steps
- Able to communicate and play cooperatively with other children (eg, shares, takes turns)
- Copes with anger and frustration

Motor
- Uses pencil, crayon, and scissors
- Runs, jumps, hops, skips, and throws ball
- Draws a person and basic shape

Box 33-2. Signs of School Difficulties

- Grade retention
- Loss of self-esteem
- Short attention span/hyperactivity
- Not able to follow directions, pay attention, or finish a task
- History of speech-language problems
- Not able to carry thoughts or ideas to paper
- Not able to read, write, or spell appropriate to age and educational level
- Requires excessive time to complete homework/excessive parental involvement with homework
- Previously tested but not eligible for special education (eg, child may be a "slow learner")
- Hates school/psychosomatic symptoms
- Has few, if any, friends or change of friends
- Sudden change in behavior
- Depression
- Substance use

Pathophysiology

Developmentally there is support for the concept of promoting **school readiness** from a young age. The developing brain continues to make new synaptic connections and "prune" away underused connections from birth to about age 5 years—well before formal schooling begins. For example, we know that children who grow up without being read to and with little exposure to books or printed language during the first 5 years of life are at an increased risk of developing reading failure and subsequent school failure (see Chapter 31). School readiness must be promoted from infancy throughout early childhood; waiting for the 4- to 5-year-old well visit is too late. Most children with learning disabilities experience language, motor skills, or behavior problems well before they encounter difficulties in the classroom. We now know that another critical period in brain development occurs during adolescence when the brain again goes through a process of synaptic pruning and myelination, especially notable in the prefrontal lobe, ie, the area responsible for reasoning, impulse control, attention, and planning.

School failure is a complex issue with a wide variety of causes. Intrinsic, or child-related, causes and extrinsic, or environmental-related, causes relating to the home or school setting must be considered (Box 33-3). In most cases, school failure is the result of a complex interaction between child, family, and school-related variables, not simply the result of a single factor (eg, ADHD). Before looking for specific learning disabilities or disorders or intellectual problems, investigate any type of external situation that may be causing the problem. Medical problems should always be considered. Neurologic, psycho-emotional, and behavioral disorders based in the central nervous system may be responsible for school failure.

Unrecognized ADHD, learning disorders, and learning disabilities are common causes of school failure. Learning disorders are defined problems within the central nervous system that prevent children from learning to their full potential. The brain has difficulty handling information (processing skills), which therefore affects the child's ability to learn or perform in school. Some of these processes include memory, language, attention, and coordination. A specific learning disability is a particular type of learning disorder that is defined as a significant difference between a child's natural ability (IQ) and his level of achievement, as defined by federal and state laws. This difference is determined by psycho-educational testing performed by psychologists and educators.

Federal law (Public Law 101-476: Individuals with Disabilities Education Act [IDEA]) defines *specific learning disability* as "a disorder in one or more of the basic psychological processes involved in understanding or in using language, spoken or written, that may manifest itself in the imperfect ability to listen, think, speak, read, write, spell, or to do mathematical calculations, including conditions such as perceptual disabilities, brain injury, minimal brain dysfunction, dyslexia, and developmental aphasia." Operationally, specific learning disabilities are characterized by a discrepancy between ability (as measured by IQ tests) and actual academic achievement (as measured by school performance). However, specific learning disability does not include children who have "learning problems that are primarily the result of visual, hearing, or motor disabilities, of mental retardation, of emotional disturbance, or of environmental, cultural, or economic disadvantage."

Another important reason for school failure is an unsatisfactory student-teacher relationship. A poor "fit" with teacher or classroom placement may cause major damage to a child's program.

Finally, there are students who are labeled "lazy" by school personnel. These students are usually found to have one or more of the

---

Box 33-3. Causes of School Failure

Intrinsic
- Low cognitive skills (intellect)
- Learning disorders
- Specific learning disabilities
- Attention-deficit/hyperactivity disorders
- Speech and language disorders
- Mood and anxiety disorders
- Low self-esteem
- Social-emotional difficulties
- Neurodevelopmental delays
- Motor coordination disorders
- Chronic or serious medical illness (eg, seizure disorders, cystic fibrosis, asthma)
- Vision, hearing, or speech difficulties
- Poor nutrition
- Sleep problems
- Substance use/abuse
- Genetic history (eg, family history of school problems)

Extrinsic
- Language/cultural differences
- Serious psychosocial concerns: parental depression, history of abuse or neglect
- Disruption in the family (eg, many moves)
- Poor school readiness/absence of enrichment prior to school entry (eg, early book exposure)
- Parental or school expectations not commensurate with child's abilities
- School, classroom placement (poor "fit" or poor teaching)

---

previously mentioned school difficulties but have never been properly diagnosed. Rarely, a student is found who has no major identifiable problem but just isn't motivated to take part in the educational experience. Alternative placement or homeschooling may be an answer for these students.

Evaluation

History

In the past, pediatricians assessed **school readiness** during the 5-year-old health maintenance visit. Clinical approaches to early identification of children at risk for school failure include risk assessments and developmental surveillance and screening. Children most at risk for school problems are those from economically and socially disadvantaged backgrounds. Developmental surveillance and screening (see Chapter 29) allow pediatricians to identify children with developmental, behavioral, and emotional delays and to provide appropriate anticipatory guidance, as well as referral to early intervention programs.

Historical factors associated with an increased risk of school-related problems include **prematurity, low birth weight, small for gestational age,** and **maternal history of tobacco, alcohol, or illicit**

substance abuse during pregnancy (Questions Box: School Readiness). Developmental risk factors especially include delays in the acquisition of language skills. Medical factors that may affect school readiness include lead poisoning, iron deficiency anemia, and failure to thrive. The presence of chronic medical conditions (eg, asthma, diabetes mellitus, seizure disorders) may affect school readiness directly or indirectly via absenteeism, medication effects, or self-esteem issues. Environmental risk factors include poverty and lower socioeconomic status, parental depression, domestic violence, substance abuse, or a family history of school problems or learning disabilities.

School Failure

When evaluating for **school failure,** historical information should be sought from parents, schools, teachers, and the children themselves (Questions Box: School Failure). A review of present and past report cards not only provides information on academic progress but also behavioral and social-emotional assessments. Teacher behavior rating forms and evaluations and results of any psycho-educational evaluations should also be reviewed.

Physical Examination

With regard to **school readiness,** the most important aspect of the 5-year-old health maintenance physical examination includes careful hearing, vision, speech, and language assessments.

The physical examination in the evaluation of **school failure** has a limited but important role. Signs of short attention span, distractibility, overactivity, sadness, or anxiety should all be noted. Special attention should be paid to head circumference, minor congenital anomalies, abnormal facies, and skin lesions suggestive of neurocutaneous disorders (eg, multiple café au lait spots, ash leaf macules). The pediatrician should assess for vision, hearing, speech and language, and other appropriate evaluations as suggested by the history.

Neurodevelopmental Assessment

School readiness assessment begins with routine pediatric surveillance and screening (see Chapter 29). Several brief school readiness tests have been developed for use by pediatricians (eg, The Pediatric Examination of Educational Readiness). However, because their reliability and ability to detect subtle learning disabilities or arrive at more complicated diagnoses is not established, it is difficult to recommend any of them for routine use. If a specific school readiness evaluation is warranted, it is best to make a referral to the school district or an independent specialist (eg, developmental and behavioral pediatrician, educational psychologist) for a full evaluation.

Neurodevelopmental assessment can help identify the etiology of **school failure.** Neurodevelopmental assessment surveys a child's abilities across the different areas of development (eg, fine motor, language, visual-spatial, and memory skills) and helps to identify areas of strength and weakness. Such an assessment can be performed by professionals such as a developmental and behavioral pediatrician or a psychologist. Psycho-educational assessment is also

Questions

School Readiness

- Has the child had any preschool or group child care experience, and how has the child responded in these settings?
- Were any behavioral, developmental, or emotional concerns raised during those group care experiences?
- Does the child play well with age-appropriate peers, or does the child seem to consistently prefer to play with younger or older children or adults?
- Is the child's speech understandable to strangers, and can the child hold a conversation about everyday topics of interest?
- Can the child sit and listen to stories or sustain attention to a quiet activity for 10 to 15 minutes?
- Can the child identify colors, shapes, and some letters and numbers?

Questions

School Failure

- How many days of school has the child missed?
- Have any behavioral or attentional concerns been raised by the classroom teacher?
- Is the child having problems in all academic areas, or are there particular subjects that are especially difficult for the child?
- Has any testing (eg, psycho-educational evaluation) been performed by the school district or privately?
- Is the child receiving any special services (eg, speech therapy) or accommodations at school?

critical in the evaluation of children with school failure. Such an assessment includes an evaluation of the children's cognitive abilities, academic achievement across subjects (eg, reading, writing, and mathematics), and assessments of perceptual strengths and weaknesses and social and emotional functioning. This can be accomplished through the public school system via the **Individualized Education Plan (IEP)** process, as mandated by federal law **(IDEA)** or privately by an educational psychologist.

Management

The first aspect of management is the counseling or demystification of parents and children. Empowering parents with knowledge gives them the confidence to interact positively with their children's schools and allows them to advocate effectively for their children's educational needs. For children, the process of demystification should begin with the assurance that all people have strengths and weaknesses—mentioning one's own weaknesses or citing famous or successful people that have dealt effectively with their own learning concerns helps humanize and destigmatize the situation for children. It is important to use an optimistic tone. In addition to addressing the needs of families and children, the physician also serves an important advisory role for the school on behavioral consequences of a child's disorder (eg, should this child have a seizure or a behavioral outburst in the classroom, how should the situation be managed?) or the educational implications of chronic medical conditions.

Early intervention is the key to success with regard to children's **school readiness.** For many at-risk children, early childhood education programs such as Head Start and other preschool compensatory programs may come too late. Programs for younger children and their families (eg, Early Head Start) that promote good parenting, language stimulation, and learning through play are valuable and available in some communities.

Reading aloud to children is one of the most important parental interventions that physicians can promote, and it builds the child's skills required for eventual success in reading (see Chapter 31). Reading promotes language mastery, and language mastery, in turn, is one of the keys to school readiness.

The pediatrician can assist families with children who have clear developmental disabilities, such as intellectual disability, cerebral palsy, or autism spectrum disorders, in accessing special education services as mandated by **IDEA of 1990 and the amendments of 1997 and 2004.** These laws require public schools to provide a free and appropriate education in "the least restrictive environment" for all children with a disability and require schools to use the IEP process (or Individualized Family Service Plan for children younger than 3 years) to identify and evaluate the educational needs of children to develop an appropriate educational program to meet each child's needs. Pediatricians should be familiar with their local laws so that they can advocate for these children at the time of school entry if needed.

Children who are at increased risk for school readiness problems because of medical, social-emotional, behavioral, or environmental concerns should be monitored carefully. If these children do not appear to demonstrate age-appropriate skills, they should be referred for further evaluation. Despite early intervention, some children may still not be ready for school at the age-appropriate time. Options for these children include delaying school entry or special educational programs. Delaying school entry may not be the best solution if children remain in the same environment that failed to produce readiness in the first place. In addition, studies have shown that students who are older than their classmates because of delayed school entry have higher rates of behavior problems, substance abuse, and other health risk behaviors in adolescence. An alternative is for these children to enter school along with their same-aged peers and provide special classrooms or programs for those having difficulties.

The recent increases in school violence and bullying remind us of the importance of looking at the social and emotional well-being of children in the school environment. A promising new educational theory, social-emotional learning, posits that children must learn to manage and cope with their emotions to reach their potential. In this model, critical coping and emotional management skills are taught in the classroom similar to the traditional academic subjects. Recent studies demonstrate that noncognitive attributes like resilience, grit, and responsibility might actually be better predictors of a person's life course than the standard academic measures; some have suggested that perhaps respect, responsibility, and resilience may be the new 3 Rs of learning.

The management of school failure requires a multidisciplinary approach. Information from the school, including school reports, teacher conferences and notes, testing that has been completed, and input from other school officials, if appropriate, should be requested. The primary care physician can assist the child and family in working with the school system to obtain appropriate services. The primary physician may also refer to appropriate resources in the community (eg, educational psychologist, developmental and behavioral pediatrician).

Not infrequently, external factors such as social, family, and school-based issues may be very difficult to alter. Knowledge of the educational laws and community services, as well as ongoing developmental surveillance and screening by the primary care physician, are necessary to build a base from which the prevention of school failure is possible.

Grade retention is often suggested as the treatment for school failure. At the end of each school year, from kindergarten through 12th grade, the question of promotion is addressed. Though school personnel may consider this decision "business as usual," its effect can be far reaching. Evidence that retention in kindergarten or first grade is helpful in affording mastery of critical reading and other skills is lacking. Retention in higher grades has not been shown to be effective because educational gaps (eg, lack of mastery of first-grade skills) are not readdressed by retention in a higher grade. It is unlikely that "more of the same" will ensure mastery of needed skills.

In fact, data suggest the effect of grade retention on most students is adverse. Most retained students do not improve and many are worse after retention. Self-esteem problems, evident in many cases, often lead to self-destructive behavior and, in later grades, problems such as substance abuse, behavior difficulties, sexual promiscuity, and early drop out from school. In addition, children characterize retention to be as bad as losing a parent.

To minimize the adverse effects of grade retention, each child's needs and strengths should be addressed and educational programs individualized. Educational alternatives to retention include extra support in the form of classroom accommodations (**Section 504 of the Rehabilitation Act of 1973** and also the **Americans with Disabilities Act**) or special education services (**IDEA**). In addition, educational therapy, counseling, or one-on-one tutoring may be beneficial for some children. Equally as important as remediating the areas of weakness is recognizing the child's areas of strength (eg, the idea of using a child's strengths to leverage his weaknesses).

Finally, the pediatrician's role in advocacy can never be underestimated. Examples of advocacy roles for physicians include involvement with assessment team processes at children's schools, consulting with local school districts, and participation in local or state early intervention interagency councils.

Prognosis

In most cases, most children who show signs of school failure fall into the group of mild to moderate learning or neurobehavioral disorders with average cognitive skills. With proper support from educational, medical, family, and psychological sources, most of these students should be able to overcome their particular problems and enjoy successful school careers. Students who may have endured major socioeconomic upheavals will often continue to struggle unless changes in their entire support system are instituted early in their lives. The progress of children who have significant cognitive, neurobehavioral, or psychological processing problems depends on the severity of their problems and the intensity and timing of the interventions they receive.

Irrespective of its cause, school failure can have lifelong consequences if not properly diagnosed and addressed. Failing students are more likely to drop out of school or engage in behaviors that are dangerous to their health as adolescents. Pediatricians can make a significant difference in outcomes by helping families advocate for their failing students to receive appropriate assessment and intervention services.

CASE RESOLUTION

The pediatrician should advise the family to request in writing a psychoeducational evaluation from the school. The pediatrician can also institute an evaluation for attention-deficit/hyperactivity disorder by gathering information from the family and school. All of this information should then be discussed with the parents so that formal diagnostic procedures and interventions may be instituted. Ideally, the pediatrician will have the time, interest, and training to guide the family through this entire process. However, if this is not possible, referral to an appropriate professional is indicated. With data from the educational evaluation and medical workup, an appropriate plan of treatment can be developed.

Selected References

Byrd RS. School failure: assessment, intervention, and prevention in primary pediatric care. *Pediatr Rev.* 2005;26(7):233–243

Byrd RS, Weitzman M, Auinger P. Increased behavior problems associated with delayed school entry and delayed school progress. *Pediatrics.* 1997;100(4): 654–661

Dworkin PH. School failure. In: Augustyn M, Zuckerman B, Caronna E, eds. *The Zuckerman Parker Handbook of Developmental and Behavioral Pediatrics for Primary Care.* 3nd ed. Philadelphia, PA: Lippincott, Williams & Wilkins: 2011:317–321

Green M, Sullivan P, Eichberg C. Helping academic underachievers become achievers in their own right. *Contemp Pediatr.* 2005;22:29–36

High PC; American Academy of Pediatrics Committee on Early Childhood, Adoption, and Dependent Care and Council on School Health. School readiness. *Pediatrics.* 2008;121(4):e1008–e1015

Kahn J. Can emotional intelligence be taught? *The New York Times.* http://www.nytimes.com/2013/09/15/magazine/can-emotional-intelligence-be-taught.html. Published September 11, 2013. Accessed November 22, 2013

Levine M. *A Mind at a Time: America's Top Learning Expert Shows How Every Child Can Succeed.* New York, NY: Simon and Schuster; 2002

Mayer JD. Emotional intelligence information. http://www.unh.edu/emotional_intelligence. Accessed November 22, 2013

Rief SF. *Ready…Start…School! Nurturing and Guiding Your Child Through Preschool & Kindergarten.* Paramus, NJ: Prentice Hall Press; 2001

Rimrodt SL, Lipkin PH. Learning disabilities and school failure. *Pediatr Rev* 2011;32(8):315–324

Shaywitz SE, Shaywitz BA. Dyslexia (specific reading disability). *Pediatr Rev.* 2003;24(5):147–153

CHAPTER 34

Immunizations

ChrisAnna M. Mink, MD

CASE STUDY

A 20-month-old boy who emigrated with his family from Botswana is brought in for a checkup. He has his World Health Organization Expanded Programme on Immunization card from his homeland showing that he received a BCG vaccine at birth; 3 doses of diphtheria, tetanus, and pertussis vaccine at 2, 4, and 6 months of age; 3 doses of live oral poliovirus vaccine at 2, 3, and 4 months of age; 3 doses of hepatitis B vaccine at birth and 2 and 9 months of age; and a monovalent measles vaccine at 9 months of age. It is August and his parents plan to enroll him in child care and have brought him for a checkup. His parents report that he is a healthy boy with no immune problems. They report that his uncle, who is infected with HIV, lives with them. The boy has had a 3-day history of a runny nose, cough, and tactile fever. His examination is normal other than mild clear coryza and a rectal temperature of 37.9°C (100.3°F). What immunizations may be given?

Questions

1. What are the different kinds of vaccines?
2. What are the mechanisms of action for live and inactivated vaccines?
3. What are the routinely recommended immunizations for *healthy* pediatric populations?
4. What are the considerations for immunizing selected pediatric populations, such as preterm infants, immunocompromised children, immigrants, international adoptees, and travelers?
5. What are reliable resources for up-to-date information about immunizations?

The Centers for Disease Control and Prevention (CDC) considered immunizations among the top 10 greatest health accomplishments of the 20th century, and vaccines continue to play a major role in the improvement of the health of the world's population. In the United States, almost all of the pathogens for which there are routine vaccinations have decreased in incidence by 95% to 100% since the early 20th century. The only exception to this is pertussis, which has had approximately an 80% reduction. In 2012 the immunization rates for children in the United States remained stable at high levels, with 82% to 90% of children aged 19 to 35 months immunized for the 4:3:1:3:3 series (4 diphtheria, tetanus, and acellular pertussis [DTaP]; 3 polio; 1 measles, mumps, and rubella [MMR]; 3 *Haemophilus influenzae* type b [Hib]; 3 hepatitis B virus [HBV]). Worldwide, the percentage of children immunized with 3 doses of diphtheria, tetanus, and pertussis (DTP) and oral polio vaccines (OPV) and a measles-containing vaccine is approaching 80%, which is greater than a 3-fold increase in the past 20 years. Since 1990 there has been a decline in the mortality rate for children younger than 5 years in every region in the world, and this is directly related to increased immunizations. Generally, immunizations are safe, well tolerated, and cost-effective, with a range of $5 to $16.50 saved for every dollar spent.

Another less recognized benefit of vaccinations is that the schedule has essentially provided the backbone for routine pediatric care in the United States, with regular visits scheduled around the recommended intervals for immunizations. These visits have afforded health care professionals opportunities for serial evaluation of newborns, infants, and young children, as well as education and anticipatory guidance for parents. Increasing availability of new vaccines targeted for older children and adolescents should permit opportunities for improved health care delivery to these older age groups, who have often been medically underserved. Additionally, health care practitioners for adults have a growing appreciation of the critical role of vaccinations for protecting their patients as well as all members of the family.

General Principles

When considering providing immunizations for an individual, 2 important factors to consider are the health status of the recipient and the type of immunization to be given. The risks and benefits of using the vaccine in the specific host should be weighed carefully. Vaccines are intended for a host who is capable of mounting an appropriate immune response, who will likely benefit from the protection provided and ideally incur little or no risks.

Types of Immunizations

The 2 major types of immunizations are passive and active.

Passive Immunization

Passive immunization refers to the delivery of preformed antibodies, usually as immune globulin (Ig), which may be a general formulation or hyperimmune Ig developed with high concentrations of antibodies against a specific disease, such as HBIg for hepatitis B.

Delivery of Ig may be useful in 3 settings.

1. A host is not able to make antibodies (eg, congenital immunodeficiency).
2. Preventive (preexposure or postexposure), especially when the host may not be able to mount an antibody response (eg, immunocompromised child with an acute exposure to hepatitis A virus).
3. Treatment—Ig may be used to ameliorate symptoms when disease is already present (eg, intravenous Ig for Kawasaki disease).

Active Immunization

With **active immunization,** all, part, or a modified product (eg, toxoid, purified antigen) of a microorganism is given to the host to elicit an immune response. The intact organisms may be inactivated (killed) or live-attenuated (weakened). The elicited immune response usually mimics the response to natural infection and, ideally, this occurs with little or no risks to the recipient.

Inactivated Vaccines

Inactivated vaccines may contain **inactivated or killed organisms,** purified components (subunit), or inactivated toxins (toxoids) of the organism. These vaccines are not capable of replication in the host. Most inactivated vaccines are delivered by the intramuscular (IM) injection. Generally, inactivated vaccines may be administered simultaneously with other inactivated vaccines, as well as live viral vaccines.

A few of the common viral vaccines are inactivated, including inactivated influenza (IIV, trivalent and quadrivalent formulations), HAV, HBV, inactivated polio (IPV), human papillomavirus (HPV), Japanese encephalitis (JE), and rabies vaccines. Toxoid vaccines that are used routinely include tetanus and diphtheria toxoids alone or in combinations with whole-cell or acellular pertussis components (eg, DTaP; DTP; tetanus, diphtheria [Td]; tetanus, diphtheria, acellular pertussis [Tdap]). The acellular pertussis vaccines are composed of one or more purified antigens of *Bordetella pertussis*, in contrast with the whole-cell pertussis vaccines, which are made with killed, whole *B pertussis* organisms. Diphtheria and tetanus toxoids combined with whole-cell pertussis (DTP) vaccines are no longer marketed in the United States but are used in most developing areas of the world. Other inactivated bacterial vaccines include capsular polysaccharide (CPS) vaccines, such as the 23-valent pneumococcal vaccine and tetravalent meningococcal CPS vaccine.

Conjugate Vaccines

Capsular polysaccharide antigens have been chemically linked to a protein carrier, which converts the T-cell independent polysaccharides to T-cell dependent antigens that can trigger an immune response, even in young infants. The first CPS-protein conjugate vaccine available was for Hib. The Hib bacterium is covered with a CPS, polyribitol-phosphate (PRP). Children younger than 2 years are not efficient at mounting antibodies to the PRP CPS, but with linkage to a protein carrier, the CPS is immunogenic. Since licensure for infants of the Hib conjugate vaccines in 1991, there has been a more than 98% reduction in Hib disease. With the success of the Hib CPS-protein conjugate vaccines, conjugation techniques have been used for other CPS pathogens, including *Streptococcus pneumoniae* and *Neisseria meningitidis*.

Live-Attenuated Vaccines

Live-attenuated vaccines are infectious agents that replicate in the host to elicit an immune response. The administration is generally not IM but by other delivery routes, such as oral, intranasal, or subcutaneous. The live vaccines are often viral, including MMR, varicella-zoster virus (VZV), rotavirus, live-attenuated influenza virus (LAIV, FluMist), OPV, and yellow fever (YF) vaccines. Two live bacterial vaccines are available: BCG used against *Mycobacterium tuberculosis* and oral typhoid (Ty21) vaccine.

Following measles vaccination, a transient suppression of T-cell immunity occurs in the 2- to 4-week postvaccination period. Because of this, when vaccinating with live viral vaccines, give 2 or more live vaccines at the same time or wait at least 4 weeks between vaccines. This principle is also true for tuberculosis skin testing; place the purified protein derivative at the same time as a live viral vaccine or wait at least 4 weeks to avoid a false-negative skin test result because of T-cell suppression. Although this has not been extensively studied with live viral vaccines other than measles, following the same guidelines with other live viral vaccines is recommended.

Vaccination Schedule

Factors for developing the schedule include

- Host ability to respond (eg, lost maternal antibody)
- Need for multiple doses (eg, IPV)
- Minimal intervals needed between serial doses
- Available products (eg, combination vaccines)

A synchronized immunization schedule is posted annually from the American Academy of Pediatrics (AAP) Committee on Infectious Diseases *(Red Book: Report of the Committee on Infectious Diseases)*, American Academy of Family Physicians, and Advisory Committee on Immunization Practices of the CDC. Since 2007, 2 immunization schedules have been posted for the pediatric age groups, one for children younger than 7 years and one for individuals 7 through 18 years of age. A separate schedule is available for adults older than 18 years. The US schedules are posted each January at www.cdc.gov/vaccines/schedules. Schedules for countries worldwide are available at http://apps.who.int/immunization_monitoring/globalsummary/schedules.

Vaccine Recipients

Healthy Pediatric Populations

Routine immunizations on the synchronized schedule are targeted for healthy newborns, infants, children, and adolescents. All licensed vaccines have undergone review by the US Food and Drug Administration (FDA) and have proven safety and immunogenicity or efficacy for the targeted population. However, no vaccine is completely free of adverse events or will provide 100% protection for every recipient. Every effort should be made to provide immunizations when the recipient is healthy and has the best chance to mount an optimal immune response without delaying vaccination or risking a missed opportunity.

Special-Risk Pediatric Populations

Although immune responses to vaccinations are likely most favorable in healthy recipients, a growing segment of the pediatric population has underlying health problems. Because of congenital or acquired immune dysfunctions, some individuals should not receive immunizations as directed by the routine schedules. Special accommodations need to be made for immunizing these individuals, such as adjusting the schedule or possibly not administering some agents. There are **no** indications for giving decreased or partial doses of vaccines. Some of the selected populations for whom special consideration is indicated are discussed as follows.

Immunocompromised Child

The plan for vaccination of a child who is **immunocompromised** should be determined by the nature and degree of immunosuppression. The health care professional should weigh risks and benefits for each child individually, keeping some general principles in mind. For example, live vaccines should not be given to severely compromised individuals because of the possible risks. Generally inactivated vaccines may be safely administered to nearly all recipients; however, immunocompromised individuals may not mount an optimal immune response. In this setting, try to adjust timing of vaccination to optimize the chance of a good immune response. Guidelines include waiting for 3 to 4 weeks' post-chemotherapy and white blood cell counts greater than 1,000 cells/mm^3 for chemotherapy patients, 4 weeks after stopping high-dose steroids (dose equivalent $\geq$2 mg/kg/day of prednisone for $\geq$14 days), and sufficient time after receipt of Ig (see AAP *Red Book*).

Types of Immunodeficiency

Newborns, infants, and children may have abnormalities of any aspect of the immune system, which may affect their ability to receive vaccinations. Weighing the risks (of the disease as well as of the vaccine) and benefits of protection is essential. A reasonable approach to developing a vaccination plan for children with immune abnormalities is to consider the mechanism of immune defense against the vaccine agents; if the needed defense mechanism is deficient, immunizing with that agent may not be appropriate. For example, **cellular immunity** is essential in defending against **viral agents.** Thus, children with abnormalities of their cell-mediated immunity (primary or acquired) may not be candidates for receipt of live viral vaccines.

Primary immunodeficiencies are generally inherited and secondary ones are acquired, such as infection with HIV, malignancy, illnesses (eg, malnutrition, uremia), or related to medications (eg, chemotherapy, immunosuppressive agents), among others. For primary humoral immunity abnormalities (not able to make antibodies), OPV is contraindicated, but MMR vaccine may be indicated for some individuals. With complement abnormalities, receipt of live viral vaccines is acceptable for most individuals. For abnormal phagocytic function, live bacterial vaccines should not be given. For individuals with asplenia (traumatic or surgical), vaccination with pneumococcal, meningococcal, and Hib vaccines is indicated and should be considered emergently in the case of trauma. Chemoprophylaxis may also have a role in protection for compromised individuals.

For immunocompromised household contacts of pediatric vaccines, it is generally acceptable to give MMR, VZV, and oral rotavirus vaccines. Some live vaccines should not be given, including OPV and LAIV in some settings. Additionally, use of some vaccines, such as IIV, is encouraged to protect the vaccinees as well as the compromised contacts.

Pregnancy

Pregnancy is associated with **some impairment of cell-mediated immunity.** With this decreased immunity, pregnant women may not have protective immune responses to some infectious agents. With this in mind, generally no live vaccines should be administered to pregnant women, though the risks and benefits should be weighed for individual cases. Rubella vaccine should not be given to pregnant women, though there have been no reported cases of rubella embryopathy following inadvertent immunization of a pregnant woman.

Two immunizations, IIV and Tdap, are recommended during the second or third trimester to provide protection for the mother and possibly the fetus. Residing with a pregnant household contact is generally not a contraindication for a child to receive live viral vaccines, a question often asked of pediatricians.

Preterm (<37 Weeks) and Low Birth Weight (<2,000 g) Newborns and Infants

In general, medically stable premature and low birth weight newborns and infants may be immunized at the same dose, schedule, and postnatal age as full-term newborns and infants.

Special consideration should be given to use of HBV vaccine in newborns and infants weighing less than 2,000 g as follows:

- Hepatitis B surface antigen (HBsAg)-positive or unknown status in mother → Give vaccine and HBIg, then give 3 additional vaccine doses.
- HBsAg-negative mother → Give HBV vaccine at 30 days (sooner if the newborn is stable for discharge), then follow the usual schedule, such that the infant receives a total of 3 doses.

Other Conditions Affecting Immunization Schedule

Child Allergic to Egg

For children with known anaphylactic reactions to eggs or egg components, special consideration is warranted for use of vaccines prepared using egg products. Current measles and mumps vaccines are prepared using chick-derived cell lines but do not contain significant amounts of proteins that cross-react with egg proteins. Children with egg allergies, including severe hypersensitivity, are at low risk of anaphylaxis from measles- or mumps-containing vaccines.

Additionally, skin testing against these antigens is not predictive of an adverse reaction. Thus, children who are allergic to egg may be immunized with measles and mumps vaccines alone or in combination preparations (eg, MMR, MMR and varicella) without skin testing.

Yellow fever and most inactivated influenza (IIV) and LAIV vaccines are prepared in eggs, may contain egg proteins, and may rarely induce an immediate allergic reaction. A history of egg allergy is no longer an absolute contraindication for immunization with vaccines prepared using eggs or egg components but requires further evaluation. For YF vaccine, skin testing before use is recommended in children with a history of anaphylaxis to eggs. A recombinant hemagglutinin influenza vaccine (egg-free) is available as a trivalent formulation (RIV3) for adults 18 to 49 years of age, including those with egg allergies. Individuals with a history of egg allergy who have experienced only hives after exposure to egg should receive influenza vaccine, with observation after vaccination. Limited data are available for use of LAIV in this setting, so use of IIV (or RIV for adults 18–49 years) is recommended with safety measures in place. These measures include administration by a health care professional familiar with the potential manifestations of egg allergy and observation of recipients for signs of a reaction for at least 30 minutes after vaccination. Individuals with a history of anaphylactic symptoms (eg, angioedema, respiratory distress, need for epinephrine) to eggs or egg components should be referred to a physician with expertise in the management of allergic conditions for further risk assessment before receiving influenza vaccine.

International Adoptees, Travelers, Immigrants, and Refugees

It is important to remember that travelers are from all socioeconomic strata, so inquiries about foreign travel should be included in routine visits in all clinical settings. In preparing patients for travel, the health care practitioner should review the child's record to ensure that all routine vaccines are up-to-date for age. The child should receive vaccinations and other preventive measures (eg, malaria prophylaxis) targeted for his or her destination. There may be a need for accelerated schedule (eg, early MMR for infants 6–12 months of age traveling to a measles-endemic area). Use of Ig prophylaxis should be considered for individuals who are susceptible to HAV and are not candidates for active immunization (eg, too young to receive HAV vaccine, immunocompromised). To help ensure healthy travel, the health care practitioner should check the current recommendations at wwwnc.cdc.gov/travel and www.who.int/ith/en.

Immigrants, refugees, and international adoptees may present with additional health care needs. A need for immunizations, underlying health status, and possible intercurrent illnesses should all be evaluated soon after arrival. Many of these children have been in poor living conditions and exposed to health hazards of environments like refugee camps and orphanages. The United States requires proof of the first dose of vaccines for entry into the country, though there are exemptions for adoptees younger than 10 years and refugees at entry. These high-risk children often have not been immunized or have missing records. Written, dated, and appropriate records (ie, age, dates, interval, and number of doses) may be considered valid, and subsequent immunization may resume according to the US schedule. Another option, especially when documentation is questionable, is to perform serologic studies for vaccine-induced antibodies.

Adolescents

Although the AAP has recommended a routine health visit at 11 to 12 years of age, historically compliance with this visit had been low. Until recently, no immunizations were routinely recommended in this age group. In the late 1990s, hepatitis B catch-up immunization was the first vaccine encouraged at this age and became required for middle-school entry in several states. Now several vaccines are available for protecting teens. One of these vaccines is Tdap for use as a single booster dose in adolescents 11 to 18 years of age who have previously received a series of DTP-containing vaccines. With recognition of waning vaccine-induced immunity to pertussis, it is probable that additional Tdap doses may be recommended in the near future.

Two kinds of meningococcal vaccines are available for use in the United States: the CPS vaccine (MPSV4, Menomune) and the CPS-protein conjugate vaccine (MCV4, Menactra and Menveo), with the latter formulation being preferred. Both vaccines contain 4 serotypes (A, C, Y, and W-135). Routine immunization with MCV4 is recommended at age 11 to 12 years with a booster dose at 16 years of age. For teens who received the first dose between 13 and 15 years, the second dose may be given at ages 16 to 18 years (up to 5 years after the first dose), but no booster dose is needed for teens who receive their first dose at 16 years or older. MCV4 is also recommended for catch-up dosing for older adolescents who have not been immunized, as well as for individuals 9 months to 55 years of age who are at increased risk of meningococcal diseases.

Two HPV vaccines are available in the United States for immunizing females against cervical cancer. Both HPV2 and HPV4 are composed of virus-like particles prepared from recombinant L1 capsid protein of HPV. One of the currently licensed vaccines is HPV2 (Cervarix, GlaxoSmithKline), containing serotypes 16 and 18, which is available for vaccinating females 10 to 25 years of age. Human papillomavirus 16 and 18 cause about 70% of cervical cancers. The other licensed vaccine is HPV4 (Gardasil, Merck), containing serotypes 6, 11, 16, and 18, which is licensed for females aged 9 to 26 years and also for males aged 9 to 26 years for protection against genital warts and anal and penile cancers. Both HPV2 and HPV4 are given in a 3-dose regimen at day 0, 1 to 2 months, and 6 months and are recommended for routine use in adolescents at 11 to 12 years of age, ideally before their sexual debut.

In addition, at adolescent visits (including precollege visits), health care professionals should review the teen's records to ensure that he or she has received all recommended vaccines, inquire about household contacts of infants or compromised hosts, and provide anticipatory guidance for safe and healthy living for the teen and parent.

Immunizations Received in Other Countries

Most vaccines used worldwide are produced with adequate quality control and may be considered reliable. Healthy individuals immunized in countries outside of the United States should receive vaccines according to the recommended schedule for age in the United States. In most cases, only written documentation should be accepted as proof of previous vaccination. Written, dated, and appropriate records (ie, correct age, dates, interval, number of doses) may be considered as valid, and immunizations may resume according to the US schedule.

Although most vaccines are acceptable, there may be some concerns for vaccine potency because of unsuitable storage and handling. Other concerns include inaccurate documentation and possibly inadequate response in some children due to other factors (eg, malnutrition, underlying illnesses). If vaccination status is uncertain, options include vaccinating with the antigen in question or checking serologic testing against the vaccine antigen, if testing is available. Generally, receipt of additional doses of diphtheria and tetanus toxoids alone or in combination with a pertussis-containing vaccine (ie, DTP, DTaP, Td, and Tdap) may lead to an increase in reactions (especially injection site reactions), and checking antibody titers against diphtheria and tetanus toxoids is encouraged. At this time, no FDA-approved assays for pertussis antibodies are available, and testing for pertussis antibodies is not recommended. For other vaccines, if the status is unknown, vaccination may be performed because extra doses are generally well tolerated. Most developing countries do not have VZV, conjugated pneumococcal, or Hib vaccines; these should be given as indicated per the US schedule.

Adverse Events and Vaccine Information

Adverse Events

As noted previously, no vaccine is completely free of adverse events, and known adverse events should be discussed with vaccinees (non-minors) or parents/legal guardians. In addition to discussing the risks and benefits of vaccination, health care professionals should include education about the risks associated with the natural disease. This is especially important in current times, when many individuals have not seen the diseases for which vaccines have been successful in controlling or eradicating.

In addition to safety information from the AAP and CDC, the manufacturer's package insert provides information about the rates of adverse events and contraindications for the specific vaccine. Most adverse events observed following routine immunizations are local injection site reactions, such as erythema, swelling, and pain, and systemic reactions, such as fever or fussiness. Although most of these adverse events are mild and self-limiting, some may be associated with significant dysfunction for the child (eg, not using a limb due to pain).

Rarely, serious adverse events may occur following immunization, and these may be associated with permanent disability or life-threatening illness. The occurrence of an adverse event after immunization does not prove a cause-and-effect relationship of the vaccine and the event but a temporal relationship. If a vaccine recipient experiences a serious adverse event, a complete evaluation for all plausible causes, including the role of the vaccine antigen, should be performed. Additionally, all clinically significant adverse events should be reported to the Vaccine Adverse Event Reporting System at http://vaers.hhs.gov, which is maintained by the CDC and FDA. Adverse event reporting is important because it helps identify possible unexpected events that were not observed in pre-licensure clinical trials.

Precautions and Contraindications

The Vaccine Information Statement (VIS) and package insert provide information for health care practitioners, vaccinees (non-minors), and parents/legal guardians about the precautions and contraindications for specific products.

A **precaution** suggests that careful analysis of risks and benefits of the vaccine should be done; if benefits outweigh risks, the vaccine may be given. A **contraindication** means that a vaccine should not be administered. An example of a contraindication is known anaphylaxis to any component of the vaccine. Breastfeeding does not interfere with oral immunization with rotavirus or OPV vaccines and is not a contraindication.

Minor illness without fever (temperature $\leq 38°C$ [100.4°F]) should not be considered a contraindication to vaccination. Temperature above 38°C (100.4°F) may not be a contraindication, depending on the physician's assessment of the child, illness, and vaccine to be given. If the child is early in the disease and the course is not predictable or the illness is moderate to severe, delaying immunization is reasonable. Deferring immunization without appropriate justification can cause a missed opportunity and may lead to inadequate immunization of the child.

Informing Vaccine Recipients and Parents and Vaccine Refusal

Vaccine recipients and parents should be informed about the risks and benefits of vaccination and the disease for which the vaccine is designed. The National Childhood Vaccine Injury Act of 1986 requires that parents receive a VIS each time a child receives a vaccine covered under this legislation, whether the vaccine was purchased with public or private funds. The VISs are available from the CDC at www.cdc.gov/vaccines/hcp/vis/index.html. Health care practitioners should document in the patient's chart the vaccine manufacturer, lot number, and date of administration and that VISs were provided and discussed with the vaccinee (non-minor) and parent/legal guardian.

In the United States, proof of immunization is required for school entry, but most states have provision for religious or philosophic exemption for individuals whose beliefs prohibit immunizations. Less than 1% of the US population of children is from families who refuse all vaccines. However, some parents will decline some or all immunizations for their child, despite best efforts to educate parents about the effectiveness of vaccines and the realistic chances of vaccine-associated adverse events. At times, parents have a genuine fear of the risks of vaccines without fear of the natural disease because many contemporary parents have not seen the diseases in the post-vaccine era. For others, their exaggerated fear of vaccine risk, without an appreciation of the benefits, results from deeply held family beliefs or has been fueled by biased information presented by unmonitored Web sites and other media outlets, promoting unsubstantiated fears. As a health care professional, a reasonable approach is to address parents' concerns in a non-condescending fashion and provide education about the known risks and benefits of immunization and risks of the natural infections. The discussion should be documented in the child's chart and the topic revisited at future encounters. Because of strong convictions that immunization benefits outweigh risks, some health care professionals choose not to provide care for children of families who refuse vaccines.

Vaccine Information

Information about current immunizations for health care practitioners and laypersons is available from many resources, including the CDC, AAP, FDA, and World Health Organization, among others (Table 34-1). Multiple apps with vaccine information are available for smart devices from the AAP and US Department of Health and Human Services (CDC, FDA, and National Institutes of Health); checking Web sites, social media, and with current carriers is recommended.

Table 34-1. Internet Sources of Vaccine Information

Source	Web Site
American Academy of Pediatrics	www.aap.org
Centers for Disease Control and Prevention	www.cdc.gov
Advisory Committee for Immunization Practices	www.cdc.gov/vaccines/hcp/acip-recs/vacc-specific/index.html
Morbidity and Mortality Weekly Report	www.cdc.gov/mmwr/preview/mmwrhtml/rr5102a1.htm
US Food and Drug Administration	www.fda.gov/BiologicsBloodVaccines/Vaccines/ApprovedProducts/UCM093833
Vaccine Adverse Event Reporting System	http://vaers.hhs.gov
American Society of Tropical Medicine and Hygiene	www.astmh.org
World Health Organization	www.who.int/en
GAVI Alliance	www.gavialliance.org

CASE RESOLUTION

The boy was appropriately immunized for Botswana recommendations through the age of 9 months, although now his immunization would be considered delayed for age on the US schedule. He is past due for the fourth dose of diphtheria, tetanus, acellular pertussis (DTaP); measles, mumps, rubella (MMR); and varicella-zoster virus vaccines. Additionally, he has not received any conjugate vaccines or hepatitis A virus (HAV) vaccine. The dose of monovalent measles vaccine does not change his need to receive 2 doses of MMR and varicella vaccines after the age of 12 months as listed on the US schedule. His uncle's immune status does not affect the use of MMR or varicella vaccines. His current respiratory illness is considered mild, and he does not have significant fever ($<$38°C [100.4°F]), so this is not problematic for receiving the needed immunizations.

During this visit, he may receive DTaP, the first dose of MMR plus varicella, one dose of *Haemophilus influenzae* type b conjugate vaccine, dose 1 of 2 of conjugate pneumococcal vaccine (2 months apart), and dose 1 of 2 of HAV (at least 6 months apart). All Vaccine Information Statements should be provided. The patient is scheduled to return in 2 months in October for his next dose of conjugate pneumococcal vaccine and dose 1 of 2 of inactivated influenza vaccine. He may not receive the live-attenuated influenza virus (LAIV) vaccine because of his young age (LAIV is licensed for children $\geq$24 months of age), as well as his uncle's immunocompromised status. He will need a fourth dose of inactivated poliovirus vaccine before school age. He is too old to receive the oral rotavirus vaccine.

Selected References

American Academy of Pediatrics. Active and passive immunization. In: Pickering LK, Baker CJ, Kimberlin DW, Long SS, eds. *Red Book: 2012 Report of the Committee on Infectious Diseases.* 27th ed. Elk Grove Village, IL: American Academy of Pediatrics; 2012:1–109

American Academy of Pediatrics. Documenting Parental Refusal to Have Their Children Vaccinated. http://www2.aap.org/immunization/pediatricians/pdf/refusaltovaccinate.pdf. Accessed January 28, 2014

American Academy of Pediatrics Committee on Infectious Diseases. Meningococcal conjugate vaccines policy update: booster dose recommendations. *Pediatrics.* 2011;128(6):1213–1218

Centers for Disease Control and Prevention. FDA licensure of bivalent human papillomavirus vaccine (HPV2, Cervarix) for use in females and updated HPV vaccination recommendations from the Advisory Committee on Immunization Practices (ACIP). *MMWR Morb Mortal Wkly Rep.* 2010;59(20):626–629. http://www.cdc.gov/mmwr/preview/mmwrhtml/mm5920a4.htm. Accessed January 28, 2014

Centers for Disease Control and Prevention. Global routine vaccination coverage, 2010. *MMWR Morb Mortal Wkly Rep.* 2011;60(44):1520–1522

Centers for Disease Control and Prevention. *Immunization Information Systems Annual Report (IISAR).* http://www.cdc.gov/vaccines/programs/iis/annual-report-IISAR. Accessed May 2, 2014

Centers for Disease Control and Prevention. Influenza vaccination of persons with a history of egg allergy. http://www.cdc.gov/flu/professionals/acip/2013-summary-recommendations.htm#egg-allergy. Accessed January 28, 2014

Centers for Disease Control and Prevention. National, state, and local area vaccination coverage among children aged 19-35 Months - United States, 2012. *MMWR Morb Mortal Wkly Rep.* 2013;62(36):733–740

Centers for Disease Control and Prevention. Updated recommendations for use of meningococcal conjugate vaccines—Advisory Committee on Immunization Practices (ACIP), 2010. *MMWR Morb Mortal Wkly Rep.* 2011;60(3):72–76. http://www.cdc.gov/mmwr/preview/mmwrhtml/mm6003a3.htm?s_cid=mm6003a3_e. Accessed January 28, 2014

Centers for Disease Control and Prevention. Vaccines & immunizations: what would happen if we stopped vaccinations? http://www.cdc.gov/vaccines/vac-gen/whatifstop.htm. Accessed January 28, 2014

James JM, Burks AW, Roberson PK, Sampson HA. Safe administration of the measles vaccine to children allergic to eggs. *N Engl J Med.* 1995;332(19):1262–1266

Kroger AT, Atkinson WL, Marcuse EK, Pickering LK; Advisory Committee on Immunization Practices, Centers for Disease Control and Prevention. General recommendations on immunization: recommendations of the Advisory Committee on Immunization Practices (ACIP). *MMWR Recomm Rep.* 2006;55(RR-15):1–48

Losonsky GA, Wasserman SS, Stephens I, et al. Hepatitis B vaccination of premature infants: a reassessment of current recommendations for delayed immunization. *Pediatrics.* 1999;103(2):E14

Markowitz LE, Dunne EF, Saraiya M, et al. Quadrivalent human papillomavirus vaccine: recommendations of the Advisory Committee on Immunization Practices (ACIP). *MMWR Recomm Rep.* 2007;56(RR-2):1–24

CHAPTER 35

Health Maintenance in Older Children and Adolescents

Monica Sifuentes, MD

CASE STUDY

Before a 13-year-old girl enters a new school, she is required to have a physical examination. She has not seen a physician in 5 years and has been healthy. Currently she has no medical complaints. Her examination is completely normal.

Questions

1. What are the important components of the history and physical examination in healthy older children and adolescents?
2. What immunizations are recommended for older children and adolescents?
3. What laboratory tests should be performed at health maintenance visits? Why?

Older children and adolescents are generally healthy individuals who infrequently visit physicians. If they are seen by a doctor, the visits are often for acute complaints, such as upper respiratory infections or sports-related injuries, and are therefore generally problem-oriented. Statistics on health maintenance visits in this age group are not readily available because patients may go to several different sites for health care and often do not receive comprehensive care at any of these places. Older children and adolescents seek treatment for acute and chronic conditions in private offices, urgent care centers, public health clinics, public hospitals, and emergency departments. It is estimated that fewer than 15% of adolescents consistently go to pediatricians for health care in general, and the same percentage probably applies to older children as well.

This all-too-common practice of inconsistent health care contributes to missed opportunities for anticipatory guidance, health education, and screening for preventable conditions. Screening tests also can be used to identify treatable conditions such as hypertension, anemia, and tuberculosis. Ideally, older children and adolescents should receive recommended immunizations beginning at 11 to 12 years of age; counseling concerning sexual activity, contraception, and sexually transmitted infections (STIs), including HIV; reassurance to address their emotional well-being; guidelines for adequate nutrition; education about tobacco, illicit drugs, and alcohol; and information about physical fitness and exercise as well as violence and injury prevention.

Guidelines for preventive child and adolescent health care have been published by the American Academy of Pediatrics (AAP) in conjunction with the Maternal and Child Health Bureau, the federal Child Health and Disability Prevention Program, the AAP Section on Adolescent Health, and the American Medical Association. Box 35-1 is a brief summary of these guidelines for older children and adolescents.

The Health Maintenance Visit

The purpose of the health maintenance visit for an older child or adolescent is to assess their general health and well-being and establish an independent relationship between the patient and health care professional for open communication and trust for future visits. Initial questions asked during this visit should be simple and focused on how the patient feels in general about his or her health, physical growth and development, and existing relationships with family and friends. More specific questions can then be formulated depending on the patient's responses. In healthy patients, medical history can be obtained using a questionnaire that parents and children complete in the waiting room. If this method is used, a separate form should be given to the adolescent if he or she is accompanied by a parent or guardian. The information is then reviewed at the start of the interview. Chronic medical conditions should be addressed at this time.

Medical History

Older children and adolescents should always be questioned directly about their medical history (Questions Box: Screening in Older Children and Adolescents). The parent or guardian should be encouraged to participate only after their child or adolescent has responded to questions or if invited by the child or adolescent himself or herself. The degree of parental participation also is influenced by the current cognitive and developmental stage of the patient.

		Box 35-1. Guidelines for Adolescent Health Maintenance Evaluation	
Screening History	*Physical Examination*	*Universal and Selective Screening Laboratory Tests/Studies*	*Anticipatory Guidance and Counseling*
Eating disorders	BMI	Snellen test	Parenting/communication
Gender identification	Blood pressure	Audiometry	Pubertal development
Sexual orientation	Comprehensive examination	Hemoglobin or hematocrit	Diet/nutrition, including calcium and vitamin D
Sexual activity (consensual and nonconsensual)	Genital examination	Tuberculin skin test	supplementation
Tobacco use	Pelvic examination[b]	Cholesterol	Exercise
Alcohol use/abuse		• If the patient is obese or there is a significant family history of hyperlipidemia, consider other laboratory tests such as fasting glucose and lipid panel.	Injury prevention
Drug use/abuse (CRAFFT questionnaire[a])			Educational or vocational plans/goals
School performance			Lifestyle modifications
Depression		If sexually active,	• Gender and sexual identity
Risk for suicide		• Urine hCG	• Abstinence
		• Urine or vaginal NAAT for GC/chlamydia	• Safe sexual activity
		• Serum HIV, RPR, hepatitis C[c]	• Other reproductive health issues
		• Papanicolaou test[b]	• Contraception
			• Avoidance of tobacco, alcohol, and illicit drugs
			• Identifying feelings of sadness/anger

Abbreviations: BMI, body mass index; GC, gonorrhea; hCG, human chorionic gonadotropin; HIV, human immunodeficiency virus; NAAT, nucleic acid amplification test; RPR, rapid plasma reagin.

[a]See Chapter 136 for CRAFFT questionnaire.

[b]A pelvic examination with a Papanicolaou test is recommended within 3 years of the onset of sexual activity (American Cancer Society) or age 21 years (American Congress of Obstetricians and Gynecologists). For indications for a pelvic examination, see Chapter 42.

[c]If patient engaged in injection drug use or young man having sex with men.

Psychosocial History

The psychosocial component of the interview should be conducted with older children or adolescents alone as well as together with parents or guardians after the issue of confidentiality has been reviewed (see Questions Box: Screening in Older Children and Adolescents). General questions about school, outside activities or hobbies, and family are often less threatening than inquiries about friends and tobacco use. More sensitive topics relating to drug use and abuse, sexuality, gender identification, sexual orientation, and sexual activity should be addressed after parents have left the room. Subjects initially discussed with parents should be reviewed once again with teenagers alone.

A useful tool for conducting the psychosocial interview has been developed and refined by physicians who specialize in pediatrics and adolescent medicine. Known by the acronym **HEADDSSS**, it reviews the essential components of the psychosocial history: *h*ome environment, *e*mployment and *e*ducation, *a*ctivities, *d*iet, *d*rugs, *s*exual activity/*s*exuality, *s*uicide/depression, and *s*afety (see Chapter 6).

Dietary History

A general dietary history should be obtained, with particular focus on eating habits, level of physical activity, and body image. Dietary restrictions, if any, should be investigated. Daily calcium, vitamin D, and iron intake also should be reviewed, especially in adolescent females. Adolescent males should be asked about nutritional supplements.

Family History

Significant illnesses, such as hypertension, hyperlipidemia, obesity, and diabetes, in first- and second-degree family members should be reviewed. Family use of alcohol, tobacco, and illegal as well as prescribed substances also should be determined. Age and cause of death in immediate family members should be recorded.

Medications and Allergies

Prescription as well as nonprescription (over-the-counter) medications, herbs, and supplements should be reviewed along with the indications and frequency of usage.

Physical Examination

The height and weight of patients should be plotted on a growth curve, with particular attention paid to the velocity of growth and body mass index (BMI = weight (kg)/[height (m)]^2). Blood pressure also should be noted and compared with age- and height-related normative values.

Aspects of the physical examination that are influenced by puberty should be emphasized. The skin should be carefully inspected for acne and hirsutism; clinicians should offer treatment whether or not patients acknowledge that they have skin problems. Tattoos, piercings, and signs of abuse or self-inflicted injury

Questions

Screening in Older Children and Adolescents

Questions for Patient and Parent

- How has the child or adolescent been doing lately? Does the parent have any complaints or concerns?
- How does the child or adolescent like school? How is he or she doing academically and socially? What are the child or adolescent's future goals?
- What activities does the child or adolescent currently participate in, including work?
- Does he or she have any hobbies?
- With whom does the child or adolescent live?
- Are there any significant illnesses in the immediate or extended family, such as hypertension, diabetes, or cancer?
- Does the child or adolescent take any medications, herbs, or supplements (prescribed or over the counter) regularly?

Questions for Child or Adolescent Alone

- Do you have any questions or concerns?
- How are things at home? Are there any problems with parents or siblings? Do you feel safe at home and school?
- Are you attending school?
- Do you like school? Who do you hang out with at school?
- Have you ever been truant, suspended, or expelled?
- What do you like to do for fun?
- See Chapter 6, Questions Box, for the rest of the interview.

(cutting) also should be noted. The oropharynx should be examined for any evidence of gingivitis or other signs of poor dental hygiene or malocclusion. The neck should be palpated for adenopathy and the thyroid gland for hypertrophy or nodules, especially in adolescent females. The back should be examined for any evidence of scoliosis, which is important to diagnose during this time of rapid growth.

Assessment of the pubertal development of the breasts and genitalia in preadolescent or adolescent females and the genitalia, including presence of pubic hair, in adolescent males is essential. The sexual maturity rating (SMR) (Tanner stage) can then be correlated with other signs of puberty, such as the appearance of acne and body odor. For example, the adolescent female with SMR 4 breasts and immature pubic hair distribution may have an underlying problem, such as complete androgen insensitivity syndrome (also called testicular feminization syndrome).

The abdomen should be palpated for organomegaly and the testicles for masses, hydroceles, hernias, or varicoceles. Lesions such as warts or vesicles also should be documented. The external female genitalia should be inspected for similar lesions and to document Tanner stage development. A speculum examination should be performed in females who are sexually active and complain of vaginal discharge, unexplained vaginal bleeding, or lower abdominal pain. (See Chapter 42 for additional indications for a pelvic examination.) In general, sexually inexperienced girls do not require a speculum examination; gentle inspection of the external genitalia is adequate in most cases, with special attention to hymenal patency. A rectal examination is generally reserved for patients with chronic abdominal pain or other specific acute gastrointestinal complaints.

Immunizations

Many recent additions have been made to the preadolescent/adolescent vaccination schedule (Table 35-1). As always, practitioners should verify that patients have completed the primary immunization series. If not, they should be given catch-up doses according to the latest Centers for Disease Control and Prevention (CDC) recommendations. The tetanus and diphtheria toxoids and acellular pertussis (Tdap) (Adacel, Boostrix), human papillomavirus (HPV) (Gardasil, Cervarix), and meningococcal conjugate (MCV4) (Menactra) vaccines should be given to preteens at the 11- to 12-year visit. The Tdap vaccine replaces the tetanus/diphtheria booster previously given at this age. Pertussis was added to the booster because immunity to pertussis has been noted to wane 5 to 8 years after vaccination, and there has been an increasing prevalence of pertussis detected in adolescents and adults with chronic cough in many communities. A conjugate vaccine against *Neisseria meningitidis* (MCV4 or Menactra) was approved by the US Food and Drug Administration in 2005. The Advisory Committee on Immunization Practices now recommends that MCV4 be given to all 11- to 18-year-olds. Finally, 2 different vaccines (Gardasil and Cervarix) are currently licensed in the United States to protect against 2 of the HPV types that cause most cervical cancers, oncogenic types 16 and 18. The quadrivalent vaccine, Gardasil, also protects against genital warts caused by non-oncogenic HPV types 6 and 11. While there has been some controversy surrounding the HPV vaccine, current recommendations state that the 3-dose series of the quadrivalent or bivalent vaccine should be given routinely at 11 to 12 years of age and to all young women and girls between the ages of 13 and 26. The vaccine is approved for patients as young as 9 years. The quadrivalent

Table 35-1. Recommended Immunization Schedule Affecting Adolescents

	Recommended Age (y)	
	11–12	*13–18*
Tetanus, diphtheria, pertussis	Tdap	Tdap (catch-up)
HPV	HPV (3 doses)	HPV (catch-up) (3 doses)
Meningococcal	MCV4	MCV4 (booster at 16 years)
Varicella	Varicella 2-dose series	
Influenza	Influenza annually	

Abbreviations: HPV, human papillomavirus; MCV4, meningococcal conjugate vaccine; Tdap, tetanus and diphtheria toxoids and acellular pertussis.

Modified from Centers for Disease Control and Prevention. Available at www.cdc.gov/vaccines/schedules.

vaccine also may be given to males between 9 and 26 years of age. Ideally, the vaccine should be administered before the initiation of sexual activity, but it also may be given to adolescents who are already sexually active.

Recommendations concerning some of the older, traditional vaccines have changed as well. If a child or adolescent has not had varicella, he or she should receive 2 doses of the vaccine. The first dose is usually administered no earlier than 12 months of age and the second dose of the varicella vaccine is now routinely administered at age 4 years prior to the start of elementary school. If an adolescent or preadolescent has received only one dose, a second dose should be administered. Routine vaccination against hepatitis B also is recommended, regardless of sexual activity, if it has not been administered previously. The 2-dose hepatitis A series should be given to all teenagers not previously vaccinated if they reside in high-incidence communities. Influenza vaccine should be given annually to all infants 6 months and older, children, and adolescents and to those who come into close contact with individuals with high-risk conditions. Pneumococcal vaccine should be offered to high-risk groups as well. In addition, a Mantoux skin test for tuberculosis should be placed if the adolescent resides in a high-risk environment. (For complete recommendations, see Chapter 34.)

Laboratory Tests

A hemoglobin level should be obtained to evaluate for anemia. Although previously included in laboratory screening, a urinalysis is no longer recommended to assess for protein, blood, and pyuria because most abnormal screens resolve spontaneously. Other suggested screening tests include hearing and vision tests and a cholesterol and lipid profile. Although cholesterol screening remains somewhat controversial, it is important to consider in patients who are overweight or obese or have a positive family history for hyperlipidemia or premature atherosclerotic heart disease.

In addition to these laboratory tests, sexually active adolescents should be screened for STIs. If a pelvic examination is performed, an endocervical specimen should be obtained for nucleic acid amplification testing (NAAT) for gonorrhea and chlamydia. However, if a pelvic examination is not indicated, routine screening for gonorrhea and chlamydia may be performed with a urine or vaginal sample alone using NAAT methods. The 2010 recommendations from the CDC state that all sexually active women younger than 25 years should be screened annually. Males should be screened if they are symptomatic, have a history of multiple partners and unprotected intercourse, or are having sex with men. In addition, a rapid plasma reagin test for syphilis and an HIV test should be obtained, especially if another STI is suspected or confirmed. All of these tests should be offered in the clinically appropriate setting after patients have received adequate education on STIs with a follow-up visit scheduled to discuss the results.

Patient Education

At the conclusion of the health maintenance visit, positive as well as negative findings should be reviewed with patients and their parents or guardians. Depending on the nature of these findings and the age of the patient, practitioners may initially choose to address these findings with the patient alone, keeping in mind issues of confidentiality. All recommended screening laboratory studies and immunizations should be reviewed before their administration, including the need for further follow-up. Subsequent vaccine doses must be outlined for patients and parents. The timing of the next visit and reasons for this visit should be discussed.

The remainder of the visit should be spent addressing any specific concerns of patients and parents or guardians, highlighting health care problems (eg, obesity, high blood pressure), and identifying any factors that may be contributing to high-risk behavior, such as drug or alcohol use. Older children or adolescents who are not participating in any deleterious activities should be praised for their positive behavior as well as provided with information about injury prevention.

Preparticipation Physical Evaluation for School-aged and Adolescent Athletes

The preparticipation physical evaluation (PPE) is essentially the "sports physical" that many schools require for participation in organized athletic programs. The primary objective of the PPE is to assess the athlete's readiness to compete safely and effectively in a given sport. Ideally, it also should identify athletes at risk for injury or sudden death, as well as those with an underlying medical condition that may preclude athletic participation.

Controversy exists about the appropriate location for performance of the PPE. Community physicians are often asked to perform limited en masse examinations at schools, or a group of clinicians is asked to perform the examinations in the gymnasium using "stations." Either way, the patient does not truly receive a complete physical examination or assessment, and neither approach lends itself to privacy. In addition, parents have a false sense of security and believe that their children have received adequate medical care. Ideally, primary care physicians should perform the PPE annually in their office during a scheduled visit at least 4 to 6 weeks before the beginning of the athletic season. Pediatricians can use this required visit as an opportunity to perform an annual comprehensive health maintenance examination on older children and adolescents, including providing important anticipatory guidance, administering catch-up immunizations, and performing the various screening tests.

History

The most challenging aspect of the PPE is reviewing the past medical and family history with the athlete to uncover abnormalities of the cardiovascular system that warrant further investigation by a cardiologist before sports participation. Red flags include a history of congenital heart disease, cardiac channelopathies such as long QT syndrome, a history of Kawasaki disease and associated coronary anomalies, and a history of myocarditis. The rest of the medical history for the PPE should focus on previous athletic participation and any current or past injuries that have required immediate evaluation and subsequent bracing, casting, surgery, or missed practice or play (Questions Box: Preparticipation Physical Evaluation). A standard questionnaire codeveloped by the AAP for this purpose may be used in the office setting. In addition, many practitioners record the results of the physical examination as well as their recommendations for the degree of athletic participation on this standard form (Figure 35-1). A review of systems should specifically include an inquiry about a history of syncope, near-syncope, chest pain, palpitations, and excessive shortness of breath or fatigue with exertion.

Physical Examination

A complete physical examination should be performed when possible. If circumstances preclude this, specific attention should be paid to the eyes, heart, abdomen, skin, and musculoskeletal system. Height, weight, blood pressure, and visual acuity also should be measured. Examination of the eyes is essential to document physiological anisocoria (different papillary diameters). A thorough cardiac evaluation should be performed for murmurs, abnormal heart sounds, or arrhythmias. The abdomen should be palpated for an enlarged liver or spleen, especially in the adolescent with a recent viral illness that could suggest mononucleosis. In males, the genitalia should be examined for sexual maturity in addition to assessing for abnormalities, such as atrophy, absence of a testis, or presence of a testicular mass or inguinal hernia. The skin should be inspected for lesions, such as tinea corporis, impetigo, or herpes simplex infection.

The 2-minute orthopedic examination consists of a head-to-toe assessment of all muscle groups and joints; any deformities, anomalies, or evidence of previous injuries should be noted (Table 35-2). Recent studies suggest expanding this examination to include a more detailed evaluation of high-risk areas for injury, such as the knee, ankle, and shoulder.

Questions

Preparticipation Physical Evaluation

- What sport(s) does the child or adolescent wish to participate in?
- Has the child or adolescent ever experienced a sports injury? If so, how much time did the athlete refrain from sports activities as a result of this injury?
- Has the athlete ever suffered a lapse of consciousness or concussion?
- Does the child or adolescent have a significant underlying health problem?
- Is the child or adolescent taking any prescribed or over-the-counter medications?
- Does the child or adolescent have any allergies?
- Has the child or adolescent ever had syncope, palpitations, or angina during exercise or at rest?
- Does the child or adolescent have a family history of sudden, early, non-traumatic deaths?

Laboratory Tests

Routine laboratory screening tests, except for those performed during the general health maintenance visit, are not recommended for the PPE. Screening young athletes for anemia or proteinuria has not been found to be particularly helpful. Such screening may be useful with highly competitive professional athletes, however. Although controversial, some groups believe that an electrocardiogram and echocardiogram should be routine components of the PPE as well.

Exclusion Criteria

The most common causes of unexpected death during athletics include undiagnosed cardiomyopathies, anomalous coronary arteries, heart valve defects, primary cardiac rhythm disorders, and pulmonary hypertension, and an important part of the PPE is geared toward determining if a patient has risk factors for any of these conditions. Medical exclusion criteria for athletic participation are based on information obtained in the medical as well as family history. Significant historical clues include a family history of sudden, nontraumatic death; premature coronary artery disease in a first- or second-degree relative; a history of palpitations, angina, or syncope during exercise; and recent, documented infection with the Epstein-Barr virus. Controversy exists concerning when athletes can return to collision sports after infectious mononucleosis. A history of a recent or suspected concussion also requires close monitoring to address when the athlete is cleared to return to participate in a given sport. Current clinical experience and neurocognitive research on adolescents and concussions support the mantra, "When in doubt, sit them out." In other words, the athlete should not be pressured to play through injuries or return to play before he or she has fully recovered. Patients with concussions should rest, physically and cognitively, until their symptoms have resolved completely at rest and with exertion, according to the AAP Council on Sports Medicine and Fitness. In most mild cases of concussion, typical recovery occurs in 7 to 10 days, although athletes with more significant injuries may require weeks to months to completely recover if the concussion is severe. The short- and long-term effects of sports-related concussions and repetitive head impacts over the life span of athletes of all ages are still under intense investigation in an effort to create appropriate return-to-play criteria and to reduce cognitive, emotional, behavioral, and neurologic consequences.

Findings discovered during the physical examination, such as stature consistent with Marfan syndrome, a cardiac arrhythmia, or the midsystolic click of mitral valve prolapse, could preclude the adolescent from participation in a particular sport. Specific conditions, such as the athlete with one eye or one kidney, should be evaluated on an individual basis by a physician qualified to assess the safety of the particular sport for the athlete (contact/collision vs limited contact).

Special circumstances to consider during the PPE are menstrual disorders and the female athlete, exercise-induced bronchospasm, anabolic steroid use, and eating disorders that may be associated with certain activities, such as gymnastics, ballet, and wrestling.

■ PREPARTICIPATION PHYSICAL EVALUATION
HISTORY FORM

(Note: This form is to be filled out by the patient and parent prior to seeing the physician. The physician should keep this form in the chart.)

Date of Exam _____

Name _____ Date of birth _____

Sex _____ Age _____ Grade _____ School _____ Sport(s) _____

Medicines and Allergies: Please list all of the prescription and over-the-counter medicines and supplements (herbal and nutritional) that you are currently taking

_____

_____

Do you have any allergies? ☐ Yes ☐ No If yes, please identify specific allergy below.
☐ Medicines   ☐ Pollens   ☐ Food   ☐ Stinging Insects

Explain "Yes" answers below. Circle questions you don't know the answers to.

GENERAL QUESTIONS	Yes	No
1. Has a doctor ever denied or restricted your participation in sports for any reason?		
2. Do you have any ongoing medical conditions? If so, please identify below: ☐ Asthma ☐ Anemia ☐ Diabetes ☐ Infections Other: _____		
3. Have you ever spent the night in the hospital?		
4. Have you ever had surgery?		

HEART HEALTH QUESTIONS ABOUT YOU	Yes	No
5. Have you ever passed out or nearly passed out DURING or AFTER exercise?		
6. Have you ever had discomfort, pain, tightness, or pressure in your chest during exercise?		
7. Does your heart ever race or skip beats (irregular beats) during exercise?		
8. Has a doctor ever told you that you have any heart problems? If so, check all that apply: ☐ High blood pressure ☐ A heart murmur ☐ High cholesterol ☐ A heart infection ☐ Kawasaki disease Other: _____		
9. Has a doctor ever ordered a test for your heart? (For example, ECG/EKG, echocardiogram)		
10. Do you get lightheaded or feel more short of breath than expected during exercise?		
11. Have you ever had an unexplained seizure?		
12. Do you get more tired or short of breath more quickly than your friends during exercise?		

HEART HEALTH QUESTIONS ABOUT YOUR FAMILY	Yes	No
13. Has any family member or relative died of heart problems or had an unexpected or unexplained sudden death before age 50 (including drowning, unexplained car accident, or sudden infant death syndrome)?		
14. Does anyone in your family have hypertrophic cardiomyopathy, Marfan syndrome, arrhythmogenic right ventricular cardiomyopathy, long QT syndrome, short QT syndrome, Brugada syndrome, or catecholaminergic polymorphic ventricular tachycardia?		
15. Does anyone in your family have a heart problem, pacemaker, or implanted defibrillator?		
16. Has anyone in your family had unexplained fainting, unexplained seizures, or near drowning?		

BONE AND JOINT QUESTIONS	Yes	No
17. Have you ever had an injury to a bone, muscle, ligament, or tendon that caused you to miss a practice or a game?		
18. Have you ever had any broken or fractured bones or dislocated joints?		
19. Have you ever had an injury that required x-rays, MRI, CT scan, injections, therapy, a brace, a cast, or crutches?		
20. Have you ever had a stress fracture?		
21. Have you ever been told that you have or have you had an x-ray for neck instability or atlantoaxial instability? (Down syndrome or dwarfism)		
22. Do you regularly use a brace, orthotics, or other assistive device?		
23. Do you have a bone, muscle, or joint injury that bothers you?		
24. Do any of your joints become painful, swollen, feel warm, or look red?		
25. Do you have any history of juvenile arthritis or connective tissue disease?		

MEDICAL QUESTIONS	Yes	No
26. Do you cough, wheeze, or have difficulty breathing during or after exercise?		
27. Have you ever used an inhaler or taken asthma medicine?		
28. Is there anyone in your family who has asthma?		
29. Were you born without or are you missing a kidney, an eye, a testicle (males), your spleen, or any other organ?		
30. Do you have groin pain or a painful bulge or hernia in the groin area?		
31. Have you had infectious mononucleosis (mono) within the last month?		
32. Do you have any rashes, pressure sores, or other skin problems?		
33. Have you had a herpes or MRSA skin infection?		
34. Have you ever had a head injury or concussion?		
35. Have you ever had a hit or blow to the head that caused confusion, prolonged headache, or memory problems?		
36. Do you have a history of seizure disorder?		
37. Do you have headaches with exercise?		
38. Have you ever had numbness, tingling, or weakness in your arms or legs after being hit or falling?		
39. Have you ever been unable to move your arms or legs after being hit or falling?		
40. Have you ever become ill while exercising in the heat?		
41. Do you get frequent muscle cramps when exercising?		
42. Do you or someone in your family have sickle cell trait or disease?		
43. Have you had any problems with your eyes or vision?		
44. Have you had any eye injuries?		
45. Do you wear glasses or contact lenses?		
46. Do you wear protective eyewear, such as goggles or a face shield?		
47. Do you worry about your weight?		
48. Are you trying to or has anyone recommended that you gain or lose weight?		
49. Are you on a special diet or do you avoid certain types of foods?		
50. Have you ever had an eating disorder?		
51. Do you have any concerns that you would like to discuss with a doctor?		
FEMALES ONLY		
52. Have you ever had a menstrual period?		
53. How old were you when you had your first menstrual period?		
54. How many periods have you had in the last 12 months?		

Explain "yes" answers here

_____

_____

_____

_____

_____

_____

_____

I hereby state that, to the best of my knowledge, my answers to the above questions are complete and correct.

Signature of athlete _____ Signature of parent/guardian _____ Date _____

©2010 American Academy of Family Physicians, American Academy of Pediatrics, American College of Sports Medicine, American Medical Society for Sports Medicine, American Orthopaedic Society for Sports Medicine, and American Osteopathic Academy of Sports Medicine. Permission is granted to reprint for noncommercial, educational purposes with acknowledgment.

HE0503   9-2681/0410

Figure 35-1. Page 1 of 4.

■ PREPARTICIPATION PHYSICAL EVALUATION
THE ATHLETE WITH SPECIAL NEEDS: SUPPLEMENTAL HISTORY FORM

Date of Exam _____

Name _____ Date of birth _____

Sex _____ Age _____ Grade _____ School _____ Sport(s) _____

		Yes	No
1. Type of disability			
2. Date of disability			
3. Classification (if available)			
4. Cause of disability (birth, disease, accident/trauma, other)			
5. List the sports you are interested in playing			
6. Do you regularly use a brace, assistive device, or prosthetic?			
7. Do you use any special brace or assistive device for sports?			
8. Do you have any rashes, pressure sores, or any other skin problems?			
9. Do you have a hearing loss? Do you use a hearing aid?			
10. Do you have a visual impairment?			
11. Do you use any special devices for bowel or bladder function?			
12. Do you have burning or discomfort when urinating?			
13. Have you had autonomic dysreflexia?			
14. Have you ever been diagnosed with a heat-related (hyperthermia) or cold-related (hypothermia) illness?			
15. Do you have muscle spasticity?			
16. Do you have frequent seizures that cannot be controlled by medication?			

Explain "yes" answers here

_____
_____
_____
_____
_____

Please indicate if you have ever had any of the following.

	Yes	No
Atlantoaxial instability		
X-ray evaluation for atlantoaxial instability		
Dislocated joints (more than one)		
Easy bleeding		
Enlarged spleen		
Hepatitis		
Osteopenia or osteoporosis		
Difficulty controlling bowel		
Difficulty controlling bladder		
Numbness or tingling in arms or hands		
Numbness or tingling in legs or feet		
Weakness in arms or hands		
Weakness in legs or feet		
Recent change in coordination		
Recent change in ability to walk		
Spina bifida		
Latex allergy		

Explain "yes" answers here

_____
_____
_____
_____
_____

I hereby state that, to the best of my knowledge, my answers to the above questions are complete and correct.

Signature of athlete _____ Signature of parent/guardian _____ Date _____

©2010 American Academy of Family Physicians, American Academy of Pediatrics, American College of Sports Medicine, American Medical Society for Sports Medicine, American Orthopaedic Society for Sports Medicine, and American Osteopathic Academy of Sports Medicine. Permission is granted to reprint for noncommercial, educational purposes with acknowledgment.

Figure 35-1. **Page 2 of 4.**

■ PREPARTICIPATION PHYSICAL EVALUATION
PHYSICAL EXAMINATION FORM

Name _____ Date of birth _____

PHYSICIAN REMINDERS

1. Consider additional questions on more sensitive issues
   - Do you feel stressed out or under a lot of pressure?
   - Do you ever feel sad, hopeless, depressed, or anxious?
   - Do you feel safe at your home or residence?
   - Have you ever tried cigarettes, chewing tobacco, snuff, or dip?
   - During the past 30 days, did you use chewing tobacco, snuff, or dip?
   - Do you drink alcohol or use any other drugs?
   - Have you ever taken anabolic steroids or used any other performance supplement?
   - Have you ever taken any supplements to help you gain or lose weight or improve your performance?
   - Do you wear a seat belt, use a helmet, and use condoms?
2. Consider reviewing questions on cardiovascular symptoms (questions 5–14).

EXAMINATION					
Height		Weight	□ Male □ Female		
BP / (/) Pulse			Vision R 20/	L 20/	Corrected □ Y □ N

MEDICAL	NORMAL	ABNORMAL FINDINGS
Appearance • Marfan stigmata (kyphoscoliosis, high-arched palate, pectus excavatum, arachnodactyly, arm span > height, hyperlaxity, myopia, MVP, aortic insufficiency)		
Eyes/ears/nose/throat • Pupils equal • Hearing		
Lymph nodes		
Heart^a • Murmurs (auscultation standing, supine, +/- Valsalva) • Location of point of maximal impulse (PMI)		
Pulses • Simultaneous femoral and radial pulses		
Lungs		
Abdomen		
Genitourinary (males only)^b		
Skin • HSV, lesions suggestive of MRSA, tinea corporis		
Neurologic^c		
MUSCULOSKELETAL		
Neck		
Back		
Shoulder/arm		
Elbow/forearm		
Wrist/hand/fingers		
Hip/thigh		
Knee		
Leg/ankle		
Foot/toes		
Functional • Duck-walk, single leg hop		

^aConsider ECG, echocardiogram, and referral to cardiology for abnormal cardiac history or exam.
^bConsider GU exam if in private setting. Having third party present is recommended.
^cConsider cognitive evaluation or baseline neuropsychiatric testing if a history of significant concussion.

□ Cleared for all sports without restriction

□ Cleared for all sports without restriction with recommendations for further evaluation or treatment for _____

_____

□ Not cleared

      □ Pending further evaluation

      □ For any sports

      □ For certain sports _____

        Reason _____

Recommendations _____

_____

I have examined the above-named student and completed the preparticipation physical evaluation. The athlete does not present apparent clinical contraindications to practice and participate in the sport(s) as outlined above. A copy of the physical exam is on record in my office and can be made available to the school at the request of the parents. If conditions arise after the athlete has been cleared for participation, the physician may rescind the clearance until the problem is resolved and the potential consequences are completely explained to the athlete (and parents/guardians).

Name of physician (print/type) _____ Date _____

Address _____ Phone _____

Signature of physician _____, MD or DO

©2010 American Academy of Family Physicians, American Academy of Pediatrics, American College of Sports Medicine, American Medical Society for Sports Medicine, American Orthopaedic Society for Sports Medicine, and American Osteopathic Academy of Sports Medicine. Permission is granted to reprint for noncommercial, educational purposes with acknowledgment.
HE0503
9-2681/0410

Figure 35-1. Page 3 of 4.

■ PREPARTICIPATION PHYSICAL EVALUATION
CLEARANCE FORM

Name _____ Sex ☐ M ☐ F Age _____ Date of birth _____

☐ Cleared for all sports without restriction

☐ Cleared for all sports without restriction with recommendations for further evaluation or treatment for _____

_____

☐ Not cleared

      ☐ Pending further evaluation

      ☐ For any sports

      ☐ For certain sports _____

      Reason _____

Recommendations _____

_____

_____

_____

_____

_____

I have examined the above-named student and completed the preparticipation physical evaluation. The athlete does not present apparent clinical contraindications to practice and participate in the sport(s) as outlined above. A copy of the physical exam is on record in my office and can be made available to the school at the request of the parents. If conditions arise after the athlete has been cleared for participation, the physician may rescind the clearance until the problem is resolved and the potential consequences are completely explained to the athlete (and parents/guardians).

Name of physician (print/type) _____ Date _____

Address _____ Phone _____

Signature of physician _____, MD or DO

EMERGENCY INFORMATION

Allergies _____

_____

_____

_____

_____

Other information _____

_____

_____

_____

_____

_____

_____

_____

_____

_____

_____

©2010 American Academy of Family Physicians, American Academy of Pediatrics, American College of Sports Medicine, American Medical Society for Sports Medicine, American Orthopaedic Society for Sports Medicine, and American Osteopathic Academy of Sports Medicine. Permission is granted to reprint for noncommercial, educational purposes with acknowledgment.

Figure 35-1. **Page 4 of 4.**

Table 35-2. The 2-Minute Orthopedic Examination	
Instructions	**Points of Observation**
Stand facing examiner.	Acromioclavicular joints, general habitus
Look at ceiling, floor, over both shoulders; touch ears to shoulders.	Cervical spinal motion
Shrug shoulders (examiner resists).	Trapezius strength
Abduct shoulders 90 degrees.	Deltoid strength
Full external rotation of arms	Shoulder motion
Flex and extend elbows.	Elbow motion
Arms at sides, elbows 90 degrees flexed; pronate and supinate wrists.	Elbow and wrist motion
Spread fingers; make fist.	Hand or finger motion and deformities
Tighten (contract) quadriceps; relax quadriceps.	Symmetry and knee effusion; ankle effusion
Duckwalk 4 steps (away from examiner with buttocks on heels).	Hip, knee, and ankle motion
Back to examiner	Shoulder symmetry, scoliosis
Knees straight, touch toes.	Scoliosis, hip motion, hamstring tightness
Raise up on toes, raise heels.	Calf symmetry, leg strength

CASE RESOLUTION

The young adolescent described in the case history should first be interviewed with the parent and then alone. Her medical and psychosocial history should be reviewed. A complete physical examination should be performed as well as a pelvic examination if she is sexually active and has a history of lower abdominal pain, abnormal vaginal bleeding, or discharge. If she is sexually active and asymptomatic or not sexually active, only general laboratory screening tests should be performed and the results reviewed with the patient. The remainder of the visit should be spent discussing issues such as nutrition, exercise, illicit substance abuse, sexuality and sexual activity, and safety. Results of the physical examination and screening tests should then be discussed with the parent who accompanied her to the office. If necessary, a follow-up visit should be scheduled. Otherwise, the adolescent should be seen annually.

Selected References

American Academy of Family Physicians, American Academy of Pediatrics, American College of Sports Medicine, American Medical Society for Sports Medicine, American Orthopaedic Society for Sports Medicine, American Osteopathic Academy of Sports Medicine. *PPE: Preparticipation Physical Evaluation.* 4th ed. Elk Grove Village, IL: American Academy of Pediatrics; 2010

American Academy of Pediatrics. *The Adolescent Preventive Care Visit.* Elk Grove Village, IL: American Academy of Pediatrics; 2009

American Academy of Pediatrics Committee on Infectious Diseases. Additional recommendations for use of tetanus toxoid, reduced-content diphtheria toxoid, and acellular pertussis vaccine (Tdap). *Pediatrics.* 2011;128(4):809–812

Centers for Disease Control and Prevention. Immunization schedules. Birth-18 years & "catch-up" immunization schedules. United States, 2014. http://www.cdc.gov/vaccines/schedules/hcp/child-adolescent.html. Accessed March 18, 2014

Demorest RA, Washington RL; American Academy of Pediatrics Council on Sports Medicine and Fitness. Athletic participation by children and adolescents who have systemic hypertension. *Pediatrics.* 2010;125(6):1287–1294

Edwards SM, Rousseau-Pierre T. Immunization in adolescents—an update. *Adolesc Med State Art Rev.* 2010;21(2):173–186

Halstead ME, McAvoy K, Devore CD, et al. Returning to learning following a concussion. *Pediatrics.* 2013;132(5):948–957

Halstead ME, Walter KD; American Academy of Pediatrics Council on Sports Medicine and Fitness. Sport-related concussion in children and adolescents. *Pediatrics.* 2010;126(3):597–615

Herman-Giddens ME, Bourdony CJ, Dowshen SA, Reiter EO. *Assessment of Sexual Maturity Stages in Girls and Boys.* Elk Grove Village, IL: American Academy of Pediatrics; 2011

Institute of Medicine, National Research Council. *Sports-Related Concussions in Youth: Improving the Science, Changing the Culture.* Washington, DC: National Academies Press; 2014

Metzl JD. Managing sports injuries in the pediatric office. *Pediatr Rev.* 2008; 29(3):75–85

Middleman AB, Rosenthal SL, Rickert VI, et al. Adolescent immunizations: a position paper of the Society for Adolescent Medicine. *J Adolesc Health.* 2006;38(3):321–327

Moscicki AB. Human papillomavirus disease and vaccines in adolescents. *Adolesc Med State Art Rev.* 2010;21(2):347–363

Peterson AR, Bernhardt DT. The preparticipation sports evaluation. *Pediatr Rev.* 2011;32(5):e53–e65

Rice SG; American Academy of Pediatrics Council on Sports Medicine and Fitness. Medical conditions affecting sports participation. *Pediatrics.* 2008;121(4): 841–848

Strasburger VC, Jordan AB, Donnerstein E. Health effects of media on children and adolescents. *Pediatrics.* 2010;125(4):756–767

CHAPTER 36

Health Care for International Adoptees

ChrisAnna M. Mink, MD

CASE STUDY

Jaxon is a 14-month-old boy adopted from Thailand. His biological mother was a 26-year-old commercial sex worker who entered a maternity house during her pregnancy to receive care and to relinquish the baby for adoption. His mom reported that she was physically and sexually abused as a child and became a street child when she was 14 years old. She used illicit drugs 5 years ago but none since. She identifies the father as a European customer but has no other information. Jaxon was born at 32 weeks' gestation and was placed in an incubator but did not have any respiratory problems. He has been in foster care in a Thai family's home with his care supervised by an internationally respected adoption organization. He was selected by his parents at the age of 4 months, and they have received monthly progress reports on his growth, development, and medical status. Reportedly, he has had several "colds" and one ear infection but otherwise has been growing and developing well. Before departure to pick up Jaxon, his adoptive parents met with you to prepare for his arrival.

From the Bangkok airport, the parents placed a call to you because Jaxon would not stop crying. They report that on the morning that his foster mom left him with them, he cried quite a bit but had settled by bedtime and seemed to be adjusting well during the week. However, over the past 12 hours he hasn't stopped crying and refuses to eat. They question if his discomfort is related to teething because he has been drooling, but they have not noticed any other symptoms. They are gravely concerned that he doesn't like them and is having attachment difficulties.

Questions

1. What factors influence the prevalence of international adoption?
2. What are some of the potential health problems of international adoptees?
3. What is an appropriate medical evaluation for international adoptees?
4. What is the pediatrician's role in caring for the child and newly formed family?

Although internationally adopted children come from a wide range of birth countries, many of their health-related issues are similar. Many of the children have lived in orphanages in impoverished areas of the developing world and have incurred the maladies associated with poverty and deprivation.

Epidemiology

From 1999 to 2012, 242,602 children were adopted internationally into the United States; this is nearly the same number as the previous 30 years combined. Through the first part of this century, most of the children (90%) were from Asia (China and South Korea most commonly), Eastern Europe, and South America (Guatemala and Colombia). From 2009 to 2012, China, Ethiopia, and Russia were the 3 leading countries of origin for children adopted into the United States. A decline in the number of international adoptions has been seen since 2009, with a nadir in 2012 of only 8,608 international adoptees entering the United States. This decline is the result of multiple factors, including economic downturn in the United States, changing geopolitical landscape in birth countries, and stricter policies governing adoption attempting to curb corruption, including the Hague Convention (an international agreement for standardizing intercountry practices to promote protection of children available for adoption).

Many factors influence adoptive parents to choose international adoption. In the United States, delays in childbearing and associated infertility have increased the demand for adoptable children. At the same time, more readily available birth control and growing acceptance of single motherhood have decreased the number of US infants available for adoption. In addition to the shortage of **adoptable** children in the United States, additional factors for parents choosing international adoptions include real and perceived risks of domestic adoption (eg, failure of birth parents to relinquish rights), fear of adopting a child with special needs from the domestic system, and limited availability of children with desired traits (eg, specific age and ethnicity). In addition, prompt termination of rights of birth parents in international adoption is cited as a factor in the choice.

The advent of **intercountry adoption** (**ICA**) in the United States occurred with World War II and the large number of orphaned children in Europe, many of whom were fathered by American soldiers. The second, and more formalized, wave of ICA occurred with the Korean War. Because of the need to care for unwanted orphans, primarily of mixed ethnicities also fathered by American soldiers, South Korea established a foster care system and the children became available for adoption to Americans. War and political turmoil are still factors for children becoming available for adoption. For example, the fall of communism was a significant factor for Russia and other states of the former Soviet Union becoming common birth countries for adoptees in the 1990s and the early part of this century. Recently, with worsening poverty and political strife, more children are being adopted from African countries.

Societal values are also factors for influencing adoption practices. China is often one of the leading birth country for **adoptees** because of the population control initiatives of the government mandating that families have only one child. With this practice and the desire to have a male heir, some newborn girls are abandoned and subsequently become available for adoption. In some countries, local laws or cultural practices are prohibitive for adoption, especially for foreigners, and, thus, these countries are infrequent birth countries. The United States is the birth country for about 500 children adopted into other countries. Absolute statistics for children adopted out of the United States are not available because the government does not track the number of exit visas issued for adopted children. These US children are often males of African American or mixed ethnicity and are adopted by families in Canada and Western Europe. They are available purportedly due to the low desire for these infants by adoptive parents in the United States.

The status of the country of origin (ie, war, turmoil, poverty, and societal values) aside, there is significant overlap in the reasons that children from foreign countries and from the United States become available for adoption, eg, parental substance use, abandonment, chronic neglect, abuse, and domestic violence.

Until the 1990s, most international **adoptees** were from South Korea, which had in place an excellent **foster care** system and health care. Since the 1990s, nearly two-thirds of **adoptees** come from institutions in poor nations without a developed foster care system, resulting in a significant decline in the health and well-being of **adoptees.**

Clinical Presentation

The majority of internationally adopted children are female (approximately 56%), in part reflecting the adoption of girls from China, as well as a preference among some adoptive parents (especially single women) to adopt a girl. International adoptees are young, with approximately 15% being younger than 1 year and 55% between 1 and 4 years of age.

Pre-adoption

Some **adoptees** become known to the US health care practitioner **"only on paper"** during the **pre-adoption stage.** Adoptive parents may ask their physician for help in assessing the child's medical status. Often parents receive a written health report (varying in the

quantity and quality of information) and photos or videos of the child they are considering adopting. The written documents may be in a foreign language or not translated by an experienced medical translator. Some countries prohibit international adoption of healthy children, so diagnoses may be embellished to improve the child's chances for adoption. Additionally, some medical records contain diagnoses that are nonsensical in US medicine but represent terms used in the country of origin. For example, **adoptees** from Russia often have neurologic diagnoses such as **perinatal encephalopathy,** which suggests serious brain injury and would carry a grave prognosis in Western medicine; in Russia, this term may reflect a minor deprivation or a lack of prenatal care and not a specific neurologic injury. However, at other times, a term may have the same meaning and intent to Russian physicians as to US physicians. These inconsistencies are therefore quite challenging when trying to evaluate the medical records of potential **adoptees.** Many physicians may not feel comfortable with reviewing medical records given so many limitations; however, even with all of the caveats, review of the records may provide valuable insight into the health status of the potential adoptee.

Also during the **pre-adoption stage,** the physician may provide information for parents and families for preventive health measures to prepare for travel to a developing area of the world. The Centers for Disease Control and Prevention (CDC) Traveler's Health Web site (www.cdc.gov/travel) is a good resource for physicians and parents. Up-to-date information may also be obtained from the World Health Organization (WHO) and the US Department of State (Table 36-1).

Table 36-1. Web Sites for International Health, Travel, and Adoption Information		
Resource	*Information*	*Web Site*
Centers for Disease Control and Prevention	Up-to-date information for travelers' health	wwwnc.cdc.gov/travel
US Department of State	Up-to-date information for travelers' risk (eg, civil unrest)	http://travel.state.gov/content/passports/english/alertswarnings.html
	Intercountry adoption procedures	http://adoption.state.gov/adoption_process.php
World Health Organization	Health status and recommendations for immunizations for each country	www.who.int/en
	Assists with interpreting foreign vaccine records	
US Department of Health and Human Services Administration for Children & Families	Adoption information and procedures	www.childwelfare.gov

Parents should be informed about the possible infections seen in international adoptees, and they should receive appropriate education and preventive measures, including vaccinations (eg, measles, hepatitis A, and hepatitis B vaccine; positive hepatitis B surface antigen [HBsAg] is seen in 1%–5% of adoptees).

During the Adoption Trip

All internationally adopted children are required by the US Department of State to have a **physical examination** before admission into the country; however, this examination is quite limited in scope and performed primarily to rule out severe impairments or certain communicable diseases that may pose a public health threat (eg, active tuberculosis [TB]). This examination should not be considered as a complete medical evaluation for an individual child. Some health care practitioners are able to provide support for families during travel via e-mail, telephone, and Internet, similar to telephone consultations performed in general practice.

Post-adoption

After the adoption, the health status of children on presentation to the US health care physician may be quite variable, ranging from well to severely ill with acute infections or chronic diseases (eg, malnutrition and TB). The adopted child should be seen by the physician within 2 to 3 weeks of arrival in the United States, or sooner if he or she has an acute illness. This 2-week period allows for the child (and parents) to recover from jet lag and become more familiar with each other, permitting a better assessment at the visit. If an acute illness visit is required, a separate appointment for a comprehensive evaluation should be scheduled at a later time.

Health Care Issues

In addition to problems commonly related to **poverty** and **deprivation,** many health issues are specific to the country of origin (eg, increased risk of **fetal alcohol spectrum disorder [FASD]** in children from Russia, malaria from Africa). Published data on health care issues are limited for children from recent countries of origins (eg, Ethiopia).

Generally, health care issues for **adoptees** are extensive, including acute illnesses (eg, respiratory infections), chronic illnesses (eg, anemia, malnutrition, poor dental hygiene, TB, asthma, parasite infestation), delayed or unknown immunizations, psychosocial challenges, and impaired growth and development.

Some children have assigned birth dates (eg, **abandoned infants** and **street children** for whom birth dates are not known), and they may have small growth parameters, making it difficult to know their true age and expected development. **Developmental delay,** most commonly language delay, is frequently identified. Assessment of development may be even more difficult in infants and young children who are nonverbal and older children who speak their native language.

Growth delay is common for **adoptees.** Many children are malnourished or have failure to thrive (FTT), and these afflictions are often multifactorial in origin, including poor prenatal environment (eg, maternal stress, malnutrition, drug and alcohol abuse), inadequate calories, inadequate nurturing, unrecognized genetic or congenital disorders (eg, FASD), and untreated chronic illnesses (eg, rickets). Institutionalized children may suffer from **psychosocial dwarfism** and may lose 1 month of linear growth for every 3 to 4 months spent in the orphanage. Delay in puberty may be observed in adolescents from deprived environments, such as **orphanages.**

Immunization records may not be available, may be incomplete, or may be in a foreign language, which hinders assessing the vaccination status of adoptees. Additionally, many vaccines available in the United States are not available in the developing world (eg, *Haemophilus influenzae* type b [Hib], pneumococcal conjugate) and, thus, children will not have had them. Adopted children immigrating to the United States who are younger than 10 years are exempt from the Immigration and Nationality Act regulations requiring proof of immunizations before arrival; however, adoptive parents are required to sign a waiver that they will comply with US recommended immunizations after arrival.

Psychosocial, emotional, and **mental health disorders** are some of the more challenging problems to assess. The spectrum of mental health problems is related to age and previous life experiences for the child. Children may have suffered from physical or sexual abuse prior to placement in an institution, and they may also be victims of abuse by older children or adult caregivers while in institutional placement. Attachment disorders are some of the most concerning abnormalities for adoptive parents, adoption professionals, and health care practitioners. Because the fundamentals for learning healthy attachments are greatly influenced by early infant-caregiver relationships, many international adoptees have difficulties bonding, in part because they have not had secure caregiver relationships. Issues for attachment and bonding may be especially problematic for children who have resided in an orphanage or had multiple caregivers from an early age. Children who have had multiple caregivers may be indiscriminately friendly; this poses risks for their safety. Other common mental health problems include depression, attention-deficit/hyperactivity disorder (ADHD), post-traumatic stress disorder, abnormal behaviors (eg, self-stimulating behaviors, hoarding food, sleep disturbances), and oppositional defiant disorder. As mentioned previously, communication with the child may be difficult because of language barriers, causing another obstacle to assessing the mental health of the child.

Sensory integration difficulties are increasingly recognized in adoptees. The children may have adverse responses to touch (eg, new clothing, hugs and kisses, bathing) or textures (eg, new foods). Individual or all of the senses (hearing, vision, taste, or smell) may be notably increased or decreased, and some children have decreased sensation to physical pain, leading to an increased risk for injuries. Dyskinesia (clumsiness or injury prone) has also been observed.

The most common identified medical issues are **infectious diseases.** These include acute illnesses (eg, upper respiratory infection, bronchitis, otitis, infectious diarrhea) as well as chronic infections, such as TB and parasite infestations (scabies and *Giardia* are common). Because of their biological mother's lifestyle and their time residing in institutions, many adoptees are at increased risk of exposure to infectious diseases such as syphilis, HIV, and hepatitis B and C.

Preventive care considered routine in the United States is unlikely to have been part of the child's care and needs to be performed as appropriate for age. This includes newborn screening laboratory studies and assessments of hearing, vision, dental, and mental health. **Anticipatory guidance** for new parents should be incorporated into pre-adoption encounters as well as all subsequent visits.

Evaluation

The initial office visit with the physician should be scheduled for an extended period because of the complexity of the evaluation and additional time needed for parental education. If the physician's schedule does not permit extended visits, ancillary staff (eg, nurses, dietitians, therapists) may perform parts of the evaluation and education.

Observation of the child's behavior, development, and interactions with the adoptive parents and physician is a critical element of the evaluation. Most physicians include such observations in their visits routinely, but particular attention is necessary for new adoptees. Things to notice include the child's demeanor and behavior: Are they easily engaged or withdrawn? Do they make eye contact with the parent or physician? Do they make any vocalizations or words, depending on the child's age? Do they play with toys? Are they too friendly or afraid of strangers? Do they seek comfort from the new parents?

History

Limited medical information is available from most birth countries, though there are some exceptions (eg, from foster care in South Korea). Family and birth history are rarely obtainable for adoptees. Immunization histories are becoming increasingly available. Previously, vaccine records were considered unreliable; however, in recent years, data have emerged to suggest that well-documented immunizations may be considered valid. Written records showing the age of the child when vaccinated, date of administration, dose given, and proper intervals between dosing that are consistent with WHO schedules or are comparable to US schedules may be considered acceptable for proof of immunization. (See Management for guidelines when vaccine records are not available.)

Dietary history is important for assessing the child's nutritional status. Questions to ask include: What food and formula/milk is the child receiving? Has he or she received adequate calories? Is there known or suspected food intolerance (eg, lactose intolerance is more common in Asian ethnicities)? Are there abnormal behaviors associated with food or eating (eg, preoccupation with food, hoarding, food refusal, gorging)?

An interim medical history may be available because many children are selected by their adoptive parents several months before immigrating to the United States. The interim medical history may be provided from the orphanage or foster care provider through the adoption agency. Parents should be encouraged to solicit as much information as possible from the child's caregivers. At a minimum,

this history should include serial growth parameters, known illnesses, hospitalizations, surgeries, allergies, and immunizations given while the child was under their care. Parents should also ask caregivers about any food preferences, special fears, toys, or friends from the current placement. If the child has a special "lovey," the parents should request to bring it with the child as a transitional object.

Physical Examination

A complete unclothed physical examination should be performed on infants and children of all ages. However, because of previous trauma, such as sexual abuse, some parts of the examination may have to be done over a series of visits to minimize the possibility of additional trauma from an examination. All aspects of the physical examination are absolutely essential. Accurate measurements of height, weight, and, depending on age and size, head circumference should be obtained. Plotting of parameters on the growth curves from WHO or the CDC (compared with birth country) should be used, with few exceptions. The child should be closely inspected for unusual scars or bruises, evidence of fractures (old or recent), rachitic changes, and genital or rectal scars. The skin should be examined for rashes, lesions, and a bacille Calmette-Guérin (BCG) scar (typically on the upper deltoid). A developmental screen should be performed, and a more complete developmental assessment should be scheduled at a separate visit (when the child is not distressed or acutely ill). A dental examination should be included and referral for a formal dental evaluation will likely be necessary. Screening evaluations of hearing and vision should be performed and formal testing may be needed, depending on the age of the child and ability to cooperate.

Laboratory Testing

Laboratory testing should include complete blood cell count, lead levels, and thyroid function testing (iodine is not in many diets in Asia) (Box 36-1). Additionally, testing for illnesses associated with specific countries of origin, findings on examination (eg, comprehensive metabolic panel for malnourished child), and as directed by the child's age (eg, newborn screening for metabolic disorders in newborns and infants) should be performed. Screening tests, if initially negative, should be repeated in 3 to 6 months, especially for children with concerns about underlying malnutrition or who are immunocompromised.

Because of the **increased risks of exposures,** laboratory screening for infectious diseases should be undertaken. Serum samples should be tested for syphilis (nontreponemal and treponemal antibodies), hepatitis B panel (HBsAg, HBsAg antibody [HBsAb], and hepatitis B core antibody), hepatitis C antibody, and HIV 1 and 2 antibodies. Human immunodeficiency virus polymerase chain reaction may be indicated in some children (eg, those who may not make specific antibodies due to malnutrition or being immunocompromised). Stool samples should be sent for ova and parasite examination and *Giardia* and *Cryptosporidium* antigen testing (see Box 36-1). Stool for bacterial pathogens (eg, *Salmonella, Shigella*) should be sent from children from some regions, such as the Indian subcontinent. Because

Box 36-1. Recommended Laboratory Testing for International Adoptees
Hepatitis A IgM
Hepatitis B virus serologic testing • Hepatitis B surface antigen • Antibody to hepatitis B surface antigen • Antibody to hepatitis B core antigen
Hepatitis C virus serologic testing
Syphilis serologic testing • Nontreponemal test (RPR, VDRL, or ART) • Treponemal test (MHA-TP or FTA-ABS)
HIV 1 and 2 serologic testing
Complete blood cell count with differential and red blood cell indices
Stool examination for ova and parasites (3 specimens)
Stool examination for *Giardia intestinalis* and *Cryptosporidium* antigen (1–3 specimens)
Additional parasite testing[a]: 1. *Trypanosoma cruzi* serology if child is from endemic area 2. If child has eosinophilia (eosinophil count >450 cells/mm^3 with negative ova and parasite stool testing): *Strongyloides* serology and *Schistosoma* serology if from endemic area
Tuberculin skin test[b]
Consider antibody testing to select vaccine antigens (if written records are unreliable).[c]
Additional testing: thyroid function tests, lead level, and others as directed by history and physical examination (see text).

Abbreviations: ART, automated reagin test; FTA-ABS, fluorescent treponemal antibody absorption; IgM, immunoglobulin M; MHA-TP, microhemagglutination test for *Treponema pallidum;* RPR, rapid plasma reagin; VDRL, Venereal Disease Research Laboratories.

[a] In conjunction with international adoption or infectious diseases specialist.

[b] Repeat at 6 months after initial testing.

[c] For children older than 6 months, may check diphtheria, tetanus, and polio; for children older than 12 months, may check measles antibodies.

Adapted from the American Academy of Pediatrics and the Centers for Disease Control and Prevention.

cytomegalovirus infection is ubiquitous, routine testing is not recommended. Testing for acute infection with hepatitis A virus (HAV) by measuring immunoglobulin M anti-HAV antibodies should be performed for adoptees from HAV-endemic areas, as infants and young children may be asymptomatic but contagious. Administering HAV vaccine, as recommended in the United States, is not problematic for children who may have had previous HAV infection.

Tuberculin skin testing (ie, purified protein derivative) should be performed on all children; history of receipt of BCG is not a contraindication to skin testing. Bacille Calmette-Guérin vaccinations are usually given at birth in most developing nations, and its influence on skin test status is controversial. Generally, BCG given within the previous 1 to 2 years may contribute to a positive PPD skin test; however, a positive PPD test is more likely reflective of true infection with *Mycobacterium* with or without active disease and merits further evaluation. For children 5 years and older, interferon gamma release assays (eg, QuantiFERON-TB Gold) are an acceptable screening alternative to PPD testing. Latent TB infection has been reported from 0.6% to 30% of international adoptees, which is not surprising because most adoptees come from TB-endemic areas.

Management

Counseling for the Transition

Education and **preparation** for the parents and all family members is a priority. Generally, countries of origin for adoptees are in the developing world, and parents should prepare for healthy travel for themselves by receiving immunizations and following travel guidelines from the CDC and the US Department of State.

Parents should provide consistent structure and boundaries in a loving milieu for adoptees. A scheduled regimen may be especially important to previously institutionalized children because it has been their way of life, but even noninstitutionalized children benefit from a predictable routine. Parents should maximize their one-on-one interactions with the adoptee while still allowing time for themselves and other family members (not an easy task with multiple children). Physical contact and affection may initially need to be tempered as directed by the child's tolerance. Parents should try to enhance bonding and attachment by frequently identifying themselves as "Mom" or "Dad." Other strategies to enhance attachment include initially limiting contact with individuals outside of the family and not "handing" the child to others, including non-household family members, because they are strangers to the child. Frequent verbal reassurances and talking to the child about the people and the new world around the child should be encouraged. In caring for the child, parents should be encouraged to meet the child at his or her developmental level and not chronologic age.

Growth and Nutrition

When children are identified as malnourished or FTT, a multidisciplinary treatment plan is recommended, including parents, physician, nutritionist, and therapists (eg, occupational therapist for feeding difficulties). The child should be offered familiar foods, if that is his or her preference, and each meal may include a new, more nutritional offering. Children should be offered frequent meals and snacks because they may not be able to eat much at one sitting. Foods should be calorie dense (eg, added butter, cheese, avocado, peanut butter, depending on age and previous dietary history). Dietary supplements, such as PediaSure, may be indicated.

Precocious puberty has been observed in female international adoptees, more than males, and is thought to be related to the rapid improvement of nutrition. If signs of precocious puberty are observed, evaluation by a pediatric endocrinologist is recommended.

Development

Because developmental delays are so common, most adoptees should have a developmental assessment. Language delays, especially expressive, are frequent and, when identified, formal audiology testing should be part of the assessment. However, performing developmental assessments of language pose difficulties, as most are conducted in English, which is rarely the child's primary language. Repeating the testing after a period of adjustment may be helpful. Language barriers do not preclude audiology testing.

Mental Health

Mental and emotional health problems are common and may manifest early or late or occur as relapses. Initial problems seen may include sleep disorders, fears and phobias, bizarre behaviors, and self-stimulating behaviors. Unless the behaviors pose a safety risk, the parents should tolerate them because most dissipate with time in a secure environment. At times of emotional distress, parents may observe a relapse of behavior problems. The physician may provide guidance for parents for milder disorders; however, moderate and severe disorders merit prompt referral to a mental health professional, ideally someone with expertise in adoption.

Immunizations

If vaccinations are considered valid, as described previously, resuming immunizations per the US schedule (see Chapter 34) is appropriate. If immunization status is unknown or incomplete, repeating immunizations or checking antibody concentrations to vaccine antigens is an acceptable option. Most areas of the world routinely administer BCG, polio (oral), and vaccines containing diphtheria and tetanus toxoids with pertussis (often whole-cell) components. Receipt of additional diphtheria, tetanus, and possible pertussis antigens may be associated with an increase in adverse events; measuring antibodies to diphtheria and tetanus is warranted to minimize adverse events. There are no US Food and Drug Administration–approved antibody tests available commercially for pertussis antibodies. Receipt of additional doses of inactivated polio vaccine is not usually associated with adverse events. Testing for HBsAb should be performed on all adoptees, and the results will guide the plan for further immunizations. Hepatitis B vaccine will only elicit HBsAb; the presence of antibodies to other hepatitis B antigens suggests natural infection. For measles, mumps, and rubella (MMR), various formulations and combinations (1- and 2-component more commonly than 3-component) vaccines are available worldwide. Checking antibodies to these antigens is possible, but likely administering a US-licensed combination (eg, MMR) may be necessary to ensure protection against all 3 antigens. Most of the other vaccines available in the United States are not available in the developing world (eg, Hib and pneumococcal conjugates, varicella, HAV), and the child should receive these vaccines as recommended for age per the US schedule.

Infectious Diseases

Any acute identified infectious disease (eg, scabies, otitis) should be treated following standard practice, keeping in mind the possibility that different antibiotic resistance patterns exist in other parts of the world. Thus, if the child does not have the predicted response to treatment, consultation with a pediatric infectious diseases specialist should be considered. For other infectious disease screening noted previously, additional evaluation and possible treatment should be initiated promptly (eg, penicillin therapy for syphilis) and pediatric infectious diseases consultation may be considered.

For TB evaluation, any positive PPD skin testing results merits further investigation for true infection with *Mycobacterium tuberculosis*. A compounding problem is that some children may be anergic due to malnutrition, giving a false-negative PPD test result. If malnutrition is suspected, consider a chest radiograph even if the PPD is negative, and consider repeating the PPD when the child's nutritional status has improved. In addition, routinely repeating the PPD 6 months after the child's arrival is advisable if the child is from an endemic area because late exposure to an infected individual is possible.

Prognosis

Being prepared for the complex needs related to international adoption has been identified as the best determinant for parents to consider the adoption experience as positive, regardless of the number or severity of the medical needs of the adoptee.

With improved nutrition and environment, most children have significant catch-up growth; however, up to one-third of adoptees may have unrecoverable loss in linear growth. For intellectual development, by 1 year of age nearly all children in orphanages have one or more areas of delay. However, their prognosis is generally good, with an increase in 2 developmental quotient points per month after arrival in the United States. After 3 years of age in an orphanage, the length of time institutionalized and delays noted at age 11 months correlate negatively with IQ (8 months in orphanage, average IQ = 90; 2 or more years in orphanage, average IQ = 69).

Many children have ongoing mental and psychosocial problems, and some disorders do not manifest until children are older (eg, ADHD or learning disorders when the child is school-aged). Ongoing attachment disorders seem to occur with greater frequency in children with lower IQs and more behavior problems and in adoptive families with a lower socioeconomic status.

Assessment of the overall outcome for children who spent 8 or more months in institutional care in Eastern Europe, when evaluated at least 3 years after adoption, showed about one-third had multiple serious problems (including IQ ≤85, insecure attachment, and severe behavior problems), about one-third had a few serious problems but were thought to be making progress, and about one-third had progressed very well. The best predictors of major problems were greater length of time in the orphanage, increased number of children adopted at the same time, younger adoptive mother, lower socioeconomic status of mother, and father alone selected the child. Although the effect of these risk factors may not be identical for all birth countries, they do provide some insight. Reviewing these risk factors with adoptive parents during the pre-adoption period may aid in their decision-making.

Pediatrician's Role

The pediatrician's role is not to tell the adoptive parent whom to adopt; parents are essentially choosing life partners, which is an individual decision. Pediatricians, however, can assist parents in reviewing available medical information, which may aid them in making an informed decision about proceeding with an adoption.

During the adoption process, the physician must assume an active role as a child advocate as well as parental advocate and educator. This may be the first parenting experience for the adoptive parents and, thus, they need the basics for child care, no matter what the age of the adoptee. This might include feeding and routine care (eg, estimate the number of diapers needed if traveling to an area with no access to supplies), as well as discipline techniques for a traumatized child. Preparation for caring for illnesses is needed because many adoptees are ill at the time of the adoption and travel. The pediatrician can facilitate emotional preparation because the parents may be isolated from their usual support systems while embarking on the new role of parent.

After the family returns home, the pediatrician has a role as primary care provider as well as serving as a referral source for other needed specialists (eg, subspecialists, mental health practitioners, post-adoption support services, developmental interventions, nutritionists).

Counseling Adoptive Parents About Expectations

Parents should be informed that it is unlikely that an institutionalized child will emerge unscathed. With this in mind, parents may make preliminary preparations for treatments and rehabilitation for the child. Families should be counseled that it is OK to say "no" to a potential adoptee. No one has benefited from adoption of children by families who do not have the resources needed to care for them. Most importantly, parents should be reassured that optimism is appropriate. Being prepared matters!

CASE RESOLUTION

In talking with the parents, they report that they have not observed any injuries and no areas seem tender when they examine Jaxon, as you have suggested. They elect to give him some diphenhydramine and take the flight home with the plan to come see you on arrival. Although they are exhausted, they come directly to your office for an acute visit. They report that he remained inconsolable and that the flight home was miserable for him (and everyone around them). On entering the examination room, Jaxon was screaming and noticeably uncomfortable but trying to find comfort in his dad's arms.

His temperature was 38.9°C (102°F) axillary; pulse rate, 144 beats per minute; and respiratory rate, 30 breaths per minute. His examination was notable for extensive oral and pharyngeal vesicular lesions with erythema, but there were no labial lesions. He had multiple shotty cervical nodes, and the rest of the examination was noncontributory. A diagnosis of herpangina was made. He was given a dose of ibuprofen, and 15 minutes later he was quiet, able to swallow electrolyte solution, and cuddling in his dad's arms. His parents were given reassurance that this was an acute infection and not an indication of poor bonding; in fact, he was already seeking comfort from them. Additional testing for infections included obtaining antibodies to HIV, rapid plasma reagin for syphilis, and hepatitis C and hepatitis B panel, especially with his biological mother's history of being a commercial sex worker. Other testing included complete blood cell count, lead level, and thyroid function tests. He was given an appointment in 2 weeks to complete the assessment, including a developmental assessment; this was deferred because he was acutely ill.

Selected References

Albers L, Barnett E, Jenista J, Johnson D. International adoption: medical and developmental issues. *Pediatr Clin North Am.* 2005;52:xiii–xv

American Academy of Pediatrics. Medical evaluation of internationally adopted children for infectious diseases. In: Pickering LK, Baker CJ, Kimberlin DW, Long SS, eds. *Red Book: 2012 Report of the Committee on Infectious Diseases.* 27th ed. Elk Grove Village, IL: American Academy of Pediatrics; 2012:191–199

Barnett ED. Immunizations and infectious disease screening for internationally adopted children. *Pediatr Clin North Am.* 2005;52(5):1287–1309

Cederblad M, Höök B, Irhammar M, Mercke AM. Mental health in international adoptees as teenagers and young adults. An epidemiological study. *J Child Psychol Psychiatry.* 1999;40(8):1239–1248

Howard CR, John CC. International travel with infants and children: international adoption. *CDC Health Information for International Travel 2014: The Yellow Book.* New York, NY: Oxford University Press; 2014. http://wwwnc.cdc.gov/travel/yellowbook/2014/chapter-7-international-travel-infants-children/international-adoption. Accessed March 4, 2014

Jones VF; American Academy of Pediatrics Committee on Early Childhood, Adoption and Dependent Care. Comprehensive health evaluation of the newly adopted child. *Pediatrics.* 2012;129(1):e214–e223

Petersen K. Preparing to meet foreign bugs. Travel, immigration, and international adoptions require special precautions. *Postgrad Med.* 2001;110(1):67–70, 73–74, 77

Saiman L, Aronson J, Zhou J, et al. Prevalence of infectious diseases among internationally adopted children. *Pediatrics.* 2001;108(3):608–612

Sloutsky V. Institutional care and developmental outcomes of 6- and 7-year-old children: a contextualist perspective. *Int J Behav Dev.* 1997;20:131–151

US Department of State Bureau of Consular Affairs. Intercountry adoption. Statistics. http://adoption.state.gov/about_us/statistics.php. Accessed March 4, 2014

Weitzman C, Albers L. Long-term developmental, behavioral, and attachment outcomes after international adoption. *Pediatr Clin North Am.* 2005;52(5):1395–1419

CHAPTER 37

Health Care Needs of Children in Foster Care

Kelly Callahan, MD, MPT; ChrisAnna M. Mink, MD; and Sara T. Stewart, MD

CASE STUDY

A 13-year-old girl is brought to your office by her foster parent for a general physical examination. The foster parent states that the girl has been living in her home for the past 2 weeks. When she was initially brought by the social worker, she was wearing dirty clothes and smelled of cigarette smoke. There are no medical records and no immunization records available for your review, and the teen is not sure the last time she saw a doctor. The girl states that she often missed school to help take care of her sick grandmother. She gets very quiet when you ask about her family. She states she misses her younger sisters but does not mention anything about her mother. When asked about her mother, she states that she doesn't care to see her because her mother "cares more about her boyfriend than she does me and my sisters." The only history known by the foster parent is that the child was failing school because of frequent absences and that there were extensive amounts of pornography and drug paraphernalia found in the home at the time of removal. The social worker also told the foster mother that there was an expired albuterol inhaler found in the home with the girl's

name on It. The foster parent states that the teen seems "sad" all the time, and 2 nights ago when asked about school, she began to cry and ran to her room.

On physical examination, the patient is sad appearing and quiet but cooperative. Her weight is in the 25th percentile and her height is in the 50th percentile for her age. She has poor dentition with multiple dental caries. She has a few basilar wheezes on lung examination and has scattered bruises on her anterior shins, but no other abnormalities were noted.

Questions

1. What are the medical, psychologic, and behavioral issues that commonly affect children in the foster care system?
2. What is the role of the primary care pediatrician in providing a medical home for the child in foster care?
3. How does a child's legal status as a child in foster care affect how medical care can be delivered?
4. What are the appropriate health care referrals and community resources to access for a patient who is in foster care?

The term **foster care** refers to the **temporary placement** of a child in the home of another caregiver or **foster parent** due to a threat to the child's safety or well-being in the original home environment. Placement of a child in foster care results from an investigation of the child's home environment by **child protective services (CPS)** and may be arranged via voluntary agreement of the parent or through court sanction. The foster parent may be related to the child or may be a nonrelative. For those children in voluntary placement, the biological parent retains the right to terminate the placement at any time. For those placed by **legal sanction,** a series of court hearings give parents, the child, and the CPS agency the opportunity to present their perspectives on the circumstances surrounding the allegations and their respective views on interventions to ensure the child has access to the best home environment.

Children in foster care may present to the primary care pediatrician soon after placement in foster care or after having been with a foster parent for a long time. In either scenario, it is recognized that as a subpopulation of pediatric patients, children in foster care have

a significant number of **unmet medical and mental health needs** and should be considered to be part of the **special needs** patient population. At the time of initial removal, the CPS worker may not be able to obtain a medical history or essential information about current medications for the child. Changes in foster care placement may interrupt continuity of care with a health care practitioner, and frequent changes in assigned social services caseworkers can create barriers to consistent communication among biological parents, foster parents, health care professionals, and caseworkers. These children have rates of medical and mental health disorders that are higher than those of children from equivalent socioeconomic backgrounds who are not in foster care. There has traditionally been a lack of appreciation within the general medical community of the complexity of the needs of this patient population, and because of low payment rates, there has been difficulty allotting sufficient time in a "routine" office visit to complete the comprehensive evaluation needed by these children. For those children with identified mental health needs, there is often a paucity of available psychiatric and psychologic resources; this is particularly true for children younger than 5 years.

These unmet needs have long-lasting effects on the well-being of children, even after exiting the foster care system, including into adulthood. Because of their complex health care issues and vulnerability to fragmented care, these children merit a medical home, providing comprehensive, multidisciplinary services and medical case management.

Epidemiology

At any point during a given year, 400,000 children nationwide will spend time in foster care. Approximately 300,000 children enter the system annually, and reasons for placement, in descending order of prevalence, include neglect, physical abuse, psychologic or emotional abuse, and sexual abuse. As a population, children in the foster care system come from home environments that experience high rates of poverty, parental mental illness, parental substance abuse, unemployment, adolescent parenthood, and frequent involvement with the criminal justice system, and low levels of education. These children have high rates of exposure to domestic violence, and many are victims of physical abuse, sexual abuse, and neglect. Their biological parents often have limited parenting skills; the children experience inconsistent parenting behaviors along with minimal developmental stimulation and emotional support. All of these factors combine to cause unpredictable, stressful, and unsafe home environments for these children, prompting their removal and placement into foster care. Children in foster care account for 25% to 41% of expenditures within Medicaid despite representing fewer than 3% of all enrollees.

Foster children are of all ethnicities, but there is disproportionate representation of children of color within the foster care population. Children younger than 5 years comprise nearly half of the children in foster care, with 11- to 15-year-olds a distant second. Over the past several decades, an increasing percentage of new entrants into foster care are infants younger than 1 year. Many of these infants are exposed to substances prenatally and are placed in foster care due to a combination of factors related to maternal drug use.

Approximately 70% of children leave foster care within 2 years of placement, with the average stay being 13 months. More than half of these children are reunited with their biological parent or primary caregiver. Seven percent remain in foster care for more than 5 years, and approximately 35% of all children leaving foster care reenter the system at some time because of a new report. Since the 1990s, the number of adoptions from foster care has increased to 20% of those leaving the child welfare system. An additional 11% of those leaving foster care are emancipating out of the system by reaching 18 years of age without attaining permanent placement. Many of these teenagers later report being incarcerated or homeless at some point after emancipation. Twenty-five percent of the children in foster care will experience 3 or more placements, which leads to further fragmentation of their health care and education. Multiple foster care placements are more common for those children with behavioral, emotional, or coping problems.

Clinical Presentation

Medical Issues

Children in the foster care system have been shown to have high rates of **acute and chronic illness** at the time of their initial medical evaluations after placement (D_x Box). In one study in Utah, more than half of children entering the foster care system had at least one medical problem. Common maladies include obesity, asthma, vision or hearing problems, neurologic disorders, gastrointestinal diseases, dental caries, and other inadequately treated chronic illnesses such as eczema and anemia. Acute infections are also common, including respiratory tract infections, skin infections, otitis media, sexually transmitted infections (STIs), and intestinal infestations with parasites. Low immunization rates are a frequent occurrence.

Many children entering foster care have growth delay with weight, height, or head circumference measurement less than the 5th percentile for their age. This may be caused by a combination of factors, including inadequate nutrition, environmental deprivation, prenatal alcohol exposure, genetic predisposition, or underlying illness such as HIV infection. Environments that are chronically stressful or lack the necessary stimulation and support for a child may also lead to behaviors such as rumination and social withdrawal. (For further discussion of failure to thrive, see Chapter 133.) Overweight (body mass index [BMI] 85%–95% for age) and obesity (BMI >95% for age) are also frequently seen among foster care children. Depression, dysfunctional coping skills, and a lack of family connectedness are thought to contribute to this chronic disease state.

Dx Common Issues of Children in Foster Care

- Acute infection
- Undiagnosed or inadequately treated chronic illnesses
- Dental caries
- Growth delay and failure to thrive
- Incomplete immunization histories
- Prenatal or perinatal exposure to sexually transmitted infections
- Effects of prenatal substance exposure
- Physical sequelae of physical and sexual abuse
- Developmental delay
- Attention-deficit/hyperactivity disorder
- Post-traumatic stress disorder
- Anxiety
- Depression
- Conduct and oppositional defiant disorders
- Attachment disorders
- Educational disabilities

Many children placed in foster care have a history of **prenatal exposure** to illicit drugs, alcohol, and tobacco. These children have high rates of premature birth and prenatal or perinatal exposure to infections such as **hepatitis C, hepatitis B, HIV, syphilis,** and **herpes simplex.** This risk of exposure to infectious agents is related to maternal drug use and its frequent association with prostitution, needle sharing, and drug use in sexual partners.

Children who have been placed in foster care may present with physical sequelae of prior physical or sexual abuse. Physical abuse may result in skin trauma, skeletal fractures, head trauma, abdominal trauma, and chest trauma. Sexual abuse may result in genital trauma or symptoms of STIs.

Developmental and Mental Health Issues

A high prevalence of developmental delay, behavioral disorders, and educational difficulties has been noted in foster children of all age groups. These disorders are more common in children with a history of neglect or abandonment than in those who have suffered other forms of child maltreatment. Of children younger than 6 years entering foster care, 38% to 65% have significant developmental delays. Speech and language difficulties, delayed fine motor skills, and poor social-adaptive skills are common, and up to one-fifth of school-aged children entering foster care had been receiving special education services prior to the time of placement.

Approximately 30% of children in foster care have behavioral difficulties, with 17% taking at least one psychotropic or antipsychotic medication, significantly higher than the national average of 5%. A disproportionate number, 29%, of children taking any psychotropic or antipsychotic drug were children placed in foster care, group homes, or residential treatment centers.

Common mental health issues in the foster care population include attention-deficit/hyperactivity disorder, depression, anxiety, and suicidal ideation. **Post-traumatic stress disorder** is common and more prevalent in those who have experienced or witnessed family violence. Adolescents in foster care may act out as a manifestation of mental health difficulties, resulting in sexual promiscuity, substance abuse, and truancy, as well as rates of conduct and oppositional defiant disorders that are higher than those in the general adolescent population.

Attachment disorders are seen more frequently in the foster care population and account for a portion of the behavioral difficulties in these children. A secure attachment to a primary caregiver is necessary to the development of emotional security and the sense that one's needs are important. Children who are removed from violent homes or who may have suffered abuse or neglect are likely to have never developed a secure attachment to a primary caregiver in that home environment and therefore may have difficulty bonding with a foster parent. This problem is then compounded if the child is moved among multiple foster homes, prohibiting development of a healthy attachment to a caregiver. In addition to their lack of emotional reciprocity, these children may exhibit self-stimulatory behaviors or sleep disturbances.

The behavioral difficulties that children in the foster care system manifest are often the result of multiple factors. These children may be predisposed to behavioral disorders by a history of prenatal drug or alcohol exposure or a history of abuse or neglect. It can also be difficult to determine whether a child's behaviors predate placement in foster care or whether they are a response to the removal from his or her home. As a result of placement in foster care, children often experience fear, sadness, and a feeling of guilt or responsibility for the family discord that resulted in their removal. Foster placements are invariably sudden and unexpected, involve the loss of a familiar caregiver, and are traumatic for children of all ages.

Evaluation

It is important for pediatricians to be familiar with the **medical consent legalities** concerning foster children in their geographic locales. While specifics vary by locality, generally foster parents have the authority to provide consent for routine medical care. The placement of a child in foster care does not supersede the right of a biological parent to participate in the medical decision-making for his or her child, and many do retain the authority to consent for medical tests and procedures. Any medical procedure or test that requires specific written consent is likely to require **authorization** by the **legally recognized parent** (eg, child welfare agency, courts, biological parent). Two common clinical scenarios that frequently require consent beyond the foster parent's authority are HIV testing and the administration of psychotropic medications.

History

Children in foster care may be brought for medical evaluation by an authorized caregiver, who may be a foster parent, a relative of the foster parent, or the social service caseworker. Often the biological parent is absent from the visit and the child's medical records are not available at the time of the evaluation. Obtaining past medical records can be difficult, but the caseworker can be of assistance in this process. It is important to ascertain the circumstances that prompted a child's placement in foster care, as this may modify portions of the evaluation.

Biological family history is useful to evaluate for the presence of genetic disorders and communicable diseases. A maternal history of drug use or STIs will assist in identifying those children who may have had prenatal exposure to infectious agents.

Birth history should include any history of prenatal care and complications such as prematurity or drug withdrawal. Results of routine newborn screening (eg, hearing, inborn errors of metabolism, thyroid function, hemoglobinopathies) should also be obtained.

A complete medical and surgical history should be gathered, including the identification of a regular health care practitioner if the child has one. Older children and adolescents may be able to provide some of their own histories. Known medications and allergies should be documented, and all available immunization records should be obtained. Documentation of a child's immunization history is frequently unavailable, so all possible sources of records, such as biological parents or school districts, should be identified.

Feeding history and nutritional assessments should include the type and amount of formula or human milk for infants and types and quantities of foods for older children.

The psychosocial history includes a child's current and prior foster placements or living arrangements and whether there was exposure to domestic violence, physical abuse, or sexual abuse (Questions Box). Verbal children may also be able to discuss their feelings about their current foster placement. Adolescents should have a confidential screening (eg, HEADDSSS [*h*ome, *e*ducation and employment, *a*ctivities, *d*rugs, *d*epression, *s*afety, *s*exuality, and *s*uicide]) (see Chapter 6) to address drug, alcohol, and tobacco use; issues related to the home and school; sexual activity; violence; and gang involvement.

The **developmental history** should include the results of prior developmental assessments as well as a listing of therapeutic or early intervention services received. The behavioral history should also include results of prior assessments, mental health services used, and any psychotropic medications prescribed. The foster parent, biological parent, or CPS caseworker may be able to provide useful observations of the child's developmental capabilities, behavioral patterns, and social interactions. The biological parent or CPS caseworker may also be able to assist in collecting records from prior assessments.

Educational history is often not available at the time of the medical evaluation. It is helpful, however, to know a child's history of prior evaluations by the school system, special education services provided, or prior therapeutic services (eg, physical, occupational, or speech therapy) received through the school district.

Physical Examination

A complete, unclothed physical examination should be performed on each child. For children who are traumatized or particularly frightened, disrobing only the immediate area being examined may help ease their discomfort. Growth parameters, including height, weight, and occipitofrontal head circumference (for children younger than 2 years) or BMI (for children 2 years and older), should be plotted on a reference chart, and a close inspection should be performed for signs of prior trauma. The child should be assessed for **dysmorphic features** consistent with prenatal alcohol exposure or other genetic syndromes. The physical examination should include a **genital examination** to assess for signs of trauma in children of all ages, and sexually active females should have a pelvic examination if there are any reports of abdominal pain, vaginal discharge, or other concerns. (See chapters 131–133 for further descriptions of physical findings.)

Immunizations

Immunizations should be given as appropriate for age, and if immunization records cannot be located in a timely fashion, the child should be considered unimmunized. In this situation, options include restarting the vaccination series or checking antibody titers for selected vaccine antigens (see Chapter 34 for further information). Other possible sources for vaccine records include state or county registry, the child's previous health care practitioner, or the school previously attended by the child. If available, the biological parent should be asked to assist with providing any vaccine record, as well as other medical records.

In addition, all children should also receive appropriate screening for tuberculosis, such as purified protein derivative skin testing or interferon-gamma release assays.

Additional Assessments

All children should undergo mental health and developmental screenings and should be referred for comprehensive testing if abnormalities are noted. Dental screening should be incorporated in the physical examination of all children older than 6 months. Vision and hearing screenings should also be performed on all children old enough to cooperate. A referral for expert vision or hearing evaluation should be made if it is indicated by history or physical examination or the patient is unable to perform the screening procedure (eg, infant, child who is developmentally delayed).

Laboratory Tests

Routine screening laboratory tests should be performed on foster children just as they are indicated for the general pediatric population. For example, hemoglobin level should be checked annually in all infants, toddlers, and preschool-aged children. Serum lead levels should be checked according to local guidelines but should be checked at least once for a child during the toddler years. A urinalysis should also be recorded at least once in all children at the time of entry into kindergarten and once during adolescence.

For infants younger than 12 months, especially those with a history of prenatal drug exposure or other known risks for maternal STI, a rapid plasma reagin, a hepatitis C antibody, a hepatitis B surface antigen and surface antibody, and an HIV test should be performed.

Adolescents who are considered to have at-risk behaviors, patients with signs or symptoms consistent with an STI, and children with a history of sexual abuse that could result in the transmission of infection should be tested for STIs. Often adolescents are able

Questions

Psychosocial Concerns

- When was the child placed in foster care?
- Why was the child placed in foster care?
- Has the child had prior foster placements? If so, when? Why did placement change?
- Was there prior exposure to domestic violence? To physical or sexual abuse?
- Does the child have siblings in foster care?
- How does the child feel about the current foster placement?
- How has the child integrated into the foster family?
- Has the child previously received mental health services or therapeutic services for developmental delay or educational difficulties?
- What is the child's social service plan (eg, parental visits, reunification, termination of parental rights)?

to sign their own consent forms for evaluations and treatment related to STIs; however, local statutes should be consulted.

Imaging Studies

If a child has a history or physical findings concerning for physical abuse, imaging such as a radiographic skeletal survey, computed tomography, and magnetic resonance imaging of the head or radionuclide bone scan may be indicated. (For more specific recommendations, see Chapter 15.)

Management

Given the breadth of health-related needs for this patient population and the frequency with which they change foster homes, **close case management** is an essential component of health care delivery to this population. There should be consistent communication with the child's caseworker to ensure that medical and mental health recommendations are incorporated into the child's social service plan. Ideally, a child should have a medical home and continuity with a primary care pediatrician over time, but changes in home placements often make this difficult. If continuity of care is broken, incorporation of the health care plan into a child's broader social service plan should ensure that medical history and medical and mental health recommendations are not lost. The use of **electronic health records** is a growing practice in many foster care systems and promotes continuity of care, even with logistical challenges.

Children and adolescents in foster care require frequent health visits. The American Academy of Pediatrics recommends a health screening within 72 hours of placement, a comprehensive medical evaluation within 30 days of placement, and a follow-up medical examination within 60 to 90 days after placement. Because of the prevalence of significant medical, social, and mental health issues affecting children in foster care, additional visits are often advisable. Anticipatory guidance should be provided to the caregiver, and age-appropriate issues should be discussed with older children and adolescents.

Children in foster care often need referral to medical subspecialists, dentists, dietitians, speech therapists, occupational therapists, mental health practitioners, and other service providers. Case management is necessary to track these referrals and to contact the foster family or caseworker if an appointment is missed.

Prognosis

Children in foster care have a spectrum of mental health and medical needs, spanning from newborns to adolescents emancipating from the child welfare system. Preliminary studies have documented improved physical health status, school performance, and adaptive functioning of young children after placement in foster care; however, these studies require replication. The strength of the bond between the foster parent and the child, as well as the consistency and predictability of the foster home environment, are significant to the development of the child's sense of safety and well-being.

To date, much of the research on the health status of children in foster care has focused on the delineation and description of the health-related issues that these children face. There has been more limited evaluation of the different models of health service delivery to the foster care population as well as of the subsequent medical, developmental, and emotional outcomes for the children in these different models.

While there is a need for continued study of health care delivery to the foster care population, it is widely accepted that children in the foster care system benefit from the establishment of medical homes with case management capabilities and physicians who are well-versed in the complex medical and mental health issues that affect this vulnerable population.

CASE RESOLUTION

This case illustrates many of the common issues that affect children when they are placed in foster care. Medical and immunization records are frequently unavailable to the medical examiner, and chronic medical needs have often gone unmet. This child's poor hygiene and frequent school absences point to a history of parental neglect, and given the presence of drug paraphernalia, her mother was likely involved with substance abuse. This child should have a thorough assessment for behavioral problems, developmental delays, and education-related disabilities. The child is able to state that she does not want to return to her parents' care, but she still misses her family members. This may be remedied through her child welfare plan, for example, by arranging for her to remain in contact with her siblings throughout their foster placement. Given her experiences in her prior home environment, she has depressive symptoms and is likely to have other unmet mental health needs, which require referral to a mental health provider. She will also require evaluation by her new school system to determine her specific educational needs and appropriate grade placement.

She has poor dentition, which is a common finding in the foster care population, so she will require a referral for dental care. The presence of mild wheezing in a child who otherwise states that she feels fine is a likely marker for untreated reactive airway disease and may be a reflection of poor continuity of medical care for the girl prior to her placement. Routine adolescent care should be initiated at this visit, including a thorough history of drug and alcohol use as well as reproductive history. Her vaccines should be updated. Anticipatory guidance on menstruation, sexuality, and drug use should be considered. She was scheduled for a revisit in 2 months for the second human papillomavirus vaccine and to talk about any concerns she may have.

Selected References

American Academy of Pediatrics. *Fostering Health: Health Care for Children and Adolescents in Foster Care.* 2nd ed. Elk Grove Village, IL: American Academy of Pediatrics; 2005

American Academy of Pediatrics Committee on Early Childhood, Adoption, and Dependent Care. Developmental issues for young children in foster care. *Pediatrics.* 2000;106(5):1145–1150

American Academy of Pediatrics Committee on Early Childhood, Adoption, and Dependent Care. Health care of young children in foster care. *Pediatrics.* 2002;109(3):536–541

American Academy of Pediatrics Task Force on Foster Care. Healthy Foster Care America. http://www.aap.org/en-us/advocacy-and-policy/aap-health-initiatives/healthy-foster-care-america. Accessed February 27, 2014

Jee SH, Tonniges T, Szilagyi MA. Foster care issues in general pediatrics. *Curr Opin Pediatr.* 2008;20(6):724–728

Mekonnen R, Noonan K, Rubin D. Achieving better health care outcomes for children in foster care. *Pediatr Clin North Am.* 2009;56(2):405–415

Oswald SH, Heil K, Goldbeck L. History of maltreatment and mental health problems in foster children: a review of the literature. *J Pediatr Psychol.* 2010;35(5): 462–472

Ringeisen H, Casanueva C, Urato M, Cross T. Special health care needs among children in the child welfare system. *Pediatrics* 2008;122(1):e232–e241

Stambaugh LF, Leslie LK, Ringeisen H, Smith K, Hodgkin D. *Psychotropic Medication Use by Children in Child Welfare.* OPRE Report #2012-33. Washington, DC: Office of Planning, Research and Evaluation, Administration for Children and Families, US Department of Health and Human Services; 2012. http://www. acf.hhs.gov/programs/opre/resource/nscaw-no-17-psychotropic-medication-use-by-children-in-child-welfare. Accessed February 27, 2014

Steele JS, Buchi KF. Medical and mental health of children entering the Utah foster care system. *Pediatrics.* 2008;122(3):e703–e709

Testimony of David Rubin, MD MSCE FAAP on behalf of the American Academy of Pediatrics. House Ways and Means Subcommittee on Income Security and Family Support hearing. Foster care and the health care system. http://www.aap.org/en-us/advocacy-and-policy/federal-advocacy/Documents/FosterChildrenandtheHealthCareSystem.pdf. Accessed February 27, 2014

US Department of Health and Human Services Administration for Children and Families; Administration on Children, Youth, and Families; Children's Bureau. *The AFCARS Report.* No. 20. http://www.acf.hhs.gov/sites/default/files/cb/afcarsreport20.pdf. Accessed February 27, 2014

Wang C, Edelstein SB, Waldinger L, Lee CM, Bath E. Care of the foster child: a primer for the pediatrician. *Adv Pediatr.* 2011;58(1):87–111

CHAPTER 38

Working With Immigrant Children and Their Families

Alejandro Diaz, MD, and Carol D. Berkowitz, MD

CASE STUDY

A 7-year-old boy presents with vomiting and clinical signs of dehydration. The family thinks he has empacho (a Latin American folk illness). You tell the family that you suspect that he has viral gastroenteritis. You want to draw some blood studies and give him fluids intravenously. The parents are skeptical; they refuse the blood work and want to leave against medical advice.

Questions

1. What are the ways that different immigrant families view illness and health?
2. What are barriers to accessing health care that children in immigrant families face?
3. What questions help the physician understand the health beliefs of immigrant families?
4. What are the considerations when dealing with parents who do not speak English?

The United States is described as a nation of immigrants. Out of a population of 314 million, current estimates are that about 40 million, or approximately 13% of the current US population, are foreign-born citizens or noncitizens. Half of these immigrants are Hispanic, and 65% of Hispanics are of Mexican descent. During the 1990s, 70% of the US population's overall growth was influenced by a wave of recent immigrants, mostly from Latin America and Asia, and by the children born to these newcomers. The vast growth in the population of children living in immigrant families, whether foreign-born (first generation) or US-born (second generation), poses a unique set of challenges. While this chapter focuses on immigrant children, children of migrant workers and children living by the US-Mexico border may face similar issues related to access to quality health care.

Immigrant children are more likely to live in families that live below the federal poverty level (FPL) and families in which at least one parent did not graduate high school or is not fluent in English. An estimated 31% of mothers and a similar number of fathers have not graduated from high school. In 2010, 30% of children in immigrant families lived below the FPL compared with 19% of children whose parents were born in the United States. They are also more likely to live in crowded housing (more than 1 person per room) and in a multigenerational household. Families of immigrant children tend to be larger, with 19% having 5 or more children, compared with US families, of which only 14% are of that size. While some immigrant children are citizens and eligible for safety net programs, their family's status directly influences whether these children will even access such care. Children of immigrant parents are twice as likely to be uninsured (15%) as children in nonimmigrant families

(8%). There is also growing concern that the health status of some immigrant children, whether foreign-born or first generation, actually declines after settling in the United States. It is expected that by 2030, Hispanic children will account for most children living in the United States.

Demographics of Immigrant Children

There are 5 general categories of immigrants in this country, each benefiting from specific entitlements and services and having certain legal rights: lawful permanent residents, naturalized citizens, refugees/asylees, nonimmigrants, and undocumented immigrants (Box 38-1).

In 2007, individuals who had become naturalized citizens included immigrants (32%), lawful permanent residents (29%), undocumented immigrants (29%), refugees (7%), and nonimmigrants (3%). From 1980 to 2000, the children of immigrants increased from 5% to 20% of school-aged children, representing approximately 10 million of the estimated 60 million school-aged children in the United States.

By far the largest category of immigrants is nonimmigrants or temporary visitors. Approximately 3 million children arrive mostly from Asia, Western Europe, and parts of North America, typically accompanying their parents, who are seeking work. A smaller percentage are students or exchange visitors. While not technically immigrants, this special group may present for care with similarly unaddressed health issues depending on their country of origin.

The next largest group, almost a quarter-million children, enter the United States as lawful permanent residents, with most

---

Box 38-1. Categories of Immigrants in the United States

Lawful Permanent Residents
- Carry a green card
- Noncitizens with permission to permanently live and work in the United States
- May apply for naturalization after 5 years (or 3 years if they marry a citizen)
- Group with the most international adoptees

Naturalized Citizens
- Born as noncitizens
- Having met certain English literacy requirements and demonstrating a basic knowledge of civics and a desirable moral character, are granted the same rights as natural-born citizens
- However, are not eligible to hold the office of president or vice president

Refugees/Asylees
- Granted permission from the US government before entry.
- Fled their country of origin for fear of persecution due to their race, religion, social group, or political opinion.
- Many unable or unwilling to return to country of origin.
- Those granted permission to remain are deemed asylees.
- After a year, both may apply to adjust their status to lawful permanent residents.

Nonimmigrants
- Carry a visa
- Granted permission to enter for a specified time and a specific purpose (usually to work or study)

Undocumented Immigrants
- Entered the country illegally or even legally but then violated the terms of their stay and remained after their visa expired
- Lack proper papers and identification to live in the United States

---

eventually becoming naturalized citizens. Although most arrive with or to meet family already residing in the United States, several thousand adolescents immigrate unaccompanied each year; most are female and many are married to a naturalized citizen at the time of immigration. Included in this group are children of refugees or asylees. More than 75,000 arrive each year, most recently from the countries of the former Yugoslavia and former Soviet Union, Vietnam, Somalia, and other war-torn regions. Numbers for the third-largest group, undocumented immigrants, are based primarily on estimates. Most are from Mexico or other Latin American states. Some entered the United States legally but have overstayed their visa or lost their status by committing a crime.

While most pediatricians are not in a position to assist families in their efforts to attain citizenship or legal status, having access to programs such as the National Center for Medical-Legal Partnership (www.medical-legalpartnership.org) may provide necessary advice and services. In addition, the pediatrician may find it helpful to be knowledgeable about programs such as the Deferred Action for Childhood Arrivals and the DREAM Act of 2013 (*D*evelopment, *R*elief, and *E*ducation for *A*lien *M*inors), which are specifically geared

to helping individuals who are foreign-born and immigrated to the United States as children.

Health Care Needs of Immigrant Children

When the child of an immigrant family presents for care, primary concerns are about the presence of an infectious disease (from exposures and possible lack of vaccination) or the presence of a hidden genetic or ethnic condition (eg, hemoglobinopathies, glucose-6-phosphate dehydrogenase [G6PD] deficiency). Investigating the health status of a child, especially from undocumented immigrant families, is paramount because these children likely have not seen a doctor prior to immigrating. Similarly, nonimmigrants, such as tourists and other temporary visitors, from many Western or Pacific Rim countries are not required to have a medical examination performed as part of their application. Only visas for permanent residency require a health examination to be performed by an approved physician, and even then the focus of the examination is to exclude certain conditions such as active tuberculosis (TB), HIV, and other severe physical or mental handicaps. In children, laboratory testing may be limited and proof of vaccination status may be exempted for certain groups, such as international adoptees.

Lack of education and poverty, which results in relative food insecurity and inadequate, crowded housing conditions, poses an ominous threat to the health of these same children. Immigrant parents of children born in the United States may be reluctant to apply for Medicaid or the Children's Health Insurance Program (CHIP) for fear of being considered a "public charge" (a person dependent on the government for expenses of living). The Patient Protection and Affordable Care Act of 2010 excluded undocumented immigrants from health care coverage. Noncitizen children must wait at least 5 years before they are able to apply for public assistance. While most refugee children may receive some form of subsidized care, such as Medicaid, many of these benefits are time-sensitive. Even US-born children of undocumented mothers, while legally eligible as US citizens for benefits such as nutritional assistance programs, may not receive these owing to parental fears of detection and deportation. Physicians should ascertain that the family has adequate housing and access to food, 2 basic human needs. Is the food available in the families' neighborhood consistent with the traditional food that the family desires? Is the food healthy or does the family live in a "food desert" where there is a plethora of fast-food restaurants and a paucity of supermarkets or grocery stores (Box 38-2)?

It has traditionally been supposed that immigration itself imposes unique stresses on these children. Mental health challenges (eg, depression, anxiety, grief) may be related to the reasons for their migration as well as to the inevitable process of acculturation. Stress is compounded by the potential loss of the immigrant's identity and separation from home support systems; inadequate language and literacy skills in a society intolerant of linguistic weakness; disparities between one's country of origin and the United States in economic, social, and professional standards and status; and the psychologic and emotional trauma of war, persecution, or exploitation in one's

---

Box 38-2. Risk Factors Affecting the Health of Immigrant Children

Social and Economic
- Inadequate or crowded housing
- Food insecurity
- Lack of insurance (due to ineligibility)
- Lack of access to insurance (eligible but unable or unwilling to apply)
- Educational level of head of household

Cultural
- Dietary preferences
- Lack of language fluency or literacy and translation/interpretation issues
- Disparate ideas about the causation and treatment of illness
- Expectations of the medical system
- Religious practices with a medical component
- Lack of access to traditional medical practitioners and treatments
- Importation drugs not approved in the United States

Physical
- Carriage of infectious disease and the possibility for repeated exposure via travel or living within one's immigrant community
- Presence of ethnic or genetic conditions
- Lack of vaccination
- Poor nutritional status

Mental Health
- Negative past living conditions, including exposure to violence or natural disaster
- Cultural adjustment (or the process of acculturation and enculturation)

Box 38-3. Questions to Consider When Evaluating Immigrant Children

1. If parents are not present, does the child's current guardian have any personal knowledge of the child's social and medical history?
2. In which countries has the child resided and under what circumstances?
3. Have the child's living conditions changed dramatically positively or negatively recently?
4. Are there verifiable birth and medical records, especially vaccination status, to be reviewed? What age is the child? What quality of care did the child seem to receive in his or her home country?
5. Has the child undergone any recent procedures or treatments?
6. Was the child exposed to any potentially toxic occupational or environmental risks?
7. What educational level did the child achieve?

---

country of origin. Sometimes children are separated from one parent or other siblings who remain in their country of origin.

Despite these challenges, epidemiologic studies indicate that children in immigrant families experience better outcomes than those in their native countries who did not immigrate, especially in some areas. The most striking example is the lower rate of low-birth-weight children born to foreign-born mothers, especially among Hispanics and non-Hispanic black immigrants, compared with women in their native countries who did not immigrate. This positive effect related to immigration has been studied less in older children due to limited availability of data samples from second-generation children that do not exclude first-generation children.

General Approach to the Initial Medical Evaluation of an Immigrant Child

Ascertaining the life history of an immigrant child, including any relevant travel history, will help determine the extent of the medical evaluation (Box 38-3).

In general, most immigrants from industrialized nations have received comprehensive medical care and the only issues facing these children are routine, such as updating immunization status. In contrast, adoptees, refugees, and undocumented children often have received little or no care. While there is no single approach to the

general medical evaluation for all immigrant children, some general principles apply.

Any and all existing medical records should be reviewed. Previous growth parameters should be obtained if available. While a complete translation is not always necessary, if an unusual diagnosis or a complicated history exists, use of clinical translational services or a nearby university's academic language department may facilitate the process. Sometimes the records suggest that a diagnosis was considered but not confirmed and it may be appropriate to reevaluate the child for any suspected condition.

It is important to screen for certain infectious diseases. The most common among immigrants are TB, intestinal parasites, hepatitis B, syphilis, and HIV. In fact, the risk for TB is more than 100 times greater in immigrant children than in US children. Fifty percent of all newly identified cases of TB in the United States are diagnosed in immigrants, many within the first 5 years of life. If not clinically apparent (incubation period) or testing is negative but clinical suspicion exists, TB testing should be repeated in 6 months. The pediatrician may be uncertain about how to interpret the results of a tuberculin skin test in a child who received BCG (Bacille Calmette-Guérin) vaccine. The pediatrician may consult with the American Academy of Pediatrics (AAP) *Red Book* for help or advice about alternative tests or the significance of the results. Intestinal parasitic infestations may be present without symptoms. Some clinics specializing in immigrant health advocate giving a single dose of albendazole as a more cost-effective approach than screening and diagnosis, but the safety and efficacy of this approach has not been substantiated in children.

Ethnic or genetic conditions should also be considered. Conditions like G6PD deficiency in Mediterraneans, Africans, and Southeast Asians may affect the child's health in the short term. Others, like hemoglobinopathies and thalassemias, while common among certain ethnic populations, such as Southeast Asians, may not be of immediate importance. Overall, anemia is extremely common among immigrant children, and the diagnostic workup of these children may uncover an underlying blood dyscrasia trait or lead intoxication. If iron therapy has been initiated empirically, repeat testing after treatment is paramount to ensure a response and confirm the diagnosis. Also, certain ritual cultural practices, such as female circumcision and tattooing, or the use of certain traditional healing techniques, such as cupping or coining, may have long-term implications. Understanding the risk for nutritional deficiencies based on the country of origin is important. For instance, nutritional disorders, such as rickets and iodine deficiency, are common in ethnic Chinese and children from the former Soviet Union.

Immunizations must be administered as appropriate and following the catch-up recommendations of the AAP and the Advisory Committee on Immunization Practices. Records of previous immunizations may be difficult to interpret. Shortened intervals or the administration of a vaccination at too early an age may not be readily apparent. Fraudulent records, especially among adoptees and children from institutional settings, often exist. In young children, it is generally considered safe and cost-effective to simply give missing vaccines; however, determining serum immunity may be more cost-effective in older children.

Cultural and Linguistic Sensitivity

Bridging language differences using professional interpreter services is required to provide adequate patient care. Such linguistic services are mandated by agencies such as the Centers for Medicare & Medicaid Services for payment from the federal government. The use of children or hospital maintenance or janitorial staff is inadequate and potentially violates federal laws, including the Health Insurance Portability and Accountability Act of 1996. Professional interpreters are taught to interpret and not carry on additional conversations with the patient or expound on the questions the physician asks. The physician should address questions directly to the patient, not the interpreter, maintaining eye contact with the patient.

Providing culturally competent care that considers cultural practices and beliefs about child health or illness when coming up with a treatment plan is also critical (see Chapter 10). Does the family access "healers" for medical problems (Box 38-4)? What are its views about medication use? Are there hierarchical structures that influence a parent's acceptance of a physician's advice (eg, father accepting advice

---

Box 38-4. Questions for Understanding Someone's Cultural Concept of the Symptoms of Illness

1. What do you call the problem?
2. What do you think caused it?
3. Why do you think it started when it did?
4. What do you think the sickness does? How does it work?
5. How severe is it? Will it have a long or short course?
6. What are the chief problems the illness has caused?
7. What kind of treatment do you think they should receive? What are the most important results you expect from this treatment?
8. What do you fear most about the illness?

Adapted from Fadiman A. *The Spirit Catches You and You Fall Down.* New York, NY: Farrar, Strauss and Giroux; 1997, quoting medical anthropologist Arthur Kleinman.

---

from a female physician, parent accepting advice from a young resident)?

Conclusion

There are numerous barriers that potentially interfere with achieving optimal health status for immigrant children. Many of these barriers are societal and relate to funding for medical services. Trust is a core component of the physician-patient relationship, and establishing trust may be more difficult when the physician and family have different cultural values and expectations. It has been stated that in medicine, the sacred trust that develops between a patient and his or her doctor should never be taken for granted. The development of trust forms the foundation of the therapeutic relationship. It provides credibility to the practitioner. The practitioner must act in a manner that elicits and fosters trust, and being knowledgeable and nonjudgmental about the beliefs and practices of one's patients is pivotal.

Health care professionals must work toward creating an atmosphere of trust so that parents feel comfortable revealing their beliefs, concerns, and fears. The threat of deportation should be considered when taking into account whether the patient or family will follow up or adhere to medical recommendations.

It is unwise not to acknowledge the cultural divide that exists between most pediatric practitioners and the families they serve. Therefore, pediatricians who are less familiar with the enrichment provided by a multicultural patient population may be less inclined to advocate for social reforms that may prove beneficial. We as physicians must approach families with an open mind, respect, and a sense of humility if we are to gain their trust, close the gaps that separate us, and promote the well-being of children.

Children are better served when their families receive information about federal, state, and community programs that provide resources to immigrant families. In addition to health care, pediatricians can provide families with information about educational programs, such as Head Start, that are not restricted by immigration status. All children, regardless of their immigration or socioeconomic status, should receive compassionate, culturally competent, and linguistically effective care services. Such care requires that health care professionals incorporate knowledge, attitudes, and skills in cultural and linguistic competence within their professional agenda.

The well-being of all children can be advanced through advocacy, especially on behalf of vulnerable children (see Chapter 2). Such advocacy addresses outreach efforts to children who are potentially eligible for Medicaid and CHIP but are not enrolled, simplifies enrollment for both programs, and expands state funding for those who are not eligible. The medical community must collaborate with legislators, families, and organizations representing underserved populations to increase the effectiveness of one's own advocacy effort. All children should receive care in a medical home (ie, the establishment of comprehensive, coordinated, and continuous health care services). This is especially critical for immigrant children with chronic health care needs and mental health problems.

CASE RESOLUTION

You reach an agreement with the family that allows a community healer to come and perform a therapeutic massage while allowing you to place an intravenous line and administer fluids. The patient is significantly improved after the massage and intravenous fluids. The family appreciates that you respected their beliefs and agrees to return for a routine well-child visit in 2 weeks.

Selected References

American Academy of Pediatrics. *Red Book: 2012 Report of the Committee on Infectious Diseases.* Pickering LK, Baker CJ, Kimberlin DW, Long SS, eds. 29th ed. Elk Grove Village, IL: American Academy of Pediatrics; 2012

American Academy of Pediatrics Council on Community Pediatrics. Providing care for immigrant, migrant, and border children. *Pediatrics.* 2013;131(6): e2028–e2034

Flores G, Brotanek J. The healthy immigrant effect: a greater understanding might help us improve the health of all children. *Arch Pediatr Adolesc Med.* 2005;159(3):295–297

Grayson J. Serving immigrant families. *Virginia Child Protection Newsletter.* 2011;90:1–20

Guendelman S, Schauffler HH, Pearl M. Unfriendly shores: how immigrant children fare in the US health system. *Health Aff (Millwood).* 2001;20(1):257–266

Jenista JA. The immigrant, refugee, or internationally adopted child. *Pediatr Rev.* 2001;22(12):419–429

Mendoza FS. Health disparities and children in immigrant families: a research agenda. *Pediatrics.* 2009;124(Suppl 3):S187–S195

National Immigration Law Center. *Guide to Immigrant Eligibility for Federal Programs.* 4th ed. Santa Monica, CA: National Immigration Law Center; 2002

CHAPTER 39

Well-Child Care for Children With Trisomy 21 (Down Syndrome)

Derek Wong, MD

CASE STUDY

A 6-month-old girl with trisomy 21 (Down syndrome) whom you have known since birth is brought to your office for well-child care. She and her parents have been doing well, although she has had several episodes of upper respiratory infections. Her medical history is significant for a small ventricular septal defect, which has since closed spontaneously, and one episode of otitis media at 5 months of age. Her weight gain has been good—along the 25th percentile on the trisomy 21 growth chart. She now sleeps through the night and has a bowel movement once a day. She has received all of the recommended immunizations for her age without any problems.

The infant smiles appropriately, grasps and shakes hand toys, and has some head control but is unable to roll from supine to prone position. Since she was 1 month old, she has been enrolled in an early intervention program. An occupational therapist visits her at home twice a month.

On physical examination, she has typical facial features consistent with trisomy 21, a single palmar crease on each hand, and mild diffuse hypotonia. Her eyes have symmetric movement, and her tympanic membranes are clear. She has no cardiac murmurs.

Questions

1. What is the prevalence of trisomy 21 (Down syndrome) in the general population? What is the association of maternal age with trisomy 21?
2. What are the clinical manifestations of this syndrome?
3. What medical conditions are associated with trisomy 21 in the newborn period, during childhood, and in adolescence? When should screening tests for these conditions be performed?
4. What is the role of early intervention services for these patients and their families?
5. What specific psychosocial issues should be included in your anticipatory guidance and health education?
6. What is the prognosis for children with trisomy 21?

Trisomy 21, or Down syndrome, is the most commonly known genetic cause of intellectual disability in children. Primary care physicians are in a unique position to offer affected children routine health care maintenance and anticipatory guidance, follow-up of intercurrent illness and chronic problems, and information on the latest recommendations for screening for conditions associated with trisomy 21. In addition, the general pediatrician has the opportunity to develop rapport with children and families that is particularly important when considering the complex medical and social implications of raising children with trisomy 21. An important goal of the well-child visit is to provide children with trisomy 21 and their families with counseling about educational, social, and financial resources and support to ensure a healthy and productive transition into adulthood.

Epidemiology

The prevalence of trisomy 21 is approximately 1 in 800 to 1,000 live births. It is estimated that trisomy 21 is responsible for up to one-third of all cases of moderate to severe intellectual disability. Trisomy 21 has a male to female ratio of 1.3:1.

Ninety-five percent of all cases of Down syndrome are caused by chromosomal nondisjunction, and most of these events occur in the mother. The chance of nondisjunction is determined by maternal age. A 25-year-old woman has a 1 in 1,240 risk of having a live baby with Down syndrome, and the risk increases to 1 in 340 at age 35 and 1 in 98 at age 40. It is estimated that approximately half of trisomy 21 embryos abort spontaneously. The risk of recurrence of nondisjunction Down syndrome in subsequent pregnancies is 1 in 100 until age 35, after which the risk determined by age takes precedence.

Other family members are generally not at increased risk of bearing children with this type of Down syndrome.

Approximately 3% to 4% of Down syndrome cases are caused by robertsonian translocations with another acrocentric chromosome (14/21, 15/21, or 21/21). Parental karyotypes should be obtained because balanced translocation carriers have an increased risk of Down syndrome in future children. Approximately 1% to 2% of Down syndrome cases are mosaic. These children are often less severely affected than those with "full" Down syndrome. A small percentage of affected children have a chromosomal rearrangement resulting in 3 copies of a portion of chromosome 21.

Recent advances in first and second trimester screening allow prenatal diagnosis of Down syndrome with a sensitivity of 80% to 90%. If a prenatal diagnosis of Down syndrome is made, and the general pediatrician is asked to participate in counseling the family, the points listed in Box 39-1 should be covered.

Clinical Presentation

Newborns, infants, and children with trisomy 21 have a characteristic appearance (D_x Box). They may be microcephalic, with flattening of the occiput and face. The eyes have an upward slant with prominent epicanthal folds, the ears are set low and small, the nasal bridge is flattened, and the tongue appears large. The feet, hands, and digits are small and stubby, and the fifth digit may be hypoplastic and turned in (brachyclinodactyly). A single palmar crease and wide spacing between the first and second toes may be evident. After the newborn period, diffuse hypotonia and developmental delay are universally seen.

Pathophysiology

Approximately 95% of cases of Down syndrome are caused by trisomy 21 resulting from meiotic nondisjunction. The remaining cases are translocations (3%–4%) and mosaics (1%–2%). Translocations are unbalanced and usually occur with another acrocentric chromosome, usually 14/21 or 15/21. Approximately 75% of these are new mutations and 25% are the result of a familial translocation. Therefore, if a child has a translocation, the parents must be evaluated for a balanced translocation. Mosaicism implies the presence of 2 cell lines, one normal and one with trisomy 21. As might be expected, children with mosaic Down syndrome are usually affected less severely than children with other types of Down syndrome.

Recent research has focused on the role of individual genes, such as *DYRK1A*, in the pathogenesis of Down syndrome. It is likely that in the near future, pharmacologic agents that mitigate the effects of excess expression of such genes will lead to new treatments for Down syndrome patients.

Evaluation

Routine health care maintenance for newborns, infants, children, and adolescents with trisomy 21 should cover the same issues in health education, prevention, and counseling that are discussed with other patients and their families. The schedule of health maintenance visits for newborns, infants, and young children with trisomy 21 is essentially the same as that recommended by the American Academy of Pediatrics (AAP) for other children, while older children with Down syndrome should be evaluated annually. The following sections will emphasize additional medical and psychosocial conditions often seen in patients with trisomy 21.

Newborn Period

Verification of the diagnosis of trisomy 21 is perhaps the single most important focus of the initial family visit. Sometimes the diagnosis has been suspected prenatally due to abnormal biochemical markers and ultrasound and verified by chorionic villus sampling or amniocentesis (see Box 39-1). If there is no prenatal testing and the diagnosis is suspected due to clinical findings, a karyotype must be sent from the nursery and reviewed at the 1- to 2-week visit. In some institutions, a FISH (fluorescence in situ hybridization) test for trisomy 21 may provide a more rapid confirmation of the diagnosis (1–3 days).

Several conditions that are associated with trisomy 21 are important to identify in the newborn period, including hearing loss,

Dx Trisomy 21

- Microcephaly, with flattening of occiput and face
- Upward slant to the eyes with epicanthal folds
- Brushfield spots
- Small ears and mouth (therefore, tongue appears large)
- Low-set ears
- Flat nasal bridge
- Broad, stocky neck with loose skin folds at the nape
- Funnel-shaped or pigeon-breasted chest
- Small, stubby feet, hands, and digits with brachyclinodactyly of the fifth digits
- Single transverse palmar crease on each hand
- Wide space between first and second toes
- Fair, mottled skin in newborns; dry skin in older children
- Hypotonia

Box 39-1. Counseling the Family After a Prenatal Diagnosis of Down Syndrom

- Review the data that established the diagnosis in the fetus.
- Explain the mechanism of occurrence and risks for recurrence.
- Review the manifestations of trisomy 21, commonly associated conditions, and the variable prognosis based on the presence of these conditions.
- Discuss other modalities that confirm the presence of associated anomalies, such as a fetal echocardiogram in the case of congenital heart disease.
- Explore treatment options and interventions for associated conditions.
- Offer resources to assist the family with decisions related to completing or terminating the pregnancy.
- Refer the family to a clinical geneticist or genetics counselor.

congenital heart disease (most commonly endocardial cushion defect), duodenal atresia, Hirschsprung disease, congenital hypothyroidism, hip dislocation, and ocular anomalies (cataracts, strabismus, and nystagmus). Hematologic abnormalities include polycythemia, leukemoid reactions that resemble leukemia but resolve during the first month of life, and, rarely, leukemia.

History

A feeding history is critical because hypotonia often leads to swallowing difficulties (Table 39-1). A history of vomiting may be indicative of gastroesophageal reflux or, less commonly, a gastrointestinal malformation. Constipation may be the first indication of Hirschsprung disease or hypothyroidism. A detailed family and social history should also be obtained if this was not done in the hospital.

Physical Examination

A detailed physical examination should reveal some common features of newborns with Down syndrome (see D_x box). All growth parameters should be recorded and compared with those obtained at birth. The size of the fontanels should be evaluated because of the increased incidence of congenital hypothyroidism. Bilateral red reflexes and conjugate gaze should be documented to exclude congenital cataracts or strabismus. A careful cardiac examination must be performed, noting any cyanosis, murmurs, irregular heart rates, abnormal heart sounds, or asymmetry of pulses. The abdomen should be palpated for organomegaly or any masses, and patency of the anus should be verified. Ortolani and Barlow maneuvers should be performed for hip laxity. Finally, the newborn should be evaluated for hypotonia.

Laboratory Tests

A karyotype is an important tool to verify the diagnosis and assess recurrence risk. Newborn screening laboratory tests must be reviewed, especially hearing evaluations and thyroid screenings. In addition, a cardiac evaluation for congenital heart disease should be performed, which may include electrocardiogram, chest radiograph, echocardiogram, and formal cardiology referral. A complete blood cell count is indicated to look for hematologic abnormalities, including leukemoid reaction, transient myeloproliferative disorder (pancytopenia, hepatosplenomegaly, and immature white blood cells), and neonatal thrombocytopenia.

Management

The primary care physician should discuss the increased propensity for respiratory infections in children with Down syndrome. Other important issues to address include those pertaining to available resources for children and families, such as early intervention programs and Down syndrome support groups in the community. Educational materials such as pamphlets and books may also be supplied at this time. Upcoming appointments with other physicians and allied health professionals should be reviewed.

Table 39-1. Health Supervision for Children With Down Syndrome

	Initial Evaluation	Subsequent Evaluations
History and Physical Examination		
Developmental assessment	Newborn	Same as regular well-child care schedule until age 5 y, then annual evaluation
Visual and hearing assessment (subjective)		
Laboratory Assessment		
Karyotype	Newborn	None
Thyroid screen	Newborn screen	6 mo, 12 mo, then annually
Complete blood cell count	Newborn	0–1 mo, then hemoglobin annually
Celiac screen	2–3 y	Obtain IgA and TTG levels in symptomatic individuals at any age.[a]
Echocardiogram	Newborn	Depends on condition
Neck radiographs	3–5 y	Obtain in symptomatic individuals with pain or neurologic abnormalities. May be required for Special Olympics entry.[a]
Audiologic evaluation	6 mo	Every 6 mo
Consultation		
Genetics	Newborn	As needed[b]
Cardiology	Newborn	Depends on condition
Ophthalmology	6 mo	Annually until age 5 y, then every 2 y until age 13 y, then every 3 y
Ear/nose/throat	As needed	As needed
Dental	By 1 y	Twice per year
Pulmonary	As needed	As needed

Abbreviations: IgA, immunoglobulin A; TTG, tissue transglutaminase.

[a]Lack of expert consensus on evaluation.

[b]Depending on experience and comfort level of primary care physician.

Infancy and Early Childhood

History

Some additional historical issues to address include a detailed developmental assessment focusing on progress made since the last visit because most affected children have motor and speech delays (see Table 39-1). It is important to review any ancillary services, such as physical, occupational, and speech therapy, in anticipation of school entry. Parents should provide their assessment of the child's vision and hearing. A history of recurrent respiratory infections should raise concern about otitis media. Many children at this age develop constipation. A history of snoring and restless sleep may indicate obstructive sleep apnea and require a sleep study. Finally, it is extremely important to document any history of neck pain, gait changes, increased clumsiness, or other neurologic symptoms that would indicate spinal cord compression from atlantoaxial dislocation.

Physical Examination

All growth parameters should be plotted on growth charts for children with Down syndrome (figures 39-1–39-4). Children with trisomy 21 are shorter than other children and may have poor weight gain in their first year. Later in life, obesity unrelated to the syndrome may become a problem. As with routine well-child visits in other infants and children, a complete physical examination should be performed at each patient encounter. Noteworthy aspects of the examination in infants and children with trisomy 21 are given in Box 39-2. In particular, the ear canals of these children are easily collapsed, making the tympanic membrane difficult to visualize. In some cases, an otolaryngologic referral may be necessary for an adequate otoscopic examination. A complete neurologic examination should be performed at each visit, including an assessment of the degree of hypotonia.

Laboratory Tests

Hearing evaluation should be performed annually, starting with the newborn hearing screen. Developmentally appropriate gross visual screening should be performed in infants between 6 and 12 months of age at each visit, and a formal ophthalmologic examination is recommended at 6 months and every 2 years thereafter. Thyroid screening tests should be repeated at 6 and 12 months and then annually.

Children with congenital heart disease should be given antibiotic endocarditis prophylaxis for dental or other procedures. In addition, these children should be considered for monoclonal antibody therapy against respiratory syncytial virus in the winter.

Children with Down syndrome have an increased risk for autoimmune disorders such as celiac disease, Graves disease, and type 1 diabetes. Because the signs of celiac disease may be subtle, some pediatric gastroenterologists recommend measuring tissue transglutaminase immunoglobulin (Ig) A antibodies, as well as an IgA level, at 2 to 3 years of age and every 5 years afterward. However, current AAP recommendations include screening only symptomatic children.

Children with Down syndrome have an increased incidence of atlantoaxial instability when screened with routine lateral cervical radiographs with flexion and extension views. Any patient with signs or symptoms of cord compression should be evaluated by computed tomography or magnetic resonance imaging and referred to an orthopedic surgeon or neurosurgeon. Symptomatic children should be kept out of any sports that involve contact or neck extension, such as swimming, gymnastics, and soccer. Experts agree that careful neurologic screening at health supervision visits is a much better predictor of serious injury. The current recommendation is to screen only symptomatic children, unless a preparticipation radiograph is required for events such as the Special Olympics.

Management

Infants with trisomy 21 should have all routine screening tests and immunizations. Growth and developmental progress should be reviewed with parents at the end of each visit, and any concerns or unmet expectations should be addressed at this time. Often the developmental delay associated with trisomy 21 is not apparent to families until infants are 4 to 6 months of age and not achieving the expected milestones of rolling over or sitting. It should also be emphasized to families that the degree of mental retardation in trisomy 21 is quite variable, ranging from mild to severe. However, social function is not necessarily related to IQ. If the child is not already enrolled in an early intervention program, the positive role of such an experience should be addressed. The availability of support groups for parents and other family members should also be discussed. Down syndrome patients with autism spectrum disorders may be especially difficult to assess.

In the early childhood years, plans for preschool attendance and future educational opportunities should be reviewed with families. The role of discipline and presence of common behavioral problems such as temper tantrums and biting should be assessed in preparation for school entry and socialization. Nutrition should be reviewed because children with Down syndrome have a reduced metabolic rate and are at increased risk for obesity. Nutritional supplements and other alternative medicines have not been proven to have any efficacy in the treatment of patients with Down syndrome.

A dental referral should be made by the age of 1 year in accordance with the latest recommendation for all children.

Older Childhood and Adolescence

History

School-aged children with Down syndrome should continue to visit their primary care physician at least annually. Educational issues should be discussed, including Individual Education Plans and transition from school. Specific medical issues to address during the history include visual or hearing deficits, evidence of hypothyroidism (decreased activity, coarse and dry hair, and constipation), skin problems including eczema, and dental problems. A careful nutritional history should also be taken because of the propensity for obesity, and children should be closely monitored for signs of obstructive sleep apnea.

Physical Examination

Height and weight should continue to be plotted. The skin should be examined closely for xerosis, acne, or syringomas (multiple papules often present on the eyelids and upper cheeks) during adolescence. A cardiac examination is important because of an increased risk of mitral valve prolapse and valvular dysfunction. The sexual maturity rating (Tanner stage) of males and females should be noted and discussed with parents. A pelvic examination is not indicated as a part of the routine visit unless there is concern about sexual abuse or a sexually transmitted infection, but a testicular examination is

Figure 39-1. Growth chart for boys with Down syndrome: 1 through 36 months. (Reproduced with permission from Cronk C, Crocker AC, Pueschel SM, et al. Growth charts for children with Down syndrome: 1 month to 18 years of age. *Pediatrics.* **1988;81[1]:102–110.)**

Figure 39-2. Growth chart for boys with Down syndrome: 2 through 18 years. (Reproduced with permission from Cronk C, Crocker AC, Pueschel SM, et al. Growth charts for children with Down syndrome: 1 month to 18 years of age. *Pediatrics.* **1988;81[1]:102–110.)**

Figure 39-3. Growth chart for girls with Down syndrome: 1 through 36 months. (Reproduced with permission from Cronk C, Crocker AC, Pueschel SM, et al. Growth charts for children with Down syndrome: 1 month to 18 years of age. *Pediatrics.* **1988;81[1]:102–110.)**

Figure 39-4. Growth chart for girls with Down syndrome: 2 through 18 years. (Reproduced with permission from Cronk C, Crocker AC, Pueschel SM, et al. Growth charts for children with Down syndrome: 1 month to 18 years of age. *Pediatrics.* **1988;81[1]:102–110.)**

Box 39-2. Physical Examination of Children With Trisomy 21 (Down Syndrome)

- Look for dry, sensitive skin and alopecia, which develops in approximately 10% of children and resolves spontaneously.
- Monitor the size of the anterior and posterior fontanels because delayed closure may indicate hypothyroidism.
- Check for visual abnormalities, such as strabismus, nystagmus, cataracts, refractive errors, and blepharitis.
- Document recurrent serous otitis media. It is estimated that 40% to 60% of children with trisomy 21 have significant conductive hearing loss and 20% to 30% have some degree of neurosensory loss.
- Examine the oropharynx carefully for delayed dentition, malocclusion, and caries.
- Auscultate for stridor, wheezing, or other abnormal breathing that may indicate airway anomalies.
- Perform a thorough cardiac examination and note any evidence of previously unrecognized congenital heart disease.
- Palpate the abdomen for distention or organomegaly. Children with trisomy 21 have a slightly increased risk of developing acute non-lymphoblastic or acute lymphoblastic leukemia.
- Perform a rectal examination in infants or children with a history of constipation.
- Evaluate any musculoskeletal abnormalities such as overall hypotonia and joint laxity (most commonly in the knees and hips) that might contribute to overall gross motor delay.

---

important due to the increased risk of testicular cancer. A complete neurologic examination should also be performed in the patient participating in sports and activities to look for signs indicating impending atlantoaxial dislocation.

Laboratory Tests

Annual thyroid screening (thyroid-stimulating hormone, thyroxine) is recommended for all school-aged children and adolescents with trisomy 21, in addition to other routine screening tests. Hearing evaluation should also occur at least once in older children and annually thereafter. Because of the risk of keratoconus, an annual ophthalmologic consultation should be arranged after the age of 10 years. In addition, children with trisomy 21 should be encouraged to continue biannual dental visits because gingivitis, periodontal disease, and bruxism (teeth grinding) are common in these individuals.

Management

The major part of the visit with school-aged and adolescent children should be spent on developmental, educational, and vocational anticipatory guidance. Educational placement and future goals should be developmentally appropriate for the child and acceptable for the parent. Activities requiring socialization and development of responsibility should continue to be encouraged; however, these events can be very stressful for parents and other family members. Injury prevention should be highlighted as well, especially because

older children are becoming more independent. In early adolescence, prevocational and vocational training within the school curriculum should be reviewed. In addition, brief discussions about independent living, group homes, transition of medical care, and financial resources (eg, community-supported employment for young adults) should begin during adolescence.

Puberty, fertility, and contraception are extremely important to address with adolescents and their parents. The patient's psychosocial development and physical sexual maturation should be discussed, including menstrual hygiene and any foreseeable problems with its management. Contraception and the potential for victimization must be addressed as well, particularly with female patients. Males with trisomy 21 are usually sterile, but females have an approximately 50% chance of having children with Down syndrome.

Prognosis

Individuals with trisomy 21 can often live well past the age of 50 years unless they are born with a congenital heart lesion, which may limit life expectancy. One major cause of morbidity and mortality is the development of symptomatic Alzheimer disease, which occurs in approximately 15% of adults after the fourth decade. Fortunately, many adults with Down syndrome remain asymptomatic, despite histopathologic evidence of the disease.

CASE RESOLUTION

In the case described at the beginning of the chapter, the family should be encouraged by the healthy progress of the patient. For this visit, anticipatory guidance should consist of a review of early intervention services, available resources, and general support services for the patient and her family. The increased risk for upper respiratory infections and otitis media should be reviewed. Medical screening should include thyroid screening, subjective hearing screening, and a formal evaluation by a pediatric ophthalmologist. If the results are normal, the next visit should take place in 3 months.

Selected References

Bull MJ; American Academy of Pediatrics Committee on Genetics. Health supervision for children with Down syndrome. *Pediatrics.* 2011;128(2):393–406

Cassidy SB, Allanson JE, eds. *Management of Genetic Syndromes.* 3rd ed. New York, NY: Wiley-Blackwell; 2010

Cohen WI. Current dilemmas in Down syndrome clinical care: celiac disease, thyroid disorders, and atlanto-axial instability. *Am J Med Genet C Semin Med Genet.* 2006;142C(3):141–148

Hickey F, Hickey E, Summar KL. Medical update for children with Down syndrome for the pediatrician and family practitioner. *Adv Pediatr.* 2012;59(1):137–157

Venail F, Gardiner Q, Mondain M. ENT and speech disorders in children with Down's syndrome: an overview of pathophysiology, clinical features, treatments, and current management. *Clin Pediatr (Phila).* 2004;43(9):783–791

CHAPTER 40

Well-Child Care for Preterm Infants

Lucinda S. Santos, MHA, and Lynne M. Smith, MD

CASE STUDY

A 2½-month-old girl was discharged from the neonatal intensive care unit 2 weeks ago, where she had been since birth. She was the 780-g product of a 26-week gestation born via spontaneous vaginal delivery to a 32-year-old primigravida. The perinatal course was complicated by premature rupture of membranes and maternal amnionitis. Several aspects of the neonatal course were significant, including respiratory distress that required surfactant therapy and 2 weeks of endotracheal intubation; a grade 2 intraventricular hemorrhage diagnosed at 1 week of life; hyperbilirubinemia, which was treated with phototherapy; several episodes of apnea, presumably associated with the prematurity; and a history of poor oral intake with slow weight gain.

The infant's parents have a few questions about her feeding schedule and discontinuing the apnea monitor, but they feel relatively comfortable caring for their daughter at home. She is feeding well (2 oz of 22 cal/oz post-discharge formula for premature infants every 2–3 hours) and is becoming progressively more alert according to the family. She sleeps on her back in a crib.

The infant's weight gain has averaged 25 g/day. The rest of the physical examination is normal, except for dolichocephaly and a left esotropia.

Questions

1. What constitutes well-child care in preterm infants?
2. What are the nutritional requirements of preterm infants in the months following discharge from the hospital?
3. What information must be considered in the developmental screening of preterm infants?
4. What immunization schedule is appropriate for preterm infants? Do they require any special immunizations?
5. What specific conditions or illnesses are more likely to affect preterm infants than term infants?

Prior to 2013, prematurity was defined as birth prior to 37 weeks' gestation. The increased frequency of adverse neonatal outcomes in neonates born at 37 and 38 weeks' gestation lead the American College of Obstetricians and Gynecologists to redefine *term* as 39 weeks' gestation to eliminate non-medically indicated deliveries prior to this time. Because advances in neonatal care have improved survival, there is an increased demand for skilled primary care physicians caring for the preterm infant. Providing primary care for these infants is an important and challenging task and often requires coordination of medical, developmental, and social services for multiple chronic conditions. Because preterm infants are at increased risk for impaired growth and developmental delay, longer visits may be necessary to evaluate their nutritional and developmental progress and to assess how families have adjusted to caring for them at home. Primary care physicians must learn to manage these and many other complex issues while providing families with comprehensive anticipatory guidance. Providing a medical home where care is accessible, comprehensive, continuous, and culturally and family oriented is essential for the optimal heath and developmental outcome of the former premature newborn patient.

Epidemiology

In the United States, 1 in 8 newborns is born prematurely, an 8% decrease since 2006. The preterm delivery rate is highest for African American women (16.7%) and lowest for white women (10.5%). The increase in preterm births over the last 3 decades has been among late preterm newborns (>34 weeks' gestation), which comprise 70% of premature births. Reasons for the increased premature delivery rates include an increased use of artificial reproductive technologies (see Chapter 23), increased interest in elective caesarian deliveries, and increased maternal age.

Although most preterm newborns are delivered at greater than 34 weeks' gestation, these neonates are at increased risk for morbidity and mortality relative to neonates born at term. In addition, many neonatologists routinely resuscitate neonates born at 23 weeks' gestation, a gestation that has a survival rate of approximately 25%. Very low birth weight (VLBW, <1,500 g) and extremely low birth weight (ELBW, <1,000 g) newborns are at risk for cerebral palsy, respiratory disease, hearing and vision problems, and intellectual disabilities. Further, learning disabilities, attention-deficit/hyperactivity disorder (ADHD), borderline to low IQ scores, psychiatric disorders or abnormalities in executive function, and visuomotor integration occur in more than 50% of VLBW infants, complicating posthospital care for these children. In 2006, the Institute of Medicine estimated the annual societal cost of prematurity at $26 billion.

Evaluation

The purpose of the health maintenance visit for preterm infants is the same as for other healthy children: to provide consistent preventive health care and education for patients and their parents. Prematurity, however, places children at risk for additional medical and neurodevelopmental conditions. Children born prematurely average nearly 3 times the number of well-child visits in the first year of life relative to those born full term.

History

Almost one-third of former premature newborns fail to keep the first outpatient appointment. Because failure to attend follow-up appointments has been associated with a higher rate of developmental delay, discussions about the importance of follow-up appointments are ideally initiated prior to discharge from the neonatal intensive care unit (NICU).

At the initial visit, it is imperative to review the entire medical history and hospital course with the family. Ideally, the NICU should provide a discharge summary that includes the following information:

1. Birth weight, gestational age, and significant prenatal and perinatal information
2. An overview of the hospital course, including significant illnesses, events, surgical procedures, and pertinent radiographic studies
3. Nutrition information and present feeding regimen
4. A list of current medications, including dosing intervals and, if appropriate, serum drug levels
5. Immunizations given during the hospitalization
6. Pertinent laboratory data, such as most recent hemoglobin, newborn screening results, ophthalmologic and hearing screening information, neurosonogram and magnetic resonance imaging (MRI) results, and highest serum bilirubin level
7. Discharge physical examination, including most recent height, weight, and head circumference
8. Problems remaining at discharge
9. Follow-up appointments

Any significant complications or concerns should be discussed with parents as soon as possible to assess their understanding of these issues as well as expectations for improvement. Specifically, growth, nutrition, and developmental issues should be addressed at each visit (Questions Box). Adequate or desirable weight gain should be explained to caregivers in terms of the infant's current weight versus discharge weight. Infants younger than 6 months should gain, on average, 20 to 40 g/day. To ensure continued weight gain, many preterm infants are discharged from the NICU on a 24-hour feeding schedule, which requires that parents feed them at least every

Questions

Well-Child Care for Preterm Infants

- How much did the infant weigh when discharged from the hospital?
- Is the infant breastfed or formula-fed? Is the infant on any special formula?
- How often and how much does the infant feed? How long do feedings take?
- Does the infant have any feeding problems (eg, pain, vomiting, gastroesophageal reflux)?
- Does the infant take dietary supplementation of vitamins and minerals?
- What developmental milestones has the infant reached? Does the infant roll over? Smile? Sit up?
- Does the infant seem to hear and see?
- Who cares for the infant?
- Where and in what position does the child sleep?
- Do the parents have any concerns about growth, development, or nutrition?
- Is the infant on an apnea monitor? Have there been any apneic episodes?

3 hours. The necessity for this practice should be reevaluated during the first few weeks following discharge after infants have demonstrated adequate weight gain.

A critical component of the health maintenance visit is developmental history. Parental expectations and observations should be noted, and any developmental concerns should be evaluated. The adjusted developmental age should be calculated by subtracting the number of weeks the infant was born prematurely from his or her current chronologic age in weeks. The adjusted age should then be used for all formal and informal developmental assessments. The importance of correcting for prematurity until children are 2 years of age must be emphasized when discussing developmental progress and giving anticipatory guidance to parents.

Physical Examination

A complete physical examination should be performed at each visit to monitor the status of associated medical conditions. All growth parameters (weight, height, and head circumference) should be plotted on the growth chart for premature newborns until approximately 50 weeks' postmenstrual age and adjusted for prematurity on standard growth charts until age 2 years. Because catch-up head growth generally precedes catch-up weight and length, preterm infants may appear to have disproportionally large heads. The onset of accelerated head growth may begin within a few weeks after birth (36 weeks' postconception) or as late as 8 months adjusted age. Average daily weight gain in grams per day should also be calculated.

The size and shape of the head must be evaluated, especially if the infant has a history of intraventricular or intracranial hemorrhage or hydrocephalus. An increase in head circumference of more than 2 cm per week should be cause for concern in these infants. In infants who have been treated neurosurgically for hydrocephalus, ventriculoperitoneal shunt and tubing may be palpated. Visual abnormalities such as strabismus must be carefully ruled out by examination as well as by history because up to 20% of preterm infants may have an ophthalmologic problem (see Chapter 79). Oropharyngeal abnormalities, such as a palatal groove, high-arched palate, or abnormal tooth formation, may occur as a result of prolonged endotracheal intubation. Baseline intercostal, substernal, or subcostal retractions; wheezing; stridor; and tachypnea in former premature babies with moderate-to-severe bronchopulmonary dysplasia (BPD) should be documented. Infants with BPD are more susceptible to pulmonary infections leading to rehospitalization and may continue to exhibit poor lung function through adolescence.

Chest scars secondary to the placement of chest tubes should be noted. Adult female breasts may be affected if scarring occurs on or close to breast tissue. The umbilicus may appear hypoplastic as a result of umbilical catheter placement and suturing. Multiple scars on the heels from blood sampling or on the distal extremities from intravenous catheters and cutdowns may be evident.

The genitalia of male and female preterm infants should be examined closely for inguinal hernias. Because of concerns about adverse neurodevelopmental outcome in children exposed to general anesthesia in the first months of life and the high rates of postoperative apnea, inguinal hernia repair is often deferred until 60 weeks' corrected gestational age unless incarceration risk is deemed high. If hernias are surgically repaired under general anesthesia, infants should be monitored for apnea for up to 24 hours postoperatively. The male scrotum should be examined for cryptorchidism because only 25% of testes are in the scrotum of prematurely delivered males at term gestation. By 1 year of age, more than 90% of testes are intrascrotal. A careful evaluation for developmental dysplasia of the hip should be performed until children are ambulatory, and a hip ultrasound should be performed at 6 weeks of age for all breech deliveries (see Chapter 104).

A thorough neuromuscular examination is essential in these children. Increased muscular tone, asymmetry, and decreased bulk should be noted along with the presence of any clonus or asymmetry of deep tendon reflexes. Inappropriate reflexes, such as a persistent Moro or fisting beyond 4 months of age, should also be documented. Other abnormalities (eg, scissoring, sustained clonus) in the neurologic examination may become more apparent as infants become older. The detection of subtle early findings is important so appropriate intervention services can begin as soon as possible.

Laboratory Tests

In addition to the standard screening tests performed on all healthy infants and children during health maintenance visits, several laboratory studies are important in preterm infants. Such tests include a complete blood cell count and reticulocyte count to check for anemia; electrolytes in infants with BPD on diuretics to detect abnormalities; and serum calcium, phosphorus, and alkaline phosphatase levels in infants with documented metabolic bone disease of prematurity.

Pulse oximetry is indicated for oxygen-dependent infants as well as those presenting with respiratory symptoms greater than baseline. Results from newborn screening tests, including auditory and ophthalmologic examinations, should be reviewed and repeated as indicated. Cranial ultrasound studies should be reviewed with caution because nearly 40% of infants born weighing less than 1,000 g with normal head ultrasound findings develop cerebral palsy or developmental delay. In addition, infants with a grade 1 or 2 intracranial hemorrhage have an increased risk for developmental delay. Brain MRI scans should be considered in infants born at less than 30 weeks' gestation or in any infant with a concerning abnormal neurologic examination or abnormal rate of head growth.

Management

Well-child care in relatively healthy preterm infants has 2 components. One is the provision of routine health care maintenance for infants and appropriate developmental anticipatory guidance for parents. The other component involves the incorporation of treatment for chronic conditions into each visit. Health care maintenance should include the psychosocial well-being of the family, nutrition counseling, developmental surveillance, immunizations, and assessment of vision and hearing in addition to standard screening tests discussed previously. Outside resources concerning developmental delay can be reviewed with parents. Care related to chronic conditions includes adjusting medication doses, such as diuretic therapy; weaning from supplemental oxygen; and discontinuing the apnea monitor.

Anticipatory Guidance

Parents should be given anticipatory guidance prior to discharge that caring for a NICU graduate is challenging (Box 40-1). The American Academy of Pediatrics (AAP) recommends parental education as 1 of 6 critical components of discharge planning for any high-risk neonate and includes not only educating parents about the patient's care but also identifying an additional caregiver who can assist with the demands of caring for the child at home. Premature newborns have poorly organized sleep-wake cycles resulting in more frequent awaking than term newborns. In addition, premature newborns have immature suck-swallow coordination, causing them to feed more frequently and for longer periods. Colic is reported twice as frequently in VLBW infants relative to term newborns, and many are described as having difficult temperament until past their first birthday. Premature infants also develop gastroesophageal reflux more often than full-term infants, which presents with such symptoms as irritability, respiratory problems, and postprandial vomiting.

The medical costs associated with the care of premature infants often strain the family finances at a time when many women decrease

---

Box 40-1. Physician Support and Education of Parents With Preterm Infants

- Understand parental expectations.
- Legitimize parental fears.
- Be a source of support and encouragement.
- Provide consistent, honest information.
- Assume the role of the overall coordinator of care.
- Provide referrals to outside resources, including respite care.

their work schedules. Additional stressors include uncertainty about the long-term outcome of the child, guilt many women feel after delivering prematurely, and anxiety about future pregnancies. The difficulty of caring for these complicated, challenging children results in significant parental stress and can interfere with parents' ability to properly bond with their babies. Those delivering primary care should be alert to signs of a parent feeling overwhelmed, as a higher caregiving burden is associated with an increased incidence of child welfare reports such as child neglect.

Nutrition

According to the AAP Committee on Nutrition, the average daily energy requirement for most hospitalized healthy preterm newborns and infants is 105 to 130 kcal/kg/day to achieve adequate growth. Energy requirements vary with individual infants depending on associated chronic conditions, such as BPD or malabsorption. Key nutrients, such as calcium, vitamin D, and phosphorus, are critical to the management of bone health in preterm infants. Growth is considered adequate in the newborn weighing more than 2,000 g if weight gain is more than 20 g/day and length and head circumference increase 0.7 to 1.0 cm/week. Feeding difficulties are common in preterm infants and lead to hospital readmission secondary to failure to thrive, dehydration, and hyperbilirubinemia.

At 40 weeks' corrected age, preterm newborns are usually smaller than term newborns. Adequate nutrition in the first year of life is critical because catch-up weight gain is unlikely to occur after age 3 years. Because human milk is insufficient for providing adequate protein and micronutrients to preterm newborns, fortifier is added to human milk.

If not receiving human milk, children born at 34 weeks or sooner or weighing less than 1,500 g are usually discharged home on a nutritionally enhanced transitional formula (eg, Similac Expert Care Neo-Sure, Enfamil EnfaCare). The calcium, phosphorous, and caloric content of these 22 cal/oz transitional formulas are between levels found in standard preterm and term formulas. Use of preterm enriched formulas is usually continued until the child reaches the fifth to 10th percentile on the growth chart or is 1 year of adjusted age. A meta-analysis showed limited evidence to demonstrate nutrient-enriched formulas improve growth rates after discharge relative to standard term formula.

Formula-fed infants require multivitamin supplementation until 750 mL/day of formula is consumed. Breastfed premature infants may benefit from continuing multivitamin solution and supplementation of oral iron drops as long as human milk is the predominant source of nutrition. Vitamin D supplementation is recommended for all breastfed infants. Because premature newborns are at increased risk for metabolic bone disease of prematurity, soy formulas are to be avoided because of low phosphate content.

The introduction of solid foods is appropriate once infants have developed acceptable oral-motor skills for swallowing solids. Recent studies have suggested that 20% of parents of preterm infants report feeding problems at age 2 years. Cow's milk should not be introduced until 12 months' adjusted age.

Developmental Surveillance

Informal and formal developmental surveillance should include referral to an early intervention program, particularly for ELBW infants, because routine screening tests are not sensitive enough to pick up subtle neurodevelopmental abnormalities (Box 40-2; see Chapter 29). The Individuals with Disabilities Education Act Part C guarantees early intervention programs for infants and toddlers with disabilities up to age 3 years. Children born weighing less than 1,200 g are automatically eligible, but any child suspected of a developmental delay is entitled to an evaluation to determine eligibility for services regardless of a family's ability to pay. Because many developmental issues do not manifest until school age, frequent developmental assessments and enrollment in preschool are especially important for infants born prematurely.

The AAP recommends that autism spectrum disorder (ASD)–specific screenings be completed for all children at 18 to 24 months of age. The prevalence of ASDs has been reported to be 8% in children born at less than 26 weeks, much higher than reported for the general population. Premature newborns have higher scores on the Modified Checklist for Autism in Toddlers, with greater social-communication difficulties and autistic-like behaviors. These increased scores may be reflective of the increased incidence of neurodevelopmental delays in the former premature newborn population, making screening for ASDs more challenging.

Immunizations

Routine immunization schedules recommended by the Centers for Disease Control and Prevention (CDC) Advisory Committee on Immunization Practices should be followed. The administration of any vaccine is determined by the patient's chronologic or postnatal age, not gestational age. Standard doses and intervals should also be used (see Chapter 34). Several studies have shown an adequate serologic response despite a history of prematurity. Absolute and relative contraindications to specific vaccine components or to live vaccines for preterm infants are identical to published guidelines for term infants and children. In addition to following the recommendation that all infants 6 months and older be vaccinated against influenza, all household contacts of premature newborns should also be strongly urged to be vaccinated. Two doses of influenza vaccine are administered 1 month apart, with subsequent immunization the following year only requiring one dose. Because the rotavirus vaccination utilizes a live virus, it is recommended only for clinically stable premature newborns if they are 6 to 14 weeks' chronologic age at discharge or have already been discharged from the NICU.

If adequate weight gain has been established, it is safe to administer hepatitis B vaccine to medically stable infants weighing less than 2,000 g as early as 30 days of age or at discharge, whichever comes first. All neonates born to mothers who are hepatitis B surface antigen positive should receive hepatitis B vaccine and hepatitis B immunoglobulin (HBIG) within 12 hours of delivery. When maternal hepatitis B status is unknown, neonates weighing less than 2,000 g should receive HBIG within 12 hours, neonates weighing more than 2,000 g should receive HBIG within 7 days, and all should be vaccinated for hepatitis B within 12 hours.

The CDC recommends that all pregnant women receive the tetanus, diphtheria, acellular pertussis (Tdap) vaccination to help protect their newborns against pertussis. Maternal vaccination results in higher concentrations of pertussis antibodies in newborns compared with unvaccinated mothers, possibly leading to increased protection from pertussis during the critical period between birth and the first diphtheria, tetanus, acellular pertussis (DTaP) dose.

Because respiratory syncytial virus (RSV) causes an increased morbidity and mortality in NICU graduates and infants with congenital heart disease, administration of RSV-specific immunoglobulin, palivizumab (eg, Synagis), is recommended every month from November to March (Box 40-3). A documented infection with RSV is not an indication to discontinue passive immunization because multiple strains may circulate during the RSV season.

Assessment of Vision and Hearing

Follow-up visits for visual and auditory sequelae of prematurity must be arranged at the health maintenance visit. An initial ophthalmologic screening examination should have been performed between 4 and 9 weeks of age in infants weighing less than 1,500 g or less than 30 weeks' gestation, irrespective of oxygen exposure. Infants between 1,500 and 2,000 g or greater than 30 weeks' gestation with an unstable clinical course should also be screened. The frequency and need for repeat examinations are determined based on initial findings. Preterm infants, regardless of the presence of retinopathy of prematurity, are at increased risk for the development of strabismus, myopia, amblyopia, and glaucoma and need an ophthalmologic examination

---

Box 40-2. Typical Speech, Play, and Physical Development

In addition to standardized tests, the following guidelines provide development milestones useful for early detection:

By 3 months' adjusted age, the infant

- Coos or vocalizes other than crying
- Visually tracks a moving toy from side to side
- Attempts to reach for a rattle held above chest
- Pushes up on arms
- Lifts and holds head up

At 6 months' adjusted age, the infant

- Begins to use consonant sounds in babbling and uses to get attention
- Reaches for a nearby toy while on tummy
- Transfers a toy from one hand to the other while lying on back
- Reaches both hands to play with feet while lying on back
- Uses hands to support self in sitting
- While standing with support, accepts entire weight with legs

At 9 months' adjusted age, the infant

- Increases variety of sounds and syllable combinations in babbling
- Looks at familiar objects and people when named
- Explores and examines an object using both hands
- Turns several pages of a chunky book at once
- Imitates others in simple play
- Sits and reaches for toys without falling

At 12 months' adjusted age, the child

- Meaningfully uses "mama" or "dada"
- Responds to simple commands (eg, "come here")
- Produces long strings of gibberish in social communication
- Finger feeds self
- Uses thumb and pointer finger to pick up tiny objects
- Pulls to stand and cruise along furniture
- Stands alone and takes several independent steps

At 15 months' adjusted age, the child

- Has a vocabulary consisting of 5–10 words
- Helps with getting undressed
- Walks independently and seldom falls
- Squats to pick up toy

At 24 months' adjusted age, the child

- Uses 2- to 4-word sentences
- Walks up and down stairs holding on for support
- Builds a tower of 4 blocks or more
- Identifies basic body parts

Modified with permission from Pathways Awareness Foundation. *Assure the Best for your Baby's Physical Development.* http://pathways.org/images/stories/Brochures/english%20brochure.pdf. Accessed February 21, 2014; and Centers for Disease Control and Prevention. Developmental milestones. http://www.cdc.gov/ncbddd/actearly/milestones/index.html. Accessed February 21, 2014.

Box 40-3. Indications for the Use of Palivizumab for Respiratory Syncytial Virus Prophylaxis

Condition	Age at Onset of RSV Season
Preterm infants with chronic lung disease requiring medical management • Oxygen • Bronchodilator • Diuretics • Chronic corticosteroids	<24 mo
Hemodynamically significant congenital heart disease • Cyanotic • Moderate to severe pulmonary hypertension	<24 mo
Significant congenital abnormalities of the airway or neuromuscular disease that compromises handling of respiratory secretions	<12 mo
Born ≤28 wk gestation	<12 mo
Born 29–31 wk 6 d gestation	<6 mo
Born 32–34 wk 6 d gestation with at least 1 of 2 risk factors • Attending child care • Sibling <5 y in the home	<3 mo

Abbreviation: RSV, respiratory syncytial virus.

between 4 and 6 months of age. Because birth before 28 weeks is associated with an increased risk of retinal detachment later in childhood and early adult life, long-term follow-up to detect and treat late-onset retinal detachment should be considered.

The AAP recommends universal hearing screening for all newborns. Neonatal intensive care unit graduates account for approximately 50% of all newborn hearing screening failures, and severe sensorineural hearing loss occurs in up to 10% of ELBW infants. Screening is recommended immediately prior to discharge, and repeat testing is recommended if speech delays develop.

Other Potential Problems

Preterm infants with chronic lung disease are at increased risk for respiratory illness, especially during the winter. Parents should be informed of this risk and counseled about symptoms such as tachypnea and wheezing associated with a simple upper respiratory infection. Physicians should have a low threshold for considering a diagnosis of pneumonia in these infants in the appropriate clinical setting.

Primary care physicians should also keep in mind that preterm infants are at increased risk for sudden infant death syndrome (SIDS; see Chapter 61). The AAP recommends that all infants sleep in the supine position. In the NICU, neonates are often placed on their stomachs if they have respiratory difficulties and on their sides if they have symptomatic gastroesophageal reflux. Neonatal intensive care unit personnel need to begin placing these babies on their backs in anticipation of discharge. Parents should also be reminded that bed sharing is not recommended and is highly associated with sudden infant death from accidental asphyxia.

Home apnea monitors are not associated with the prevention of SIDS and should be reserved for infants who are considered to have extreme cardiorespiratory instability. Discontinuation of home monitoring may be considered at 42 weeks' postmenstrual age and when significant apneic events have ceased, whichever comes later.

Preterm survivors who were critically ill can be particularly at risk for developing **vulnerable child syndrome** because their parents often perceive them as fragile and vulnerable. Features of this syndrome include abnormal separation difficulties for mother and child, sleep difficulties, parental overprotectiveness and overindulgence, lack of appropriate discipline, tolerance of physical abusiveness by the child toward the parent, and excessive preoccupation with the child's health. Serious behavioral problems may arise as a result of such parent-child interactions, and recent studies suggest higher parental perception of child vulnerability correlated with worse developmental outcomes. Primary care physicians must be cognizant of early signs of this syndrome and should try to prevent its occurrence by reassuring parents about the child's well-being. Once vulnerable child syndrome is suspected, connecting the child's history of critical illness with ongoing parent concerns is important as many parents are unaware that current concerns may stem from their unresolved anxiety. Every effort should be made to normalize the family's schedule once the infant is stable and to encourage parent-child interactions unrelated to health care.

Prognosis

Neurodevelopmental impairment is a concern for physicians who care for preterm infants. Risk factors for developmental delay include postnatal steroid exposure, necrotizing enterocolitis, BPD, and small for gestational age. Chorioamnionitis is a risk factor for cerebral palsy in term infants and possibly in infants born prematurely. Extremely low birth weight infants and those born between 20 and 25 weeks' gestation have significant risk for developmental issues. Surviving infants born at less than 26 weeks' gestation in the United Kingdom in 1995 had median Bayley mental and psychomotor scores at 30 months of age of 80, with comparable cognitive score deficits at age 6 years. Furthermore, an assessment of the effect of extremely preterm birth on academic attainment at age 11 years demonstrated a higher prevalence of learning difficulties, including lower reading and mathematics scores, than in term peers.

During adolescence, 50% of former VLBW infants will have an IQ in an abnormally low range, and 30% will have ADHD. Though former premature newborns experience higher rates of chronic medical and neurodevelopmental problems, their self-perception of health and well-being in adolescence, relative to their normal birth weight peers, was the same. In addition, increased systolic blood pressure, insulin resistance, and impaired glucose tolerance has also been reported in VLBW adults. Parents should also understand that long-term follow-up information may not accurately reflect the outcome for their child because these adolescents were managed prior to advances in prenatal and neonatal care.

CASE RESOLUTION

In the case presented at the beginning of the chapter, the infant's current feeding schedule should be continued because appropriate weight gain has occurred. Iron and multivitamin supplementation is recommended until 750 mL/day of formula is consumed. Discontinuation of the apnea monitor can be considered after the infant reaches term gestation and has been event-free. The first set of immunizations should be administered at this visit, and any questions the family has should be answered. A follow-up visit should be scheduled in 3 to 4 weeks. Formal developmental testing should be arranged in 1 to 2 months, and the parents should be encouraged to continue having the infant sleep on her back.

Selected References

Abrams SA; American Academy of Pediatrics Committee on Nutrition. Calcium and vitamin D requirements of enterally fed preterm infants. *Pediatrics.* 2013;131(5):e1676–e1683

American Academy of Pediatrics. *Pediatric Nutrition.* Kleinman RE, ed. 7th ed. Elk Grove Village, IL: American Academy of Pediatrics; 2014

American Academy of Pediatrics. *Red Book: 2012 Report of the Committee on Infectious Diseases.* Pickering LK, ed. 29th ed. Elk Grove Village, IL: American Academy of Pediatrics; 2012

American Academy of Pediatrics Committee on Fetus and Newborn. Hospital discharge of the high-risk neonate. *Pediatrics.* 2008;122(5):1119–1126

American Academy of Pediatrics Section on Ophthalmology, American Academy of Ophthalmology, American Association for Pediatric Ophthalmology and

Strabismus, American Association of Certified Orthoptists. Screening examination of premature infants for retinopathy of prematurity. *Pediatrics*. 2013;131(1):189–195

American Academy of Pediatrics Task Force on Sudden Infant Death Syndrome. The changing concept of sudden infant death syndrome: diagnostic coding shifts, controversies regarding the sleeping environment, and new variables to consider in reducing risk. *Pediatrics*. 2005;116(5):1245–1255

Ballantyne M, Stevens B, Guttmann A, Willan AR, Rosenbaum P. Transition to neonatal follow-up programs: is attendance a problem? *J Perinat Neonatal Nurs*. 2012;26(1):90–98

Bonamy AK, Holmström G, Stephansson O, Ludvigsson JF, Cnattingius S. Preterm birth and later retinal detachment: a population-based cohort study of more than 3 million children and young adults. *Ophthalmology*. 2013;120(11):2278–2285

Cortese MM, Parashar UD; Centers for Disease Control and Prevention. Prevention of rotavirus gastroenteritis among infants and children: recommendations of the Advisory Committee on Immunization Practices (ACIP). *MMWR Recomm Rep*. 2009;58(RR-2):1–25

Hack M, Flannery DJ, Schluchter M, Cartar L, Borawski E, Klein N. Outcomes in young adulthood for very-low-birth-weight infants. *N Engl J Med*. 2002;346(3):149–157

Hovi P, Andersson S, Eriksson JG, et al. Glucose regulation in young adults with very low birth weight. *N Engl J Med*. 2007;356(20):2053–2063

Institute of Medicine. *Preterm Birth: Causes, Consequences and Prevention*. Behrman RE, Butler AS, eds. Washington, DC: National Academies Press; 2007

Johnson S, Wolke D, Hennessy E, Marlow N. Educational outcomes in extremely preterm children: neuropsychological correlates and predictors of attainment. *Dev Neuropsychol*. 2011;36(1):74–95

Kelly KB, Ponsky TA. Pediatric abdominal wall defects. *Surg Clin North Am*. 2013;93(5):1255–1267

LaHood A, Bryant CA. Outpatient care of the premature infant. *Am Fam Physician*. 2007;76(8):1159–1164

Lapillonne A, O'Connor DL, Wang D, Rigo J. Nutritional recommendations for the late-preterm infant and the preterm infant after hospital discharge. *J Pediatr*. 2013;162(3 Suppl):S90–S100

Marlow N, Wolke D, Bracewell MA, Samara M; EPICure Study Group. Neurologic and developmental disability at six years of age after extremely preterm birth. *N Engl J Med*. 2005;352(1):9–19

Martin JA, Hamilton BE, Ventura SJ, Osteran M, Wilson EC, Mathews TJ. Births: final data for 2011. *National Vital Statistics Report*. 2013;62(1)

Melville JM, Moss TJ. The immune consequence of preterm birth. *Front Neurosci*. 2013;7:79

Moster D, Lie RT, Markestad T. Long-term medical and social consequences of preterm birth. *N Engl J Med*. 2008;359(3):262–273

Nandyal R, Owora A, Risch E, Bard D, Bonner B, Chaffin M. Special care needs and risk for child maltreatment reports among babies that graduated from the neonatal intensive care. *Child Abuse Negl*. 2013;37(12):1114–1121

Tyson JE, Parikh NA, Langer J, Green C, Higgins RD; National Institute of Child Health and Human Development Neonatal Research Network. Intensive care for extreme prematurity—moving beyond gestational age. *N Engl J Med*. 2008;358(16):1672–1681

Wang KS; American Academy of Pediatrics Committeee on Fetus and Newborn, Section on Surgery. Assessment and management of inguinal hernia in infants. *Pediatrics*. 2012;130(4):768–773

Wood NS, Marlow N, Costeloe K, Gibson AT, Wilkinson AR. Neurologic and developmental disability after extremely preterm birth. EPICure Study Group. *N Engl J Med*. 2000;343(6):378–384

Woodward LJ, Anderson PJ, Austin NC, Howard K, Inder TE. Neonatal MRI to predict neurodevelopmental outcomes in preterm infants. *N Engl J Med*. 2006;355(7):685–694

Young L, Morgan J, McCormick FM, McGuire W. Nutrient-enriched formula versus standard term formula for preterm infants following hospital discharge. *Cochrane Database Syst Rev*. 2012;3:CD004696

CHAPTER 41

Care of Children With Special Health Care Needs

Julie E. Noble, MD

CASE STUDY

A 5-year-old girl with a physical disability is brought to your office for her first visit for a routine physical examination for school entrance. She was the result of a full-term pregnancy complicated by an elevated screening α-fetoprotein and a subsequent fetal ultrasound that demonstrated a lumbar myelomeningocele and no hydrocephalus. Delivery was elective cesarean with Apgar scores of 9 at 1 minute and 9 at 5 minutes to a 25-year-old gravida 1, para 0–1 mother. The mother used no illicit drugs, alcohol, or any other medications during pregnancy but was not on vitamins or folate supplementation at the time of conception. At delivery, a low lumbar spinal malformation was noted without other malformations. The quadriceps muscles were strong, but the feet demonstrated a rocker-bottom deformity.

Shortly after birth the myelomeningocele malformation was closed by neurosurgery. The girl has had orthopedic surgical release of Achilles tendon contractions and is ambulatory with ankle-foot orthotics. She has a neurogenic bladder and requires intermittent catheterization.

She also has chronic constipation treated with a bowel regimen. Her cognitive function is age-appropriate.

She will be entering a school program for the first time since moving to this community and has not established care with any specialists.

Questions

1. Why is early identification and intervention important for newborns, infants, and children with special health care needs (SHCN)?
2. What are the unique needs of newborns, infants, and children with SHCN?
3. What role do primary care practitioners play in the care of children with SHCN?
4. What are the appropriate referrals and resources for families of children with SHCN?
5. What specific psychosocial issues should be addressed whenever children with SHCN visit their primary care practitioners?

Children and youth with special health care needs (SHCN) have physical, developmental, emotional, or behavioral conditions that require special health-related services. These conditions must last longer than 1 year and have 1 of 5 consequences: prescription medications; increased medical care; mental health or educational limited ability; special therapy; or counseling. Children with SHCN are defined by the International Classification of Functioning, Disability and Health as *disabled* if they are limited from doing what children of the same age can do. Most information on children with SHCN combines the group with and the group without disabilities. These conditions can range from mild to severe, depending on the nature and extent of the conditions and their effect on daily living. Frequently, care requirements of families and health care professionals for children diagnosed as having SHCN are dramatically increased. For parents, the diagnosis of a condition in their child can be initially overwhelming and disappointing. Support of the parents is essential as they transition from disappointment to acceptance and assume the role of facilitator of their child's treatment plans.

Early identification of a health condition by physicians can lead to appropriate, definitive treatment for many diagnoses. Early intervention can sometimes even prevent secondary conditions (eg, early management of hearing loss with hearing aids may minimize speech abnormalities). Even when such corrective treatment is not available, prompt identification improves children's long-term outcome and allows families to obtain appropriate resources for their children. Through early intervention, newborns, infants, and children with irreversible conditions can be introduced to medical, educational, and psychosocial services available in the community that serve to help each child maximize and reach his or her full potential.

Epidemiology

The prevalence of children in the United States with SHCN is difficult to assess. Studies report that approximately 17% of children younger than 17 years have at least one medical condition, including deafness or hearing loss, blindness, cerebral palsy, physical malformations, speech impediments, developmental delay, and other learning problems. Comorbid conditions, such as epilepsy, and secondary conditions, such as behavior problems, have a very high incidence. An estimated 30% of children with disabilities have more than one disability. A single sensory disability, such as deafness, affects approximately 3.5% of children; blindness occurs in 1% of children. The prevalence of cerebral palsy is 1.5 to 2 per 1,000 live births. Advances in medical technology, as well as improved survival of low birth weight newborns and children with malformations, have increased the number of children living with such disabilities. When mental health issues and obesity are added, the incidence of SHCN increases to 22.3% of US children (2007 data). Environmental exposures have also increased the incidence of chronic medical conditions such as asthma.

The presence of SHCN has a profound effect on the health and education of affected children. Studies show that children with SHCN have 1.5 times more doctor visits and spend 3.5 more days in the hospital than children without these conditions. Children in this group miss twice the number of school days and are twice as likely to repeat a grade compared with children without medical conditions.

In addition, numerous associated conditions occur more commonly in children with SHCN. These include mental retardation, growth failure, and nutrition problems. Problems with dentition, respiratory infections, and bowel and bladder continence may also develop. Significant emotional disturbances may occur as a child adapts to his or her condition.

Clinical Presentation

Children with SCHN can present in a variety of ways depending on their diagnosis. Many physical disabilities may be readily apparent at birth on the newborn examination or through newborn screening. Some diagnoses, such as cerebral palsy, may be detected later, as the motor impairment becomes more evident. Following development at routine health maintenance visits is essential for early detection of developmental delay. Implementing the Bright Futures program from the American Academy of Pediatrics (AAP) can help in early detection of many conditions. Children with SHCN can also present with chronic illness, such as asthma or diabetes, or with specific complaints, such as poor vision or hearing. Their presentation may be for a more general concern, such as growth failure (D_x Box).

Dx **Children With Physical and Sensory Disabilities[a]**

- Growth failure
- Microcephaly
- Abnormal neurologic examination, including hypertonicity, spastic diplegia or quadriplegia, and brisk deep tendon reflexes
- Developmental delay
- Speech or hearing deficit
- Visual deficit
- Physical malformations

[a]May not be present in all children.

Behavioral problems or difficulties in school may precipitate the initial visit.

Pathophysiology

Pathophysiology of a medical condition is totally dependent on the specific diagnosis. Conditions may be secondary to an embryologic defect, such as myelomeningocele, or an infection, such as congenital cytomegalovirus (CMV), which interferes with cochlear development and leads to hearing loss. Etiologies are often multifactorial. For some conditions, such as autism spectrum disorders (ASDs), the pathophysiology is unknown and may have several different etiologies.

Special health care needs may be classified as *acquired* or *congenital* and *static* or *progressive*. **Cerebral palsy,** for example, is a group of nonprogressive neuromotor disorders resulting from a central nervous system insult prenatally or in the first 2 years of life. It is characterized by abnormal motor movements and posturing and may be accompanied by other problems. Causes of cerebral palsy include prematurity, low birth weight, asphyxia, prenatal abnormalities (eg, placental insufficiency), congenital infections (eg, toxoplasmosis, CMV), and biochemical abnormalities (eg, severe hyperbilirubinemia). Other causes are environmental (eg, alcohol) and genetic (eg, inborn errors of metabolism). Severe postnatal injuries or infections can also lead to cerebral palsy (eg, abusive head trauma, meningitis). However, an estimated 25% to 50% of cases of cerebral palsy have no discernible cause.

Diagnosis

The term **SHCN** is used in a broad sense to include conditions that require additional medical care and supervision. It was defined by the US Department of Health and Human Services Maternal and Child Health Bureau. As previously noted, children that fall into the group of having SHCN may have significant physical, sensory, or developmental disabilities that may result from prematurity, congenital infections such as CMV, or exposure in utero to alcohol or illicit substances. Some children are born with congenital malformations or inborn errors of metabolism that mandate special diets and occupational or physical therapy. Other children with SHCN include those with chronic medical conditions such as asthma, obesity, and sickle cell anemia. All of these medical conditions alter lifestyle, require increased medical care including subspecialty care, increase medication usage, and use community services beyond the general pediatric population.

Evaluation

History

When initially evaluating children with newly diagnosed SHCN, practitioners should first determine any specific parental concerns. A complete medical history should be obtained, including information about the pregnancy and birth. The history should also include any possible exposures as well as significant infections. General screening questions about development are important to ask (Questions Box) so that the child's developmental progress can be assessed. Specific questioning is warranted if parents are concerned about delayed development or if any of their responses indicate that their child is not attaining age-appropriate developmental milestones.

In cases of children with known sensory or physical disabilities, families should be asked directly at each visit about daily activities and the child's ability for self-help skills. Because many children with disabilities are also on daily medication for seizures or other chronic conditions, it is important to ask about the presence of any drug side effects.

Behavioral or emotional problems that the child might be having should be identified. In addition, an overall assessment of family dynamics should be made. It is important to inquire about the relationships between children with SHCN and their siblings, as well as the effect these children have on the parents' marriage/relationship.

Physical Examination

In general, a complete physical examination, including an oral health assessment and a detailed neurologic assessment and neuromotor examination, should be performed at each visit. Height, weight, and head circumference should be plotted on the growth chart and compared with previous measurements. Failure of adequate growth as measured by any of these parameters should be examined closely. For example, microcephaly, nutritional problems, and growth failure are not uncommon in children with cerebral palsy. Depending on the specific diagnosis, the examination

should focus on physical findings associated with the particular condition. For children with physical disabilities such as congenital or acquired amputations, for instance, assessment of the skin that comes in contact with prosthetic devices is a pertinent aspect of the physical examination. Pressure sores may be found in nonambulatory children with cerebral palsy. In children with sensory disabilities such as unilateral hearing loss, the evaluation of middle ear effusion or infection in the unaffected ear should be a priority. If a child has a tracheostomy or gastrostomy tube, inspection of the site is essential at each visit to look for erosions or skin infections.

Overall, for most children with SHCN, the neurologic examination is extremely important. The following questions should be addressed: Are normal primitive reflexes such as Moro and rooting reflexes present in neonates? Have all primitive reflexes been extinguished in older children? Do newborns and infants appear to visualize and track objects appropriately? Are there any abnormal movements of the trunk or extremities at rest? Is muscle tone normal? Is any hypertonicity or hypotonicity evident? Is any asymmetry of the upper and lower extremities apparent? Are deep tendon reflexes normal and symmetrical? Is the gait appropriate for age?

An age-appropriate developmental assessment is also an essential part of the examination at all health maintenance visits.

Laboratory Tests

Laboratory evaluation of newborns, infants, and children with physical or sensory disabilities depends on their specific conditions. Not all patients need a costly array of diagnostic procedures. A **chromosomal karyotype or comparative genomic hybridization** using peripheral blood is helpful in children with suspected genetic disorders (eg, abnormal facies, a major anomaly and developmental delay). Routine testing for fragile X syndrome in all boys with mental health disabilities and in girls with a family history should be strongly considered. Other testing should be specific, relating to the suspected diagnosis (see Chapter 72).

Metabolic screening for inborn errors of metabolism should be performed on children with mental health disabilities and any of the following symptoms: intermittent vomiting or lethargy, loss of developmental milestones, or seizures. Such screening is not needed in the routine evaluation of children with developmental delay and no other symptoms.

A screening test for visual acuity (Snellen test) and hearing (audiogram) should be performed in all children suspected of having sensory deficits, even mild ones. For infants or toddlers, a brain stem auditory evoked response or behavioral audiogram is a more appropriate screening test for hearing. A visual evoked response can be performed to test vision.

Psychometric testing may be helpful in certain school-aged children to assess intellectual function.

An electroencephalogram is indicated in all patients who have a history of seizures or seizure-like episodes.

Questions

Children With Special Health Care Needs

- Were there any perinatal complications, such as premature rupture of membranes or fetal distress?
- Was the child born prematurely? If so, how long did the child remain in the hospital and for what reasons?
- Was the child exposed to any toxins (eg, alcohol, illicit drugs) in utero?
- Is there any history of infection during the perinatal period or infancy?
- What developmental milestones has the child mastered?
- Is the child attending school or some type of early intervention program?
- How does the child get there?
- What does the child do on returning from school?
- Who feeds and bathes the child?
- Can the older child use the toilet without assistance?
- How is the child sleeping? Does the child take naps at school and home?
- Has respite care been arranged for the family?
- Does the caregiver seem overwhelmed or excessively tired, especially one who is caring for a child with multiple disabilities?
- Do other family members help care for the child?
- Is extended family available to help with siblings?
- Are there any other people with disabilities in the family?
- Does the family receive any financial assistance for care of the child?

Imaging Studies

Brain imaging studies, such as magnetic resonance imaging scans of the head, can be informative when intrauterine infection, intraventricular hemorrhage, or genetic disorders with associated developmental delay and even isolated global developmental delay are suspected. An electromyogram can be used to differentiate cerebral palsy from a congenital myopathy.

Management

Caring for children with SHCN can be a rewarding and challenging task for primary care pediatricians. The pediatrician should be cognizant that these patients will take increased practice time and paperwork to ensure that they receive all services necessary. Case management services are an essential aid to their management. The primary care pediatrician needs to supervise acute and chronic medical care, provide anticipatory guidance, monitor growth and development, coordinate subspecialty involvement, make educational referrals, and offer community services. Sometimes a subspecialist will provide comprehensive care if the diagnosis, such as cystic fibrosis, encompasses most of the child's health care needs. Although all cases should be handled individually, general guidelines have been developed for the provision of pediatric services for newborns, infants, and children with SHCN. They include recommendations for establishing a medical home with the primary care pediatrician, medical services, suggestions for parental involvement, assistance from community agencies, and fulfillment of specific federal requirements for educational opportunities for children with disabilities. Pediatricians who care for children with SHCN should be familiar with the principles of care, published by the AAP, and should incorporate these principles into the overall treatment plan. Pediatricians should also be knowledgeable about the rights of such individuals as established by various legislation, including the Americans with Disabilities Act and the Individuals with Disabilities Education Act Part C. Coordination of intervention services and the use of adaptive or assistive technology are essential components of management.

General Considerations

The major role of primary care pediatricians who care for children with SHCN is 4-fold: provide primary medical care; serve as the patient and family advocate in evaluating therapeutic options; inform families of available community resources; and most importantly, serve as a proactive coordinator of care. The first task of the pediatrician is to establish the diagnosis and recognize comorbid conditions. Whether the diagnosis is an obvious physical malformation or one that is not readily apparent, physicians are placed in the challenging position of breaking the news to families. Parents should be informed of the diagnosis as soon as possible, but care should be taken to refrain from discussing the prognosis, especially if it is still unknown. The cause of any disability and the possible complications of the condition should be reviewed with parents. *The primary goal is to help children with disabilities reach their full potential.*

Health care professionals are in a unique position to establish a treatment plan with families that includes medical, psychosocial, and educational services. A multidisciplinary team that includes the pediatrician, a member of the school system, a social worker, and a representative of an early intervention program should be identified. Federally funded, nonprofit, regional centers can provide an organized treatment plan and entry into an early intervention program to some children with disabilities. To qualify, children must be diagnosed with an eligible condition, such as cerebral palsy, epilepsy, ASDs, or global developmental delay. In addition, newborns and infants considered at risk for developing disabilities qualify for assistance (eg, premature newborns with bronchopulmonary dysplasia and intraventricular hemorrhage). For children who do not qualify, similar services can be coordinated on an individual basis by the physician's office or the school district.

Children with severe physical and sensory disabilities are often cared for by many medical subspecialists in addition to primary care pediatricians. Referrals to pediatric orthopedic surgeons, plastic surgeons, geneticists, ophthalmologists, otolaryngologists, child neurologists, and psychologists may be necessary. Special comprehensive clinics, such as craniofacial or spina bifida, are established in some children's referral centers to facilitate care of patients, with multiple subspecialists forming a multidisciplinary team in the same clinic setting. In addition, speech and language, occupational, and physical therapists are often an integral part of the medical team. Initial and ongoing therapeutic services provided by each of these individuals must be monitored periodically to assess the progress and overall effectiveness of the treatment plan. Ideally, services should be coordinated so that children as well as parents miss a minimum number of school days and workdays (eg, Saturday and after-school appointments, visits to several practitioners on one day). All information from diagnostic studies and initial evaluations should be shared among each of the health care practitioners. The AAP has produced a *Building Your Medical Home* toolkit (www.pediatricmedhome.org), which can be very helpful to the primary pediatrician.

The primary care physician should also offer counseling to parents on ethical issues as they pertain to their child's condition. These issues include palliative care decisions, decision-making in critical care situations, limiting non-beneficial interventions at the end of life, and advance directives. Because of the pediatrician's relationship with the family, he or she may be in the best position to engage parents in conversations concerning these topics. Coordinated conferences with the primary care physician, specialists, social workers, and the family may be effective in counseling.

The family has a vital role in caring for the child with SHCN, and that care can frequently be stressful and emotionally draining. Family support and counseling should be readily available. The sociocultural context of the family and needs of the other children in the family should to be considered when the care of the child with SHCN is addressed.

With improved medical care and services, 90% of children with SHCN reach adulthood. Transition into adult services can be challenging. Preparation for this transition should begin as early as

11 years of age to ensure success. The goal should be independence to the degree that is possible. The individual should be prepared for a work environment if possible and financial independence. The family and child should be evaluated to determine whether the child is capable of independent living or will need support in a group home or an institution or to remain with the family. If necessary, guardianship issues must be addressed. A successful transition to adult health care professionals must be ensured, and insurance coverage must be arranged. The Patient Protection and Affordable Care Act of 2009 has greatly improved insurance coverage for these patients, including extending the age of coverage for dependent children until 26 years, preventing exclusion from coverage based on preexisting conditions, and prohibiting lifetime caps on medical expenses.

Psychologic Concerns

Children with SHCN have more mental health issues than their peers. These conditions include behavioral problems, depression, anxiety, low self-esteem, peer relationship problems, school performance problems, and absenteeism. Children with SHCN that include a disability have even higher rates of psychologic comorbidity. It is important that primary care physicians screen for these disorders and refer for counseling when appropriate.

Economic Concerns

The cost of care for children with SHCN places a significant financial burden for as many as 40% of these families in the United States. Families with an affected child are more likely to have a single income, have a single parent, live in poverty, and have poor-quality housing. Economic evaluation should be performed by caseworkers to determine the eligibility of children with SHCN for financial support through Supplemental Security Income and medical insurance under Medicaid. Caseworkers can then assist families to apply for the appropriate assistance or to other programs such as the Supplemental Nutrition Assistance Program and the Low Income Home Energy Assistance Program, which can help extend a family's resources.

It is apparent that children with SHCN from low-income families have decreased access to health, educational, and social services. Recent studies have been undertaken to determine the best strategy to improve access to services and availability of services for underserved communities. It is recognized that early intervention services can decrease the economic burden of these patients and their families.

Specific Medical Conditions

A number of medical conditions commonly occur in children with moderate to severe disabilities. While providing children with comprehensive well-child care, general pediatricians can also address and treat these conditions.

Problems with adequate nutrition, which usually result from insufficient caloric intake, are manifested by growth failure. Depending on the degree of disability and amount of oropharyngeal dysfunction, the placement of a nasogastric or gastrostomy tube may be necessary. Caloric needs may be 10% to 50% higher than normal basal needs to ensure growth.

Respiratory illness is not uncommon among these children. Close observation and conservative treatment of viral illnesses are often necessary. Aspiration pneumonia is likely to occur, especially in children with severe developmental delay because of poor handling of oral secretions or severe oral dyspraxia. To help minimize respiratory infections, influenza vaccine should always be administered during the winter months.

Maintaining good oral hygiene is another challenge because some children with disabilities do not clear oral secretions well and retain food in their mouths, predisposing to cavity development. In addition, many children are treated with anticonvulsants and antibiotics that can cause gingival and enamel dysplasia. Abnormal oromotor coordination, tone, and posturing also contribute to the development of oropharyngeal deformities, such as high-arched palate and overcrowded teeth. As with other children, fluoride supplementation and consistent preventive dental care are recommended.

Bowel and bladder continence is important to attain for several reasons. It allows children to function in a socially acceptable fashion, provides independence, and prevents the development of complications such as recurrent urinary tract infections, diaper dermatitis, and decubitus pressure sores. Behavior modification techniques coupled with positive reinforcement are associated with complete or partial success for bowel training.

Community Resources

Optimal care for children with SHCN depends on maximum use of community agencies and resources. An assessment of parental and patient needs should first be performed and prioritized. The appropriate resources should then be identified for individual children. Early intervention services should be used. Primary care physicians may need to help determine the appropriateness of specific services for patients and families. Emphasis should be placed on integrating each child into support services. Parent-to-parent support and support groups can be very helpful in relieving stress, helping parents to understand the diagnosis, and avoiding feelings of isolation. Support groups for siblings as well as parents are available. Respite care to give parents a break from caregiving and in-home health service programs should also be investigated. Hospice care in the home is now available for children near the end of life; it can be an excellent support for the patient and family. Physicians should act as liaisons between all agencies. Case conferences are occasionally necessary to review the progress of individual children with each member of the health care team.

Education

By federal law, every child with a disability is entitled to an education. Every effort should be made to enroll children with disabilities in conventional schools and to provide opportunities for socialization at an early age. The concepts of structured independence and mainstreaming, the placement of children with disabilities in classes with children who are not disabled, can be very productive for a child as well as his or her schoolmates.

Mainstreaming may not be available in some areas, and the severity of some disabilities may not allow attendance on a regular school campus. Several other educational possibilities can be considered, and each case should be evaluated on an individual basis. Options include special education classes in designated schools (full or part time), special education classes in regular schools (full or part time), part-time special education classes and part-time regular classes, or home education. The decision can be facilitated through the development of an Individual Education Plan by a multidisciplinary team at the school. Parents and primary care physicians are encouraged to participate in this evaluation (see Chapter 33).

Prognosis

The prognosis for children with SHCN is dependent on the diagnosis, severity and extent of any disability, medical and supportive intervention, and environment of the child. It may be impossible to establish a prognosis at the time of diagnosis. Children can adapt differently to the same diagnosis. It is important to establish realistic goals to determine the best intervention. With comprehensive care, many affected children are able to lead productive, independent lives, and maximal potential can be realized in all cases.

CASE RESOLUTION

Although the girl's medical condition of low lumbar spina bifida seems stable, the physician should inquire about any ongoing problems or concerns. A complete examination should be done. Routine screening laboratory tests and immunizations required for school entry should be performed. The family should be evaluated for financial stability and support services. The mother should be placed on folate supplementation for prevention of recurrence in future children. The patient should be referred to the local spina bifida clinic for comprehensive specialist care by orthopedists, urologists, and physical therapists. Integration into the regular classroom should be recommended. The school should be contacted to arrange for adaptive physical education and for intermittent catheterization by school nursing personnel. A follow-up visit is scheduled with the primary care physician in 2 months to review the child's integration into services.

Selected References

Adams RC, Tapia CA; American Academy of Pediatrics Council on Children With Disabilities. Early intervention, IDEA Part C services, and the medical home: collaboration for best practice and best outcomes. *Pediatrics.* 2013;132(4):e1073–e1088

American Academy of Pediatrics, American Academy of Family Physicians, American College of Physicians–American Society of Internal Medicine. A consensus statement on health care transitions for young adults with special health care needs. *Pediatrics.* 2002;110(Suppl 3):1304–1306

American Academy of Pediatrics Council on Children With Disabilities. Care coordination in the medical home: integrating health and related systems of care for children with special health care needs. *Pediatrics.* 2005;116(5):1238–1244

American Academy of Pediatrics Council on Children With Disabilities. Supplemental Security Income (SSI) for children and youth with disabilities. *Pediatrics.* 2009;124(6):1702–1708

Anderson D, Dumont S, Jacobs P, Azzaria L. The personal costs of caring for a child with a disability: a review of the literature. *Public Health Rep.* 2007;122(1):3–16

Burdo-Hartman WA, Patel DR. Medical home and transition planning for children and youth with special health care needs. *Pediatr Clin North Am.* 2008;55(6):1287–1297

Houtrow AJ, Okumura MJ, Hilton JF, Rehm RS. Profiling health and health-related services for children with special health care needs with and without disabilities. *Acad Pediatr.* 2011;11(6):508–516

Kogan MD, Strickland BB, Newacheck PW. Building systems of care: findings from the National Survey of Children With Special Health Care Needs. *Pediatrics.* 2009;124(Suppl 4):S333–S336

Kuo DZ, Turchi RM. Best practices: kids with special health care needs. *Contemp Pediatr.* 2010;27:36–40

McPherson M, Arango P, Fox H, et al. A new definition of children with special health care needs. *Pediatrics.* 1998;102(1 Pt 1):137–140

Norwood KW Jr, Slayton RL; American Academy of Pediatrics Council on Children With Disabilities, Section on Oral Health. Oral health care for children with developmental disabilities. *Pediatrics.* 2013;131(3):614–619

Okun A. Children who have special health-care needs: ethical issues. *Pediatr Rev.* 2010;31(12):514–517

Palfrey JS, Foley SM, Huntington NL, eds. Children and youth with disabilities and special health care needs from traditionally underserved communities. *Pediatrics.* 2010;126(Suppl 3):S107–S196

Perrin JM, Bloom SR, Gortmaker SL. The increase of childhood chronic conditions in the United States. *JAMA.* 2007;297(24):2755–2759

Perrin JM, Gnanasekaran S, Delahaye J. Psychological aspects of chronic health conditions. *Pediatr Rev.* 2012;33(3):99–109

Strickland BB, van Dyck PC, Kogan MD, et al. Assessing and ensuring a comprehensive system of services for children with special health care needs: a public health approach. *Am J Public Health.* 2011;101(2):224–231

CHAPTER 42

Reproductive Health[1]

Monica Sifuentes, MD

CASE STUDY

An 18-year-old female college student in good health comes in for a routine health maintenance visit during her spring break. She is unaccompanied by her parents and has no complaints, stating that she just needs a checkup. She enjoys college, passed all of her fall and winter classes, and has some new friends. She denies tobacco use but says most of her friends smoke. She occasionally drinks alcohol and has tried marijuana once. Although she is not sexually active, she is interested in discussing oral contraception. Her last menstrual period, which occurred 2 weeks ago, was normal. She is taking no medications. Her physical examination is entirely normal.

Questions

1. What issues are important to discuss with adolescents at reproductive health maintenance visits?
2. What are the indications for a complete pelvic examination?
3. When is a Papanicolaou test (Pap smear) indicated as a part of the reproductive health visit?
4. What methods of contraception are most successful in adolescent patients? What factors about each method should be considered?
5. What are the legal issues involved in prescribing contraception to minors in the absence of parental consent?

Adolescent visits to primary care physicians are relatively infrequent by the time teenagers reach puberty. At most, healthy adolescent patients are seen once or twice during high school for preparticipation sports or camp physicals. If adolescents are not involved in athletics or if their schools do not require periodic assessments, these teenagers will probably never visit their health care professionals again while in high school except for an acute illness. Therefore, it is extremely important to use any interaction with an adolescent as a unique opportunity to provide anticipatory guidance and health education, particularly reproductive health education.

Reproductive health can be defined as sexuality-related services, screening, and counseling. Such services should be included as a part of the routine health maintenance examination for male and female adolescents for several reasons. The high incidence of sexually transmitted infections (STIs) in this age group, the risk of acquiring HIV, and the reality of an unplanned pregnancy make reproductive health issues increasingly important for teenagers. In addition, adolescents rarely schedule appointments with primary care physicians prior to the initiation of coitus. Experimentation with drugs and alcohol at this time in their lives also contributes to early, unplanned sexual experiences (Box 42-1).

Aside from issues of sexual activity, adolescents also may have questions about their progression through puberty. Normal variants in body habitus or certain physical characteristics can be a source of unnecessary anxiety for uninformed teenagers. Health education to alleviate these fears is ideal. Adolescents who come for physical examinations should be allotted extra time so that topics such as puberty, abstinence, sexual identity, sexual behaviors and activity, STIs, and contraception can be discussed. In addition, during more acute, problem-oriented visits, adolescents should be encouraged to voice any other concerns they may have. Depending on the nature of these issues, follow-up appointments can be scheduled.

Normal Secondary Sexual Development

Puberty begins during early adolescence with the development of secondary sexual characteristics. Because there can be tremendous variation with regard to the age, duration between pubertal stages, and somatic growth of adolescents, a sexual maturity rating (SMR) scale (Tanner staging) is used to describe breast and pubic hair development in females and genital development and pubic hair growth in males (figures 42-1, 42-2, and 42-3). The average age of menarche in the United States is 12.5 years, which, for most females, occurs during SMR 3 and 4. In contrast, spermarche occurs early in pubertal development in boys, at approximately 13 years of age, with little to no pubic hair development. Full fertility is generally achieved by age 15 years, or mid-adolescence, in most boys and girls.

---

[1]This chapter is largely devoted to a discussion of the reproductive health of adolescent females. However, Evaluation is divided into 2 sections, one for females and one for males. The reader is referred to Chapter 101 for more information on reproductive health.

Box 42-1. Reproductive Health: Sexual Activity

Statistics on sexual activity among adolescents in the United States have changed over the last decade. Previously, it was reported that 1 in 4 females and 1 in 3 males had had sexual intercourse by 15 years of age. Currently, only 13% of teens have ever had vaginal intercourse by age 15, according to the Guttmacher Institute. Most adolescents are now waiting until later to initiate sexual activity; by their 19th birthday, 7 in 10 teens of both sexes have had sexual intercourse. Contraceptive use at first premarital sexual encounter has increased to almost 80% in adolescent females and 87% in adolescent males; however, unintended pregnancy and sexually transmitted infections (STIs) continue to be a major public health concern for this age group. While the pregnancy rate among teenagers has dropped steadily over the past 10 years, each year almost 850,000 adolescent females younger than 20 years become pregnant. Most of these pregnancies are unintended and occur premaritally, especially among certain racial and ethnic minority groups. The outcome of these pregnancies in 15- to 19-year-olds varies. An estimated 50% to 60% of these pregnancies result in live births, 30% end in abortion, and 10% to 15% are miscarried or stillborn.

Unprotected sexual activity among adolescents has several adverse health consequences, the most obvious being teenage pregnancy. Of the adolescents who continue their pregnancies, prematurity (<37 weeks' gestation) and low birth weight (<2,500 g) are 2 of the most frequently reported neonatal complications. Long-term maternal psychosocial sequelae of adolescent pregnancy include under-education/school failure, limited vocational training and skills, economic dependency on public assistance, subsequent unwanted births, social isolation, depression, and high rates of separation and divorce among teenaged couples.

In addition to unintended pregnancy, the risk of contracting an STI, such as chlamydia, human papillomavirus, herpes, and HIV, is increased. In cases of pelvic inflammatory disease from gonorrhea or chlamydia, future problems with fertility and an increased risk of ectopic pregnancy can occur. Human papillomavirus, which is associated with the development of genital warts, cervical dysplasia, and cancer, accounts for about half of STIs diagnosed in adolescents and young adults. The prevalence rates of other STIs, such as chlamydia and gonorrhea, are still highest among 15- to 19-year-old females compared with older age groups in the United States. More alarming, however, is the relationship between AIDS in young adults aged 20 to 29 years and probable exposure to HIV during adolescence.

Many factors have been associated with the initiation of early coitus in adolescents. They include male gender; race/ethnicity; poverty; a large, single-parent family; previous teen pregnancy in the household (mother or sibling); poor academic achievement; discrepancy between the onset of physical puberty and cognitive development; peer group encouragement; and problem behaviors such as drug use. In addition, religious affiliation and cultural norms probably influence this decision. The role of hormonal changes during puberty and their influence on behavior is yet to be determined.

An estimated 10% to 20% of adolescents have limited typical functioning because of a disability or chronic illness by the age of 20 years. However, most of these adolescents experience normal pubertal development and fertility because of advances in medical treatment for conditions such as diabetes and sickle cell disease. Like their healthy peers, many of these adolescents begin sexual intercourse at an early age. Unintended pregnancy and childbirth can exacerbate some illnesses and increase risks significantly for adolescents and fetuses. The genetic implications and specific patterns of inheritance of certain chronic conditions must also be considered. For this reason, attention to sexual issues is essential for adolescents with chronic medical illness.

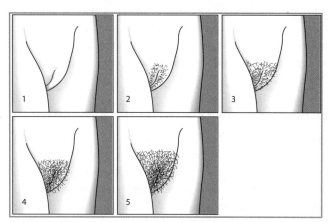

Figure 42-1. Female pubic hair development. Sexual maturity rating 1: prepubertal, no pubic hair. Sexual maturity rating 2: straight hair is extending along the labia and between ratings 2 and 3, begins on the symphysis pubis. Sexual maturity rating 3: pubic hair is increased in quantity; is darker, coarser, and curlier; and is present in the typical female triangle. Sexual maturity rating 4: pubic hair is more dense, curled, and adult in distribution but is less abundant. Sexual maturity rating 5: abundant, adult-type pattern; hair may extend on the medial aspect of the thighs.

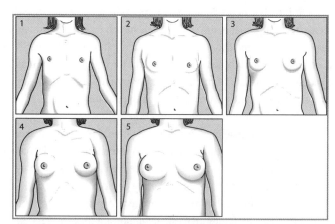

Figure 42-2. Female breast development. Sexual maturity rating 1: prepubertal, elevations of papilla only. Sexual maturity rating 2: breast buds appear, areola is slightly widened and projects as small mound. Sexual maturity rating 3: enlargement of the entire breast with no protrusion of the papilla or of the nipple. Sexual maturity rating 4: enlargement of the breast and projection of areola and papilla as a secondary mound. Sexual maturity rating 5: adult configuration of the breast with protrusion of the nipple, areola no longer projects separately from remainder of breast.

Figure 42-3. Male genital and pubic hair development. Sexual maturity rating 1: prepubertal, no pubic hair, genitalia unchanged from early childhood. Sexual maturity rating 2: light, downy hair develops laterally and later becomes dark; penis and testes may be slightly larger; scrotum becomes more textured. Sexual maturity rating 3: pubic hair is extended across pubis; testes and scrotum are further enlarged; penis is larger, especially in length. Sexual maturity rating 4: more abundant pubic hair with curling, genitalia resemble those of an adult, glans has become darker. Sexual maturity rating 5: adult quantity and pattern of pubic hair, with hair present along the inner borders of the thighs. The testes and scrotum are adult in size.

Evaluation

History

The history obtained at a reproductive health visit should include 2 parts: the medical history, which focuses primarily on the gynecologic history in females, and the psychosocial interview. Regardless of the type of visit scheduled, practitioners should take a few moments at the beginning of the interview to address routine health maintenance issues with the adolescent (Questions Box: Reproductive Health). The primary care physician should find out whether the female adolescent has ever had a genital or pelvic examination. In addition, current methods of contraceptive use, if any, should be reviewed (Questions Box: Contraceptive Use). If the adolescent female has just started taking oral contraceptives, compliance, common side effects, and a review of the more emergent complications of birth control pills is warranted, especially at an initial visit. **ACHES** (*a*bdominal pain, *c*hest pain, *h*eadaches, *e*ye problems, *s*evere leg pain) is a useful acronym to remember life-threatening reactions that can be associated with hormonal contraceptive use (Box 42-2), although they occur uncommonly in otherwise healthy adolescent girls.

The rest of the psychosocial history, otherwise known as the **HEADDSSS** interview (*h*ome environment, *e*mployment and education, *a*ctivities, *d*iet, *d*rugs, *s*afety, *s*exual activity/sexuality, *s*uicide/depression), should be completed whether or not the adolescent is currently sexually active (see Chapter 6). Risk factors for an unplanned pregnancy or unintentional exposures to STIs should be kept in mind when formulating health care plans with the teenager.

Questions

Reproductive Health

For Males and Females
- How is the adolescent feeling overall?
- Has the adolescent had any recent illnesses or conditions that the health care practitioner should know about?
- When was the last physical examination performed? Did it include a genital or pelvic examination?
- Is the adolescent sexually active?
  — If so, when was the last episode of vaginal intercourse?
  — Was the last episode of sexual intercourse protected or unprotected?
  — Does the adolescent have anal or oral sex?
  — How old was the adolescent when he or she began having sexual relationships? Was it consensual? Coerced? Forced?
  — How many sexual partners does the patient have currently? How many sexual partners has the patient had in his or her lifetime? What gender are they (all contacts may not be heterosexual)?
- Is there any history of or ongoing physical or sexual abuse?
- Has the adolescent or any of his or her partners ever been treated for a sexually transmitted infection or tested for HIV?

For Females Only
- What was the age at menarche?
- What was the date of the last menstrual period and the duration and amount of flow?
  — Are any symptoms such as cramping, bloating, or vomiting associated with menses?
  — Are any of these symptoms incapacitating? Do they cause the adolescent to miss school or work?
  — Does the mother or siblings have similar problems? If so, how do they manage them, if at all?

Questions

Contraceptive Use

- Does the adolescent use condoms never, sometimes, or always?
- Is any other method, such as spermicidal foam or jelly, also used?
- Is the adolescent female currently using oral contraceptives?
  — If so, what particular type is she taking, and how long has she been using this method of contraception?
  — How often does she forget to take the pill? What does she do when she forgets to take the pill?
  — Does she experience common minor side effects such as breakthrough bleeding, headache, or nausea?
- Is the adolescent female using a long-acting progestin, such as Depo-Provera? If so, has she experienced irregular bleeding, weight gain, hair loss, headache, or acne?
- Is there another method of contraception that the adolescent has used or might be interested in discussing or starting?
- What does the adolescent know about emergency contraception?

Box 42-2. Danger Signs Associated With Oral Contraceptive Use

A	Abdominal pain (severe)
C	Chest pain (severe) with shortness of breath
H	Headaches
E	Eye problems (visual loss or blur)
S	Severe leg pain (calf/thigh)

Physical Examination

A complete physical examination should be performed on all adolescents, with particular attention paid to their SMR. Chaperones are strongly encouraged, with the permission of the patient, even when the patient and examiner are the same gender, particularly during the breast and genital examination.

Males

The genitalia should be examined closely for penile and testicular size, distribution of pubic hair, and presence of any ulcerative, vesicular, or wart-like lesions. Any urethral erythema or discharge should be noted. Testicular masses require further evaluation. Ideally, clinicians should use this opportunity to teach male adolescents how to perform a testicular self-examination.

Females

Prior to performing the physical examination, the physician should determine whether a full-speculum examination is indicated (Box 42-3). This decision should be based on the details of the individual case and not solely on the basis of sexual activity. With the advent of noninvasive screening methods for STIs, a routine pelvic examination is often unnecessary. Most experts now recommend the use of urine-based nucleic acid amplification tests (NAATs) to screen for gonorrhea or chlamydia instead of endocervical swabs. However, if a speculum examination is indicated, proper preparation of the adolescent is imperative. This should include an explanation of the procedure and the physical sensations felt while the speculum is being inserted and the endocervical specimen is being obtained. The choice of who should be present during the examination (eg, parent or friend who may have accompanied the patient) and a discussion of the desired positioning (ie, supine vs semi-sitting) are also

---

Box 42-3. Indications for a Complete Pelvic Examination

- Pregnancy
- Request by the adolescent
- Unexplained lower abdominal pain
- Persistent abnormal vaginal discharge
- Unexplained vaginal bleeding
- Dysmenorrhea, unresponsive to nonsteroidal anti-inflammatory medications
- Suspected or reported sexual assault
- Perform a Pap test

---

important points to review. In addition, the speculum, specimen swabs, and other equipment should be shown to the adolescent before she is draped. The goal is to minimize the adolescent's fears, anxieties, misconceptions, and discomfort regarding the examination.

A breast examination should be performed on female adolescents, and any breast tenderness, nodularity, or masses should be noted. Again, this portion of the examination can be used to educate patients about the purpose and importance of breast self-examinations and to document breast SMR.

The external genitalia should be examined in all adolescent females whether or not they are sexually active. The SMR and any congenital anomalies, such as asymmetric enlargement of the labia minora or an imperforate hymen, should be identified. In sexually active adolescents, the external genitalia should be carefully examined for warts, ulcers, and vesicular lesions. Any urethral erythema, edema, or discharge that may indicate an otherwise asymptomatic chlamydial infection should be noted. If a pelvic examination is indicated, a vaginal discharge may be appreciated prior to inserting the speculum, but, ideally, the cervix should be examined for cervical ectopia, friability, and any lesions or discharge from the os. The vaginal mucosa should also be inspected as the speculum is withdrawn.

During the bimanual examination, the cervix should be palpated for any cervical motion tenderness. Uterine size and position should be appreciated, and adnexal tenderness or masses should be noted. Because normal ovaries are approximately the size of almonds, they are often not palpated by many clinicians. A rectovaginal examination is necessary to rule out fistulas, especially in postpartum adolescents. If the practitioner is unable to perform a vaginal bimanual examination, a rectoabdominal examination can be done to assess uterine size and position and the presence of adnexal masses.

Laboratory Tests

Because most *Chlamydia trachomatis* and *Neisseria gonorrhoeae* infections in adolescents are asymptomatic, screening noninvasive urine-based or vaginal NAATs should be sent annually in all sexually active adolescents and more frequently in those who have a history of unprotected intercourse or a new sexual partner. If the adolescent has a vaginal discharge or cervical friability noted on speculum examination, the specimen should be obtained directly from the endocervix and sent for NAAT. A saline and potassium hydroxide wet mount should also be collected in symptomatic patients. A Pap smear should be performed in sexually active females who are 21 years or older. The Pap smear can also help detect *Trichomonas vaginalis* or the cytological changes associated with human papillomavirus (HPV). A NAAT (eg, polymerase chain reaction) for human herpesvirus should be performed if painful vesicles are noted on examination. Additionally, a fresh vesicle can also be unroofed and a specimen sent for human herpesvirus culture.

Other laboratory tests include a rapid plasma reagin test for syphilis and an HIV screening test in the adolescent identified as high risk. Baseline complete blood cell count, liver function tests, cholesterol, and fasting glucose may be indicated as part of the health maintenance visit but are not required before starting contraception. A pregnancy test is warranted in sexually active females if the practitioner chooses to begin oral contraceptives or another method of hormonal contraception mid-cycle.

Management

Reproductive Health Education

All management plans during reproductive health visits should include a frank **discussion of puberty, gender identification, sexual orientation, sexual behavior, and STIs** regardless of current sexual activity. The adolescent should be counseled about abstinence as an acceptable choice. Ideally, preventive health care measures such as **breast and testicular self-examinations** have been reviewed during the physical examination. It is hoped that by encouraging adolescents' familiarity with these self-examinations, they will continue to perform them throughout their adult lives. The use of posters, plastic models, and electronic or written materials to support the discussion is greatly encouraged. The goal of education should be to assist adolescents in identifying and communicating their thoughts and feelings about sexual abstinence as well as sexual activity and to aid in the prevention of unintended pregnancy, parenthood, and STIs. Prevention programs offered by schools must be supplemented by open parental communication in the home about sexuality.

Legal Issues

The issue of **confidentiality** is important to consider when providing reproductive health care for adolescents. Parental involvement should be strongly encouraged, but health care practitioners are not required to disclose any information to parents except in cases of suicidal ideation, harmful intent to others, and sexual or physical abuse. In most states, contraceptive services can be provided to adolescents of any age without specific parental knowledge or consent. The complex issue of parental consent and pregnancy termination varies from state to state and should be reviewed by the individual health care practitioner. Of note, all 50 states, including the District of Columbia, explicitly allow minors to consent for their own health services for STIs and do not require parental consent for STI care. Providing confidential care for adolescents enrolled in private health insurance plans, however, continues to be a difficult issue because many states mandate that health plans provide a written statement to the beneficiary about the services covered and received, including clinical services provided confidentially to teens.

Pap Smear

The 2009 recommendation of the American College of Obstetricians and Gynecologists (ACOG) is that cervical cancer screening should begin at 21 years of age in young women. However, the American Cancer Society continues to recommend that young women start cervical screening with Papanicolaou tests 3 years after the onset of vaginal intercourse and no later than age 21 years. After the initiation of screening, a Pap smear for average-risk women aged 21 through 29 years should be performed every 2 years, and every 3 years for women 30 years and older with 3 consecutive normal cervical cytology test results. The rationale for the most recent changes in cervical cancer screening by ACOG is that there seems to be little risk in not treating abnormal cervical cytology in adolescents because 90% to 95% of low-grade lesions, as well as many high-grade lesions, in this age group regress to normal without treatment. Screening prematurely can lead to an overdiagnosis of cervical dysplasia and an overtreatment of lesions with potentially harmful procedures such as excision or ablation of the cervix. Because the incidence of cervical cancer is very low among adolescents, the benefits of Papanicolaou testing are offset by the potential harm of unnecessary procedures and treatments in this age group.

Contraceptive Methods

The appropriate method of contraception should be individualized. Barrier methods include condoms (male and female), diaphragms, and cervical caps. Vaginal spermicides such as nonoxynol-9 are available in a variety of forms (foams, gels, films, and suppositories) and should be used in conjunction with a barrier method because there are general concerns that these products in high doses can increase the risk of genital ulceration and irritation, thereby facilitating STI acquisition. Hormonal contraceptive methods include oral contraceptives, transdermal methods, the intravaginal ring, injectable long-acting progestin agents, and long-acting reversible contraceptives. Although previously not recommended for teens, a levonorgestrel intrauterine device (IUD) may be indicated in postpartum teenagers as well as for the treatment of severe dysfunctional uterine bleeding in nulliparous adolescents. The withdrawal method, or coitus interruptus, and natural family planning are ineffective methods for adolescents for protection against pregnancy.

Hormonal Contraception

Combined oral contraceptives (COCs) are an effective means of birth control for adolescents, with most pills containing 30 to 35 μg ("low-dose") to 20 μg ("very low-dose") of ethinyl estradiol (estrogen) and a progestin. Monophasic pills contain a fixed dose of estrogen and progestin throughout the 21-day pill cycle. Biphasic preparations contain a lower dose of the progestin component during the first 10 days of the cycle but are rarely used in teens. In triphasic pills, the doses of estrogen and progestin, or the progestin component alone, are varied 3 times throughout the cycle. This contraceptive was created to decrease the overall progestin-related side effects, such as hypertension, acne, and lipid abnormalities, but has not been shown to have any great advantage over a monophasic pill. Most recently, very low-dose monophasic estrogen (20 μg) pills have been developed to minimize estrogen-related side effects and decrease discontinuation rates. However, 20-μg estrogen pills may be associated with a higher rate of intermenstrual bleeding and less bone mass acquisition than 30- to 35-μg pills, especially in young patients. With this in mind, monophasic pills with 30 to 35 μg of ethinyl estradiol are considered the first-line therapy for most teens. There may be specific instances, however, in which their lower efficacy must be taken into account and the ethinyl estradiol dose increased to 50 μg, such as in patients concurrently receiving medications that increase the metabolism of synthetic steroids, such as anticonvulsants.

Another COC regimen is 3-month continuous hormonal therapy followed by 1 week of withdrawal bleeding for young women who prefer to menstruate only 4 times a year (an extended-cycle pill). To lessen the frequency of breakthrough bleeding often experienced by users of the extended-cycle pill, another product is now available that replaces the placebo pills with 7 days of low-dose estrogen. Progestin-only pills, referred to as minipills, also are available and particularly useful in postpartum and lactating teen mothers.

Clear benefits associated with COC use include prevention of pregnancy, protection against ovarian and endometrial cancers, decreased risk of functional ovarian cysts and benign breast conditions, improvement of acne, and decreased menstrual blood loss and menstrual symptoms, such as dysmenorrhea. The most common side effects of COCs include breakthrough bleeding, nausea, and breast tenderness, which generally resolve after 3 cycles. Although potential risks of COC include venous thromboembolic (VTE) phenomena, hypertension, and changes in the lipid profile, actual risks are minimal in most healthy adolescents compared with the morbidity and mortality associated with teenage pregnancy and childbirth.

Other combined hormonal contraceptive methods for the adolescent include the vaginal ring (NuvaRing) and the transdermal patch (Ortho Evra). Approved in 2001, the vaginal contraceptive ring is a soft, flexible device that contains estrogen and progestin, which is released directly through the vaginal wall into the bloodstream. The ring is inserted into the vagina for 3 weeks, then removed for 1 week to allow for a withdrawal bleed. Systemic side effects are similar to other low-dose combined hormonal methods (headache, breast tenderness, nausea, breakthrough bleeding/spotting); specific local effects include vaginal discharge and discomfort secondary to local irritation. Sensation of a foreign body and expulsion of the ring during coitus may also occur. The teenager must be comfortable with insertion and removal of the device for this method to be used successfully.

The transdermal adhesive patch is a thin, beige, 3-layered plastic patch that contains estrogen and progestin and is applied weekly to specific areas of the body (lower abdomen, upper torso, upper arm, or buttocks) followed by 1 week off. Although well tolerated, high detachment rates in teens have been documented. In addition, adolescents may have concerns about the visibility of the patch. Side effects are similar to other combined hormonal methods of contraception; local effects include skin irritation, redness, and rash at the site of application. Reduced effectiveness has been reported in women weighing more than 198 lb (90 kg). Additionally, concerns have been cited by the US Food and Drug Administration (FDA) about the risk of VTE events associated with the patch, although conflicting data have been reported. The reader is referred to the article by Trenor et al in Selected References for a comprehensive review of this topic.

The long-acting injectable progestin depot medroxyprogesterone acetate (DMPA) (Depo-Provera) is given intramuscularly every 3 months to inhibit ovulation, thicken cervical mucus, and induce an atrophic endometrium; a subcutaneous formulation is also available. The most common side effect is irregular menstrual bleeding, especially in the first few months, and eventual amenorrhea with prolonged use. Weight gain remains a significant issue for some patients and clinicians, particularly in obese adolescents in whom exaggerated increases in weight can be seen. Breast tenderness and mood disturbances also can occur but less frequently. In 2004, the FDA issued a black box warning for DMPA about possible irreversible bone loss in women with long-term use of DMPA and a potential reduction in overall bone mineral density (BMD) in teenagers that may contribute to the development of osteoporosis later in life. The FDA therefore recommends that DMPA should not be used in adolescents for longer than 2 years; however, many experts believe that the risk for pregnancy using an inferior method of birth control far outweighs the risk for the development of osteoporosis in a healthy teenager. Ongoing studies suggest that although adolescents may not increase their BMD while receiving DMPA and do experience bone loss, the effects appear to be temporary and reversible with the discontinuation of DMPA. Adolescents desiring this method of contraception should be made aware of the black box warning and receive adequate calcium and vitamin D.

A subdermal implant (Nexplanon) originally received approval by the FDA in 2006 under the name Implanon and is available for young women who desire a long-acting reversible method of contraception. It is designed to deliver a low, steady dose of continuous progestin for 3 years via a single plastic polymer rod placed below the skin. Formal instruction for insertion and removal is required for the health care professional interested in providing this form of contraception. The subdermal implant is highly effective, but, as with other long-acting progestin-only contraceptives, it is associated with bleeding abnormalities, especially during the first year of use.

Other long-acting reversible contraceptives include levonorgestrel intrauterine systems (Mirena, Skyla) and the copper IUD (ParaGard). Although previously not recommended for nulliparous women, including teens, Mirena was approved in 2009 for treatment of severe menorrhagia and dysmenorrhea and is effective for up to 5 years. Skyla releases a lower dose of levonorgestrel and is approved for 3 years. An increased risk of pelvic inflammatory disease was previously thought to be associated with IUDs in teenagers, but this is no longer supported by the literature.

Emergency Postcoital Contraception

Emergency contraception (EC), or the morning-after pill, is an effective way to prevent unintended pregnancy in adolescents. It requires, however, that the physician educate teens about its availability and usage and that teens feel comfortable contacting their health care physician, if necessary, within 72 to 120 hours of unprotected or inadequately protected intercourse. Although not meant to be used repeatedly as the sole method of contraception, EC is useful for the "unplanned" sexual encounter, which is often the case with adolescents, or a failed current contraceptive method. The most frequently used EC contains a total dose of 1.5 mg of levonorgestrel in a 1- or 2-dose regimen (Plan B One-Step, Next Choice One Dose). Emergency contraception acts primarily by preventing follicular rupture and therefore inhibiting ovulation. Levonorgestrel-based EC does not interrupt or disrupt an already-established pregnancy and is not an abortifacient.

Another EC product, ulipristal acetate (Ella), is a progestin receptor agonist and antagonist whose mechanism of action is similar to levonorgestrel. However, unlike levonorgestrel-based EC, existing pregnancy must be excluded prior to prescribing ulipristal because of the risk of fetal loss if used in the first trimester of pregnancy. Patients also must be counseled to seek immediate medical attention if they experience severe lower abdominal pain after its use because ectopic pregnancy can occur. Currently, ulipristal is available only with a prescription, regardless of age.

The original EC regimen was a combination of high-dose estrogen and progestin, known as the Yuzpe method; however, nausea and vomiting occurred in about 25% to 30% of patients. Two-pill formulations of levonorgestrel-based EC such as Plan B and Next Choice currently require a prescription for adolescents younger than 17 years and are kept behind the pharmacy counter. This type of EC consists of 2 doses of 0.75 mg of levonorgestrel, which should be taken 12 hours apart within 3 days of unprotected intercourse. Based on data reported by the World Health Organization, this regimen has been modified to *take both pills at once up to 5 days after unprotected or inadequately protected intercourse.* Plan B One-Step is a single pill regimen available without a prescription without an age restriction in the United States. Emergency contraception is most highly effective when used within the first 24 hours after unprotected coitus. Although less common than with the Yuzpe method, side effects of Next Choice and Plan B One-Step include nausea, vomiting, breast tenderness, and irregular bleeding patterns such as spotting; shortened interval to menses; and lighter or heavier menses. Because EC is safe and highly effective in preventing pregnancy, physicians should consider providing the sexually active teen with a prescription or advance supply of EC at the health maintenance visit.

The patient should be given a follow-up office or clinic appointment 2 to 3 weeks after using EC so that a pregnancy test can be performed, treatment failures can be identified early, STI screening can occur, and issues of contraception can be discussed.

Nonhormonal Contraception

Numerous studies and clinical experience have shown that nonhormonal methods are less effective in adolescents. However, latex condoms in conjunction with a spermicide have become crucial as a method of contraception since the emergence of AIDS. Although they help prevent transmission of some STIs, such as gonorrhea, chlamydia, trichomoniasis, and HIV, condoms do not protect against HPV and human herpesvirus infection overall because the genital area is not completely covered. A few moments, therefore, should be taken during the visit to explain these details and demonstrate proper use of condoms. Risks of condom use are minimal, except for allergic reactions to the spermicide, latex, or lubricants. Although available, the female condom is not widely used by adolescents but may be helpful in situations in which a male partner refuses to wear a condom. The inner ring is inserted into the vagina up to 8 hours prior to intercourse, and a prescription or physician visit is not necessary to obtain a female condom. Some teenagers, however, may be uncomfortable with its insertion and the fact that the outer ring remains on the vulva during vaginal intercourse. Similar issues are encountered when considering the diaphragm as a contraceptive method for teens; therefore, it is not recommended as a first-line contraceptive method for most adolescents. Other nonhormonal methods should be reviewed with adolescents as they become available.

Sexually Transmitted Infections

All STIs should be treated according to the most recent guidelines published by the Centers for Disease Control and Prevention based on current epidemiology. See Chapter 101 for details on the diagnosis and management of STIs in adolescents.

CASE RESOLUTION

In the case study presented at the beginning of the chapter, a more detailed history should be obtained about the adolescent's menstrual history and daily activities (eg, with whom does she spend most of her time? What does she like to do in her spare time?). In addition, the indications for a pelvic examination should be reviewed because most teens are not familiar with the new recommendations to delay the Pap smear until 21 years of age. Because the new indications do not apply in this case, the pelvic examination can be deferred. A discussion should then follow about barrier and hormonal methods of contraception and their role in the prevention of pregnancy and sexually transmitted infections. Emergency contraception should also be reviewed with the patient. Written information as well as useful Web site addresses should be given to the adolescent for future reference. A follow-up visit should be scheduled in the next few months, especially if she decides to begin oral contraception.

Selected References

American Academy of Pediatrics Committee on Adolescence. Condom use by adolescents. *Pediatrics*. 2013;132(5):973–981

American Academy of Pediatrics Committee on Adolescence. Contraception and adolescents. *Pediatrics*. 2007;120(5):1135–1148

American Academy of Pediatrics Committee on Adolescence. Emergency contraception. *Pediatrics*. 2012;130(6):1174–1182

American College of Obstetrics and Gynecologists Committee on Gynecologic Practice. ACOG Committee Opinion No. 415: depot medroxyprogesterone acetate and bone effects. *Obstet Gynecol*. 2008;112(3):727–730

Braverman PK, Breech L; American Academy of Pediatrics Committee on Adolescence. Gynecologic examination for adolescents in the pediatric office setting. *Pediatrics*. 2010;126(3):583–590

Burkett AM, Hewitt GD. Progestin only contraceptives and their use in adolescents: clinical options and medical indications. *Adolesc Med Clin*. 2005;16(3):553–567

Cavanaugh RM Jr. Screening adolescent gynecology in the pediatrician's office: have a listen, take a look. *Pediatr Rev.* 2007;28(9):332–342

Centers for Disease Control and Prevention. Reproductive health. United States Medical Eligibility Criteria (US MEC) for Contraceptive Use, 2010. http://www.cdc.gov/reproductivehealth/UnintendedPregnancy/USMEC.htm. Accessed March 24, 2014

Cromer BA, Scholes D, Berenson A, et al. Depot medroxyprogesterone acetate and bone mineral density in adolescents—the black box warning: a position paper of the Society for Adolescent Medicine. *J Adolesc Health.* 2006;39(2):296–301

Duffy K, Wimberly Y, Brooks C. Adolescent contraceptive care for the practicing pediatrician. *Adolesc Med State Art Rev.* 2009;20(1):168–187

Feucht C, VandenBussche H. Pharmacology update in adolescents: contraception and human papillomavirus vaccination. *Adolesc Med State Art Rev.* 2013;24(1):57–89

Ford C, English A, Sigman G. Confidential health care for adolescents: position paper for the Society for Adolescent Medicine. *J Adolesc Health.* 2004;35(2):160–167

Gold MA, Delisi K. Motivational interviewing and sexual and contraceptive behaviors. *Adolesc Med.* 2008;19:69–82

Gupta N. Advances in hormonal contraception. *Adolesc Med Clin.* 2006;17(3):653–671

Gupta N, Corrado S, Goldstein M. Hormonal contraception for the adolescent. *Pediatr Rev.* 2008;29(11):386–397

Guttmacher Institute. In brief: fact sheet. Facts on American teens' sexual and reproductive health. http://www.guttmacher.org/pubs/FB-ATSRH.html. Published June 2013. Accessed March 24, 2014

Guttmacher Institute. State policies in brief. An overview of minors' consent law. http://www.guttmacher.org/statecenter/spibs/spib_OMCL.pdf. Published March 1, 2014. Accessed March 24, 2014

Klein JD; American Academy of Pediatrics Committee on Adolescence. Adolescent pregnancy: current trends and issues. *Pediatrics.* 2005;116(1):281–286

Levine SB. Adolescent consent and confidentiality. *Pediatr Rev.* 2009;30(11):457–459

Morgan Mulchahey K. Practical approaches to prescribing contraception in the office setting. *Adolesc Med Clin.* 2005;16(3):665–674

Murphy NA, Elias ER. Sexuality of children and adolescents with developmental disabilities. *Pediatrics.* 2006;118(1):398–403

Trenor CC 3rd, Chung RJ, Michelson AD, et al. Hormonal contraception and thrombotic risk: a multidisciplinary approach. *Pediatrics.* 2011;127(2):347–357

Upadhya KK. Contraception for adolescents. *Pediatr Rev.* 2013;34(9):384–394

Providing Culturally Competent Care to Diverse Populations: Sexual Orientation and Gender Expression

Lynn Hunt, MD

CASE STUDY

The mother of an 11-year-old boy makes an appointment with you to discuss her son's "behavior problems." He is the youngest of 4 children and is doing well in fifth grade, but she is concerned that her son does not like typical "male" activities. He dropped out of Little League, won't join other sports teams, and prefers riding his bike. In addition, he still likes dressing up in costumes and prefers playing with girls rather than boys. She finally mentions that she is worried that he will be gay and is wondering what she can do to help her son develop "normally."

Questions

1. What is meant by gender expression, sexual orientation, and gender identity?
2. What is the role of the pediatrician in counseling parents and patients about gender expression, sexual orientation, and gender identity?
3. What are some of the consequences of discrimination of sexual minority populations?
4. Are there programs that can change sexual orientation?

Every pediatrician and health care professional needs a basic understanding of lesbian, gay, bisexual, transgender, and questioning (LGBTQ) populations. Each of us has contact with sexual and gender minority individuals. They are among our patients and parents of our patients. Every day we encounter family members of someone who is LGBTQ, whether or not we are aware of it. Furthermore, the Joint Commission and Association of American Medical Colleges, among other professional organizations, call for nondiscrimination and proactive cultural competence as markers of quality, appropriate patient care, and key content for health care profesisonal education. Additionally, Healthy People 2020, which provides a science-based plan for improving the health of all Americans, included lesbian, gay, bisexual, and transgender health among the listed objectives.

Incidence

The US census and other large-scale surveys indicate that approximately 5% of the adult population identifies as LGBTQ or reports same-sex relationships. The prevalence of sexual minority persons is impressively consistent across all ethnic and socioeconomic groups.

The number of adolescents who identify as LGBTQ tends to increase with age. However, in one survey, more than twice as many youth reported same-sex sexual experiences as those who eventually identified as gay. These data reinforce the important distinction between sexual orientation and sexual behavior. There is a wide range of sexual behavior in teens, and sexual identity formation is a dynamic developmental process. Teens who eventually identify as gay may have had heterosexual sexual contact, and those who identify as straight may have had same-sex partners.

Lesbian, Gay, Bisexual, Transgender, and Questioning (LGBTQ) Youth

Despite an increase in public dialogue and recent changes in some discriminatory laws, LGBTQ youth continue to suffer stigmatization and its consequences. All too often, LGBTQ youth are the objects of bullying, isolation, and family rejection. Individuals at particular risk are those whose gender expression or identity does not meet societal expectations. In national surveys of LGBTQ youth, verbal, electronic, and physical harassment in schools are commonplace and associated with school avoidance and other far-reaching consequences.

Additionally, sexual minorities are by far the group most targeted for violent hate crimes in the United States. More murders motivated by antigay bias occurred in 2011 than any year since data were first tracked by the National Coalition of Anti-Violence Programs.

Gender-Variant Youth

Gender identity, gender expression, and sexual orientation are 3 separate concepts that sometimes become confused (see Glossary, page 266). **Sexual orientation** describes to whom we are attracted and love. **Gender expression** refers to the way we outwardly manifest masculinity or femininity through, for example, clothing, hair, and mannerisms. **Gender identity** refers to a person's internal sense of being male, female, or something else. Gender identity is a spectrum completely distinct from sexual orientation. For most people, gender identity coincides with biological or natal sex. For some, gender identity and biological sex are discordant. While many young people are aware of their lesbian, gay, or bisexual sexual orientation by puberty, we know that gender identity generally develops earlier. Some children who are gender variant, whose gender identity is discordant with their natal sex, will later identify as transgender. Others will desist and may later identify as straight, bisexual, or gay. Regardless, all of these children will be under your care during childhood and adolescence, and we know that adult outcomes are dependent on the level of nonjudgmental support each child receives.

Health Consequences of Discrimination

Most LGBTQ youth are resilient and develop into healthy adults, yet they are at increased risk as a group. There are data documenting increased suicide attempts, substance use, and risky sexual behavior among LGBTQ youth, but it is important to understand the key mediators of these adverse health outcomes. Youth who have been victimized or perceive discrimination are more vulnerable to engaging in high-risk behaviors.

Family support is particularly important. In one study, LGBTQ young adults who experienced higher levels of family rejection during adolescence were 8 times more likely to report suicide attempts, 6 times more likely to report significant depression, and 3 times more likely to use illegal drugs or engage in unprotected sexual intercourse compared with those who did not experience family rejection. Conversely, families that are highly supportive are more likely to have children who are resilient and well adjusted. Family acceptance during adolescence is associated with better general health, self-esteem, and social support in LGBTQ young adults.

Lesbian, gay, bisexual, transgender, and questioning youth are also significantly overrepresented among homeless youth. Studies estimate that up to 40% of homeless youth identify as sexual minorities. Youth become homeless usually as a result of family conflict about their sexual orientation or gender expression. Sexual minority youth are more likely to suffer negative outcomes associated with living on the streets. Physical assault, sexual victimization, substance abuse, and high-risk sexual behavior are all more common for LGBTQ than heterosexual homeless youth.

Important Role of Pediatricians

Pediatric health care professionals have a unique opportunity to model acceptance of each patient (Box 43-1) and provide appropriate family support and risk-reduction counseling. Yet studies have shown that many adolescents are reluctant to share information about their sexuality or gender identity with their health care professional for various reasons. Lesbian, gay, bisexual, transgender, and questioning adolescents want the same attributes in their health care professionals as studies document for other groups of teens: confidentiality, honesty, respect, competence, and a nonjudgmental approach to history taking and guidance.

Box 43-1. Ways for Clinicians to Indicate Support for Lesbian, Gay, Bisexual, Transgender, and Questioning Youth

Waiting or Examination Room Environment
- Signal a welcoming environment with lesbian, gay, bisexual, transgender, and questioning (LGBTQ) SafeZone or rainbow stickers.
- Assess the images and literature available in your office. Much available information for teens assumes that the consumer is heterosexual. Consider including some posters or brochures that are not exclusively heterosexual in character.

Office Forms
- Review standard intake and history forms for assumptions that every patient (or parent) is heterosexual and consider modifying them to be more inclusive. Instead of only "single," "married," and "divorced," consider "partnered" and "other." Instead of "mother's name" or "father's name," consider simply using "parent's name."

Patient Interview
- Stress the importance of privacy and confidentiality. Concerns about possible disclosure of sexual orientation or behavior are often reasons mentioned by LGBTQ youth as a reason to avoid seeking health care.
- Use gender-neutral language. Questions like "Are you dating?" or "Are you currently in a relationship?" are more inclusive than "Do you have a boyfriend/girlfriend?" Other approaches, such as "What types of sexual experiences have you had?" or "Have you been attracted to/had sex with boys, girls, or both?" are useful no matter what the self-identified orientation of the patient may be. Discuss "protection" rather than just "birth control."
- As with any adolescent, a nonjudgmental attitude from the health care professional will help elicit honest and relevant information.

Physical Examination
- General primary care for LGBTQ youth, including examination and laboratory evaluation, should follow the recommendations for all adolescent health care as outlined by the American Academy of Pediatrics *Bright Futures* health supervision guidelines.

Family Counseling
- Help families understand that parental rejection or attempts to change their child have long-term negative health consequences. Reinforce that all the evidence supports the power of acceptance in helping young people thrive.
- Do not tolerate bullying at school or anywhere else the child is mistreated. Meet with appropriate personnel; encourage development or implementation of anti–LGBT-bullying education and policies.

"Reparative" or Conversion Therapy

Some religiously and politically motivated groups use outdated and discredited medical theories to justify trying to "cure" the natural sexual orientation or gender identity of those who are lesbian, gay, bisexual, and transgender. "Reparative therapy" does not work, and the process can severely damage self-esteem, leading to depression and self-destructive and suicidal behaviors. In 2001, the *Surgeon General's Call to Action to Promote Sexual Health and Responsible Sexual Behavior* asserted that homosexuality is not "a reversible lifestyle choice." Reparative therapy is considered inappropriate and dangerous by many professional organizations, including the American Academy of Pediatrics (AAP).

Children With LGBTQ Parents

As many as 6 million American children and adults have a lesbian, gay, bisexual, or transgender parent, and combined data suggest that almost 2 million children younger than 18 years are being raised by at least one gay or lesbian parent in the United States. Children join families with same-sex parents in a variety of ways; for example, adoption, assisted reproductive technologies, or from previous heterosexual contact as step or blended families. It is surprising to some that the "typical" same-sex–parent families are not all upper or middle class. Parents in same-sex couples are more likely to be racial minorities; their children are more likely to have disabilities and to be adopted; and same-sex parents tend to have lower household incomes than opposite-sex couples.

Child Outcomes

Multiple longitudinal and cross-sectional studies indicate that children with same-sex parents do well in domains of social, academic, and total competence. In study after study, children in same-sex–parent families turn out remarkably similar to children in heterosexual families. In a 2013 technical report, the AAP stated that "…more than 100 scientific publications over 30 years, taken together, have demonstrated that children's well-being is affected much more by their relationships with their parents, their parents' sense of competence and security, and the presence of social and economic support for the family than by the gender or the sexual orientation of their parents." The report concluded that "children growing up in households headed by gay men or lesbians are not disadvantaged in any significant respect relative to children of heterosexual parents." Suggestions for how families can support their lesbian, gay, bisexual, or transgender child's well-being are noted in Box 43-2.

How to Be an Ally

An ally is someone straight (or gay) who acknowledges and supports sexual diversity, acts accordingly to challenge homophobic or transphobic remarks and behaviors, and works to understand these forms of bias within oneself. Following are some concrete next steps health care professionals can take to be allies:

- Register as an ally provider in the Gay and Lesbian Medical Association (GLMA) online provider directory (www.glma.org).

Box 43-2. Supportive Behaviors That Help Families Promote Their Lesbian, Gay, Bisexual, or Transgender Child's Well-being

- Talk with your child about his or her lesbian, gay, bisexual, or transgender (LGBT) identity.
- Express affection when your child tells you or when you learn that your child is LGBT.
- Support your child's LGBT identity even though you may feel uncomfortable.
- Advocate for your child anywhere he or she is mistreated because of an LGBT identity.
- Insist that all family members respect your LGBT child.
- Bring your child to LGBT organizations or events.
- Connect your child with an LGBT adult role model to show your child options for the future.
- Work to make your faith community supportive of LGBT members, or find a supportive faith community that welcomes your family and LGBT child.
- Welcome your child's LGBT friends and partner to your home and family events and activities.
- Support your child's gender expression.
- Believe your child can have a happy future as an LGBT adult.

From Ryan C. *Supportive Families, Healthy Children: Helping Families with Lesbian, Gay, Bisexual & Transgender Children.* San Francisco, CA: Marian Wright Edelman Institute, San Francisco State University; 2009

Joining the directory is a great way to signal your support in health care. This is an easy way to let LGBTQ people in your community who are looking for health care professionals to know that you are a supportive ally.

- Visit the Parents, Families and Friends of Lesbians and Gays (PFLAG) Web site (www.pflag.org) and review its program for health care professionals, Straight for Equality (www.straightforequality.org).
- Learn more at any of the resources listed on page 266.

CASE RESOLUTION

This child is displaying behaviors that do not meet his parent's expectation for male gender expression. The pediatrician should let the mother know that gender expression, sexual orientation, and gender identity are separate and distinct and that there is a broad range of normal for all of these. There is no way to predict sexual orientation or gender identity from the behaviors described.

Many adolescents go through a period of questioning their sexuality. The child's mother should be informed that whether her son grows up gay, straight, transgender, or typically male, a major risk factor for him engaging in unsafe behaviors as an adolescent is parental rejection. Programs designed to change a person's sexual orientation don't work and are actually dangerous; they are associated with significant depression and thoughts of suicide. For her son to develop normally, he will need supportive adults in his life who accept and love him—ideally, his parents.

It would be important to determine if her son has been a victim of bullying at school or on sports teams. Schedule an appointment for the son (and of course, spend some time during the visit without his parents present). You will have the opportunity to evaluate the child's strengths and note if he is displaying any signs of anxiety or depression. Questions about sexuality would be those appropriate for all children at his age and stage of development. An ongoing dialogue with the mother will also help to know if or when referrals to Parents, Families, and Friends of Lesbians and Gays or other support and educational groups are appropriate.

Online Resources

For LGBTQ Youth

It Gets Better Project
www.itgetsbetter.org
See hundreds of videos of encouragement. This Web site is a place where young people who are LGBTQ can see how love and happiness can be a reality in their future. It's a place where straight allies can visit and support their friends and family members.

The Trevor Project
www.thetrevorproject.org
The Trevor Project is a national organization focused on crisis and suicide prevention efforts among LGBTQ youth. Trained counselors are ready 24/7 at 866/488-7386.

Gay, Lesbian & Straight Education Network (GLSEN)
www.glsen.org
Gay, Lesbian & Straight Education Network strives to ensure that each member of every school community is valued and respected regardless of sexual orientation or gender identity or expression.

National Runaway Safeline
www.1800runaway.org
1-800-RUNAWAY is a confidential and anonymous crisis hotline for runaway and homeless youth available 24 hours a day, 365 days a year.

Go Ask Alice!
www.goaskalice.columbia.edu
This Web site contains sexual health information by and for youth.

For Children With LGBTQ Parents

COLAGE: People With a Lesbian Gay Bisexual Transgender or Queer Parent
www.colage.org
COLAGE is a national movement of children, youth, and adults with one or more LGBTQ parents.

For Parents and Others

Family Acceptance Project
http://familyproject.sfsu.edu
A research-based, culturally grounded approach to help ethnically, socially, and religiously diverse families decrease rejection and increase support for their LGBTQ children.

Glossary	
Ally	A friend or supporter of LGBTQ communities.
Bisexual	A person who develops romantic, physical, and emotional attraction regardless of the other's sex.
Gay	The adjective used to describe people whose enduring romantic, physical, and emotional attractions are to people of the same sex. Often refers to men but also used more generically as well.
Gender expression	Outward expression of maleness or femaleness.
Gender identity	Knowledge of oneself being male, female, or something else along the spectrum.
Gender nonconforming	A person who by nature or choice does not conform to gender-based expectations of society. These children and adolescents are among the most vulnerable to bullying and violence.
Homosexual	A dated clinical term that is considered abrasive by some gay people.
Intersex	Also known as *disorders of sex development* or *differences of sex development (DSD)*. A general term used for the variety of conditions in which a person has atypical external or internal genitalia. These conditions may be apparent at birth and can cause difficulty assigning gender, or they may be diagnosed later due to infertility or other pubertal clues. Many adults with DSD say that is it important to avoid genital plastic surgery in newborns and to be open to the fact that children may develop a gender identity different than the one assigned at birth, no matter how thoughtful and caring the parents and physicians were.
Lesbian	A woman whose enduring romantic, physical, and emotional attraction is to other women.
Partner/spouse	A way to talk about someone's boyfriend, girlfriend, husband, or wife without mentioning gender. Using these words instead of gendered words allows you to be more inclusive, putting LGBTQ patients or parents at ease.
Queer	Traditionally a pejorative term, queer currently is used by some LGBTQ people, particularly among younger people, to describe themselves. Some value the term for its defiance and because it can be inclusive of the entire LGBTQ community; others find it to be an appropriate term to describe their identities in a less categorical way. Straight health care professionals should generally avoid using the term.
Sexual behavior	Refers to the way one chooses to express one's sexual feelings. Sexual behavior does not necessarily correlate with sexual orientation. Heterosexually identified individuals may have same-gender sexual experiences, and homosexually identified youth may have opposite-gender sexual experiences.
Sexual orientation	Permanent emotional, romantic, or sexual feelings toward other people. Straight individuals experience these feelings primarily for people of the opposite sex. Gay or lesbian individuals experience these feelings primarily for people of the same sex. Bisexual individuals can experience these feelings for people regardless of sex.
Transgender	A term describing a person whose gender identity does not necessarily match his or her assigned gender at birth or, more generally, who experiences or expresses gender differently from what people expect. Transgender individuals can be gay, straight, lesbian, or bisexual. Gender identity is a spectrum completely distinct from sexual orientation.

Parents, Families and Friends of Lesbians and Gays (PFLAG)

www.pflag.org

Parents, Families and Friends of Lesbians and Gays promotes the health and well-being of LGBTQ persons, their families, and friends through support, education, and advocacy.

Gender Spectrum

www.genderspectrum.org

Gender Spectrum provides education, training, and support to help create a gender-sensitive and inclusive environment for all children and teens. It provides resources to help families, educators, professionals, and organizations understand and address the concepts of gender identity and expression.

For Professionals

Gay and Lesbian Medical Association (GLMA)

www.glma.org

The mission of GLMA is to ensure equality in health care for LGBTQ individuals and health care professionals. The GLMA Web site features an online provider directory and educational materials.

Fenway Institute

www.fenwayhealth.org

The Fenway Institute is dedicated to advancing the skills, attitudes, and knowledge of clinicians and other health care professionals by providing professional development, educational materials, and resources on LGBTQ health topics. There are several online educational modules for physicians.

Suggested References

Dibble SL, Robertson PA. *Lesbian Health 101:A Clinician's Guide.* San Francisco, CA: University of California, San Francisco Nursing Press; 2010

Dowshen N, Garofalo R. Optimizing primary care for LGBTQ youth. *Contemp Pediatr.* 2009;26:58–66

Gartrell N, Bos H. US National Longitudinal Lesbian Family Study: psychological adjustment of 17-year-old adolescents. *Pediatrics.* 2010;126(1):28–36

Institute of Medicine. *The Health of Lesbian, Gay, Bisexual, and Transgender People: Building a Foundation for Better Understanding.* Washington, DC: National Academies Press; 2011

Kaiser Permanente National Diversity Council and Kaiser Permanente National Diversity. *A Provider's Handbook on Culturally Competent Care: Lesbian, Gay, Bisexual and Transgendered Population.* 2nd ed. Oakland, CA: Kaiser Permanente National Diversity; 2004

Levine DA; American Academy of Pediatrics Committee on Adolescence. Office-based care for lesbian, gay, bisexual, transgender, and questioning youth. *Pediatrics.* 2013;132(1):e297–e313

Makadon HJ, Mayer KH, Potter J, Goldhammer H, eds. *Fenway Guide to Lesbian, Gay, Bisexual, and Transgender Health.* Philadelphia, PA: American College of Physicians; 2008

Olson J, Forbes C, Belzer M. Management of the transgender adolescent. *Arch Pediatr Adolesc Med.* 2011;165(2):171–176

Perrin EC. *Sexual Orientation in Child and Adolescent Health Care.* New York, NY: Kluwer Academic/Plenum Publishers; 2002

Perrin EC, Siegel BS; American Academy of Pediatrics Committee on Psychosocial Aspects of Child and Family Health. Promoting the well-being of children whose parents are gay or lesbian. *Pediatrics.* 2013;131(4):e1374–e1383

Ryan C, Huebner D, Diaz RM, Sanchez J. Family rejection as a predictor of negative health outcomes in white and Latino lesbian, gay, and bisexual young adults. *Pediatrics.* 2009;123(1):346–352

CHAPTER 44

Injury Prevention

Sarah J. Atunah-Jay, MD, MPH, and Iris Wagman Borowsky, MD, PhD

CASE STUDY

A 16-year-old girl was brought to the emergency department after being rescued from her submerged vehicle. The girl was texting a friend while driving and crashed into a pond. After several weeks in the intensive care unit, she was transferred out for rehabilitative care from her injury.

Questions

1. How extensive is the injury problem in children?
2. What are the different methods of injury prevention? How could this particular injury have been prevented?
3. What injury prevention program has been developed by the American Academy of Pediatrics?
4. What are some general guidelines for effective injury prevention counseling?

Traditionally, unintentional injuries have been called "accidents." The problem with that term, however, is that it implies unpredictability, carrying with it connotations of chance, fate, and unexpectedness. The perception that injuries are chance occurrences that cannot be predicted or prevented has been a major barrier to progress in injury prevention and the study and control of injury as a scientific discipline. According to the modern view of injury, accidents must be anticipated to be prevented. Specialists in injury prevention have tried to replace the word *accident* with *injury* and have developed the idea of reducing injury risk. Thus, injuries are not random events at all; they occur in predictable patterns determined by identifiable risk factors. For example, if a 16-year-old girl is texting while driving, which has been shown to be a dangerous driving distraction, the resulting injury can hardly be called an accident. On the contrary, the injury is entirely predictable.

Epidemiology

Unintentional injuries are the leading cause of death among people aged 1 to 44 years in the United States. In 2010, unintentional injuries claimed the lives of more than 15,000 Americans younger than 24 years. The leading causes of unintentional injury-related deaths by age are suffocation (newborns and infants), drowning (1- to 4-year-olds), and motor vehicle crashes (5- to 24-year-olds). Fires and burns are another major cause of unintentional injury–related death in young people.

Intentional injuries are also a major cause of mortality in young people. Homicide ranks second among all causes of death for 15- to 19-year-olds, with 85% being firearm related. Suicide ranks third for 15- to 24-year-olds, the majority also being firearm related.

In addition to deaths, in 2011, nonfatal unintentional injuries led to almost 12 million hospital emergency department (ED) visits in persons younger than 24 years in the United States. In the same year,

almost 1 million young people visited EDs due to a violence-related injury. The most common causes of nonfatal unintentional injuries in people aged 1 to 24 years are falls, followed by injuries from being struck by or against something, bites, cuttings/piercings, overexertion, and motor vehicle occupancy.

Several epidemiologic factors are associated with higher rates of pediatric injuries. These include male gender, low income, and family stressors (eg, death in the family, new residence, birth of a sibling). There is a bimodal age distribution of injuries, with newborns/infants and adolescents at greatest risk. Females are most likely to experience rape or assault. American Indian/Alaska Native and black children have higher rates of total injury-related deaths than other racial/ethnic age-matched populations. Geography influences injury rates: Drowning deaths tend to be higher in coastline states (Alaska and California) or states with a higher number of swimming pools (Texas); injury-related deaths are higher in rural areas and may be related to decreased access to emergency medical care; and homicide occurs more frequently in urban areas.

Strategies for Injury Prevention

During this century, efforts to prevent injuries have shifted from changing the behavior of individuals to modifying the environments in which injuries occur. William Haddon, a medical epidemiologist, devised 2 useful frameworks for developing injury prevention strategies.

Haddon Matrix

This matrix relates 3 factors (host, vector, and environment) to the 3 phases of an injury-producing event (pre-event, event, and post-event). The 3 factors interact over time to produce injury. Table 44-1 shows a Haddon matrix of motor vehicle crash injuries. The precrash phase describes elements that determine whether a crash will occur; the crash phase describes the variables that influence the nature and

Table 44-1. The Haddon Matrix			
Phase	*Host (Human)*	*Vector (Vehicle)*	*Environment*
Precrash	Driver vision Alcohol consumption	Brakes Tires Speed	Speed limit Road curvature Road signs
Crash	Use of safety belts Osteoporosis	Vehicle size	Median barriers Laws about use of car seats and safety belts
Postcrash	Age Physical condition	Fuel system integrity	EMS personnel training

Abbreviation: EMS, emergency medical services.

Adapted from the National Committee for Injury Prevention and Control. Injury prevention: meeting the challenge. *Am J Prev Med.* 1989;5(3 suppl):1–303

severity of the resultant injury; and the postcrash phase describes the factors that determine the degree to which the injury is limited and repaired after the crash occurs. By describing the "anatomy" of an injury, the Haddon matrix illustrates the numerous characteristics that determine an injury and the many corresponding strategies for interfering with the production of an injury.

Haddon also developed a list of **10 countermeasures to prevent injuries** or reduce the severity of their effects.

1. Prevent creation of the hazard (eg, stop producing poisons, toys with small parts, and non-powder firearms; do not participate in dangerous sports; support community centers that engage children in safe after-school activities).
2. Reduce the amount of the hazard (eg, package drugs in nonlethal amounts; reduce speed limits).
3. Prevent the release of the hazard (eg, use child-resistant caps for medications, toilet locks, and safety latches on cabinets and drawers; pass and enforce distracted driving laws; implement restrictions on handgun purchases).
4. Modify the rate or spatial distribution of release of the hazard (eg, require air bags in cars; use child safety seats and seat belts; make poisons taste bad).
5. Separate people from the hazard in space or time (eg, make sidewalks for pedestrians, bikeways for bicyclists, and recreation areas separated from vehicles).
6. Separate people from hazards with material barriers (eg, use bicycle helmets and protective equipment for athletes; install fences around swimming pools; build window guards).
7. Modify relevant basic qualities of the hazard (eg, place padded carpets under cribs; require guns to have safety locks; develop inter-vehicle communication systems).
8. Increase resistance to damage from the hazard (eg, train and condition athletes; make structures more earthquake-proof; use flame-retardant sleepwear).
9. Limit the damage that has already begun (eg, use fire extinguisher; begin cardiopulmonary resuscitation).
10. Stabilize, repair, and rehabilitate injured individuals (eg, develop pediatric trauma centers and physical rehabilitation programs; improve emergency medical services).

Haddon's work serves as a practical guide for thinking about ways to prevent injury. It emphasizes the importance of considering injuries as a result of a sequence of events, with many opportunities for prevention. The shift of emphasis away from changing human behavior to preventing injury is particularly appropriate for injuries in children because inhibiting children's curiosity is impractical as well as undesirable.

Passive and Active Interventions

Interventions to prevent injuries can also be categorized as passive or active. **Passive or automatic strategies** protect whenever they are needed, without the action of parents or children. An example is the automobile air bag that automatically inflates to cushion occupants during a crash. Other examples of automatic strategies are water heater temperatures set to 120°F or lower, not having guns in the home, and energy-absorbing surfaces under playground equipment. In contrast, **active interventions** require action to become effective, such as in the case of nonautomatic safety belts, which require individuals to "buckle up" every time they enter an automobile. Supervision of swimming children is another example of an active injury prevention strategy.

Some strategies are partially automatic, requiring some action by individuals. Smoke detectors can be very effective in preventing injury and death in house fires, but roughly one-third of smoke detectors do not have working batteries. Batteries should be changed once a year and ideally tested once a month. As might be expected, the greater the effort required for children to be protected, the smaller the chance that protection occurs. Therefore, whenever possible, passive measures are preferable because they are the most effective.

Several approaches have been used successfully to prevent childhood injuries, including engineering, education, legislation, and enforcement. An engineering intervention, the car safety seat, is extremely effective (Table 44-2). When used correctly, child safety

Table 44-2. Pediatric Car Safety Seat Guidelines		
Age Group	*Type of Car Seat*	*General Guidelines*
Term newborns/infants	Rear-facing	Until 2 years of age or until they reach the highest weight or height allowed by car seat manufacturer.
Toddlers/preschoolers	Rear-facing and forward-facing	Rear-facing as long as possible. A full harness should be used as long as allowed by car seat manufacturer.
School-aged children	Belt-positioning booster seat	When weight exceeds limit for car seat. Use until adult belt fits correctly (usually at 4'9" and between 8 and 12 years of age).
Older children	Seat belts	When old enough and large enough to use the vehicle seat belt alone.
All children younger than 13 years should be restrained in the rear seats of vehicles.		

Adapted from American Academy of Pediatrics. Car seats: information for families for 2013. http://www.healthychildren.org/English/safety-prevention/on-the-go/Pages/Car-Safety-Seats-Information-for-Families.aspx. Accessed October 17, 2013 seats in passenger cars reduce the risk of death by 71% for infants and 54% for toddlers aged 1 to 4 years. Booster seats reduce injury risk by 59% for children aged 4 to 7 years compared with safety belts alone. Unfortunately, studies indicate that between one-third and two-thirds of car safety seats are used incorrectly. To address this, newborn care units often have car safety seat education programs, and some require possession of an infant car safety seat prior to hospital discharge. Police departments and private motor companies hold free public events to teach and manually check appropriate car seat use. In addition to engineering and education, passage and strict enforcement of child restraint laws are essential to compliance. All 50 states and the District of Columbia have child restraint laws (www.iihs.org/iihs/topics/laws/safetybeltuse). Nevertheless, loopholes still exist, such as exemptions in some states for seat belt use if older children are riding in rear seats; for seat belt use in school buses, taxis, and police vehicles; and if all safety belts are already in use. Such exemptions reinforce parental misconceptions, particularly that the lap of an occupant (ie, the "child crusher" position) is a safe position.

Counseling by Pediatricians

Although the existence of significant gaps in parental knowledge about injury prevention has been clearly established, studies have shown that pediatricians spend surprisingly little time counseling parents about childhood safety. One survey found that only 42% of caregivers of children younger than 15 years who had a medical visit in the past year recalled receiving injury prevention information. Another survey found that while 55% of pediatricians responded that they provided injury prevention information, only 19% of their patients recalled receiving this information. Reasons for limited discussion of safety issues may include lack of emphasis on preventive medical care in medical schools and pediatric training programs, inadequate time or payment, and lack of perceived self-efficacy or effectiveness. Research, however, has shown that injury prevention counseling in primary care settings is effective, resulting in increased knowledge and improved safety practices. Parents report that they would listen to physicians much more than any other group about child safety.

TIPP–The Injury Prevention Program was developed in 1983 by the American Academy of Pediatrics (AAP) to firmly establish injury prevention as a cost-effective standard of care for pediatricians. The AAP suggests that health care professionals focus their safety counseling on a few topics targeted to individual risk factors (eg, age, gender, location, season of the year, socioeconomic status of family). Table 44-3 shows the age-specific counseling schedule of TIPP, which indicates the minimum topics to cover at each visit. Topics are scheduled for discussion before children reach a particular developmental milestone. For example, a discussion of falls is scheduled for the 2- or 4-week visit, before newborns normally begin to roll over, and a discussion of choking is scheduled for 4 months, before infants can grasp and put things in their mouths. Specific preventive measures should be reinforced at each visit. Areas of injury prevention guidance recommended for adolescents include traffic safety (eg, seat belts, alcohol use, motorcycle and bicycle helmets), water safety (eg, alcohol use and diving injuries), sports safety, and firearm safety.

Table 44-3. TIPP–The Injury Prevention Program Safety Counseling Schedule for Early and Middle Childhood		
Visit	*Introduce*	*Reinforce*
Prenatal/newborn	Infant car seat, smoke detector, crib safety	
2 d–4 wk	Falls	Car safety seat
2 mo	Burns—hot liquids, choking/suffocation	Car safety seat, falls
4 mo	Water safety—bathtubs	Car safety seat, falls, burns, choking/suffocation
6 mo	Poisonings, burns—hot surfaces	Falls, burns, choking
9 mo	Water/pool safety, toddler car safety seat, firearms	Poisonings, falls, burns
1 y		Water/pool safety, falls, burns
15 mo		Car safety seat, poisonings, falls, burns
18 mo		Car safety seat, poisonings, falls, burns, firearm hazards
2 y	Falls—play equipment, tricycles, pedestrian safety	Car safety seat, water/pool safety, burns, firearm hazards
3 y		Car safety seat, pedestrian safety, falls, burns, firearm hazards
4 y	Booster seat use	Pedestrian safety, falls—play equipment, firearm hazards
5 y	Water/pool safety, bicycle safety	Firearm hazards, pedestrian safety, booster seat
6 y	Fire safety	Bicycle, booster seat, pedestrian, and firearm hazards
8 y	Sports safety, seat belt use	Bicycle
10 y	Firearm hazards	Sports, seat belt use, bicycle safety

Adapted from the American Academy of Pediatrics Council on Injury, Violence, and Poison Prevention. *TIPP–The Injury Prevention Program: A Guide to Safety Counseling in Office Practice.* Elk Grove Village, IL: American Academy of Pediatrics; 1994

Connected Kids: Safe, Strong, Secure is a violence prevention tool introduced by the AAP in 2006 to augment TIPP. Acknowledging that injury and violence prevention are intertwined, it uses an asset-based approach to engage parents in understanding and fostering healthy child development. An emphasis is put on support and open communication to promote emotional and physical safety.

Health care professionals should involve parents and patients in educational efforts (eg, have a bicycle helmet in the office for children to try on). Safety counseling is most effective if limited to 2 or 3 topics per visit. Advice should be well defined and practical rather than general information (eg, write the Poison Help number on the phone; never leave children unattended in water). Advice should be tailored to each family after exploring individual situations through open-ended questions (eg, "Where does your baby spend awake time during the day?"; "What do you think is the biggest safety risk for your child?"). Health care professionals should be aware of different levels of health literacy and confirm understanding rather than rushing through a prepared statement. Access to interventions should be considered, such as cost and accessibility of helmets and child safety seats. Whenever possible, pediatricians should coordinate their educational efforts with current community injury prevention efforts (eg, bicycle helmet campaigns; handgun regulation).

Recent Recommendations

The AAP has multiple safety recommendations. Following are newer and revised recommendations:

- Motor vehicle crashes are the leading cause of death for children 5 years and older. Comprehensive legislation and education promoting 3-stage graduated driver's license programs should be encouraged. The AAP recommends that pediatricians know their state laws addressing teenage drivers, encourage seat belt use, discourage distractions when driving, encourage restrictions on nighttime driving and limits on number of passengers, and counsel teenagers about the dangers of driving while impaired (2006).
- Pedestrian injuries are a significant traffic-related cause of morbidity and mortality. Emphasis should be given to community- and school-based strategies to reduce exposure to high-speed and high-volume traffic, improvements in car engineering, and driver education to reduce pediatric pedestrian injury (2009).
- The most effective measure to prevent suicide, homicide, and unintentional firearm-related injuries to children and adolescents is the absence of guns from homes and communities. Guns should be subject to consumer product regulations addressing child access, safety, and design. The AAP supports law enforcement activities that trace the origins of firearms used in the commission of crimes and that these data be used to enforce regulations aimed at preventing illegal sales to minors (2012).
- Pediatricians should assess water exposures and provide targeted counseling addressing supervision, swimming ability, medical conditions, and alcohol use. Four-sided fences around swimming pools and drain covers are examples of passive strategies to reduce water-related injuries (2010).

- Health care equity is fundamental to child health. Children should be protected from injury within their built environment and provided with access to quality, patient-centered, and culturally effective medical care (2010).
- Improving pediatric trauma services will decrease injury-related morbidity and mortality. The AAP recommends an integrated public health approach to trauma, starting at preventive care and continuing through long-term follow-up (2008).
- Increased efforts should be made to prevent food-related choking among children through federal agency surveillance and regulation, food manufacturer design, and health care professional counseling efforts (2010).
- Sports-related concussions are common yet underreported; any pediatric or adolescent athlete who sustains a concussion should be evaluated by a health care professional and receive medical clearance before returning to play (2010).

Additional guidelines can be found at www.aappolicy.org using the key words "injury prevention."

Pediatricians as Advocates

As advocates for child safety, pediatricians can play a major role in injury prevention outside of the clinical setting. Pediatricians have started community programs or provided support to ongoing programs. Safe Kids Worldwide (www.safekids.org) is an organization made up of safety experts, educators, corporations, foundations, governments, and volunteers whose mission is to prevent childhood injury through education and advocacy. Safe Kids and other issue-specific organizations, such as the Children's Defense Fund (www.childrensdefense.org) and Farm Safety For Just Kids (www.farmsafetyforjustkids.org), can provide resources to support pediatricians in local or national projects and provide avenues for legislative participation. Through community pediatrics programs (www.aap.org/commpeds), the AAP provides grants to pediatricians and pediatric residents who want to create innovative community projects promoting child health.

Legislative advocacy is an exciting opportunity for health care professionals to effect wide-reaching change. States have enacted laws covering many aspects of injury prevention, including car safety seats, poison centers, cribs, playgrounds, amusement parks, protective gear for sports, swimming pools, and school buses. Dramatic reductions in injuries often follow safety legislation. For example, infant walker–related injuries have decreased by 76% since the introduction of the ASTM International F977 Consumer Safety Performance Specification for Infant Walkers in1997 and the introduction of stationary activity centers as alternatives to mobile infant walkers. Other examples of product-related legislation include federal crib standards of 1974 mandating close spacing of vertical slats to reduce the risk of entrapment, the Child Safety Protection Act of 1994 requiring toy safety labels on any balls with a diameter less than 1¾ inches (4.44 cm), window blinds manufactured with tassels instead of loops and children's clothing without drawstrings to prevent strangulation, and toy boxes manufactured with safer lids and airholes in case a child is trapped within. Similarly, in December 2010, the Consumer Product Safety Commission voted to ban drop-side cribs, citing the recall of more than 9 million cribs over the previous 5 years and the entrapment and death of 30 babies over the previous 10 years. The ban went into effect in June 2011 and prohibits the sale of such cribs even at garage sales.

Pediatricians can heighten awareness about the magnitude of childhood injuries through calls or letters to legislators, testifying about the benefits of specific safety legislation, or partnering to introduce new legislation. Pediatrician legislative involvement is critical to ensuring evidence-guided local and national injury prevention.

CASE RESOLUTION

Some of the factors that influenced the injury suffered by the girl in the case history are the age of driver's licensure, passage and enforcement of laws pertaining to cell phone use in cars, design of the car, road conditions, and availability of emergency rescue services and specialized pediatric care.

Health care professionals have the opportunity to teach injury prevention to children and their parents as well as to influence the individuals who manufacture the products and pass the laws that affect children's risk of injury.

Selected References

Bernard SJ, Paulozzi LJ, Wallace DL; Centers for Disease Control and Prevention. Fatal injuries among children by race and ethnicity—United States, 1999–2002. *MMWR Surveill Summ.* 2007;56(5):1–16

Centers for Disease Control and Prevention. Injury prevention & control: data & statistics (WISQARS). http://www.cdc.gov/injury/wisqars. Accessed October 17, 2013

Chen J, Kresnow MJ, Simon TR, Dellinger A. Injury-prevention counseling and behavior among US children: results from the second Injury Control and Risk Survey. *Pediatrics.* 2007;119(4):e958–e965

Eaton DK, Kann L, Kinchen S, et al. Youth risk behavior surveillance—United States, 2011. *MMWR Surveill Summ.* 2012;61(4):1–162

Gardner HG; American Academy of Pediatrics Committee on Injury, Violence, and Poison Prevention. Office-based counseling for unintentional injury prevention. *Pediatrics.* 2007;119(1):202–206

Gittelman MA, Pomerantz WJ, Schubert CJ. Implementing and evaluating an injury prevention curriculum within a pediatric residency program. *J Trauma.* 2010;69(4 Suppl):S239–S244

Hunter WM, Helou S, Saluja G, Runyan CW, Coyne-Beasley T. Injury prevention advice in top-selling parenting books. *Pediatrics.* 2005;116(5):1080–1088

National Center for Injury Prevention and Control. *CDC Injury Fact Book.* Atlanta, GA: Centers for Disease Control and Prevention; 2006. http://stacks.cdc.gov/view/cdc/11438. Accessed October 17, 2013

Peden M, Oyegbite K, Ozanne-Smith J, et al. *World Report on Child Injury Prevention.* Geneva, Switzerland: World Health Organization; 2008. http://www.who.int/violence_injury_prevention/child/injury/world_report/en. Accessed October 17, 2013

CHAPTER 45

Fostering Self-esteem

Rick Goldstein, MD

CASE STUDY

A 4-year-old girl is brought to the office for her annual physical examination. She has been healthy. Her mother expresses concern that her daughter is shy and does not always play well with other children. She has never participated in a child care program or group activities out of the home. She spends most of her time with her mother, grandmother, and 7-year-old sister, with whom she gets along fairly well. Both parents work outside the home, her father full-time and her mother part-time.

The girl's medical history is unremarkable except for an episode of bronchiolitis at 8 months of age. She has reached all of her developmental milestones at appropriate ages, currently speaks well in sentences, is able to dress herself without supervision, and can balance on one foot with no difficulty.

The physical examination is entirely normal. However, numerous times during the visit, the mother tells her daughter to "sit up straight," "stop fidgeting," and "act your age." The mother rolls her eyes as she tells you, "She doesn't know how to act."

Questions

1. What is self-esteem?
2. How do parents or other caregivers affect the development of their children's self-esteem positively and negatively?
3. What role does discipline play in the development of self-esteem?
4. How does illness affect self-esteem?
5. What suggestions can primary care physicians give parents and other caregivers to help foster positive self-esteem in children?

A parent worries that her spouse is too sarcastic with their son. Another worries that indiscriminate praise at school inflates his child's sense of ability while setting her up for "a rude awakening" and failure. There is a plea that a child's obesity not be discussed in front of him. You are asked to intervene when a school fails to address bullying. Embedded in these scenarios, and countless others, is a concern that a child's self-esteem is malleable and fragile and that its preservation is crucial to that child's success. What should a primary care pediatrician know about how a child's self-concept affects his or her thoughts, feelings and behavior?

Self-esteem: Basic Concepts

Parents often use the term *self-esteem* to describe their child's confidence, with an implied sense of agency and feelings of self-worth. *Agency* is considered the capacity to act in the world, the notion that what an individual thinks, wants, and does has importance. A person of high self-esteem has a sense of self-respect, purpose, and self-awareness, while those with low self-esteem are self-questioning, defensive, and overly self-critical, even when receiving positive feedback. As a concept, self-esteem is based on the confidence a child has for success as well as the child's confidence that difficulties, failures, and disappointments are tolerable and can be met while still feeling whole and supported. It is also grounded in the fact that success with other people is fundamental to a sense of who we are. Most would agree that it is essential to a child's health and well-being and

influences the development of relationships and identity during childhood and adulthood.

Self-esteem is the product of how one understands the effect of one's actions (efficacy) and how one *believes* they are seen by others (self-worth). Whether a child's self-estimate is inflated, overly negative, or accurate is not of importance to the concept of self-esteem per se; there is no "objective yardstick." In this regard, it is important to understand that there is a difference between high self-esteem and narcissism. A child can have a healthy self-regard without a sense of entitlement, grandiosity, and feelings of superior worth. This distinction is important when critically reading research finding correlations between bullies and high self-esteem, for example (studies also find high self-esteem in those who tend to intervene). Alternatively, a child's disfigurement or disability should not preclude that child from possessing feelings of positive self-esteem. Self-esteem is a phenomenological construct, and its importance lies in how a child's self-concept shapes his or her actions.

While the appearance of what is understood as self-esteem requires the development of certain cognitive abilities, it springs from an accumulated experience with parents and other caregivers. Preschool-aged children become much more independent and spend more time away from primary caregivers. This newly acquired independence, however, does not remove the need for attention, interest, and approval from their parents. Agency must be nurtured, and not simply controlled, to feed self-esteem. Opportunities to demonstrate the competence of children can be seen in the autonomy that appropriate parenting affords and heard as a source of pride in parents taking note of it. Preschoolers also enjoy playing alongside other children, although not necessarily in cooperative play (eg, helping each other in addition to playing together).

The emergence of self-esteem can be framed in terms of Erik Erikson's conceptualization of a child's social development. In the "industry versus inferiority" stage, the task of a child is to demonstrate his or her agency and for his or her efforts to be acknowledged and appreciated. The joy of autonomy and initiative are suffused with a need to live up to expectations—part of feeling she is a big girl is feeling she is a good girl. The first stirrings of conscience and the confidence to manage measured responsibility can be seen. The complex interaction of temperament, developmental stage, the family's security, the parental style of discipline, sibling and peer interactions, and school experiences coalesce in the experience of a uniquely competent child. For her caregivers, the desire to encourage a kind of fearlessness is balanced by the very real need to keep the child safe and appropriate. All of these aspects of her life contribute to the development of her competence, autonomy, and relatedness and animate her self-esteem. Its development can be seen when children at the age of 5 years begin to experiment with identity roles, when they demonstrate an awareness of social comparison at 7 or 8 years in their peer play and activities, and most clearly when they develop a sense of global self-esteem around the age of 8 years.

Much of a child's self-concept is established and reinforced by those around them, especially primary caregivers. While important activities occur when the child is alone and engaged in individual pursuits, much of a child's self-concept develops in a context of relatedness. This continues into the school years, with peers and teachers eventually assuming a more influential role in the continued development and reinforcement of self-esteem. The development of self-esteem is transactional, built by the responses children receive to their increasing initiative and abilities, resting on a foundation of security. A secure interpersonal environment is essential to exploration and correction. This transactional nature is at the core of self-esteem interventions and their enthusiasm for effects on individuals as well as society.

All parents hope that their children will develop a positive self-concept that will aid them throughout their lives. Unfortunately, discussions related to self-esteem are usually held as a result of a crisis or an observation by worried parents or teachers. Primary care physicians should bring the parents' focus to this important aspect of their child as a normal part of anticipatory guidance. Pediatricians and child health practitioners are in a unique position to offer specific recommendations for fostering self-esteem that may affect their patients' lives. During health maintenance visits with the child, they should model respect for the child's self-concept and growing capabilities in the child's interactions.

Research

Researchers have examined global self-esteem, a measure of the overall assessment of the self, and domain-specific self-esteem, measures of self-assessment with regard to performance and attributes, eg,

academic competence, physical appearance. The most widely used measure for self-esteem, the Rosenberg Self-Esteem Scale, assesses global self-esteem. One complexity in the self-esteem literature is that interventions meant to address specific performance areas may be assessed with global self-esteem measures and vice versa. It is no surprise that a child's feeling better about himself is not sufficient to improve his performance on a spelling quiz.

Research suggests a biological element in self-esteem. For example, twin studies conclude that approximately 40% of variability in self-esteem can be explained by genetic factors. At the same time, self-esteem is a concept with cultural underpinnings that resonates especially in contemporary American culture. It can be left to speculation whether the prominence of self-esteem is somehow rooted in the US national identity, but it is clear that its importance is not universally shared in all populations; for example, it is hard to detect it as a motivating factor in more collectivist cultures like Japan. This stands in broad contrast to its importance, however waning, in US classroom reform or claims by psychologists in the 1990s that "self-esteem has profound consequences for every aspect of our existence". There is debate over its proper conceptualization and importance.

At first glance, associations exist between levels of self-esteem and important outcomes. However, a debate among researchers, and one that undermines many studies, is whether the demonstrated outcomes associated with levels of self-esteem are actually caused by them. Does self-esteem lead to higher performance, or does better performance lead to higher self-esteem? This question can be applied to correlations that have been found between self-esteem and academic performance and motivation, task performance, aggression, gender differences, racial differences, and health outcomes. Credible research concludes that high self-esteem predicts lower rates of depression and more happiness. Adolescents with higher self-esteem have better mental and physical health, higher graduation rates, and lesser criminal records. Lower levels of self-esteem are found in obesity, drug abuse, and tobacco use. Inconsistent or harsh parenting and authoritarian as opposed to authoritative parenting styles detrimentally affect levels of self-esteem. Higher self-esteem predicts improved persistence when confronting failure.

Whether interventions promoting enhanced self-esteem cause improved outcomes is debatable. Recent research seems to have tipped the scales toward benefit from such programs when the programs include 3 specific elements: attributional feedback (helping children attribute outcomes to effort), goal feedback (promoting realistic attainable goals), and contingent praise (praise based on effort and improvements in performance). This seems to underscore the central importance of examining domain-specific interventions and self-estimation.

Parental Guidance

Vulnerabilities for Some

There are instances in which a child's self-esteem can be particularly vulnerable. The primary care physician should be cognizant of circumstances in which a child may feel shame, confusion, or guilt for problems occurring in the child or her family. Negative experiences in school and at home can predispose a child to feelings of shame and worthlessness. Marital conflict, divorce, or the abuse of a parent may negatively influence the self-esteem of children who may feel complicit or responsible for the problem. In such circumstances, parents are often concerned about the impact on the child, which provides an opportunity to work together to minimize negative effects. Honest, open communication with parents will reinforce the need for sensitive support of the child and help them set priorities or rehearse how they will talk with the child about the matters at hand (see Chapter 140).

Physical and psychiatric illness can challenge a child's sense of competence, autonomy, and relatedness. A child can be left uncertain of his standing, expecting failure, or feeling he stands apart. It is worth mentioning the challenge of supporting self-esteem regularly confronted by pediatricians when dealing with "new morbidities." The diagnoses of obesity, attention-deficit/hyperactivity disorder, and learning disabilities can have in common the taint of personal judgment and the threat of undermining self-worth. This aspect of a child's care is present in disclosure of diagnosis, the response of the parent and the child, determining a realistic treatment plan, following what can be a frustrating lack of progress, and ultimate outcomes. Parents and patients will benefit from careful modeling when representing the problem and how to talk about it by the pediatrician.

In the clinical setting, it can be challenging to provide practical advice that reflects research in this area. One helpful model for understanding self-esteem is the *self-determination theory*. In the self-determination theory, a child's general self-concept is understood as an organization of complex, hierarchically interrelated components. Self-esteem is the evaluative aspect of self-concept and is linked to and rests on intrinsic motivation. Research has demonstrated that optimal challenges, effectance-promoting feedback, and freedom from demeaning critique; parenting that promotes autonomy rather than control; and a secure interpersonal environment of relatedness are all essential contributions to intrinsic motivation and, by extension, self-esteem.

Optimal Challenges

Successful parenting creates opportunities for the child to safely extend her boundaries while ensuring the child's feeling of personal control. An overly critical or controlling style of parenting constrains the emergence of a child's young sense of competence and, by extension, affects the child's self-esteem. Being handed a scribble drawing by a preschooler and told what it represents is emblematic. An appreciative, interested, positive response to the disordered marks is sustaining; disinterest and immediate correction or criticism undermine.

It may be important to discuss the difference between encouragement and pressure with parents, and many may benefit from an introduction to the concept of positive communication. To support positive self-esteem, children need encouragement at all levels of their development (Box 45-1). This is communicated verbally and

Box 45-1. Encouraging Self-esteem
Don'ts
Have negative expectations.
Focus on mistakes.
Expect perfection.
Overly protect children.
Dos
Show confidence in children's abilities.
Build on children's strengths.
Value children as they are.
Stimulate independence.

nonverbally and should be distinguished from overt pressure. For example, a first grader learning to spell should be praised for his early, if flawed, application of phonemes when he spells "winter" as "wntur" and may not need correction at that point. In general, children should be allowed to develop at their own rate and not be coaxed into activities before they are ready or judged too harshly for earnest, early attempts.

When pressure occurs, it may be due to parents having unrealistic expectations of how a child learns and develops or an improper sense that lack of success is due to laziness or a character flaw. Inadvertent pressure can be detrimental and cause tremendous frustration when, for example, parents try to lead a toddler into toilet training when the child has shown few signs of readiness, even if many of the children in his preschool class are out of diapers. Pressuring young children to give up pacifiers or another security object without giving thought to the child's readiness may also be quite anxiety provoking to them.

While children may not know what is best for their ultimate development, well-intentioned pressure can also be harmful as children grow older. Forcing children to participate in rigid, structured play and, sometimes, classes or lessons does not foster individual creativity or independence. The acquisition of technical skill is only part of learning, and the absence of intrinsic motivation can lead to the effort feeling meaningless or inauthentic. Children ought to, but should not merely, do what parents have arranged. Encouragement to explore and occasionally take risks should build on their "islands of competence." Mistakes should be put into the context of a sincere effort and seen in terms of what can be learned rather than as a humiliation. Pressuring children to do things "right" or "perfectly" discourages normal, healthy, risk-taking behavior and interferes with future efforts by children to participate in activities unless they are certain they can succeed.

A variation on this theme is overprotection, where the parent controls the child's environment so as to reduce any risk of failure or discomfort to the child. This generally comes at the cost of sacrificing the experience of novel achievement and developing the competence to work through frustrations and disappointments. Indiscriminate, unanchored praise is a corollary to this. Parents should be cautioned against always speaking in the superlative to their child and staying blind to any shortcomings. Children are adept at seeing the world as it is. A failure to see themselves reflected realistically by parents or caregivers may feed a kind of insecurity in which despite the glowing language of parents, the children feel uncertain of their actual worth. It avoids opportunities for children to make accommodations. Both have a negative effect on self-esteem.

Effectance-Promoting Feedback and Freedom From Demeaning Critique

Specific ways to communicate that support self-esteem include active listening, use of positive language, discarding "labels," use of encouragement rather than pressure, and use of the "I" method of communication (Box 45-2). The pediatrician should coach parents that this is not a rigid code to be followed at all times and at great hazard, but rather that the goal is a "good-enough" environment where well-intended parents put up a fairly consistent effort to be mindful of how they deal with their children. A useful way to set the correct tone with parents and caregivers is the use of strength-based counseling, in which advice grows out of a focus on what parents are doing right.

The purpose of active listening is to hear the child's message and understand its meaning. Its success rests on a centered approach to important parenting moments; parents should strive to be attentive and present at these moments. They should stop what they are doing and look directly at children. They should be aware of nonverbal cues, such as body posture and facial expression. If children are having trouble understanding their feelings, the parent should repeat what they hear them saying ("It sounds like…").

A nonjudgmental response, validating and non-dismissive, should be the goal of communication between primary caregivers and children. The basic message should be stated simply, clearly, and at a level that respects the maturity of the child. Words should be easily understood and spoken in a moderate tone, especially when discipline is necessary. Facial expression and body language should also be consistent with the message parents or caregivers are trying to convey.

Many parenting courses teach primary caregivers to use the "I" method of communication, which requires that parents explain their feelings to children rather than blame them for their actions. This approach is believed to be less threatening and demeaning for children, especially in situations requiring discipline. The "I" method has 4 recommended steps.

1. Statement of behavior or situation to be addressed (eg, "When you…")
2. Statement in specific terms of how one feels about the effect of the situation on oneself (eg, "I feel…")
3. Statement of reason (eg, "Because…")
4. Statement of expectations (eg, "I would like…"; "I want…")

Using this approach, a parent's statement might be, "When you speak so unkindly, I feel upset because I would never speak with you in that way. It makes you seem like the kind of person that you are not. I would like you to speak with me in the way we all try to speak with you, no matter how angry you feel."

Parents should be encouraged to reflect on the complex relationship between discipline and self-esteem, and they should be questioned about their impressions of their child's independence and competence. Promoting the growth of healthy autonomy should be a goal for all parents. As children grow, so does their ability to act responsibly and maintain greater self-control. This central insight is an important way to help parents see beyond discipline in simply punitive terms.

The poorer outcomes associated with authoritarian parenting show the importance of positive language, even when disciplining children (see Chapter 49). For instance, when children are playing kickball in the house, it is understandable that a parent might yell, "Don't play ball in the house!" or "Haven't I told you before? No ball playing inside!" While emotionally honest parenting in a loving context is the best parenting, parents should be mindful of when they are speaking in a reprimanding and negative fashion or transmitting their frustration. Parents or other adults should attempt to tell children clearly what they can do, what the limits are, and the reason for these rules. For example, a calm, more positive response might be, "You have to stop playing ball right now. If you kick the ball inside, you may break a window or hurt yourself or someone else. You may kick the ball outside in the backyard." Communicating in a clear manner changes the tone of the interaction from a reprimand for being bad to one where rules are clarified to a child who wants to do the right thing.

Parents should praise their children for successes and achievements. Failures should be put into context whenever possible, although the acknowledgment of mistakes can be important. A forgotten jacket or a careless job with homework can be frustrating but are not worthy of a demeaning critique. Negative labels have no helpful role. If children hear themselves referred to pejoratively by their primary caregivers, not only is an undesirable behavior modeled, but they will feel undermined and wonder about the truth of such statements, no matter how innocuous they may initially seem to parents.

Promoting Autonomy

Children do best when they are provided with clear, consistent guidelines for their behavior while at the same time being encouraged to do well, pursue their interests, and increase their abilities. They do this even better when they see this modeled in the adults around them. Parents and other caregivers should remember that certain methods of discipline, particularly if harsh or shame provoking, can be detrimental to a child's self-esteem. Several different approaches to discipline have been adapted by various ethnic, cultural, religious, and socioeconomic groups. While a discussion of each of these meth-

---

Box 45-2. Communication That Builds Self-esteem
Active listening
Use of positive language
Discarding "labels"
Use of encouragement
Use of the "I" method of communication

ods is beyond the scope of this chapter (see Chapter 51), it is important to explore strategies with parents and caregivers.

Talents and abilities should be recognized and highlighted. Children should know that parents have confidence in their abilities and that any display of effort is appreciated. Even small successes should be noted and not overshadowed by the large ones or the failures. Children thrive on the joy and pride they see in the eyes of their parents. Lack of encouragement can limit their optimism for continued success.

No parent wants their child to feel badly about themselves. Indeed, from the perspective of most parents, self-esteem is in itself an important goal. Children with high self-esteem are happier, less likely to be depressed, and better able to persist in the face of challenges and failure. But this will not be achieved by withholding all criticism and praising without merit. In many ways, the importance of self-esteem lies in its role in the discussion about criticism and praise in careful parenting. The point is that children need to feel good and confident about themselves while also perceiving themselves accurately and with self-awareness. There may be broad agreement about the goals, but there is not one way to parent, nor a single prescription for how to talk with sons and daughters. Pediatricians have a special role in putting all of these elements together as they advocate for the children under their care and the people they are becoming.

CASE RESOLUTION

In the case history, the health maintenance visit provides the perfect opportunity for promoting parental support of the child's self-esteem. The shy child should be approached by giving sincere general compliments (eg, "My goodness, you are so big"; to a carefully dressed girl, "What a beautiful pink outfit!") and, in the interview, inviting her to tell you some things about herself (eg, "What are your favorite things?" "What is your favorite color?"), while employing humor and enthusiasm to engage her in some details. This models interactions, which allows the child to demonstrate her autonomy, with the hope that this approach will be repeated by the parent at home. The health care professional can reassure the girl and her mother that the child's overall health and development are normal. In addition, once the careful, protective experience the parent has managed for the child is appreciated, the physician should attempt to normalize the child's behavior for the parent. While it may be important to directly discuss shyness in a developmental context, whether she is shy is not certain, and the parent's sense of deficiencies should be challenged by a view of developing competencies. Concrete suggestions should be offered for positive communication, such as minimizing "don't" and "no" phrases and being cognizant of how one speaks about the daughter. The parent should be encouraged to think about the child's temperament when considering involvement in multiple school activities but reminded that the parent has not yet seen the child in an independent setting, where she may negotiate very well and show sociability not yet evident at home.

Selected References

American Academy of Pediatrics Committee on Psychosocial Aspects of Child and Family Health. Guidance for effective discipline. *Pediatrics.* 1998;101(4):723–728

Baumeister RF, et al. Does high self-esteem cause better performance, interpersonal success, happiness or healthier lifestyles? *Psychol Sci Pub Int.* 2003;4(1):1–44

Brooks R. *The Self-Esteem Teacher.* Circle Pines, MN: American Guidance Service; 1981

Deci EL, Ryan RM. Human autonomy: the basis for true self-esteem. In: Kemis M, ed. *Efficacy, Agency and Self-esteem.* New York, NY: Plenum Press; 1995:31–49

Howard BJ. Discipline in early childhood. *Pediatr Clin North Am.* 1991;38(6):1351–1369

Kendler KS, Gardner CO, Prescott CA. A population-based twin study of self-esteem and gender. *Psychol Med.* 1998;28(6):1403–1409

O'Mara AJ et al. Do self-concept interventions make a difference?. *Educ Psychol.* 2006;41(3):181–206

Ryan RM, Deci EL. Self-determination theory and the facilitation of intrinsic motivation, social development, and well-being. *Am Psychol.* 2000;55(1):68–78

Sieving RE, Zirbel-Donisch ST. Development and enhancement of self-esteem in children. *J Pediatr Health Care.* 1990;4(6):290–296

Trzesniewski KH, Donnellan MB, Moffitt TE, Robins PW, Poulton R, Caspi A. Low self-esteem during adolescence predicts poor health, criminal behavior, and limited economic prospects during adulthood. *Dev Psychol.* 2006;42(2):381–390

CHAPTER 46

Sibling Rivalry

Carol D. Berkowitz, MD

CASE STUDY

An 8-year-old boy is brought to the office for an annual checkup. During the course of the evaluation, his mother complains that her son and his 6-year-old sister are always fighting. She says her son hits his sister and pulls her hair, and nothing she does prevents them from fighting. The boy is a B+ student and has no behavior problems in school. The medical history and physical examination are completely normal.

Questions

1. What is sibling rivalry?
2. What is the physician's role in counseling a family about sibling rivalry?
3. What is the role of anticipatory guidance in preparing older children for the birth of a new sister or brother?
4. How does birth order and gender affect sibling rivalry?
5. What are some of the unique considerations related to sibling rivalry between step-siblings?
6. What are some practical suggestions to share with parents about sibling rivalry?

Sibling relationships are important in helping children shape peer and, later, adult interactions. Moderate levels of sibling rivalry are a healthy indication that each child is assertive enough to express his or her needs or wants. Siblings educate and socialize together and mediate parental demands. Siblings often spend more time interacting with each other than with either parent. The sibling relationship is characterized by continuity and permanence, but the relationship is not without turmoil.

Sibling rivalry refers to the competitiveness between siblings based on the need for **parental love** and **esteem.** The rivalry is often characterized by jealousy, teasing, and bickering. The term was introduced in 1941 by David Levy, who described it as "a common feature of family life." Historical examples of sibling rivalry include relationships between the biblical figures Cain and Abel, Joseph and his brothers, Jacob and Esau, and Leah and Rachel. Sibling rivalry is also noteworthy in pairs of celebrities, such as actresses Joan Fontaine (Academy Award winner for *Suspicion*) and her older sister, Olivia de Havilland (Academy Award winner for *To Each His Own* and *The Heiress*). Their relationship was termed one of the most dysfunctional sibling relationships in Hollywood and may have had its roots in their simultaneous nomination for an Academy Award in 1942. By 1975, the sisters were no longer in communication with each other. Other siblings whose performances are often compared include football players Peyton and Eli Manning, tennis stars Venus and Serena Williams, musicians Liam and Noel Gallagher of Oasis and Ray and Dave Davies of the Kinks. Many Shakespearean plays have battling siblings. Television has included the issue of sibling rivalry in sitcoms, sometimes trivializing the challenges for parents. On the other hand, some shows portray unrealistic compatibility between children. Shows such as *Good Luck Charlie* and *Jessie* show

large families in which conflicts are easily and humorously resolved. This may perpetuate unrealistic expectations in families.

Sibling rivalry is a **universal phenomenon** occurring even in the animal kingdom. For instance, the firstborn eaglet pushes the other eaglets out of the nest as soon as they are hatched as a way of ensuring an adequate food supply. A similar phenomenon is noted in the blue-footed booby, especially in times of food shortages. Studies in animals show variation depending on brood or litter dominance and sex dominance (male or female) within the species. On the other hand, among wolves, older siblings help to feed and guard younger ones. In humans, the fear of displacement, dethronement, and loss of love occurs with the birth of a new brother or sister, leading to sibling rivalry. Older children fear they are not good enough and need to be replaced. Such feelings lead to a **fear of abandonment.** Jealousy also plays a role, and older children may be angry with younger siblings for displacing them within the family.

Sibling rivalry frequently has a negative effect on parents because it is hard for them to see one of their children hurt, even if it is by a sister or a brother. The challenge for parents is to know when, and when not, to intervene and what strategies to use to minimize conflicts. Physicians can help by offering **anticipatory guidance** to all parents and specific recommendations to parents who are experiencing such individual problems.

Epidemiology

Sibling rivalry is a universal phenomenon, and a number of factors influence its development. Time interval between children affects the degree of rivalry, as does the age of the older children. Toddlers who are entering the **"terrible 2s"** may have a particularly hard time mastering independence and tolerating the presence of their younger sibling. Close spacing results in more problems, particularly when the children are fewer than 2 years apart. In such situations, older children still have dependency needs, often feel less secure, and experience a need for maternal attention. They stay closer to mothers, are less playful, and are tenser. Closely spaced children engage in less spontaneous play, seem angrier, and issue sterner commands to their playmates. Sex of a new sibling also influences the relationship. There tends to be greater rivalry between same-sex siblings. Additionally, child's temperament affects sibling relationships. The 3 components of temperament include emotional intensity, activity level, and sociability. It is also important to remember that children are egocentric, which, according to Erich Fromm, lasts through 8 years of age. This contributes to a child's willingness to share (including toys and parental attention) and to act unselfishly.

Position in the family also influences sibling rivalry. Middle children experience what is referred to as **middle-child syndrome**; they lack the prestige of older children or the privileges of younger ones. These children are often least secure and strive hardest to gain affection. Special difficulties may develop if middle children are the same gender as older ones. Middle children grow up to be flexible, adaptable, and good negotiators. In myths and folklore, youngest children are "favorites." They are often the ones defended by parents when there are bouts of fighting.

Twins rarely present a problem of sibling rivalry; instead, they have a problem maintaining their individuality. However, sets of twins create problems for older siblings because they are not as unique as the pair of twins.

Step-siblings also present a unique problem in sibling rivalry. Children of divorce frequently feel abandoned by one parent and in competition for the time and love of the custodial parent (see Chapter 140). Competition with step-siblings is especially difficult if the step-siblings are in the same home.

There are also unique considerations when one child has a chronic or potentially terminal illness or long-term disability. Similarly, being the sibling of a gifted child (see Chapter 32) places unique challenges on sibling relationships. The unique strengths of each child need to be acknowledged.

Issues of sibling conflict change over time. Toddlers are protective of their toys and belongings and are particularly upset when a younger sibling touches their possessions. Sharing is a challenging theme of the toddler years. Children during their school-aged years are concerned about equity and fairness. They may be upset by what they construe as preferential treatment, eg, when a 1-year-old sibling is not expected to put his or her toys away. Sibling competitiveness is said to peak between the ages of 10 and 15 years. Adolescents, with their additional responsibilities, including minding younger siblings, may resent the siblings for imposing on their time. Sibling rivalry can persist into adulthood, and one-third of adults describe their relationship with a sibling as distant or rivalrous. After age 60 years, 80% of siblings report being close.

Clinical Presentation

Parental complaints related to sibling rivalry consist of fighting between siblings, including physical violence and verbal abuse, bickering, and regression to immature behavioral patterns. Although such immature behavior occurs most often following the birth of a new baby, it may also be apparent if one sibling is receiving more attention, such as during an illness or after a major accomplishment. Regressive behavior includes bed-wetting, drinking from a bottle, and wanting to be carried to bed. Substitution behavior, such as nail-biting in place of biting the new sibling, may occur after the birth of a new baby.

Before the birth of a new baby, parents may complain that their children exhibit temper tantrums, irritability, and solemness. They may mimic the pregnancy by eating a lot and putting a pillow under their clothes. In addition, children may have psychosomatic complaints such as stomachaches or headaches. Risk factors for maladjustment following the addition of a sibling include family discord, physical or emotional exhaustion in parents, and housing insecurity. Conversely, a good marital relationship and family support facilitates the adjustment to new siblings.

Differential Diagnosis

Dilemmas concerning the correct diagnosis of sibling rivalry most often relate to the appearance of behavioral changes, such as regressive or aggressive patterns after the birth of a new sibling. For example, a child who was previously toilet trained may become incontinent of urine. Although urinary tract infection may be considered in the diagnosis, a careful history concerning the birth of the sibling reveals the correct etiology.

Evaluation

The evaluation of children with suspected sibling rivalry involves a history of the problem and parental strategies for dealing with the difficulties. The parent should be particularly queried about one-on-one opportunities between parents and individual children. Physical examination and laboratory assessment are noncontributory.

Management

The focus of management is to allow parents to recognize the normalcy of sibling rivalry while helping them define the behaviors that are acceptable and not acceptable within the family context. Children fight more often in families when parents condone fighting and aggression between siblings as normal behavior. Likewise, children of parents who are angry may interact with their siblings through anger. Parents should be counseled about this. Parents may not appreciate their child's fear of loss of parental love as the basis of the sibling conflicts. They should be reminded that many children think, "If I am so good, why do I have to be replaced?" Parents should be asked to empathize by imagining how they would feel if their spouse brought home another mate, even if they were reassured about being loved. Physicians can also help parents deal with sibling rivalry by having them consider their treatment of children in terms of uniqueness versus uniformity and quality versus inequality. In general, parents should be advised to set the ground rules for acceptable behavior. Such rules include no hitting, punching, hair pulling, name-calling, cursing, or door slamming. There may be a neutral area in the home that can be set aside for arbitration should disagreements arise. Moving to a neutral area also allows for some time to cool off. Parents should be reminded that children who are hungry, tired, or bored are more easily frustrated and may start fights more readily.

Birth of New Siblings

Parents may notice behavioral changes in their children before the birth of the new sibling. These changes depend on the age of the children and presence of other siblings. Children should be told about the upcoming birth. The timing depends on the children's age; younger children do not need much lead time. Some studies have evaluated the inclusion of older children in the birthing process. The results of these studies vary, but they suggest that children younger than 4 years need their mother for emotional support and are concerned about her physical exertion during the birthing process. Some older children may also want to distance themselves from the actual events.

Physicians should suggest that older children be involved in planning for the arrival of the new baby as a means of minimizing their feelings of exclusion. For example, they can help purchase clothes or prepare the baby's room. Physicians should also suggest that parents purchase a gift for older children that represents a present from the new baby, such as T-shirts that announce the older sibling's new status, such as "big sister" or "big brother." In addition, older siblings may be given a doll to serve as a baby they can care for. Parents should point out the advantages of being older with comments such as, "You can stay up later," or "You can walk and play with all these toys." Frequently, the birth of a new baby is met with regressive behavior in older siblings. Regressive behavior should be handled with tolerance and a realization that symptoms resolve with time.

Once the mother goes to the hospital, she should be advised to maintain contact with older children by telephoning. Many hospitals now allow for visitation by siblings. At present, hospital stays are so brief that this period of separation is much shorter than previously. Household changes that may be necessitated by the birth of the new baby, such as room changes, the substitution of a bed for a crib, and entrance into nursery school, should be made before the arrival of the new baby.

Rivalry Between Older Children

Physicians need to consider individual parenting techniques when counseling parents of older children. Parents who compare one child with the other may foster contentious behavior, and those who strive to treat all children equally may inadvertently perpetuate rivalry. Children need to feel that they are unique rather than ordinary. For example, parents who buy both children the same presents may think they are preventing rivalry from developing, but they are actually depriving each child of a sense of uniqueness. The harder parents try to be uniform, the more vigilantly children may look for inequality. Each child needs a parent's undivided attention, time alone together. Siblings also need time apart from each other, and they should be encouraged to hold separate playdates and individual activities. Not all children in a family need piano lessons and soccer practice. Individuality and uniqueness are important. The more agreeable a parent-child relationship is, the more agreeable a sibling-sibling relationship is because each child has good self-esteem. Practitioners should recommend uniqueness and quality in each parent-child relationship.

Parents sometimes have to deal with sibling rivalry between older children. Physicians should reassure parents that these older children should be allowed to vent their negative feelings toward each other. For example, if a girl refers to her brother by saying, "I hate him," the parents should respond by validating these emotions and saying something like, "It sounds as if he's done something to really annoy you." Parents should also be advised not to take sides. They should examine how they usually respond to squabbling between siblings. Is one child's name always called first during a fight? Do they perpetuate sibling rivalry by using certain nicknames (eg, "turkey brain") or other derogatory terms? Parents should assume that both parties are at least partially guilty and should not allow themselves to be drawn into the fight as referees. Parents can respond to a request for arbitration with a statement such as, "I wasn't here when things started, so I don't know who is right or wrong." The parents should also advise siblings that they do not have to be friends with one another, but they should not hurt each other's feelings.

Anticipatory guidance helps parents anticipate conflictual situations, such as who sits where during long car rides and who holds the remote control. Family meetings can be held to determine the ground rules that may avoid such battles. If conflicts arise, children should be allowed to work out a solution by themselves, with the stipulation that the parents will solve the problem if the children do not reach an agreement. If fights between siblings have recurrent themes (eg, which television shows to watch [who controls the remote] or video games to play), parents can devise a weekly schedule. Failure to abide by the schedule means both children forfeit the activity. If borrowing is the source of disputes, children who borrow from their siblings should leave collateral, which gets given back when the borrowed item is returned. Box 46-1 lists suggestions for parents who are seeking advice about fighting between children.

Siblings of Children With Special Health Care Needs

Nearly 1 in 5 children in the United States is a child with special health care needs (see Chapter 41). Caring for such children places increased demands on parents and their resources, and there is less parental attention or time available for siblings. Integrating the unaffected sibling into the families' care plan and activities can be empowering for the child and positively influence his or her self-esteem. As with all children, time alone between the unaffected child and parent should be strongly encouraged. Support groups for siblings of children with special health care needs have been

---

Box 46-1. Coping With Rivalry Between Siblings: Physicians' Advice to Parents

Dos
- Allow children to vent negative feelings.
- Encourage children to develop solutions.
- Anticipate problem situations.
- Foster individuality in each child.
- Spend time with children individually.
- Compliment children when they are playing together.
- Tell children about the conflicts you had with your siblings when you were children.
- Define acceptable and unacceptable behavior.

Don'ts
- Take sides.
- Serve as a referee.
- Foster rivalry.
- Use derogatory names.
- Permit physical or verbal abuse between siblings.

---

demonstrated to help youngsters cope and deal with their often conflicted feelings of anger at the special attention their brother or sister receives and their guilt about being healthy.

Prognosis

Although sibling rivalry may last for years, most siblings become good friends as adults. Rarely, mental health services are needed, especially if the sibling conflict has led to marital discord, there is concern about physical or severe emotional harm, or there is evidence of another psychiatric disorder such as depression. Learning how to negotiate with one's siblings enables children to develop skills to collaborate with peers and colleagues as adolescents and adults.

CASE RESOLUTION

In the case history presented at the beginning of the chapter, the mother should be advised not to serve as a referee. She should learn how to validate each child's feelings about the other. The physician can help her by talking to her son about his feelings. The mother should be advised to have a discussion with her children during which each child has the opportunity to define areas of conflict and the means to resolve them. The mother has the right and responsibility to prohibit physical fighting and encourage verbal dialogue.

Selected References

Adams MM. *Sister for Sale*. Grand Rapids, MI: ZonderKidz; 2002

Alderfer MA, Long KA, Lown EA, et al. Psychosocial adjustment of siblings of children with cancer: a systematic review. *Psychooncology*. 2010;19(8): 789–805

Anderson JE. Sibling rivalry: when the family circle becomes a boxing ring. *Contemp Pediatr*. 2006;23:72–90

Benhaiem S, Hofer H, Kramer-Schadt S, Brunner E, East ML. Sibling rivalry: training effects, emergence of dominance and incomplete control. *Proc Biol Sci*. 2012;279(1743):3727–3735

Dunn J. Sibling influences on childhood development. *J Child Psychol Psychiatry*. 1988;29(2):119–127

Goldenthal P. *Beyond Sibling Rivalry: How to Help Your Child Become Cooperative, Caring and Compassionate*. New York, NY: Henry Holt and Company; 2000

Hass E, Light P. Talking about the new baby. *Parents Magazine*. 1983;58:68–70

Leung AK, Robson WL. Sibling rivalry. *Clin Pediatr (Phila)*. 1991;30(5): 314–317

Nolbris M, Abrahamsson J, Hellström AL, Olofsson L, Enskär K. The experience of therapeutic support groups by siblings of children with cancer. *Pediatr Nurs*. 2010;36(6):298–305

Okun A. Children who have special health-care needs: ethical issues. *Pediatr Rev*. 2010;31(12):514–517

Pakula LC. Sibling rivalry. *Pediatr Rev*. 1992;13(2):72–73

Samalin N, McCormick P. How to cure sibling fights. *Parents Magazine*. 1993;68:147–150

Schmitt BD. Sibling rivalry toward a new baby. *Contemp Pediatr*. 1990;7: 111–112

Schmitt BD. When siblings quarrel. *Contemp Pediatr*. 1991;8:73–74

CHAPTER 47

Toilet Training

Sabrina D. Diaz, MA, MMFT, and Lynne M. Smith, MD

CASE STUDY

A 2-year-old boy is brought to the office for a well-child visit. His mother, who is about to begin toilet training her son, asks your advice. The mother says that by the time her daughter was 2 she was already toilet trained, and she wants to know if training her son will be any different. The boy was the product of a full-term pregnancy and a normal delivery. He has been in good health, and his immunizations are up-to-date. He is developmentally normal, uses some 2-word phrases, and has been walking since the age of 13 months. His physical examination is normal.

Questions

1. When should physicians begin discussing toilet training with parents?
2. What factors help determine children's readiness to begin toilet training?
3. Is toilet training in boys different from toilet training in girls?
4. What are some of the methods used to toilet train children?

The age at which toilet training is carried out is culturally determined. Some cultures train children at a very early age. For example, in the East African Digo culture, some children between 2 and 3 months of age are conditioned to urinate or defecate when placed in certain positions. Similar conditioning practices are carried out in China. Chinese children are kept without diapers, and when caregivers who are holding them sense a change in their bodies in response to a need to eliminate, they place their children in an appropriate position. In addition, children are dressed in clothing that facilitates toileting. Split pants, with the back and bottom portion missing, are used so that children can squat and eliminate without removing complicated clothing.

American culture has emphasized the learning aspects of toilet training as opposed to the conditioning aspects. This training focuses on the cognitive development of children and children's readiness to learn the complexity of the task. It has been demonstrated that infants as young as 6 months can be trained to signal the need to urinate or defecate and suppress emptying for brief periods.

Toilet training is potentially a rewarding and frustrating experience for children and parents. Parents may have unrealistic expectations of their children's capability or may be very intolerant of normal accidents that occur in the training process. It is important for physicians to introduce the topic of toilet training early on to prevent these unrealistic expectations. Refusal by a child to toilet train or accidents related to toilet training are often cited as a precipitating event for child physical abuse. It is recommended that the issue of toilet training be introduced and anticipatory guidance provided by the age of 18 to 24 months to help parents develop reasonable expectations.

Epidemiology

The age at which children are toilet trained varies depending on social considerations and pressures. Prior to the 1920s, the American approach to toilet training was permissive. This attitude then changed, and the methods became more rigorous, requiring that children be trained at an earlier age. In 1947, only 5% of children were not trained by 33 months of age, but by 1975, this figure had increased to 42%. Currently, approximately 25% of typically developing American children are daytime toilet trained at 24 months and 98% by 48 months, although many parents expect their child to be trained by 18 months. Cultural and socioeconomic factors also influence parental beliefs about toilet training. Horn and colleagues found that white race and higher family income were associated with parents favoring later initiation of toilet training. There has been a renewed interest in earlier toilet training in the United States. This has been attributed to 3 societal factors: the lower cost and increased options for child care and schooling associated with children once toilet trained, concerns about contagious illnesses such as hepatitis and infectious diarrhea in child care facilities where diapers are changed, and the adverse environmental effects of nonbiodegradable disposable diapers. There may be some reversal in these trends related to the development of highly absorbent, biodegradable disposable diapers that are also flushable and the marketing of nighttime training pants (eg, Pull-Ups) to children as old as 4 years.

As a general rule, girls are trained a bit earlier than boys, but only by a matter of a few months. Additionally, younger siblings often require less time to achieve daytime continence than firstborn children. Most children (80%) are trained simultaneously for bladder and bowel control. Approximately 12% are trained first for bowel control and about 8% for bladder control. Girls achieve nighttime continence at a younger age than boys.

Pathophysiology

Toilet training involves the ability to inhibit a normal reflex release action and then relax the inhibition of the involved muscles. For the process to be successful, a certain degree of neurologic and biological development is essential. Although a recent literature review found no consensus on which or how many readiness signs are ideal to start toilet training, following are several factors that affect a child's toilet-training readiness. Myelination of the pyramidal tracts and conditioned reflex sphincter control are necessary. Voluntary control is evidenced by myelination of the pyramidal tracts by the age of 12 to 18 months. Conditioned reflex sphincter control occurs by 9 months of age and voluntary cooperation between 12 to 15 months of age. In assessing the neurologic development of children, walking is viewed as one of the milestones that indicate motor readiness for toilet training. Appropriate motor skills, including getting to the bathroom, being able to remove clothing, and sitting on the toilet, are also key skills required for successful toilet training.

Toilet training depends on physiological and psychologic readiness. Cognitive development is assessed by a child's ability to follow certain instructions and understand what the potty is used for. Two years of age has been suggested as the appropriate age to initiate toilet training in most children given that the developmental and physiological skills necessary for successful toilet training begin maturing at this time. Some researchers suggest toilet training should not be attempted until after 27 months of age and argue that training will be delayed as a result of starting sooner. Toilet training usually takes 2 weeks to 2 months to master, although training may occur in less time using more intense conditioning methods. Achieving nighttime continence is often separate from daytime continence. Although culturally dependent, nighttime wetting is considered normal in the United States up to 6 years of age.

A child's temperament can also affect the success of toilet training. Children who struggle with inflexibility, are less persistent, or have a more negative mood often experience delays in toilet training. Unlike physiological or psychologic readiness, temperament is not likely to change after a 2-month delay in training, but understanding a child's temperament can better assist parents in supporting their child through the process of toilet training.

Differential Diagnosis

The differential diagnosis of toilet-training difficulties focuses on factors that contribute to a delay in acquisition of skills. Physicians should look for associated symptoms such as dysuria, a weak urinary stream, constantly wet underwear, or fecal soiling when assessing children who continue to manifest signs of urinary or stool incontinence. In addition, it is important to determine if children are essentially toilet trained but are having intermittent accidents.

Voiding dysfunctions involve an abnormal voiding pattern stemming from a problem with the bladder filling or emptying. They are characterized by urine leakage, an increase in urgency, and an increase in frequency and often result in frequent urinary tract infections (UTIs). The most common cause of isolated daytime wetting in previously trained children is UTI (see Chapter 56). **Chemical urethritis** may also

be associated with urinary incontinence. **Stress incontinence,** which has also been called *giggle incontinence,* may result in wetting. **Urgency incontinence** occurs when children delay going to the bathroom and then are unable to hold urine any longer. Some children have ectopic ureters, which can empty into the lower portion of the bladder, vagina, or urethra and cause a constant dribble of urine. **Labial fusion** with **vaginal reflux of urine** may also be associated with daytime wetting. Urine pools behind the fused labia or labia that do not separate sufficiently to allow natural egress during voiding, and when children stand up, the urine exits. Children with **neurogenic bladders** may also have symptoms of daytime enuresis.

Stooling accidents may be associated with chronic **constipation** and overflow incontinence or with congenital megacolon (Hirschsprung disease) (see Chapter 57). Stool toileting refusal occurs when a child is trained to urinate in the toilet but refuses to defecate in the toilet for at least one month. While many parents view stool toileting refusal as insignificant, it is often associated with developing encopresis, constipation, painful bowel movements, and delayed completion of toilet training. Children who prefer to stand in a corner to defecate should be commended for recognizing their physiological urge. However, parents should be aware that children who hide while stooling in their diaper are more likely to exhibit stool toileting refusal and be constipated. Successful treatment of constipation may decrease the incidence of toileting refusal.

Evaluation

History

Typically developing toddlers should be assessed for their physiological and psychologic readiness to initiate toilet training, as well as for any underlying medical conditions that may affect their ability to learn toileting skills at the customary age. Physicians should provide anticipatory guidance to parents about toileting readiness. Affirmative answers should be obtained to the following 3 questions:

1. Do children exhibit bladder control as evidenced by periods of dryness that last up to 2 hours and facial expressions that show their physiological response to the elimination process?
2. Do children have the motor skills necessary to get around? This essentially involves the children's ability to walk and remove their clothing.
3. Do children have the cognitive ability to understand the task at hand?

Cognitive ability can be assessed by giving children 10 one-step tasks and seeing if they are able to carry out at least 8 of the 10 tasks (Box 47-1). The ability to carry out these tasks does not ensure a willingness to be toilet trained.

Stress in the home may negatively affect a toddler's ability to master the task of toilet training. The physician might counsel a family to delay toilet training if the family has moved recently, the birth of a new baby is expected, or there has been a major family crisis, such as a death or serious illness.

Children who have had difficulties with toilet training need to undergo a similar assessment.

Box 47-1. Requests or Imperatives Used to Help Assess Toilet-Training Readiness	
Bring me the ball.	Give the pen to your mom.
Go to the door.	Put the ball on the table.
Sit on the chair.	Put the doll on the floor.
Pick up the doll.	Take off your shoes.
Open the door.	Open the book.

Physical Examination

A physical examination to rule out underlying problems such as spina bifida occulta, which may be associated with a neurogenic bladder, should be performed. A neurologic examination may reveal nerve damage impeding muscles from relaxing or tightening at the right time. A careful examination of the genitalia is important in children who are having urinary incontinence to determine if conditions such as labial fusion, meatal stenosis, or posterior urethral valves are evident. In children who are having stooling problems, physicians should check for an abdomen with feces-filled intestines, a sign of obstipation. In addition, a rectal examination should be considered to determine the presence of hard or impacted stools or any other abnormalities in the anal area.

Laboratory Tests

Although a laboratory assessment is not indicated in normal toddlers who are being toilet trained, diagnostic studies may be appropriate in children who are having problems with training. In older children, urinalysis may show evidence of a UTI.

Management

Physicians should help parents understand the appropriate approach to the toilet-training process. Unfortunately, most parents do not obtain the necessary advice from physicians. In one report, no parents attending a clinic and only 7% of parents in a private practice received advice about toilet training from their physicians. Therefore, it is important for physicians to initiate the discussion early enough to prevent the development of any problems.

There are 2 main contrasting styles of toilet training, although reliable efficacy studies are lacking. The first method, described by Azrin and Foxx, is parent-oriented and uses intense operant conditioning methods and a potty doll to assist with learning. The 6 components of the method include increasing the amount of fluids consumed; regularly scheduled times for toileting starting with 15-minute intervals; positive reinforcement for asking about, approaching, or sitting on the potty chair; grasping pants and successful urinating or defecating in the potty chair; time-out from positive reinforcement/cleanliness training following accidents; and teaching the child to differentiate between wet and dry pants, checking for dry pants every 5 minutes. Though this method has been effective in training children, including those individuals with intellectual disabilities, it is not recommended for training typically developing children.

The second method, endorsed by the American Academy of Pediatrics (AAP), is a child-oriented approach that stresses the child's physiological and psychologic readiness to toilet train. There are 3 versions of this approach: Brazelton's, AAP guidelines, and Dr Spock's. All versions use the same components with only minor deviations. This method involves gradual training and emphasizes the use of **rewards,** not punishments. Children with autism spectrum disorders (ASDs) who do not understand the social reward system advocated by this method may benefit from the intense conditioning methods described by Azrin and Foxx.

When toilet training typically developing children, parents should be advised to take the following approach:

1. Teach children the **appropriate vocabulary** related to the toilet-training process. This could include words such as "pee," "poop," "urine," "stool," "dry," "wet," "clean," "messy," and "potty."

2. Tell children what the **purpose of the potty** is. Placing the contents of a soiled diaper into the toilet can educate them on the purpose of the potty. In general, a child potty chair should be purchased. The potty chair has a number of advantages over the toilet. Parents can encourage children to decorate the potty and put their names on it. The potty can be kept in a place where children spend much of their time, not necessarily in the bathroom. Children can sit on the potty and have their feet on the floor, which is more physiologically sound and gives them a greater sense of security. Parents should suggest that children stand fully clothed in the bathroom as an initial step in encouraging their use of a potty. Children should be allowed to sit on the potty with their clothes on for about a week before the process of toilet training begins. Then children should sit on the potty without their clothes on, but no attempt to catch stool or urine should be made. Boys should learn to urinate in the seated position because they may otherwise resist sitting for defecation.

   When away from home, the potty chair should be packed to maintain the established routine. It is important that all individuals caring for the child (eg, grandparents, babysitters) understand the parents' plans for toilet training.

   Toilet adapter rings can be used if the family is resistant to using a potty chair or if the transition from a potty chair to the toilet is likely to be stressful, as is true for many children with ASDs. Adapter rings fit directly onto the toilet and do not require emptying, as do separate potty chairs. They require that the toddler climb up on the toilet, and they need to be removed for others to use the toilet. A stool should be used to aid in climbing onto the toilet as well as to provide more leverage while defecating.

3. Encourage cleanliness and dryness by **changing children frequently.** Parents should ask their children whether they need to be changed using the appropriate vocabulary. This phase is important to continue as the toilet-training process proceeds. Some parents mistakenly do not change their soiled children as a means of punishing them for having accidents. This gives children a confusing message about the need for cleanliness.

4. Explain the **connection between dry pants and going to the potty** to children. Children should understand that dry pants feel good and that they can keep their pants dry by going to the potty.

5. Help children understand the **physiological signals** for using the toilet. Parents can facilitate this by observing children's behavior around the time of elimination and making comments such as, "When you jump up and down like that, Mommy knows you have to go to the bathroom."

6. Children must have the physiological ability to postpone the "urge to go." This usually occurs when children have the ability to delay voiding for at least 2 hours. Parents then can initiate toilet training by taking children to the bathroom at 2-hour intervals. In addition, children should sit on the toilet immediately after naps and 20 minutes after meals. Children should not be left on the toilet for more than 5 minutes and should be permitted to get up if they want. While sitting on the potty, they can be entertained with reading a story or playing games. It is helpful to have designated toys or books enjoyed only when the child is sitting on the potty. Parents are encouraged to rotate the toys so toilet training continues to be interesting to the child.

Additional suggestions involve allowing children to have their clothes off and keeping the potty chair near them during play. This facilitates using the potty and is reminiscent of the practice of using split pants in China.

Children who use the potty successfully should be rewarded. Rewards can be in the form of verbal comments such as "Mommy is so proud of you," hand clapping, or the use of star charts that can be redeemed for rewards. Children can be consulted about what rewards they like. The AAP recommends using praise rather than treats for reinforcement. Punishment should not be used, particularly physical punishment. One report indicates that 15% of parents of clinic patients believe that spanking their children for accidents is acceptable. Parental disapproval of accidents can be articulated; however, parents should understand that accidents may continue to occur for months. Regression, being no longer willing or able to execute their toilet-training skills, may also occur with stressors such as a recent move, a new sibling, or divorce. Consistent parental reminders and a consistent schedule can assist with eliminating regression. It is important to normalize regression and encourage parents to focus on regression as sometimes a temporary step on the way to being successfully toilet trained.

There are 2 additional conditioning methods less commonly used in North America. The first is assisted newborn toilet training, which begins when the newborn is 2 to 3 weeks of age. The baby is placed over a toilet after feeding or if showing signs of elimination and is rewarded with food or affection for voiding or stooling. The second method focuses on elimination communication and begins at birth. The parent learns baby's body language, noises, and elimination patterns. The parent also makes noises, such as the sound of running water, to associate with voiding while the newborn is placed in positions to facilitate elimination. Interest in these conditioning methods has increased over the past few years.

If children are trained on a potty chair, they can generally begin using a toilet between 2½ and 3½ years of age. Children should wash their hands following sessions sitting on the toilet. Children can also use training pants, which are thickened underwear, or Pull-Ups, which are diaper-like underwear, rather than diapers. Pull-Ups are now marketed to children as old as 4 to 5 years, and there is anecdotal evidence to suggest that the age of completion of toilet training may be delayed by the use of Pull-Ups. Regular underwear is promoted as advantageous because it feels different from diapers and encourages the use of the potty. Using a bigger size or snipping the waistband facilitates children's ability to remove their underpants and can be recommended.

Some children seem fearful of certain aspects of the toilet-training process. These include fear of falling into the toilet (this is circumvented with the use of a potty or toilet adapter rings) or fear of the noise of the flush. Allowing children to flush the toilet without using it may dispel the fear. Toilet phobias can cause children to hold their urine until the last moment, resulting in wetting, or cause children to hurry and not fully empty their bladder, resulting in possible infections. Some children become fascinated with flushing or unrolling toilet paper, and parents should discourage children from wasting water or paper.

One of the major components of toilet training children is **modeling.** Children should be allowed to enter the bathroom with parents and even sit on the potty chair as one or the other parent sits on the toilet. Some children who are very strong-willed and independent, coupled with perfectionist parents, may have problems with toilet training.

Special considerations have to be made for children attending child care. Their teachers should be advised about toilet training. Children should have open bathroom privileges, which means that they should be permitted to leave the room to go to the bathroom without raising their hands or other reminders. Child care offers the advantage of peer modeling and peer pressure during the toilet-training process. Potty chairs should not be used in child care settings because of the risk of infectious diseases.

Children with special needs generally encounter more obstacles when mastering toileting. Communication delays, decreased motor skills, sensitivity to stimulation, and preference for routine are just a few of the additional challenges that make it difficult to ascertain whether the child is ready to toilet train. Although incontinence was once thought to be inevitable for children with special needs, it is important for parents to understand that continence can be achieved but that expectations need to modified (ie, may take until age 5 to achieve, and standard toilet training methods rarely are successful).

Medications have a limited role in toilet training. Some physicians recommend the use of drugs to increase bladder capacity. Although tolterodine and oxybutynin (Ditropan) increase bladder capacity and decrease the frequency of bladder contraction, they should not be used because they do not assist children with the toilet-training process. However, children who are constipated may require stool softeners, such as mineral oil, or the addition of fiber bulk to their diet and increased fluid consumption to facilitate the stooling process. Physicians should see children who seem to have particularly challenging toilet-training problems on a weekly or biweekly basis until they show improvement.

Parents can also be referred to the many books on toilet training, particularly if problems develop. Many books are geared for children to help them understand their body and the elimination process. Videos are available to help children with toilet training. Children may also have the opportunity to practice with dolls designed to wet or poop after being fed.

Prevention

If children demonstrate resistance to toilet training, the process should be delayed for 1 to 2 months. Children who learn how to withhold need additional time to learn how to relax their sphincter when sitting on a potty. It is important for parents to avoid an aggressiveness/resistance struggle because this may become the source of future bowel problems, including constipation. Children who are regular, particularly those who have a bowel movement at the same time every day, are more easily toilet trained. Creating a regularly scheduled toilet sitting session can assist with decreasing or stopping withholding.

Prognosis

All typically developing children are eventually toilet trained. The age when this occurs varies and is significant only if it restricts children from participating in school.

CASE RESOLUTION

The mother in the case history should be advised that this is a good time to initiate the toilet-training process. She should be told that boys, as a group, are successfully toilet trained at a later age than girls. Her son can be assessed to see if he can follow at least 8 out of 10 instructions (Box 47-1). If he can, the mother should be given the stepwise approach to initiating the toilet-training process. The mother should be informed that nighttime continence could take months to years after daytime continence is achieved.

Selected References

Physicians

Blum NJ, Taubman B, Nemeth N. During toilet training, constipation occurs before stool toileting refusal. *Pediatrics.* 2004;113(6):e520–e522

Choby BA, George S. Toilet training. *Am Fam Physician.* 2008;78(9):1059–1064

Harris A. Toilet training children with learning difficulties: what the literature tells us. *Br J Nurs.* 2004;13(13):773–777

Horn IB, Brenner R, Rao M, Cheng TL. Beliefs about the appropriate age for initiating toilet training: are there racial and socioeconomic differences? *J Pediatr.* 2006;149(2):165–168

Kaerts N, Van Hal G, Vermandel A, Wyndaele JJ. Readiness signs used to define the proper moment to start toilet training: a review of the literature. *Neurourol Urodyn.* 2012;31(4):437–440

Kiddoo D, Klassen TP, Lang ME, et al. *The Effectiveness of Different Methods of Toilet Training for Bowel and Bladder Control.* Rockville, MD: Agency for Healthcare Research and Quality; 2006. No.07-E003

Macias MM, Roberts KM, Saylor CF, Fussell JJ. Toilet concerns, parenting stress, and behavior problems in children with special health care needs. *Clin Pediatr (Phila).* 2006;45(5):415–422

Mota DM, Barros AJ. Toilet training: methods, parental expectations and associated dysfunctions. *J Pediatr (Rio J).* 2008;84(1):9–17

Taubman B, Blum NJ, Nemeth N. Children who hide while defecating before they have completed toilet training: a prospective study. *Arch Pediatr Adolesc Med.* 2003;157(12):1190–1192

Toilet training guidelines: clinicians—the role of the clinician in toilet training. *Pediatrics.* 1999;103(Suppl 3):1364–1366

Toilet training guidelines: day care providers—the role of the day care provider in toilet training. *Pediatrics.* 1999;103(Suppl 3):1367–1368

Toilet training guidelines: parents—the role of the parents in toilet training. *Pediatrics.* 1999;103(Suppl 3):1362–1363

Vermandel A, Van Kampen M, Van Gorp C, Wyndaele JJ. How to toilet train healthy children? A review of the literature. *Neurourol Urodyn.* 2008;27(3):162–166

Weissman L. Toilet training: how to foster success and manage pitfalls. *Consultant for Pediatricians.* 2012;11:307–315

Parents and Children

American Academy of Pediatrics. *Guide to Toilet Training.* Wolraich ML, ed. Elk Grove Village, IL: American Academy of Pediatrics; 2003

Azrin NH, Foxx RM. *Toilet Training in Less Than a Day.* New York, NY: Simon & Schuster; 1974

Bennett HJ. *It Hurts When I Poop! A Story For Children Who Are Scared to Use the Potty.* Washington, DC: Magination Press; 2007

Berger S. *Princess Potty.* New York, NY: Cartwheel Books; 2010

Berry R. *It's Potty Time for Boys.* La Jolla, CA: Penton Overseas Inc; 2009

Brooks JG. *I'm a Big Kid Now.* Neenah, WI: Kimberly-Clark Corporation; 1990

Foote T. *My Potty Reward Stickers for Boys: 126 Boy Potty Training Stickers and Chart to Motivate Toilet Training.* New York, NY: Tracy Trends; 2006

Foote T. *My Potty Reward Stickers for Girls: 126 Girl Potty Training Stickers and Chart to Motivate Toilet Training.* New York, NY: Tracy Trends; 2006

Frankel A. *Once Upon a Potty.* Hauppauge, NY: Barron's Educational Series, Inc; 1980

Gomi T. *Everyone Poops.* La Jolla, CA: Kane/Miller; 2001

Hochman D. *The Potty Train.* New York: NY: Simon & Schuster; 2008

Katz K. *A Potty for Me! A Lift-the-Flap Instructional Manual.* New York: NY: Little Simon; 2004

Mack A. *Toilet Learning: The Picture Book Technique for Children and Parents.* Boston, MA: Little, Brown and Company; 1978

Mayer G, Mayer M. *The New Potty.* New York, NY: Golden Book Publishing Company, Inc; 1992

Miller V. *On Your Potty.* Cambridge, MA: Candlewick Press; 1994

Patricelli L. *Potty.* Somerville, MA: Candlewick Press; 2010

Pinnington A. *Big Girls Use the Potty!* New York, NY: DK Publishing; 2008

Rogers F. *Going to the Potty.* New York, NY: Penguin Putnam Books for Young Readers; 1986

Smith DC, McClure D. *Monkey Learns to Potty.* Knoxville, TN: PottyMD LLC; 2004

CHAPTER 48

Crying and Colic

Geeta Grover, MD

CASE STUDY

The parents of a 2-week-old bring their son to the emergency department because he has been crying persistently for the past 4 hours. He has no history of fever, vomiting, diarrhea, upper respiratory tract infection, or change in feeding. The newborn is breastfed.

On physical examination, the neonate appears well developed and well nourished. His weight is 7 lb, 7 oz—7 oz more than when he was born. Although he is fussy and crying, he is afebrile with normal vital signs. The remainder of the physical examination is within normal limits.

Questions

1. What is the normal crying pattern in newborns and young infants?
2. What is colic?
3. What conditions are associated with prolonged crying in newborns and young infants?
4. What are key factors in the history of crying newborns and infants?
5. What laboratory tests are indicated in crying newborns and infants?
6. What are a few of the management strategies that can be used by parents to soothe their crying or colicky newborns and infants?

Crying, an important method of communication between babies and caregivers, is nonspecific, and many stimuli can produce the same response (eg, hunger, fatigue, pain). Parents report that they can discriminate among various types of cries in their babies. Crying can be divided into 3 categories: normal or physiological crying, excessive crying secondary to distress (eg, hunger) or disease, and excessive crying without an apparent cause.

The difference between normal and excessive crying may be more qualitative than quantitative. Some investigators have used the mnemonic **PURPLE** to characterize crying during early life, focusing on the qualities that make the crying particularly frustrating to caregivers: **P,** peak pattern (increases weekly until 2 months of age); **U,** unexpected bouts of crying; **R,** resistance to soothing measures; **P,** pain-like facial grimacing; **L,** long periods of crying; **E,** evening clustering. Deciding whether crying is excessive varies with parents' expectations and thresholds. Expressed parental concern about extreme crying or fussiness requires attention. If parents complain that newborns and infants cry inconsolably or continuously as well as excessively, the crying may have an underlying organic etiology.

Colic, a poorly understood, benign, self-limited condition, falls into the third category. It manifests as unexplained crying or fussing in newborns and infants that usually occurs in the late afternoon or evening. During an episode of colic, babies cry and may draw the knees up to the chest or rigidly stiffen the legs, flex the elbows, clench the fists, and turn red (Figure 48-1). Although neonates and infants may appear to be totally miserable during an episode of colic, they are otherwise healthy, eat well, and demonstrate good weight gain.

Figure 48-1. Colicky baby

Epidemiology

Qualitatively, **excessive crying** is any amount of crying that concerns or worries parents. Quantitatively, definitions of excessive crying have been based on the results of Brazelton's study of normal newborns and infants. Excessive crying begins at 2 weeks of age (median daily crying time: about 2 hours per day), peaks at 6 weeks of age (median daily crying time: about 3 hours per day), and decreases to less than 1 hour per day by 12 weeks of age. Apparently, more crying occurs during the evening hours, especially between the ages of 3 and 6 weeks.

Although many neonates and infants exhibit a fairly similar pattern of fussiness that peaks at about 6 weeks of age, those with colic tend to be inconsolable for longer periods and cry with more intensity. Colic affects 10% to 20% of newborns and infants younger than 3 months. There is no seasonal variation in its occurrence, and breastfed and formula-fed babies are affected equally. Colic usually begins at 2 to 3 weeks, peaks at 6 to 8 weeks, and resolves by 3 to 4 months of age. In studies of colic, the definition of colic that is cited most frequently is the definition from Wessel et al, which describes colicky babies as having unexplained paroxysmal bouts of fussing and crying that last for more than 3 hours a day, for more than 3 days a week, and for more than 3 weeks' duration (rule of 3s).

Clinical Presentation

Colicky babies are otherwise healthy newborns and infants younger than 3 months who cry or fuss inconsolably for extended periods, usually during the afternoon or evening. The crying usually resolves within a few hours.

Pathophysiology

Crying is a complex vocalization that changes during the first year of life as babies develop. In the first few weeks of life, crying is a signal that newborns are experiencing a disturbance in homeostatic regulation (eg, hunger, discomfort). As babies mature and begin to differentiate internal from external stimuli, crying may also be an indication of too little or too much environmental stimulation. During the second half of the first year, as infants mature neurologically and gain voluntary control over vocalizations, crying can be an expression of different affects (eg, frustration, fear).

A variety of explanations for the etiology of colic have been proposed. Some authorities believe that colic may not be a pathologic entity but simply an extreme variant of normal crying. The condition may result from an allergy, cow's milk intolerance, abnormal intestinal peristalsis, or increased intestinal gas, which are some of the more frequently associated factors. Others have proposed that colic is caused by problems in the interaction between babies and their environment, specifically their parents. This interactional theory requires not only excessive crying on the part of the newborn or infant but also an inability of the parents to soothe the crying baby. The "missing fourth trimester" theory of colic posits that babies cry because they are born "3 months too soon" (ie, human gestation should last 3 months longer). There is no scientific evidence to support this hypothesis. Whether maternal anxiety has any role in colic remains a controversial issue. More than one of these factors may contribute to the pathogenesis of colic.

Differential Diagnosis

An acute episode of excessive crying may be secondary to disease (eg, fever, otitis media). An organic etiology should be suspected in newborns and infants who present with inconsolable crying of acute onset. Box 48-1 lists the most common causes. Some conditions occur in a more chronic or recurrent pattern, particularly if the condition is not treated.

Box 48-1. Most Common Causes of Acute, Unexplained, Excessive Crying in Newborns and Infants

Idiopathic[a]

Colic[a]

Infectious
  Otitis media
  Urinary tract infection
  Stomatitis
  Meningitis

Gastrointestinal[a]
  Constipation
  Anal fissure
  Gaseous distention
  Peristalsis problems
  Reflux
  Intussusception

Trauma
  Corneal abrasion
  Foreign body in eye
  Hair tourniquet syndrome

Behavioral[a]
  Overstimulation
  Persistent night awaking

Drug Reactions
  Immunization reactions (previously common with diphtheria-tetanus-pertussis vaccine)
  Neonatal drug withdrawal (narcotics)

Child Abuse
  Long bone fractures
  Retinal hemorrhage
  Intracranial hemorrhage

Hematologic[a]
  Sickle cell crisis

Cardiovascular
  Arrhythmia (supraventricular tachycardia)
  Congestive heart failure
  Anomalous left coronary artery[a]

[a]May present as acute or recurrent episodes of excessive crying.

The differential diagnosis of newborns and infants who experience recurrent episodes of excessive crying or recurrent night awakenings associated with crying focuses more on behavior and temperament. Colic, neonatal drug withdrawal, or difficult temperament (eg, extreme fussiness) may cause recurrent crying. Recurrent night awaking and difficult temperament are discussed in chapters 27 and 50, respectively.

Evaluation

A thorough history and physical examination usually provide clues to the diagnosis in instances of acute onset of crying.

History

The focus of the history should be on determining the presence of any associated symptoms. In addition, circumstances surrounding the crying (eg, occurrence during day or night) should be ascertained (Questions Box).

Physical Examination

A thorough physical examination is required for accurate diagnosis. Particular attention should be given to the following aspects of the examination:

1. Careful inspection of the skin after all clothing has been removed to look for any suspicious bruises or marks
2. Palpation of all long bones to detect occult fractures
3. Examination of all digits and the penis to check for hair tourniquets (ie, single strands of hair wrapped around digits or the penis)
4. Examination of the retina to look for retinal hemorrhages (may indicate prior head injury)
5. Eversion of the eyelids to check for ocular foreign bodies
6. Fluorescein staining of the cornea to look for corneal abrasion

Laboratory Tests

Except for urinalysis, most screening laboratory tests are probably not useful. Test selection can be guided by the history and physical examination (eg, newborns and infants with fever without an apparent cause should have a septic workup, with an examination of blood, urine, and cerebrospinal fluid). Urinalysis, which may provide clues to an underlying metabolic deficiency, is sometimes helpful. Even when the initial history and physical examination are nondiagnostic, babies who persist in crying inconsolably should be suspected of having a serious underlying condition (eg, intracranial hemorrhage, drug ingestion). Such newborns and infants may warrant an extended period of observation or a more extensive workup that includes laboratory assessment.

Imaging Studies

Roentgenographic studies such as long bone radiographs may be necessary in some situations (eg, newborns and infants with long bone pain on palpation, suspicion of child abuse). Neonates and infants with retinal hemorrhages should have a computed tomography scan.

Management

Management and treatment depend on identification of the cause of the crying. Underlying organic conditions (eg, urinary tract infection, fractures) should be treated. Management of colic depends on presumptions about its etiology. It is important for physicians to **reassure** parents about the benign nature of colic and its resolution over time. Physicians should provide a caring and supportive environment in which parents may express their concerns and frustrations. Reassurance along with practical suggestions of feeding and handling techniques (eg, cuddling, swaddling, rocking) may often suffice.

Questions

Crying and Colic

- Is this the first time the newborn/infant has cried inconsolably, or does this happen on a recurring basis?
- Has the newborn/infant had a fever?
- Does the newborn/infant have any cold symptoms, vomiting, or diarrhea?
- Is the newborn/infant having any difficulty feeding? Is the newborn/infant formula-fed or breastfed?
- Has the newborn/infant had a recent fall or accident?
- What do you do when your newborn/infant cries?

Some management strategies have specifically been developed to reduce the risk that a newborn or infant will be injured by a frustrated caregiver. Educational materials in the form of booklets and instructive videos have been used to prevent the risk of abusive head trauma.

Management suggestions for colic should be customized for babies and their families. Common management techniques are listed in Box 48-2. Complementary and alternative medicine therapies have been used historically to treat colic. Evidence from recent small clinical trials and pilot studies have shown that some natural health products, nutritional modulation, cranial osteopathy, newborn/infant massage, and parental behavioral training have some promise in the treatment of infantile colic, but larger confirmatory trials are needed to address concerns about safety and efficacy.

Changes in sensory input (eg, soothing sounds or motions) may resolve crying and soothe colicky babies. According to the "missing fourth trimester" theory of colic, re-creating the sensory environment of the womb calms babies by triggering a soothing response—the calming reflex—and promotes relaxation. Five maneuvers that mimic uterine sensations are noted to activate this calming reflex: swaddling, side or stomach position, shushing, swinging, and sucking; ie, the 5 Ss. It is further recommended by proponents of this theory that 3 to 5 of these maneuvers should be performed simultaneously and vigorously to activate the calming reflex.

Prophylactic measures to prevent the passage of swallowed air through the pylorus can also be useful. Such techniques include feeding in an upright position and limiting the period of sucking at

---

Box 48-2. Management of Colic

Parental reassurance

Parental education

Alteration in techniques of newborn/infant feeding and handling

Alteration of sensory input to newborn/infant

Prevention of swallowed air from passing through pylorus

Dietary alterations

Medication

Complementary and alternative medicine therapies

Increased carrying

Responding quickly to crying

the breast or bottle to about 10 minutes (after this time, greater amounts of air are swallowed relative to the amount of milk ingested). Some newborns and infants eat very fast and swallow a lot of air. Burping these babies every 5 to 10 minutes during feeds may help alleviate discomfort due to excessive air swallowing (aerophagia). Decreasing the size of the opening of a nipple in a bottle-fed baby may reduce the amount of air-swallowing.

Methods to decrease intestinal spasm (eg, abdominal massage, warm baths, avoidance of overfeeding) may be helpful. The use of suppositories or rectal thermometers to break up rectal spasm and thereby release retained gas should be discouraged.

Data on **dietary changes,** such as the use of hypoallergenic diets by breastfeeding mothers, have been inconclusive but suggest that there may be some therapeutic benefits. Similarly, the use of soy-based or hypoallergenic infant formulas also seems to have beneficial effects on the symptoms of colic. Generally, these dietary modifications should be reserved for newborns and infants with additional symptoms of allergy (eg, wheezing, rash) or intolerance (eg, vomiting, diarrhea, hematochezia, weight loss).

Various drugs, including anticholinergics, motility-enhancing agents, barbiturates, laxatives, and antiflatulents, have limited success and are best avoided. Currently, antiflatulents (eg, simethicone) are prescribed most commonly. Despite lack of scientific evidence to support their efficacy, parents indicate that they are effective.

As long as no adverse effects are evident, limited amounts (eg, 1–2 oz per day) of **herbal remedies** (eg, chamomile tea) can be supported if parents report satisfaction. Over-the-counter homeopathic preparations are also innocuous and have no scientifically demonstrated efficacy but may be advocated as helpful by some parents.

Finally, physicians should encourage parents to respond to their baby's cries quickly and carry the baby as much as possible (eg, at least 3–4 hours daily). Parents should be advised that they cannot "spoil" babies younger than 4 months and that they might actually improve behavior by their own increased responsiveness.

Presently, the best evidence-based approaches to the management of colic include holding, swaddling, and comforting a newborn or infant; a trial of dietary modifications; limited amounts of herbal teas; and attempting to minimize environmental stimulation levels.

Prognosis

Fortunately, the natural history of persistent crying during infancy is resolution over time. Mothers of colicky newborns and infants are more likely to stop breastfeeding early and are also at higher risk for postpartum depression. Excessively fussy babies are at higher risk for child abuse. Although there have been some suggestions about the possible relationship between colic and later development of irritable bowel syndrome or increased levels of externalizing behavior problems in childhood (eg, hyperactivity, conduct concerns, decreased adaptability), there are no systematic studies to support these assertions at present.

CASE RESOLUTION

The newborn described in the case history is experiencing an acute episode of unexplained crying. Despite a normal physical examination, he was observed for 1 hour in the emergency department because his crying persisted. Subsequently, a septic workup was initiated, which revealed that a urinary tract infection was present.

Selected References

Barr RG, Paterson JA, MacMartin LM, Lehtonen L, Young SN. Prolonged and unsoothable crying bouts in infants with and without colic. *J Dev Behav Pediatr.* 2005;26(1):14–23

Barr RG, Rivara FP, Barr M, et al. Effectiveness of educational materials designed to change knowledge and behaviors regarding crying and shaken-baby syndrome in mothers of newborns: a randomized, controlled trial. *Pediatrics.* 2009;123(3): 972–980

Brazelton TB. Crying in infancy. *Pediatrics.* 1962;29:579–588

Cohen GM, Albertini LW. Colic. *Pediatr Rev.* 2012;33(7):332–333

Garrison MM, Christakis DA. A systematic review of treatments for infant colic. *Pediatrics.* 2000;106(1 Pt 2):184–190

Herman M, Le A. The crying infant. *Emerg Med Clin North Am.* 2007;25(4): 1137–1159

Iacovou M, Ralston RA, Muir J, Walker KZ, Truby H. Dietary management of infantile colic: a systematic review. *Matern Child Health J.* 2012;16(6): 1319–1331

Karp H. The "fourth trimester": a framework and strategy for understanding and resolving colic. *Contemp Pediatr.* 2004;21:94–116

Rosen LD, Bukutu C, Le C, Shamseer L, Vohra S. Complementary, holistic, and integrative medicine: colic. *Pediatr Rev.* 2007;28(10):381–385

Waddell L. Management of infantile colic: an update. *J Fam Health Care.* 2013;23(3):17–22

Wessel MA, Cobb JC, Jackson EB, Harris GS Jr, Detwiler AC. Paroxysmal fussing in infancy, sometimes called colic. *Pediatrics.* 1954;14(5):421–435

CHAPTER 49

Discipline

Carol D. Berkowitz, MD

CASE STUDY

A 3-year-old boy is being threatened with expulsion from preschool because he is biting the other children. His mother states that he is very active and aggressive toward other children. In addition, his language development is delayed. She is at her wit's end about what to do. The birth history is normal, and the mother denies the use of drugs or cigarettes, but she drank socially before she realized she was pregnant. The medical and family histories are noncontributory, and the physical examination is normal.

Questions

1. What is the definition of discipline?
2. What are the 3 key components of discipline?
3. What strategies can parents use to discipline children?
4. What are the guidelines for using time-out?
5. What is meant by parental monitoring?
6. What is the relationship between corporal punishment and child abuse?

Discipline can be defined as an educational process in which children learn how to behave in a socially acceptable manner. The word is derived from *disciplinare,* meaning to teach or instruct. It involves a complex set of interactions of attitudes, models, instructions, rewards, and punishments. Discipline is not synonymous with punishment. The goal is to help children gain self-control and respect for others and to learn behavior that is appropriate for given situations. It also serves to ensure a child's safety in the environment. Proactive discipline is action taken by parents to encourage good behavior, and reactive discipline is parental action following misbehavior. To be effective, child discipline must have 3 components: a learning environment with a positive, supportive parent-child relationship; a refined strategy for teaching and reinforcing desired behaviors; and a defined strategy for decreasing or extinguishing undesired behaviors. Children thrive in a supportive environment in which they are praised for socially appropriate behavior and are able to participate in the responsibilities and activities of the household. Appropriate discipline teaches a child empathy and to consider how other children feel when they are hit or teased. Parents, however, are more focused on eliminating unwanted behaviors and may bring these specific concerns to their pediatrician.

Parental monitoring relates to the oversight of children's activities at home, in school, and in the community. The extent and form of parental monitoring varies with the age of the child. Parental monitoring occurs when parents ask their children: "With whom are you going to be? Where are you going? What will you be doing?" Parental oversight involves children's access to and use of the Internet and social media (Chapter 9). Inadequate parental monitoring has long-term sequelae, including a greater incidence of risk-related behaviors. Parental monitoring must be coupled with parental discipline to promote desirable behaviors and eliminate undesirable ones.

Physician-Parent Interactions Concerning Discipline

Practitioners can assist parents by giving them guidelines for appropriate childhood discipline related to routine and problem development and to counsel about the scope of monitoring. The age and temperament of the child are important factors to consider. In addition, pediatricians can discourage corporal punishment as the major method of discipline. Pediatricians may also have a role in advising against corporal punishment in schools. While most states have banned corporal punishment in the school setting, 19 states, mostly in the south, still permit it.

It is important to encourage parents to establish a positive interactive environment with verbal communication, monitoring children's behavior and commending desirable behavior, ignoring trivial problems, and consistently applying predetermined consequences for misbehavior. Psychologist Marshall B. Rosenberg promotes the concept of compassionate communication, using the analogy of the language of the giraffe, which is a language of requests, versus the language of the jackal, one of demands. Identifying feelings is integral to the language of giraffes. Rules should be simple, clear, and established ahead of time. Frequently, physicians fail to inquire about children's behavior. Unless parents bring up the topic, it is not discussed during the physician visit. On average, physicians spend only 90 seconds per visit on anticipatory guidance and counseling. However, one survey of mothers in a physician waiting room showed that up to 90% were concerned about one aspect of behavior. Sixty percent of mothers surveyed found physician intervention quite helpful. The American Academy of Pediatrics recommends anticipatory guidance about discipline at each health maintenance visit between 9 months and 5 years and studies report that physicians counsel parents about discipline about 40% of the time. Such counseling is especially important to help parents understand the value of appropriate discipline in shaping their children's self-esteem. Information about discipline in the media may be confusing and contradictory and often supports the unfounded approaches of nonprofessionals. Starting when a child is 5 years old, physician-parent discussions should include the notion of monitoring.

Early in the physician-parent relationship, physicians may express their interest in behavioral problems by saying, "I am interested not only in your child's physical well-being but also in his [or her] growth and development and how he [or she] gets along with friends and family." They may then question parents about how children spend their days. During subsequent visits, pediatricians may say, "Parents of children of [child's name]'s age frequently worry about discipline. I wonder if you have any concerns." In making these inquiries, the physician may establish what factors, such as religious or ethnic beliefs, or family influences are shaping parents' decisions about discipline. Certain tools exist that can assist the primary care physician with counseling parents. One such model, Play Nicely, involves a multimedia educational program in English and Spanish that presents videos of hypothetical scenarios and has parents select from a list of options how they would manage the behavior. The program helps augment parents' repertoire of responses to their child's behaviors.

Problem Behaviors

Behavioral problems can be placed in 5 major categories.
1. **Problems of daily routine.** Such problems refer to the refusal of children to go about their daily activities, such as eating, going to bed, awakening at a certain time, and toilet training.
2. **Aggressive-resistant behavior.** This behavior is characterized by negativism and includes temper tantrums and aggressive responses to siblings and peers. Some undesirable behavior can place children or those around them in danger or at risk for injury.
3. **Overdependent or withdrawal behavior.** Such behavior is typical of children who are very attached to their mothers. These clingy children find separation difficult, especially in a preschool setting.
4. **Hyperactivity or excessive restlessness.**
5. **Undesirable habits,** which include thumb sucking, nail biting, throat clearing, and playing with genitals (see Chapter 53).

Some of the behaviors listed are age appropriate, and physicians can help parents by counseling them about stage-related behavior, such as oppositional behavior in a 2-year-old and independence-dependence problems in a 3- to 5-year-old. Parents may be more tolerant of a particular behavior if they understand what is normal at a given age. Just because something is normal, however, does not mean that it should be tolerated. Physicians can suggest to the parents ways of dealing with age-appropriate behavior (eg, placing breakable objects out of reach of toddlers).

Certain behavioral problems reflect differences in childhood temperaments. Temperament is the biological predisposition to a style of behavior. Carey has compiled a series of temperament scales to assess children and adolescents of different ages. For example, some children are shy and have a hard time adjusting to new situations. If parents anticipate such problems, they are often less angry when difficulties arise. Parental expectations can vary with a child's gender. Boys may be permitted to act a certain way ("He's all boy!") that would be disapproved of in girls. Physicians can discuss such expectations at health maintenance visits.

Physicians can also be particularly helpful in detecting and advising parents about disparities in the achievement of different developmental skills. Some children acquire motor skills before verbal skills, yet parents expect their children to be equally versatile in speech and movement.

Psychophysiology

All behaviors are modified by the responses and reactions of other individuals. The basic premise of discipline is to discourage unwanted behavior and to encourage desired behavior. This is accomplished by using techniques that are based on conditioning modalities.

Several factors contribute to an increased incidence of behavioral problems in children. Ten percent to 15% of all preschool children are raised in grossly disrupted family situations. These homes are affected by divorce, death, separation, violence, parental substance abuse, mental illness, or extreme poverty. Parental insecurity may also be a factor. In addition, families may have fewer social contacts than they once did because of greater mobility within society. As a result, families face greater social isolation.

Differential Diagnosis

In addition to providing anticipatory guidance about discipline, physicians must make 2 diagnostic decisions. First, they must determine whether a specific behavioral problem represents normal childhood behavior or an abnormality in behavior that warrants more specific intervention. Between 8% and 18% of behavioral disturbances may deserve physician intervention. More intensive management may be necessary for problems related to aggressive-resistant behavior and hyperactivity. Hyperactive behavior, which may exist as part of attention-deficit/hyperactivity disorder (ADHD), may be a sign of a significant underlying problem that warrants one-on-one intervention or the use of neuropharmacologic agents (see Chapter 129).

Second, physicians must differentiate between legally permitted corporal punishment and child abuse. Some individuals feel that any form of physical punishment is unacceptable and note studies that suggest that violence in the form of physical punishment is prone to escalate. Despite this, the use of physical punishment remains widely accepted in our society and is legally condoned in the home setting, though there may be guidelines about what exceeds legal limits. Fractures and bruises are not acceptable, and physical abuse should be suspected in children who present with such injuries.

Evaluation

History

The key component in the evaluation process is the assessment of the means parents use to discipline children (Questions Box). To obtain this information, physicians may simply ask parents, "How do you get your child to mind you?" This question is designed to lead to a discussion of how parents interact with their children. If parents have specific complaints, such as oppositional behavior, they should be questioned about the strategies they have used in their effort to discipline their children. It may also be useful to ask parents how they were disciplined as children to better understand their personal experience.

Physical Examination

Children's behavior should be assessed during the office visit. A general physical examination is useful to check for any signs of physical abuse as well as to evaluate children's well-being. A developmental assessment is also helpful because it may delineate disparities in the achievement of certain skills. Some hyperactive children may warrant a more extensive psycho-developmental assessment to look for findings consistent with ADHD. Behavioral checklists may be used to evaluate children's temperament.

Laboratory Tests

No specific laboratory or imaging studies are indicated for children with discipline problems. Such studies are indicated if child abuse is suspected (see Chapter 131).

Management

Physicians should assist parents in establishing appropriate guidelines for disciplining their children and reinforce the role of parents as the source of authority (Box 49-1). It is important for parents to realize that total freedom results in uncontrollable anxiety. Children mimic behavior, and **parents should act as role models.** If parents have temper tantrums when they are frustrated, their children may act in a similar manner. **Consistency** is also important. A system with a limited number of enforced rules is better than one with many different rules. In families in which both parents are working, especially if they have overlapping time schedules, consistency is sometimes difficult to attain, particularly if children are supervised by non-parental caregivers.

Box 49-1. Advice for Parents About Discipline

Set rules.

Set limits.

Define consequences.

Be consistent.

Ignore trivial problems.

Compliment desirable behavior.

Take time out when angry.

Physicians should emphasize to parents that it is best to **avoid power struggles.** Children engaged in a struggle often win because they have final control (eg, refusing to eat). Children should always be given the opportunity to graciously back out of a situation and save face. It is easier to avoid situations that lead to head-on confrontations than to get out of them once the confrontation has occurred. Parents should be the source of information for physicians. This helps strengthen parents' egos and validates their ability to handle their children appropriately.

In the past, specific methods of dealing with children with discipline problems concerned the issues of permissiveness versus over-permissiveness and accommodation versus strict punishment. Over-permissiveness refers to the allowing of undesirable acts and may exacerbate anxiety and increase demands for privilege.

Physicians should remind parents that preventing many behavioral disorders is easier than treating them. Reasoning is a useful modality, but it is unrealistic to expect infants and toddlers to have the cognitive skills to understand adult reasoning or to consistently respond to verbal commands or reprimands. Discipline should not only discourage bad behavior but also reinforce good behavior. Following are 5 examples of reactive discipline.

Redirection

Redirection is a simple and effective method in which the parent removes the problem and distracts the child with an alternative. This technique is frequently used to remove some object (eg, a valued knickknack) from the hands of an infant, replacing it with a toy. Parental patience, ingenuity, and enthusiasm facilitate this approach. This approach is also important in teaching children what is acceptable behavior. For instance, one cannot draw on the wall but can draw on a piece of paper. Children also respond to making tedious routines into a game. For instance, children can be challenged to see who can get their clothes on faster or who can brush their teeth first. Parental creativity and energy often avert confrontations.

Spanking

Spanking involves inflicting physical pain, which is usually successful in bringing about the immediate cessation or a decrease in problem behavior. Spanking is highly prevalent as a form of discipline, with between 70% and 94% of parents reporting using the practice. Spanking is used more often for younger children and for boys and correlates with parental attributes such as age, education, socioeconomic status, and religious orientation. Spanking is often employed

---

Questions

Discipline

- What does the child do that the parents wish he or she would not do?
- What do the parents do to stop unwanted behavior?
- Does the child usually obey the parents?
- When and where does most of the unwanted behavior occur? Does it occur mainly if a child is tired?
- Which parent is responsible for disciplining the child?

when other methods of discipline have failed to abort the unwanted behavior. Spanking tends to clear the air and get the punishment over with rather than producing a lingering guilt. To be truly effective, however, physical punishment must immediately follow the act. The "wait until Daddy comes home" approach is less effective because of the lack of temporal association. In addition, spanking tends to become situation-specific so that children associate a particular action with being spanked. This learning does not generalize to other situations. Spanking can teach children to be afraid of adults rather than to respect them.

Spanking may actually be damaging to the parent-child relationship and have a long-term effect on a child's self-esteem. Many parents feel remorseful after having spanked a child, and some acknowledge that they spank out of anger and frustration and question the efficacy of this modality. Most pediatricians discourage spanking as a means of disciplining children. Differentiation of physical punishment from child abuse is often difficult. In general, punishment with the hands is acceptable, but punishment with objects and spanking on parts of the body other than the buttocks or thighs is unacceptable. Spanking may be an early precursor of later physical violence and subsequent abuse. Again, parents act as role models. Children should never be allowed to hit their parents. This makes children feel extremely insecure.

Devices that are marketed for child discipline and inflict physical pain on a child, such as a sudden sting (modified stun gun), are never appropriate.

Scolding

Scolding involves the excess use of reasoning and explanations and is used by most parents as part of the discipline process. In families in which communication or interaction is minimal, scolding or verbal reprimands may result in an initial increase in inappropriate behavior because this is the only way children receive any attention. Verbal reprimands are more effective if used infrequently. Verbal reprimands should not be used during time-outs because they reinforce undesirable behavior.

Scolding, because of its negative focus, can be damaging to children's self-esteem. Scolding would be categorized as "jackal language."

Ignoring

Ignoring represents the opposite of explaining and reasoning. This form of discipline is difficult to use successfully because parents must totally ignore children's behavior. If even the least flicker of recognition occurs, then activity increases. A brief initial increase in unwanted behavior, a so-called response burst, may occur with ignoring. This disciplinary method works better in younger children.

Time-out and Removal of Privileges

Time-out, the form of discipline most recommended, refers to time out from positive reinforcement. In sports, teams call a time-out to rethink what they are doing and to replan their strategies. Children are placed in a neutral or boring environment whenever they engage in inappropriate behavior. The time-out technique can be used to discourage undesired habits. For example, parents may say, "You can suck your thumb, but you may only do it in such and such a room." This type of discipline is better than ignoring, especially if "ignored" children are receiving attention from siblings and peers. Children should understand the rules ahead of time and why the behavior is unacceptable. Once this is accomplished, time-out may occur without any warning.

A timer should be used, and children should stay in the time-out area for 1 minute per 1 year of age. An appropriate area must be selected. This area should be fairly boring, so children's rooms are often not appropriate. A laundry room, a corner, or a specific chair may be better. If children act unacceptably during the time-out, the timer should be reset. If children have to go to the bathroom during the time-out, they are allowed one trip. After they return from the bathroom, the timer is reset.

The use of the time-out method is sometimes difficult. If the inappropriate behavior occurs in the morning when children are getting ready for school, time-out just encourages children's desire to delay. "Beat the buzzer" is another idea that may be used in such situations. With "beat the buzzer," the timer is set. If children are dressed before the timer goes off, they may be rewarded for the behavior by being allowed to go to bed half an hour later. If the buzzer "beats" them, then they have to go to bed half an hour earlier.

Inappropriate behavior away from home presents the greatest difficulty. These situations can be dealt with in numerous ways, particularly if the behavior problem involves temper tantrums. When children are crying or screaming uncontrollably, it is best to remove them from the embarrassment of the situation. This "manual guidance" often occurs in a supermarket, where children select something that parents do not wish to buy. Parents can often circumvent this problem easily by walking into the supermarket and saying, "If you are a good boy [or girl] during the whole trip, then I will get you something at the checkout counter." If children still have temper tantrums, they should be removed from the area and brought to a neutral place, such as the automobile or a restroom, and allowed to finish their crying and screaming. In the past, some have said that a glass of cold water splashed in a child's face might sometimes be beneficial because it rapidly aborts the behavior, although there is now disagreement by experts on the use of this approach. If the inappropriate behavior does not develop into a temper tantrum, then "marking" time-out is helpful. This consists of putting a mark with a colored water-soluble marker on the child's wrist every time he or she engages in an inappropriate behavior. When the child returns home, the marks are totaled, and the time-out method is used.

Removal of privileges is a strategy applied in older children. Classically this involves grounding a child, prohibiting television or video games, or loss of driving privileges. The privilege must be something of value to the child for this method to be effective.

Parents who complain about inappropriate behavior should be asked to keep a record of children's behavior for 1 to 2 weeks. This helps determine if the behavior is really inappropriate and what is motivating it. Parents should be encouraged to talk to their children in a reasonable manner and to verbalize what they think children are feeling. They might say something like this: "It's terrible to be 3 years old and get so upset. You feel that you can't get the things you want, but some day you will grow up and then you will be in charge. I am really sorry it is so hard for you right now." Physicians should tell parents that it is important to set limits for children and to avoid threatening, judging, and constantly criticizing children. Frequent threats such as, "If you don't stop hitting your sister, you'll get a time-out," that are not carried out undermine the entire discipline process. To help foster compassionate communication, parents should ask themselves, "If someone said this to me, how would I feel?" Many parents have themselves been disciplined only with spanking and know no other means, and the advice that physicians offer is valuable.

Prognosis

Children raised in a supportive environment that teaches respect for others and self-control grow up as caring adults. Children who have been exposed to excessive physical punishment show aggressive behavior later.

CASE RESOLUTION

In the case presented at the beginning of the chapter, further history should be elicited about the mother's disciplining techniques. It is also significant that the child's speech is delayed. The boy's ability to articulate his feelings may be limited, and a formal speech and hearing assessment is warranted. The preschool should be advised that the evaluation is underway. A report from the preschool concerning the boy's behavior would be appreciated.

Selected References

American Academy of Pediatrics Committee on Psychosocial Aspects of Child and Family Health. Guidance for effective discipline. *Pediatrics.* 1998;101(4):723–728

American Academy of Pediatrics Committee on School Health. Corporal punishment in schools. *Pediatrics.* 2000;106(2):343

Barkley RA. *Defiant Children: A Clinician's Manual for Assessment and Parent Training.* 2nd ed. New York, NY: The Guilford Press; 1997

Burke MG. Is a 12-month-old too young to be disciplined? *Contemp Pediatr.* 2006;23:109–110

Carey WB. Pediatric assessment of behavioral adjustment and behavioral style. In: Levine MD, Carey WB, Crocker AC, eds. *Developmental-Behavioral Pediatrics.* 2nd ed. Philadelphia, PA: WB Saunders; 1992:609–612

Larzelere RE. To spank or not to spank. *Pediatrics.* 1999;103(3):696–697

Regalado M, Sareen H, Inkelas M, Wissow LS, Halfon N. Parents' discipline of young children: results from the National Survey of Early Childhood Health. *Pediatrics.* 2004;113(6 Suppl):1952–1958

Rosenberg MB. *Nonviolent Communication; A Language of Life.* 2nd ed. Encinitas, CA: Puddledancer Press; 2003

Runyan DK, Shankar V, Hassan F, et al. International variations in harsh child discipline. *Pediatrics.* 2010;126(3):e701–e711

Schmitt BD. Discipline: rules and consequences. *Contemp Pediatr.* 1991;8:65–69

Schmitt BD. Time-out: intervention of choice for the irrational years. *Contemp Pediatr.* 1993;10:64–71

Schmitt BD. When a child hurts other children. *Contemp Pediatr.* 1990;7:81–82

Scholer SJ. Parental monitoring and discipline in middle childhood. *Pediatr Rev.* 2009;30(9):366–367

Scholer SJ, Hudnut-Beumler J, Dietrich MS. A brief primary care intervention helps parents develop plans to discipline. *Pediatrics.* 2010;125(2):e242–e249

Socolar RR, Stein RE. Maternal discipline of young children: context, belief, and practice. *J Dev Behav Pediatr.* 1996;17(1):1–8

Straus MA, Sugarman DB, Giles-Sims J. Spanking by parents and subsequent antisocial behavior of children. *Arch Pediatr Adolesc Med.* 1997;151(8):761–767

Trumbull DA. To spank or not to spank. *Pediatrics.* 1999;103(3):696

Vittrup B, Holden GW, Buck J. Attitudes predict the use of physical punishment: a prospective study of the emergence of disciplinary practices. *Pediatrics.* 2006;117:2055–2064

Waterson T. Giving guidance on child discipline. *BMJ.* 2000;320:261–262

Wolraich M. To spank or not to spank. *Pediatrics.* 1999;103(3):697–698

CHAPTER 50

Temper Tantrums

Geeta Grover, MD

CASE STUDY

During a routine office visit, the parents of a 3-year-old boy express concern about his recent behavior. They report that whenever he is asked to do something he does not want to do, he throws a "fit." He cries fiercely, falls to the floor, bangs his hands, and kicks his feet until his parents give in. He often displays such behavior at bedtime or mealtime if he is asked to turn off the television or eat foods that he does not want. He has 2 to 3 such episodes per week. The parents state that their home life has not changed, and the boy's teacher reports that he displays no such behaviors at preschool.

Questions

1. At what age are temper tantrums common in children?
2. How do parents' reactions encourage or discourage temper tantrums?
3. What appropriate management strategies may help control such oppositional behavior?
4. What factors or aspects of such oppositional behavior indicate underlying pathology?

Temper tantrums are common, normal, age-related behaviors in young children. To a certain degree, oppositional behaviors such as negativism, defiance, and tantrums are part of the normal progression toward self-reliance and independence. Toddlers need to assert their freedom and explore their environment, which often puts them at odds with the limitations imposed by society and well-meaning parents. Young children cannot appreciate that rules and limitations have been established in the interest of their own safety and well-being. They see only that their own desires have been thwarted, and they may react to this disappointment with intense emotions. Children are not simply upset because they cannot have their way. They are angry and frustrated, and they lose control over their emotions. During tantrums, children cry and scream uncontrollably. They may fall to the floor, bang their heads, kick their feet, pound their hands, and thrash about wildly. Some children may throw things, try to hit one another, or destroy property.

Such intense displays of anger may be a terrifying experience for children and parents. Some children use tantrums to gain attention, whereas others use them to achieve something or avoid doing something. Recurrent temper tantrums may strain relationships among parents, children, and other family members.

Epidemiology

Temper tantrums are noted most often in children who are 2 to 3 years of age, but they may occur any time between the ages of 12 months and 5 years. Parental surveys reveal that about 20% of 2-year-olds, 18% of 3-year-olds, and 10% of 4-year-olds have at least one tantrum per day. Most children are able to express their feelings verbally by 3 to 4 years of age, so temper tantrums begin to taper off. Children who are not able to express their feelings well with words (eg, children with developmental delays, especially those with speech and language delays or autism spectrum disorders) are more likely to continue to have tantrums. Boys and girls are affected equally. Although temper tantrums are unusual in school-aged children, they often reappear in the form of verbal tantrums during adolescence, when autonomy and independence once again become developmental issues.

Pathophysiology

Temperament, or adaptability and emotional style, affects the ease with which children adjust to environmental inputs and their reactions to these inputs. Temperament is the "how" of behavior, as opposed to "why." It is innate rather than learned. Although inherent from birth, temperament may be modified in the early years of life by children's experiences and interactions. Stella Chess and Alexander Thomas identified 9 major temperamental traits based on their study of children's behavioral characteristics during the 1950s: activity level, rhythmicity (regularity), approach or withdrawal, adaptability, intensity, mood, persistence and attention span, distractibility, and sensory threshold. Three common patterns of temperament based on whether a child shows a greater or lesser degree of each of these traits are easy (high rhythmicity and adaptability with a positive mood), slow to warm up or shy (slow adaptability slowly and tendency to withdraw initially in new situations), and difficult or challenging (low rhythmicity and adaptability resulting in negative and intense reactions to the environment).

Appreciation of children's temperament allows parents to anticipate and understand their children's reactions, thereby giving them the opportunity to rethink how they interpret and respond to their behaviors. Ultimately, this knowledge allows parents to guide children in ways that respect their individual differences. Temperament does not excuse children's unacceptable behaviors, but it does provide some insight into the origins of problematic behaviors such as tantrums. For example, allowing extra time in the morning for the high–activity-level child with high distractibility and low attention span to get ready for school may avoid the daily negative interactions between parent and child. A discussion of temperament is not complete without noting that ultimately it is the "goodness of fit" between parental and child temperaments that is the key issue. What may appear to be a behavioral problem may actually be a mismatch between parental and child temperaments (eg, a high-energy and high-intensity child may be quite challenging for the slow to warm up or shy parent.). It is important to help parents appreciate that such mismatches in temperamental traits between themselves and their children do not necessarily represent problems in their children's personality.

Appreciation of children's level of maturity and the developmental tasks normally associated with the toddler and preschool years, when temper tantrums occur most often, facilitates further understanding of tantrum behavior. Young children who are exploring the world and developing a sense of autonomy think primarily in egocentric terms. They view reality from their own perspective and are unable to appreciate the perspective of other individuals. Only as they mature and enter school do they learn to recognize the position of others and begin to develop a sense of morality, of right and wrong. Toddlers may become frustrated or angry because of their lack of control over the world, their inability to communicate, or limitations of their cognitive and motor abilities, which do not allow them to accomplish desired tasks. Unlike adults, who have the ability to verbalize frustrations or simply walk away from unpleasant situations, young children have neither the sophisticated ability to articulate their feelings nor the freedom to walk away. Therefore, they may react to disappointments with temper tantrums.

Temper tantrums may be classified as normal or problematic based on their cause, frequency, and characteristics. Normal tantrums can simply be demands for attention or signs of frustration, anger, or protest. In the interval between tantrums, the child's disposition and mood are normal. The well-behaved 3-year-old boy who has an occasional tantrum following the birth of a sibling, the 2½-year-old girl who throws a tantrum to express frustration because no one understands what she is trying to say, and the 2-year-old boy who cries uncontrollably because he cannot complete the puzzle he has started or run fast enough to keep up with his 4-year-old brother are all examples of normal tantrums. A typical reason for an avoidance-type tantrum is not wanting to go to bed at bedtime. All types of tantrums are more common when children are tired, ill, or hungry because their ability to cope with disappointment and frustration is limited under these circumstances.

Frequent tantrums (>5 per day) or tantrums that result in destruction of property or physical harm to the child or others are signs of problematic tantrums (Box 50-1). These tantrums result from factors that are beyond the child's control, such as parental problems, school difficulties, or health-related conditions (Box 50-2). For example, the child with unrecognized hearing loss may be performing poorly at school and resort to tantrum behavior in frustration. Marital discord or domestic violence may create anxiety for a child, which may manifest as frequent or destructive tantrums.

Differential Diagnosis

Temper tantrums are readily recognizable because of their classic pattern in which a child becomes frustrated, reacts physically, and cries or screams. Sometimes temper tantrums are indicative of more significant problems, such as speech or language delays or ASDs (see Chapter 128).

Box 50-1. Features of Problematic Tantrums

- Tantrums that persist or get worse beyond 5 years of age
- Frequent tantrums (>5 per day)
- Persistent negative mood or behavior in intervals between tantrums
- Recurrent tantrums at school
- Destruction of property during tantrums
- Harm to self or others during tantrums
- Other behavioral problems (eg, sleep disorders, aggressive behaviors, enuresis)

Box 50-2. Underlying Causes of Problematic Tantrums

Parent-Related Factors
- Marital discord
- Abusive behavior toward children
- Domestic violence
- Substance abuse
- Depression
- Inappropriate parental expectations

Child-Related Factors
- Developmental or learning disabilities
  —Hearing loss
  —Speech and language delays
  —Autism spectrum disorders
- Mood disorders (eg, depression)
- Attention-deficit/hyperactivity disorder
- Temperament (eg, high persistence and intensity of response and slow adaptability)
- Illness
  —Unrecognized illness (eg, otitis media, sinusitis)
  —Chronic or recurrent illness

Evaluation

History

Thorough history taking is essential (Questions Box). Frequency of temper tantrums, circumstances that provoke them, a description of actual tantrums, and parental reaction must be ascertained. In some instances, this reaction may provide insight as to why tantrums recur. In addition, parental expectations should be assessed. Expectations that are inappropriate for children's age and developmental maturity may create unnecessary tensions between parents and children and lead to tantrum behavior. Factors associated with problematic tantrums should also be assessed (Box 50-2).

Tantrums that are frequent (>5 per day), severe, or persist after the age of 5 years may be a sign of underlying conditions, such as depression or low self-esteem. Frequent tantrums may also be associated with attention-deficit/hyperactivity disorder (ADHD). Children with a history of impulsivity, hyperactivity, and inattention that are inappropriate for age should be evaluated for ADHD. Children who hurt themselves or others or destroy property during tantrums may have significant emotional problems. Peer pressure may inhibit tantrum behavior; if tantrums occur frequently at school, the presence of learning disabilities or speech and hearing deficits should be considered.

It is important to remember that physicians usually see children whose tantrums are frequent, severe, or cannot be controlled by parents. First, pediatricians must determine whether any underlying pathology may be contributing to the behavior and, if so, what parental or child factors may be provoking it. Second, they must differentiate between normal and problematic tantrums. Identification and remediation of the cause of problematic tantrums are the first steps toward cure. Children with suspected underlying conditions such as ADHD or mood disturbances should be referred to the appropriate specialist for further evaluation.

Physical Examination

A thorough physical examination is appropriate, as is a developmental assessment to determine if there are findings such as speech delay or behavioral signs consistent with ASDs. Most often, the physical examination is normal.

Laboratory Tests

There are no laboratory tests indicated in the assessment of the child with temper tantrums. Routine tests that are age-appropriate and suggested as part of health maintenance are appropriate.

Management

Punishment is not the solution to temper tantrums (see Chapter 49). Health maintenance visits are an ideal time to provide **anticipatory guidance** on tantrums and discuss strategies to prevent or minimize this behavior. Parents typically report that their children become defiant and difficult to manage during the "terrible 2s." At the 12- and 15-month visits, physicians should alert parents that this period is approaching and remind them that it is a normal part of development. Preventive strategies, such as **childproofing** the home to minimize unnecessary conflicts, should be discussed. In addition, parents can give young children **frequent opportunities to make choices** (eg, which color shirt to wear; which of 2 foods to have for lunch). These opportunities allow children to exercise independence and autonomy in a positive rather than a negative manner. Physicians can provide **reassurance** that this unpleasant stage will pass; children will eventually become more cooperative and agreeable.

Parents may inadvertently reinforce negative behaviors by primarily giving attention to their children during the moments they are misbehaving. Setting aside **special time** between parent and child on a regular basis gives children a close connection with parents without having to misbehave. Similarly, **time-in** is a strategy in which the parent, upon noticing that the child's behavior is beginning to escalate, spends 5 to 10 minutes soothing and comforting the child in an effort to mitigate the emerging negative behavior.

Parents should be told that helping children learn self-control and how to handle anger are keys to management. To expect that children will never get angry is unrealistic. Children should be taught how to **vent their anger and frustration in an acceptable manner** (eg, articulating their feelings, hitting a designated punching bag or pillow). As children mature, their ability to verbalize their feelings increases, but even young children can say, "Me angry." Physicians should emphasize that it is **important for parents to remain calm** during children's temper tantrums. Shouting and spanking indicate to children that parents are also out of control. Children feel more secure if the adults around them are calm and in control.

Different types of temper tantrums may require specific treatment and management strategies. Parents should **be supportive** of children who are having tantrums resulting from frustration or fatigue by letting the children know that they understand. Children's energy should be redirected into activities they can do well. Parents should be encouraged to **praise positive behavior** (eg, completing tasks properly, handling anger in an acceptable fashion). They should **ignore some tantrums,** such as those for purposes of attention seeking or wanting something. If children have no audience, they have no need to perform. **Time-outs** may also be used in such situations (see Chapter 49). Parents should not give in to children's wishes; this may reinforce tantrum behavior. **Physical movement** of children to

Temper Tantrums **Questions**

- How often does the child have temper tantrums?
- What circumstances provoke the tantrums?
- How does the child behave during the tantrums? What does the child do?
- How does the child behave in the interval between tantrums?
- How do the parents react to the child during the tantrums? What do they do or say?
- Are parental expectations consistent with the child's developmental stage?
- Have there been any changes at home or school (eg, birth of a sibling, new school)?
- Is the child having any other behavioral or development-related problems (eg, enuresis, sleep difficulties)?

where they belong may be necessary if they are refusing to do something (eg, bed for the child who is refusing to go to sleep at bedtime) or in danger of hurting themselves. **Holding children** who are raging may give them a sense of security and help calm them. If temper tantrums occur outside the home, it may be necessary to accompany children to a **quiet, private place,** such as an automobile, until they calm down. Distracting children by suggesting another activity or pointing out something of interest in the environment may also interrupt the unwanted behavior.

CASE RESOLUTION

The child in the case scenario seems to be having normal, age-appropriate tantrums. The boy's tantrums occur when he is asked to do something that he does not want to do. In these situations, the parents should try to ignore the tantrums as much as possible and not give in to the child's wishes.

Selected References

American Academy of Pediatrics. How to understand your child's temperament. http://www.healthychildren.org/English/ages-stages/gradeschool/pages/How-to-Understand-Your-Childs-Temperament.aspx. Accessed October 18, 2013

Beers NS. Managing temper tantrums. *Pediatr Rev*. 2003;24(2):70–71

Belden AC, Thomson NR, Luby JL. Temper tantrums in healthy versus depressed and disruptive preschoolers: defining tantrum behaviors associated with clinical problems. *J Pediatr*. 2008;152(1):117–122

Degnan KA, Calkins SD, Keane SP, Hill-Soderlund AL. Profiles of disruptive behavior across early childhood: contributions of frustration reactivity, physiological regulation, and maternal behavior. *Child Dev*. 2008;79(5):1357–1376

Harrington RG. Temper tantrums: guidelines for parents. http://www.nasponline.org/resources/behavior/tantrums_ho.aspx. Accessed October 18, 2013

Potegal M, Davidson RJ. Temper tantrums in young children: 1. Behavioral composition. *J Dev Behav Pediatr*. 2003;24(3):140–147

Potegal M, Kosorok MR, Davidson RJ. Temper tantrums in young children: 2. Tantrum duration and temporal organization. *J Dev Behav Pediatr*. 2003;24(3):148–154

Zahrt DM, Melzer-Lange MD. Aggressive behavior in children and adolescents. *Pediatr Rev*. 2011;32(8):325–332

CHAPTER 51

Breath-Holding Spells

Geeta Grover, MD

CASE STUDY

A 15-month-old girl is brought to the office because of parental concern about seizures. In the last month she has passed out momentarily 3 times. Each episode seems to be precipitated by anger or frustration on her part. Typically she cries, holds her breath, turns blue, and passes out. Each time she awakens within a few seconds and seems fine. The medical history and family history are unremarkable, and the physical examination is entirely within normal limits.

Questions

1. What are breath-holding spells (BHS)?
2. What is the differential diagnosis of BHS?
3. What, if any, laboratory studies are indicated in the evaluation of BHS?
4. What measures can be taken to prevent BHS? Are anticonvulsants necessary?
5. What, if any, are the long-term sequelae of BHS?

Breath-holding spells (BHS) are a benign, recurring condition of childhood in which anger or pain produce crying that culminates in noiseless expiration and apnea. The frequency of BHS, which are involuntary phenomena, is variable and ranges from several episodes a day to only several episodes per year. Although the spells are innocuous, they usually provoke parental fear and anxiety because children often turn blue and become limp. The diagnosis can usually be made on the basis of a characteristic history and description of the episode, but the possibility of seizures should be considered.

Epidemiology

Breath-holding spells occur in about 5% of all children between the ages of 6 months and 6 years, but they are most common in children between 12 and 18 months of age. Most children have experienced their first episode by 18 months and virtually all by 2 years of age. Although BHS have been described in children younger than 6 months, occurrence in such young infants is uncommon. Boys and girls are affected equally. A positive family history is found in about 25% of cases.

Clinical Presentation

See "Pathophysiology" and D$_x$ Box for the typical clinical sequence of the major types of BHS. After the spells, children may experience a short period of drowsiness.

Pathophysiology

Breath-holding spells may be classified as one of the non-epileptic paroxysmal disorders of childhood. These recurrent conditions, which have a sudden onset and no epileptiform focus, resolve spontaneously. Other disorders in this heterogeneous group include syncope, migraine, cyclic vomiting, benign paroxysmal vertigo,

Dx Breath-Holding Spells

- Identifiable precipitating event or emotion
- Brief duration
- Color change, if present, prior to loss of consciousness and rhythmic jerking of extremities
- Rapid restoration of full activity
- Normal neurologic examination

---

paroxysmal torticollis, sleep disorders (eg, narcolepsy, night terrors, somnambulism), and shudder attacks.

Types of Breath-Holding Spells

The 2 major types of BHS are **cyanotic** and **pallid.** The cyanotic type is more common. Approximately 60% of children with BHS have cyanotic spells, 20% have pallid spells, and 20% of affected children have both types. Most commonly, affected children experience several spells per week. Approximately 15% of children with BHS have complicated features. Complicated BHS are defined as typical BHS followed by seizure-like activity or rigid posturing of the body. Unlike the postictal period of epileptic seizures, prolonged periods of lethargy or drowsiness following spells are uncommon.

Pallid spells are similar to cyanotic BHS with some exceptions. Pallid episodes are more commonly provoked by minor injury, pain, or fear rather than frustration or anger; the initial cry is minimal prior to apnea and loss of consciousness; and children become pale rather than cyanotic. In pallid BHS, children often lose consciousness or tone after only a single gasp or cry, whereas in the cyanotic form, the period of apnea prior to loss of consciousness is much longer.

Etiology

Although the spells are triggered by identifiable stimuli, they are involuntary phenomena. It is believed that loss of consciousness in the cyanotic and pallid forms is caused by cerebral anoxia. The actual mechanisms of the 2 types of BHS are different. The processes involved in cyanotic BHS are not clear. Proposed mechanisms include centrally mediated inhibition of respiratory effort and altered lung mechanics, which may inappropriately stimulate pulmonary reflexes, resulting in apnea and hypoxia. In the pallid form, the pale coloration and loss of tone are thought to result from vagally mediated severe bradycardia or asystole. Pallid spells have been spontaneously induced in the electroencephalogram (EEG) laboratory using ocular compression to trigger the oculocardiac reflex. Vagally mediated bradycardia or asystole lasting more than 2 seconds has been produced by this maneuver.

An association between iron deficiency anemia and BHS has been recognized for many years but is poorly understood. It may be related to iron's importance in the function of various enzymes and neurotransmitters in the central nervous system or because children with anemia have decreased cerebral oxygenation, making them more susceptible to BHS.

Differential Diagnosis

The differential diagnosis primarily includes seizures and syncope secondary to cardiac arrhythmia or a vasovagal episode. Although vasovagal syncope, like BHS, may be provoked by fear or pain, it is uncommon in children younger than 12 years. Three factors may help differentiate BHS from true epileptic seizure activity. First, spells are usually provoked by some upsetting event or emotion, unlike seizures, which generally do not have a recognizable precipitating event. Second, episodes are brief in duration and followed by rapid restoration of full activity. Third, color change precedes loss of consciousness and rhythmic jerking of the extremities, whereas in the typical epileptic seizure, convulsive activity and loss of muscular tone usually precede change in color. Box 51-1 contains the differential diagnosis of BHS.

Evaluation

History

History alone may be diagnostic (Questions Box). A family history of BHS should be obtained. It is essential to record a detailed history of the suspected breath-holding episode. The sequence in which the events occurred may help differentiate BHS from epileptic seizures.

Physical Examination

Children should have a complete physical examination, including a thorough neurologic evaluation. Focal neurologic signs or evidence of structural lesions such as meningomyelocele or hydrocephalus may lead the physician away from a diagnosis of BHS.

Box 51-1. Differential Diagnosis of Breath-Holding Spells
Central Nervous System
Seizures (epilepsy)
Occult or overt brain stem lesions (causing dysfunction within the pontomedullary area)
Benign paroxysmal vertigo
Cardiovascular
Cardiac arrhythmia (eg, long QT syndrome)
Syncope (orthostatic or vasovagal)
Miscellaneous
Gastroesophageal reflux/Sandifer syndrome
Cataplexy (transient loss of muscle tone associated with narcolepsy; rare before adolescence)
Central or obstructive apnea
Munchausen syndrome by proxy

Breath-Holding Spells **Questions**

- What happened before the episode?
- Was the child crying?
- What was the child's color before and during the episode?
- Was the child lethargic after the episode?
- Does the family have a history of breath-holding spells?

Laboratory Tests

If the history is consistent with BHS and the physical examination is normal, laboratory evaluation is usually unnecessary. Because of the association of BHS with iron deficiency anemia in some children, it is appropriate to determine a hemoglobin level. An EEG may be performed if the physician is concerned about the possibility of epileptic seizures. In both forms of BHS, the EEG shows generalized slowing followed by flattening (a pattern characteristic of cerebral anoxia) during attacks, although it is unusual to record the EEG during BHS. Simultaneous EEG and video recordings can be very useful in helping to distinguish BHS from seizures, especially in children having frequent episodes. The interictal EEG is normal in children with BHS, whereas it may often be abnormal in children with epilepsy. An electrocardiogram may be obtained if there is any question about cardiac arrhythmia (eg, long QT syndrome).

Management

Management of BHS includes **parental support and reassurance.** Breath-holding spells may be extremely frightening for parents to witness, especially if the episodes are routinely associated with loss of consciousness or seizure-like activity. Parents should be told about the involuntary nature of the attacks and cautioned against reinforcing the spells by giving in to the child's wishes. They should be advised to avoid unnecessary confrontations with the child. Similarly, it is impossible to ensure that the child will never be frustrated or injured. Instead, parents should be encouraged to handle the episodes in a "matter-of-fact" manner and continue age-appropriate discipline. They should be reassured that the long-term prognosis is excellent.

Referral to a neurologist, cardiologist, or psychiatrist may be considered for children with frequent episodes or complex cases. Pharmacologic therapy is usually not necessary, but atropine sulfate may be considered in the management of children with frequent pallid BHS because of atropine's anticholinergic action. Anticonvulsants are not effective. For a subset of children with iron-deficiency anemia and BHS, iron therapy may be effective in the treatment of cyanotic and pallid BHS. Successful cardiac pacemaker implantation has been performed for complex cases of pallid BHS with severe and frequent spells associated with seizures, life-threatening bradycardia, or asystole. Finally, recent case reports have noted the successful treatment of pallid BHS with fluoxetine or a combination of glycopyrrolate and theophylline in small cohorts of patients.

Prognosis

Breath-holding spells resolve spontaneously in most children by 5 to 6 years of age. About 50% of cases resolve by 4 years of age, and 90% resolve by 6 years of age. Neither pallid nor cyanotic BHS are associated with an increased risk of development of epilepsy, although children with pallid BHS do have an increased incidence of developing syncopal attacks during adulthood.

CASE RESOLUTION

The child presented in the case scenario has a history and physical examination suggestive of breath-holding spells (BHS). The girl's episodes are consistent with cyanotic BHS. The episodes are preceded by an identifiable emotion, brief in duration, and followed by a rapid recovery of normal consciousness and activity. Assessment of the hemoglobin level revealed mild iron deficiency anemia. The child received iron therapy, and the parents were reassured about the benign nature of BHS.

Selected References

Anderson JE, Bluestone D. Breath-holding spells: scary but not serious. *Contemp Pediatr.* 2000;17:61–72

Benbadis S. The differential diagnosis of epilepsy: a critical review. *Epilepsy Behav.* 2009;15(1):15–21

Carano N, Bo I, Zanetti E, Tchana B, Barbato G, Agnetti A. Glycopyrrolate and theophylline for the treatment of severe pallid breath-holding spells. *Pediatrics.* 2013;131(4):e1280–e1283

Daoud AS, Batieha A, al-Sheyyab M, Abuekteish F, Hijazi S. Effectiveness of iron therapy on breath-holding spells. *J Pediatr.* 1997;130(4):547–550

DiMario FJ Jr. Prospective study of children with cyanotic and pallid breath-holding spells. *Pediatrics.* 2001;107(2):265–269

Kelly AM, Porter CJ, McGoon MD, Espinosa RE, Osborn MJ, Hayes DL. Breath-holding spells associated with significant bradycardia: successful treatment with permanent pacemaker implantation. *Pediatrics.* 2001;108(3):698–702

Mocan H, Yildiran A, Orhan F, Erduran E. Breath holding spells in 91 children and response to treatment with iron. *Arch Dis Child.* 1999;81(3):261–262

Walsh M, Knilans TK, Anderson JB, Czosek RJ. Successful treatment of pallid breath-holding spells with fluoxetine. *Pediatrics.* 2012;130(3):e685–e689

CHAPTER 52

Fears, Phobias, and Anxiety

Carol D. Berkowitz, MD

CASE STUDY

A 5-year-old girl is brought into the office by her mother, who complains that her daughter has been afraid to sleep alone since the occurrence of an earthquake. The house did not sustain any significant damage, but the entire family was awakened. The mother says that the girl has become more timid. As nighttime approaches, she becomes particularly fearful. She will not stay in her bed, and she is comforted only by sleeping with her parents. In addition, the girl has begun bed-wetting since the earthquake, and the mother wonders whether she should put her daughter in diapers. The physical examination, including vital signs, is normal, except for the observation that the child is very clingy and whiny.

Questions

1. What are normal childhood fears?
2. When do these fears commonly occur?
3. What strategies are used to deal with these fears?
4. What are simple phobias? What are social phobias?
5. What is school phobia, and how is it best handled?
6. What are common anxiety disorders in children and adolescents?
7. How can families deal with childhood disturbances that emerge after natural and artificial disasters?

Fears are normal feelings that cause emotional, behavioral, and physiological changes that are essential for survival. Fears are associated with psychologic discomforts, such as a negative, unpleasant feeling. Children may develop fears in response to actual events (eg, earthquakes) or as a result of the temporal association of 2 events (eg, seeing a scary movie on a rainy day and then becoming afraid of rain). Some fears seem to be innate, and others seem to be developmental. Children fear different things at different ages. For example, school phobia is sometimes particularly problematic in young, school-aged children. Worry is the cognitive manifestation of fear and anxiety.

Phobias are overwhelming, intense, highly specific, and often irrational fears. The *Diagnostic and Statistical Manual of Mental Disorders, Fifth Edition,* defines a phobia as excessive anxiety accompanied by worry occurring more often than not, for at least 6 months and associated with one or more of the following: restlessness, easy fatigability, difficulty concentrating, irritability, tense muscles, and disturbed sleep. Childhood phobias can be divided into 5 categories: animals (eg, spiders, snakes, dogs), natural environment (eg, heights), medical related (eg, doctors, dentists, injections), situations (eg, flying), and other (eg, loud noises, rain, thunder). Specific phobias are often managed by avoidance and may not present to the physician for treatment. Social phobias (also called social anxiety disorders) are specific to social situations that arouse intense concerns about humiliation or embarrassment. Fear of speaking in public may represent a social phobia. Selective mutism involves children who are able to speak but are unable to do so in certain settings, such as school. This probably represents one form of a social phobia. When these fears are combined with avoidance behavior, they may be incapacitating. Anxiety refers to fear without a definable source.

It is characterized by a physiological response and may be perceived as a vague feeling of uneasiness, apprehension, and foreboding of impending doom. A child may experience an anxiety **problem** where there is significant but not severe distress and an anxiety **disorder** when the distress is excessive or functioning is impaired. Up to 8% to 10% of children and adolescents have anxiety disorders; these may be referred to as generalized anxiety disorders. Girls are twice as likely to develop anxiety disorders as boys. There is often a positive family history of anxiety disorders, which is felt to be related to a genetic predisposition and environmental factors.

Different strategies are useful for dealing with different fears. It is important for parents not to trivialize these fears or reinforce them but to empower children to deal with them.

It is also important to realize that parents sometimes foster fears by using threats with children, such as, "The doctor will give you a shot unless you eat your spinach," or "The boogie man will get you." By fostering fears, the parents are also fostering dependency. Parents lack the imagination that children have and find it difficult to understand the degree of fear that children experience.

The opportunities for primary care physicians to counsel families about childhood fears has increased over the past decade related to a number of catastrophic events, such as the terrorist attacks of 9/11, the tsunami in Asia, hurricane Katrina, and the earthquake in Haiti. Acts of violence, such as the shootings at Columbine High School and Virginia Tech, also create fear and anxiety in children who witness these events on the television. It is important to recognize the pervasiveness of mental health sequelae following disasters and the factors that influence the prevalence of these disturbances. One percent of children in New York, NY, lost a relative on 9/11.

There is a greater risk of mental health sequelae if there are poor social supports or a prior history of psychopathology or if the child is fearful or shy by nature. Natural disasters have less of an effect than intentional ones. While many of the recent disasters have been acute and unexpected, there are children who are continuously exposed to what has been called "process trauma" in the form of war and child abuse.

Epidemiology

Fears follow a developmental pattern (Box 52-1). Neonates are believed to have no fear, although young infants whose faces are covered with a blanket struggle to toss off the blanket. Infants who are 6 months of age exhibit what is known as **stranger anxiety** in response to unfamiliar persons, places, or objects. To combat this anxiety, infants seek refuge with a parent. Stranger anxiety becomes equated with separation anxiety and reaches a peak at 2 years of age. Children between 6 months and 2 years of age are also frightened by loud noises and falling or quickly moving objects.

Children between the ages of 2 and 5 years are in what is termed the **age of anxiety.** They fear many things, including animals, abandonment, loud noises, and darkness. Children in this age group are particularly fearful of physicians, hospitals, and getting hurt. Young children are afraid of the physically disabled, who represent bodily injury, and monsters and scary movies. They sometimes displace their anger onto monsters and witches and attribute to these imaginary characters the bad feelings they are experiencing. Children in this age group have strong imaginations, which makes it difficult for them to differentiate fantasy from reality.

Children between 6 years of age and adolescence tend to have more abstract thoughts, and their fears are less relevant to physical immediacy. These children are afraid of the death of their parents or the burning of their home. They also fear war, growing up (expressed as "How will I know what to do?"), going into the next grade, being alone or kidnapped, and the divorce of their parents. Children in this age group are often reluctant to bother their parents with their fears, and they can easily misinterpret parental concerns when they overhear parental conversations. Childhood anxiety disorders are reported in 6% to 20% of children.

Separation anxiety, which may manifest as school phobia and may be referred to as separation anxiety disorder, may occur in school-aged children. The prevalence is estimated at 3.2% to 4.1%, though up to 50% of third graders report separation anxiety symptoms. Separation anxiety disorder is defined as developmentally inappropriate, excessive anxiety precipitated by actual or anticipated separation from home or family. Affected children develop physical complaints (eg, stomachaches) on school days. The mother-child relationship is often disturbed, and the child is fearful of leaving the parent alone. Childhood school phobia and parental history of panic attacks and agoraphobia may be associated.

Fears during adolescence relate to social functioning, such as public speaking or talking to members of the opposite sex. Older children are also concerned about school failure and physical injury. They have many of the same fears expressed by younger school-aged children, although phobias are uncommon. Social phobia is a distinct entity and different from shyness, as reported in a recent study of adolescents. Social phobia is a potentially impairing psychiatric disorder. Overall, phobias occur in less than 1.7% of the general population but are reported in 13% of children with other emotional or behavioral problems.

Anxiety disorders are rare in childhood but more common during adolescence. They may include panic attacks, which involve the sudden onset of intense fear or discomfort associated with physiological symptoms such as palpitations and shortness of breath. Fear about a panic attack may lead to agoraphobia, the avoidance of going away from home. Post-traumatic stress disorder (PTSD) involves a set of symptoms that recurs after a person has experienced a traumatic event. Symptoms include intense fear, helplessness, or a sense of horror. The person reexperiences the trauma, avoids circumstances that are reminiscent of the trauma, and is in a state of hyperarousal. It is estimated that 5% of men and 10% of women have a lifetime prevalence of PTSD.

Pathophysiology

Fear has its basis in a series of psychophysiological reactions, which are mediated through a series of neurotransmitters. The reaction is often referred to as the fright/flight response and is critical for survival. The response is regulated through the limbic system. Elevated levels of certain transmitters, such as γ-aminobutyric acid and norepinephrine, are associated with feelings of anxiety. Excess serotonin has also been related to anxiety disorders. Patients with panic attacks and anxiety disorders have disturbances in neurotransmitter regulation.

Differential Diagnosis

The challenge for physicians is to assess the etiology of the fear and to differentiate normal fears from those that may be signs of unusual stresses or signs of psychopathology. Appropriate fears represent a real reaction to a real danger. As a rule, children are more resilient than adults and recover more rapidly from traumatic events. On the other hand, children are prone to inappropriate fears, which may develop for a number of reasons.

Inappropriate fears may occur because of operant conditioning, in which a conditioned stimulus becomes associated with another

---

Box 52-1. Common Fears During Childhood
Neonates: no fears
6 months–2 years: separation anxiety, loud noises, quickly moving objects, the dark
2–5 years (age of anxiety): animals, abandonment, loud noises, darkness, physicians, hospitals, getting hurt, monsters, witches, ghosts, storms
6 years–adolescence: death (parental death), parental divorce, natural and artificial disasters, growing up, school performance (going into the next grade), war
Adolescence: social situations, school performance, health, public speaking

object. Fear of the other object becomes reinforced through this association. Inappropriate fears may also develop in a child whose parent has the fear (modeling) or through witnessing a fearful event in the media (informational). True phobias represent neuroses and may occur in more than one family member.

School phobia, also called school refusal, may occur under 3 distinct conditions. Not uncommonly, young children who are entering school for the first time are frightened. This fear is a normal component of separation anxiety, which usually resolves within a few days of starting school. This is also referred to as adaptive anxiety. In contrast, older children may experience school phobia because they are truly afraid of a school situation. They may fear a teacher, violence, or a bully. To avoid the problem, children may actually request to change classrooms or schools. It is important to talk with children to find out what is behind their fear of school.

On the other hand, some children who seem fearful of school are actually concerned about parental separation (ie, separation anxiety). Frequently, these children enjoy school and miss it when they are absent. Absences occur when feelings of separation from parents are so intense that they do not allow children to function well in school settings. Children are worried that something bad will happen to them or to their parents when they are apart. This separation anxiety disorder may result from parental illness or parents' fostering dependency in children. Children then see parents as vulnerable and are uncomfortable about leaving them alone. To qualify as an anxiety disorder, the symptoms must last at least 4 weeks.

School refusal is the third leading cause of school absenteeism after transient illness and truancy. Fifty percent of children with school refusal have other problems, including depression (28%), tantrums (18%), sleep disturbances (17%), obsessive-compulsive behavior (11%), other fears (10%), enuresis (3%), and learning disabilities (3%). Overall, school refusal has a good prognosis, although adolescents do not do as well as younger children, and individuals with a higher IQ have a poorer outcome. Twenty percent of parents of children with school refusal have a diagnosable psychiatric disorder. Issues of mother-child dependency are often a concern.

Another type of childhood fear concerns physicians and hospitals. Children have many concerns about what happens to them at the doctor's office. They are particularly fearful of needles. To children, needles represent possible mutilation. When asked to represent needles in drawings, children often portray needles as larger than themselves and very pointed. They comment that needles are sharp (eg, "Needles can make you pop, just like a balloon"; "Needles can also take out all your blood until you die"). In addition, children are preoccupied with what happens to their blood. One youngster commented, "They check out your blood to see if it's good or bad, and if your blood is bad, then it means that you need to have more tests." Another youngster thought that physicians were doing a "blood taste" rather than a blood test.

Hospitalization raises other issues concerning parental separation as well as painful procedures. As children adjust to hospitalization, they progress through 3 stages: protest, during which they complain about the hospital and cry; despair, during which they have given up hope that their parents will return; and detachment, during which they seem to be adjusting but actually have distanced themselves from their parents. Unrestricted visitation by family members and involvement of child life specialists mitigates much of the distress.

Evaluation

Physicians should explore the area of childhood fears and phobias at routine health maintenance visits, even if parents do not have specific concerns. Sometimes parents are embarrassed by children's fears (eg, the fear of an older child to sleep without a night-light; the fear of dogs, which may preclude the child from visiting certain friends). Parents may not report children's fears unless these fears seem to be unusually intense. Practitioners may ask children, "What is the scariest thing you can think of?" If children are having difficulty providing details, physicians may ask them to name things that other children fear or to complete the sentence, "I feel afraid when…." Alternatively, practitioners may suggest things that other children may fear: "Do the kids you know seem to be worried about kidnapping?"

There are a number of instruments that have been used to assess the level of anxiety in children. These include the Multidimensional Anxiety Scale for Children, 2nd Edition; Spence Children's Anxiety Scale; and Screen for Child Anxiety Related Emotional Disorders. The latter instrument is in the public domain and readily available.

History

The evaluation of children with specific fears demands a careful history that provides information about situations in which children are fearful (Questions Box). Physicians should consider fears within a developmental context because many childhood fears are normal and experienced by all children. It is also important to look at changes in the family situation. Children sometimes develop what seem to be fears but in fact are behaviors designed to manipulate other family members. For instance, young children who sense marital discord may insist on sleeping with their parents as a way of ensuring that the parents are together rather than separate.

Physical Examination

A routine examination is warranted, but findings are usually normal. Such an evaluation, however, is particularly important if

---

Questions

Fears and Phobias

- What fear does the child have? Exactly what does the child fear?
- Under what circumstances was the fear originally expressed? Did any changes in the child's life occur around the time that the fear appeared?
- Under what conditions is the fear currently expressed?
- How long has the child had the fear?
- How does the fear affect the daily living of the child and family?
- What has the family done to help the child deal with the fear?

presenting complaints include symptoms such as abdominal pain, headache, or palpitations.

Laboratory Tests

As a rule, laboratory tests are not required unless the symptoms suggest an organic etiology, such as hyperthyroidism, as the cause of palpitations.

Management

The management of the fear or phobia is determined by the degree to which children are incapacitated. As a general rule, **children should be empowered to conquer their fears.** Children's books that address the issues of certain fears can help achieve this empowerment; for example, *The Berenstain Bears in the Dark* discusses specific worries such as fear of lightning and thunder (see Parents and Children on page 313 for more examples). These books often explain the basis of such natural phenomena in easy-to-understand terms. Books also normalize particular fears and show how one character is fearful. Parents can re-create some of the sounds that children fear. For example, children who are afraid of the noise the wind makes are shown a teakettle from which hot steam blows through the whistle, creating the same noise as the wind. For fears about nuclear war, empowering children to become active, such as joining a nuclear protest group, may be useful.

Parents may feel helpless because they do not know how to deal with children's fears. Physicians should give them the necessary information. Children's fears should not be trivialized. Even if the **fears** are unfounded, they **should be validated.** In general, children should be questioned about whether they are fearful about a situation. The following 2 examples illustrate the proper handling of fears in children:

If children are visiting the dentist for the first time, it is appropriate for parents to ask, "Are you afraid?" If children reply, "Yes, a little bit," parents can say, "Almost everybody is afraid. Tell me what it is you're afraid of. Fear is a normal emotion, and I'm glad you told me about it."

Parents of children who express fear of imaginary characters can reassure children that they do not exist. In addition, parents can tell children what the parents would do if such characters did exist. For instance, the father of a little girl who was afraid of witches told her, "There are no such things as witches. But if there were, and they came into your room, I would punch them in the nose and punch them in the stomach and beat them up, and then there would be no more witches to hurt you." For those who would opt for a less violent approach, the parent could state: "I would tell any witch who came into your room, 'STOP! Go away. No witches allowed in here.' And the witch would run away and I would slam the door!" By doing this, parents establish the reality of the situation and then also create a plan to deal with the problem should it actually happen.

Parents can also help to limit or reduce children's fears by **minimizing** their **exposure to fear-provoking situations** such as television shows or scary movies. These programs can be particularly frightening for some children, who should not watch them without

adult supervision. Minimizing exposure to television is particularly important following a disastrous event. The recurrent images of planes flying into buildings on 9/11 were interpreted by children as repeated different attacks.

When dealing with children who have school phobia because of problems in school, it is important to determine if a change in school would be appropriate to facilitate their school attendance. This may be particularly appropriate in children whose schools are plagued with violence.

Cognitive-behavioral therapy (CBT) is reported to have the highest rate of success for dealing with anxiety-related conditions. Cognitive-behavioral therapy includes psycho-education, somatic management (eg, relaxation techniques), cognitive restructuring (modifying negative thoughts), and exposure methods including desensitization. The goal of the therapist is to teach the child alternative ways of viewing the feared object and of coping with the fear itself. Medications such as antidepressants, anxiolytics, sedatives, and β-blockers have an unsubstantiated role in managing phobic disorders in children but may be indicated in other conditions such as anxiety disorders.

When school refusal is linked to separation anxiety, a program of **desensitization or habituation (graded exposure)** is recommended. Desensitization may involve the participation of mothers in the classroom for a time. When children acclimate and can tolerate some separation, mothers move to another area in the school, such as the principal's office. Next they go outside the school grounds. As children reestablish a sense of well-being in spite of the separation, the mothers gradually move farther and farther away. This solution is somewhat problematic for mothers who work outside the home. There is some research to suggest that children adjust more readily if they resume school immediately without the gradual withdrawal of their parent. Children with significant school refusal may need the assistance of child psychologists or psychiatrists.

Phobias may be treated using the concept of **flooding,** which consists of rapid, prolonged exposure to the feared item. For example, a child who is afraid of dogs is exposed to a friendly, docile, small dog while in the company of his or her parents. Alternatively, systematic desensitization, during which children are exposed to the feared objects over a series of weeks, coupled with relaxation techniques, is also used. Phobias usually require the help of mental health specialists. Selective serotonin reuptake inhibitors (see Chapter 130) have been found to be beneficial in the management of certain anxiety disorders in children and adolescents. They are noted to be effective for panic disorders, social phobia, generalized anxiety disorder, obsessive-compulsive disorder, and PTSD. Benzodiazepines are safe and generally used on a short-term basis. Sedation is a frequent side effect, and there is the potential for abuse, tolerance, and drug dependence. Propranolol lessens the peripheral autonomic nervous system symptoms of social phobias and may be used for specific instances. Combined therapy involving CBT and medication is beneficial in some patients.

Children who must undergo hospitalization benefit from a prehospital visit, when possible. This visit familiarizes the child with the facilities and explains proposed procedures. Many hospitals have child life specialists who ease the adjustment of children as well as their parents to the hospital stay.

Prognosis

Most childhood fears resolve with time, nurturing, and reassurance. Most fears last only several weeks, and then new fears may develop. As a rule, specific fears should not last longer than 2 years, and the younger the child, the shorter the duration of the fear.

Prognosis is good for children with true phobias, with 100% resolution of monosymptomatic phobias. More significant anxiety disorders may persist into adulthood, at which time similar management involving CBT and medications may be indicated.

CASE RESOLUTION

In the case study, the girl's fear of sleeping in her bed was triggered by a significant environmental event. Although earthquakes are uncontrollable, the girl can be empowered to deal with manageable aspects of an earthquake as much as possible. She should be assured that in the same situation, many adults probably would also fear sleeping alone. The parents should stock a box with shoes, a flashlight, a radio, and water and place the box under the child's bed. In addition, they may have their daughter get into her bed and then shake it, simulating the jiggling that she would experience during an earthquake. The girl should also practice getting out of bed and standing in the doorway. To combat the child's fear of separation during times of natural disaster, the parents should reassure their daughter that they will all be together.

Selected References

Physicians

American Psychiatric Association. *Diagnostic and Statistical Manual of Mental Disorders.* 5th ed. Washington, DC: American Psychiatric Association; 2013

Bagnell AL. Anxiety and separation disorders. *Pediatr Rev.* 2011;32(10): 440–446

Benun J, Lewis C, Siegel M. Fears and phobias. *Pediatr Rev.* 2008;29(7): 250–251

Bothe D, Olness K. Worried sick. Anxiety among youth. *Contemp Pediatr.* 2007;24:58–63

Brown EJ. Clinical characteristics and efficacious treatment of posttraumatic stress disorder in children and adolescents. *Pediatr Ann.* 2005;34(2):138–146

Burstein M, Ameli-Grillon L, Merikangas KR. Shyness versus social phobia in US youth. *Pediatrics.* 2011;128(5):917–925

Compton SN, March JS, Brent D, Albano AM, Weersing R, Curry J. Cognitive-behavioral psychotherapy for anxiety and depressive disorders in children and adolescents: an evidence-based medicine review. *J Am Acad Child Adolesc Psychiatry.* 2004;43(8):930–959

Emotions and moods. In: Wolraich ML, ed. *The Classification of Child and Adolescent Mental Diagnoses in Primary Care: Diagnostic and Statistical Manual for Primary Care (DSM-PC) Child and Adolescent Version.* Elk Grove Village, IL: American Academy of Pediatrics; 1996:145–149

Hanna GL, Fischer DJ, Fluent TE. Separation anxiety disorder and school refusal in children and adolescents. *Pediatr Rev.* 2006;27(2):56–63

Jurbergs N, Ledley DR. Separation anxiety disorders. *Pediatr Ann.* 2005;34(2):108–115

Kendall PC, Chu BC, Pimentel SS, Choudhury M. Treating anxiety disorders in youth. In: Kendall PC, ed. *Child and Adolescent Therapy: Cognitive Behavioral Procedures.* 2nd ed. New York, NY: The Guilford Press; 2000

Klein RG, Last CG. *Anxiety Disorders in Children.* Newbury Park, CA: Sage Publications; 1989

Sarafino EP. *The Fears of Childhood.* New York, NY: Human Sciences Press; 1986

Walsh KH. Welcome advances in treating youth anxiety disorders. *Contemp Pediatr.* 2002;19:66–82

Williams TP, Miller BD. Pharmacologic management of anxiety disorders in children and adolescents. *Curr Opin Pediatr.* 2003;15(5):483–490

Parents and Children

Berenstain S, Berenstain J. *The Berenstain Bears and the Bully.* New York, NY: Random House; 1993

Berenstain S, Berenstain J. *The Berenstain Bears in the Dark.* New York, NY: Random House; 1982

Berenstain S, Berenstain J. *The Berenstain Bears Visit the Dentist.* New York, NY: Random House; 1981

Mayer M. *There's a Nightmare in My Closet.* New York, NY: Penguin Books; 1992

Ziefert H, Brown R. *Nicky's Noisy Night.* New York, NY: Penguin Books; 1986

CHAPTER 53

Thumb Sucking and Other Habits

Carol D. Berkowitz, MD

CASE STUDY

A 5-year-old boy is brought to the office because of thumb sucking. His mother claims that she has tried nearly everything, including tying his hands at night and using aversive treatments on his thumbs, but nothing has worked. She reports that her son has been teased at school and has few friends. He is in good general health, and his immunizations are up-to-date.

His growth parameters are at the 50th percentile. Except for a callus on the right thumb, the physical examination is normal.

Questions

1. What are common habits in children?
2. What is the significance of transitional objects?
3. What are the consequences of common habits in children?
4. What are strategies used to break children of habits?
5. How does one differentiate benign habits from self-injurious behaviors?

Habits are defined as somewhat complicated, repetitive behaviors that become automatized, fixed, and carried out easily and effortlessly. They are different from tics, which are rapid, repetitive muscle twitches involving the head, face, or shoulders. Tics are also referred to as habit spasms (see Chapter 121). Children have many socially unacceptable habits, including thumb sucking, nail biting, skin picking, nose picking, hair pulling (trichotillomania), rocking, biting other children, and teeth grinding (bruxism). Some habits, such as pica, are potentially harmful. Children engage in most of these habits because of their soothing potential. In recent years, cutting, a form of self-injury in adolescents, has received attention. While not a habit in a traditional sense, cutting is described by teens as a way of dealing with stress and alleviating anxiety. One-third of children use transitional objects for comfort. Blankets or favorite toys are traditional transitional objects that represent an age-appropriate coping strategy. Most transitional objects are stroked, and the stroking often occurs in association with thumb sucking. Transitional objects sometimes present a problem because children experience distress if these objects are lost or misplaced or need cleaning.

Epidemiology

Thumb sucking probably represents the most common habit of children. A reported 50% to 87% of children engage in this habit. The median age for the onset of hand sucking is 54 minutes of life, and 90% of newborns show hand-sucking behavior by the age of 2 hours. Forty percent of children between the ages of 1 and 3 years, 33% of children between the ages of 3 and 5 years, and 25% of children at the age of 5 years still suck their thumbs. Some children suck their fingers rather than thumbs. Other oral behavior may involve lip sucking, lip biting, and toe sucking. Lip sucking and biting begin at about 5 to 6 months of age and occur in about 90% of infants. It is unusual for these actions to persist as habits. Toe sucking is noted in infants who are 6 to 7 months of age and is reported in 80% of normal infants.

Trichotillomania is a disorder once believed to be uncommon but now thought to affect 8 million Americans (about 5 in 1,000). The term, first coined in 1889 by French dermatologist Hallopeau, is derived from the Greek *thrix* (hair), *tillein* (pull), and *mania* (madness). The condition is an impulse control disorder in which alopecia develops from compulsive hair pulling. Hair pulling may involve hair from the head, eyebrows, eyelashes, or pubic area. Although trichotillomania seems to peak during early childhood and adolescence, the disorder is reported from infancy to adolescence. In young children, boys and girls are equally affected, but in older children and adolescents, females outnumber males. The disorder is not associated with comorbid psychopathology, but there may be some association with mood disorders or attention-deficit/hyperactivity disorder. There is a condition in infants, called "baby trich," in which infants pull their mother's hair when they are being held or nursed. This is considered normal exploratory behavior.

Rhythmic habits are stereotypical, repetitive behaviors that usually occur in infants younger than 1 year. These habits are reported in 15% to 20% of the population. Rhythmic habits include rocking (about 19% of infants), when infants rock back and forth; jouncing (5%–10%), when they move up-and-down on their hands and knees so that the whole crib rocks; head rolling (8%); and head banging (5%). Rhythmic habits are seen more commonly in boys; the male-female ratio is 3:1. These habits usually occur with a frequency of 60 to 80 movements per minute, often when infants are tired, and last for less than 15 minutes before they fall asleep.

Rhythmic movements have been equated with **sleep tics.** These tics are reported in 20% of children, most often between the ages of 6 and 10 years. As a rule, tics are 3 times more common in boys than girls. They tend to be noted with increased frequency in children who are shy or overly self-conscious or have obsessive-compulsive tendencies. Tics usually occur when children are under stress.

Biting, an aggressive habit noted in toddlers, may be related to teething. It occurs more often in children with slow verbal skills.

Nail biting (onychophagia) is usually believed to be a sign of internal tension. The disorder affects 10% to 40% of children. Nail biting begins between the ages of 3 and 6 years , and the peak age is 13 years. One-third of adolescents bite their nails, but 50% of these adolescents break the habit by the time they reach adulthood. Nail biting in adults is regarded as a sign of emotional and social immaturity and regression. The family history for nail biting is often positive. Identical twins are concordant for the condition in 66% of cases. In contrast, the incidence in dizygotic twins is 34%.

Nose picking, noted in children and adults, is reported in more than 90% of individuals. In general, adults and older children limit nose picking to when they are unobserved, but younger children will pick their noses in public. There are no gender-based differences in the incidence of nose picking. Epistaxis is the most common complication of nose picking.

Pica, which is not a normal behavior, is defined as the ingestion of nonfood products. The peak incidence of pica is between the ages of 1 and 3 years. The incidence is increased in children from lower socioeconomic levels, and the behavior occurs in 10% of children who present with lead poisoning.

Teeth grinding (bruxism) is reported in 5% to 15% of children. Boys are more commonly affected than girls, and the disorder seems to regress later in life. It is reported with increased incidence among developmentally delayed children, including those with autism spectrum disorder (ASD). The cause is unknown, although it may be associated with malocclusion in some children. The disorder may contribute to temporomandibular joint dysfunction and pain.

Self-injury has been reported in up to 20% of adults with intellectual disabilities. Autism spectrum disorders and the absence of speech are the highest associated risk factors. Nail biting, head banging, and self-biting are frequently described associated behaviors. Severe self-injury related to biting is seen in Lesch-Nyhan syndrome.

Clinical Presentation

Children with common habits, such as thumb sucking or rhythmic movements, may be brought to the physician with these particular complaints because the parent wants advice about stopping the behavior. Other children may present with consequences of habits, such as alopecia (trichotillomania), paronychia (nail biting), or lead intoxication (pica). Whitlow (also called felon; infection of the tip of the finger) and, rarely, osteomyelitis of the distal phalanx have also been reported with nail biting. Osteomyelitis should be considered in a nail-biting child who presents with an abscess of the finger. Hair pulling can be associated with hair ingestion, also referred to as trichophagia. Trichobezoars that can complicate trichotillomania associated with trichophagia may present with gastric outlet or bowel obstruction. Symptoms then include abdominal pain, anorexia, early satiety, nausea, vomiting, halitosis, and weight loss (D$_x$ Box).

Pathophysiology

Children engage in habits to reduce stress and provide comfort. Thumb sucking is related to nonnutritive sucking. Although the initial purpose of sucking is nutritional, the pleasure associated with sucking reinforces the behavior. Infants who are served from a cup from birth develop no interest in sucking. Humans and other primates spend more time in nonnutritive than in nutritive sucking. Monkeys use a 5-point hold, with 2 hands, 2 feet, and mouth (holding on to their mother's nipple) for attachment. Universal thumb sucking is noted even in orphan monkeys, and sucking is thought to be an important aspect of environmental adaptation. Nonnutritive sucking occurs even in the absence of fatigue, hunger, or discomfort and has a purpose in itself—to provide comfort and be self-soothing. The maximum intensity of sucking occurs at 7 months. For older children (>3 years), sucking is also a way of dealing with boredom.

In bottle-fed infants, thumb sucking seems to commence when feeding stops. Some infants, described as "type A," seem to be satisfied only when their thumb is in their mouth. As infants spend more time engaged in motor activity, they spend less time thumb sucking. Placid infants who cry less also do less sucking. Some studies have shown that thumb sucking is less common in breastfed infants and that thumb suckers as a group feed less frequently (every 4 hours rather than 3 and for 10 minutes rather than 20).

Nail biting is related to thumb sucking, a form of oral gratification, and children may progress from thumb sucking to nail biting. The pattern of nail biting usually involves placement of the hand in the vicinity of the mouth, tapping of the fingers along the teeth, quick spasmodic bites with the fingers around the central incisors, and the

Dx Childhood Habits

- History of a habit
- Callus on thumb or fingers
- Short, chewed nails
- Alopecia
- Lead intoxication
- Iron deficiency anemia

removal and inspection of the hands. Other oral habits, such as pencil gnawing, gum chewing, lip biting, and nail picking, are related activities, as is nose picking. The cause of teeth grinding is unclear.

Rocking habits are believed to be kinesthetically pleasing and soothing and a means of autostimulation. The etiology of hair pulling is less apparent. The *Diagnostic and Statistical Manual of Mental Disorders, Fifth Edition,* defines trichotillomania as chronic hair pulling often associated with hair ingestion. In recent years, investigators have linked trichotillomania to disorders of serotonin reuptake and placed it in the category of obsessive-compulsive behavior. Some individuals who engage in trichotillomania have abnormal head positron emission tomography. Although the etiology of trichotillomania is unclear, affected children share certain features, which have been characterized as fiddling SHEEP (*s*ensation, *h*ands, *e*motion, *e*nvironment, *p*erfectionism). The overriding factor is a need for tactile stimulation. Pica, which is also considered abnormal, may be associated with intellectual disability, environmental deprivation, or inadequate nutrition, particularly iron deficiency.

Differential Diagnosis

The differential diagnosis of most habits is not difficult. Tics or habit spasms should be differentiated from Tourette syndrome, which is a neurologic disorder, reported in 1 in 3,000 children, characterized by severe, frequent, and multiple tics. These tics are also often vocal and consist of sounds such as hissing, barking, grunting, or coprolalia (repeating profanities). Some rhythmic habits may be mistaken for seizures but can be easily distinguished because of the stereotypical, repetitive nature of the behavior.

Trichotillomania usually has a classic physical appearance that has been referred to as *tonsure (Friar Tuck)* pattern baldness, with baldness around the vertex of the head. Unilateral temporal baldness is also a consequence of trichotillomania. The differential diagnosis of trichotillomania includes alopecia areata, tinea capitis, syphilitic alopecia, and androgenic alopecia (see Chapter 123). Broken hairs of variable length usually characterize alopecia secondary to trichotillomania. Other disorders in the differential diagnosis include traction alopecia, related to tight braids or hair brushing; atopic eczema; seborrheic dermatitis; hypothyroidism; systemic lupus erythematosus; and dermatomyositis. When trichotillomania is associated with a trichobezoar and signs of gastric outlet obstruction, the differential diagnosis includes neuroblastoma, lymphoma, and gastric carcinoma.

Cutting is not a benign habit, but it can provide stress relief, a feature of many benign childhood habits. It is usually associated with a wide range of psychopathology, including depression; anxiety; eating disorders, especially bulimia nervosa; a history of prior sexual abuse; and obsessive-compulsive symptoms. The mechanism by which cutting alleviates stress and anxiety has not been elucidated, but the role of endogenous endorphins has been suggested. Cutting is felt not to represent suicidal behavior, but some studies differentiate the site of cutting as predictive of suicidality: Wrist cutters as opposed to arm cutters have a higher rate of suicide ideation and attempts. All cutters are at greater risk for suicide than the general population. Management generally involves referral to a mental health specialist and the use of psychotherapy. Other forms of self-injury are reported with increased frequency among children with developmental disabilities, including ASDs (see Chapter 128).

Evaluation

History

Children who present with thumb sucking, nail biting, and teeth grinding usually do not require an assessment other than a routine health maintenance history and physical examination. The history should determine the specific circumstances when the habit is manifest. Is the habit more likely to emerge when the child is tired or stressed? Habits must also be evaluated in the context of the child's developmental level and home situation. Understanding the effect of the habit on the child and family is important. Children who present with movements that resemble tics should be carefully questioned about the frequency and duration of the tics, the effect of the tics on their behavior, and whether coughing is associated with the tics (sign of Tourette syndrome). The occurrence of obsessive-compulsive mannerisms should also be noted (Questions Box).

Physical Examination

A routine physical examination should be performed. The physical examination may reveal the sequelae of the habit, such as thumb calluses, candidal infection of the nails, or evidence of malocclusion with an overbite (Figure 53-1). Children with suspected trichotillomania should have a thorough assessment of their scalp in an effort to differentiate other causes of alopecia (see Chapter 123). A careful neurologic examination should be performed in children with tics, and referral to a child neurologist may be indicated in children with suspected neurologic disorders.

Laboratory Studies

Routine laboratory studies are not needed in children diagnosed with habit disorders. Studies are indicated if the children have experienced complications from the habit. For instance, if osteomyelitis is suspected in a nail-biting child, magnetic resonance imaging would be the study of choice.

Children with trichotillomania should be evaluated for the disorders listed previously. An easy evaluation process for trichotillomania

---

Questions

Childhood Habits

- What about your child's habit concerns you?
- Is your child experiencing any adverse consequences (eg, being teased at school) as a result of the habit?
- Does the habit interfere with your child's routine activities?
- Can you identify stressors in your child's life?
- Is your child comforted by the habit?

Figure 53-1. Anterior open bite associated with thumb sucking.

involves shaving the hair in the middle of the area of baldness. The growth of these small hairs is uniform because children are unable to pull them out. Head shaving may not be acceptable, however, to the parent or child. Disorders such as syphilis and collagen vascular diseases can be ruled out using appropriate laboratory studies. Fungal infections can be differentiated by the use of appropriate cultures. A Wood light examination may reveal fluorescence noted with certain fungal infections.

Children who present with pica should be evaluated for the presence of iron deficiency anemia and lead poisoning.

Management

The management of childhood habits should be directed at specific symptoms. For older children, self-monitoring and relaxation training may be helpful as alternative means for dealing with stress. The issue of thumb sucking versus the use of pacifiers can be addressed by anticipatory guidance. **Pacifiers,** which were previously discouraged, are now believed to have some advantages over thumb sucking. A report from the American Academy of Pediatrics noted a decrease in the incidence of sudden infant death syndrome in infants who used a pacifier. With pacifiers, the risk for dental disturbances is lower because the pacifiers are softer and are accompanied by a plastic shield that puts counter pressure on the teeth. Pacifiers are also detachable and cleanable.

Pacifiers can be lost, however. Parents should be advised not to attach a pacifier to the child's shirt with a string because of risk of strangulation. For children who are pacifier dependent and are unable to go back to sleep if they lose their pacifier at night, multiple pacifiers can be placed in the crib to make finding one easier. For infants who desire pacifiers because they complete their feeding in less than 20 minutes, a nipple with a smaller hole can be used or the cap can be screwed on the bottle more tightly to prolong the time spent in nutritive sucking. Dental problems may develop when pacifiers are used upside down, all day long, or after the eruption of permanent dentition.

It is suggested that parents do not try to stop thumb-sucking behavior until children have reached the age of 4 years. Dental problems in late thumb suckers include anterior open bite, increased horizontal overlap (protruding upper incisors), intruded and flared upper incisors, lingually flipped lower incisors, and warped alveolar ridge. When thumb sucking persists to school age, tongue thrust is noted, as are articulation problems, specifically with consonants s, t, d, n, z, l, and r. The physician should reassure parents that children who stop sucking their thumbs prior to the eruption of the secondary dentition are not at risk for poor dentition.

Numerous devices have been proposed to help with the cessation of thumb sucking, but reported success has been variable. The use of arm restraints, particularly at night, is not recommended and may result in rumination. Bitter paints seek to reduce thumb sucking by subjecting children to a bitter, aversive taste. This medication consists of 49% toluene, 19% isopropyl alcohol, 18% butyl acetate, 11% ethyl cellulose, and 0.3% denatonium benzoate. A ¾-oz bottle is toxic if ingested in its entirety. Nocturnal application is needed if children suck their thumbs during the night. The principle of retraining, in which thumb sucking becomes a duty and children are required to suck all 10 fingers one at a time, has also been recommended. Some recommend that elastic bandages be put on the hand of nocturnal thumb suckers. Problems associated with thumb sucking include sore thumbs, calluses, and candidal infections. Dentists may fashion a reminder appliance, called a palatal crib or rake, making it difficult for children to suck their thumbs. Such devices are usually applied for a minimum of 3 months. A fixed appliance is preferable to a removable one and treatment should be initiated in spring or summer when children are engaged in numerous physical activities. Some dental devices are available commercially or online. They may consist of a plastic covering for the thumb and hand. This covering eliminates the pleasurable sensation created by the interaction of thumb, saliva, and mouth. Such devices cost about $80 and success is variable.

Encouragement works better than nagging, as a rule, and a **reward system** is particularly useful in children who are 5 to 6 years of age. Parents may be referred to books such as *Danny and His Thumb* and encouraged to talk to their children about how good it feels not to suck their thumbs. A star chart and diary are also useful. Sometimes, telling children something like, "Mommy would be so proud of you if you didn't suck your thumb now that you're such a big girl or a big boy," is effective. In addition, the pressure to stop thumb sucking becomes greater during the school years. Children who suck their thumbs are regarded by their peers in first grade as less intelligent, less happy, less likable, and less desirable as friends.

In children who suck their thumbs and twirl their hair at the same time, the hair twirling stops once the thumb sucking ends. The phenomenon is referred to as *habit covariance*. Hair pulling in young children seems to often resolve spontaneously but is more problematic in adolescents and adults. Management of trichotillomania usually involves non-pharmacologic treatments. In children, behavior modification, including putting socks on the hands and the use of time-out for hair pulling, in addition to extra attention for not pulling the hair, is recommended. Substituting behavior is also encouraged. For instance, children should be advised to sit on their hands, wear gloves, pull rubber bands, or squeeze a ball whenever they have an urge to pull their hair. In older individuals, hair pulling may be related to obsessive-compulsive disorders. A form of cognitive-behavioral therapy referred to as habit reversal therapy is said to have significant empirical support. This therapy involves an understanding of the hair pulling by the patient and then a combination of awareness training, self-monitoring, stimulus control, and competing response procedures. Habit reversal therapy is more appropriate for older children and adolescents. Trichotillomania may lead to the presence of bezoars (hair balls) from swallowed hair. Sometimes, hair balls can extend through the gastric outlet into the small intestine, a phenomenon referred to as Rapunzel syndrome. Gastric hair balls can be dissolved enzymatically or with the installation of a cola soda through a nasogastric tube. If such maneuvers fail, they are removed endoscopically or through surgery. Pharmacologic therapy for trichotillomania is not routinely recommended for the management of affected children. In adults, selective serotonin reuptake inhibitors, bupropion, and risperidone have been used. Children whose symptoms have not improved with behavioral interventions should be referred to a mental health professional for additional management.

Nail biting also often responds to behavior modification. Olive oil may be put on the nails to make them soft so there are fewer jagged edges to bite. In the children's book, *The Berenstain Bears and the Bad Habit,* collecting pennies is suggested as a habit substitution for nail biting.

Rhythmic habits are less easy to modify. For the most part, reassurance is all that is available. The use of metronome-like devices has had no demonstrable effect. Children older than 3 years who disturb the family's sleep with their rhythmic habits may be given mild sedatives, such as diphenhydramine or hydroxyzine. Medications to reduce head banging include transdermal clonidine and thioridazine (eg, Mellaril). Other maneuvers involve placing the crib or bed on carpeting or bolting the crib to the wall to decrease the amount of noise from movement.

Children who engage in biting behavior should be managed with behavior modification, including praising of good behavior and time-out for inappropriate behavior. Aversive conditioning involves the placement of some non-palatable food, such as a lemon or onion on a necklace, and having the child bite on that object rather than biting another child. Biting behavior is reported to be extinguished with this technique. Another option is the placement of a whistle. The child blows the whistle rather than biting the other child.

Nose picking is a common habit in children and adults. One suggestion to extinguish or minimize this habit involves letting children look in a mirror and pick their nose or videotaping the child while nose picking. Their reaction is that nose picking looks "gross" and the habit may decrease in frequency.

Iron deficiency related to pica requires iron supplementation. Lead intoxication should be managed with chelation and environmental manipulation.

Prognosis

Most habits are not harmful to children's health. The major problem is social acceptability. Parents should be encouraged to stop a habit before it becomes ingrained. This can often be done by praising good behavior and encouraging activities during which the unwanted behavior does not appear. Habits that do not respond to parental influence often resolve spontaneously under peer pressure.

CASE RESOLUTION

In the case history presented at the beginning of the chapter, it is important for the physician and the mother to empower the boy to stop thumb sucking before he finds himself ridiculed by his classmates. He might be allowed to suck his thumb at certain times and in certain places (eg, "You can suck in your room after school for 15 minutes."). Books geared at children and parents to help stop thumb sucking are recommended, and the boy is rewarded for times when he is not sucking his thumb.

Selected References

Balighian E, Tuli SY, Tuli SS, et al. Index of suspicion. Case 1: persistent fever and cough following episodes of emesis in a 7-year-old girl. Case 2: blurry vision and unilateral dilated pupil in a 14-year-old girl. Case 3: swelling, pain, and erythema of the thumb in a 10-year old girl with habits of nail biting and thumb sucking. *Pediatr Rev.* 2012;33(1):39–44

Blum NJ, Barone VJ, Friman PC. A simplified behavioral treatment for trichotillomania: report of two cases. *Pediatrics.* 1993;91(5):993–995

Brazelton TB. Sucking in infancy. *Pediatrics.* 1956;17(3):400–404

Collacott RA, Cooper SA, Branford D, McGrother C. Epidemiology of self-injurious behaviour in adults with learning disabilities. *Br J Psychiatry.* 1998; 173:428–432

Davidson L. Thumb and finger sucking. *Pediatr Rev.* 2008;29(6):207–208

Dimino-Emme L, Camisa C. Trichotillomania associated with the "Friar Tuck sign" and nail-biting. *Cutis.* 1991;47(2):107–110

Flessner CA, Lochner C, Stein DJ, Woods DW, Franklin ME, Keuthen NJ. Age of onset of trichotillomania symptoms: investigating clinical correlates. *J Nerv Ment Dis.* 2010;198(12):896–900

Friman PC, Barone VJ, Christophersen ER. Aversive taste treatment of finger and thumb sucking. *Pediatrics.* 1986;78(1):174–176

Friman PC, McPherson KM, Warzak WJ, Evans J. Influence of thumb sucking on peer social acceptance in first-grade children. *Pediatrics.* 1993;91(4): 784–786

Friman PC, Schmitt BD. Thumb sucking: pediatricians' guidelines. *Clin Pediatr (Phila).* 1989;28(10):438–440

Golomb RG, Vavrichek SM. *The Hair Pulling "Habit" and You: How to Solve the Trichotillomania Puzzle.* Silver Spring, MD: Writers' Cooperative of Greater Washington; 2000

Johnson ED, Larson BE. Thumb-sucking: literature review. *ASDC J Dent Child.* 1993;60(4):385–391

Koç O, Yildiz FD, Narci A, Sen TA. An unusual cause of gastric perforation in childhood: trichobezoar (Rapunzel syndrome). A case report. *Eur J Pediatr.* 2009;168(4):495–497

Morris SH, Zickgraf HF, Dingfelder HE, Franklin ME. Habit reversal training in trichotillomania: guide for the clinician. *Expert Rev Neurother.* 2013;13(9): 1069–1077

Panza KE, Pittenger C, Bloch MH. Age and gender correlates of pulling in pediatric trichotillomania. *J Am Acad Child Adolesc Psychiatry.* 2013;52(3): 241–249

Peterson JE, Schneider PE. Oral habits. A behavioral approach. *Pediatr Clin North Am.* 1991;38(5):1289–1307

Repetitive behavioral patterns. In: Wolraich ML, ed. *The Classification of Child and Adolescent Mental Diagnoses in Primary Care: Diagnostic and Statistical Manual for Primary Care (DSM-PC) Child and Adolescent Version.* Elk Grove Village, IL: American Academy of Pediatrics; 1996:269–275

Rosenberg MD. Thumbsucking. *Pediatr Rev.* 1995;16(2):73–74

Schmitt B. Helping the child with tics (twitches). *Contemp Pediatr.* 1991;8: 31–32

Tay YK, Levy ML, Metry DW. Trichotillomania in childhood: case series and review. *Pediatrics.* 2004;113(5):e494–e498

CHAPTER 54

Enuresis

Carol D. Berkowitz, MD

CASE STUDY

A 9-year-old boy who is in good general health is evaluated for a history of bed-wetting. He is the product of a normal pregnancy and delivery, and he achieved his developmental milestones at the appropriate time. The boy was toilet trained by the age of 3 years, but he has never been dry at night for more than several days at a time. Enuresis occurs at least 3 to 4 times a week even if he is fluid-restricted after 6:00 pm. The boy never wets himself during the day, has normal stools, and is an average student. His father had enuresis that resolved by the time he was 12 years old.

The boy's physical examination is entirely normal.

Questions

1. What conditions account for the symptoms of enuresis?
2. What is the appropriate evaluation of children with enuresis?
3. What is the relationship between enuresis and emotional stresses or psychosocial disorders?
4. What management plans are available for enuresis?
5. How do physicians decide which management technique is appropriate for which patients?

Enuresis is defined as involuntary or intentional urination in children whose age and development suggest achievement of bladder control. Voiding into the bed or clothing occurs repeatedly (at least twice a week for at least 3 consecutive months). Urinary continence is reached earlier in girls than in boys, and the diagnosis of enuresis is reserved for girls older than 5 years and boys older than 6 years. The term *diurnal enuresis,* wetting that occurs during the day, has been replaced by *daytime incontinence.* The International Children's Continence Society promotes a new standardization for enuresis-related terminology. It prefers the use of the term *incontinence* to denote uncontrollable leakage of urine, intermittent or continuous, that occurs after continence should have been achieved. *Nocturnal* or *sleep enuresis* refers to involuntary urination or incontinence that occurs during the night. The term **primary nocturnal enuresis (PNE)** is used when children have never achieved sustained dryness, and **secondary enuresis** is used when urinary incontinence recurs after 3 to 6 months of dryness. Monosymptomatic nocturnal enuresis means that nighttime wetting is the only complaint. Children who experience urgency, frequency, dribbling, or other symptoms have poly-symptomatic enuresis. Such symptoms may be related to inappropriate muscle contraction, are usually associated with constipation, and are termed *dysfunctional elimination syndrome.*

Physicians can be particularly helpful by routinely questioning parents about bed-wetting during health maintenance visits. Many families are otherwise reluctant to bring up this embarrassing complaint because enuresis is viewed as socially unacceptable. It poses particular difficulties if children wish to sleep away from home. In addition, enuresis may be a marker for other behavioral or developmental problems.

Epidemiology

Enuresis affects 5 to 7 million patients in the United States. It is one of the most common conditions of childhood, affecting 10% to 20% of first-grade boys and 8% to 17% of first-grade girls. By age 10 years, 5% to 10% of boys have enuresis (1% of army recruits are enuretic). Seventy-four percent of affected children have nocturnal enuresis, 10% daytime incontinence, and 16% both. Primary enuresis affects the majority (75%–80%) of children with enuresis, and 80% to 85% of these children have monosymptomatic nocturnal enuresis. Although the overall incidence of secondary enuresis is lower (20%–25%), it increases with age; secondary enuresis makes up 50% of cases of enuresis in children 12 years of age.

Several epidemiologic factors have been associated with enuresis, including low socioeconomic level, large family size, single-parent family, low birth weight, short height at 11 to 15 years of age, immature behavior, relatively low IQ, poor speech and coordination, and encopresis (fecal incontinence; 5%–15% of cases). Enuresis has been associated with obstructive sleep apnea in which an increased level of atrial natriuretic factor has been reported. Atrial natriuretic factor inhibits the renin-angiotensin-aldosterone pathway, causing diuresis. Correcting obstructive sleep apnea with tonsillectomy or adenoidectomy leads to an elimination of the enuresis. Enuresis occurs more often in institutionalized children. Enuresis has a familial basis, with 44% being enuretic if one parent was enuretic and as many as 77% of children being enuretic if both parents were similarly affected. Concordance for enuresis is reported in up to 68% of monozygotic twins and between 36% and 48% of dizygotic twins.

Clinical Presentation

A history of enuresis may be obtained as a presenting complaint or elicited by physicians during a health maintenance visit. Medical complaints such as encopresis, obstructive sleep apnea (nighttime snoring), or attention-deficit/hyperactivity disorder (ADHD) may be associated with enuresis (D_x Box). Children with ADHD have a 30% greater risk of being enuretic. The physical examination is usually normal.

Pathophysiology

Delayed control of micturition has several possible causes (Box 54-1).

1. **Faulty toilet training.** Faulty toilet training may perpetuate diurnal and nocturnal enuresis but is not expected to selectively perpetuate the latter. Parental expectations are believed to play a role in the toilet-training experience. Parents who allow children to sleep in diapers may be delaying the achievement of nighttime dryness, but it is unlikely that the use of diapers causes nocturnal enuresis. Poor toilet habits, particularly infrequent voiding or constipation, may be associated with urinary tract infections (UTIs).

Dx **Enuresis**

- Bed-wetting
- Old enough to be toilet trained
- Precipitating problem such as diabetes or urinary tract infection
- Encopresis
- Attention-deficit/hyperactivity disorder
- Family history of enuresis

Box 54-1. Causes of Enuresis

Primary Enuresis
- Faulty toilet training
- Maturational delay
- Small bladder capacity
- Sleep disorder/impaired arousal
- Allergens
- Nocturnal polyuria/relative vasopressin deficiency
- Dysfunctional bladder contraction

Secondary Enuresis
- Urinary tract infection
- Diabetes mellitus
- Diabetes insipidus
- Nocturnal seizures
- Genitourinary anomalies
- Sickle cell anemia
- Medication use
- Emotional stress

2. **Maturational delay.** The development of the inhibitory reflex of voiding may be delayed in some children, which may contribute to enuresis until the age of 5 years. This is similar to the range in which children achieve other developmental milestones. It is unlikely that maturational delay persists as a cause of enuresis beyond this age. Experts believe that maturational delay is not a reasonable explanation if children can achieve dryness in the daytime but not at night.

3. **Small bladder capacity.** Evidence suggests that some children with enuresis have smaller bladder capacities. Bladder capacity in ounces is estimated as the age in years plus 2. For example, 5-year-old children have a bladder capacity of 7 oz (210 mL). Adult bladder capacity is 12 to 16 oz (360–480 mL). Small bladder capacity is associated with diurnal frequency or incontinence.

4. **Sleep disorder/impaired arousal.** It has been suggested that children with enuresis are in "deep sleep" and do not sense a full bladder. This is often the parent's perception of their child's sleep pattern. However, studies have shown that enuresis occurs during all stages of sleep, particularly in the first one-third of sleep and in transition from non–rapid eye movement stage 4 to rapid eye movement sleep. During this period, body tone, respiratory rate, and heart rate increase, and erection and micturition occur. Studies suggest that the arousal center in the brain fails to respond (ie, the child does not awake) to full bladder sensation. Children with enuresis do not seem to sleep more deeply than other children. However, enuretic children may have diminished arousal during sleep. In one study, 40% of enuretic children, compared with only 8.5% of non-enuretic children, failed to awaken to an 80-decibel noise.

5. **Allergens.** No evidence confirms the notion that exposure to certain foods (eg, food additives, sugar) contributes to enuresis. However, some parents believe that bed-wetting is decreased if certain foods, such as sodas and sweets, are eliminated from the diet. The ingestion of caffeine-containing beverages may exacerbate nocturnal enuresis.

6. **Nocturnal polyuria/relative vasopressin deficiency.** Research has shown that although non-enuretic children exhibit a diurnal variation in vasopressin secretion, this rhythm is disturbed in some children with enuresis, resulting in nocturnal polyuria.

7. **Dysfunctional bladder contraction.** In cases of daytime incontinence, contractile disturbances of the bladder affect normal voiding. Children with an "uninhibited bladder" have not learned to inhibit bladder contraction. They may assume a certain posture, called Vincent curtsy, in an effort to prevent micturition. Some children exhibit uncoordinated, incomplete voiding and the urine exits the urethra in a staccato stream. Trabeculations or bladder wall thickening may be noted on imaging studies.

Daytime incontinence can be related to problems with bladder filling and storage or to bladder emptying. Each of these functions is under different neurologic control, with filling and storage under the sympathetic nervous system and bladder emptying related to the action of acetylcholine and the parasympathetic system. Effective voiding requires the coordinated effort of these 2 phases.

Management of daytime incontinence is dependent on which phase is malfunctioning.

Differential Diagnosis

Primary nocturnal enuresis is usually related to the conditions discussed in Pathophysiology on page 322. An organic problem is rarely the cause. However, secondary enuresis may result from an organic problem, such as UTI, diabetes mellitus, diabetes insipidus, nocturnal seizures, genitourinary anomalies (eg, ectopic ureter), sickle cell anemia, medication (eg, diuretics, theophylline), or emotional stress. When primary enuresis is diurnal and nocturnal, some of these conditions should be considered. Additional diagnoses include neurogenic bladder, which may occur in association with cerebral palsy; sacral agenesis; or myelomeningocele. Some children experience urinary frequency, a benign self-limited condition characterized by the sudden need to urinate very frequently, often 25 to 30 times a day. Rarely, there is nocturia without other urinary symptoms. The condition occurs most often in children between 3 and 8 years of age, is self-limited, and is felt to be stress related. A urinary diary, noting time and amount of voiding, is sometimes helpful in diagnosing the condition.

Evaluation

History

A thorough history should be obtained when evaluating children with enuresis (Questions Box).

Questions

Enuresis

- Is the enuresis primary or secondary?
- Is the enuresis diurnal, nocturnal, or both?
- How old was the child when he or she was toilet trained?
- How old was the child when he or she achieved daytime and nighttime dryness?
- How often does the child urinate and defecate during the average day?
- Is the child's urinary stream forceful or dribbling?
- Does the child dribble before or after voiding?
- Does the child experience symptoms such as polydipsia, polyuria, dysuria, urgency, frequency, or problems with stooling?
- Who changes the bed and who washes the bedclothes after bed-wetting occurs?
- Does the child wear diapers or training pants or use incontinence pads?
- Does the child seem to delay using the toilet?
- Does the child assume any unusual or distinct postures to avoid being incontinent?
- What is the attitude of the family toward the child with enuresis? Are family members accepting or ashamed?
- Has the family tried any treatments yet?
- Is there a family history of enuresis?
- Does the child have other symptoms such as encopresis, attention-deficit/hyperactivity disorder, or obstructive sleep apnea?

Physical Examination

A general physical examination should be performed, with particular attention to certain areas. The pattern of growth should be plotted. Blood pressure should be obtained. The abdomen should be assessed for evidence of organomegaly, bladder size, and fecal impaction. An anal examination should be performed to evaluate rectal tone.

If possible, physicians should watch children void. Practitioners should determine whether children can start and stop micturition and whether the stream is forceful. Dribbling in girls may indicate an ectopic ureter. A more sophisticated approach involves the uroflow test in which the patient voids into an apparatus that electrically senses the rate of flow. A graph is generated that notes the flow rate and quantity. This study is most useful in children with diurnal incontinence. The appearance of the genitalia should be assessed. A rash in the genital area may be secondary to wetness from urinary incontinence. The skin may be macerated, erythematous, or hyperpigmented secondary to persistent moisture and irritation.

Labial fusion in girls may trap urine, allow reflux into the vagina, and lead to dribbling. Meatal stenosis, epispadias, hypospadias, or cryptorchidism may be present in boys. Any of these conditions suggests a possible underlying genitourinary anomaly.

Neuromuscular integrity of the lower extremities should be evaluated. This may provide a clue to a disorder such as spina bifida occulta. The presence of some anomaly in the sacral area, such as a sacral dimple or a tuft of hair, may also be a sign of this condition.

Laboratory Tests

Only a minimal laboratory evaluation is indicated in most children with primary enuresis. Urinalysis, including specific gravity, is usually indicated. A complete blood cell count, hemoglobin electrophoresis, serum electrolytes, and blood urea nitrogen should also be considered. Studies such as urine culture and blood glucose are more often indicated in cases of secondary enuresis.

Imaging Studies

In cases in which urinalysis is abnormal, the culture is positive, or genitourinary anomalies are apparent on physical examination, a renal ultrasound and vesicoureterogram may be warranted. Vertebral radiographs or magnetic resonance imaging is appropriate in the diagnosis of spina bifida. Magnetic resonance urography is helpful in girls suspected of having an ectopic ureter. An electroencephalogram is indicated if nocturnal epilepsy is suspected. Urodynamic studies to evaluate bladder contractility are controversial but are recommended by some urologists in children who do not respond to traditional therapy or are suspected of having spina bifida occulta.

Management

Primary Enuresis

Family counseling about enuresis should be part of all management plans. Issues related to psychosocial stress should be explored, particularly in cases of secondary enuresis. Families should be advised that the wetting is not intentional and that punishing children for accidents is inappropriate. However, children may take some responsibility for the consequences of their actions, such as removing soiled bedding or helping with the laundry. They should be rewarded for dry nights. Star charts, in which a sticker or gold star is applied to a calendar for each dry night, have traditionally been used. Star charts and rewards are part of motivational therapy, which is a recommended first-line intervention for younger children (5- to 7-year-olds) who do not wet the bed every night. Success as defined by a 2-week period of dry nights occurs in 25%, and improvement is reported in more than 70%. The exclusive use of these charts without other interventions, however, has limited success and suggests that the enuresis may have a volitional component. Star charts should be used in conjunction with other management strategies.

Two treatment modalities are acceptable for managing enuresis. Most studies do not support the use of fluid restriction as a reliable isolated means of controlling enuresis. Some children benefit from sequential or combination therapy.

Conditioning therapy involves the use of an alarm that is triggered when children void during the night. Children are awakened by the sounding of the alarm, and further urination is inhibited. Eventually, bladder distention is associated with inhibition of the urge to urinate. When conditioning therapy is used for 4 to 6 months, it is associated with a success rate of 70%. If the alarm is used for 4 more weeks with sustained dryness, relapses are uncommon.

Because patient cooperation is needed with the alarm system, its use is reserved for children older than 7 years. A newer system is a transistorized version of the original device that contains a small sensor in the underwear and an alarm on the wrist or collar. Some systems use vibrations so other family members are not disturbed by loud alarms.

Overall, conditioning devices have a cure rate of 70% to 85% and a relapse rate of 10% to 15%. They incur a one-time cost of $50 to $75. Conditioning devices may be covered by insurance companies if the alarm is prescribed by a physician as a medical device. Approximately 30% of families discontinue use of the alarm before the recommended period for various reasons. Conditioning without the use of auxiliary alarms may also be undertaken. One proposed method involves instituting a self-awakening program. Older school-aged children practice lying in bed during the daytime and simulating the experience of awaking, sensing a full bladder, and going to the toilet. Another dry-bed training program involves parents awaking their children first hourly and then at longer intervals over the period of about 1 week. Children eventually learn to self-awake. A 92% success rate with a relapse rate of 20% is reported with this program.

Pharmacologic agents include tricyclic antidepressants and desmopressin. Generally, medications produce a more rapid response but have a higher rate of relapse. Tricyclic antidepressants, especially imipramine, have been successfully used to treat nocturnal enuresis, although the mechanism of action is uncertain. The antidepressant action of the drug, its effect on sleep and arousal, and its anticholinergic properties may all play a role. There is also some evidence that imipramine increases concentrations of antidiuretic hormone. The bladder capacity of individuals with enuresis treated with imipramine may be increased by 34%, which indicates that the anticholinergic effects of the drug may be the most significant.

Imipramine should not be prescribed for children younger than 6 or 7 years because of potential adverse effects. The recommended dosage is 0.9 to 1.5 mg/kg/day. In general, children younger than 8 years are given 25 mg 1 to 2 hours before bedtime, and older children are given 50 to 75 mg. Beneficial results usually occur within the first few weeks of therapy. Medication is usually continued for 3 to 6 months to prevent relapses, which are reported in up to 75% of cases. The drug should be tapered by reducing the dose or using an alternate-night regimen. Side effects are rare and include insomnia, nightmares, and personality changes. Acute overdoses are potentially fatal secondary to cardiac complications. The initial cure rate is 10% to 60% with a relapse rate of 90%. The monthly cost of imipramine is about $5.

Desmopressin, an analog of vasopressin, the antidiuretic hormone, is another pharmacologic agent used for enuresis. Desmopressin most likely works by decreasing nocturnal urine production. Most patients respond rapidly to desmopressin and become dry within 1 to 2 weeks of the initiation of therapy. The medication is taken orally as a 0.2-mg tablet 1 hour before bedtime. The dose may be increased by 1 tablet at weekly intervals (maximum dose: 0.6 mg). Desmopressin in nasal spray is no longer recommended for the treatment of enuresis because of the risk of severe hyponatremia, seizures, and even death. Hyponatremia has also been reported with oral desmopressin in the face of high fluid intake sometimes associated with habit polydipsia. Fluid restriction is recommended from 1 hour before until 8 hours after desmopressin administration. While some recommend a 6-month course of the medication, others suggest a shorter trial period. If patients achieve a 2-week period of dryness, the dose can be tapered at 2-week intervals. The cure rate is 40% to 50% with a relapse rate of 90% off medication. Desmopressin is expensive, with an average monthly cost of $150 to $250.

Oxybutynin is an antispasmodic, anticholinergic agent used in the management of daytime incontinence or poly-symptomatic nocturnal enuresis. The dosage is 5 mg at bedtime for children 6 to 12 years of age and 10 mg at bedtime for children older than 12 years. The response rate is 33%, and the major side effects include drowsiness, flushing, dry mouth, constipation, and hyperthermia. Hyoscyamine sulfate and flavoxate hydrochloride are 2 other medications used for daytime incontinence.

Treatment of enuresis in children with small bladder capacities includes bladder retention training. Such children are fluid loaded and asked to delay voiding for 5 to 10 minutes. This strategy is generally reserved for children with daytime incontinence.

Associated symptoms, particularly constipation and encopresis, should be adequately addressed.

Secondary Enuresis

The management of secondary enuresis should focus on the treatment of the causal disorder, such as a UTI or diabetes mellitus.

Prognosis

The prognosis for children with enuresis is good. Spontaneous cure rate is 15% per year. Medical management results in a reduction in symptoms in more than 70% of affected children.

CASE RESOLUTION

The boy in the case scenario has primary nocturnal enuresis. The history of childhood enuresis in the father is significant. Two management options, behavior modification and treatment with desmopressin or imipramine, can be discussed with the family. The child's symptoms will probably spontaneously improve over time.

Selected References

Alloussi SH, Mürtz G, Lang C, et al. Desmopressin treatment regimens in monosymptomatic and nonmonosymptomatic enuresis: a review from a clinical perspective. *J Pediatr Urol.* 2011;7(1):10–20

Bennett HJ. *Waking Up Dry: A Guide to Help Children Overcome Bedwetting.* Elk Grove Village, IL: American Academy of Pediatrics; 2005

Graham KM, Levy JB. Enuresis. *Pediatr Rev.* 2009;30(5):165–173

Joinson C, Heron J, von Gontard A. Psychological problems of children with daytime wetting. *Pediatrics.* 2006;118(5):1985–1993

Mercer R. *Seven Steps to Nighttime Dryness: A Practical Guide for Parents of Children with Bedwetting.* Ashton, MD: Brookeville Media; 2004

Nevéus T, von Gontard A, Hoebeke P, et al. The standardization of terminology of lower urinary tract function in children and adolescence: report for the Standardisation Committee of the International Children's Continence Society. *J Urol.* 2006;176(1):314–324

Perrin N, Saver L, While A. The efficacy of alarm therapy versus desmopressin therapy in the treatment of primary mono-symptomatic nocturnal enuresis: a systematic review. *Prim Health Care Res Dev.* 2013;19:1–11

Robson WL. Clinical practice. Evaluation and management of enuresis. *N Eng J Med.* 2009;360(14):1429–1436

Robson WL. Enuresis. *Adv Pediatr.* 2001;48:409–438

Robson WL, Leung AK. An approach to daytime wetting in children. *Adv Pediatr.* 2006;53:323–365

Robson WL, Leung AK, Van Howe R. Primary and secondary nocturnal enuresis: similarities in presentation. *Pediatrics.* 2005;115(4):956–959

Treatment of childhood enuresis. *Clin Pediatr (Phila).* 1993;32

van Dommelen P, Kamphuis M, van Leerdam FJ, et al. The short- and long-term effects of simple behavioral interventions for nocturnal enuresis in young children: a randomized controlled trial. *J Pediatr* 2009;154(5):662–666

CHAPTER 55

Encopresis

Carol D. Berkowitz, MD

CASE STUDY

A 7-year-old boy presents with the complaint of soiling his underpants. His mother states that he has never been completely toilet trained and that stooling accidents occur at least 2 to 3 times a week, mainly during the day. The boy rarely has a spontaneous bowel movement without assistance. He sits on the toilet for just a few minutes and passes small, pellet-like stools. His mother has never sought medical care before for this problem.

The boy is very fidgety during the physical examination. His vital signs are normal and the child's height and weight are at the 25th percentile. His abdomen is soft but distended, with palpable loops of stool-filled bowel. A small amount of stool is present around the anus and in the boy's underpants. Digital examination of the rectum reveals hard stool. The rectal tone is normal, as is the rest of the physical examination.

Questions

1. What is the definition of encopresis?
2. What is the difference between retentive and non-retentive encopresis?
3. What are some physiological conditions that contribute to encopresis?
4. What conditions may be mistaken for encopresis?

Encopresis is the repeated passage of stool into inappropriate places (eg, clothing), voluntary or involuntary, in children who should be toilet trained on the basis of age (usually at least 4 years, the age at which 95% of children have achieved stool continence) and developmental level and who have no primary organic pathology. One such encopretic event occurs each month for at least 3 months. The term *encopresis*, coined in 1926 by Weissenberg and originally used for children with psychogenic soiling, is similar to enuresis. Unlike enuresis, encopresis rarely occurs at night. Now, encopresis is used in a broader sense to refer to all types of fecal incontinence. Fecal incontinence is the currently preferred term as recommended by the Multinational Working Teams to Develop Diagnostic Criteria for Functional Gastrointestinal Disorders.

Retentive encopresis, also referred to as functional fecal retention with encopresis or retentive fecal incontinence, occurs in the face of constipation (obstipation), in which chronic rectal distention leads to the seepage of liquid stool around hard, retained feces. Sometimes this is called overflow, fecal soiling, or pseudo-incontinence because the individual has the potential for bowel control. Onset of symptoms is usually about 4 years of age. Approximately 95% of cases of fecal incontinence are retentive. **Non-retentive fecal incontinence** is characterized by the passage of soft stool without colonic distention or retention of stool. It is fecal incontinence in the absence of constipation. Some have recognized 2 categories of children with non-retentive fecal incontinence: those who can control defecation but stool in inappropriate places, and those who have true failure to achieve bowel control. Primary encopresis occurs when children have never been completely toilet trained. Secondary encopresis occurs in children who have had a period of complete continence of stool. Most encopretic children have secondary encopresis.

Epidemiology

Encopresis is reported in approximately 1.5% of school-aged children, and boys are reported to be affected 2 to 6 times more often than girls. This gender ratio reverses in the elderly, in which the prevalence of fecal incontinence is twice as high in females as in males. An association between encopresis, enuresis, attention-deficit/hyperactivity disorder (ADHD), and autism spectrum disorder is sometimes present. About 15% of children with enuresis also have encopresis. Family history for encopresis may also be positive; 16% of affected children have one affected parent, usually the father. An association between encopresis and child sexual abuse has been reported in a small number of children. There is no reported relationship between socioeconomic status, parental age, child's birth order, or family size.

Clinical Presentation

Children with encopresis have a history of staining of the underpants, which may be hidden in drawers or under beds by embarrassed children. Occasionally, parents are unaware of the problem. Stooling accidents occur more frequently at home than in school. Some children have a history of constipation. Other children may initially be misdiagnosed as having diarrhea and are inappropriately placed on antidiarrheal medications, which exacerbate their problem. Parents may complain that their children exude a fecal odor, but children are unaware they are malodorous (D_x Box). Some children may complain of abdominal pain, which may be vague and nonspecific or severe and crampy.

Encopresis

- Incontinence of stool
- Constipation
- Hyperactivity
- Distended abdomen
- Stool-filled loops of bowel
- Lax rectal tone
- Soiled clothing or bedding
- Fecal odor

Pathophysiology

There are 3 identified milestones when children may be at risk for the development of functional constipation: when dietary solids are introduced into an infant's diet, with toilet training, and with the start of school. Constipation, if associated with painful defecation, may be associated with the development of retentive fecal incontinence. With time, the colon distends and liquid feces seep around impacted stool (Figure 55-1). In 30% to 50% of children, anal spasm, referred to as animus, occurs and contraction rather than relaxation occurs during evacuation of feces. In another 40%, rectal hyposensitivity is apparent so that the children are unaware of the presence of stool. Some children have an evacuation release disorder in which the presence of stool does not result in relaxation and stool evacuation. In such cases, the rectum is chronically distended by stool, water is absorbed, and stool becomes harder and drier. The distended rectum fails to sense the presence of the stool. When evacuation is attempted, the process is painful, leading to further retention (see Chapter 115).

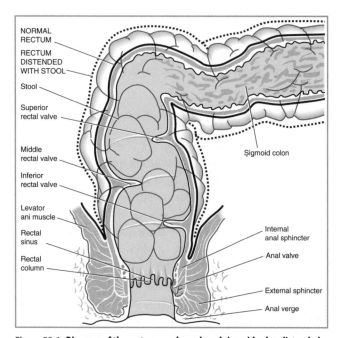

Figure 55-1. Diagram of the rectum, anal canal, and sigmoid colon distended with stool.

Encopresis has been associated with a short attention span and a high level of motor activity. Affected children are unable to sit on a toilet for more than a few minutes and do not adequately attend to the task of stool evacuation. As a result, they get off the toilet after the incomplete evacuation of only small amounts of stool. In some toddlers, constipation is related to the struggle of toilet training and an unwillingness to sit on the toilet (see Chapter 47).

The pathophysiology of non-retentive encopresis seems to be psychogenic. Some children who have been chronically sexually abused have lax anal tone, which may contribute to fecal incontinence. Animus, abnormal anal sphincter contraction, has been reported in up to 30% of children with constipation.

Differential Diagnosis

The differential diagnosis of encopresis focuses on organic conditions associated with chronic constipation. Organic conditions account for 5% to 10% of fecal incontinence. These conditions include congenital megacolon (Hirschsprung disease), disorders of intestinal motility (eg, pseudo-obstruction), disorders of anal tone and anal anatomy (eg, imperforate anus with fistula), disorders of the lumbosacral spine (eg, meningomyelocele), and previous surgeries (eg, repair of imperforate anus). Neurofibromatosis, lead poisoning, and hypothyroidism are also associated with constipation. Congenital anorectal anomalies, which are reported in 1 in 5,000 live births, are rare.

Most of these conditions can be ruled out on the basis of a careful history and physical examination. In some cases, specific testing, such as anal manometry or rectal biopsy, may be necessary to exclude a particular disorder.

Evaluation

History

The age of onset of the problem, as well as the age of initiation of toilet training, should be determined. In general, affected children are 4 years and older. A detailed history of the stooling pattern should be obtained as well as a dietary history (Questions Box). The frequency and consistency of stools as well as quantity of stools should also be noted. In addition, the presence of nocturnal episodes of fecal incontinence should be determined. In cases of secondary encopresis, the duration of fecal continence and the occurrence of any events, such as the birth of a sibling or the start of school, that may have precipitated the episodes of encopresis should be noted. Some children experience the onset of encopresis when they start school. Because of "toilet phobia," they are unwilling to use the public toilet in the school setting.

Physical Examination

The next step involves the performance of a comprehensive physical examination, paying particular attention to the abdomen to check for the presence of distended, stool-filled loops of bowel. The rectal area should be assessed for rectal tone, an anal wink, and the

Questions

Encopresis

- At what age was the child toilet trained?
- Does the child have spontaneous bowel movements (without enemas or suppositories)? If so, how frequently?
- Does the child have large, dry, hard stools that clog the toilet?
- Does the child pass blood with the stool?
- Did the child pass meconium within the first 24 hours after birth?
- Has the child had any surgery in the anogenital area, spine, or bowel?
- Is the child taking any medications, such as aspirin, iron, methylphenidate, imipramine, calcium channel blockers, or anticholinergics?
- Does the child seem to resist the urge to defecate (eg, squeezes legs together and rocks back and forth)?
- Does the child have a history of enuresis or attention-deficit/hyperactivity disorder?
- What is the pattern of encopresis (ie, is the encopresis primary or secondary)?
- When and where does the child soil (eg, nocturnal, at home)?
- Have there been changes or stresses in the home or family?
- What happens to the child's stained underwear?
- What has the family done to manage the problem?
- What is the child's diet? How much milk does the child drink? Does the child eat fruits and vegetables?

presence of hard stool. To elicit an anal wink, the skin adjacent to the anus should be stroked using a cotton swab. Children with a patulous anus may have a neurologic disorder and should have a thorough neurologic examination. Rectal prolapse, if present, may be indicative of chronic constipation or another condition, such as cystic fibrosis. Perianal fissures may reflect passage of large, hard stools. Hemorrhoids are unusual in children and can indicate chronic constipation. Location of the anus should also be noted, and anterior displacement may suggest incomplete forms of imperforate anus. Children with retentive encopresis have normal or tight anal tone on rectal examination because they are frequently contracting their external anal sphincter to prevent the seepage of liquid stool.

Dysmorphic features should be noted and may suggest a syndrome in which constipation is a feature. Abnormalities around the anus, such as fistulas, should also be noted. Fistulas are found in Crohn disease. The underpants should be evaluated for the presence of stool, mucus, or pus. A sensory and motor examination of the lower extremities helps determine if any signs of spinal cord dysfunction are evident. An evaluation of the skin over the spinal area may reveal abnormalities such as sacral dimples or tufts of hair.

Children who do not exhibit abdominal distention may have soft stool on rectal examination, which indicates non-retentive encopresis. If patulous anal tone is noted, spinal cord abnormalities or prior child sexual abuse should be suspected.

Laboratory Tests

Most children with encopresis require few laboratory studies. Studies focus on eliminating organic causes of encopresis, such as congenital

megacolon (Hirschsprung disease) or spinal cord anomalies. Urinalysis and urine culture are recommended in children with fecal impactions to exclude urinary tract infection. Encopresis is reported to be an independent risk factor for urinary tract infections. Thyroid function studies, a lead level, and a serum calcium level have been suggested, particularly in children with refractory constipation. Anorectal manometry, which may be used to measure the pressure generated by the anal sphincter, may also reveal abnormalities of anal tone or evidence of aganglionosis. The Child Behavior Checklist is useful to determine if certain behavior problems exist. Such problems may potentiate the encopresis or result from it.

Imaging Studies

In most encopretic children, imaging studies are not necessary. If radiographs of the abdomen are taken in children with retentive encopresis, distended, stool-filled bowel may be noted. A contrast enema with barium or a hydrosoluble substance is useful if congenital megacolon (Hirschsprung disease) or an anorectal malformation is suspected. Strictures, which may occur following necrotizing enterocolitis, will also be detected. Electromyogram to determine whether the innervation of the external anal sphincter is intact is recommended for children with encopresis who fail to respond to routine treatment.

Management

The management of encopresis focuses on complete rectal evacuation and patient and parent education and counseling. Regaining muscle tone of the anal canal usually requires 2 to 6 months. Children with anorectal malformations or prior gastrointestinal tract surgery may require additional surgical procedures to help them achieve fecal continence.

Rectal evacuation requires **pharmacologic management** to ensure an adequate cleaning out of retained stools. The decision about which laxatives to use depends on the degree of constipation. If the degree of fecal retention is mild, a high-fiber diet and stool-bulking agents or oral laxatives, such as senna derivatives, bisacodyl, or lactulose syrup, may be used in association with stool softeners or lubricants, such as mineral oil. The amount of mineral oil may be titrated up to ensure success. Some practitioners recommend that mineral oil be given until it oozes from the rectum. The amount may then be titrated back to a lower level. Magnesium sulfate is also recommended to relieve constipation. Magnesium citrate can be used but should be administered cautiously and with the admonition to drink plenty of fluids to prevent dehydration. Polyethylene glycol 3350 has a very high success rate in the management of constipation and encopresis.

If the degree of retention is more severe, suppositories or enemas may be needed. Occasionally, children have to undergo manual disimpaction. Alternative methods to manual disimpaction include 2 to 3 sodium phosphate enemas over 1 to 2 days or 8 oz of mineral oil a day for 4 days. Pulsed irrigation–enhanced evacuation involves the insertion of a rectal tube and the installation of pulses of warm irrigating solution, simultaneously draining rectal contents. If these modalities are not successful, children may need to be admitted to the hospital for oral lavage using polyethylene glycol-electrolyte solution at 30 to 40 mL/kg/hour until successful evacuation has occurred. This procedure often requires insertion of a nasogastric tube and 6 to 8 hours of treatment. Once the fecal accumulation has been relieved, every effort should be made to keep children regular. This can be accomplished with the combined use of toilet retraining, stool softeners or laxatives, and enemas or suppositories. Prokinetic agents such as metoclopramide may also be used.

Dietary manipulation is important to ensure sustained regular stooling. Parents should be told that children require a high-fiber diet with fruit juices, such as pear or peach juice, and decreased milk (≤16 oz/day). It has been suggested that a "team and coach" approach is the most successful route and that bowel training be likened to fitness training.

The toilet retraining process, sometimes referred to as enhanced toilet training, requires that children sit on the toilet at least 2 or 3 times a day, usually after meals, for about 10 minutes or until they have had a bowel movement. Some practitioners recommend the use of an egg timer to ensure that children spend the appropriate amount of time on the toilet. Children should be requested to maintain a diary of their evacuation, which may take the form of a star chart. Stars or other rewards are given for successful bowel movements in the toilet.

If children skip a day between bowel movements, they may be treated with a suppository, such as a glycerin or bisacodyl suppository. If they still have not succeeded in having a bowel movement, an enema may be appropriate. This sequence should be maintained until children are having bowel movements in the toilet and not soiling for at least 1 month. In general, stool softeners are required for at least 3 to 6 months. The regimen may have to be modified, particularly in younger children.

Behavior modification and biofeedback, such as using external anal sphincter electromyography, are 2 other modalities that can be used to help manage encopresis. Consultation with specialists such as pediatric gastroenterologists may be required.

Thirty percent of children with encopresis may need psychologic consultation. Psychologic intervention in the form of interactive parent-child family guidance has been reported as successful when standard gastroenterologic intervention has failed. Children with evidence of child sexual abuse or non-retentive encopresis should be referred to a psychologist early in the course of therapy. The underlying psychosocial problems of children with non-retentive encopresis must be adequately addressed before their condition can improve.

Prognosis

The prognosis for children with retentive encopresis is reportedly good with appropriate intervention. In one study, children who were able to defecate a rectal balloon filled with 100 mL of water within 5 minutes were twice as likely to recover from constipation and encopresis. It is estimated that about 30% to 50% of affected children experience long-lasting remission after 1 year and up to 75% are in remission by 5 years.

The prognosis for children with non-retentive encopresis is less predictable and highly dependent on the underlying psychopathology.

CASE RESOLUTION

In the case study, the boy exhibits typical manifestations of retentive encopresis. His condition should be managed with the use of laxatives, stool softeners, and toilet retraining with a star chart. The possible attention-deficit/hyperactivity disorder should be addressed separately but may be contributing to his inability to attend to the task of toileting.

Selected References

Borowitz SM, Cox DJ, Sutphen JL, Kovatchev B. Treatment of childhood encopresis: a randomized trial comparing three treatment protocols. *J Pediatr Gastroenterol Nutr.* 2002;34(4):378–384

Burket RC, Cox DJ, Tam AP, et al. Does "stubbornness" have a role in pediatric constipation? *J Dev Behav Pediatr.* 2006;27(2):106–111

Fishman L, Rappaport L, Cousineau D, Nurko S. Early constipation and toilet training in children with encopresis. *J Pediatr Gastroenterol Nutr.* 2002;34(4): 385–388

Fishman L, Rappaport L, Schonwald A, Nurko S. Trends in referral to a single encopresis clinic over 20 years. *Pediatrics.* 2003;111(5 Pt 1):e604–e607

Har AF, Croffie JM. Encopresis. *Pediatr Rev.* 2010;31(9):368–374

Levitt MA, Peña A. Pediatric fecal incontinence: a surgeon's perspective. *Pediatr Rev.* 2010;31(3):91–101

Loening-Baucke V. Encopresis. *Curr Opin Pediatr.* 2002;14(5):570–575

Loening-Baucke V. Functional fecal retention with encopresis in childhood. *J Pediatr Gastroenterol Nutr.* 2004;38(1):79–84

Pashankar DS, Bishop WP, Loening-Baucke V. Long-term efficacy of polyethylene glycol 3350 for the treatment of chronic constipation in children with and without encopresis. *Clin Pediatr (Phila).* 2003;42(9):815–819

Peeters B, Noens I, Philips EM, Kuppens S, Benninga MA. Autism spectrum disorders in children with functional defecation disorders. *J Pediatr.* 2013;163(3): 873–878

Reid H, Bahar RJ. Treatment of encopresis and chronic constipation in young children: clinical results from interactive parent-child guidance. *Clin Pediatr (Phila).* 2006;45(2):157–164

Setty R, Wershil BK. In brief: fecal overflow incontinence. *Pediatr Rev.* 2006;27(8):e54–e55

Acute and Emergent Problems

CHAPTER 56

Fever and Bacteremia

Eric R. Schmitt, MD, MPH

CASE STUDY

An 8-month-old girl is brought to the emergency department with a 2-day history of fever and increased fussiness. She is irritable but consolable by parents. Her parents believe that her immunizations are up-to-date, but they do not have the immunization record with them. On examination, she has a rectal temperature of 39.5°C (103.1°F). The rest of the physical examination is within normal limits, and no source for the fever is apparent.

Questions

1. What are the serious bacterial infections in febrile newborns and infants?
2. What has been the effect of conjugated vaccines against *Haemophilus influenzae* and *Streptococcus pneumoniae* on the incidence of bacteremia and meningitis in febrile newborns and infants?
3. What are the challenges in differentiating between serious and benign febrile illnesses in young children?
4. What diagnostic studies are recommended in the evaluation of febrile newborns, infants, and children?
5. When are empiric antibiotics indicated and when should febrile newborns and infants be hospitalized?

Fever is one of the most common chief complaints among pediatric patients seeking medical attention in physician offices, urgent care centers, and emergency departments and accounts for up to 20% to 30% of these visits. Most of these patients will have a benign, self-limited viral illness. Some patients, however, will have a **serious bacterial infection** (SBI), defined as meningitis, urinary tract infection (UTI)/pyelonephritis, pneumonia, bacteremia, septic arthritis, osteomyelitis, cellulitis, or deep tissue infection. **Bacteremia** is a bacterial infection within the bloodstream; it is considered to be **occult** when there is no apparent source of infection after a thorough physical examination in an otherwise healthy-appearing child.

Epidemiology

Historically, management decisions concerning febrile children have been largely dictated by age. Children have been broken down into age-defined categories: newborns and infants younger than 90 days, infants and young children 3 to 36 months of age, and children older than 3 years. Febrile newborns and young infants (ie, <90 days) have higher rates of SBIs than older children and often represent a diagnostic challenge. They have relatively immature immune systems rendering them particularly susceptible to bacterial infections and have not yet received most of their immunizations. Furthermore, they often have limited responses in the face of bacterial infections and exhibit relatively nonspecific signs and symptoms. In addition, newborns and young infants have different bacterial pathogens that can cause these serious infections, including *Escherichia coli*; *Streptococcus agalactiae* (group B streptococci); less commonly, *Streptococcus pneumoniae*; and,

rarely, *Listeria monocytogenes* and other gram-negative organisms (Box 56-1). The overall prevalence of an SBI among febrile newborns and infants younger than 90 days with a temperature of 38.0°C (100.4°F) or higher is about 10%, with the rate approaching 20% in newborns younger than 28 days. Urinary tract infections are by far the most common source, with a smaller percentage having pneumonia, bacteremia, or meningitis. Recent studies have demonstrated that febrile newborns and young infants with diagnosed viral infections have lower rates of SBI than those without viral infections (4% vs 12%).

Box 56-1. Organisms Implicated in Serious Bacterial Infection/Occult Bacteremia in Children

Newborns and Infants Younger Than 3 Months
- *Escherichia coli*
- Group B streptococcus
- *Streptococcus pneumoniae*
- *Listeria monocytogenes*
- *Salmonella* species (infants >1 month)
- *Haemophilus influenzae* type b (Hib)[a] (infants >1 month)

Children Between 3 and 36 Months of Age
- *Streptococcus pneumoniae*
- *Neisseria meningitidis*
- *Salmonella* species
- *Staphylococcus aureus*
- Hib[a]

[a] Hib disease has been virtually eliminated with the routine use of Hib conjugate vaccines.

In these studies, none of the febrile newborns and young infants with viral infections by diagnostic testing had meningitis, but some did have UTIs and, rarely, bacteremia.

Febrile infants and children aged 3 to 36 months are at a higher risk for bacteremia than older children but less so than febrile newborns and young infants. The physical examination is more reliable in this age group than in newborns and younger infants, but there are still many patients whose examination will be normal without any localizing source of infection. These individuals may, in turn, have occult bacteremia. Vaccine development and widespread immunization programs have dramatically changed the epidemiology and clinical course of bacteremia among this age group within the United States over the last several decades. Prior to the introduction of the *Haemophilus influenzae* type b (Hib) and pneumococcal vaccines, the prevalence rates of bacteremia were around 3%. During this time, *Haemophilus* was considered the most significant organism causing bacteremia because of its invasiveness and ability to cause localized infection, particularly meningitis. In the mid-1980s, the Hib vaccine was introduced, which has now virtually eliminated this particularly invasive organism. In the post-Hib but pre-pneumococcal conjugate vaccine era, the rates of occult bacteremia ranged from 1.6% to 1.9% in children with a temperature of 39.0°C (102.1°F) or higher and no obvious source of infection. More than 90% of the cases of occult bacteremia in this age group were caused by *S pneumoniae*, with the remainder being caused by *Salmonella, Neisseria meningitides, Staphylococcus aureus,* and a few other rare organisms. Pneumococcus is not as virulent a microorganism as some other bacteria. Most cases of occult pneumococcal bacteremia resolved spontaneously without any intervention. If untreated, a small percentage (3%–5%) went on to develop pneumococcal meningitis, which has the most serious complication and fatality rate. In 2000, the heptavalent pneumococcal conjugate vaccine was licensed by the US Food and Drug Administration for use within the United States. This vaccine provided coverage against the 7 main serotypes of *S pneumoniae* responsible for approximately 80% of the cases of invasive pneumococcal disease in the United States and Canada at the time. Following the introduction of this vaccine, the rate of invasive pneumococcal disease (including bacteremia) and carriage for the serotypes covered by the vaccine dropped considerably. In addition, there was evidence suggestive of herd immunity in that there was a decline in invasive pneumococcal disease among older individuals who had not received the vaccine. Consequently, there has been a selective pressure that has increased the prevalence of invasive pneumococcal disease caused by strains not covered by the heptavalent vaccine, although the overall magnitude of this effect appears to be relatively small. In addition, other bacteria, such as *E coli, Salmonella,* and *S aureus,* appear to have increased in relative frequency as a source of bacteremia. In 2010, a new 13-valent pneumococcal conjugate vaccine (PCV13) was licensed and is manufactured in the same way as the heptavalent vaccine. This vaccine expanded coverage to include 6 different serotypes that have emerged with increasing frequency as a cause of invasive pneumococcal disease following the introduction of the heptavalent vaccine. The American Academy of Pediatrics and the Advisory Committee on Immunization Practices currently recommends the pneumococcal conjugate vaccine for all infants in a 4-dose regimen to be given at 2, 4, 6, and 12 to 15 months of age. Continued surveillance of invasive disease will be necessary to ascertain what effect the changes in epidemiology of these newer vaccines may have on the diagnosis and management of bacteremia in young febrile children. Preliminary data have shown a 42% decrease overall in the incidence of invasive pneumococcal infection in 2011 after the implementation of routine PCV13 immunization and a 53% decrease in the incidence in children younger than 24 months compared with 2007–2009.

Clinical Presentation

In many febrile children, fever is the only complaint or manifestation of disease. These children may look fine and behave normally. Young children, especially newborns and infants younger than 3 months, have fewer and subtler behavioral signs with bacterial infections. Physicians must, therefore, maintain a high index of suspicion for the presence of an SBI even in the absence of localizing signs (D_x Box). Occult bacteremia, by definition, has no abnormal physical manifestations aside from fever.

Pathophysiology

Fever is an elevation in the thermoregulatory set point of the body. The thermoregulatory center is located in the preoptic region of the anterior hypothalamus, and an elevation in the hypothalamic set point above the normal body temperature initiates the physiological changes that lead to fever. Exogenous pyrogens (eg, bacteria, viruses, antigen-antibody complexes) stimulate host inflammatory cells (eg, macrophages, polymorphonuclear cells) to produce endogenous pyrogens (EPs). Interleukin 1 is currently regarded as the prototypical EP. Endogenous pyrogens cause the hypothalamic endothelium to increase intermediary substances, such as prostaglandins and neurotransmitters, which then act on the preoptic neurons of the anterior hypothalamus to produce an elevated set point. The body uses physiological mechanisms (eg, peripheral vasoconstriction, shivering) and behavioral actions (eg, bundling up, drinking hot tea) to increase body temperature to reach and maintain this higher set point, thus producing fever (Figure 56-1).

Dx | Serious Bacterial Illness

- Lethargy, irritability, or change in mental status
- Tachycardia disproportionate to the degree of temperature elevation
- Tachypnea or labored respirations
- Bulging or depressed anterior fontanelle
- Nuchal rigidity
- Petechiae
- Localized erythema, pain, or swelling
- Abdominal or flank pain
- Fever

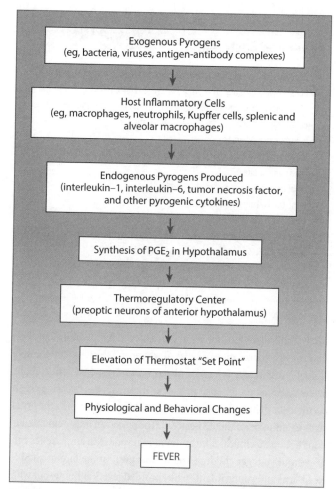

Figure 56-1. Pathophysiology of fever production. Antipyretics work by blocking the synthesis of prostaglandin E$_2$ (PGE$_2$).

Box 56-2. Risk Factors for Occult Bacteremia

- Age 36 months or younger
- Temperature 39.5°C (103.1°F) or higher
- White blood cell count 15,000/μL or higher or 5,000/μL or lower
- Total band cells 1,500/μL or higher
- Erythrocyte sedimentation rate 30 mm/h or higher
- Underlying chronic disease (malignancy, immunodeficiency, sickle cell disease, malnutrition)
- Clinical appearance (irritability, lethargy, toxic appearance)

Box 56-3. Common Infectious Causes of an Acute Episode of Fever in Children

Upper Respiratory Tract
- Upper respiratory infection (common cold)
- Otitis media
- Sinusitis

Pulmonary
- Bronchiolitis
- Pneumonia

Oral Cavity
- Gingivostomatitis
- Pharyngitis
- Dental abscess

Gastrointestinal Tract
- Acute gastroenteritis (bacterial or viral)
- Appendicitis

Genitourinary Tract
- Urinary tract infection
- Pyelonephritis

Musculoskeletal
- Septic arthritis
- Osteomyelitis

Central Nervous System
- Meningitis

Miscellaneous (Including Noninfectious Causes)
- Bacteremia
- Immunization reaction
- Viral exanthems (eg, chickenpox, measles)
- Neoplasia
- Collagen vascular disease

In contrast, the thermoregulatory set point of the body is normal in hyperthermia. Due to abnormal physiological processes, heat gain exceeds heat loss, and the body temperature rises in spite of efforts to return to the control set point.

Differential Diagnosis

In most cases, the duration of fever in children is short, and signs and symptoms are localized. Fever without a source involves an acute episode of fever that lasts 1 week or less in children in whom history, physical examination, and preliminary laboratory tests fail to reveal a source. Most affected children are eventually diagnosed with an acute, generally self-limited, infectious illness. Occult bacteremia has been a major concern in young children, primarily in infants younger than 36 months. High-risk factors for occult bacteremia are presented in Box 56-2. Fever of unknown origin (FUO) is fever of at least 8 days' duration in infants or children in whom routine history, physical examination, and laboratory assessment fail to reveal a source.

The differential diagnosis of children with an acute febrile illness is primarily infectious (Box 56-3), including benign and generally self-limited illnesses (eg, upper respiratory infections) and less common but more serious illnesses (eg, meningitis, osteomyelitis). Occasionally, a child with a fever without a source turns out to have a noninfectious illness such as collagen vascular disease or neoplasia. By comparison, the differential diagnosis of children with FUO is quite broad (Box 56-4) and contains infectious and noninfectious disorders.

Box 56-4. Common Causes of Fever of Unknown Origin in Children

Infectious Diseases

Bacterial

- Localized infection: mastoiditis, sinusitis, pneumonia, osteomyelitis, pyelonephritis, abscess (eg, abdominal, pelvic)
- Systemic disease: tuberculosis, brucellosis, salmonellosis, leptospirosis, tularemia

Viral

- Hepatitis viruses
- Cytomegalovirus
- Epstein-Barr virus (infectious mononucleosis)
- HIV

Fungal

- Disseminated coccidioidomycosis
- Disseminated histoplasmosis

Miscellaneous

- Malaria
- Rocky Mountain spotted fever
- Syphilis
- Lyme disease

Neoplasia

- Leukemia
- Lymphoma
- Hodgkin disease
- Neuroblastoma

Collagen Vascular Diseases

- Juvenile idiopathic arthritis
- Systemic lupus erythematosus
- Rheumatic fever

Miscellaneous

- Inflammatory bowel diseases
- Kawasaki disease
- Thyroiditis
- Drugs
- Factitious fever

Evaluation

History

The medical history can provide a great deal of valuable information in the evaluation of children with fever (Questions Box). The history should focus on the duration and severity of the fever. The presence of associated symptoms that may be signs of specific organ system involvement should also be noted.

Physical Examination

Rectal temperatures should be performed in all newborns, infants, and young children. An elevation in rectal temperature in a newborn or an infant should not be attributed to over-bundling. Vital signs in addition to temperature may provide important diagnostic clues.

Questions

Fever and Bacteremia

- How long has the child had fever? How high has the temperature been?
- Does the child have any other symptoms, such as rash, vomiting, diarrhea, abdominal pain, or dysuria; cough, rhinorrhea, or other respiratory symptoms; or lethargy, irritability, or change in mental status?
- Is anyone sick at home?
- Has the child's activity level changed (eg, more sleepy than usual) or is the child more irritable?
- What immunizations has the child received?
- Is the child taking any medications?
- Do any pets live in the house?
- Has there been any history of recent travel, especially outside the country?
- Has the child ever been hospitalized for an infectious illness?
- Does the child have any medical problems, especially asthma, sickle cell anemia, congenital heart disease, or immunodeficiency?

Tachycardia disproportionate to the degree of temperature elevation may suggest dehydration or sepsis. Tachypnea, which is often the only sign of a respiratory infection, also occurs in response to metabolic acidosis secondary to sepsis or shock. These changes may suggest an occult focus of infection. Response of the temperature and other vital signs to antipyretics should be noted. The physician must remain cautious because a clinical improvement in response to antipyretics can be seen in younger children and infants even in the face of an SBI. Newborns and young infants with recorded fevers at home, but who are afebrile on physician evaluation, should be managed as if they have a fever present. The report of a tactile fever without a recorded temperature is sensitive, but not specific, and therefore overestimates the true likelihood of a fever. However, in newborns and young infants in whom the risk of SBI is relatively high, the report of a tactile temperature should be taken seriously and these patients should be managed as if they had a documented fever.

Observation of the overall hydration and activity of newborns, infants, and children is extremely important. An attempt should be made to determine whether they are behaving and responding in an age-appropriate fashion. Physicians should look for eye contact, spontaneous motor movements, negative responses to adverse stimuli, and positive responses to pleasant stimuli.

All febrile children should receive a complete physical examination. This is important even when the history may suggest involvement of one organ system. For example, in young children, vomiting and fever may be the only signs of viral illness, or possibly a more serious infection, such as a UTI or central nervous system (CNS) infection. The underlying condition may go undiagnosed unless a thorough examination and diagnostic evaluation are performed.

The anterior fontanel should be palpated. It may be normal, bulging as a result of CNS infection, or depressed secondary to dehydration. The ears should be examined carefully and pneumatic otoscopy performed. Careful inspection may reveal otitis media as the source of fever, especially in children younger than 3 years. The occurrence of otitis media should not preclude further workup for invasive bacterial disease in children who do not appear well (see Chapter 75). The oropharynx should also be examined carefully. Dry mucous membranes may indicate dehydration. Enlarged, inflamed, or exudative tonsils may signal the presence of a viral infection or group A streptococcal infection in older children. Respiratory symptoms such as retractions, nasal flaring, grunting, stridor, rales, rhonchi, or wheezing may all be clues to respiratory tract infections. Enanthems on the buccal mucosa or exanthems on the skin are often signs of viral infections. The presence of petechiae in association with fever is usually benign but, in rare cases, may indicate a serious underlying infection such as meningococcemia. The capillary refill time, quality of peripheral pulses, and the general temperature of the extremities assess perfusion. Localized areas of pain, erythema, swelling, induration, or fluctuation may point to cellulitis, septic arthritis, osteomyelitis, or the presence of an abscess. Nuchal rigidity can be an important clue to the presence of meningitis. This clinical finding is rarely present in children younger than 15 to 18 months, and physicians must rely on other clinical factors and maintain an index of suspicion for meningitis in febrile children of this age.

Laboratory Tests

Newborns and Infants 90 Days or Younger

Because the physical examination alone cannot reliably identify an SBI in all febrile newborns and infants 90 days or younger with a temperature of 38.0°C (100.4°F) or higher, a thorough evaluation for a bacterial source of infection is required. This evaluation includes a complete blood cell count (CBC) with differential, urinalysis with microscopic evaluation, and blood and urine cultures. Cerebrospinal fluid (CSF) studies and cultures should be performed on all newborns and infants younger than 60 days and strongly considered between 60 to 90 days. Peripheral white blood cell (WBC) counts, while possibly helpful in older infants and children, do no reliably predict UTIs, bacteremia, or meningitis in febrile newborns and young infants. Decisions about whether to send blood and urine cultures or to perform a lumbar puncture should not be based on the screening peripheral WBC count in this age group. In addition, the standard urinalysis has a sensitivity of only around 85% in this age group and should not be used to determine the need for urine culture.

Rapid viral diagnostic techniques that can reliably identify several of the more common viral pathogens (eg, respiratory syncytial virus, influenza, adenovirus, parainfluenza) are becoming increasingly available. The presence of a positive viral test result, however, does not automatically preclude further diagnostic testing in this age group. Studies have identified a small but significant number of patients with UTIs who also happen to have a positive viral test result, and for this reason, urine culture should still be routinely obtained. However, the risk of bacteremia and meningitis is significantly decreased, and in well-appearing patients older than 1 month with a positive viral test result, further testing may not be indicated or cost effective.

If empiric antibiotics are to be administered, a lumbar puncture must be performed so as not to obscure the possibility of partially treated meningitis should pleocytosis be discovered on a subsequent CSF specimen. Stool analysis and culture should be reserved for those febrile newborns and young infants with diarrhea. Routine diagnostic radiographic studies (eg, chest) are not necessary and should be reserved for infants with respiratory symptoms or examination findings (eg, tachypnea, hypoxia, rales, wheezes, increased work of breathing).

Infants 3 to 36 Months

The diagnostic approach to older infants and young children has changed following the introduction of pneumococcal conjugate vaccines. Prior to widespread vaccine use, the standard of care involved an aggressive diagnostic approach looking for occult bacteremia in febrile children 3 to 24 months with temperature higher than 39.0°C (102.2°F) and in febrile children 2 to 3 years with temperature higher than 39.5°C (103.1°F) without any apparent source of infection. This historical approach included a screening CBC, blood cultures, and empirically treating infants and children with an elevated WBC count greater than 15,000/mm³ or an absolute neutrophil count (ANC) greater than 10,000/mm³ because they were at higher risk for occult bacteremia. The ANC was generally considered to be the best predictor of risk for occult bacteremia. More recently, other acute phase reactants, such as erythrocyte sedimentation rate, C-reactive protein, and procalcitonin, have been studied. These are all commonly elevated in serious infections but have not been shown to be reliably better predictors for occult bacteremia than the peripheral WBC count or ANC. Other laboratory tests, including antigen testing, serum cytokine measurements, and polymerase chain reaction, are not particularly useful because of their limited availability, relatively high false-positive rates, or cost. Currently, there is no single test that has been able to reliably identify all young febrile children with occult bacteremia.

With the declining prevalence of invasive pneumococcal disease post-licensure of the heptavalent conjugate vaccine and the further decrease with PCV13, the need for routine screening, culturing, and selective antibiotic use for occult bacteremia has been challenged. The peripheral WBC count is no longer as useful a screening tool in the face of such low rates of invasive disease. In addition, the rates of contaminated blood cultures are now much higher than actual cases of bacteremia, which often results in unnecessary additional testing, hospitalization, antibiotic administration, and family stress. *Infants and children who have received at least 2 doses of the vaccine can be safely managed without blood tests because this is no longer a cost-effective strategy.* Individuals who are at higher risk because they are unimmunized, whose vaccine status is uncertain, or who have received only 1 dose of the vaccine may need screening evaluation with CBC, blood, and urine cultures and expectant antibiotics if they are found to have an elevated WBC count or ANC. The increase in herd immunity and change in epidemiology of bacteremia following the widespread use of the pneumococcal vaccine may warrant reconsideration of this in the future following long-term surveillance of invasive disease.

Infants with temperature higher than 39.0°C (102.1°F) warrant urine testing, especially in girls younger than 2 years, uncircumcised boys younger than 12 months, and circumcised boys younger than 6 months. Chest radiograph should be considered in infants with significant respiratory symptoms or auscultatory findings suggestive of pneumonia. In infants with temperatures higher than 39.5°C (103.1°F) and WBC counts greater than 20,000/mm³, chest radiographs should also be obtained to detect occult pneumonias, reported in up to 25% of these patients, even in the absence of significant respiratory symptoms or auscultatory findings.

Children Older Than 3 Years

The laboratory evaluation of children older than 3 years is individualized and influenced by the history and physical examination; most patients do not need any testing. Healthy children in this age group are not at high risk for occult bacteremia. In addition, their physical examination is more reliable and they are better able to communicate their symptoms than younger children. Routine screening tests are not generally indicated in healthy individuals and should be reserved for those who look toxic or have an underlying disease that puts them at increased risk for bacterial infections (eg, sickle cell disease, cancer, immunodeficiency, nephrotic syndrome).

Imaging Studies

As noted previously, chest radiographs are the most common imaging study done in the routine evaluation of a newborn, infant, or child with fever and symptoms consistent with lower respiratory infection or with fever and no apparent source. Other imaging studies, such as bone scans, gallium scans, magnetic resonance imaging, and computed tomography scans, are indicated if there are suspected infections, such as an occult abscess or osteomyelitis, and if positive imaging findings will change patient management.

Management

Management of children with fever includes controlling the fever and treating the underlying process causing the fever. There is no evidence that fever itself is harmful. To the contrary, animal studies have suggested that fever may have some survival advantage. Despite the possible beneficial effects of fever, febrile children may still feel uncomfortable. Fever should be reduced to relieve the associated discomfort and malaise. **Antipyretics** such as acetaminophen and ibuprofen can be used. The use of both of these medications concurrently can lead to dosing errors; therefore, in most cases, families should be advised to use only a single medication. Aspirin should not be used for fever control in children because of the association with Reye syndrome and viral illnesses. **Sponging** or **bathing** with tepid water and **unbundling** children aid in fever reduction. Ice water or alcohol baths should be avoided.

All toxic-appearing febrile newborns, infants, and children, regardless of age, require hospitalization and administration of broad-spectrum antibiotics. Hospitalization and the initiation of empiric intravenous (IV) antibiotics are recommended for all febrile newborns 28 days or younger pending culture results. Ampicillin and gentamicin are the most commonly used initial antibiotics within this age group, but careful consideration must be made to resistance patterns and local practice within a particular region. With the onset of standard GBS surveillance during pregnancy and the use of intrapartum antibiotics, more gram-negative organisms and increased gentamicin resistance have been reported, necessitating the use of a third-generation cephalosporin, such as cefotaxime, for initial empiric coverage. Ceftriaxone is generally avoided in this age group, particularly among jaundiced newborns, because of its ability to displace bilirubin from albumin, thereby increasing the risk of kernicterus.

Well-appearing febrile infants aged 29 to 90 days may be managed as outpatients with antibiotics (ceftriaxone 50 mg/kg intravenously or intramuscularly) or close observation alone, provided they meet established low risk for SBI criteria (Box 56-5). For this approach to be safe, however, parents must be reliable and have means of communication and transportation in the event of a positive culture result, so that they can be notified to return the infant for reevaluation and possible admission. All febrile infants aged 29 to 90 days need very close follow-up, typically within 24 hours. Most pathogens will be isolated from cultures within the first 24 hours, and hospitalization with IV antibiotics is generally warranted for any young infant with a positive culture result consistent with a pathogen and not a contaminant. The addition of vancomycin must be considered if resistant pneumococcus is a possibility.

The management of well-appearing febrile infants and children between 3 to 36 months of age is based on the results of any diagnostic studies. Antibiotics should be administered for any bacterial infection identified. Those well-appearing infants who are tolerating oral fluids well and have no significant respiratory distress or hypoxia can be managed as outpatients, even if they have a UTI or pneumonia. Clinicians may administer a dose of ceftriaxone for the first 24 hours and transition to an oral antibiotic thereafter. Continued close follow-up is necessary, usually within 24 to 48 hours. Infants who have received one dose or less of the pneumococcal vaccine can receive a dose of ceftriaxone pending culture results if the WBC count is greater than 15,000/mm³ or the ANC is greater than 10,000/mm³.

Healthy and well-appearing febrile children older than 3 years can be managed as outpatients if they are well hydrated and have no

---

Box 56-5. Low-Risk Criteria for Serious Bacterial Infection in Young Febrile Infants

1. Well-appearing
2. No focal bacterial infection on examination
3. Previously healthy term infant with unremarkable neonatal course
4. White blood cell (WBC) count between 5,000 and 15,000/mm³
5. Absolute band cell count less than 1,500/mm³ or a band-to-neutrophil ratio of less than or equal to 0.2
6. Normal cerebrospinal fluid examination with less than 8 WBCs per high-power field and negative Gram stain
7. Normal urinalysis with less than 10 WBCs per high-power field
8. Stool studies with less than 5 WBCs per high-power field (if diarrhea present)
9. Normal chest radiograph (if respiratory signs/symptoms present)

respiratory distress or hypoxia. Children with underlying medical conditions or at risk for bacterial infections may need to be managed in the hospital with IV antibiotics regardless of age, depending on their individual circumstances.

Children with occult pneumococcal bacteremia who are afebrile and well-appearing at follow-up can probably continue to be managed as outpatients. Additional dosing of ceftriaxone may be necessary; transition to an oral antibiotic can be considered if sensitivity testing has been performed. Repeat blood cultures are probably not necessary if the child is afebrile, as the likelihood of persistent bacteremia is low. Those who are younger than 90 days, are still febrile at follow-up, or have clinically worsened warrant hospitalization and IV antibiotics. In addition, a lumbar puncture should be considered if not previously performed in a child with a positive blood culture. All individuals with occult *N meningitides* bacteremia warrant hospitalization and IV antibiotics. A lumbar puncture should also strongly be considered if not previously performed given the substantial risk for meningitis with this particular microorganism. In general, most other cases of occult bacteremia warrant hospitalization and IV antibiotics. Consultation with an infectious disease specialist may be indicated to determine appropriate antibiotic selection and duration of therapy.

Prognosis

Occult bacteremia may resolve without therapy and have no sequelae, but it may persist or produce localized infections such as meningitis or septic arthritis. In children with bacteremia who do not receive antimicrobial therapy, the risk of persistent bacteremia is approximately 20% and the risk of meningitis is about 5% to 10%. These risks vary depending on which organism is isolated from the blood. In general, the risk of developing serious sequelae is greater with bacteremia caused by *H influenzae* than *S pneumoniae* (25% vs 5%). Concern about SBI related to either of these organisms is now significantly diminished with the introduction of the conjugate vaccines.

Acknowledgment

Special thanks to Paul Bryan for his contributions to the previous edition of this chapter.

CASE RESOLUTION

The infant presented in the case study is irritable and has a high fever of unknown source. Her vaccine status is uncertain. Her physical examination fails to reveal a source of her infection. Because her fever is 39.5°C (103.1°F), she is irritable, and her immune status is uncertain, a complete laboratory assessment, including a lumbar puncture, should be performed. Management should be determined after all laboratory data are available. If laboratory assessment reveals a focus of infection, such as a urinary tract infection, she should be managed with antibiotics. If laboratory assessment fails to reveal a source for the fever and her white blood cell count is greater than 15,000/mm³ or her absolute neutrophil count is greater than 10,000/mm³, she can receive an intramuscular injection of ceftriaxone as expectant management for occult bacteremia and be reevaluated in 24 hours or be managed without antibiotics.

Selected References

Alpern ER, Alessandrini EA, McGowan KL, Bell LM, Shaw KN. Serotype prevalence of occult pneumococcal bacteremia. *Pediatrics.* 2001;108(2):e23

American College of Emergency Physicians Clinical Policies Committee and Clinical Policies Subcommittee on Pediatric Fever. Clinical policy for children younger than three years presenting to the emergency department with fever. *Ann Emerg Med.* 2003;42(4):530–545

Bachur RG, Harper MB. Predictive model for serious bacterial infections among infants younger than 3 months of age. *Pediatrics.* 2001;108(2):311–316

Baraff LJ. Management of infants and young children with fever without source. *Pediatr Ann.* 2008;37(10):673–679

Biondi E, Evans R, Mischler M, et al. Epidemiology of bacteremia in febrile infants in the United States. *Pediatrics.* 2013;132(6):990–996

Bonsu BK, Chb M, Harper MB. Identifying febrile young infants with bacteremia: is the peripheral white blood cell count an accurate screen? *Ann Emerg Med.* 2003;42(2):216–225

Brik R, Hamissah R, Shehada N, Berant M. Evaluation of febrile infants under 3 months of age: is routine lumbar puncture warranted? *Isr J Med Sci.* 1997;33(2): 93–97

Byington CL, Enriquez FR, Hoff C, et al. Serious bacterial infections in febrile infants 1 to 90 days old with and without viral infections. *Pediatrics.* 2004;113(6): 1662–1666

Centers for Disease Control and Prevention. Direct and indirect effects of routine vaccination of children with 7-valent pneumococcal conjugate vaccine on incidence of invasive pneumococcal disease—United States, 1998–2003. *MMWR Morb Mortal Wkly Rep.* 2005;54(36):893–897

Gajdos V, Foix L'Hélias L, Mollet-Boudjemline A, Perreaux F, Trioche P, Labrune P. Factors predicting serious bacterial infections in febrile infants less than three months old: multivariate analysis [in French]. *Arch Pediatr.* 2005;12(4): 397–403

Grijalva CG, Poehling KA, Nuorti JP, et al. National impact of universal childhood immunization with pneumococcal conjugate vaccine on outpatient medical care visits in the United States. *Pediatrics.* 2006;118(3):865–873

Huppler AR, Eickhoff JC, Wald ER. Performance of low-risk criteria in the evaluation of young infants with fever: review of the literature. *Pediatrics.* 2010;125(2): 228–233

Isaacman DJ, Burke BL. Utility of the serum C-reactive protein for detection of occult bacterial infection in children. *Arch Pediatr Adolesc Med.* 2002;156(9): 905–909

Isaacman DJ, Zhang Y, Reynolds EA, Ehrlich GD. Accuracy of a polymerase chain reaction–based assay for detection of pneumococcal bacteremia in children. *Pediatrics.* 1998;101(5):813–816

Joffe MD, Alpern ER. Occult pneumococcal bacteremia: a review. *Pediatr Emerg Care.* 2010;26(6):448–457

Kaplan RL, Harper MB, Baskin MN, Macone AB, Mandl KD. Time to detection of positive cultures in 28- to 90-day-old febrile infants. *Pediatrics.* 2000;106(6):e74

Kaplan SL, Barson WJ, Lin PL, et al. Early trends for invasive pneumococcal infections In children after the introduction of the 13-valent pneumococcal conjugate vaccine. *Pediatr Infect Dis J.* 2013;32(3):203–207

Kaplan SL, Mason EO Jr, Wald ER, et al. Decrease of invasive pneumococcal infections in children among 8 children's hospitals in the United States after the introduction of the 7-valent pneumococcal conjugate vaccine. *Pediatrics.* 2004;113(3 Pt 1):443–449

Krief WI, Levine DA, Platt SL, et al. Influenza virus infection and the risk of serious bacterial infections in young febrile infants. *Pediatrics*. 2009;124(1):30–39

Kuppermann N. Occult bacteremia in young febrile children. *Pediatr Clin North Am*. 1999;46(6):1073–1109

Lee GM, Fleisher GR, Harper MB. Management of febrile children in the age of the conjugate pneumococcal vaccine: a cost-effectiveness analysis. *Pediatrics*. 2001;108(4):835–844

Levine DA, Platt SL, Dayan PS, et al. Risk of serious bacterial infection in young febrile infants with respiratory syncytial virus infections. *Pediatrics*. 2004;113(6): 1728–1734

Manzano S, Bailey B, Gervaix A, Cousineau J, Delvin E, Girodias JB. Markers for bacterial infection in children with fever without source. *Arch Dis Child*. 2011; 96(5):440–446

Newman TB, Bernzweig JA, Takayama JI, Finch SA, Wasserman RC, Pantell RH. Urine testing and urinary tract infections in febrile infants seen in office settings: the Pediatric Research in Office Settings Febrile Infant Study. *Arch Pediatr Adolesc Med*. 2002;156(1):44–54

Nigrovic LE, Kuppermann N, Malley R; Bacterial Meningitis Study Group of the Pediatric Emergency Medicine Collaborative Research Committee of the American Academy of Pediatrics. Children with bacterial meningitis presenting to the emergency department during the pneumococcal conjugate vaccine era. *Acad Emerg Med*. 2008;15(6):522–528

Pulliam PN, Attia MW, Cronan KM. C-reactive protein in febrile children 1 to 36 months of age with clinically undetectable serious bacterial infection. *Pediatrics*. 2001;108(6):1275–1279

Rudinsky SL, Carstairs KL, Reardon JM, Simon LV, Riffenburgh RH, Tanen DA. Serious bacterial infections in febrile infants in the post-pneumococcal conjugate vaccine era. *Acad Emerg Med*. 2009;16(7):585–590

Singleton R, Hammitt L, Hennessy T, et al. The Alaska *Haemophilus influenzae* type b experience: lessons in controlling a vaccine-preventable disease. *Pediatrics*. 2006;118(2):e421–e429

Strait RT, Kelly KJ, Kurup VP. Tumor necrosis factor-alpha, interleukin-1 beta, and interleukin-6 levels in febrile, young children with and without occult bacteremia. *Pediatrics*. 1999;104(6):1321–1326

Wilkinson M, Bulloch B, Smith M. Prevalence of occult bacteremia in children aged 3 to 36 months presenting to the emergency department with fever in the postpneumococcal conjugate vaccine era. *Acad Emerg Med*. 2009;16(3): 220–225

CHAPTER 57

Emerging Infectious Diseases

Christian B. Ramers, MD, MPH, and Thomas R. Hawn, MD, PhD

CASE STUDY

A previously healthy 8-year-old boy is brought to his pediatrician's office in late August with 2 days of fever, fatigue, headache, myalgia, nausea, and gingival bleeding. On the morning of the visit his mother noted a rash on his legs. He lives with his family in the Northeastern United States but recently returned from a 1-week vacation in Key West, FL. He engaged in extensive outdoor activities, including snorkeling, hiking, and several evening boat trips, and sustained multiple mosquito bites during the trip. He received all routine childhood immunizations, denies any allergies, and takes no medications. No other family members are ill.

On physical examination, his temperature is 101.7°F (38.7°C) and he is generally ill-appearing. He has photophobia and mild meningism, and a petechial rash is noted on his trunk and lower extremities. Laboratory studies sent from the office reveal microscopic hematuria, leukopenia (white blood cell count 2.8), and thrombocytopenia (platelets 85,000).

Questions

1. What is an emerging or reemerging infection?
2. What pathogens are associated with emerging infections?
3. What are some common or emerging infectious diseases that may cause the clinical syndrome in the case scenario?
4. What types of exposures should be considered when assessing acute febrile illnesses such as that described in the case scenario?
5. How does recent travel influence the differential diagnosis?
6. What are appropriate steps in initial management?
7. What resources can a primary care physician access to help in making a diagnosis?
8. When do isolation and reporting procedures need to be considered?

Introduction

Emerging and *reemerging* infectious diseases are defined as those whose incidence in human populations has increased in the past 2 decades or threaten to do so in the near future. They may represent the resurgence of an ancient human scourge, a novel zoonosis that has broadened its host range, a common pathogen that has acquired a new antimicrobial resistance profile, or, in some cases, a previously unidentified or unknown microorganism. A startling diversity of organisms have met these criteria, including viral, fungal, parasitic, and bacterial pathogens. Likewise, a variety of factors have been implicated in the process of emergence or reemergence related to range and susceptibility of human hosts, evolution and antigenic shift of the pathogen, and ecologic and environmental changes, such as vector amplification or breakdown of public health measures. Although a select few of these emerging pathogens represent malicious propagation or bioterrorism, most appear spontaneously at ambulatory or emergency health facilities and are thus relevant to the practicing primary care physician. It has only been through astute clinical observation, targeted outbreak investigation, and a coordinated public health response that many emerging infectious diseases have been identified.

In this chapter we will review the factors involved in the emergence and reemergence of infectious diseases of public health significance, discuss several specific examples that are likely to be most relevant to pediatric practice, summarize regional and global outbreaks of emerging infectious diseases, and provide practical steps for the primary care physician to access local diagnostic and public health support.

Contributing Factors

The spectrum of infectious diseases has always changed and evolved along with societal and environmental changes. Literature supports the supposition that throughout human history, several general driving forces influence the emergence or reemergence of certain infectious diseases. The most important factors are human migration, environmental and ecologic changes, changing patterns of human host susceptibility and immunity, and more recently, the use and overuse of antimicrobial agents. Table 57-1 shows some of the mechanisms identified in recent emerging infectious diseases and provides illustrative examples from the United States and abroad. In reality, there are often many simultaneous contributing factors at play, and diseases may emerge or retreat within human populations without clear drivers. Common themes that lead to recognizable emergence events typically couple a vulnerable host population with a pathogen to which that population lacks immunity or prior exposure.

Table 57-1. Factors Contributing to Infectious Disease Emergence/Reemergence		
Contributing Factor	**Examples**	**Illustrative Pathogens**
Societal change	Economic impoverishment Population growth or migration Globalization of food distribution Urban decay	Cholera, malaria, salmonella
Advances in health care	New medical devices Organ transplantation Drugs causing immunosuppression Use of antimicrobial agents	Aspergillosis, cytomegalovirus, methicillin-resistant *Staphylococcus aureus*
Human behavior	Worldwide travel Injection drug use Sexual activity Outdoor recreation activities	HIV/AIDS, hepatitis C virus, histoplasmosis
Environmental changes	Deforestation/reforestation Flood/drought Global warming	*Cryptococcus gattii*, dengue, *Burkholderia pseudomallei*
Public health infrastructure and control	Reduction of prevention programs Inadequate surveillance Waning immunization rates	*Mycobacterium tuberculosis* (multidrug-resistant and extensively drug-resistant), measles, mumps, pertussis
Microbial adaptation and change	Antigenic drift/shift Changes in virulence factors Development of drug resistance	H1N1, H5N1, H7N9 influenza, chloroquine-resistant malaria, vancomycin-resistant enterococci

Adapted from Morens DM, Folkers GK, Fauci AS. The challenge of emerging and re-emerging infectious diseases. *Nature.* 2004;430(6996):242–249

Pediatric populations are particularly susceptible to emerging and reemerging diseases in several of these categories. After immunity from acquired maternal antibody wanes, children develop adaptive immunity on their own and may experience up to 12 upper respiratory or diarrheal diseases per year. In some cases an unexplained increase in pediatric mortality from a typical clinical syndrome, such as upper respiratory or flu-like illness, may be the harbinger of an emerging pathogen. Large institutional settings, such as child care centers and schools, place children at high risk for exposure to infectious agents via close contact, respiratory system, and droplet spread. Similarly, differing hygiene practices, such as hand washing, cough etiquette, sharing of fomites, and fecal or urinary incontinence, place infants and children at particular risk of exposure.

Antimicrobials are commonly prescribed in primary care settings for otitis media, pharyngitis, or respiratory infections, and overuse of antibiotics in these settings has been associated with a higher risk of colonization and infection with drug-resistant organisms. In many cases, what was once a first-line therapy for a particular clinical syndrome must be reconsidered due to the emergence of altered antibiotic susceptibility patterns. Advances in medical care have expanded the number of vulnerable hosts through increased survival of premature newborns, cancer chemotherapy, organ transplantation, and the use of immunosuppressive or immunomodulatory agents. Lastly, due to access, parental belief systems, or personal choice, immunization rates in certain regions remain suboptimal, placing children at risk of acquiring vaccine-preventable disease.

Special Situations

Increasingly, primary care physicians find themselves in settings that demand careful consideration of the risks of emerging or reemerging infectious diseases. Following is a collection of some unique clinical settings in which less common or emerging infectious diseases should warrant consideration:

Expanded International Travel

With increasing accessibility of long-distance international travel, children are more frequently being included in tourist trips or, in the case of immigrant families, visits to friends or relatives back in their home country. Children are less likely to seek pretravel advice and consequently less likely to adhere to recommended travel guidelines. A report from the GeoSentinel surveillance network, a large group of worldwide travel clinics, found that only 32% of children visiting friends and relatives in developing countries received recommended travel vaccines or prophylactic medications, yet they were more likely to present with illness and require hospital admission after travel. Primary care physicians evaluating returning travelers must consider detailed travel history, prophylaxis or protective measures taken (if any), risk profile of the region visited, and incubation period of the suspected pathogen. Although by far the most common travel-related illnesses are self-limited diarrheal disease, emerging infections, such as dengue, chikungunya, or H5N1, H7N9, or H1N1 influenza, must be considered along with other infectious diseases, such as malaria or tuberculosis.

Immigration and International Adoption

Increasing rates of international adoption or recent immigration may result in primary care physicians evaluating children with unknown or unavailable birth, early childhood, or immunization histories (see chapters 36 and 38). Vaccine schedules vary by country of origin, including some vaccines that are no longer given in the United States (eg, BCG, oral polio). There is a wide range of reliability among medical reporting in these situations, with some reaching or exceeding developed world standards but most providing dubious quality. Many physicians specializing in "adoption clinics" or working in settings with large immigrant populations obtain serologic evidence of prior immunization (eg, measles, mumps, varicella, polio, diphtheria, tetanus). Physicians must also be aware of infections with clinically silent latent phases (viral hepatitis, latent tuberculosis, intestinal helminth infections, even HIV). Several emerging or reemerging infectious diseases in the United States may be endemic in the countries of origin of adopted or recently arrived immigrant children.

Immune Suppression and Immunomodulation

Therapeutic advances in pediatric oncology, organ transplantation, rheumatology, and care of chronic congenital conditions have resulted in an increasing population of immunosuppressed children. Although typically under the care of specialists, these children may have a medical home in a primary care facility and thus can present with an opportunistic or emerging infectious disease to their primary care physician. The spectrum of risk for infectious diseases varies considerably depending on the type of immunosuppression. For example, tumor necrosis factor α-inhibitors, now commonly used in the treatment of juvenile idiopathic arthritis, convey a particularly high risk of fungal and mycobacterial infection. Neutropenia from cytotoxic chemotherapy is associated with an increased risk of bloodstream bacterial infection, among others. Similarly, lymphocytopenia related to solid organ transplantation portends a particular vulnerability to viral infections, ranging from widespread community respiratory viruses to reactivation of common agents such as varicella-zoster virus. Emerging infectious diseases such as new coronaviruses (eg, Middle East respiratory syndrome [MERS-CoV], severe acute respiratory syndrome [SARS]), human metapneumovirus, or H1N1 influenza may have particularly severe clinical manifestations in immunosuppressed children when compared with the general population.

Unvaccinated or Under-vaccinated Child

Despite the ongoing efforts of public health authorities, some regions have noted a worrisome downward trend in immunization rates. Although the most widely cited study linking autism spectrum disorders (ASDs) to measles, mumps, rubella (MMR) vaccination was retracted by the *Lancet* in February 2010, several recent parental surveys indicate persistent beliefs surrounding a suspected vaccine-ASD link. In 2004, the Institute of Medicine Immunization Safety Review Committee published a comprehensive report that found no convincing evidence of a causal link between the MMR vaccine or any thimerosal-containing vaccine and ASDs. However, in a survey of 1,552 parents conducted in 2009, 25% agreed with the statement, "Some vaccines cause autism in healthy children" (Freed et al). Decreasing vaccination rates have led to in increased risk for outbreaks of reemerging infectious diseases. In 2011, a total of 222 cases of measles were reported to the Centers for Disease Control and Prevention, occurring in 17 distinct outbreaks. The median age of these patients was 14 years, and 86% were unvaccinated or had unknown vaccination status. This compares with a median 60 cases reported annually every year from 2001 through 2011. Similarly, a 2010–2011 pertussis epidemic in California is the largest since 1955, affecting more than 9,000 individuals and causing 10 infant deaths. It is crucial for clinicians to include vaccination status and exposure history when evaluating children with an infectious syndrome. Increasingly, the differential diagnosis and diagnostic workup must include emerging and reemerging diseases, some of which may be unfamiliar to the physician from training or clinical experience.

Select Emerging Pathogens

Major emerging and reemerging infectious diseases (Figure 57-1) in the last 20 years are listed in Table 57-2. This table is not meant to be an exhaustive list but rather a sampling of emerging pathogens most likely to present to a primary care office.

Viruses

Measles

Caused by a virus from the *Paramyxoviridae* family, measles began to decline as a major threat in the United States after a safe and effective vaccine was developed in 1963. However, a significant resurgence occurred between 1989 and 1991, due largely to a pool of vulnerable unvaccinated preschoolers. Nearly 55,000 cases and 130 deaths occurred in the United States, prompting a renewed effort at prevention through vaccination. A second dose of vaccine for school-aged children was also recommended after this outbreak. Since 2004, there has been another resurgence of new cases but with new epidemiologic features; 90% of the cases were directly imported from travelers or immigrants or were associated with importation from outside the United States. Large outbreaks in the United States have been reported in 2008, 2011, and 2013, typically with most outbreaks originating from imported cases and affecting unvaccinated individuals. Of those sickened in the 2013 outbreak, 72% were 19 years or younger, and unvaccinated school-aged children compose a large pool of at-risk hosts.

Measles is known as a highly contagious pathogen passed via respiratory droplets. Secondary transmission is thought to be greater than 90% among susceptible household contacts. Roughly 10 days after exposure, clinical illness is characterized by a distinctive febrile

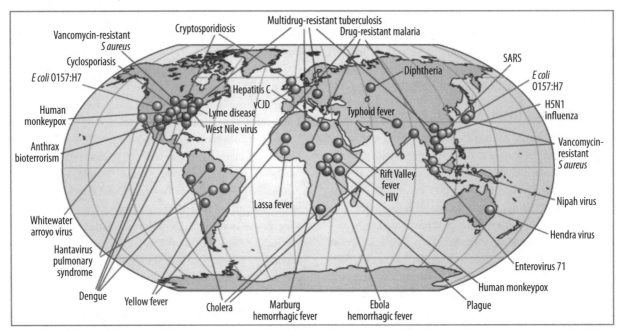

Figure 57-1. Global examples of recently emerging and reemerging infectious diseases. This figure does not demonstrate recently increased West Nile virus, methicillin-resistant *Staphylococcus aureus*, and measles. (Reprinted with permission from Fauci AS. Infectious diseases: considerations for the 21st century. *Clin Infect Dis*. 2001;32[5]:675–685.)

prodrome (conjunctivitis, coryza, cough), followed by Koplik spots (blue-gray enanthema on buccal mucosa) and, ultimately, the classic maculopapular erythematous eruption. Diagnosis is usually ascertained on clinical grounds alone given the distinct clinical presentation; however, for confirmatory testing, the immunoglobulin (Ig) M serology is nearly 100% sensitive if performed after the onset of rash. Respiratory droplet isolation should occur until 4 days following appearance of the rash in immunocompetent patients and until the clinical illness resolves in those who are immunocompromised. Treatment is largely supportive; however, respiratory and neurologic complications can occur in 6% and 0.1% of patients, respectively. Further control of this reemerging infectious disease will likely depend on renewed attention to domestic vaccination efforts and the rollout of vaccination worldwide.

Mumps

Although the clinical syndrome of the mumps virus is distinct from that of measles, the 2 members of the *Paramyxoviridae* family share a similar history of initial control and recent reemergence. A live, attenuated mumps vaccine was licensed in 1967 and incorporated into the Advisory Committee on Immunization Practices recommended schedule by 1977. Because of high vaccination rates, mumps had declined by more than 99% by 2005. However, there have been 2 major resurgences in the United States. In 2005–2006, a total of 6,584 cases were reported in a multistate outbreak in the midwestern United States. Although numerically most of these cases occurred among college students who had been previously vaccinated, attack rates were considerably higher in unvaccinated individuals. In 2009–2010, an outbreak involving more than 1,500 reported cases occurred in New York and New Jersey.

Clinical presentation of mumps typically involves fever, malaise, and parotitis. Complications are rare, but in some studies up to 10% of patients had aseptic meningitis, of which hearing loss is an important sequela. Up to 37% of adolescent and adult males can present with orchitis, which may result in sterility. Diagnosis is typically made based on a compatible clinical syndrome with confirmation by isolation or polymerase chain reaction (PCR)-based detection of the virus from saliva, cerebrospinal fluid, urine, or seminal fluid. Immunoglobulin M serology is also a useful confirmatory method.

Treatment is generally supportive, with analgesics used for the pain of parotitis or orchitis. For severe cases, intravenous Ig has been used to mitigate immune-mediated post-infectious complications, and interferon α-2b has been used to alleviate orchitis.

There has been much scrutiny of these outbreaks as indicators of vaccine effectiveness and community vaccination rates. Based on extensive analyses, MMR vaccine effectiveness is still considered 80% to 90% after 2 doses. This, however, leaves a significant portion of the population still vulnerable to sustain occasional outbreaks. No change was made to immunization schedules or interim recommendations after these outbreaks.

Dengue

Dengue virus is a member of the *Flaviviridae* family and is known to occur in 4 serotypes. It is transmitted via a vector, usually *Aedes aegypti*, and is present in more than 100 countries throughout the Americas, Asia, and Africa. Although historically confined to tropical and subtropical regions roughly overlapping with malarial zones, the range of dengue virus is expanding. In the United States, there were no cases of locally acquired dengue reported between 1946 and 1980. Since 1980, sporadic cases have been reported along the US-Mexico

Table 57-2. Sampling of Recent Emerging Infectious Diseases

Pathogen	Clinical Syndrome	Diagnosis	Management
Measles virus	Measles Pneumonia Post-infectious encephalitis	Clinical Confirm with IgM.	Supportive Consider antibiotics for bacterial superinfections.
Mumps virus	Parotitis Orchitis Encephalopathy	Serology Culture PCR	Supportive NSAIDs
Dengue virus	Unspecified febrile illness Dengue Hemorrhagic dengue	Serology	Supportive Aggressive fluid management
Influenza virus (H1N1, 2009; H5N1, 2007; H7N9, 2013)	Fever, respiratory symptoms	PCR or antigen	Oseltamivir, zanamivir, amantadine, rimantadine
Coronavirus (SARS, MERS-CoV)	Fever, respiratory symptoms	PCR	Supportive
Chikungunya virus	Febrile syndrome with arthralgia, rash, conjunctivitis	Clinical Confirm with serology, viral culture, or PCR.	Supportive, NSAIDs
WNV	Asymptomatic West Nile encephalitis (flaccid ascending paralysis)	Serology WNV antigen or PCR IgM in CSF	Supportive (Ribavirin and interferon α-2b are experimental.)
MRSA	Skin and soft tissue infections, bacteremia, pneumonia	Culture and susceptibility	Antibiotics
Resistant gram-negatives	Pneumonia, UTI, bacteremia, sepsis	Culture and susceptibility	Antibiotics
Resistant *Streptococcus pneumoniae*	Pneumonia, meningitis, otitis media	Culture and susceptibility	Antibiotics
Ehrlichiosis/anaplasmosis	Fever, headache, myalgia, rash	PCR or peripheral blood smear	Doxycycline
Cryptococcus gattii	Pneumonia, meningitis	Culture or cryptococcal antigen	Amphotericin, 5-FC, fluconazole

Abbreviations: 5-FC, 5-fluorocytosine; CSF, cerebrospinal fluid; Ig, immunoglobulin; MERS-CoV, Middle East respiratory syndrome–coronavirus; MRSA, methicillin-resistant *Staphylococcal aureus;* NSAID, nonsteroidal anti-inflammatory drug; PCR, polymerase chain reaction; SARS, severe acute respiratory syndrome; UTI, urinary tract infection; WNV, West Nile virus.

border, and in 2009–2010, a small outbreak of locally acquired dengue occurred in Key West, FL. The worldwide incidence of dengue has increased at least 4-fold in the past 3 decades for unclear reasons.

Clinical manifestations occur over a wide spectrum, from asymptomatic seroconversion to severe, even fatal disease. Headache and petechial rash are commonly seen. Classically, the disease is thought to occur in 3 forms: undifferentiated febrile illness, dengue, and hemorrhagic dengue. However, in reality, clinical manifestations are diverse and may include hepatitis, myocarditis, pericarditis, and encephalopathy. Leukopenia and thrombocytopenia are common laboratory findings and, in severe cases, coagulopathy and bleeding manifestations seem to be the most dangerous sequelae. Diagnosis can be made with a compatible clinical history and confirmed with serology. Unfortunately, there are no direct-acting antivirals, nor is a vaccine available. Care is generally supportive.

Influenza viruses

In 2009, a novel strain of influenza A known as H1N1 caused the first global influenza pandemic since 1968 with an estimated 59 million illnesses and 12,000 deaths in the United States alone. Although

early in the year it seemed that "bird flu" or H5N1 influenza would be the greatest concern to public health, it was a different strain of swine origin that led to a global pandemic. In April 2013, a different strain of bird flu known as H7N9 emerged in China with a disturbing 28% case fatality rate. However, like the related H5N1 strain, human-to-human transmission was not observed, and outbreaks have been limited to clusters of individuals with very high levels of exposure to poultry.

Influenza viruses have a segmented genome and thus are able to adapt and evolve quite rapidly to evade slower adaptive immune responses. Through antigenic drift, small changes occur in cell surface genes through time, resulting in subtle structural changes to cell surface proteins (neuraminidase and hemagglutinin) and less recognition by the immune system. In antigenic shift, genome segments from diverse strains recombine in a single new virus particle, creating abrupt and substantial changes in antigenic variation. Typically, shifts are more likely to cause pandemics because there are more nonimmune hosts in the population.

The clinical manifestations of H1N1 influenza seemed to be similar to prior influenza outbreaks; however, there were more severe cases and higher mortality in previously healthy young people than in typical influenza epidemics. Testing for H1N1 most commonly involves antigen-based PCR methods with variable sensitivities and specificities. Treatment for severe cases consists of oral oseltamivir or inhaled zanamivir. Although there have been reports of oseltamivir resistance outside the United States, this currently remains the drug of choice. Of note, the circulating H1N1 strains identified in 2009 were mostly resistant to older adamantanes (amantadine, rimantadine).

The more recently recognized H7N9 strain seems to be more virulent than H1N1, with a high proportion of patients presenting with severe pulmonary manifestations. In the preliminary reports of the first 111 patients in China, 77% were admitted to an intensive care unit and 28% died. Thus far, human-to-human spread of H7N9 has not been observed, and the outbreak appears to have died down after April 2013. Because of the ability of influenza virus to change rapidly with genetic drift and shift, health officials are on alert for any increase in H7N9 activity in the fall influenza season.

Chikungunya

A vector-borne disease transmitted primary by *Aedes* species mosquitoes, chikungunya was first described in Tanzania in 1953. It often occurs in epidemic outbreaks rather than steady endemic patterns and is most commonly seen in tropical Africa and Asia. More recently, outbreak ranges have expanded slightly, occurring in Italy and Madagascar. In 2006, there were an unprecedented 37 cases diagnosed in the United States; however, all of these were determined to be imported. The clinical hallmark of chikungunya is the presence of intense arthralgia and occasionally frank arthritis after a febrile illness with rash and conjunctivitis. Whereas the clinical illness of malaise and fever may last days to weeks, joint symptoms may last months to years. Other than the possibility of persistent and nagging arthralgia, severity is typically mild, and fatality is rare. Treatment of chikungunya is generally supportive, as there are no specific antivirals available.

Coronaviruses: Severe Acute Respiratory Syndrome and Middle East Respiratory Syndrome

From 2002 through 2004, an epidemic of severe pneumonia caused by a previously unrecognized coronavirus (SARS-CoV) caused considerable international concern due to its highly infectious nature and high mortality rate. Epidemiologic studies led to identification of palm civets as the main reservoir of transmission to humans from contact in the marketplace. Further studies suggested that horseshoe bats were the likely natural reservoir. The epidemic, which originated in China, eventually spread to 29 countries with an overall mortality rate of 9.6%, which included numerous health care workers. Clinical features included a mean incubation period of 4.6 days with a presentation of severe pneumonia with a high rate of respiratory failure. Additional clinical manifestations included watery diarrhea and hepatitis. Common laboratory features included lymphocytopenia,

neutropenia, and disseminated intravascular coagulation. The cornerstone of treatment was supportive care. Although many subjects received ribavirin, there was no proven role for it or any antiviral agents during the outbreak. Despite the impressive nature of this epidemic, it subsided rapidly and there has not been evidence of ongoing SARS-CoV transmission. This epidemic highlighted an agent with high transmissibility, morbidity, and mortality, yet only a transient global effect.

In 2012, a second emerging coronavirus was identified as the cause of a severe acute respiratory infection in a patient in Saudi Arabia. From 2012 to 2013, 130 cases were reported and all had direct or indirect travel or residence in 4 countries: Saudi Arabia, Qatar, Jordan, and the United Arab Emirates. The reservoir has not been conclusively established yet, although a zoonotic origin has been suggested because of the identification of related coronaviruses in bats and camels. Clinical features include an incubation period of 5.2 days with symptoms that range from none or mild to severe disease, including death in 45% of the reported cases. A large proportion of patients (96%) have underlying comorbidities, and 80% required ventilatory support.

Bacteria

Drug-Resistant Bacteria

Community-Acquired Methicillin-Resistant Staphylococcus aureus

Methicillin-resistant *Staphylococcus aureus* (MRSA) strains were recognized shortly after the introduction of methicillin in the 1960s and have been a substantive problem in health care settings for several decades. Hospital-acquired MRSA (HA-MRSA) has well-established risk factors, which include exposure in the health care setting (eg, hospital, nursing facility) and the presence of comorbid medical conditions (eg, malignancy, chronic liver or lung disease, indwelling catheters). In the 1990s, a new strain of community-acquired MRSA (CA-MRSA) appeared that was not associated with these traditional risk factors; it often was found in otherwise healthy individuals with no health care–related exposure. Furthermore, CA-MRSA carries the *mecA* resistance gene on a type 4 or 5 chromosomal cassette in contrast with HA-MRSA, which belongs to type 1 through 3. Community-acquired MRSA is also more likely to contain Panton-Valentine leukocidin genes, which may encode virulence factors that influence clinical symptoms. These genotypic differences have facilitated epidemiology studies that suggest that CA-MRSA is a distinct MRSA strain that has increased in frequency throughout the United States and is a bona fide emerging pathogen. In addition to genotypic differences, CA-MRSA is less likely to have a multidrug-resistant susceptibility pattern. Treatment of CA-MRSA follows similar principles to HA-MRSA with the exception that more antibiotic choices are generally available. For an uncomplicated cutaneous abscess, incision and drainage without antibiotics is often sufficient. For deeper or more severe infections, empiric treatment with trimethoprim-sulfamethoxazole, clindamycin, tetracycline (doxycycline or minocycline), or linezolid are options while awaiting antibiotic susceptibilities. Although linezolid is an effective drug, it is far more expensive than the other choices. Tetracycline should not be used in children younger than 8 years. For impetigo and other minor infections, topical mupirocin can be used.

Resistant Gram-negative Bacteria and Streptococcus pneumoniae

Similar to CA-MRSA, there are other resistant bacteria that have established significant niches. For example, *Streptococcus pneumoniae* was previously uniformly sensitive to penicillin. Currently, penicillin- and ceftriaxone-resistant strains of *S pneumoniae* are now common and circulating in the community. Similarly, a number of gram-negative bacteria, such as *Escherichia coli* and *Klebsiella pneumoniae*, are highly resistant because of a variety of plasmid and chromosomally encoded mechanisms, such as β-lactamases, cephalosporinases, carbapenamases, porins, and efflux pumps. These strains are mostly seen in the nosocomial setting, although community circulation of these strains has also occurred. Although the emergence of these strains is not as extensive or as clearly delineated as CA-MRSA, each of these strains has similarly "emerged" to a prevalence level in the population that substantially affects human health.

Ehrlichiosis and Anaplasmosis

Ehrlichia chaffeensis (agent of human monocytic ehrlichiosis) and *Anaplasma phagocytophilum* (agent of human granulocytic anaplasmosis), formerly human granulocytic ehrlichiosis, are examples of infections that emerged because of new diagnostic tests. Both infections were initially recognized as infections of the veterinary world until the application of molecular methods to humans with undiagnosed febrile illnesses. They have likely caused human disease for a long time, although the incidence may have increased with the recent resurgence of populations of some animal reservoirs, such as the white-tailed deer. In the early 1990s, *E chaffeensis* and *A phagocytophilum* were identified as human pathogens that are transmitted by ticks. *Ehrlichia chaffeensis* is transmitted by several ticks *(Amblyomma americanum, Dermacentor variabilis,* and *Ixodes pacificus)* and is found in the southeastern and south central United States as well as California. *Anaplasma phagocytophilum* is transmitted by *Ixodes scapularis* and is found in the northern United States. Both agents cause a febrile illness with headache, myalgia, and malaise that is often accompanied by thrombocytopenia, leukopenia, and transaminitis. Rash, which is found in 90% of subjects with Rocky Mountain spotted fever (caused by *Rickettsia rickettsii),* is less often found with HME (31%) and rarely with HGA. Diagnosis of these infections can be made by PCR and less commonly with direct microscopy because the latter methods are insensitive (<10% for HME and 25%–75% for HGA). However, due to the potential severity of the illness, empiric treatment should be initiated if clinical suspicion is high while awaiting the diagnostic workup. The drug of choice for treatment of HGA and HME is doxycycline. Because of a lack of reliable alternative drugs, doxycycline is also recommended for children younger than 8 years.

Fungi

Cryptococcus gattii

Cryptococcus gattii (formerly *Cryptococcus neoformans* var *gattii)* and *Cryptococcus neoformans* are yeast that cause pneumonia and central nervous system infections in hosts who are immunocompetent and immunocompromised. Although *C neoformans* is present in most regions of the world, *C gattii* has a restricted geographic distribution and previously had been identified in tropical and subtropical countries such as Australia, New Zealand, and Papua New Guinea. In the early 2000s, *C gattii* was identified as a cause of meningoencephalitis for the first time on Vancouver Island in British Columbia. From 1999 to 2007, 218 cases were reported with a case fatality rate of 8.7%. Subsequent studies identified its presence in the Pacific Northwest, including Washington and Oregon. Similar to many emerging pathogens, the increased numbers of cases may be caused by improved diagnostics and surveillance as opposed to the actual emergence of a new infection to a region. However, some molecular evidence suggests that the strain on Vancouver Island is novel. Clonal analysis suggests that it arose from an unusual type of sexual mating that generated a strain that is hypervirulent. This mechanism of emergence suggests that a species endemic to an original location (eg, tropics) can emerge in a new geographic region (Vancouver Island) in a clonal manner. The clinical presentation of *C gattii* is similar to *C neoformans,* although there may be an increased frequency of cryptococcoma in the lungs and central nervous system caused by *C gattii.* Treatment principles are the same for both species and include initial treatment with amphotericin B and 5-fluorocytosine for meningitis followed by consolidation therapy with fluconazole. For uncomplicated pulmonary disease, fluconazole is the cornerstone of treatment. *Cryptococcus* species, including *gattii,* infect children; treatment principles are similar to those for adults.

Summary

Contrary to myopic claims that public health would conquer infectious diseases in the 20th century, new pathogens have continued to emerge and old ones have reemerged time and time again, making for a challenging future of disease identification and control. The tools employed by public health include surveillance and response, yet most of the major epidemics identified in the last 20 years began with astute clinical observation at the primary care level. It is thus essential for primary care physicians and others caring for children to remain vigilant to the constant and unpredictable nature of emerging infectious diseases. With astute primary care clinicians, attentive scrutiny of new outbreaks, and collaboration with regional and national public health laboratories and officials, the medical field will hopefully keep pace with emerging and reemerging pathogens.

CASE RESOLUTION

The patient was hospitalized and underwent an extensive diagnostic workup for infectious causes of fever and rash. A lumbar puncture revealed a mild lymphocytic pleocytosis. He received 2 days of empiric antibiotic therapy, which was discontinued when cultures were negative for 48 hours. The pediatrician notified the local health department, which facilitated laboratory testing performed by the state public health laboratory, and the Centers for Disease Control and Prevention (CDC).

Serologic testing at the state health department was positive for immunoglobulin M antibodies against dengue virus. This was confirmed on samples sent to the CDC; in addition, cerebrospinal fluid sent to the CDC was positive by reverse-transcriptase polymerase chain reaction for dengue virus serotype 1. The patient recovered uneventfully over the following 2 weeks, but a public health investigation was launched that eventually resulted in the identification of 27 total cases of dengue acquired in Key West, FL. Subsequently, an adult serosurvey was conducted indicating recent exposure to dengue in 5.4% of adults.

This outbreak, which occurred in 2009–2010, represented the first reported cases of dengue acquired in Florida since 1934. Although dengue is the most common virus transmitted by mosquitoes in the world, no cases had been acquired in the continental United States between 1946 and 1980 and, subsequently, only sporadic cases were known along the Texas-Mexico border. Reported dengue cases have increased 4-fold in Latin America since 1980, and incidence has risen steadily among returning US travelers. Dengue represents a truly reemerging infectious disease and primary clinicians should be aware of its rising incidence.

Internet Resources

Centers for Disease Control and Prevention: home page, www.cdc.gov; dengue, www.cdc.gov/dengue; seasonal influenza, www.cdc.gov/flu/weekly

Selected References

Assiri A, Al-Tawfiq JA, Al-Rabeeah AA, et al. Epidemiological, demographic, and clinical characteristics of 47 cases of Middle East respiratory syndrome coronavirus disease from Saudi Arabia: a descriptive study. *Lancet Infect Dis.* 2013;13(9):752–761

Centers for Disease Control and Prevention. Addressing emerging infectious disease threats: a prevention strategy for the United States. Executive summary. *MMWR Recomm Rep.* 1994;43(RR-5):1–18

Centers for Disease Control and Prevention. Locally acquired dengue—Key West, Florida, 2009–2010. *MMWR Morb Mortal Wkly Rep.* 2010;59(19):577–581

Centers for Disease Control and Prevention. Measles—United States, January 1-August 24, 2013. *MMWR Morb Mortal Wkly Rep.* 2013;62(36):741–743

Centers for Disease Control and Prevention. Preventing emerging infectious diseases: a strategy for the 21st century. Overview of the updated CDC plan. *MMWR Recomm Rep.* 1998;47(RR-15):1–14

Centers for Disease Control and Prevention. Update: chikungunya fever diagnosed among international travelers—United States, 2006. *MMWR Morbtal Wkly Rep.* 2007;56(12):276–277

Centers for Disease Control and Prevention. Update: mumps outbreak—New York and New Jersey, June 2009-January 2010. *MMWR Morb Mortal Wkly Rep.* 2010;59(5):125–129

Centers for Disease Control and Prevention. Updated information on the epidemiology of Middle East respiratory syndrome coronavirus (MERS-CoV) infection and guidance for the public, clinicians, and public health authorities, 2012-2013. *MMWR Morb Mortal Wkly Rep.* 2013;62(38):793–796

Centers for Disease Control and Prevention, American Academy of Family Physicians, American Academy of Pediatrics. Diseases and the vaccines that prevent them: information for parents. Measles. http://www.cdc.gov/vaccines/vpd-vac/measles/downloads/PL-dis-measles-bw-office.pdf. Updated February 2013. Accessed January 30, 2014

Datta K, Bartlett KH, Baer R, et al. Spread of *Cryptococcus gattii* into Pacific Northwest Region of the United States. *Emerg Infect Dis.* 2009;15(8):1185–1191

David MZ, Daum RS. Community-associated methicillin-resistant *Staphylococcus aureus:* epidemiology and clinical consequences of an emerging epidemic. *Clin Microbiol Rev.* 2010;23(3):616–687

Feikin DR, Lezotte DC, Hamman RF, Salmon DA, Chen RT, Hoffman RE. Individual and community risks of measles and pertussis associated with personal exemptions to immunization. *JAMA.* 2000;284(24):3145–3150

Fraser JA, Giles SS, Wenink EC, et al. Same-sex mating and the origin of the Vancouver Island *Cryptococcus gattii* outbreak. *Nature.* 2005;437(7063):1360–1364

Freed GL, Clark SJ, Butchart AT, Singer DC, Davis MM. Parental vaccine safety concerns in 2009. *Pediatrics.* 2010;125(4):654–659

Gao HN, Lu HZ, Cao B, et al. Clinical findings in 111 cases of influenza A (H7N9) virus infection. *N Engl J Med.* 2013;368(24):2277–2285

Hagmann S, Neugebauer R, Schwartz E, et al. Illness in children after international travel: analysis from the GeoSentinel Surveillance Network. *Pediatrics.* 2010;125(5):e1072–e1080

Hui DS, Chan PK. Severe acute respiratory syndrome and coronavirus. *Infect Dis Clin North Am.* 2010;24(3):619–638

Hviid A, Rubin S, Mühlemann K. Mumps. *Lancet.* 2008;371(9616):932–944

Institute of Medicine Immunization Safety Review Committee. *Immunization Safety Review: Vaccines and Autism.* Washington, DC: National Academies Press; 2004. http://www.iom.edu/Reports/2004/Immunization-Safety-Review-Vaccines-and-Autism.aspx. Accessed January 30, 2014

Liu C, Bayer A, Cosgrove SE, et al. Clinical practice guidelines by the Infectious Diseases Society of America for the treatment of methicillin-resistant *Staphylococcus aureus* infections in adults and children. *Clin Infect Dis.* 2011;52(3):e18–e55

Morens DM, Folkers GK, Fauci AS. The challenge of emerging and re-emerging infectious diseases. *Nature.* 2004;430(6996):242–249

Morse S. Factors in the emergence of infectious diseases. *Emerg Infect Dis.* 2005;1(1):7–15

Perfect JR, Dismukes WE, Dromer F, et al. Clinical practice guidelines for the management of cryptococcal disease: 2010 update by the Infectious Diseases Society of America. *Clin Infect Dis.* 2010;50(3):291–322

Sabella C. Measles: not just a childhood rash. *Cleve Clin J Med.* 2010;77(3):207–213

Walker DH, Paddock CD, Dumler JS. Emerging and re-emerging tick-transmitted rickettsial and ehrlichial infections. *Med Clin North Am.* 2008;92(6):1345–1361

CHAPTER 58

Febrile Seizures

Kenneth R. Huff, MD

CASE STUDY

A 12-month-old girl is brought to the emergency department by paramedics because she is having a seizure. She is unresponsive and hypertonic, with arched trunk and extended arms and legs that are jerking rhythmically. Her eyes are open, but her gaze is directed upward. She has bubbles of saliva around her lips as well as circumoral cyanosis. Her vital signs are a respiratory rate of 60 breaths/min, heart rate of 125 beats/min, blood pressure of 130/78 mm Hg, and temperature of 105.8°F (41.0°C). An assessment of her respiratory status discloses that she is moving air in all lung fields, and there is no evidence of upper airway obstruction.

The paramedics inform you that the girl has been convulsing with varying intensity of tone and movements but remaining unresponsive for approximately 6 minutes. Glucometer testing reveals a normal serum glucose. Blood samples for other tests are sent to the laboratory, and urine is collected. An intravenous (IV) line is started, and the girl is given lorazepam by IV push. Within 2 minutes, the movements cease, and her respirations become slow and even. Her physical examination shows no signs of trauma. Her only abnormality other than her unresponsive mental status is an inflamed and bulging right tympanic membrane.

The girl's parents tell you that she has had a mildly stuffy nose for 2 days but has been afebrile and has seemed to be her usual self. While she was playing, she became cranky, and her parents put her in her crib for her nap. Thirty minutes later they heard grunting noises, found her in the midst of a seizure, and called the paramedics. The girl has never had a seizure before. Her father recalls that his mother once told him that he had several "fever seizures" as an infant.

Questions

1. What are the characteristics of simple febrile seizures?
2. What is the appropriate evaluation of children with febrile seizures, whether it is the first one or a recurrence?
3. What is the recurrence risk for febrile seizures and the risk of developing unprovoked seizures following a febrile seizure?
4. What are the treatment options for children with febrile seizures?

Febrile seizures are easily recognized, dramatic, generalized convulsions. These seizures are defined by the presence of a fever or an acute inflammatory illness (often sudden) from a source outside the nervous system; patient age of about 5 years or younger; absence of chronic brain pathology, including developmental delay; and absence of metabolic or structural abnormalities of the brain. Frequently, familial predisposition to similar seizures or a history of similar events in other family members is present. Despite the relatively uniform presentation of the seizure, genetic abnormalities in channels, neurotransmitter receptors, or hippocampal damage may influence prognosis, and individual clinical variables and social factors may play a part in the treatment.

Epidemiology

Febrile seizures occur in children between the ages of 6 months and approximately 5 years but are more common in those who are younger than 3 years. Some studies indicate that as many as 5% of all children experience at least one febrile seizure. The recurrence rate is 30% to 50% in children younger than 1 year but drops to 25% between 1 and 3 years and is only 12% after 3 years. Seizures usually occur with the rise in temperature and often so suddenly that the febrile illness is not recognized by the family prior to the seizure. Frequently, the febrile illness is eventually diagnosed as an upper respiratory tract or influenza infection or follows immunization. Human herpesvirus 6 infections may produce a somewhat higher incidence of complex febrile seizures. Febrile seizures are seen often in children who have a first-degree relative who experienced the problem at the same age.

Clinical Presentation

Simple febrile seizures are characterized by a single episode of generalized, symmetric, tonic posturing and clonic movements of a few minutes' duration that occur suddenly in children whose developmental progress is generally normal. Fever or an acute inflammatory illness is present, although it may not have been recognized before the seizure, and its source is outside the nervous system. A short time after the seizure (after usually 1–2 hours of postictal sleepiness), children become neurologically normal again (D$_x$ Box).

Recently described generalized epilepsy with febrile seizures plus (GEFS+) is characterized by the association of generalized febrile

Dx Febrile Seizures

- Sudden unresponsiveness, tonic posturing, and generalized rhythmic jerking
- Fever or acute inflammatory illness source outside nervous system
- Age 6 months to approximately 5 years
- Normal neurodevelopmental history

seizures beyond the age of 6 years and afebrile generalized convulsions, a positive family history of epilepsy with variable phenotypes, and a benign prognosis in most cases. The same families may have simple febrile seizures, febrile seizures beyond the age of 6 years, febrile seizures and absences, atonic or myoclonic seizures, and myoclonic-astatic epilepsy or Dravet syndrome.

Pathophysiology

The susceptibility of young children to febrile seizures may be related to an increased incidence of sudden high fevers in this age group, a developmental genetic factor that may lower the seizure threshold, or both. Animal models indicate that the immature brain has a lower seizure threshold than the adult, and seizures in the immature brain are more likely to occur by a different mechanism than those in the adult. A sudden increase in temperature to a sufficiently high level can provoke seizures regardless of age. Cultured neurons subjected to hyperthermia show epileptiform activity. Seizures occur more frequently with fever in many seizure-prone patients who have seizures of different etiologies, including genetic epilepsies. Perhaps circulating pyrogens or interleukins interact with a brain cellular circuitry mechanism or susceptible ion channels, causing hyper-synchronous depolarization and a seizure. The multigenerational familial history that is often seen suggests a dominantly expressed genetic transmission.

The precise definition of the genetic markers and mechanisms of generalized seizures in all cases are not yet fully understood. Recent work suggests possible mechanisms. Mutations in γ-aminobutyric acid (GABA) A receptor genes have been found to be associated with febrile seizures and GEFS+ pedigrees. GABA A receptors transmit inhibitory signals and are composed of combinations of 5 subunits. The γ-2 subunit is critical for receptor trafficking, clustering, and synaptic maintenance, and mutations in this subunit have been associated with febrile seizure families. It has also been found that the trafficking of mutant receptors with γ-2 subunit mutations was more highly temperature dependent than mutations of other subunits and impaired membrane insertion or accelerated receptor endocytosis when brief increases of 37°C to 40°C occurred. In families with these mutations, febrile seizures may be caused by a fever-induced change in the status of a dynamic membrane receptor system, producing reduced numbers of available GABA A receptors.

In other families with GEFS+, it has been found that mutations in the *SCN1A* sodium channel genes have occurred. Mutations in this same gene may occur in sequences that encode for the critical

"pore" region of the subunit protein that participates in ion selectivity and results in a more severe phenotype with early prolonged resistant seizures and later, a severe myoclonic epilepsy of infancy and intellectual disability, the Dravet syndrome. A less severe GEFS+ phenotype is associated with a less functionally critical position of the missense mutation in the *SCN1A* gene. A rat model of hyperthermic seizures has a comparable mutation and may provide additional pathophysiologic clues.

Differential Diagnosis

When a young child presents with a fever and a seizure, the possibility that the seizure is symptomatic of meningitis, encephalitis, or brain abscess must be considered, although other clinical signs are virtually always present. However, signs of meningeal irritation may not be reliable in infants younger than 12 months, and these and other signs of the illness may be obscured in the postictal period. If there is a history of lethargy or persistent vomiting; the seizure is focal in onset, prolonged, or multiple; or the postictal depression is prolonged, an examination of the cerebrospinal fluid (CSF) should be done. In addition, if the patient is deficient in *Haemophilus influenza* type b or *Streptococcus pneumoniae* immunizations or the patient has been pretreated with antibiotics, which could mask meningeal signs or symptoms, a CSF examination should be considered. It is rare that febrile seizures would cause CSF pleocytosis. The fever also could be provocative or coincidental to a seizure of different etiology, such as trauma, toxic ingestion, metabolic derangement, degenerative or neurocutaneous disorder, or stroke.

A useful concept for the physician caring for a child with a febrile seizure has been the differentiation of simple febrile seizures from complex febrile seizures (Table 58-1). A question that has prognostic implications is whether children in the appropriate age range have had a true febrile seizure or a seizure with fever, which may be an early fever-provoked episode of a nonfebrile seizure disorder. The factors defining a complex febrile seizure also predict an increased likelihood of later unprovoked nonfebrile seizures. A complex febrile seizure may be longer than 15 minutes. Most febrile seizures are shorter than 90 seconds, although a significant number present in status epilepticus. More than one febrile seizure during the same infectious illness or 24-hour period makes these recurrent seizures complex febrile seizures. The history of a focal or partial onset or the presence of postictal focal neurologic signs makes the febrile seizure

Table 58-1. Simple Versus Complex Febrile Seizures

Feature	Simple	Complex
Onset of clonic movements	Generalized	Focal
Length	<15 min (usually <90 s)	>15 min
Number of seizures per 24-h febrile illness	1	Recurrent
Neurodevelopmental history	Normal	Abnormal
Parent-sibling history of febrile seizure	Often positive	Often negative

complex. The presence of an abnormal neurodevelopmental history prior to the febrile seizure or abnormal neurologic examination or brain imaging study before or after the seizure also increases the likelihood of later unprovoked seizures.

Evaluation

History

After the seizure has been controlled and the child has been stabilized, a more detailed history relating to the circumstances of the seizure (the child's state leading up to the seizure; prenatal, birth, and developmental histories; and family seizure history) should be obtained (Questions Box).

Physical Examination

Children should be examined completely after stabilization, noting the possibility that the fever may be coincidental and signs from an unrelated cause inciting the seizure could be present. Physicians should look for bruises, fractures, retinal hemorrhages, or other signs of trauma. The presence of dysmorphic features, enlarged organs, or bony changes should be noted. The skin should be examined for abnormal, pigmented, or textured spots. Lateralized signs of tone or strength should be assessed. An appropriate examination to determine the etiology of the fever should also be performed (see Chapter 56).

Laboratory Tests

If the seizure is prolonged, focal, or multiple; if there is a history of lethargy, stupor, or persistent vomiting before the seizure; or if the patient still appears ill after the postictal period, cultures should be obtained and metabolic and toxicologic blood and urine studies sent. A lumbar puncture for CSF examination for meningitis or encephalitis should be done unless there are signs of increased intracranial pressure or a lateralized neurologic examination, in which case antibiotics should be given and an imaging study obtained prior to the lumbar puncture.

If the seizure is a simple febrile seizure, without history or signs of dehydration, blood tests are of low yield. Likewise, an electroencephalogram (EEG) has limited usefulness. The record is often abnormal in a nonspecific way and not helpful in predicting future simple febrile seizures or epilepsy. If the patient does not fully recover after the postictal period, the EEG may be useful to help define the nature of the encephalopathy.

Imaging Studies

Computed tomography and magnetic resonance imaging scans have a low yield of abnormal results in children with simple febrile seizures. However, children who have a persistently abnormal neurologic examination or signs of increased intracranial pressure, or who have had an abnormal neurodevelopmental history or a focal or partial onset to their seizure, should have an imaging study to detect a structural lesion that may be acute and the source of the present or chronic seizures and serve as a nidus for future seizures.

Management

If children are still convulsing on presentation and have been for at least 5 minutes, their condition should be managed as for status epilepticus (see Chapter 151). The airway must be secure, blood drawn and sent to the laboratory for testing, an intravenous line started, and lorazepam administered in the appropriate dose to stop the seizure.

If children are not in status epilepticus, management decisions are made on a more long-term basis (Box 58-1). Whether or not to recommend **anticonvulsant prophylaxis** for children who have experienced febrile seizures is controversial. Factors that must be considered include (1) the benign, age-limited nature of the condition; (2) the morbidity of the anticonvulsant treatment; (3) the chance of recurrence of febrile or nonfebrile seizures; (4) the risk of overmedication during an acute recurrence; and (5) the family's reaction and social disruption caused by the seizures. Given the combination of these factors, particularly the weight of the first two, many physicians do not recommend antiepileptic drug prophylaxis for febrile seizures.

Daily doses of phenobarbital or valproic acid are effective prophylactic anticonvulsants. The most commonly used regimen is daily phenobarbital, but its potential side effects include attention-deficit/hyperactivity disorder and depressed cognition and learning. Valproic acid can produce thrombocytopenia and may have the potential of provoking acute liver dysfunction in a patient younger than 2 years who is taking other medications. Fever control measures should be instituted to make the patient more comfortable but have not been found effective as prevention for seizures. Intermittent anticonvulsant

---

Questions

Febrile Seizures

- What were the child's symptoms for the few days before the seizure?
- Where was the child and what was he or she doing immediately before the seizure?
- Were there any pregnancy-related or perinatal complications?
- Has the child's development been normal or similar to that of siblings?
- Have any other family members had seizures of any kind, including during infancy?

Box 58-1. Treatment Options for Febrile Seizures

- Cooling measures during febrile illness (antipyretics or bathing in tepid water)
- Family reassurance and education
- Diazepam, 0.3 mg/kg orally or 5–10 mg rectal gel (Diastat) every 8 h (during febrile illness only)
- Phenobarbital, 3–5 mg/kg orally daily, for prophylaxis
- Valproic acid (divalproex), 30 mg/kg orally divided twice daily, for prophylaxis

therapy with diazepam has the advantage of reducing side effects but relies on recognizing the fever prior to the seizure and mandates greater vigilance for compliance during each fever. Because prolonged febrile seizures tend to recur as repeated prolonged seizures, this group may benefit by having rectal diazepam or intranasal midazolam to administer at home as an abortive drug to stop the seizure earlier in its course while paramedics are being called.

Recommendations for prophylactic anticonvulsant treatment are often individualized. Anticonvulsants are usually not recommended unless the child has presented in status epilepticus, has experienced marked respiratory compromise (perhaps needing ventilatory support) during the seizure, or has had complex febrile seizures. There is no definitive evidence yet that anticonvulsant prophylaxis for simple febrile seizures prevents the development of unprovoked seizures. Children who have had frequently recurring seizures that are extremely disruptive for the family and deleterious to parent-child interactions despite educational efforts by medical caregivers may also be candidates for prophylactic anticonvulsant treatment.

Prognosis

Febrile seizures are a common age-limited problem. The prognosis for children with simple febrile seizures is generally good; the incidence of seizure episodes later in life is 3 to 6 times higher than in the general population at the same age but is still low—2% to 3%. Those who have a complex presentation have a higher likelihood of developing a nonfebrile seizure disorder, but this risk is only 6% if 2 of the first 3 factors (see Table 58-1) are present or 17% if they are neurodevelopmentally abnormal. Overall, one-third of children with febrile seizures experience a recurrence. The risk of febrile seizure recurrence is most dependent on age: 50% of infants younger than 1 year at the time of their first seizure will have a recurrence, but only 20% of children older than 3 years will have a recurrence. Other factors that have a lesser influence on the recurrence risk include family history of seizures, temperature at the initial seizure, time since the previous seizure, and history of previous recurrences.

Animal models suggest that seizures, even status epilepticus episodes, in the immature brain are less often associated with neuronal death, but that seizures, particularly hyperthermic seizures, can modify brain development by altering cortical motor maps and the expression of ion channels and inhibitory receptor subunits regulating neuronal excitability; in addition, epileptogenic mechanisms may be more robust than in the adult. However, children with febrile convulsions have shown no difference in later academic progress or behavior compared with control children.

Among patients who had surgery for intractable temporal lobe epilepsy, mesial temporal sclerosis (MTS) was the most frequent pathology, and 30% of these patients had antecedents of prolonged complex febrile seizures compared with 6% in those who did not have MTS. It is possible that MTS is the etiologic consequence of a prolonged febrile seizure when the hippocampus is developmentally vulnerable. Mesial temporal sclerosis is frequently unilateral, and focal complex febrile seizures can actually originate in the temporal lobe in some children, suggesting causality. An alternative explanation is that some preexisting hippocampal malformation, genetic predisposition, or subsequent damage may be present in patients with hippocampal sclerosis and prolonged febrile seizures, and the complex febrile seizure is a collateral phenomenon.

A small percentage of infants with febrile seizures may develop Dravet syndrome, a phenotype influencing neuro-cognition as well as later resistant epilepsy, if they carry a particular channel subunit gene mutation.

CASE RESOLUTION

In the case history presented, the girl had a somewhat prolonged simple febrile seizure, a diagnosis supported by a family history positive for febrile seizures. Her family is educated about treatment options. They are comfortable with a decision to use intermittent therapy with oral diazepam for her subsequent febrile illnesses, realizing that a fever may not be recognized before the seizure occurs.

Selected References

American Academy of Pediatrics Subcommittee on Febrile Seizures. Febrile seizures: guideline for the neurodiagnostic evaluation of the child with a simple febrile seizure. *Pediatrics.* 2011;127(2):389–394

Baram TZ, Shinnar S, eds. *Febrile Seizures.* San Diego, CA: Academic Press; 2002

Cendes F. Febrile seizures and mesial temporal sclerosis. *Curr Opin Neurol.* 2004;17(2):161–164

Jensen FE. Pediatric epilepsy models. *Epilepsy Res.* 2006;68(1):28–31

Kanai K, Hirose S, Oguni H, et al. Effect of localization of missense mutations in SCN1A on epilepsy phenotype severity. *Neurology.* 2004;63(2):329–334

Kang JQ, Shen W, Macdonald RL. Why does fever trigger seizures? GABA-A receptor gamma2 subunit mutations associated with idiopathic generalized epilepsies have temperature-dependent trafficking deficiencies. *J Neurosci.* 2006;26(9):2590–2597

Korff CM, Nordli DR Jr. Epilepsy syndromes in infancy. *Pediatr Neurol.* 2006;34(4):253–263

Nelson KB, Ellenberg JH. *Febrile Seizures.* New York, NY: Raven Press; 1981

CHAPTER 59

Respiratory Distress

David B. Burbulys, MD

CASE STUDY

A 6-month-old boy has been coughing and breathing fast for the past day. This morning he refused feeding and has been irritable. On examination, the infant is fussy. He has an oxygen saturation of 92%, a respiratory rate of 60 breaths/min, a pulse of 140 beats/min, and a normal blood pressure and temperature. In addition, he has nasal flaring, intercostal and supraclavicular retractions, and occasional grunting.

Questions

1. What are the causes of respiratory distress in infants and children?
2. What are the signs and symptoms of respiratory distress in infants and children?
3. What are the signs and symptoms of impending respiratory failure in infants and children?
4. What are the critical interventions for infants and children in respiratory distress?

Respiratory distress and respiratory failure may cause significant morbidity and mortality in infants and children. The signs and symptoms of respiratory compromise may be subtle, particularly in small infants. Decompensation may occur rapidly if ventilation or oxygenation is inadequate but may be prevented by prompt recognition and treatment. **Respiratory distress** is defined as increased work of breathing, and it usually precedes respiratory failure. **Respiratory failure** occurs when ventilation or oxygenation is not sufficient to meet the metabolic demands of the tissues. Thus, oxygenation of the blood is inadequate or carbon dioxide is not eliminated. This may be caused by diseases of the airway, inadequate gas exchange in the lungs, or poor respiratory effort (Box 59-1). Respiratory failure may lead to cardiopulmonary arrest if not corrected promptly.

Epidemiology

Primary care physicians frequently care for children in respiratory distress in offices and emergency departments. Respiratory distress continues to be the most common reason for hospital admission. Such admissions usually involve young infants with acute infections such as bronchiolitis or croup. Reactive airway disease (asthma) accounts for respiratory distress–related admission commonly in older children.

Clinical Presentation

Increases in respiratory rate and work of breathing are the most common signs of respiratory disease. Effortless tachypnea may be a sign of respiratory compensation for metabolic acidosis rather than an indication of pulmonary pathology. Similarly, hypoxia that fails to improve with supplemental oxygen may suggest a primary cardiac lesion. Tachycardia is often present, although bradycardia, if present, may be an ominous sign of impending cardiopulmonary failure. Signs of poor oxygenation include alterations in mental status, head bobbing, and change in skin color. Pallor, mottling, and cyanosis are often late signs indicating respiratory failure and shock. Children who are severely hypoxemic may first appear dusky or pale. If children are anemic, cyanosis may not be evident, although oxygen saturation is low (Box 59-2).

Pathophysiology

The adequacy of respiration depends on effective gas exchange of carbon dioxide and oxygen and the ability to move an adequate volume of gas in and out of the airways. Infants and children generally breathe with minimal effort. In very young children, the **diaphragm** and abdominal musculature are primarily used for ventilation, and the tidal volume is approximately 6 to 8 mL/kg. If the tidal volume is decreased because of obstruction, children compensate by increasing the respiratory rate, thus attempting to maintain adequate **minute ventilation** (minute ventilation = rate × tidal volume). If the minute ventilation is still insufficient for adequate gas exchange or the child can no longer sustain the increased work of breathing, respiratory failure ensues. Respiratory failure may then lead to acidosis, myocardial dysfunction, and shock and may progress to complete cardiopulmonary arrest.

Box 59-1. Common Causes of Respiratory Distress in Infants and Children	
• Infection	• Submersion injuries
• Epiglottitis	• Pneumothorax or hemothorax
• Croup	• Pulmonary contusion
• Bronchiolitis	• Smoke inhalation
• Pneumonia	• Toxin exposure
• Reactive airway disease (asthma)	• Cardiac disease
• Foreign body aspiration	• Metabolic disease with acidosis
• Allergic reactions	• Neuromuscular disease
• Congenital anomalies	

Box 59-2. Respiratory Distress

• Increased respiratory rate	• Production of sounds with respiration (eg, gurgling, stridor, rhonchi, grunting)
• Changes in tidal volume or minute ventilation	
• Presence of retractions: intercostal, substernal, diaphragmatic, or supraclavicular	• Diaphoresis
	• Alterations in mental status
	• Poor feeding
• Nasal flaring	• Inability to speak in sentences
• Decreased or absent breath sounds	• Presence of pale or cyanotic skin
• Changes in inspiratory-expiratory ratio	• Presence of central cyanosis

Infants and children are more prone than adults to respiratory distress because of the differences between their respiratory systems (Box 59-3).

Differential Diagnosis

The differential diagnosis of children with respiratory distress can include abnormalities with the pulmonary, cardiovascular, or metabolic systems or be related to a reduction in the central nervous system drive. It is also important to make an initial differentiation between upper and lower airway disease based on the presence or absence of stridor, rhonchi, rales, or wheezes on examination. Many common causes are shown in Box 59-1.

Evaluation

History

A brief history should be taken (Questions Box) while physical examination proceeds and initial treatment is begun.

Box 59-3. Comparison of Respiratory Systems in Children and Adults

- The head in children is proportionally larger and has less muscular support.
- The tongue in children is larger in relation to the mouth, is poorly controlled, and can cause airway obstruction.
- The airway diameter is smaller in children and collapses easily. Reductions in size due to secretions or inflammation cause greater resistance to air flow (resistance is proportional to $1/radius^4$).
- The larynx is higher and more anterior in children and the epiglottis is floppy, which makes visualization of the vocal cords more difficult.
- The narrowest part of the airway in children is at the cricoid ring, unlike in adults, in whom the narrowest point is at the vocal cords.
- The trachea in children is short. In newborns it is 4 cm long; in 18-month-old infants, 7 cm long; and in adults, 12 cm long.
- The major muscle of respiration in children is the diaphragm. Any interference with diaphragmatic motion in young children impedes respiratory function. Intercostal muscles are immature in children and fatigue easily.
- Children have less pulmonary reserve and higher metabolic demands.
- Normal respiratory rates are higher in children and vary by age.

Questions

Respiratory Distress

- For how long has this problem been occurring? Has a similar problem ever occurred before?
- Did the problem begin while the child was eating or playing?
- Has the child had any recent infections?
- Are any members of the household ill?
- Is the child taking any medications?

Physical Examination

Before a complete assessment can proceed, critical interventions that may change children's clinical status should be made. Children should be placed in a position of comfort and oxygen should be applied. **Ventilation** and **oxygenation** should be assessed.

Respiratory and heart rates should be determined for a period of at least 30 seconds. In infants, abdominal excursions should be counted; in older children, chest excursions should be counted. **Respiratory rates** in children are higher than in adults; infants may breathe 40 times per minute, 1-year-olds 25 times per minute, and 10-year-olds 18 times per minute (Table 59-1). These rates vary with age and changes of activity, emotion, and illness. Abnormal respiratory rates are defined as being faster than normal (**tachypnea**), slower than normal (**bradypnea**), or absent (**apnea**). Neonates may exhibit **periodic breathing**, with periods of regular respirations alternating with irregular breathing. This is a normal variant for age. True apnea (cessation of respiration) is accompanied by change in skin color or tone or altered level of consciousness.

The depth of respiration should be noted. Whether breaths are deep, gasping, or shallow should be determined. Rapid, shallow respirations may not provide enough **inspiratory time** for adequate gas exchange. The heart rate may also reflect respiratory compromise. Breath sounds should first be listened to in the axillae and then at the bases and apices. The absence of breath sounds may be an ominous sign. Children's breath sounds are usually well transmitted across the thorax because of the thin chest wall. It is common to hear upper airway noises when auscultating the lungs.

Table 59-1. Vital Signs by Age

Age	Respiration (breaths/min)	Pulse (beats/min)	Systolic Blood Pressure (mm Hg)
Newborn	30–60	100–160	50–70
1–6 wk	30–60	100–160	70–95
6 mo	25–40	90–120	80–100
1 y	20–40	90–120	80–100
3 y	20–30	80–120	80–110
6 y	12–25	70–110	80–110
10 y	12–20	60–90	90–120

Abnormal sounds are caused by turbulent air passing through a narrowed airway. Resistance to flow through a hollow tube increases exponentially. Thus, the smaller the airway, the greater the resistance to flow generated by even small changes in the radius (as with, eg, edema, secretions, foreign bodies). The nature of the sounds produced depends on the location of the narrowing in the airway. **Gurgling, snoring,** and **stridor** come from the upper airway; **rales, rhonchi,** and **wheezing** from the lower airway. If no abnormal sounds are evident and breath sounds are absent or decreased, the upper or lower airways may be totally obstructed. **Grunting** is caused by turbulent air coming in contact with a partially closed glottis. Children who grunt are generating their own partial obstruction of the upper airway and positive end-expiratory pressure to increase oxygenation.

The physician should also observe the effort children expend in breathing. Increased work of breathing occurs when intercostal, subcostal, or supraclavicular **retractions** are present, the **accessory muscles** of respiration are used, breathing is abnormally noisy, or **nasal flaring** is seen. The normal work of breathing consumes 2% to 3% of total oxygen consumption. The increased work of breathing in children with severe respiratory distress can potentially increase total oxygen consumption to 50%. Increased work of breathing can also be manifested by feeding difficulties and diaphoresis in young infants.

In addition, the physician should observe the inspiratory-expiratory ratio while assessing the work of breathing. The ratio is approximately 1:1 in most patients. Prolonged expirations are most often seen with reactive airway disease.

Oxygen saturation should be measured by pulse oximetry in all children with respiratory complaints. Levels below 93% while awake indicate significant hypoxemia.

Laboratory Tests

Although the physical examination is the most important tool for assessing children in respiratory distress, laboratory tests such as complete and differential blood cell counts and blood cultures may help in the diagnosis of infection. It should be remembered that meningitis, sepsis, and metabolic derangement may present with effortless tachypnea not associated with increased work of breathing. Arterial or venous blood gases may be beneficial in this situation but, in general, should be reserved for patients in impending respiratory failure.

Peak expiratory flow or forced expiratory volume in 1-second determinations can be helpful in assessing compliant older children with reactive airway disease. Oxygen saturation measurements can also be helpful in these children because reduced levels (below 100%) often correlate with the severity of disease.

Imaging Studies

Chest radiographs can aid in assessing children in respiratory distress but should not be routinely performed in patients with known reactive airways disease unless children have a fever or are in status asthmaticus. A patient with significant respiratory distress should not be moved from a monitored setting to the radiology suite; rather, portable radiographs should be obtained, if needed.

Management

All infants or children in respiratory distress should be managed emergently. As stated earlier, in such situations, assessment and intervention often occur simultaneously. All children in respiratory distress should be reassessed frequently. The highest possible oxygen concentration should be delivered. Children who are able to maintain their own airway should never be forced to use an airway adjunct because this may cause increased anxiety and distress. Patients with clear airways can be maintained with simple interventions such as **oxygen** blown by the face or given by mask or nasal prongs. More advanced airway management such as bag-valve-mask ventilation or endotracheal intubation may be necessary for children who need assisted ventilation, airway protection, or hyperventilation.

Position

Children in respiratory distress who are alert and breathing spontaneously should be allowed to choose a **position of comfort.** Small infants who are incapable of positioning themselves are best placed upright with care taken not to flex or extend the neck. Children and their caregivers should be kept together to reduce anxiety.

The proper position for unconscious children is the "sniffing position," with the neck slightly flexed and the head extended to open the airway. This can be facilitated by placing a towel under the occiput of the head or shoulders. If simple positioning does not relieve an obstruction, the airway should be opened using the chin lift or jaw thrust. If spinal trauma is a possibility, only the jaw thrust should be used. If this fails, **airway adjuncts**, such as nasopharyngeal or oropharyngeal airways, can be placed to help prevent the soft tissue of the oropharynx from collapsing against the posterior pharyngeal wall.

Monitoring

All infants and children in respiratory distress should be carefully monitored. Pulse oximetry will assist the clinician in determining the degree of oxygen saturation, and, if available, a cardiac and respiratory monitor will provide constant readings of respirations and heart rate. Frequent assessments of the patient are critical to ensure a good outcome.

Oxygen Administration

Oxygen should be delivered by any method tolerated by children. **Nasal prongs** have 2 advantages: They are noninvasive and allow maintenance of a constant gas flow even when talking and eating. The concentration of oxygen delivered is limited, however, and irritation and drying of the mucous membranes may result.

Oxygen masks deliver a higher concentration of humidified oxygen. Disadvantages include obstruction of children's visual field, potential for carbon dioxide retention, and anxiety because the face is covered. Various types of masks are available.

The **simple mask** can deliver 30% to 60% oxygen concentration at flow rates of 6 to 10 L/min. Room air is drawn into the mask through the exhalation ports in the side of the mask.

A **non-rebreathing mask** has valves that allow only oxygen (85%–95%) to flow from the reservoir bag to the patient on inhalation and additional valves on the exhalation ports of the mask that prevent entrapment of room air (Figure 59-1).

The **face tent** is a soft plastic bucket shaped to the chin that is well tolerated by children. The face tent allows up to 40% oxygen to be delivered, and it has the advantage of allowing access to the face and mouth (Figure 59-2).

A **Venturi mask** is rarely used in children but has the advantage of precisely titrating the oxygen concentration to be delivered from 24% to 60%.

Children with potential respiratory failure require **assisted ventilation** with **bag-valve-mask** devices or **endotracheal intubation**. Masks of the proper size should be used. The upper edge of the mask should fit snugly over the bridge of the nose without touching the eyes. The lower edge should rest directly on or just above the mandible. An oropharyngeal airway should be inserted in unconscious children to prevent the tongue from obstructing the upper airway. An appropriately sized oropharyngeal airway should reach from the patient's earlobe to the corner of the mouth (Figure 59-3). A nasopharyngeal airway may be inserted if the patient has an intact gag reflex to achieve the same goal. Measure the nasopharyngeal airway from the child's earlobe to the tip of the nostril. If a bag-valve-mask is not available, assisted ventilation can be given with a **pocket mask** with a one-way valve. Oxygen can be attached to the mask at the side port (Figure 59-4). Endotracheal intubation is indicated in those children who require control of the airway, need airway protection, or require hyperventilation.

Figure 59-3. A, Oropharyngeal airways. B, Nasopharyngeal airways.

Figure 59-1. A non-rebreathing mask can deliver a high concentration of oxygen to a patient in respiratory distress.

Figure 59-4. A pocket mask with a one-way valve and side oxygen port that can be used for assisted ventilation in the office setting.

Figure 59-2. Use of a face tent.

Prognosis

Respiratory failure and resulting cardiopulmonary arrest are preventable in most infants and children if their condition is carefully assessed and appropriate critical interventions are made. Careful attention to ventilation and oxygenation of patients usually results in a good outcome.

CASE RESOLUTION

The fussy infant discussed in the case history has obvious signs of respiratory distress, including tachypnea, tachycardia, grunting, nasal flaring, and retractions. The differential diagnosis includes foreign body, infection such as croup or bronchiolitis, and reactive airway disease. It is important to place the infant in a position of comfort and provide supplemental oxygen before any diagnostic studies, such as chest radiograph, are performed. Appropriate treatment, such as albuterol, should be initiated while further evaluation proceeds. Pulse oximetry should be monitored. The clinical status of the infant should be reassessed periodically to prevent further deterioration.

Selected References

American Heart Association. Pediatric Advanced Life Support (PALS). http://www.heart.org/HEARTORG/CPRAndECC/HealthcareProviders/Pediatrics/Pediatric-Advanced-Life-Support-PALS_UCM_303705_Article.jsp. Accessed March 10, 2014

American Heart Association. Pediatric Emergency Assessment, Recognition and Stabilization (PEARS). http://www.heart.org/HEARTORG/CPRAndECC/HealthcareProviders/Pediatrics/Pediatric-Emergency-Assessment-Recognition-and-StabilizationPEARS_UCM_308135_Article.jsp. Accessed March 10, 2014

Berg MD, Schexnayder SM, Chameides L, et al. Part 13: pediatric basic life support: 2010 American Heart Association guidelines for cardiopulmonary resuscitation and emergency cardiovascular care. *Circulation*. 2010;122(18 Suppl 3):S862–S875

Choi J, Lee GL. Common pediatric respiratory emergencies. *Emerg Med Clin North Am*. 2012;30(2):529—563

CHAPTER 60

Stridor and Croup

David B. Burbulys, MD

CASE STUDY

A 2-year-old boy has been breathing noisily for 1 day. For the past 3 days he has had a "cold," with a runny nose, fever (temperature up to 100.4°F [38°C]), and slight cough. The cough has gradually become worse and now has a barking quality.

On examination, the child is sitting up and has a respiratory rate of 48 breaths/min with marked inspiratory stridor and an occasional barking cough. His other vital signs include an oxygen saturation of 95%, heart rate of 100 beats/min, and temperature of 101.2°F (38.4°C). He has intercostal retractions, his breath sounds are slightly decreased bilaterally, and his skin is pale. The remainder of the examination is normal.

Questions
1. What is stridor?
2. What are the common causes of stridor?
3. What is the pathophysiology of viral croup?
4. How are children with stridor managed?

Noisy breathing is a common symptom that often accompanies respiratory infections in children. The presence of **stridor,** a high-pitched crowing sound, often concerns children's caregivers. Some parents try home remedies to alleviate the symptoms, whereas many others immediately seek help in the office or emergency department setting. **Croup** is an inflammation of the larynx, trachea, and upper bronchioles (laryngotracheobronchitis) that causes noisy breathing and stridor. It is one of the most common causes of a seal-like barking cough and stridor in children.

Epidemiology

Croup most commonly affects children between 6 months and 3 years of age, generally in the fall or early winter. Children younger than 1 year make up 26% of cases. The condition is more common in boys than girls; two-thirds of all hospitalized children with croup are boys.

Stridor, which may be indicative of croup, may also be a sign of epiglottitis. The incidence of epiglottitis in children has dramatically decreased since 1988 following the development and widespread use of the vaccine against *Haemophilus influenzae* type b (Hib). Many young children may be incompletely immunized, and there are other bacteria that may cause epiglottitis; therefore, epiglottitis should still be considered in *toxic-appearing* children with *rapid onset* of symptoms of upper airway obstruction. Prior to Hib immunization, the ratio of cases of epiglottitis to croup was 1:100. Today, epiglottitis in children is exceedingly rare.

Pathophysiology

Stridor

Stridor is generally caused by obstruction of the airway between the nose and larger bronchi. Obstruction at the level of the nose or pharynx may produce snoring or gurgling sounds. Turbulence of airflow in the laryngeal area or upper trachea causes the high-pitched crowing sound characteristic of stridor. Edema and inflammation at the vocal cords and subglottic areas result in **inspiratory stridor,** whereas obstruction below the cricoid cartilage may lead to inspiratory and **expiratory stridor.**

Some of the more common causes of stridor are listed in Box 60-1.

The sounds produced at various levels of obstruction can give the primary care physician clues as to the etiology of the problem. The most common cause of stridor that begins shortly after birth is tracheomalacia, a condition secondary to the immaturity of the cartilage of the trachea. Laryngomalacia, which is caused by floppy supraglottic structures, resolves after several months.

The upper airway of infants and children is more susceptible to obstruction as a result of anatomic differences between children and adults. The tongues of children are relatively large and the epiglottis is floppy and shaped somewhat like the Greek letter omega (Ω). The angle between the epiglottis and glottis is more acute in children, which makes direct visualization of the airway more difficult. Cartilaginous structures are less rigid in infants. During inspiration, negative intraluminal pressure is generated below the level of obstruction, which leads to narrowing of the airway and turbulence of the airflow. This occurs more often in children because the tracheal rings are not well formed. In addition, the smaller size of the airway in children makes resistance to airflow greater when obstruction is present.

Box 60-1. Causes of Stridor	
Congenital Anomalies	*Trauma*
Tracheomalacia	Direct trauma to the upper airway
Laryngomalacia	Post-intubation subglottic stenosis
Choanal atresia	*Neurogenic*
Laryngeal web	Laryngeal paralysis
Laryngocele	Poor pharyngeal muscle tone
Subglottic stenosis	*Caustic or Thermal Injury*
Vascular ring	Lye or caustic ingestion
Macroglossia (Beckwith syndrome)	Hot gas or liquid
Tracheal web or cyst	*Foreign Body*
Inflammatory/Infectious Lesions	Neoplasm
Viral croup	
Epiglottitis	
Abscess (retropharyngeal, peritonsillar, parapharyngeal)	
Tracheitis	
Bronchitis	
Severe tonsillitis	
Angioedema	
Infectious mononucleosis	
Diphtheria	

The smaller the airway, the greater the resistance to flow (resistance increases exponentially). Alterations in the diameter of the airway are most often caused by edema and inflammation from a variety of conditions, including congenital anomalies, infection, allergic and anaphylactic reactions, cysts, tumors, and trauma. Even small localized areas of airway narrowing in infants and children can lead to respiratory distress because the airway is so small, particularly at the cricoid ring, which is the narrowest portion of the airway in children.

Croup

Croup is most often caused by an infection with **parainfluenza virus** (type 1 or 2). Several other causes include respiratory syncytial virus (RSV), influenza virus A or B, adenovirus, rhinovirus, coxsackievirus, measles, and herpes simplex virus. Metapneumovirus and novel coronavirus, which more commonly cause bronchiolitis, have also been implicated. Co-viral infections are common. Particularly severe disease may be associated with influenza A, RSV, or adenovirus infection. Infection occurs via respiratory droplets spread from other infected individuals.

The virus first attacks the nasopharynx and subsequently spreads to the larynx and upper trachea. The infection causes inflammation and edema of the airway that often involves the vocal cords and subglottic areas producing the typical barking cough, hoarseness, and inspiratory stridor. Uncommonly, in severe cases, the lower airways also may be involved, leading to impaired alveolar ventilation and wheezing. In some children, secondary bacterial superinfection may rarely occur with bacterial tracheitis or extension of infection to the lower airway producing pneumonia. Airways of infants are small

and particularly susceptible to obstruction because of the narrow subglottic region and laxity of the cartilaginous structures.

Spasmodic croup, an entirely different disease, is common, frequently occurs at night, and may be recurrent. It is characterized by the sudden onset of hoarseness, barking cough, and stridor. This condition may resolve when children are exposed to cool or humid air. The etiology is unknown but is probably a reaction to a viral infection or an allergic phenomenon. There may be a family history of recurrent stridor in children with spasmodic croup, and it tends to occur in older children.

Differential Diagnosis

The differential diagnosis of stridor is presented in Table 60-1.

Evaluation

History

A complete history should be obtained (Questions Box).

Physical Examination

It is important to assess the degree of respiratory distress and to place children in a position of comfort; monitor heart rate, ventilation, and oxygenation; and deliver oxygen (see Chapter 59). The stridor sounds produced are usually inspiratory but may be inspiratory and expiratory if the disease progresses to the lower airway. The presence of stridor at rest or with sleep should be assessed as well as the severity of retractions with breathing. Breath sounds may be decreased bilaterally, and severe tachypnea, with respiratory rates from 40 to 80 breaths/min, may occur. Peripheral or central cyanosis and alterations in mental status associated with severe disease should be noted. Assessment of the croup score may be helpful to direct initial therapy in mild, moderate, or severe cases as well as monitor response to treatment (Table 60-2).

Laboratory Tests

Investigations, such as a complete blood cell count and cultures, are rarely helpful unless the physician is concerned about secondary bacterial infection. The white blood cell count may be normal or mildly elevated, and the differential count may show a predominance

---

Questions

Stridor and Croup

- Did the child have an antecedent respiratory infection?
- Does the child have a fever? If so, how high is the temperature?
- Was the onset of stridor abrupt?
- Is there stridor at rest/sleep or only with agitation?
- Does the child have any ill contacts?
- Does the child have any associated symptoms such as vomiting, diarrhea, or rash?
- Is the child feeding normally?
- Is the child drooling?

Table 60-1. Differential Diagnosis of Stridor

Data	Viral Croup	Spasmodic Croup	Bacterial Tracheitis	Epiglottitis	Foreign Body
Age	3–36 mo	3–36 mo	1–10 y	1–8 y	All Ages
Prodrome	Upper respiratory infection symptoms; onset over 2–5 d	None; sudden onset at night	Upper respiratory infection symptoms for days followed by rapid onset fever and respiratory distress	Usually none; rapid onset over several hours	None; sudden onset
Fever	Low grade	None	Low grade initially, then higher	Usually temperature above 102.2°F (39°C)	None
Cough	Barking	Barking	Dry initially, then barking	None or dry	May or may not be present
Respiratory distress	Present	Present	Absent or mild initially, then severe	Present and severe	Usually present
White blood cell count	Normal or slightly elevated	Normal	Normal initially, then elevated	Elevated	Normal
Blood culture	No growth	No growth	Growth uncommon	*Haemophilus influenzae*	No growth
Radiograph	Subglottic narrowing; steeple sign	(±) Subglottic narrowing	Subglottic narrowing; steeple sign and ragged trachea	Swollen epiglottis	Air trapping; may show a foreign body

of polymorphonuclear cells. If epiglottitis is being considered, no blood should be drawn until the airway has been visualized and secured.

Imaging Studies

Radiographs of the soft tissues of the upper airway are often helpful. In children with croup, lateral neck radiographs may reveal ballooning of the hypopharynx, a normal epiglottis, and narrowing of the subglottic area (Figure 60-1). The frontal view shows the classic steeple sign of the subglottic area where the airway narrows like a church steeple or pencil tip. Radiographic studies should not delay the management of children with suspected epiglottitis; nor should children with respiratory compromise be taken from a monitored area for radiographs. Thickening of the epiglottis (thumbprint-shaped) and obliteration of the vallecular space may be seen on lateral neck films in patients with epiglottitis if radiographs are obtained.

Other imaging studies, such as a barium swallow or computed tomography scan of the thorax, are helpful in diagnosing congenital anomalies (eg, vascular ring).

Management

Most children with croup and stridor can be managed as outpatients. Caregivers should be given careful instructions so that they understand the course of the illness, know what to expect, and realize when emergency care is needed. Children with a prolonged or recurrent history of stridor may require consultation with a head and neck specialist. If a specific cause of stridor, such as a foreign body, is identified, appropriate management should be instituted.

Children with croup should be treated with gentleness and should not be upset. They should remain with their caregivers and be allowed to assume a position of comfort. Agitation and crying

Table 60-2. Croup Score

	0	1	2	3
Stridor	None	Only with agitation	Mild at rest	Severe at rest
Retraction	None	Mild	Moderate	Severe
Air entry	Normal	Mild decrease	Moderate decrease	Marked decrease
Color	Normal	Normal	Normal	Cyanotic
Level of consciousness	Normal	Restless when disturbed	Restless when undisturbed	Lethargic

Disease Category by Score

Score	Degree	Management
≤4	Mild	Consider mist therapy and dexamethasone 0.6 mg/kg orally. Outpatient observation.
5–6	Mild to moderate	Dexamethasone 0.6 mg/kg orally and consider mist therapy. If child improves after observation, is >6 mo, and has a reliable family, outpatient observation.
7–8	Moderate	Dexamethasone 0.6 mg/kg orally or intramuscularly; consider racemic epinephrine and admission.
≥9	Severe	Racemic epinephrine, dexamethasone 0.6 mg/kg orally or intramuscularly, oxygen, and admit to intensive care unit.

Modified from Taussig LM, Castro O, Beaudry PH, Fox WW, Bureau M. Treatment of laryngotracheobronchitis (croup). Use of intermittent positive-pressure breathing and racemic epinephrine. *Am J Dis Child.* 1975;129(7):790–793, with permission from the American Medical Association.

Figure 60-1. Lateral neck radiograph of viral croup. Note the ballooning of the hypopharynx and narrowing in the subglottic area. (Courtesy of Dr J. S. Seidel, Division of General and Emergency Pediatrics, Harbor-UCLA Medical Center.)

increase respiratory distress and oxygen demand. Procedures should be kept to a minimum. The heart rate, respiratory status, and oxygen saturation should be continuously monitored while the patient is being treated and observed. Airway adjuncts that cause increased agitation should not be used.

Cool mist may be provided by blowby or mask. **Humidified oxygen or air,** which is thought to decrease the viscosity of secretions and reduce the edema of the airway, has been the mainstay of therapy for croup for quite some time. This treatment is currently controversial. Several randomized, controlled trials have questioned this practice, demonstrating no benefit of cool humidified mist therapy. Many find it difficult not to continue this treatment practice at this time though. Symptoms of spasmodic croup usually resolve within 6 hours of the onset without treatment, but cool, humidified mist is often employed as the sole therapy in this disorder.

Treatment of croup with **corticosteroids** is less controversial. A number of studies have demonstrated that dexamethasone given as a single dose of 0.6 mg/kg is effective in shortening the course and severity of mild, moderate, and severe croup if given in the first 3 days. Several smaller randomized trials have also suggested that half the dose of dexamethasone may be equally effective with fewer adverse effects. It should be given orally but may be given as an intramuscular injection for children who are unable to take oral medication or have persistent emesis. Use of the tablet preparation ground

up in applesauce is often recommended because the liquid preparation does not taste good and is not well tolerated. Recent studies using nebulized budesonide also demonstrate the same efficacy in reducing respiratory distress and lowering of the croup score but at considerably more cost. Continuous or long-term therapy with steroids does not seem to alter the clinical course of the disease or the period of hospitalization and is not recommended. Treatment with antibiotics is not indicated unless infection with bacteria is evident.

Use of **racemic epinephrine** has also been somewhat controversial. Several older studies have shown that there was no difference in the long-term outcome between those children who were treated with epinephrine and those who received a placebo. Other studies have clearly demonstrated an acute effect of the drug when given via nebulizer. This effect lasts a few hours, and repeat respiratory distress after the drug effects have worn off has been reported in the literature. It is therefore prudent that if racemic epinephrine is used on patients who are going to be discharged, they be observed for 3 to 4 hours after treatment for return or worsening of stridor. The anti-inflammatory effects of dexamethasone take several hours for onset, and racemic epinephrine may have more benefit in reducing symptoms during this period.

Hospitalization should be considered for children in severe respiratory distress or with significant stridor at rest who are unable to eat and those whose parents are unable to cope with the tasks required to manage children at home. It is always indicated for children with a bacterial infection, such as epiglottitis or tracheitis.

About 10% of infants and children with croup may need **controlled ventilation with endotracheal intubation.** Indications for intubation include severe respiratory distress, altered mental status, hypoxia, and hypercapnia. A major complication of endotracheal intubation in children with croup is subglottic stenosis, which develops because the endotracheal tube may traumatize the inflamed airway, leading to permanent damage. Patients should be extubated as soon as possible.

Direct laryngoscopy may be necessary in some children in whom the etiology of the stridor is not clear. This procedure should be done by a practitioner who is experienced in managing the airway.

Prognosis

Stridor is a serious sign indicative of upper airway obstruction and potential respiratory compromise. Although it has many causes, prognosis is usually determined by the rapidity of diagnosis and institution of appropriate therapeutic measures, particularly stabilizing the patient and ensuring patency of the airway. Certain conditions such as croup often resolve spontaneously within a few days, although some children require hospitalization and, rarely, assisted ventilation. Other conditions, such as foreign bodies or tumors, necessitate aggressive intervention to prevent death from airway obstruction.

CASE RESOLUTION

In the case history at the beginning of this chapter, the 2-year-old with the antecedent infection and stridor has the classic signs of croup and a croup score of 6. First, adequate ventilation and oxygenation should be ensured. As soon as the assessment and management of airway, breathing, and circulation are completed, other diagnostic studies and specific therapy, such as dexamethasone, racemic epinephrine, or both, can be considered. A period of posttreatment observation is warranted.

Selected References

Bjornson C, Russell KF, Vandermeer B, Durec T, Klassen TP, Johnson DW. Nebulized epinephrine for croup in children. *Cochrane Database Syst Rev.* 2011;(2): CD006619

Cherry JD. Clinical practice. Croup. *N Engl J Med.* 2008;358(4):384–391

Choi J, Lee GL. Common pediatric respiratory emergencies. *Emerg Med Clin North Am.* 2012;30(2):529–563

Everard ML. Acute bronchiolitis and croup. *Pediatr Clin North Am.* 2009;56(1): 119–133

Russell KF, Liang Y, O'Gorman K, Johnson DW, Klassen TP. Glucocorticoids for croup. *Cochrane Database Syst Rev.* 2011;(1):CD001955

CHAPTER 61

Sudden Infant Death Syndrome and Apparent Life-Threatening Events

Lynne M. Smith, MD

CASE STUDY

A 4-month-old boy is brought to the emergency department by paramedics after being found blue and not breathing by his mother. He had previously been well except for a mild upper respiratory infection. His mother fed him at 2:00 am, and when she checked on him at 6:00 am she found him blue and lifeless. Although the mother smoked cigarettes during pregnancy, the pregnancy and delivery were otherwise normal. The infant received the appropriate immunizations at 2 months of age.

Questions

1. What factors are associated with sudden infant death syndrome (SIDS)?
2. How are SIDS and apparent life-threatening events (ALTEs) related?
3. How are SIDS and sudden unexpected infant deaths (SUIDs) related?
4. What is the appropriate evaluation of infants who present with an ALTE?
5. What services are available to families who have lost infants to SIDS?
6. What should parents be advised to help prevent SUIDs?

Sudden infant death syndrome (SIDS), previously referred to as **crib death,** is defined as the sudden, **unexpected death** of an apparently well infant younger than 1 year that is not adequately explained by a comprehensive medical history of the infant and family, a thorough postmortem examination, and a death scene investigation. The syndrome has been known since biblical times; parents were advised not to lie with their children for fear of suffocating them. In the United States, SIDS is the most common cause of death in children younger than 1 year beyond the neonatal period. Research suggests that infants who died of SIDS had **serotonin-mediated dysregulation** of the autonomic nervous system, which increased their vulnerability to exogenous stressors such as prone sleep position and environmental overheating.

Sudden infant death syndrome–like events associated with successful resuscitation were once described as **near-miss SIDS** or **aborted crib death.** The term that is now used is **apparent life-threatening event (ALTE)** and was adopted in 1987 at a National Institutes of Health Consensus Development Conference on Infantile Apnea and Home Monitoring. Apparent life-threatening events are characterized by some combination of **apnea, color change,** **marked change in muscle tone,** and **choking** or **gagging.** Though some have theorized ALTEs are precursors to SIDS, only approximately 5% to 10% of SIDS victims experienced a previous ALTE. In an attempt to establish the efficacy of home monitoring, the **Collaborative Home Infant Monitoring Evaluation (CHIME)** study followed more than 1,000 healthy term infants as well as infants at varying risks for SIDS. The CHIME study found that 43% of term infants experienced apnea or bradycardia episodes, indicating these cardiorespiratory events are common in all infants and unlikely to be precursors to SIDS. Further, SIDS usually occurs during infant sleep, whereas an estimated 50% of ALTEs occur during wakefulness, which may explain why the Back to Sleep campaign has successfully decreased SIDS but not affected the incidence of ALTEs. Thus, SIDS and ALTE should not be considered varying manifestations of a similar disease process.

With expanded and more thorough home scene investigations, exogenous contributing factors have been increasingly noted in these deaths and are found in the vast majority of what is now referred to as **sudden unexplained or unexpected infant death (SUID).** The term *unexpected* is preferred because a careful death scene investigation usually reveals an explanation, such as unsafe sleep.

Sudden unexpected death in childhood occurs in children older than 12 months. Sudden unexplained death in childhood is rare, with a reported incidence in the United States in 2002 of 1.3 deaths per 100,000 children, compared with 57 deaths per 100,000 live-birth infants younger than 12 months.

Epidemiology

Sudden unexpected infant death accounts for 2,000 to 3,000 deaths per year in the United States, with an overall incidence of 0.57 per 1,000. These figures were dramatically higher prior to the campaign of the American Academy of Pediatrics (AAP) to place babies in the supine position for sleep. Prior to the institution of the **Back to Sleep** campaign, the annual death rate from SIDS was approximately 5,000 to 8,000, with an incidence of approximately 2 per 1,000. Sudden infant death affects boys more commonly than girls and occurs more often in the winter months. This seasonality may be related to infection with respiratory syncytial virus (RSV). The highest incidence of SIDS occurs at 2 to 3 months of age, with 90% occurring before the age of 6 months.

The frequency of SIDS differs in different populations in the United States and other countries. Although the incidence of SIDS is decreasing among all groups, SIDS rates in African American and American Indian/Alaska Native children is 2 to 3 times the national average. One factor contributing to the higher SIDS rate is the higher incidence of non-supine sleeping in African American infants. In 2001, the prevalence of prone positioning was 11% for white infants and 21% for African American infants.

Numerous epidemiologic, maternal, and infant factors have been associated with SIDS, including **prematurity** and **intrauterine growth restriction** (Box 61-1). Mothers of children with SIDS are frequently young and unwed, smoke cigarettes, and have had fewer doctor visits during the prenatal and postpartum periods. Parental alcohol use is also a risk factor for SIDS. Sudden infant death syndrome rates in one study were 33% higher on New Year's Day, suggesting parents under the influence of alcohol are less able to safely monitor their infants. Despite initial reports and significant research efforts, no clear data have established a causal relationship of ALTEs, apnea, immunizations, or repeated episodes of cyanosis with SIDS.

Box 61-1. Risk Factors for Sudden Infant Death Syndrome

• Male gender	• Poor prenatal care
• Maternal youth	• Family previously reported to child protective services
• Socioeconomic disadvantage	• Sleeping in prone or side position
• Maternal smoking	• Soft bedding
• Prematurity	• Overheating
• Low birth weight	• Bed sharing

Clinical Presentation

Victims of SIDS present in **cardiopulmonary arrest,** with a history of previous good health or antecedent upper respiratory infection. They often present in the early morning hours, having succumbed during sleep.

Infants who have experienced an ALTE at home may appear well without any need for medical intervention or resuscitation or may appear in the emergency department (ED) pale, cyanotic, hypotonic, lethargic, and with bradycardia. They often present between the hours of 8:00 am and 8:00 pm, a different time of day than for SIDS victims. If resuscitation is successful en route, infants may look normal and be fully alert.

Pathophysiology and Risk Factors for Sudden Infant Death Syndrome

Sudden infant death syndrome is related to the interaction of a number of factors. Sudden infant death syndrome occurs in infants with an underlying vulnerability at a critical time during development when they are exposed to known risk factors such as sleeping in a non-supine position. The AAP recommends only the supine sleep position because side sleeping increases the risk of SIDS 2-fold relative to back sleeping.

A firm crib mattress covered by a fitted sheet is the recommended sleep surface for infants. Soft bedding such as water beds, couches, stuffed toys, pillows, quilts, and comforters are to be avoided. Though **bed sharing** has been promoted as enhancing breastfeeding, **accidental suffocation** and sudden infant deaths are associated with this practice. The AAP recommends parents sleep in a separate but proximate sleeping environment from their infant (room sharing but not bed sharing). The importance of a safe sleep environment is underscored by the work of Kemp and colleagues, who investigated 119 SIDS cases over a 4-year period following the initiation of the Back to Sleep campaign. Only 8.4% of these SIDS victims were found in a non-prone position, alone in their bed, without any potential obstructions of the external airway by bedding. Overheating can increase the risk of SIDS, so dressing babies in light clothing during sleep and keeping the room temperature at a comfortable level for adults is recommended.

Because approximately 20% of SIDS cases in the United States occur while in the care of someone other than the parent, there is a critical need to educate secondary caregivers and child care centers on the need for babies to sleep on their backs. Another group of infants likely to sleep in a non-supine position are infants born weighing less than 1,500 g. These infants are twice as likely to be placed to sleep in the prone position at home than infants weighing 1,500 to 2,500 g. During the first weeks of hospitalization, premature newborns are often placed in a non-supine position because of respiratory complications and gastroesophageal reflux. The newborns become accustomed to this position, and the parents learn from the hospital staff's modeling to place them in this unsafe position. The AAP Task Force on SIDS encourages neonatologists and nurses to begin placing premature newborns on their backs "significantly before the infant's anticipated discharge."

One unintended consequence of supine sleep positioning is the increased incidence of **positional plagiocephaly.** To minimize the risk for head deformities and foster appropriate motor development, parents are encouraged to vary the head position at sleep times, avoid swing and bouncy seats that increase pressure on the back of the head, and encourage adult-observed **tummy time** during waking hours starting from birth. One can suggest tummy time at every diaper change, even for only a minute or two.

In addition to being exposed to an environment that increases the infant's risk for SIDS, most theories suggest that there is an underlying vulnerability in SIDS victims. The brain stems in infants who died of SIDS have significantly lower concentrations of serotonin and tryptophan hydroxylase, a key biosynthetic enzyme of serotonin; higher **serotonergic neuron** counts; decreased **serotonin 1A receptor** binding; and reduced **serotonin transporter** binding in the medulla. Further, there is a significant increase in monoamine oxidase A gene polymorphism allele 4 in females and allele 3 in male SIDS cases. These findings suggest that abnormalities in serotonin synthesis, release, and clearance impair the infant's ability to appropriately regulate arousal and respiratory drive in response to potential life-threatening challenges during sleep. Numerous other associations with SIDS have been reported, including altered polymorphisms of proinflammatory cytokines, small mandibular size, disorders of fatty acid oxidation, and cardiac channelopathies including long QT syndrome. Findings from a SIDS mouse model suggest postnatal hypoxia can delay maturation of the cardiac conduction system, resulting in an increased risk of developing cardiac arrhythmias. However, the AAP does not currently recommend universal electrocardiogram (ECG) screening at birth to identify potential SIDS victims.

The association between SIDS and **fatal child abuse** has also received attention, though infanticide is estimated to be the cause in less than 5% of suspected SIDS cases. The evaluation of the home environment of SIDS victims, referred to as *death scene investigations,* may reveal factors that contributed to the death of some of these infants. Unsafe sleeping environments (eg, sofas) and parental drug paraphernalia may identify such factors. A complete postmortem examination may reveal prior or recent trauma. Autopsy should include an assessment for long bone fractures as well as intracranial hemorrhage, which establish inflicted trauma as the cause of the sudden death. In some municipalities, child fatality boards review each case of reputed SIDS to determine whether an etiology other than SIDS is present. Infants with parents who have Munchausen syndrome by proxy (MSBP) may present with SIDS or ALTE. Such infants are suffocated by the parents until they become apneic or die. Because distinguishing between SIDS and intentional suffocation is very difficult pathologically, the AAP Committee on Child Abuse and Neglect has cited factors that should heighten the clinician's suspicion for possible child abuse (Box 61-2). The use of in-hospital covert video surveillance has facilitated the recognition of apnea secondary to MSBP.

Differential Diagnosis

The physician is usually not charged with determining the cause of death of the deceased infant; that is the role of the coroner. The major challenge for physicians is to evaluate infants who have experienced an ALTE and determine if any underlying condition caused the episode (Box 61-3). In most cases, no etiology for an ALTE episode is established and the episode represents an isolated event.

Sepsis, respiratory infections, seizures, gastroesophageal reflux, inborn errors of metabolism, infantile botulism, cardiac anomalies, and child abuse should all be considered. The circumstances surrounding ALTEs suggest which of these conditions is suspect. A sepsis evaluation is particularly warranted in children who have symptoms such as fever, vomiting, or diarrhea or appear toxic at presentation. Infants with respiratory symptoms such as tachypnea and wheezing may have **RSV** infection, which is associated with apneic episodes, particularly during the first week of illness in infants younger than 3 months who had been premature and experienced apnea of prematurity. Young infants with pertussis do not exhibit the classic cough with whoop and may present with respiratory distress and apnea. Overuse or misuse of over-the-counter cough and cold medication has been associated with drowsiness and seizures, which can present as an ALTE. Infants with abnormal movements or ALTEs when awake may be experiencing seizures. The apnea may represent the seizure or a postictal event. Infantile botulism causes decreased muscle tone and weakness. Apnea may also accompany gastroesophageal reflux. In general, affected infants have a history of eating, regurgitating, and then developing apnea. As previously

---

Box 61-2. Circumstances in Which the Clinician Should Be Alert to the Possibilities of Child Abuse

- Previous recurrent cyanosis, apnea, or apparent life-threatening event (ALTE) while in the care of the same person
- Age at death older than 6 months
- Previous unexpected or unexplained deaths of one or more siblings
- Simultaneous or nearly simultaneous deaths of twins
- Previous death of infants under the care of the same unrelated person
- Discovery of blood on the infant's nose or mouth in association with ALTE

Box 61-3. Differential Diagnosis of an Apparent Life-Threatening Event

• Gastroesophageal reflux	• Inborn errors of metabolism
• Lower respiratory tract infection	• Child abuse
• Sepsis	• Intracranial hemorrhage
• Pertussis	• Airway anomalies
• Respiratory syncytial virus	• Aspiration
• Infantile botulism	• Breath-holding spell
• Seizures	• Cardiac arrhythmias/anomalies
• Incorrect medication dose or overdose	

noted, child abuse, particularly with intracranial hemorrhage or MSBP, may result in apnea or SIDS.

Inborn errors of metabolism are reported in 4% to 8% of cases of ALTE. Inborn errors of metabolism should be considered in infants with other symptoms, such as vomiting or failure to thrive, or in the context of a positive family history. Symptoms may first appear when a previously well infant is metabolically stressed as by an acute infectious illness. Rarely, cardiac arrhythmias, most notably long QT syndrome, are associated with apnea or sudden episodes of bradycardia.

Evaluation

History

The history may provide the clue to the etiology of SIDS or ALTE (Questions Box).

Physical Examination

A complete examination should be conducted. If infants are floppy and have poor color or have required mouth-to-mouth resuscitation or vigorous stimulation, significant events are likely. Physicians should check for the presence of bruises, retinal hemorrhages, dysmorphic features, growth impairment, and abnormal neurologic or developmental findings, which may suggest an alternative etiology. The presence of tachypnea, retractions, wheezing, or cough is consistent with a respiratory infection such as RSV or pertussis.

Laboratory Tests

In general, the laboratory workup is guided by the findings of the history and physical examination (Box 61-4). A sepsis evaluation, including a complete blood cell count, blood culture, lumbar puncture, and urine culture, is appropriate to rule out sepsis in febrile or toxic-appearing infants. Serum electrolytes, serum ammonia, and glucose are important to check because they may indicate an inborn error of metabolism or other abnormalities (eg, hypoglycemia), which may be associated with apnea with or without the presence of a seizure. Hypotonic infants should be evaluated for infantile botulism by sending a stool specimen for testing. All infants with a history of apnea or ALTE should be admitted to the hospital for observation, workup, and monitoring. A pilot study has identified a subset of well-appearing, low-risk patients presenting with ALTEs that may be safe to discharge home after a thorough evaluation. However, these data need to be validated in a large study that includes children of all ethnicities. In addition, one must be certain that the family is comfortable with this course of action and knows what to do should there be a recurrence.

Imaging Studies

A chest radiograph should be performed to rule out pneumonia if respiratory symptoms are present or sepsis is suspected. If the history and physical examination suggest other etiologies, computed tomography and barium swallow may also be indicated, though the risks of radiation exposure need to be carefully considered.

Diagnostic Studies

An electroencephalogram should be obtained if a seizure disorder is suspected. In-hospital covert video surveillance is a complex procedure that may be undertaken if MSBP is suspected. Multichannel pneumograms detect apnea and bradycardia but are not able to identify infants at risk for SIDS. They are no longer considered in the routine assessment of infants presenting with ALTE. An ECG may be useful in the rare infant with long QT syndrome.

Management

Infants who have not been fully resuscitated in the field should be resuscitated, stabilized, and admitted. Any identifiable conditions such as sepsis, seizures, and reflux should be appropriately managed. In general, infants who experienced an ALTE but do not have an

---

Questions

Sudden Infant Death Syndrome and Apparent Life-Threatening Event

- What were the events leading up to the episode?
- Was the infant awake and eating, indicating that gastroesophageal reflux should be considered?
- Was the infant awake and did the eyes roll back or the body stiffen or jerk, suggesting that a seizure may have occurred?
- How serious was the event? Did breathing resume spontaneously or did cardiopulmonary resuscitation have to be initiated?
- Have similar events occurred in the past?
- Is the infant basically well? Has the infant been ill recently?
- Has the infant had respiratory symptoms such as wheezing or cough?
- Was the infant given an over-the-counter cough and cold product?
- Do siblings have a history of sudden infant death syndrome or apparent life-threatening event that would suggest the presence of a familial disorder or child abuse?
- Were there any problems with the pregnancy or delivery?
- Is there a history of maternal smoking?
- Does the infant sleep in a supine, prone, or side-down position?

Box 61-4. Laboratory Studies to Consider in Evaluating Infants With Apparent Life-Threatening Event	
Often Indicated	*Sometimes Indicated*
Complete blood cell count	Electroencephalogram
Blood culture	Computed tomography scan
Lumbar puncture	Barium swallow
Urine culture	Electrocardiogram
Chest radiograph	Skeletal survey
Serum electrolytes	
Blood sugar	
Serum ammonia	

identifiable precipitating condition are also admitted for monitoring and observation. Recent evidence suggests that infants older than 30 days who have not had multiple ALTEs and have no identifiable medical condition may be safely discharged from the ED. Prior to discharge from the hospital, the parents of infants who experienced an ALTE should receive cardiopulmonary resuscitation training and be advised to eliminate tobacco smoke exposure.

In the past, home apnea monitoring was prescribed for newborns at risk for apnea. Based on a plethora of studies, the AAP does not recommend home apnea monitors for the prevention of SIDS. Home apnea monitoring may be indicated for premature newborns and infants at risk for repeated episodes of apnea of prematurity on discharge from the hospital. Discontinuation should be considered at approximately 43 weeks' gestation.

Home monitoring may be indicated for individuals who are technology-dependent (home ventilators, tracheostomy) or those with ALTEs if the physician wants to monitor episodes of apnea or respiratory failure. The family of an infant who experienced an ALTE should clearly be informed that a home apnea monitor has not been shown to prevent SIDS and is not indicated for that purpose.

Pacifier use has been associated with a lower incidence of SIDS. The AAP recommends that caregivers consider offering a pacifier at nap time and bedtime throughout the first year of life. The pacifier should not be reinserted once the infant falls asleep or coated in any sweet solution. The pacifier should be cleaned often and replaced regularly. Breastfed infants should have pacifier introduction delayed until 1 month of age to ensure that breastfeeding is well established.

In addition to managing infants with ALTE, physicians must provide care to families whose infants have succumbed to SIDS. In most jurisdictions, cases of SIDS must be reported to the coroner's office. The AAP recommends a prompt death scene investigation; appropriate use of available medical specialists by medical examiners and coroners, including pediatricians; and a postmortem examination within 24 hours of death, including radiographic skeletal surveys and toxicologic and metabolic screening. A complete review of the medical records of the victim is essential. It is important for physicians to tell families when they think the cause of death is probable SIDS even before definitive autopsy results are available. A timely information session with parents is recommended when the results of the investigation conclude SIDS or a medical causation for death.

Parents of children who have succumbed to SIDS should be guided through issues such as planning the funeral and ending lactation. For ongoing support, they should be referred to groups and agencies to help them deal with the loss of their child. Information about these organizations can be obtained from First Candle (800/221-7437; www.firstcandle.org).

Prognosis

Prevention of SIDS has become a focus of public health measures. Improving maternal risk factors involves smoking cessation and access to prenatal care. Parents must be instructed to avoid soft bedding for their infants, not to bed share with their infants, not to place their infants on a sofa for sleep, to avoid overheating, and to place their infants in the supine position in a crib. The prognosis for children who have experienced an ALTE varies and depends on predisposing conditions. Parents can be assured that most ALTEs are isolated events and the risk of a chronic condition, such as seizure disorders, is rare. Abnormal neurodevelopmental conditions are generally associated with a poor prognosis when associated with apnea.

CASE RESOLUTION

The infant presented in the case history succumbed to sudden infant death syndrome (SIDS). In spite of resuscitative efforts by the paramedics, he could not be revived. The mother is advised of the diagnosis of suspected SIDS and referred to appropriate agencies and support groups. The coroner is notified about the case and the presence of any associated physical findings, such as bruises. The mother is advised that a coroner investigator will visit her to learn more about the circumstances surrounding the sudden death of her infant.

Selected References

American Academy of Pediatrics Task Force on Sudden Infant Death Syndrome. SIDS and other sleep-related infant deaths: expansion of recommendations for a safe infant sleeping environment. *Pediatrics.* 2011;128(5):1030–1039

Blair PS, Mitchell EA, Heckstall-Smith EM, Fleming PJ. Head covering—a major modifiable risk factor for sudden infant death syndrome: a systematic review. *Arch Dis Child.* 2008;93(9):778–783

Claudius I, Keens T. Do all infants with apparent life-threatening events need to be admitted? *Pediatrics.* 2007;119(4):679–683

Courts C, Grabmüller M, Madea B. Monoamine oxidase A gene polymorphism and the pathogenesis of sudden infant death syndrome. *J Pediatr.* 2013;163(1):89–93

Duncan JR, Paterson DS, Hoffman JM, et al. Brainstem serotonergic deficiency in sudden infant death syndrome. *JAMA.* 2010;303(5):430–437

Esani N, Hodgman JE, Ehsani N, Hoppenbrouwers T. Apparent life-threatening events and sudden infant death syndrome: comparison of risk factors. *J Pediatr.* 2008;152(3):365–370

Farrell PA, Weiner GM, Lemons JA. SIDS, ALTE, apnea, and the use of home monitors. *Pediatr Rev.* 2002;23(1):3–9

Franco P, Kato I, Richardson HL, Yang JS, Montemitro E, Horne RS. Arousal from sleep mechanisms in infants. *Sleep Med.* 2010;11(7):603–614

Fu Ly, Moon RY. Apparent life-threatening events: an update. *Pediatr Rev.* 2012;33(8);361–369

Horn MH, Kinnamon DD, Ferraro N, Curley MA. Smaller mandibular size in infants with a history of an apparent life-threatening event. *J Pediatr.* 2006;149(4):499–504

Kemp JS, Unger B, Wilkins D, et al. Unsafe sleep practice and an analysis of bed-sharing among infants dying suddenly and unexpectedly: results of a four-year, population-based, death-scene investigation study of sudden infant death syndrome and related deaths. *Pediatrics.* 2000;106(3):E41

Kinney HC, Thach BT. The sudden infant death syndrome. *N Engl J Med.* 2009;361(8):795–805

Klintschar M, Rothämel T, Läer K. Monoamine oxidase A and sudden infant death syndrome. *J Pediatr.* 2013;163(5):1533

Neary MT, Breckenridge RA. Hypoxia at the heart of sudden infant death syndrome? *Pediatr Res.* 2013;74(4):375–379

Phillips DP, Brewer KM, Wadensweiler P. Alcohol as a risk factor for sudden infant death syndrome (SIDS). *Addiction.* 2011;106(3):516–525

Putnam-Hornstein E, Schneiderman JU, Cleves MA, Magruder J, Krous HF. A prospective study of sudden unexpected infant death after reported maltreatment. *J Pediatr.* 2014;164(1):142–148

Ramanathan R, Corwin MJ, Hunt CE, et al. Cardiorespiratory events recorded on home monitors: comparison of healthy infants with those at increased risk for SIDS. *JAMA.* 2001;285(17):2199–2207

Trachtenberg FL, Haas EA, Kinney HC, Stanley C, Krous HF. Risk factor changes for sudden infant death syndrome after initiation of Back-to-Sleep campaign. *Pediatrics.* 2012;129(4):630–638

CHAPTER 62

Syncope

David Atkinson, MD

CASE STUDY

A 15-year-old girl comes to your office a week after her quinceañera because she fainted after the ceremony. The celebration was on a hot summer's day, and she was so nervous that she had nothing to eat or drink the entire day. Though the girl thinks she has never fainted before but has gotten dizzy momentarily after standing up "too fast and sometimes in the shower," her mother reports that she fainted about a year ago while having blood drawn. In addition, at age 18 months, she fell off her parents' bed. She cried, gasped, stopped breathing, became pale, and passed out for about 30 seconds. She was diagnosed with a breath-holding spell. There is no family history of sudden death or seizures.

Prior to fainting, she had completed the quinceañera mass and entry into the celebration hall with her family and was standing while her godfather began his toast. She remembers feeling "light-headed"; the next thing she recalls is awaking on the ground with her family and friends around her. Her mother states that she had passed out for about 10 to 15 seconds. She denies taking any medications or using any illicit drugs and denies sexual activity. The mother wants to know if it is safe for her daughter to go to the local amusement park with her friends next week. She has read about sudden death in high school athletes and asks if it is safe for her daughter to continue to play for the high school soccer team.

The girl's physical examination is unrevealing, and her vital signs are all normal. Electrocardiogram shows normal sinus rhythm with normal voltages and intervals for her age.

Questions

1. What are the causes of syncope?
2. What type of workup is done primarily to evaluate for syncope?
3. When should patients who experience syncope be referred to a subspecialist?
4. Which pediatric subspecialists assist in the evaluation of a patient with syncope?
5. Which patients presenting with syncope are at the greatest risk for sudden death?

Syncope, or **fainting,** is a transient loss of consciousness and tone and a very common clinical problem in pediatrics, particularly during puberty and adolescence. The most common causes of syncope in pediatrics are benign neurocardiogenic events; however, syncope may rarely be a harbinger of sudden death caused by arrhythmia, obstruction of aortic outflow, or other serious cardiovascular events.

There are 3 general categories of syncope: **neurocardiogenic** (also called vasovagal syncope), **cardiac syncope,** and **noncardiac syncope** (Box 62-1). The workup for syncope can easily become expensive and time-consuming and may provide little information beyond that gleaned by the initial history and physical examination. It is the role of the pediatrician to appropriately direct the evaluation for syncope so that a cost-effective evaluation may occur without missing the patient who may be at risk for a sudden death event.

Epidemiology

Syncope is defined as a temporary, transient loss of consciousness and muscle tone, usually associated with a rapid recovery. It is the result of a decrease in cerebral blood flow that can occur through many different mechanisms. Syncopal events are very common in the pediatric population; up to 50% of college undergraduates have reported experiencing syncope or near syncope, and it accounts for about 1% of all pediatric emergency department visits. Females are more commonly affected than males, and the mean age at presentation is 10 to 12 years. Syncope is uncommon in children younger than 5 years. Many cases of syncope resolve quickly and medical attention is not sought, so the true incidence of syncope is almost certainly underestimated.

Clinical Presentation

The clinical presentation of syncope varies with the etiology. In **vasovagal syncope** there is often a prodrome of symptoms, including light-headedness, visual disturbances, nausea, and diaphoresis. The patient has usually been standing for a long period or has suddenly gone from the supine or sitting position to standing. Other forms of **neurally mediated syncope** include **hair-grooming syncope,** which occurs mostly in girls while combing, brushing, or blow-drying their hair. Micturition syncope, while more common in the elderly, may occur in all ages of patients. Younger patients tend to be male; predisposing factors may include reduced food intake, fatigue, alcohol ingestion, and recent respiratory infection. Micturition syncope events often occur at night when voiding after awakening from sleep (ie, while standing immediately after being recumbent). Recurrences of micturition syncope are rare in young patients. **Breath-holding**

Box 62-1. Causes of Syncope

Neurocardiogenic (Vasovagal Syncope)
Cardiac
- Tachyarrhythmia
  —Supraventricular tachycardia
  —Ventricular tachycardia
- Bradyarrhythmia
  —Second- or third-degree heart block
  —Sinus node dysfunction
- Left or right ventricular outflow tract obstruction
  —Hypertrophic cardiomyopathy
  —Aortic stenosis
- Idiopathic pulmonary hypertension
- Coronary artery disease
  —Acquired coronary artery disease
    • Kawasaki disease
  —Congenital coronary anomaly
    • Intramural coronary artery
    • Anomalous origin of coronary artery
- Primary cardiac dysfunction
  —Dilated cardiomyopathy
  —Non-compaction syndrome
- Secondary cardiac dysfunction
  —Viral or idiopathic myocarditis
  —Restrictive cardiomyopathy
Noncardiac
- Orthostatic hypotension
- Neurologic (seizures, atypical migraine, dysautonomia)
- Breath-holding spells
- Psychogenic (hysteria, hyperventilation)
- Self-induced (hyperventilation, the "choking game")
- Metabolic abnormality (hypoglycemia, anemia)
- Drug or medication effect

spells (BHS) in toddlers brought on by anger, pain, fear, or frustration may be associated with syncope; this is an infantile form of cardioinhibitory neurally mediated syncope. Infants who suffer syncopal BHS are more likely to grow up and have neurally mediated syncope (see Chapter 51).

Syncope of cardiac etiology will often lack the prodrome of vasovagal syncope. The main cardiac causes of syncope are arrhythmia and left ventricular outflow obstruction. Patients may complain of palpitations, chest pain, or chest tightness. Cardiac syncope commonly occurs during physical activity and may be accompanied by a complete loss of body tone.

Syncope related to **seizures** generally has a longer recovery time associated with the postictal phase; witnesses may describe the patient as being dazed or "having a blank look on face" prior to fainting. These episodes may occur whether the patient is recumbent or upright.

Pathophysiology

Autonomic

Autonomic causes of syncope are the most common etiology, accounting for up to 80% of cases of syncope that come to medical attention. They are also referred to as neurally mediated reflexive syncope, vasovagal syncope, neurocardiogenic syncope, and, in toddlers, pallid BHS. They have in common disturbances in autonomic control of heart rate and blood pressure in response to postural changes, bodily functions, pain, fear, or other strong emotional events. Vasovagal syncopal events usually occur when the patient is upright, resulting in decreased venous return, decreased arterial blood pressure, and decreased left ventricular volume. There is a resultant reflex stimulation of vagal fibers leading to bradycardia, vasodilation, and worsening hypotension (Bezold reflex). There are 3 clinical types of neurally mediated syncope: vasodepressor, which starts and is primarily marked by profound hypotension; cardioinhibitory, marked by severe bradycardia or even brief asystole; and mixed response, which is a mixture of vasodepressor and cardioinhibitory.

Cardiac

Cardiac causes of syncope are more likely to be associated with sudden death, so it is important to identify and treat these abnormalities. Cardiac mechanisms of syncope are mainly related to arrhythmias or obstructive lesions. Obstructive lesions lead to decreased ventricular outflow, resulting in decreased cerebral perfusion; arrhythmia may lead to decreased ejection volume, also leading to cerebral hypoperfusion and syncope.

Left-sided obstructive lesions, including aortic stenosis and hypertrophic cardiomyopathy, are the most likely cause of obstructive syncope. Rarely, syncope can be caused by pulmonary stenosis or severe primary pulmonary hypertension, mitral stenosis, atrial myxoma, or cardiac tamponade. Cardiac syncope, unlike routine vasovagal syncope, often occurs during exertion because of the inability of the heart to increase cardiac output to meet the demands placed on it by increased physical activity. Increased diastolic pressure caused by an obstructive lesion may also decrease myocardial perfusion, leading to cardiac ischemia, dyskinesis, or ventricular arrhythmias, further decreasing ventricular output.

Anomalous origin of the coronary arteries, though not an obstructive lesion, may also cause syncope with exercise. The left coronary artery may arise from the pulmonary artery, delivering deoxygenated blood to the left coronary system, or the left coronary artery may arise from the right coronary cusp and course between the aorta and pulmonary arteries. When the patient is in a high cardiac output state, such as during exercise, the left coronary artery may be compressed between the great arteries, leading to ischemia or arrhythmias.

Primary arrhythmias causing syncope are a rare but important cause of syncope. Chest radiograph, echocardiogram, and other imaging modalities will generally be normal, with no evidence of structural heart disease or pulmonary edema. Supraventricular tachycardia may cause syncope or near syncope. In most pediatric patients, the tachycardia is propagated through a concealed pathway, and the resting electrocardiogram (ECG) will be normal if the tachycardia is not occurring while the ECG is being obtained. Supraventricular tachycardia may also be associated with Wolff-Parkinson-White (WPW) syndrome. Wolff-Parkinson-White syndrome is characterized by a short P-R interval followed by an abnormally wide QRS complex with an initial delta wave.

Ventricular tachycardia is rare in children with no underlying structural heart disease but may be brought on by infection (especially myocarditis or pericarditis), cardiomyopathies, drugs (eg, cocaine, amphetamines), drug interactions (nonsedating antihistamines taken with erythromycin or ketoconazole), and long QT syndrome.

Patients with long QT syndrome have prolonged cardiac repolarization, which will usually manifest on the resting ECG as a prolongation of the corrected QT interval. The prolongation of the repolarization period of the heart puts patients with long QT syndrome at risk for torsades de pointes, a malignant form of ventricular tachycardia. Genetic forms of long QT syndrome result from mutations in genes that code for ion transport channels or related proteins. Romano-Ward syndrome is an autosomal-dominant form of long QT syndrome that is associated with congenital deafness. Autosomal-recessive long QT syndrome has historically been referred to as Jervell and Lange-Nielsen syndrome. Although the clinical diagnosis of long QT syndrome is based on a QTc that is prolonged for the patient's age, it is estimated that 20% of patients with a gene mutation associated with long QT syndrome will have a normal resting ECG; therefore, a critical part of the evaluation of the syncopal patient is obtaining a family history of long QT syndrome, sudden death or near sudden death, seizures, or a history of torsade de pointes. Long QT syndrome may also be brought on by electrolyte imbalance, increased intracranial pressure, or medications (Table 62-1).

Noncardiac

Noncardiac causes of syncope include neurologic etiologies (seizures, migraines), metabolic disturbances (hypoglycemia), hyperventilation (panic attacks or self-induced), and hysteria. Low iron stores have been associated with neurally mediated syncope in children and adolescents and may provide a partial explanation for the higher incidence of neurocardiogenic syncopal events in adolescent girls than boys. Seizures may be difficult to distinguish from vasovagal events because both can have tonicoclonic movements. Unlike vasovagal or cardiac syncope, seizures result in unconsciousness secondary to neurologic dysfunction. Syncope associated with hypoglycemia is caused by insufficient substrate being delivered to the brain. Cerebral vasoconstriction secondary to arterial hypocapnia produces syncope with hyperventilation that may be secondary to panic attacks or self-induced. The "choking game" or "fainting game" refers to intentional cutting off of oxygen to the brain, with the goal of inducing a "high" or euphoric feeling, usually resulting in syncope and occasionally in serious injury or death. Hysterical syncope lacks a true prodrome, and patients usually suffer no injury when they fall.

Table 62-1. Drugs Known to Increase the Risk of Ventricular Arrhythmia in Patients With Long QT Syndrome[a]

Drug	Class/Clinical Use
Amiodarone	Antiarrhythmic/abnormal heart rhythm
Arsenic trioxide	Anticancer/leukemia
Bepridil	Antianginal/heart pain
Chloroquine	Antimalarial/malaria infection
Chlorpromazine	Antipsychotic/schizophrenia Antiemetic/nausea
Cisapride	GI stimulant/heartburn
Clarithromycin	Antibiotic/bacterial infection
Disopyramide	Antiarrhythmic/abnormal heart rhythm
Dofetilide	Antiarrhythmic/abnormal heart rhythm
Droperidol	Sedative/anesthesia adjunct Antinausea/nausea
Erythromycin	Antibiotic/bacterial infection GI stimulant/increase GI motility
Halofantrine	Antimalarial/malaria infection
Haloperidol	Antipsychotic/schizophrenia, agitation
Ibutilide	Antiarrhythmic/abnormal heart rhythm
Mesoridazine	Antipsychotic/schizophrenia
Methadone	Opiate agonist/pain control, narcotic dependence
Pentamidine	Anti-infective/pneumocystis pneumonia
Pimozide	Antipsychotic/Tourette tics
Procainamide	Antiarrhythmic/abnormal heart rhythm
Quinidine	Antiarrhythmic/abnormal heart rhythm
Sotalol	Antiarrhythmic/abnormal heart rhythm
Sparfloxacin	Antibiotic/bacterial infection
Thioridazine	Antipsychotic/schizophrenia

Abbreviation: GI, gastrointestinal.

[a]For a complete list of drugs to avoid in patients with long QT syndrome, visit www.crediblemeds.org.

This form of syncope is thought to be related to Munchausen syndrome by proxy.

Differential Diagnosis

The differential diagnosis of syncope is presented in Box 62-1. Events that precede and follow the syncopal event are key in determining the etiology of syncope.

Evaluation

History

A thorough history should be obtained from the family and patient, focusing on the patient's symptoms, situation surrounding the event, and family history (Questions Box). A primary goal of the history is

Questions

Syncope

- What was the patient doing when the episode occurred?
- What was the position of the patient?
- Did the patient have any symptoms before the syncopal event?
- Did the patient have any chest pain or palpitations during the event?
- How long did it take for the patient to recover from the syncopal event?
- Were any residual symptoms present after the syncopal event?
- Has the patient recently been ill, dehydrated, or fatigued?
- Does the patient have a history of underlying cardiac disease?
- Is the patient taking any type of medication (eg, prescribed, over the counter, illicit)?
- Does the patient have a history of breath-holding or pallid spells?
- Is there a family history of sudden death, seizures, deafness, or cardiac abnormalities?

to identify any underlying cardiac problems because these patients are at the greatest risk for sudden death.

Physical Examination

The patient with syncope needs a thorough physical examination. Vital signs should assess blood pressure to screen for hypotension and hypovolemia. The cardiac examination should include palpation of the chest for the point of maximal intensity, thrills and lifts, and auscultation to assess the intensity of the heart sounds and detect the presence of murmurs or other adventitial sounds. Upper- and lower-extremity pulses should be palpated for their presence and quality. The remainder of the examination should focus on identifying any abnormal neurologic findings.

Laboratory Tests

The history and physical examination should guide which laboratory tests are necessary. In general, few tests are needed. Serum glucose shortly after the syncopal event may reveal hypoglycemia. Fasting glucose or glucose tolerance tests are usually normal, and such testing is not indicated. In pubertal females, a pregnancy test should be obtained as well as a hemoglobin level. Iron levels may be low in patients with neurally mediated syncope.

Imaging Studies

Every patient who is being evaluated for syncope requires an ECG. The ECG may reveal WPW or long QT syndrome, neither of which can be diagnosed by history and physical examination alone. These studies can also be useful in identifying underlying structural abnormalities such as right ventricular hypertrophy secondary to pulmonary hypertension, left ventricular hypertrophy secondary to hypertrophied cardiomyopathy, or Q waves associated with anomalous origin of the coronary arteries. Patients with findings suggestive of cardiac disease (ie, positive history, physical findings, or an abnormal ECG) require referral to a pediatric cardiologist for further evaluation. The cardiac workup of syncope may include a Holter monitor or an event recorder. The Holter monitor is worn for

24 hours and continuously records the heart rhythm. Because this is a limited window of observation, the Holter monitor will capture arrhythmia less than 20% of the time, even in patients with known arrhythmias. Event recorders are worn for longer periods, often up to several weeks. They can record and retain the cardiac rhythm prior to, during, and following an event. When the patient activates the monitor, the recording is saved for download to the cardiologist. If the monitor is not activated, the event recorder will not save the information but will record over it. Although the event recorder has a higher probability of capturing an arrhythmia if one is present than does a Holter monitor, the tracings are generally lower quality. Exercise stress testing is often used to evaluate the patient's response to exertion and to allow for replication of symptoms in a monitored setting. Electrophysiology studies may be ordered if an arrhythmia is uncovered during the evaluation.

The workup for patients without evidence of cardiac disease (negative family history of cardiac disease and sudden death and no exertional symptoms such as chest pain) should focus on the noncardiac or autonomic causes of syncope. Patients with prolonged recovery time or persistent neurologic symptoms following an event should be referred to a neurologist and may require an electroencephalogram to rule out seizure disorders.

A tilt test may be used to aid in the diagnosis of vasovagal syncope, although in most cases the history will be sufficient. The patient receiving a tilt test is placed on a table that is then tilted to simulate standing in an upright position, a condition that is commonly associated with vasovagal syncope. Unfortunately, there is great variability in the tilt test, with an incidence of up to 20% of false-positives. Factors that influence test results include the time of day, whether the patient has fasted, hydration status, and whether the test was augmented with isoproterenol. There are very few false-negative tilt tests, but because of the high number of false-positives, the tilt test should be reserved only for refractory, recurrent, or unexplained syncope.

Management

Management of syncope depends on its cause. Recurrent vasovagal syncope may be treated simply by having the patient increase fluid intake (including carrying a water bottle in school) and increasing salt intake. Fludrocortisone, a mineralocorticoid, is the most common medical intervention for vasovagal syncope, although the efficacy is not well established. Other treatments include β-blockers (propranolol or atenolol), vagolytic drugs (disopyramide), or centrally acting drugs (imipramine, fluoxetine). These medications have varied benefits, and results between small controlled trials are not consistent.

Patients with neurologic syncope secondary to seizures should be treated with anticonvulsants. Patients with hyperventilation, hysteria, or hypoglycemia are most amenable to behavioral interventions. Patients with syncope secondary to a cardiac etiology should be referred to a cardiologist for further evaluation and correction of the underlying problem. These types of syncopal episodes may require more aggressive management, such as surgery or cardiac pacing, because they are more likely to result in sudden death.

Prognosis

The prognosis for autonomic and noncardiac syncope is good. Patients with vasovagal syncope will often suffer only a single event, and those with recurrent events can be treated with increased fluid intake or medication. One subgroup to be aware of is children with pallid BHS; while most will have resolution of these spells by 5 years of age, up to 17% may continue to have syncope in adulthood. Patients who have syncope with an underlying cardiac etiology are at the greatest risk for sudden death, and it is only through identification and treatment of these structural or rhythm abnormalities that sudden death may be prevented.

CASE RESOLUTION

The adolescent girl in the opening scenario describes symptoms consistent with vasovagal syncope. Her family history, physical examination, and electrocardiogram do not suggest any underlying cardiac disease. The patient and her family should be informed that certain factors, such as dehydration, fatigue, and hunger, can precipitate syncope. Behavioral changes, such as eating breakfast and drinking plenty of water, should be implemented to prevent or limit recurrence of syncope. The patient should be encouraged to carry a water bottle in school and a note written to the school to allow her to do so, if necessary. Management with medications is not indicated at this time.

Selected References

Evans WN, Acherman R, Kip K, Restrepo H. Hair-grooming syncope in children. *Clin Pediatr (Phila).* 2009;48(8):834–836

Fischer JW, Cho CS. Pediatric syncope: cases from the emergency department. *Emerg Med Clin North Am.* 2010;28(3):501–516

Goble MM, Benitez C, Baumgardner M, Fenske K. ED management of pediatric syncope: searching for a rationale. *Am J Emerg Med.* 2008;26(1):66–70

Grubb BP. Clinical practice. Neurocardiogenic syncope. *N Engl J Med.* 2005; 352(10):1004–1010

Jarjour IT, Jarjour LK. Low iron storage in children and adolescents with neurally mediated syncope. *J Pediatr.* 2008;153(1):40–44

Khositseth A, Martinez MW, Driscoll DJ, Ackerman MJ. Syncope in children and adolescents and the congenital long QT syndrome. *Am J Cardiol.* 2003;92(6): 746–749

Krongrad E. Syncope and sudden death. In: Emmanouilides GC, ed. *Moss Adams Heart Disease in Infants, Children and Adolescents, Including the Fetus and Young Adult.* 5th ed. Baltimore, MD: Williams & Wilkins; 1995:1604–1619

Kumpf M, Sieverding L, Gass M, Kaulitz R, Ziemer G, Hofbeck M. Anomalous origin of left coronary artery in young athletes with syncope. *BMJ.* 2006; 332(7550):1139–1141

Massin MM, Malekzadeh-Milani S, Benatar A. Cardiac syncope in pediatric patients. *Clin Cardiol.* 2007;30(2):81–85

Petko C, Bradley DJ, Tristani-Firouzi M, et al. Congenital long QT syndrome in children identified by family screening. *Am J Cardiol.* 2008;101(12):1756–1758

Piccirillo G, Naso C, Moisè A, et al. Heart rate and blood pressure variability in subjects with vasovagal syncope. *Clin Sci (Lond).* 2004;107(1):55–61

Ramowski SK, Nystrom RJ, Rosenberg KD, Gilchrist J, Chaumeton NR. Health risks of Oregon eighth-grade participants in the "choking game": results from a population-based survey. *Pediatrics.* 2012;129(5):846–851

Salim MA, Di Sessa TG. Effectiveness of fludrocortisone and salt in preventing syncope recurrence in children: a double-blind, placebo-controlled, randomized trial. *J Am Coll Cardiol.* 2005;45(4):484–488

Stewart JM. Postural tachycardia syndrome and reflex syncope: similarities and differences. *J Pediatr.* 2005;154:481–485

Strickberger SA, Benson DW, Biaggioni I, et al. AHA/ACCF scientific statement on the evaluation of syncope: from the American Heart Association Councils on Clinical Cardiology, Cardiovascular Nursing, Cardiovascular Disease in the Young, and Stroke, and the Quality of Care and Outcomes Research Interdisciplinary Working Group; and the American College of Cardiology Foundation: in collaboration with the Heart Rhythm Society: endorsed by the American Autonomic Society. *Circulation.* 2006;113(2):316–327

Sun BC, Emond JA, Camargo CA Jr. Inconsistent electrocardiographic testing for syncope in United States emergency departments. *Am J Cardiol.* 2004;93(10): 1306–1308

CHAPTER 63

Shock

Kelly D. Young, MD, MS

CASE STUDY

A 7-month-old boy is brought in by his parents with a history of vomiting and diarrhea for 2 days. He also has had a low-grade fever and, according to his parents, has become progressively more listless. Vital signs show a heart rate of 200 beats/min, respiratory rate of 30 breaths/min, and blood pressure of 72/35 mm Hg. The infant is lethargic and mottled. Capillary refill time is 3 seconds. His anterior fontanelle is sunken, and his mucous membranes are dry. The abdomen is flat and non-tender and displays hyperactive bowel sounds.

Questions

1. What is shock, and what clinical signs can help in the recognition and assessment of shock?
2. What are the stages of shock?
3. What different types of shock are there, and what are the possible causes for each type?
4. What are the management priorities in treating shock?

Shock is defined as a state of circulatory dysfunction resulting in insufficient delivery of oxygen and other metabolic substrates to the tissues. Shock is not a disease but rather an abnormal physiological state that may result from many disease processes. Early recognition and prompt therapy of shock are critical to avoid permanent end-organ damage or death.

Epidemiology

The most common type of shock in children is hypovolemic shock, and the most common causes are dehydration from gastrointestinal infections that cause vomiting and diarrhea, and hemorrhage from traumatic injury. However, in a case series of 147 pediatric patients with shock (excluding trauma patients) from Children's Hospital of Nevada, septic shock was the most common etiology, accounting for 57% of patients. Of the remaining patients, 24% had hypovolemic shock, 14% distributive shock, and 5% cardiogenic shock. Shock may be seen in any age group, but it is more difficult to recognize the early stages in young children because early clinical signs of shock in children are subjective and may be attributed to other causes. By the time young children have developed more typical signs, such as thready pulses and hypotension, they are in the late stages of shock.

Clinical Presentation

Early signs of shock include tachycardia; cool, clammy, pale, or mottled skin; and delayed capillary refill time. There may be a history of decreased urine output. In this early **compensated** stage, perfusion to vital organs such as the brain and heart is maintained by compensatory physiological processes. As the shock state progresses, it becomes **uncompensated,** resulting in impairment of vital organ perfusion. Signs of uncompensated shock include hypotension; altered mental status (irritability, lethargy, decreased interactivity);

weak, thready, or absent pulses (although pulses may be bounding in "warm" septic shock); and severely mottled or cyanotic skin (D$_x$ Box). In the Nevada epidemiologic study, young children commonly presented with poor extremity perfusion and poor pulses, while adolescents presented with hypotension. **Irreversible** shock occurs when multiple organs fail and death occurs.

Pathophysiology

Shock occurs when oxygen delivery to tissues is impaired. Adequate oxygen delivery depends on sufficient blood oxygen content and adequate circulatory blood flow (Figure 63-1). The oxygen content in blood depends primarily on the concentration of hemoglobin and the amount of oxygen bound to hemoglobin. In children, oxygen consumption by end organs depends most on oxygen delivery, while in adults it depends on oxygen extraction by the tissues.

Blood flow, or cardiac output, is determined by heart rate and stroke volume. Stroke volume depends on preload, contractility, and

 Shock

Compensated	**Uncompensated**
• Tachycardia	• Tachycardia or bradycardia
• Normal blood pressure	• Hypotension
• Normal or bounding pulses	• Weak, thready, or absent pulses
• Normal or cool, clammy skin	• Cool, clammy skin
• Pale or mottled skin color	• Severely mottled or cyanotic skin color
• Alert, anxious mental state	
• Mildly delayed capillary refill time	• Altered mental state, lethargic
	• Delayed capillary refill time
• Decreased urine output	• Decreased or absent urine output

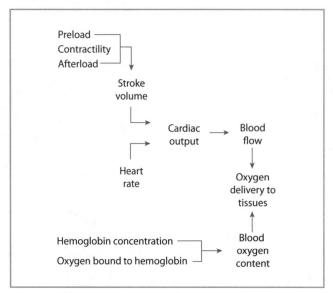

Figure 63-1. Pathophysiology of shock. Factors affecting oxygen delivery to tissue.

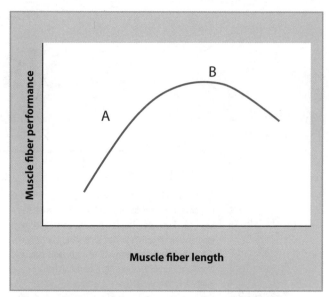

Figure 63-2. Starling curve of cardiac output. A, As muscle fiber length increases, performance increases. B, Muscle fiber reaches its optimal length, after which performance declines.

afterload. Preload refers to the amount of blood entering the heart from the systemic vasculature. Increasing preload, for example, via administration of intravenous (IV) fluid boluses, will increase cardiac output until a point of optimal heart muscle fiber length is reached. The Starling curve demonstrates that increased stretching of a muscle fiber results in improved performance of that muscle fiber (ie, improved stroke volume and cardiac output), but after the point of optimal stretching is reached, there is decreased performance (Figure 63-2).

Contractility, or inotropy, is the heart's intrinsic ability to contract and pump blood to the body. Afterload refers to the systemic vascular resistance impeding ejection of blood from the ventricles. Optimal cardiac output depends on sufficient preload, unimpaired cardiac contractility, and the ability of the heart to overcome any afterload. During states of decreased cardiac output leading to decreased tissue perfusion, adults compensate primarily by decreasing systemic vascular resistance, increasing cardiac contractility, and increasing heart rate, whereas children compensate primarily by increasing their heart rate and by vasoconstriction. The vasoconstriction in children may make hypotension a late sign of shock. Irreversible septic shock in adults is often due to vasomotor collapse, while in children cardiac failure plays a larger role.

Differential Diagnosis

There are several types of shock depending on the underlying pathophysiology (Table 63-1).

Hypovolemic shock is the most common type seen in children and usually results from dehydration or traumatic hemorrhage. Hypovolemia results in inadequate preload, which leads to impaired cardiac output and impaired perfusion. Other causes of hypovolemic shock include diabetic ketoacidosis (dehydration due to osmotic diuresis) and peritonitis and burns leading to third spacing of fluids (shifting from intravascular to extravascular sites) with resultant

Table 63-1. Types of Shock		
Type of Shock	**Physiological Mechanism**	**Common Causes**
Hypovolemic	Decreased preload	Dehydration Traumatic hemorrhage Nontraumatic hemorrhage Diabetic ketoacidosis Peritonitis Burns
Distributive	Relative hypovolemia due to vasodilation	Sepsis Anaphylaxis Neurogenic Toxin-mediated
Cardiogenic	Decreased contractility	Congestive heart failure from congenital lesions Myocarditis Tachydysrhythmias
Obstructive	Impaired cardiac output to systemic circulation	Pulmonary embolus Pericardial tamponade Tension pneumothorax Ductal-dependent cardiac lesions
Dissociative	Abnormal hemoglobin—inadequate oxygen bound	Carbon monoxide poisoning Methemoglobinemia

intravascular hypovolemia. Nontraumatic hemorrhage may occur from entities such as epistaxis, gastrointestinal bleeding, and vessel fistula formation.

Distributive shock is a relative hypovolemia; vasodilation results in inadequate circulating blood volume relative to the vasodilation (ie, the "tank" has been made larger by vasodilation, and now there is insufficient fluid to fill the tank). Causes include anaphylaxis and sepsis, which result in the release of vasoactive mediators that cause vasodilation. Spinal cord injury (**neurogenic shock**) may result in loss of sympathetic nerve–mediated vascular tone and subsequent vasodilation. Finally, certain intoxications such as iron, barbiturates, and tricyclic antidepressants can cause vasodilation and distributive shock.

Cardiogenic shock is an uncommon but important cause of shock in children. Congestive heart failure from a congenital heart lesion, myocarditis, or cardiomyopathy results in impaired cardiac contractility and decreased cardiac output. Tachydysrhythmias, such as supraventricular tachycardia, do not allow sufficient time for the ventricles to fill with blood, resulting in decreased stroke volume.

Rare causes of shock in pediatric patients include obstructive and dissociative types. In **obstructive shock,** cardiac output to the systemic circulation is obstructed due to pulmonary embolus, cardiac tamponade, or tension pneumothorax. Closure of the ductus arteriosus in a neonate with a ductal-dependent congenital heart lesion is another cause of insufficient cardiac output and obstructive shock. In **dissociative shock,** abnormal hemoglobin such as methemoglobin or carboxyhemoglobin from carbon monoxide poisoning results in decreased oxygen bound to hemoglobin and decreased oxygen delivered to tissues.

Septic shock combines elements of distributive, hypovolemic, and cardiogenic shock. Vasoactive mediators lead to decreased systemic vascular resistance and a relative hypovolemia. Third spacing of fluid leads to a true intravascular hypovolemia as well. In addition, mediators of sepsis cause impaired cardiac function.

Because shock is a physiological state resulting from a variety of etiologies, and because it is recognized through clinical findings, it is important to interpret individual findings in the context of the patient as a whole. Heart rate may be elevated for many reasons, including fear, anxiety, fever, and other reasons. Capillary refill may appear delayed in the extremities of a child who is cold. Blood pressure may appear artificially low when too large a cuff is used to measure it. The clinician must consider whether the child's history is consistent with risk for shock and whether the physical examination taken as a whole supports the diagnosis.

Evaluation

Early recognition and prompt treatment of shock is the goal. A rapid, focused history and physical examination should be performed to identify patients in shock, and early therapy should be instituted before returning for a more complete evaluation. Recognition of shock depends on history and physical examination alone; therapy should never be withheld while awaiting results of diagnostic tests.

History

A history of vomiting with or without diarrhea, decreased oral intake, and decreased urine output, especially in infants, should alert the clinician to possible hypovolemic shock. Children presenting with major trauma should be evaluated for hemorrhagic shock. A history of fever, lethargy, or irritability, and sometimes a rash, may point toward septic shock. Patients with asplenia, sickle cell disease, or indwelling catheters and those who are immunocompromised (eg, young infants or children on chemotherapy) are at increased risk for sepsis. Children in cardiogenic shock may have a history of a murmur, poor feeding, sweating with feeds, cyanosis, tachypnea, dyspnea, and in the older child, palpitations.

Physical Examination

A brief examination to identify shock focuses on mental status, vital signs, pulses, and skin signs. Impaired level of consciousness, such as lethargy or lack of recognition of parents, occurs later in shock. Earlier, children are anxious or fussy but alert. Tachycardia occurs early in shock but must be interpreted in the context of other signs of shock because tachycardia may also result from fever, pain, or simply the child's fear of the examination process. Bradycardia is a late, ominous sign in shock and often results from hypoxemia. Hypotension is also a late sign in pediatric shock. It is important to remember that normal values for heart rate and blood pressure vary by age. The lower limit of acceptable systolic blood pressure in a neonate from birth to 1 month is 60 mm Hg and in an infant from 1 month to 1 year is 70 mm Hg. For a child 1 year or older, the lower limit can be estimated using the formula $70 + (2 \times \text{age in years})$ mm Hg; the lower limit is 90 mm Hg for children 10 years or older. Systolic blood pressures lower than these guidelines represent hypotension and late uncompensated shock. Heart rate and blood pressure values requiring immediate attention are shown in Table 63-2.

Presence and quality of pulses should be checked. Weak, thready, or absent peripheral pulses are indicative of shock. However, in warm septic shock, pulses may be bounding. Skin color, moisture, and temperature give valuable clues to diagnosis. Children in shock may have pale, cyanotic, or mottled skin. Early in shock, however, skin color may be normal. Some infants may also have mottled skin normally. As with tachycardia, isolated signs must be correlated with the bigger clinical picture to diagnose shock. Decreased perfusion in shock leads to cool and clammy skin. This is often best appreciated in the hands and feet initially.

Capillary refill is tested by compressing the capillary bed of a fingertip, palm, or dorsal foot with gentle pressure until it blanches. On release, color should return in 2 seconds or less; a capillary refill time of 3 seconds or more is abnormal and indicative of shock. Children

Table 63-2. Critically Abnormal Heart Rate and Blood Pressure

Age	Bradycardia	Tachycardia	Hypotension
Neonate 0–28 d	<100 bpm	>180 bpm	<60 mm Hg
Infant 1–12 mo	<90 bpm	>160 bpm	<70 mm Hg
Child 1–10 y	<60 bpm	>140 bpm	<70 + (2 × age) mm Hg
Child >10 y	<60 bpm	>120 bpm	<90 mm Hg

Abbreviation: bpm, beats per minute.

in warm septic shock may display "flash" (ie, shortened) capillary refill time. Capillary refill should be tested with the extremity elevated above the heart so that arterial, not venous, perfusion is tested. Also, cool ambient temperatures can falsely delay capillary refill times.

In hypovolemic shock caused by dehydration, look for signs of dehydration such as dry mucous membranes, lack of tears, sunken eyes, sunken anterior fontanelle in infants, and tenting of the skin. The degree of dehydration can often be estimated clinically (see Chapter 69). Patients with hemorrhage, traumatic or nontraumatic, must be examined thoroughly to locate the source of hemorrhage.

Children with congestive heart failure and cardiogenic shock may demonstrate dyspnea on exertion, tachypnea, orthopnea, rales, hepatomegaly, gallop rhythm, and a heart murmur. Jugular venous distention and peripheral edema are appreciated less often in children compared with adults. Other signs may include a cardiac murmur, hepatomegaly, cardiomegaly on chest radiograph, and a differential in pulses or blood pressure between upper and lower extremities.

Ductal-dependent cardiogenic shock should be suspected in the newborn in the first few weeks of life presenting with severe cyanosis unresponsive to oxygen therapy, and shock. Cardiac tamponade is suspected when there are muffled or decreased heart tones, paradoxical pulse (decrease in systolic blood pressure >10 mm Hg during inspiration), and distended neck veins. Tension pneumothorax is suspected in patients with deviated trachea (away from the affected side), decreased breath sounds and hyperresonance to percussion on the affected side, and distended neck veins. Pulmonary embolism is rare in pediatric patients, and signs are subtle. It is mainly suspected when there are predisposing factors.

Approximately 20% of children with septic shock present with the classic adult form of warm shock, including increased cardiac output, hypotension, decreased systemic vascular resistance, warm non-mottled skin, bounding pulses, and flash capillary refill. Children are more likely (60%) to present with cold septic shock, including decreased cardiac output; increased systemic vascular resistance; normal blood pressure to hypotension; cool, clammy, or mottled skin; thready pulses; and delayed capillary refill. The remaining 20% of children with septic shock present with both decreased cardiac output and decreased systemic vascular resistance. Petechiae or purpura point toward meningococcemia as the etiology of septic shock. A sunburn-like rash may be seen in toxic shock syndrome due to streptococcus or staphylococcus.

Laboratory Tests

The suspected cause of the shock will determine which laboratory tests are performed. In hypovolemic shock secondary to dehydration, a chemistry panel should be obtained for electrolyte abnormalities and acidosis. Serial hematocrit determinations and a type and crossmatch are important studies in traumatic and nontraumatic hemorrhage, known or suspected. In septic shock, a complete blood cell count and blood cultures should be obtained, as well as cultures of other potential sources of infection (eg, urine, cerebrospinal fluid, wound, indwelling venous access line). Results of coagulation studies including panels to evaluate for disseminated intravascular coagulopathy, and electrolyte studies including calcium and magnesium levels, are frequently abnormal in sepsis. Hypoglycemia is a common finding in any type of shock, and a rapid bedside glucose determination should be performed. Arterial blood gases can demonstrate adequacy of oxygenation and degree of acidosis and are necessary to diagnose elevated carboxyhemoglobin and methemoglobin levels. Initial lactate levels, particularly for septic shock and trauma patients, may be correlated with overall prognosis and can be followed serially to chart progress. Procalcitonin is another increasingly popular biomarker followed in suspected sepsis. Troponins may be useful in determining severity of disease and following patients with cardiogenic shock. D-dimer assay is useful in patients with suspected pulmonary embolism.

Other Studies

Chest radiography, electrocardiogram, and echocardiogram may be obtained in cardiogenic or ductal-dependent obstructive shock to further elucidate the specific etiology. Workup of stabilized trauma patients may include bedside ultrasound, radiographs, or computed tomography scans. Imaging studies contribute to the diagnoses of cardiac tamponade, tension pneumothorax, and pulmonary embolism. Invasive monitoring with arterial lines for systemic arterial blood pressure and central venous lines for central venous pressure or pulmonary artery wedge pressure may be helpful in the ongoing management of shock, particularly fluid-resistant shock.

Management

The first management priority in the treatment of any critically ill child is attention to airway patency and ventilation. If there is significant respiratory compromise, bag-and-mask ventilation followed by endotracheal intubation is performed. Usually, however, patients in compensated shock do not require initial advanced airway management. Instead, the immediate priorities are administration of **oxygen** and initiation of **cardiorespiratory monitoring.** Oxygen by mask or nasal cannula, preferably heated and humidified, should be administered immediately. Elective, rather than emergent, endotracheal intubation should be considered to reduce metabolic demands caused by increased work of breathing. When intubating and sedating patients in shock, agents with fewer hemodynamic effects such as ketamine are preferred over those that may contribute to hypotension, such as opiates, benzodiazepines, and propofol. Etomidate, however, although its effects are hemodynamically neutral, is not recommended in septic shock because of its effect of cortisol suppression. Mechanical ventilation settings should emphasize a lung-protective approach.

Almost concurrently, the next priority is achieving **intravascular access** and, in most cases, administering fluids. Peripheral IV access should be attempted. If this is unsuccessful after 3 attempts or 90 seconds, an intraosseous line may be placed, or IV access may be obtained by placement of a central venous catheter or by cutdown technique. Ultrasound-guided vascular access is another option. Intraosseous lines have been demonstrated to provide much more rapid vascular access compared with central line placement. Umbilical venous lines can sometimes be placed in neonates within the first 1 to 2 weeks of life. More than one intravascular line is usually needed for managing patients in shock.

Decreased preload and hypovolemia (actual or relative) are present in the most common causes of pediatric shock. Only cardiogenic shock may not benefit from increasing preload via a fluid bolus. Generally, an **initial fluid bolus of 20 mL/kg isotonic crystalloid fluid,** such as normal saline or lactated Ringer solution, should be rapidly infused over 5 to 10 minutes (this may require manually pushing the fluid using a large syringe). Fluid boluses can be hand pushed into an intraosseous line. Colloid fluid (eg, albumin) theoretically has the advantage of staying intravascular longer, but this has not been proven to result in a measurable benefit. Crystalloid fluid is recommended for initial boluses because it is less expensive and more readily available. If a patient with traumatic hemorrhage is still hemodynamically unstable after 2 crystalloid fluid boluses, packed red blood cells at 10 mL/kg may be required. The patient should be assessed for improvement in mentation, vital signs, peripheral pulses, and skin signs after each fluid bolus. **Repeat fluid boluses** of 20 mL/kg to a total of 80 mL/kg or more may be necessary to restore intravascular volume. Patients should be reassessed after each bolus prior to ordering another bolus. Development of hepatomegaly or rales may indicate fluid overload and the need to begin other therapies such as vasoactive infusions. This is particularly true for cardiogenic and septic shock.

A well-designed and executed trial carried out in Africa, the Fluid Expansion as Supportive Therapy (FEAST) trial, has called into question aggressive fluid resuscitation in septic shock. While patients randomized to rapid fluid therapy showed earlier improvement in circulatory parameters, their mortality was consistently higher. It has been suggested that the results of this trial may not be generalizable to patients in developed countries due to differences in malaria infection, nutritional status, and other factors. The authors suggest that aggressive fluid therapy is particularly associated with increased mortality in highly acidotic patients, especially in developing countries where inotropic support and mechanical ventilation may not be available. Currently, expert guidelines still recommend early aggressive fluid therapy for septic shock in developed countries where inotropes and mechanical ventilation are available.

The mnemonic SHOCKED may be used to recall overall management (Table 63-3). Further management in addition to fluids depends on the specific etiology. Patients in septic shock should receive empiric broad-spectrum antibiotic coverage within the first hour after presentation. Patients with toxic shock syndrome should receive antibiotics to include clindamycin. A surgeon must assist in identifying the source of hemorrhage and controlling the bleeding in patients with traumatic hemorrhage and may be required for non-traumatic hemorrhage as well depending on the specific etiology. Blood transfusions may be required. Spinal cord injury is treated with supportive care in consultation with a neurosurgeon. Anaphylactic shock is treated with IV epinephrine, IV diphenhydramine, antihistamine H_2 receptor blockers, glucocorticoids, and nebulized

\multicolumn{2}{l}{**Table 63-3. SHOCKED Mnemonic for Management**}
S	**Sound the alarm:** Obtain help from consultants, intensivists, ancillary personnel. Move the patient to a monitored room and place on cardiorespiratory monitor, automated blood pressure measurement, and pulse oximetry.
H	**Help hypovolemia:** Get intravascular access and start 20 cc/kg crystalloid fluid bolus. Reassess after each bolus, and continue giving boluses unless hepatomegaly or rales develop. Patients may require 80 cc/kg of fluids or more.
O	**Optimize oxygenation:** Give supplemental oxygen regardless of pulse oximetry values. Consider elective intubation and artificial ventilation to reduce metabolic demands as indicated. Transfusion may be required if hemoglobin is low ($<$8–10 g/dL).
C	**Constrict and contract:** Use inotropic and vasoconstrictive agents as needed for fluid-refractory shock.
K	**Keep in mind underlying causes:** Give or apply therapies specific to the underlying cause.
E	**Electrolytes and glucose normalized:** Measure and normalize electrolytes (especially calcium) and glucose. Control hyperglycemia with a target of $\leq$180 mg/dL.
D	**Decrease metabolic demand:** Treat hyperthermia and pain to reduce metabolic demand on the patient. Consider elective intubation. Keep patient nil per os (nothing by mouth).

albuterol. Pericardial tamponade is relieved by pericardiocentesis, tension pneumothorax by needle or tube thoracostomy, and pulmonary embolus with supportive care and thrombolytics. Carbon monoxide poisoning is treated with 100% oxygen and, if severe, hyperbaric oxygen therapy. Patients with methemoglobinemia appear cyanotic even while receiving 100% oxygen and may be treated with methylene blue. Supraventricular tachycardia should be treated with adenosine if the patient is hemodynamically stable and with synchronized cardioversion if the patient is unstable. Ductal-dependent obstructive shock should be treated with prostaglandin E_1 (PGE_1) infusion.

Patients with cardiogenic shock require **inotropic agents** to increase cardiac contractility and improve tissue perfusion. Patients in the later stages of other forms of shock (eg, hypovolemic, distributive, septic) may also suffer cardiac dysfunction. In such patients, only after adequate fluid resuscitation has been performed and there are still signs of shock or hypotension (fluid-refractory shock) should inotropic agents be started. Central venous pressure monitoring may be needed to determine whether fluid resuscitation is adequate. Patients with septic shock may require **vasoactive agents** to reduce or increase systemic vascular resistance.

Epinephrine or dopamine is often the first-line inotropic agent. Guidelines recommend beginning inotropic agents when indicated in a peripheral line until a central line is available; ie, do not delay. At low doses (2–5 µg/kg/min), dopamine improves renal blood flow and enhances urine output. At mid-range doses (5–10 µg/kg/min), dopamine exerts primarily a β-adrenergic effect, improving contractility and increasing heart rate. At higher doses (10–20 μg/kg/min), dopamine's α-adrenergic effects cause peripheral vasoconstriction to improve hypotension. Because of recent (primarily adult) data showing increased mortality in patients receiving dopamine as first-line inotrope, many centers prefer epinephrine. **Epinephrine** has predominantly β-adrenergic effects at lower doses (0.05–0.1 μg/kg/min) and α-adrenergic effects at higher doses (up to 1.0 μg/kg/min). Because epinephrine is a strong inotrope, it is recommended for dopamine-resistant cold septic shock. **Norepinephrine** (0.01–1.0 μg/kg/min) has predominantly α-adrenergic vasoconstrictive effects and is therefore preferred for warm septic shock with low systemic vascular resistance and for distributive shock states (eg, anaphylaxis, neurogenic shock, certain toxin-induced shock states). **Dobutamine** (1–20 μg/kg/min) may be the most useful drug for cardiogenic shock because it is selective for β-adrenergic effects, increasing cardiac contractility. However, if hypotension is present, dobutamine-mediated peripheral vasodilation may be detrimental. Dobutamine is typically used in a range of 10 to 20 μg/kg/min. Combinations of inotropic agents may be beneficial to maximize improvements in cardiac contractility and cardiac output without compromising renal perfusion or worsening hypotension. Dopamine and dobutamine may be less effective in infants younger than 12 months. This is another reason that some centers recommend epinephrine as the first-line inotropic agent.

Patients in cardiogenic shock or cold septic shock may also benefit from afterload reduction using systemic vasodilators such as **nitroprusside** (0.5–5 μg/kg/min). If these are used, blood pressure should be continuously monitored, typically in the setting of the intensive care unit. Cold septic shock refractory to epinephrine may also be treated with type 3 phosphodiesterase inhibitors (**inamrinone** 1–20 μg/kg/min; **milrinone** 0.25–1.0 μg/kg/min), which exert inotropic and vasodilator actions. Typically, a pediatric intensive care specialist should be involved in the care of the patient, and central venous pressure monitoring should be begun before vasodilator agents are started.

Neonates with ductal-dependent lesions present with a sudden onset of shock and cyanosis in the second half of the first week of life. Common lesions include hypoplastic left heart syndrome, aortic coarctation, and tricuspid atresia. **Prostaglandin E$_1$** (0.1 μg/kg/min, titrated to effect), which acts to keep the ductus arteriosus open, should be immediately infused if a ductal-dependent lesion is suspected as the cause of shock. Apnea may result from PGE$_1$ therapy, and attention to airway management is key.

It used to be common to mix vasoactive infusions using the **rule of 6 and 0.6.** For dopamine, dobutamine, and nitroprusside, mix 6 μg/kg of drug with enough dextrose 5% in water (D5W) to produce a final volume of 100 mL. Infusion at 1 mL/hour provides a dose of 1 μg/kg/min. For epinephrine, norepinephrine, and PGE$_1$, mix 0.6 μg/kg of drug with enough D5W to produce a final volume of 100 mL. Infusion of 1 mL/h provides a dose of 0.1 μg/kg/min. However, calculations such as these are error prone, and computerized order forms with automatic error alerts or "smart" pumps that

automatically calculate doses based on the patient's inputted weight are better choices.

Treatment of patients in shock must include attention to conditions that increase metabolic demand. Acidosis should be assessed and medical therapy and ventilator management aimed to improve acid-base status. Temperature should be kept neutral with use of antipyretics and cooling measures as needed. Electrolyte abnormalities, particularly hypocalcemia, and hypoglycemia must be assessed and corrected. If a hypothyroid state is suspected, thyroid hormone replacement therapy is important. Blood products may be required for patients with septic shock and disseminated intravascular coagulation. Packed red blood cells, 10 cc/kg at a time, should be given to maintain hemoglobin of at least 10 g/dL for unstable, hypoxemic, or hemorrhaging patients, and 7 to 9 g/dL for stable patients. Fresh frozen plasma may be given to correct abnormalities in prothrombin and partial thromboplastin times but should not be pushed due to its propensity to cause further hypotension. Cryoprecipitate should be reserved for documented hypo-fibrinogenic states.

An expert panel from the American College of Critical Care Medicine created **clinical practice parameters for the treatment of pediatric septic shock** (Figure 63-3). Recommended therapy is divided between therapies for the first hour (the "golden hour") and therapies beyond the first hour (often with critical care specialists involved). In the first 15 minutes after recognition of septic shock, practitioners should attend to the airway and establish intravascular access, begin fluid boluses in 20 cc/kg increments, and diagnose and correct any hypoglycemia and hypocalcemia. The goal of therapy is normalization of heart rate, blood pressure, and capillary refill (<2 seconds), no difference between peripheral and central pulses and warm extremities, urine output greater than 1 mL/kg/h, normal mental status, cardiac index between 3.3 and 6.0 L/min/m^2, and superior vena cava (SVC) oxygen saturation (O$_2$ sat) 70% or higher. Patients who are responsive to fluid may be observed in the pediatric intensive care unit. Dopamine therapy should be started for those who are still hypotensive after fluid resuscitation. Once dopamine therapy is titrated up to 20 μg/kg/min, epinephrine should be added for dopamine-resistant cold septic shock, while norepinephrine should be added for dopamine-resistant warm septic shock. The updated guidelines emphasize that inotropic therapy should not be withheld because there is no central line and can be given peripherally if there are no other options. Two studies of patients transferred into a tertiary pediatric medical center showed significantly reduced mortality and morbidity for patients cared for by community practitioners who followed these guidelines for the first hour of care.

Corticosteroids are controversial in the treatment of sepsis. Guidelines suggest administering "stress doses" of hydrocortisone 2 mg/kg or 50 mg/m^2 body surface area beyond the first hour of therapy for catecholamine-resistant septic shock when adrenal insufficiency is suspected. Adrenal insufficiency may be suspected in patients with a history of a central nervous system abnormality or pituitary abnormality, a known adrenal gland disorder, recent surgery, history of chronic steroid therapy (eg, for asthma, inflammatory bowel disease, a rheumatologic condition), and in purpura

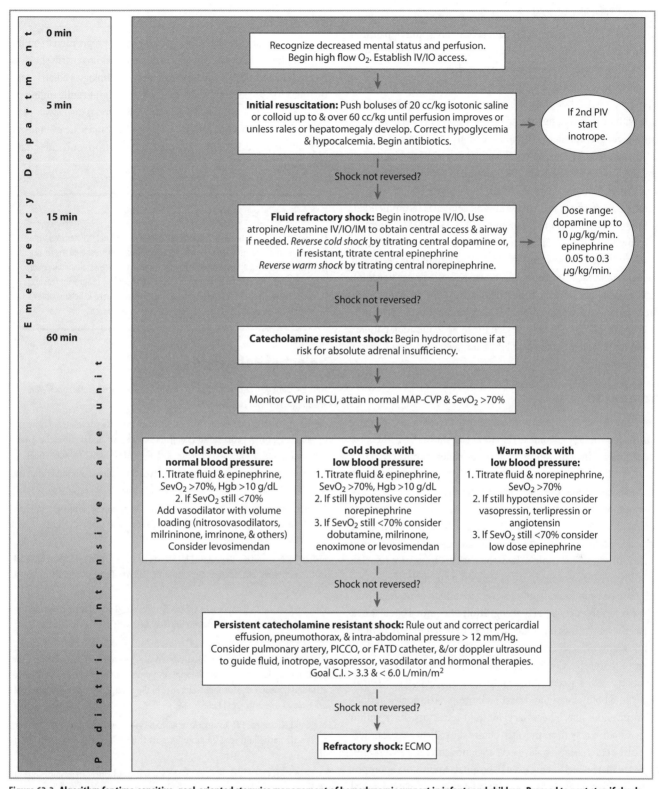

Figure 63-3. Algorithm for time-sensitive, goal-oriented stepwise management of hemodynamic support in infants and children. Proceed to next step if shock persists. (1) First-hour goals: Restore and maintain heart rate thresholds, capillary refill ≤2 seconds, and normal blood pressure in the first hour/emergency department. Support oxygenation and ventilation as appropriate. (2) Subsequent intensive care unit goals: If shock is not reversed, intervene to restore and maintain normal perfusion saturation >70%, and CI >3.3, <6.0 L/min/m² in pediatric intensive care unit (PICU). Abbreviations: CI, cardiac index; CRRT, continuous renal replacement therapy; ECMO, extracorporeal membrane oxygenation; FATD, femoral arterial thermodilution; Hgb, hemoglobin; IM, intramuscular; IO, interosseous; IV, intravenous; PICCO, pulse contour continuous cardiac output. (Adapted with permission from Society of Critical Care Medicine and Lippincott Williams and Wilkins. Brierley J, Carcillo JA, Choong K, et al. Clinical practice parameters for hemodynamic support of pediatric and neonatal septic shock: 2007 update from the American College of Critical Care Medicine. *Crit Care Med.* 2009;37[2]:668–688.)

fulminans. "Shock doses" of hydrocortisone (50 mg/kg) may be given in catecholamine-resistant fulminant septic shock and dopamine-resistant purpura fulminans. It is suggested that a baseline cortisol level be drawn prior to giving corticosteroids.

Following the first hour of therapy, a vasodilator (nitroprusside) or type 3 phosphodiesterase inhibitor (inamrinone or milrinone) along with further volume loading may be helpful in catecholamine-resistant cold septic shock with normal blood pressure and SVC O_2 sat less than 70%. In cases of "cold" septic shock with low blood pressure and SVC O_2 sat less than 70%, continued titration of epinephrine and volume is recommended. For "warm" septic shock, continued titration of norepinephrine and volume is recommended, with the possible addition of vasopressin (0.0003–0.0008 U/kg/min) or terlipressin. Vasopressin and terlipressin have not been well studied in children but show promise in adults. Finally, for persistent catecholamine-resistant shock (particularly septic or cardiogenic), consideration may be given to ventricular assist devices or extracorporeal membrane oxygenation. Recombinant activated protein C (drotrecogin alfa) was recommended for some septic adult patients but not for pediatric patients, and the commercial product Xigris is no longer available.

Prevention

Improving outcomes focuses primarily on early recognition and early appropriate therapy of shock. Carcillo et al showed significantly reduced morbidity and mortality in shock patients transferred to a tertiary pediatric medical center if community hospital physicians recognized shock and used pediatric advanced life support (PALS)–recommended interventions early. Appropriate PALS-recommended therapy was defined as more than 20 mL/kg of fluids (except in those with cardiac conditions) and use of inotropes in fluid-refractory shock. Unfortunately, while 37% of the patients transferred during the study period were in shock, as defined by prolonged capillary refill time or hypotension, only 7% were identified as in shock during the referral process. **Early recognition of compensated shock** is a key preventive measure to reduce mortality. In the study, of those in shock, only 36% received appropriate PALS-recommended therapy prior to transfer. Community practitioners must concentrate on obtaining vascular access (with an intraosseous needle, if necessary), giving fluid boluses early, and starting inotropes (through a peripheral intravenous line, if necessary) for fluid-refractory shock within the first hour. **Early therapy,** often before the patient reaches a tertiary care center, is also a key preventive measure. Rapid response teams are increasingly being used in hospitals to institute appropriate medical therapy for inpatients with concerning symptoms or vital signs. At a minimum, community pediatricians should have the ability to obtain intravascular or intraosseous access and administer rapid fluid boluses in their offices.

Prognosis

Children in shock are critically ill and at risk for progression to multi-organ failure and death. Prognosis depends on how early shock is recognized and treated and on the underlying etiology. Pediatric septic shock carries a 9% mortality rate, which is significantly improved from 60% in the 1980s and 97% in the 1960s and is also lower than the adult septic shock mortality rate. Mortality rates are even lower (6% in one study) with prompt recognition and adequate treatment.

CASE RESOLUTION

The boy in the case history is in barely compensated (he is not hypotensive) hypovolemic shock due to diarrhea, vomiting, and dehydration. He should receive oxygen and cardiorespiratory monitoring, and intravenous access should be rapidly established. Isotonic fluid boluses of 20 mL/kg should be given with reassessment between each bolus. As much as 80 mL/kg may be needed before improvements in mentation, vital signs, pulses, and skin signs are seen.

Selected References

Aneja R, Carcillo J. Differences between adult and pediatric septic shock. *Minerva Anestesiol.* 2011;77(10):986–992

Brierley J, Carcillo JA, Choong K, et al. Clinical practice parameters for hemodynamic support of pediatric and neonatal shock: 2007 update from the American College of Critical Care Medicine. *Crit Care Med.* 2009;37(2):666–688

Carcillo JA, Kuch BA, Han YY, et al. Mortality and functional morbidity after use of PALS/APLS by community physicians. *Pediatrics.* 2009;124(2):500–508

Dellinger RP, Levy MM, Rhodes A, et al. Surviving sepsis campaign: international guidelines for management of severe sepsis and septic shock: 2012. *Crit Care Med.* 2013;41(2):580–637

Fisher JD, Nelson DG, Beyersdorf H, Satkowiak LJ. Clinical spectrum of shock in the pediatric emergency department. *Pediatr Emerg Care.* 2010;26(9):622–625

Han YY, Carcillo JA, Dragotta MA, et al. Early reversal of pediatric-neonatal septic shock by community physicians is associated with improved outcome. *Pediatrics.* 2003;112(4):793–799

Kissoon N, Orr RA, Carcillo JA. Updated American College of Critical Care Medicine–pediatric advanced life support guidelines for management of pediatric and neonatal septic shock: relevance to the emergency care clinician. *Pediatr Emerg Care.* 2010;26(11):867–869

Maitland K, George EC, Evans JA, et al. Exploring mechanisms of excess mortality with early fluid resuscitation: insights from the FEAST trial. *BMC Med.* 2013;11:68

Mtaweh H, Trakas EV, Su E, Carcillo JA, Aneja RK. Advances in monitoring and management of shock. *Pediatr Clin North Am.* 2013;60(3):641–654

Wheeler DS, Basu RK. Pediatric shock: an overview. *The Open Pediatric Medicine Journal.* 2013;7:2–9

Yager P, Noviski N. Shock. *Pediatr Rev.* 2010;31(8):311–319

CHAPTER 64

Approach to the Traumatized Child

David B. Burbulys, MD

CASE STUDY

A 6-year-old boy is brought to the emergency department after being struck by an automobile while crossing the street. He was found unconscious at the scene. Initial evaluation shows that he has an altered level of consciousness, shallow respirations, ecchymosis across the upper abdomen, and a deformed, swollen left thigh. The pediatric emergency physician is called in to discuss an initial assessment and management plan for the injured child with the trauma surgeon.

Questions

1. What are the most common mechanisms of injury responsible for trauma in children?
2. What are some of the physiological differences between adults and children that make children more susceptible to certain types of injuries?
3. Which areas of the body are most likely to be injured in a typical automobile versus pedestrian collision?
4. What are the components of a primary survey in pediatric trauma patients?
5. What radiographic and laboratory studies should be performed in children with multiple injuries?

Trauma is often referred to as the neglected disease of modern society. Childhood trauma, in particular, is poorly understood and studied. Death from trauma is higher in pediatric patients than in adult patients. Mechanisms of injury may be similar in adults and children, but children have particular anatomic differences and physiological responses to injury. Health care professionals should realize that children have unique anatomic and physiological features compared with adults (Box 64-1). Evaluation and management of traumatized children requires specialized knowledge, training, and equipment. Recognition of such facts, coupled with expertise in the performance of emergency procedures, should improve the outcome of children who sustain major injuries.

Epidemiology

Traumatic injuries are the most common cause of death in children aged 1 to 14 years. This number peaks at 8 years of age. Approximately 1.5 million pediatric injuries result in a quarter-million to half-million hospitalizations and 15,000 to 25,000 deaths each year. Adolescents are most likely to die in motor vehicle crashes, and school-aged children are most likely to die after being struck by automobiles. This figure, unfortunately, may be an underestimation, as most childhood injury fatalities occur in the field prior to arrival at a health care facility. The magnitude of the problem becomes even more evident when morbidity is considered. Between 50,000 and 100,000 children per year become permanently disabled as a result

Box 64-1. Characteristics of Children That Lead to Increased Susceptibility to Injury

Anatomic Characteristics

- Smaller body size allows for the greater distribution of force with trauma, so multiple system injury is common.
- A prominent occiput, exaggerated head-to-body ratio, weak neck muscles, and higher center of gravity predispose younger children to head injury.
- Cranial bones are thinner and the brain is less myelinated, resulting in more serious head injury.
- Skeletal and ligamentous structures have increased flexibility, which results in greater transmission of force to internal organs.
- Less protective muscle and subcutaneous tissue over internal organs expose them to injury.
- Growth plates are not yet fused, which leads to Salter-Harris–type fractures and possible bone growth abnormalities with healing.

Physiological Characteristics

- High body surface area-to-weight ratio predisposes children to hypothermia, which may complicate shock and worsen acidosis and coagulopathy if it is not corrected.
- Hypoxia and respiratory failure are increasingly likely in children.
- Hemorrhagic shock is initially well tolerated by increasing heart rate and peripheral vascular resistance without significant changes in systolic blood pressure.

of their injuries. Such disabilities have an enormous effect on society; they result in financial and emotional losses for families and many years of lost productivity for individuals.

Blunt trauma, which is more common than penetrating injury in children, represents about 87% of all childhood injuries. Head injuries, followed by thoracoabdominal injuries, are the leading causes of death in this group. In adolescents, however, penetrating injury (suicide and homicide) accounts for a higher percentage of the total, especially among minority populations in urban areas. Causes of non-penetrating trauma are motor vehicle crashes (>40%), falls (25%–30%), drowning (10%–15%), and burns (5%–10%). Included in the remainder are bicycle-related and automobile versus pedestrian injuries. These numbers vary somewhat by locale. Boys are injured twice as often as girls. Different mechanisms of injury predominate in different age groups; these figures refer to overall causes of trauma. Perhaps as many as 25% to 35% of trauma deaths are related to child abuse in some centers.

Clinical Presentation

Children who sustain severe trauma present with multiple organ system injury manifested by shock, respiratory failure, or altered mental status (singly or in combination). Those with mild to moderate injury may present in this way or simply with localized signs and symptoms in the injured area.

Pathophysiology

Patterns of injury are important to identify to develop strategies for injury prevention as well as anticipate injuries during patient management. One common pattern is the triad of injuries that result from an automobile versus pedestrian collision (Waddell triad) (Figure 64-1).

Multisystem injury is the rule rather than the exception in children. Internal injury must always be suspected, even if no evidence suggestive of external trauma is apparent when the mechanism of injury warrants. Because children are anatomically and physiologically different from adults, they are more susceptible to different types of injuries (see Box 64-1). The most striking physiological differences between adults and children concern responses to acute blood loss. Children have a tremendous capacity to maintain systolic blood pressure despite 25% to 30% acute blood loss.

Hypovolemic shock secondary to acute blood loss is the most common cause of shock in pediatric trauma patients. In general, hemorrhagic shock is a clinical state in which cardiac output is unable to meet the metabolic demands of tissues for oxygen and nutrients; it is not defined by any absolute blood pressure value.

Acute blood loss stimulates peripheral and central receptors and results in an increased production of catecholamines and corticosteroids. The body responds by increasing peripheral vascular resistance, stroke volume, and heart rate. Children are able to dramatically increase heart rate and peripheral vascular resistance, and they often may exhibit normal blood pressure in the presence of hypovolemic shock. By the time their blood pressure falls, they commonly have

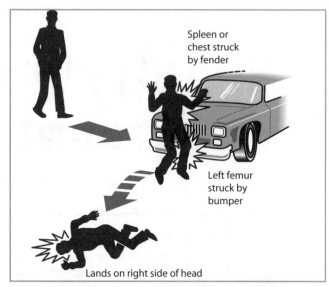

Spleen or chest struck by fender

Left femur struck by bumper

Lands on right side of head

Figure 64-1. The Waddell triad. Femur, abdominal, and contralateral head injuries (Waddell triad) should be expected to result from automobile versus pedestrian collisions in the United States. A child crossing the street is struck on the left side of the body by an automobile traveling on the right side of the road. The left femur is likely to be injured by the bumper, and the abdomen or chest strikes the grille as the child is lifted into the air and lands on the opposite side of the head, sustaining blunt head trauma. The Waddell triad illustrates the necessity of having a high degree of suspicion for a complex of injuries based on a well-known mechanism.

lost 20% to 25% of their circulating blood volume. In adults, blood pressure tends to decline after a less significant blood loss and therefore may be recognized sooner (Figure 64-2). Subtle changes in heart rate, blood pressure, pulse pressure, and capillary refill may indicate impending cardiovascular collapse in children who have been traumatically injured and should not be overlooked. Indicators of end organ perfusion such as lactic acid levels or calculated base deficit may also be helpful.

Another obstacle to the recognition of shock in children is the lack of knowledge on the part of many health professionals of age-appropriate vital signs, particularly blood pressure. Table 64-1 gives the normal blood pressure ranges for children of different ages.

Three stages of shock correspond to the progression of volume loss. In the first stage, **compensated shock,** mechanisms for preserving blood pressure are still effective. Decreased capillary refill, diminished pulses, cool extremities, and tachypnea may be apparent, but blood pressure is normal and accompanied by tachycardia. Unrecognized, untreated compensated shock rapidly progresses to **uncompensated shock.** Examination reveals decreased level of consciousness, pallor, reduced urine output, and lower blood pressure with weak, thready pulses and marked tachycardia. With inadequate therapy, uncompensated shock becomes **irreversible shock,** resulting in irreparable organ damage and often unpreventable death. (See Chapter 63 for a more extensive discussion.)

Shock has several causes, and it is important to emphasize that in trauma patients, it should always be initially attributed to hemorrhage. Shock due to obstructive cardiac output causes, such as

Figure 64-2. Cardiovascular response to hypovolemia in children. Blood pressure does not begin to decline until the volume deficit is more than 25% because of the compensatory increase in vascular resistance. Cardiac output drops earlier and is manifested clinically as delayed capillary refill; cool, clammy skin; and tachycardia.

Table 64-1. Normal Vital Signs for Children of Different Ages

Age	Respiration (breaths/min)	Pulse (beats/min)	Blood Pressure (Systolic)
Newborn	30–60	100–160	50–70
1–6 wk	30–60	100–160	70–95
6 mo	25–40	90–120	80–100
1 y	20–40	90–120	80–100
3 y	20–30	80–120	80–110
6 y	12–25	70–110	80–110
10 y	12–20	60–90	90–120

tension pneumothorax or cardiac tamponade, are much less common. Shock due to spinal cord injury is exceedingly rare. Shock should never be attributed solely to head trauma. The pathways resulting in decreased blood pressure in patients with head trauma are present only at the terminal stages. Therefore, the possibility of blood loss from internal organs should be pursued promptly.

Evaluation and Management

Because of the high potential for serious morbidity and mortality in trauma patients, evaluation and management are performed simultaneously. This care is best handled using an organized, multidisciplinary team approach, with preestablished criteria for activation of the trauma team. History of the event provides important information when implementing these criteria. For example, the entire team responds for all pedestrians struck by an automobile. The types of subspecialists that make up a trauma team are decided by individual institutions and commonly include pediatric emergency and critical care specialists, anesthesiologists, trauma surgeons, surgical subspecialists, emergency nurses, respiratory therapists, social workers, and radiograph technicians.

Several approaches to the assessment of trauma patients have been developed by professional organizations. The Advanced Trauma Life Support (ATLS) course of the American College of Surgeons and the International Trauma Life Support (ITLS) course of the American College of Emergency Physicians (formerly Basic Trauma Life Support) are 2 such approaches. The ATLS and ITLS methods stress the importance of a primary evaluation, or primary survey, to identify and treat immediate life-threatening injuries and a more detailed regional examination, or secondary survey, after stabilization to identify and treat all other injuries. In addition, they both adhere to the principles of serial examination and reassessment after each intervention. The primary survey and initial resuscitation efforts

must occur simultaneously and within the first several minutes of the evaluation. The secondary survey is meant to enhance the primary survey. Vital signs should be repeated every 5 minutes during the primary survey and every 15 minutes during the secondary survey until the trauma team feels the patient has been adequately stabilized. The reader should understand the rationale for the trauma examination and its parts. (See Selected References for articles that explain the rationale for trauma examination and provide detailed descriptions of evaluation and management techniques.)

Physical Examination

The **primary survey** begins with an assessment of **level of consciousness,** patency of the **airway** (Box 64-2), and quality of **breathing** (Box 64-3). When evaluating injured patients, physicians should always assume that the cervical spine has been injured and should use in-line immobilization to secure it. Basic airway maneuvers for positioning should be performed. The safest method is the jaw thrust to avoid moving the cervical spine (Figure 64-3). The oral cavity should be examined for foreign bodies, blood, or secretions. The most common form of airway obstruction in children is a posteriorly displaced tongue, which is relieved by good airway positioning. Advanced airway maneuvers (bag-valve-mask ventilation or endotracheal tube intubation) are performed during the primary survey if children have apnea, significant respiratory distress, severe head trauma, or an airway that cannot be maintained with basic techniques. All trauma patients are initially given supplemental oxygen

Box 64-2. Airway Assessment and Treatment

Assessment
- Airway patency and ability to protect it
- Level of consciousness
- Stridor

Treatment
- Spinal immobilization.
- Jaw thrust and suctioning.
- 100% oxygen by non-rebreathing mask.
- Intubate for Glasgow Coma Scale score <9, no gag reflex.

Figure 64-3. **Correct method for positioning the head with chin lift or jaw thrust.**

Box 64-3. Breathing Assessment and Treatment

Assessment
- Respiratory rate and depth
- Chest wall compliance, symmetry, and movement
- Tracheal deviation

Treatment
- 100% oxygen by non-rebreathing mask.
- Intubate for respiratory failure, severe flail chest.
- Compress obvious bleeding sites.
- Seal open pneumothorax with occlusive dressing.
- Needle decompress tension pneumothorax.
- Place chest tube for pneumothorax or hemothorax.

Box 64-4. Circulation Assessment and Treatment

Assessment
- Identify obvious bleeding sites.
- Peripheral pulses and capillary refill.
- Heart rate.
- Level of consciousness.

Treatment
- Compress obvious bleeding sites.
- 100% oxygen by non-rebreathing mask.
- 2 large-bore intravenous lines.
- Fluid resuscitation; 20 mL/kg normal saline.
- Packed red blood cells; 10 mL/kg after 60 mL/kg normal saline and still in shock.

Box 64-5. Glasgow Coma Scale Modified for Pediatric Patients

Eye-Opening Response
4   Spontaneous
3   To verbal command/shout[a]
2   To pain
1   None

Motor Response
6   Obeys commands/spontaneous[a]
5   Localizes pain
4   Withdraws to pain
3   Decerebrate posturing to pain (flexion)
2   Decorticate posturing to pain (extension)
1   None

Verbal Response
5   Oriented and conversant/appropriate words[a]
4   Confused/inappropriate words[a]
3   Inappropriate words/persistent crying or screaming[a]
2   Incomprehensible sounds/grunts or moans[a]
1   None

Scoring
14–15 Mild
9–13 Moderate
<9 Severe

[a]Younger than 1 year.

---

by non-rebreathing mask at a concentration of 100% and the adequacy of ventilation is assessed by a general evaluation of the respiratory rate, depth, chest movement and symmetry, and tracheal deviation.

After a patent airway and adequate ventilation have been established, **circulatory status** is assessed. All pediatric trauma patients require placement of the largest bore intravenous catheter obtainable for that patient; these should be placed, if possible, in each antecubital fossa. In life-threatening situations, peripheral vascular access is attempted 3 times or for 90 seconds, whichever comes first. If peripheral attempts fail, intraosseous infusion or central venous access should be used. A bolus of 20 mL/kg of an isotonic fluid (normal saline or lactated Ringer solution) should be given. This may be repeated, if necessary, to treat hypovolemic shock. After 60 mL/kg, administration of 10 mL/kg of blood should be considered, and the likelihood of surgical exploration is high. Acutely exsanguinating wounds are treated using direct pressure bandages (Box 64-4).

A brief neurologic assessment to assess patient **disability** is also performed during the primary survey. One rapid assessment technique is the **AVPU** system (**a**lert; responds to **v**erbal stimuli; responds to **p**ainful stimuli; **u**nresponsive). Subsequently, a Glasgow Coma Scale or Children's Coma Scale score should be calculated (Box 64-5).

Once life-threatening conditions are stabilized, more information can be collected. The **secondary survey** involves a complete and thorough head-to-toe examination of the child, fully exposed, to identify additional injuries, while taking great care to maintain normothermia. It also includes a **SAMPLE** history (**s**ymptoms, **a**llergies, **m**edications, **p**ast history/hospitalizations/surgeries, **l**ast meal, **e**vents preceding trauma). A detailed history of events preceding trauma should ensure that injuries are consistent with the causal mechanism. Health care professionals should be prepared to consider abuse when specific diagnoses do not correlate with the history given by the caregiver or the developmental ability of the child. Measurement of vital signs should occur as previously described and other devices, such as Foley catheters, nasogastric tubes, and pulse oximetry, should be used at this time. Every time an intervention is performed, repeat reassessments that incorporate the elements of the primary survey are made.

Laboratory Tests

Most institutions have a standardized trauma panel (complete blood cell count with differential, electrolytes, blood urea nitrogen, creatinine, glucose, amylase, lipase, prothrombin time, partial thromboplastin time, urine analysis, and blood typing and crossmatching). In addition, drug and alcohol screens may provide important information, particularly in the child with altered mental status. Female children of potential childbearing age should have a point-of-care pregnancy test performed as well.

Imaging Studies

When major trauma is suspected, imaging of at least the chest, pelvis/abdomen, and cervical spine should be obtained. This prevents missing injuries in children who may be unconscious or who need lifesaving procedures during resuscitation, which obscure an area of injury from examination. Additional radiographs of the extremities, for example, may be indicated when other areas of injury are detected on secondary survey. Children are often initially distracted from one injury because of the presence of a more painful one.

More sophisticated imaging techniques, such as computed tomography scans and ultrasound, are a usual part of the evaluation of the seriously injured pediatric trauma patient. The choice of test depends on the experience of the trauma team and individual characteristics of the patient.

Prognosis

The highest survival rates for seriously injured children have been found among those who are brought to the operating room for treatment within 1 hour of the injury. Definitive care for trauma takes place in the operating room, and initial stabilization takes place in the emergency department. Absolute indications for surgery include hemodynamic instability despite aggressive resuscitation, transfusion of more than 50% of the total blood volume, pneumoperitoneum, intraperitoneal bladder rupture, severe renovascular injury, gunshot wounds to the abdomen, evisceration, and peritonitis. Other injuries, often in contradistinction to similarly injured adult patients, are frequently treated more conservatively in the intensive care unit after complete consultation with all involved practitioners.

An organized, preestablished, multidisciplinary approach to care is essential. Studies have shown that the single most important element for any hospital treating injured children is the commitment on the part of the institution and its surgeons. Regional pediatric trauma centers have increased resources for dealing with severely injured patients that include long-term care and rehabilitation. Other non-designated hospitals may do an excellent job in the initial stabilization phase of care. Indications for transfer to a specialty center include inability to provide definitive surgical intervention, inability to provide an appropriate intensive care environment, presence of multisystem injuries or injuries requiring extensive orthopedic or plastic surgery procedures, or major burns. Health care professionals who treat children should not only become adept at the recognition and initial stabilization of injuries but should also serve as advocates for injury prevention and coordinated pre-hospital care services in the community.

CASE RESOLUTION

The 6-year-old boy in the case study sustained multiple trauma from an automobile versus pedestrian collision. He presents with altered level of consciousness; respiratory failure (shallow respirations); potential internal organ injury, which may lead to shock; and probable fracture of the left femur, which may also contribute to the development of shock. These injuries are identified by performance of a primary and secondary survey. Proper management includes stabilization of the cervical spine, airway management, aggressive early shock treatment with fluid replacement, and a vigilant search for additional injuries. Continued reassessment is also an integral part of emergency department stabilization. Due to the presence of multisystem injuries, after initial stabilization, the patient should be transferred to a regional pediatric trauma center for extended care.

Selected References

American College of Surgeons. Advanced Trauma Life Support. http://www.facs.org/trauma/atls/index.html. Accessed February 21, 2014

American College of Surgeons. *Advanced Trauma Life Support (ATLS) Student Manual.* 9th ed. Chicago, IL: American College of Surgeons; 2012

Avarello JT, Cantor RM. Pediatric major trauma: an approach to evaluation and management. *Emerg Med Clin North Am.* 2007;25(3):803–836

Kenefake ME, Swarm M, Walthall J. Nuances in pediatric trauma. *Emerg Med Clin North Am.* 2013;31(3):627–652

Kleinman ME, Charneides L, Schexnayder SM, et al. Pediatric advanced life support: 2010 American Heart Association guidelines for cardiopulmonary resuscitation and emergency cardiovascular care. *Pediatrics.* 2010;126(5):e1361–e1399

Leeson K, Leeson B. Pediatric ultrasound: applications in the emergency department. *Emerg Med Clin North Am.* 2013;31(3):809–829

CHAPTER 65

Abdominal Trauma

David B. Burbulys, MD

CASE STUDY

An 8-year-old boy who was riding quickly on a bicycle unintentionally crashed into a tree and is transported to the pediatric emergency department by emergency medical services. On arrival at the trauma center, the paramedics report that the bike handlebars struck the child's stomach, "knocking the wind out of him." The boy complains of dizziness and vomits several times. Initial vital signs show a heart rate of 135 beats/min, blood pressure of 105/60, oxygen saturation of 98% on room air, and a respiratory rate of 24 breaths/min. The abdomen is flat but tender to palpation in the mid-epigastric region and left upper quadrant.

Questions

1. What are the most frequent types of intra-abdominal trauma in children?
2. What are the diagnostic studies used to evaluate abdominal trauma?
3. What are the basic components of the treatment of shock that occurs following abdominal trauma?
4. What is a simple rule for establishing the lower limit of normal blood pressure in children?

Abdominal trauma is the leading *preventable* cause of fatal injury in trauma patients. Death results when the extent and nature of abdominal injuries are neither appreciated nor appropriately managed, fluid replacement is inadequate, and airway maintenance and surgical intervention are not implemented soon enough. Abdominal trauma is the third leading cause of traumatic death, following head and thoracic injury. Clinicians should be knowledgeable about mechanisms of injury that result in abdominal trauma, early manifestations of shock, and methods for aggressive treatment of hemorrhagic shock.

Epidemiology

Twenty-five percent of children who sustain multisystem trauma have significant abdominal injury and 9% die from abdominal-associated trauma. When head and abdominal injury occur simultaneously, the risk of death is higher than when either occurs alone. Blunt-force mechanisms are responsible for almost 85% of abdominal injuries; the remainder result from penetrating injuries. Examples of blunt-force mechanisms, presented in order of frequency, include motor vehicle crashes (also the most lethal), pedestrian versus automobile collisions, falls, bicycle injuries, sports injuries, and direct blows from abuse and assault. Injuries to the spleen and liver predominate, followed by injuries to the kidney, bowel, and pancreas. In multiple injuries, the incidence of trauma involving pelvic bones and organs (bladder, ureter, iliac vessels) is also high. A straddle injury (eg, fall that occurs when climbing over a fence) can also result in abdominal and pelvic trauma.

Clinical Presentation

Pain, tenderness, ecchymoses, and peritoneal signs tend to be more reliable signs of pathology, whereas distension or the absence of bowel sounds is less consistent as a marker for injury. (See D_x Box for signs and symptoms suggestive of abdominal trauma.) It is particularly important to note that no sign is completely reliable and that acute hemorrhage into the abdomen does not lead to irritation initially. A high index of suspicion must be maintained when the severity of the mechanism of injury warrants, despite minimal initial physical findings. Unexplained hypotension or shock mandates further investigation to assess for intra-abdominal hemorrhage.

Pathophysiology

Blunt trauma largely involves injury to solid, not hollow, intra-abdominal organs (ie, spleen and liver rather than small bowel) for a variety of reasons. First, the rib cage is flexible in children. Therefore, rib fractures are less likely to occur, reducing the potential for penetration of abdominal organs by broken ribs. Second, children have less well-developed abdominal musculature and less adipose

Dx Abdominal Trauma

- Pain
- Tenderness
- Distention
- Peritoneal signs (absent or diminished bowel sounds, rebound tenderness)
- Ecchymoses
- Tire tracks
- Seat belt marks
- Urine, stool, or nasogastric aspirate positive for blood
- Unexplained hypotension or other signs of hypovolemic shock

tissue than adults and relatively larger organs. Blunt force is therefore transmitted to the solid organs more easily and more diffusely. Third, because the diaphragm is oriented more horizontally in children than in adults, the liver and spleen lie more anteriorly and caudally within the abdomen.

It is important to emphasize that abdominal injury may lead to excessive blood loss. The pathophysiology of hemorrhagic shock is discussed in detail in chapters 63 and 64. The liver and spleen are highly vascularized organs that bleed profusely when lacerated. Even the accumulation of subcapsular hematomas without rupture may cause a profound drop in hematocrit. Because intra-abdominal organs are not directly visible when a patient is examined, signs and symptoms of injury are not always obvious. Therefore, hemorrhagic shock should always be suspected with abdominal trauma. Likewise, large volumes of blood can accumulate in the pelvis and retroperitoneum, and because of their proximity to the abdomen, they should always be considered as a reservoir for hemorrhage in abdominal as well as pelvic trauma.

Differential Diagnosis

Physicians should be familiar with the most common patterns of abdominal injury and should consider the possibility of specific injuries. Any solid abdominal organ can be injured by any mechanism, blunt or penetrating. The spleen is the most common intra-abdominal organ injured by a blunt force. **Hepatic injuries** are the most common fatal abdominal injuries, although they are less frequent than **splenic injuries.** The right lobe of the liver is injured more frequently than the left lobe.

Injuries to **hollow viscera** such as the stomach and intestines, which represent only about 5% to 15% of injuries from blunt forces, are difficult to diagnose and often present late. Three mechanisms lead to injuries of hollow structures: (1) "crush" between the anterior wall of the abdomen and the vertebral column; (2) deceleration, which causes shearing of the bowel from its mesenteric attachments; and (3) "burst," which occurs when an air-filled or fluid-filled loop of bowel is closed at both ends at the time of impact. Peritonitis may develop in 6 to 48 hours secondary to fecal spillage or devascularization as a consequence of any of these mechanisms. Occasionally, a diagnosis of hollow viscera injury is made incidentally or may be delayed more than 48 hours, highlighting the need for serial examinations. **Duodenal** and **pancreatic** injuries are examples of potentially delayed diagnoses that can have grave consequences. Leakage of bile and enzymes may activate autolysis of the pancreas and result in sepsis syndrome.

Evaluation

Determining which organ or organs may be injured from abdominal trauma is difficult. Children are often uncooperative or unable to assist with the physical examination. Physicians tend to focus on injuries to the extremities, pelvis, face, or chest that are painful and distracting to children and more clinically obvious to the examiner.

Initial clinical impressions may be incorrect, causing delay in diagnosis or unnecessary surgical exploration.

History

The history should focus on the mechanism of injury and the physiological response of the child, especially in the pre-hospital setting (eg, initial hypotension, tachycardia, cyanosis) (Questions Box). A poor history concerning the circumstances of the injury may contribute to a delayed diagnosis.

Physical Examination

An abnormal physical examination may not always be indicative of pathology. Clinicians should avoid relying on physical examination alone as a predictor of abdominal injury. Studies have demonstrated that patients with and without proven injuries often showed no significant differences with respect to physical findings. In particular, children with abusive abdominal trauma often have no cutaneous evidence of bruising, especially immediately after the injury is inflicted (see Chapter 131). Definitive evaluation of the abdomen is therefore mandated with significant mechanism of injury and often includes rapid computed tomography (CT) scan, ultrasound, diagnostic peritoneal lavage, laparoscopy, or laparotomy.

Vital signs should be monitored. In children, the range for normal heart rate, respiratory rate, and blood pressure is age-dependent. A simple rule for calculating the lower limit of normal systolic blood pressure is $70 + (2 \times \text{age in years})$. Physicians should always remember that a drop in blood pressure is a very late sign in the development of shock in children (see chapters 63 and 64).

Serial abdominal examinations increase the likelihood of detecting a previously missed condition. Inspection of the abdomen to look for ecchymoses, distention, tire tracks, penetrations, or paradoxical motion should occur first. Auscultation for bowel sounds follows this inspection, and palpation should come last. Palpation should be done in all 4 quadrants to elicit tenderness, rebound, and guarding. If a hepatic or splenic injury is initially suspected, palpation should be minimized to avoid further hemorrhaging.

Laboratory Tests

Laboratory evaluation should be guided by the history and physical examination. A urinalysis to look for hematuria and check for associated genitourinary injuries is helpful. Elevated serum transaminases, amylase, lipase, and alkaline phosphatase may be

Questions

Abdominal Trauma

- How was the child injured?
- How long ago did the injury occur?
- What parts of the body were injured?
- Has the child received any treatment prior to coming to the hospital, and what was the response?

indicative of injury, but normal values do not exclude pathology. A comprehensive trauma panel, which usually includes a complete blood cell count and differential, serum electrolytes, blood urea nitrogen, creatinine, glucose, prothrombin time, partial thromboplastin time, urinalysis, lactic acid, and blood type and crossmatch, should be carried out for all patients with serious or multiple injuries (see Chapter 64).

Imaging Studies

Multiple imaging modalities are available to assess the pediatric trauma patient with suspected abdominal injuries. The time to perform an imaging study is after the patient is responding appropriately to resuscitation (ie, fluid therapy). Unstable patients require surgical exploration for definitive treatment of abdominal or pelvic injury.

Computed tomography scanning remains the standard of care for imaging the injured abdomen of a pediatric trauma patient. Computed tomography scans have greater than 97% accuracy in identifying abdominal or retroperitoneal injury, are noninvasive, and most notably provide detailed specific information about injuries. The images are also routinely extended to include the pelvis, as necessary. Disadvantages of CT scanning may include the lack of proximity to the trauma suite, which may not be ideal for unstable patients; the length of time it takes to perform the procedure; and the need for an intravenous (IV) contrast, which has inherent risks such as allergic reactions and renal toxicity.

The use of ultrasonography has become very popular, with encouraging results for the identification of abdominal injury, though its use in pediatric trauma patients remains unclear. Ultrasound can rapidly and noninvasively document the presence of intraperitoneal and pelvic fluid (blood). While it is as effective as CT scanning for documenting the **presence of injury,** it does not provide as much specific information about the **nature** of the injury and does not image the **retroperitoneal space.** Ultrasound has a few additional advantages: It is relatively inexpensive; does not require contrast or radiation exposure; can be performed in 5 to 10 minutes in the trauma room, thus minimizing the risk to an unstable patient; and can be used many times for serial assessments.

Over the last several decades, diagnostic peritoneal lavage had been a dependable method of detecting intra-abdominal hemorrhage. However, its use may be largely replaced by ultrasound and it is limited in the pediatric population because many children with blunt trauma to the abdomen are now managed without surgery, as stated previously.

Management

Management of abdominal trauma in children occurs simultaneously with evaluation. The stabilization of children with abdominal trauma, especially in the context of multiple trauma, requires a multidisciplinary team approach that includes surgeons, pediatricians, and emergency physicians. A discussion on approach to trauma management can be found in Chapter 64.

Hypovolemic shock, if present, is the primary complication of abdominal trauma on which to focus because the leading unrecognized cause of death in affected children is profound blood loss. **Airway problems** and **breathing difficulties** should be addressed initially, followed by **vascular access** and **fluid replacement.** No more than 3 attempts at peripheral vascular access should be made (≥90 seconds) before moving on to more invasive procedures.

The intraosseous route should be used for the next vascular access attempt. The flat, medial portion of the proximal tibia is most commonly used for the procedure, which is performed with an intraosseous, bone marrow, or spinal needle (Figure 65-1). Fluids and medications, delivered into the marrow cavity, flow into the venous circulation. Intraosseous cannulation is rapid and simple and may be lifesaving. It is limited by low flow rates (approximately 30 mL/min), which can be augmented by using pressure on the IV bag or by pushing fluid by hand through a syringe. Complications associated with intraosseous line placement are rare. All physicians who care for pediatric trauma patients should be familiar with this technique.

A variety of central venous access sites, such as femoral, subclavian, and internal jugular, may be used in older children. Upper and lower saphenous vein cutdowns are also possible access sites. The Seldinger technique, with insertion of a large-bore catheter over a guidewire, is often used. A description of these procedures is beyond the scope of this book but may be found in many other publications, including the 2010 American Heart Association guidelines for cardiopulmonary resuscitation and emergency cardiovascular care of pediatric and neonatal patients (see Selected References). Intravenous access above the diaphragm is preferred in patients with blunt or penetrating abdominal trauma who have the potential for disruption of the vena cava or other large veins.

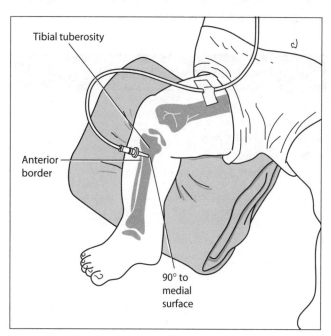

Figure 65-1. Intraosseous cannulation technique.

Fluid replacement begins with a 20- to 40-mL/kg bolus of crystalloid solution, either warmed normal saline or lactated Ringer solution. If no improvement in circulation occurs, additional 10- to 20-mL/kg boluses may be given, and type-specific blood should be considered. In most scenarios, type-specific blood is given after 60 mL/kg of crystalloid has failed to improve circulatory parameters. Frequent hematocrits or hemoglobins should be determined to monitor ongoing blood loss. Vital signs should be repeated frequently. Serial examinations, which detect the signs and symptoms of shock (Box 65-1), are the most important gauge of hemodynamic recovery and stability. All children require close hospital observation, preferably in a pediatric trauma center and pediatric intensive care unit.

Orthostatic fall in blood pressure and supine hypotension (late sign) must be aggressively managed. If hemodynamic stabilization is not achieved after appropriate vascular access and fluid resuscitation, the trauma surgeon will most likely perform an exploratory laparotomy. If children have been stabilized with initial airway and circulatory support, diagnostic procedures such as CT scans can be performed as part of the emergency department evaluation. Once identified, specific organ injury can be managed.

Other specific management concerns for pediatric patients with abdominal injury are early decompression of the stomach with a nasogastric or orogastric tube to prevent respiratory compromise and urinary catheter insertion to decompress the bladder. Before inserting a urinary catheter, the trauma team should evaluate for possible urethral trauma and check for the presence of blood in the urine, which may indicate other genitourinary trauma.

Nonoperative management of minor to moderate liver or spleen injuries is common in children. More severe injuries, including bowel rupture, require surgical intervention.

Box 65-1. Signs and Symptoms of Hemorrhagic Shock in Children
• Tachycardia
• Delayed capillary refill (>2 s)
• Cool and mottled skin, pallor
• Respiratory distress
• Anxiety, irritability, decreased responsiveness
• Thirst

Prognosis

Morbidity and mortality related to abdominal trauma depend on the specific organ injury and style of management. More than 40% of patients with major liver injuries die in the pre-hospital setting. However, a large number of minor liver injuries can be managed without surgery. Currently, an increasing number of injuries to the spleen and liver are managed with observation in the pediatric intensive care unit. Surgical exploration and repair are performed only if patients become hemodynamically unstable. Reduction in anesthetic-related mortality, post-splenectomy sepsis, and a decrease in other postoperative complications have resulted from this shift in practice style. Without surgical intervention, however, a severe injury such as complete splenic rupture has a 90% to 100% mortality rate.

CASE RESOLUTION

The boy in the case study sustained isolated abdominal trauma. Initial presenting signs and symptoms are consistent with internal organ injury, specifically splenic hematoma, pancreatic injury, internal hemorrhage, and compensated shock (eg, tachycardia, tachypnea). The child should undergo initial resuscitation with attention to the airway, breathing, and circulation, especially fluid repletion. Serial hemodynamic measurement and hematocrits, if stable, permit diagnosis of specific injuries by CT scanning. Surgical consultation with expectant observation is the likely management choice. If the child deteriorates, surgical intervention would ensue. Trauma to the small intestine, particularly a duodenal hematoma, must also be suspected because of the mechanism of injury.

Selected References

American College of Surgeons. Advanced Trauma Life Support. http://www.facs.org/trauma/atls/index.html. Accessed February 21, 2014

American College of Surgeons. *Advanced Trauma Life Support (ATLS) Student Manual.* 9th ed. Chicago, IL: American College of Surgeons; 2012

Gaines BA. Intra-abdominal solid organ injury in children: diagnosis and treatment. *J Trauma.* 2009;67(2 Suppl):S135–S139

Hom J. The risk of intra-abdominal injuries in pediatric patients with stable blunt abdominal trauma and negative abdominal computed tomography. *Acad Emerg Med.* 2010;17(5):469–475

Kleinman ME, Charneides L, Schexnayder SM, et al. Pediatric advanced life support: 2010 American Heart Association guidelines for cardiopulmonary resuscitation and emergency cardiovascular care. *Pediatrics.* 2010;126(5):e1361–e1399

Leeson K, Leeson B. Pediatric ultrasound: applications in the emergency department. *Emerg Med Clin North Am.* 2013;31(3):809–829

Schonfeld D, Lee LK. Blunt abdominal trauma in children. *Curr Opin Pediatr.* 2012;24(3):314–318

Sivit CJ. Abdominal trauma imaging: imaging choices and appropriateness. *Pediatr Radiol.* 2009;39(Suppl 2):S158–S160

CHAPTER 66

Acute Abdomen (Appendicitis)

Steve L. Lee, MD

CASE STUDY

A 10-year-old girl presents with abdominal pain for 24 hours. The pain began in the periumbilical area and is now located in the right lower quadrant (RLQ). She had one bout of emesis but no diarrhea. She has no fevers or chills. She also has some pain with voiding. On physical examination, she has a low-grade fever and tachycardia. She is lying still in bed. Her abdomen is non-distended, but she is tender to palpation in the RLQ. She also has rebound tenderness and guarding in this area.

Questions

1. What is the differential diagnosis for patients with acute abdominal pain?
2. What is the appropriate workup for children with suspected appendicitis?
3. What is the current management for children with appendicitis?
4. What is the expected postoperative course and possible complications following appendectomy?

Appendicitis is one of the most common surgical emergencies in children. Pediatricians play a key role in the diagnosis and management of patients with abdominal pain and must be able to distinguish appendicitis from other causes of abdominal pain. When patients present with the classic signs and symptoms of appendicitis, the diagnosis is simple. Unfortunately, roughly 50% of patients will present with atypical signs and symptoms of appendicitis, making the diagnosis difficult. Until recently, there has been controversy in nearly every aspect of the diagnosis and management of children with appendicitis. Thus, it is important for primary care physicians, emergency department physicians, and surgeons to communicate effectively to provide the highest level of care and cost efficiency.

Epidemiology

More than 70,000 cases of appendicitis in children are seen each year in the United States. The lifetime risk of appendicitis is 9% in boys and 7% in girls.

Pathophysiology

The 2 main causes of abdominal pain are distention of the viscera (visceral pain) or irritation of the peritoneum (somatic pain). Distention of any hollow organ in the abdomen will cause crampy and intermittent abdominal pain. Examples include distention of the biliary tree, small or large intestine, urinary structures (bladder or ureters), or gynecologic structures (uterus or fallopian tubes). This visceral pain is poorly localized and will tend to be reported in the midline. Distention of any foregut structure will localize to the epigastric region. Foregut structures derive their blood supply from the celiac trunk and include the stomach, duodenum, and biliary tree. Distention of midgut structures will localize to the periumbilical

region and hindgut structures to the suprapubic region. Midgut structures are supplied by the superior mesenteric artery (duodenum to transverse colon) and hindgut structures by the inferior mesenteric artery (transverse colon to rectum). Unlike visceral pain, somatic pain is well localized. Irritation of the parietal peritoneum leads to sharp pain and localized tenderness on examination. Anything that causes the irritated peritoneum to move or stretch will make the pain and tenderness worse.

The classic example of these 2 types of pain is seen with appendicitis. The basic pathophysiology of appendicitis is obstruction of the lumen of the appendix followed by infection. Obstruction may be caused by fecal material (appendicolith or fecalith), lymphoid hyperplasia, foreign body, tumor, or parasites. Following obstruction, the appendix becomes distended from accumulation of mucus and proliferation of bacteria. This distention leads to vague, periumbilical pain. As intraluminal pressure increases, lymphatic and venous drainage are impaired, resulting in edema of the appendicular wall. As the overlying parietal peritoneum becomes progressively more irritated, the pain localizes to the right lower quadrant (RLQ). This stage is known as *acute appendicitis*. A further increase in pressure will limit arterial inflow and ultimately lead to tissue necrosis and perforation. Although the natural history of untreated appendicitis is usually perforation and abscess, not all patients will progress to perforation.

Clinical Presentation

Abdominal pain is the most common symptom and is present in nearly every patient with appendicitis. The classic presentation of a child with appendicitis includes a history of initial periumbilical pain migrating to the RLQ. The pain is gradual in onset and progressively worsens. Anorexia, nausea, and vomiting are typically associated with appendicitis. In most cases, these associated symptoms develop after the onset of abdominal pain. Intermittent, crampy pain that develops after the onset of vomiting or diarrhea is less commonly associated with appendicitis. The inflamed appendix irritates the overlying peritoneum by direct contact. This leads to focal peritonitis and localized RLQ pain. However, the symptoms vary based on the location of the appendix. When the appendix is retrocecal, a dull ache is often described. When the tip of the appendix is located in the pelvis, atypical pain is described. Children may complain of dysuria and urinary frequency due to the inflamed appendix irritating the bladder. Diarrhea or tenesmus may occur if the appendix is adjacent to the rectum. Fever, tachycardia, and leukocytosis develop as a consequence of systemic inflammatory mediators released by ischemic tissues, white blood cells, and bacteria. Higher fevers are associated with perforated appendicitis.

On physical examination, the patient is usually lying still, as movement worsens the pain. The most common finding is focal tenderness in the RLQ. Only gentle pressure is required to elicit wincing, moving, or guarding. Narcotic analgesics improve the comfort level of the patient but do not alter the inflammatory process; thus, tenderness will still persist. Rebound tenderness is difficult to elicit in children. An easier and more accurate method for determining the degree of peritoneal irritation is to ask the patient to walk or jump. Palpating a mass is difficult and often impossible to detect due to the level of discomfort and guarding.

Differential Diagnosis

Acute appendicitis can mimic nearly any intra-abdominal process and should be high on the differential in all children complaining of abdominal pain. Other causes of RLQ pain that are often indistinguishable from acute appendicitis include mesenteric adenitis, viral gastroenteritis, regional bacterial enteritis, tubo-ovarian pathologic processes, inflammatory bowel disease, Meckel diverticulum, cecal diverticulitis, and constipation. Other causes of lower abdominal pain include urinary tract infection, kidney stone, uterine pathologic process, bowel obstruction, and malignancy (lymphoma). Vague abdominal pain can be caused by right lower lobe pneumonia, sigmoid diverticulitis, pancreatitis, hepatitis, and cholecystitis.

Evaluation

History

A careful history is required to distinguish acute appendicitis from other causes of abdominal pain (Questions Box). In most patients with acute appendicitis, pain is often the first symptom. Associated symptoms such as nausea, vomiting, and diarrhea present after the onset of pain. It is important to distinguish between intermittent crampy pain versus constant and progressively worsening pain. If patients have nausea, vomiting, or diarrhea followed by intermittent crampy pain, the diagnosis of gastroenteritis is more likely than appendicitis. Patients may develop low-grade fevers within 24 hours of the pain. Higher fevers develop later and are seen more frequently

---

Questions

Abdominal Pain

- When did the pain start?
- Can you describe the nature of your pain?
- Is your pain constant or intermittent?
- Where is your pain?
- What makes your pain worse? Better?
- Do you have any fevers or chills?
- Do you have any nausea, vomiting, or diarrhea?
- When was your last bowel movement?
- Is there any pain with urinating?
- Are you hungry?
- When was the last time that you ate? Drank?
- Have you had any sick contacts?
- Have you had any upper respiratory symptoms?

---

with perforated appendicitis. If fever is the first sign/symptom of the patient, appendicitis is less likely.

Physical Examination

A thorough examination is required to rule out other sources of infection. Upper respiratory infections may lead to mesenteric adenitis, causing abdominal pain. Patients with acute appendicitis usually lie still, as movement worsens the pain. The most common finding is focal tenderness in the RLQ. Applying pressure to a stethoscope while listening to the abdomen is a subtle way to palpate the abdomen in frightened children in whom it is difficult to obtain an accurate examination. Because of the level of discomfort, it may be difficult to elicit rebound tenderness and palpate for a mass. Asking the child to walk or jump is an easier and more accurate way of determining the degree of peritoneal irritation. Localized tenderness is dependent on peritoneal irritation; thus, obesity, a retrocecal appendix, or a walled-off appendix by omentum, mesentery, or small bowel may make the diagnosis of appendicitis more challenging.

Laboratory Tests

Laboratory studies often show a mild leukocytosis. A markedly elevated leukocyte count suggests perforation or another diagnosis. A left-shifted differential count may be a better diagnostic indicator for appendicitis. Other inflammatory markers including C-reactive protein, procalcitonin, and lactic acid have also been investigated but have not been routinely used in workup for patients with suspected appendicitis. A urinalysis should also be obtained and is usually free of bacteria, but a few or moderate number of red or white blood cells may be found as the inflammatory process of the appendix may locally irritate the bladder or ureter.

Imaging Studies

Appropriate use of diagnostic imaging can minimize negative appendectomy and perforation rates.

Plain Radiography

In general, plain films of the abdomen and chest may be more useful to evaluate for other disease processes when the suspicion for appendicitis is low. Specific to appendicitis, plain radiography can show fecaliths in 10% to 20% of patients. Other helpful findings include lumbar scoliosis and obliteration of the psoas shadow.

Ultrasonography

Ultrasound is an efficient bedside study that is noninvasive, requires no contrast, and emits no radiation. Ultrasound should be the first study used in the workup of patients with suspected appendicitis. Common ultrasound findings consistent with appendicitis include a fluid-filled, noncompressible tubular structure; a diameter greater than 6 mm; appendicolith; and periappendicular or pericecal fluid (Figure 66-1). In experienced hands and ideal situations, ultrasound has sensitivity greater than 85% and specificity greater than 90%. Results are also influenced by patient factors such as bowel gas pattern, obesity, and guarding or movement. When a normal appendix is identified, it is a reliable study to rule out appendicitis. Unfortunately, only 10% to 50% of children with normal appendixes can be identified. Furthermore, there is still a risk of appendicitis despite an otherwise normal ultrasound when the appendix is not identified.

Computed Tomography

When ultrasound is unable to exclude or confirm appendicitis, additional imaging with computed tomography (CT) scan or observation is warranted. Findings consistent with appendicitis on CT scan include an enlarged appendix (>6 mm), appendicular wall thickening (>1 mm), periappendicular fat stranding, and appendicular wall enhancement (Figure 66-2). The sensitivity and specificity of CT are around 95%. There are, however, several concerns with CT scans: there can be significant delay in obtaining the study if oral contrast is administered; younger children may require sedation to complete the study; and there is also growing concern for the increased radiation exposure from the CT scan (see Chapter 15). Developing tissues are more sensitive to the effects of radiation, as evidenced by an increased risk of radiation-induced malignancy in patients exposed at a younger age.

Observation

When the history, physical examination, laboratory studies, and ultrasound are unable to exclude or confirm appendicitis, additional imaging with CT scan or observation is indicated. Given the radiation risks associated with CT scans, admission to the hospital for intravenous (IV) fluids and serial examinations is a safe alternative. Diets should be withheld and a repeat complete blood cell count with manual differential should be obtained the next morning. In most instances, patients who do not have appendicitis will improve and can be safely given a diet and discharged home. In children with appendicitis, their pain will increase and IV antibiotics should be administered while arrangements for appendectomy are made.

Figure 66-1. Ultrasound images consistent with acute appendicitis: A, transverse view. B, longitudinal view. The arrows are used to measure the diameter of the appendix in both images.

Figure 66-2. Computed tomography scan image consistent with appendicitis. Arrow points to inflamed appendix.

Management

The treatment of appendicitis begins with IV fluids and broad-spectrum IV antibiotics. Single-agent or double-agent therapy has been shown to be as effective and more cost-efficient than triple-agent antibiotics. Management after initiating antimicrobial therapy is based on whether patients are likely to have non-perforated or perforated appendicitis. This distinction is not always clear, even if preoperative imaging studies have been obtained. For patients presenting with symptoms than have been present less than 24 hours, the risk of having perforated appendicitis is low. These patients should be adequately resuscitated with IV fluids and antibiotics and scheduled for appendectomy. Once antibiotic therapy has been started, it is likely that the progression of disease has been halted or even reversed. Thus, the likelihood of non-perforated appendicitis progressing to perforated appendicitis is highly unlikely once appropriate antibiotics have been started. For this reason, appendectomy may be considered a semi-elective operation rather than an urgent or emergent procedure as it has been considered in the past. When the duration of symptoms is longer than 24 hours, the risk of perforation increases. For the most part, patients with fewer than 5 to 7 days of symptoms are treated as described previously. Patients with more than 7 days of symptoms will likely have perforated appendicitis with or without an abscess. In patients with prolonged duration of symptoms, appendectomy can be more technically challenging and associated with higher postoperative complications. To potentially decrease these risks, nonoperative management has been employed. Nonoperative management includes administration of IV antibiotics and drainage of intra-abdominal abscess (if present) using interventional radiologic techniques. Initial nonoperative management is successful in approximately 85% of patients. Once clinically stable, patients are discharged and elective interval appendectomy is typically performed in 6 to 8 weeks. If patients fail nonoperative management, appendectomy will be performed. Nonoperative management remains a controversial topic, and many surgeons will not attempt this treatment plan but proceed to immediate appendectomy once the patient is adequately resuscitated.

McBurney first described open appendectomy through a traditional RLQ incision and muscle-splitting technique in 1893. Laparoscopic appendectomy was introduced more than 30 years ago and has, for the most part, replaced open appendectomy. Laparoscopic appendectomy is associated with lower wound infection rates, shorter lengths of hospitalization, less postoperative outpatient visits, and earlier return to routine activity. While earlier studies associated laparoscopic appendectomy with higher postoperative abscess rates and longer duration of operation, more recent studies show no difference in both of these areas. In fact, some studies have shown shorter operative and lower abscess rates with laparoscopic appendectomy.

For patients with non-perforated appendicitis, antibiotics should be administered for 24 hours or less. A single preoperative dose of antibiotics has shown to decrease the risk of wound infection and abscess. For patients with perforated appendicitis, IV antibiotics should be administered until resolution of clinical symptoms. This includes resolution of fever, normalization of physical examination,

full return of gastrointestinal function, and normalization of leukocyte count and differential. If this duration of IV antibiotic therapy is for fewer than 5 days, patients can be safely discharged on oral antibiotics to complete a 7-day course.

Prognosis

Overall complication rates are less than 3% for non-perforated appendicitis and 16% to 18% for perforated appendicitis. The common complications following appendectomy are infection-related. With respect to wound infections, this complication occurs in less than 1% of patients with non-perforated appendicitis and up to 16% of patients with perforated appendicitis. Rates of postoperative abscess are less than 1% for non-perforated appendicitis and less than 15% for perforated appendicitis. Mortality related to appendicitis is rare.

CASE RESOLUTION

This patient was found to have an elevated white blood cell count with a left shift and a small number of white blood cells in the urinalysis. Ultrasound findings were consistent with acute appendicitis. She was administered intravenous fluids and antibiotics and underwent laparoscopic appendectomy. Her postoperative course was unremarkable and she was discharged the next day. She was doing well in follow-up and cleared for full activity 2 weeks after laparoscopic appendectomy.

Selected References

Blakely ML, Williams R, Dassinger MS, et al. Early vs interval appendectomy for children with perforated appendicitis. *Arch Surg*. 2011;146(6):660–665

Chen C, Botelho C, Cooper A, Hibberd P, Parsons SK. Current practice patterns in the treatment of perforated appendicitis in children. *J Am Coll Surg*. 2003; 196(2):212–221

Jaremko JL, Crockett A, Rucker D, Magnus KG. Incidence and significance of inconclusive results in ultrasound for appendicitis in children and teenagers. *Can Assoc Radiol J*. 2011;62(3):197–202

Lee SL, Islam S, Cassidy LD, Abdullah F, Arca MJ; 2010 American Pediatric Surgical Association Outcomes and Clinical Trials Committee. Antibiotics and appendicitis in the pediatric population: an American Pediatric Surgical Association Outcomes and Clinical Trials Committee systematic review. *J Pediatr Surg*. 2010;45(11):2181–2185

Lee SL, Yaghoubian A, Kaji A. Laparoscopic vs open appendectomy in children: outcomes comparison based on age, sex, and perforation status. *Arch Surg*. 2011;146(10):1118–1121

Martin AE, Vollman D, Adler B, Caniano DA. CT scans may not reduce the negative appendectomy rate in children. *J Pediatr Surg*. 2004;39(6):886–890

CHAPTER 67

Head Trauma

Joseph Ravera, MD

CASE STUDY

A 2-year-old girl is playing on a window ledge unsupervised. She pushes the screen out and falls onto the concrete sidewalk below, striking her head. A neighbor reports that she is unconscious for 10 minutes. When paramedics arrive, the girl is awake but lethargic. She is transported to the emergency department. Her vital signs are normal. A scalp hematoma is present, and a depressed area of cranial bone is palpated.

Questions

1. What are the priorities in the initial stabilization and management of pediatric head trauma?
2. What is the difference between primary and secondary brain injury?
3. What are the common structural injuries sustained by children with head trauma?
4. What are the various modalities available for treatment of increased intracranial pressure?
5. What are the scoring systems used in the evaluation of mental status in children with head trauma?

Although most childhood head injuries are minor and can be treated on an outpatient basis, it is important for clinicians to become adept at recognizing and managing concussions and more severe forms of head injury. Health care professionals can also help lower mortality from head trauma by actively promoting injury prevention to patients and communities.

Epidemiology

Head trauma is one of the most common pediatric injuries and the leading cause of morbidity and mortality among pediatric trauma patients. Pediatric head trauma accounts for more than 500,000 emergency department (ED) visits, 95,000 hospital admissions, 7,000 deaths, and 29,000 permanent disabilities per year in the United States. Hospital care costs exceed a billion dollars annually. In multiple-injured pediatric patients, 70% of the deaths that occur within 48 hours of hospitalization are the result of trauma to the head. Rates of intracranial injuries in children with only minor head trauma, however, are low, with the largest numbers occurring in young children and infants with an incidence of 3% to 6%. Only 0.4% to 1% of children require surgical intervention after minor closed head injury.

Falls account for most cases of pediatric head trauma. Other major causes include motor vehicle crashes, vehicle versus pedestrian collisions, bicycle crashes, sports-related injuries, and recreational activities. Non-accidental trauma (ie, child abuse) must be recognized as another important cause of head injury in children, particularly among those younger than 2 years.

Clinical Presentation

Children who have sustained head trauma may present with a history of an antecedent event (eg, fall, collision with another child) or signs and symptoms related to the injury. These include external bruises or lacerations, alterations in the level of consciousness, and neurologic findings, including seizures. Vital signs may be altered; in particular, deep or irregular respirations, hypertension, or bradycardia may be apparent (D_x Box). These changes are indicative of elevated intracranial pressure (ICP).

Pathophysiology

Children have significant anatomic differences from adults that predispose them to head trauma and certain types of intracranial injuries. They have a higher center of gravity, an increased head-body ratio, and weaker neck muscles compared with adults. In addition, children have thinner cranial bones and less myelinated brain tissue, predisposing them to intraparenchymal injuries. Whereas adults are more likely to have focal intracranial

---

Dx | Head Trauma[a]

- Loss of consciousness
- Somnolence
- Pallor
- Emesis/nausea/anorexia
- Irritability
- Lethargy
- Seizure
- Ataxia
- Weakness
- Pain
- Paresthesias
- Amnesia
- Headache
- Visual changes
- Confusion/altered mental status

[a]All of these symptoms may not be present in head trauma.

hematomas, children are more likely to develop diffuse cerebral edema. Cerebral edema can disrupt cerebral blood flow, resulting in ischemic injury.

Normally, blood flow to the brain is maintained at a constant rate by a process known as *autoregulation*. With severe brain injury, autoregulation is disrupted and blood flow to the brain is determined by cerebral perfusion pressure (CPP), which is a measure of the mean arterial pressure (MAP) minus ICP (CPP = MAP − ICP). Cerebral blood flow is therefore compromised when the MAP is too low (ie, hypotension) or the ICP is too high (ie, cerebral edema). Several of the management strategies in children with severe brain injuries focus on maintaining MAP and reducing ICP, but control of CPP after head injury can be quite difficult. Children have a greater capacity for recovery than adults, especially infants and very young children, whose open sutures and fontanels permit expansion of the skull in response to edema and blood.

In head trauma, primary and secondary brain injury can occur (Figure 67-1). Primary injury is the structural damage that occurs to the cranium and its contents at the time of injury. Secondary injury is damage to the brain tissue after the initial event. Such damage may result from hypoxia, hypoperfusion, hypercapnia, hyperthermia, and altered glucose or sodium metabolism. The main management strategies for head trauma victims focus on the prevention of secondary brain injury. Primary brain injury can only be prevented through education and safety.

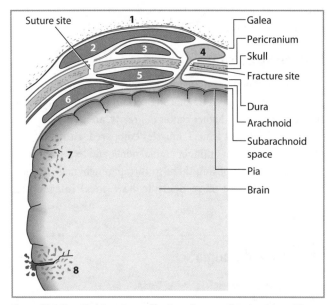

Figure 67-1. Functional anatomy of brain and surrounding structures with sites of pathology. 1, Caput succedaneum. 2, Subgaleal hematoma. 3, Cephalhematoma. 4, Porencephalic or arachnoid cyst. 5, Epidural hematoma. 6, Subdural hematoma. 7, Cerebral contusion. 8, Cerebral laceration. (From Tecklenburg FW, Wright MS. Minor head trauma in the pediatric patient. *Pediatr Emerg Care.* 1991;7[1]:40–47, with permission from Wolters Kluwer Health.)

Types of Head Injuries

Even minor head trauma in children can result in fractures to the skull or intracranial injuries. Most skull fractures are simple and linear. Other fracture types are comminuted, diastatic, basilar, and depressed. Comminuted fractures occur when there are multiple skull fragments. Diastatic fractures occur when there is a wide separation at the fracture site. Basilar fractures occur at the base of the skull and often have characteristic findings on physical examination (ie, bilateral periorbital ecchymosis, hemotympanum, postauricular ecchymosis [Battle sign]). Depressed fracture occurs when fragments of the skull are displaced inward, potentially damaging intracranial structures.

Head trauma may result in a **concussion** or mild traumatic brain injury. A concussion is defined as a trauma-induced impairment of neurologic function. This may occur with or without a loss of consciousness (LOC). Neurologic examination is usually normal, but patients may experience somatic symptoms (eg, headache), physical signs (eg, LOC, amnesia), behavioral changes, cognitive impairment, or sleep disturbances. Some of these minor and subtle neurologic sequelae can last for months following the injury (postconcussion syndrome). Most resolve over a relatively short period, typically 7 to 10 days.

A **cerebral contusion** is essentially a bruise of the brain tissue and typically occurs with a more severe injury, such as a high-speed motor vehicle crash. A coup-contrecoup–type injury may be produced when the brain strikes the skull on direct impact, bruising one portion of the brain, and then injury occurs to the opposite portion of the brain when rapid deceleration occurs. Clinical manifestations depend on the location of the contusion but often include altered mental status, excessive sleepiness, confusion, and agitation. Small intraparenchymal hemorrhages and swelling of the surrounding tissues are often seen on computed tomography (CT) scan.

Epidural hematomas are collections of blood that accumulate between the skull bone and the tough outer covering of the brain (dura mater). They are often the result of tears in the middle meningeal artery caused by skull fractures. Classically, patients have initial LOC followed by a lucid interval and then rapid deterioration secondary to brain compression. On CT scan, an epidural hematoma appears as a large collection of blood with convex borders next to the skull (Figure 67-2A). Surgical evacuation is required in most cases.

Subdural hematomas accumulate between the dura and the underlying brain tissue. They are associated with skull fractures and contusions. On CT scan, they appear to have crescent-shaped borders (Figure 67-2B). Large subdural hematomas usually require surgical evacuation. In infants and young children, these are often the result of non-accidental trauma.

Diffuse axonal injury (DAI) occurs when there is extensive damage to the axonal white matter of the brain that results from shearing forces that typically occur with rapid acceleration or deceleration of the brain (Figure 67-2C). Children who suffer DAI may have normal or nonspecific CT scans.

Figure 67-2. A, Epidural hematoma, marked by the asterisk. Note convex borders and midline shift. B, Subdural hematoma. Note crescent shape. C, Diffuse axonal injury. Note ground-glass appearance and tightly compressed ventricles. (Reproduced with permission from Harris JH Jr, Harris WH, Norelline RA. *The Radiology of Emergency Medicine*. 3rd ed. Baltimore, MD: Williams & Wilkins; 1993:15, 16, 17.)

Evaluation

History

Historical data are obtained during the secondary survey or reassessment phase of evaluation. Prehospital health care practitioners or witnesses to the injury should be asked about details of the event and the child's status following the event (Questions Box).

Physical Examination

Careful attention to the vital signs of children with head injuries is important. The presence of hypertension, bradycardia, and an irregular breathing pattern **(Cushing triad)** suggests a significant intracranial injury with associated increased ICP.

Secondary survey actions include palpation and inspection of the scalp for soft-tissue swelling, step-offs, lacerations, and fullness of the fontanel. Facial bones should be tested for stability and deformities. Other clues to possible head trauma include the presence of a septal hematoma, draining blood or fluid from the nose or ears, dental injury, and malocclusion of the mandible. The tympanic membranes should be visualized for the presence of hemotympanum or cerebrospinal fluid (CSF) otorrhea, which, along with postauricular

ecchymosis **(Battle sign),** periorbital ecchymosis, or cranial nerve palsies, suggests a basilar skull fracture. Funduscopic examination should be performed if possible to look for the presence of papilledema associated with increased ICP or **retinal hemorrhages** that indicate non-accidental trauma.

A comprehensive neurologic examination is the most important part of the secondary survey. This examination should include a mental status assessment, cranial nerve evaluation, presence and quality of deep tendon reflexes, muscle tone, muscle strength, sensation, and cerebellar function. When describing mental status, imprecise terms such as *altered, lethargic,* and *obtunded* should be avoided. Several widely used scoring systems are available for mental status assessment of children who have suffered head trauma that are useful predictors of intracranial injury. A number of scales exist for assessment of the level of consciousness. The most universally accepted and widely used of these scales is the **Glasgow Coma Score** (GCS). It is used routinely in children older than 5 years but can be modified for younger children. Each scoring system has 3 measured responses (eye opening, verbal, and motor) to a variety of stimuli. Scores should be tabulated when children first present to establish a baseline. They can then be used for reassessment on a regular basis until patients have stabilized or returned to normal mental status. Use of these scores helps promote consistent and accurate communication among health care practitioners. Tables 67-1 and 67-2 show how to calculate the GCS and modified GCS.

Table 67-1. Glasgow Coma Score		
Elements		*Points*
1. Eye opening		
	a. Spontaneous	4
	b. To command	3
	c. With pain	2
	d. No response	1
2. Verbal response[a]		
	a. Oriented, converses normally	5
	b. Disoriented, confused	4
	c. Utters inappropriate words	3
	d. Incomprehensible sounds	2
	e. No response	1
3. Motor response		
	a. Obeys commands	6
	b. Localizes pain	5
	c. Flexes with pain	4
	d. Flexes abnormally with pain	3
	e. Extensor response	2
	f. None	1
Maximum score		*15*

[a]Assessment of verbal response is modified in children (see Table 67-2).

Head Trauma — Questions

- What was the mechanism of injury (eg, motor vehicle crash, ejection from motor vehicle, fall, assault)?
- What was the height of the fall?
- What was the type of impact surface?
- What was the shape of the object(s) striking the head?
- What was the child's immediate status after injury?
- What changes in status occurred before arrival at the hospital?
- Did the child lose consciousness? If so, for how long?
- Did the child vomit?
- Did the child have a seizure? If so, when did it occur in relation to the injury, and does the child have an underlying seizure disorder?

Table 67-2. Modified Glasgow Coma Score for Younger Children		
Elements		**Points**
1.	**Eye opening**	
	a. Spontaneous	4
	b. To command	3
	c. With pain	2
	d. No response	1
2.	**Verbal response**[a]	
	a. Coos and babbles	5
	b. Irritable cry	4
	c. Cries to pain	3
	d. Moans to pain	2
	e. None	1
3.	**Motor response**	
	a. Normal spontaneous movement	6
	b. Withdraws to touch	5
	c. Withdraws to pain	4
	d. Abnormal flexion	3
	e. Abnormal extension	2
	f. None	1
Maximum score		**15**

[a]Assessment of verbal response is modified in children.

The secondary survey should be completed to identify any additional life- or limb-threatening injuries.

Laboratory Testing

All pediatric patients with significant head trauma should have a complete blood cell count and serum electrolytes performed. Bedside glucose should be performed in any child with a head injury with an altered level of consciousness. Toxicologic evaluation may be indicated in adolescents who appear to be intoxicated or have an altered level of consciousness. Those infants and children with an intracranial hemorrhage should have screening coagulation studies performed (ie, prothrombin time, activated partial thromboplastin time), as well as a type and screen or crossmatch, should surgery be required.

Imaging Studies

In cases of acute pediatric blunt or penetrating trauma, a noncontrast CT of the head is currently the diagnostic study of choice. It is very sensitive for the detection of acute hemorrhages and skull fractures. It can also provide additional information on the severity of injury indicating increased ICP, cerebral edema, or pending herniation. Some of the findings on CT scan that indicate severe brain injury are the shift of midline structures, effacement of the sulci, ventricular enlargement or compression, and loss of normal gray-white matter differentiation.

All children with altered mental status, a GCS below 14, penetrating trauma, or focal neurologic deficits warrant an emergent head CT scan. The question of which children with minor head trauma should receive a CT scan was evaluated in a study of 17,000 children from the Pediatric Emergency Care Applied Research Network database. In this study, a decision rule was retrospectively derived and then prospectively validated as a method to identify children at very low risk for intracranial injury. These criteria can be found in Box 67-1. If children are otherwise healthy and meet these criteria, their risk of intracranial injury is extremely low and they can be safely discharged from the ED or clinic without a CT and with appropriate return precautions. It should be noted that this decision rule was validated as "rule out" only and meant to identify those children at very low risk. All children who fail the rule do not necessarily need a head CT scan. In cases in which a child meets all but one or otherwise looks well, the practitioner may consider a period of observation to monitor for progression of symptoms. The optimal time of observation has not been well studied, but 6 hours from time of injury is usually considered standard in most EDs.

With the speed and widespread availability of CT scanners, skull radiographs have relatively little role in the acute evaluation of pediatric head trauma patients. Current CT scans can be performed very quickly, often with little or no need for sedation. Although sensitive for the detection of skull fractures, plain radiographs do not provide any information about associated intracranial injuries. In addition, several studies have demonstrated that intracranial injuries occur in the absence of a skull fracture, particularly among young pediatric patients. The role of plain radiographs is limited to part of the skeletal survey in suspected cases of non-accidental trauma.

Magnetic resonance imaging (MRI) has little role in the management of the acutely injured head trauma victim. Computed tomography scan is often more sensitive at detecting acute intracranial hemorrhages and is sufficient to guide most immediate patient care issues. Magnetic resonance imaging may be superior to CT for identifying DAI and subtle brain injuries. In general, MRI takes longer to complete and often requires sedation, and the scanners are frequently located away from the ED where the child cannot be monitored appropriately.

One important consideration of any trauma victim is the possibility of a cervical spine injury. Although cervical spine injuries are

Box 67-1. Low-Risk Criteria for Pediatric Intracranial Injury	
Age <2 y	**Age >2 y**
• Normal mental status	• Normal mental status
• No scalp hematoma except frontal	• No loss of consciousness
• No loss of consciousness, or loss of consciousness for <5 seconds	• No vomiting
• Non-severe injury mechanism	• Non-severe injury mechanism
• No palpable skull fracture	• No signs of basilar skull fracture
• Acting normally according to parents	• No severe headache

rare in children, the clinician must maintain a high index of suspicion when presented with a child who has suffered significant head trauma, particularly from a high-energy mechanism such as an unrestrained motor vehicle crash. All children with an altered level of consciousness; significant, painful, distracting injuries; an inability to communicate; focal neurologic deficits; or localized pain, swelling, or ecchymosis of the cervical spine require careful evaluation and imaging of the cervical spine. Younger children (<8 years) have a larger occiput-body ratio and consequently a higher fulcrum; thus, most cervical spine injuries in this age group tend to be at higher levels (C1, C2, C3). Furthermore, due to increased flexibility and lack of ossification, children are at risk for ligamentous or direct cord injury in the absence of a bony injury. Clinicians should maintain a high index of suspicion with severely injured children, even if there is no bony injury evident on radiographs or CT.

Management

Assessment and management occur simultaneously when an acutely injured child presents. A primary survey is initially performed with attention to airway, breathing, circulation, and cervical spine immobilization. Prompt neurosurgical consultation should be obtained for all children with significant head trauma to assess the need for operative management and ICP monitoring. The primary management goal of significant acute head trauma is the prevention of secondary brain injury by maximizing oxygenation and ventilation, supporting circulation to maximize cerebral perfusion, decreasing elevated ICP, and decreasing cerebral metabolic demands.

Individuals with significant intracranial injuries will often require intubation for airway protection. Those individuals with a GCS of 8 or lower should undergo **rapid sequence intubation** to control the airway. These individuals should be premedicated with etomidate, a sedative that is cardiovascular neutral with minimal effect on blood pressure. Most other sedatives can result in hypotension, thereby lowering MAP and reducing CPP. Although there is little evidence to support improved outcomes, lidocaine may be considered as an adjuvant to potentially blunt the transient increase in ICP often associated with orotracheal intubation. When intubation is indicated, steps should be taken to minimize desaturations, as several studies have demonstrated worse outcomes with hypoxia in children with severe traumatic brain injury.

In the past, moderate hyperventilation was advocated to reduce ICP. Hyperventilation lowers arterial carbon dioxide partial pressure (Pco_2), leading to cerebral vasoconstriction and decreased cerebral blood flow, lowering ICP. This has been shown to have the unwanted effect of disrupting cerebral metabolism and possibly exacerbating ischemic injury. Currently, normal ventilation is recommended with the goal of maintaining Pco_2 no lower than 34 mm Hg. Moderate hyperventilation may have a role in the transient management of serious or acute life-threatening elevations in ICP (ie, acute herniation).

Circulation and MAP should be aggressively supported with fluids to prevent hypoperfusion to the brain. Hypovolemia or hypotension should never be assumed to result from head trauma alone.

Children should be examined carefully for evidence of additional injury. Central venous pressure monitoring is often necessary to accurately assess volume status. Pressors may be necessary to maintain MAP in euvolemic patients. Morbidity has been shown to significantly increase with subsequent episodes of hypotension that occur.

Elevations in ICP may impede cerebral blood flow and exacerbate ischemic injury. Administration of hypertonic solutions is indicated in the management of increased ICP, particularly with signs of herniation. In the most recent guidelines, hypertonic (3%) saline is the first-line agent as opposed to mannitol. In addition, elevation of the head of the bed to 30 degrees to promote venous drainage is an example of a method used to reduce ICP. Use of mannitol and other diuretics is contraindicated in patients with borderline blood pressures because they can cause hypotension, which can in turn lower MAP, worsening cerebral perfusion. Paralytic agents, sedatives, and analgesics may be needed to prevent agitation, which also leads to increased ICP and increases cerebral metabolic demands. Painful procedures (eg, suctioning) should receive adequate premedication with sedatives and analgesics. Intraventricular pressure catheters are often necessary to allow for close monitoring of ICP. In addition, they can be used to drain CSF to help lower elevated ICP.

Hyperthermia and seizure activity should be managed aggressively because they increase cerebral metabolic demands. Hyperthermia should be managed with antipyretics and active cooling measures. There is conflicting evidence on controlled hypothermia in children with severe brain injuries. Future studies will hopefully determine if this is of some benefit, as has been shown in certain animal models. Anticonvulsant prophylaxis should also be considered in children with severe brain injuries, especially within the first 7 days. It is important to remember that the ability to detect clinical seizure activity is lost if the child is paralyzed.

Serum electrolytes should be followed closely, and any alterations should be minimized. Patients with head injuries should be monitored closely for the development of diabetes insipidus or syndrome of inappropriate secretion of antidiuretic hormone.

Children with large epidural and subdural hematomas will frequently require surgical evacuation. Individuals with depressed skull fractures often require operative management to lift the depressed fragment away from the underlying brain. Children who have suffered significant penetrating head trauma warrant antibiotic and antiepileptic prophylaxis and may need angiography to assess for vascular injury. They should all have their tetanus status updated if necessary.

Children with minor head injuries (GCS = 14–15) with no LOC or a brief witnessed period of LOC, no focal deficits on neurologic examination, no skull fractures, and without persistent vomiting who demonstrate improvement and normal mental status (GCS = 15) after 4 to 6 hours of observation can be discharged with written instructions if they have adequate transportation back to the hospital, a telephone, and a reliable parent or guardian. Children should be admitted if these criteria cannot be met. Younger children (<2 years) are more difficult to assess accurately and consistently and are at higher risk for intracranial injuries. Admission should be strongly considered if their mental status is not completely normal or at baseline. Physicians should be wary of discharging children whose conditions have not improved to baseline following minor injuries or who have persistent emesis, even if their CT scans are normal.

More moderate head injuries (initial GCS = 9–12) necessitate a longer period of evaluation, probably in a monitored setting along with neurosurgical consultation. Severe head injuries (GCS <8) require aggressive stabilization in the ED with the measures described previously and admission to a pediatric intensive care unit.

Children who have suffered a concussion warrant close observation and reevaluation before resuming sporting activities because there is mounting evidence that multiple, sequential concussions can have long-term debilitating effects. The American Academy of Neurology has guidelines for the evaluation and return-to-play parameters. These recommendations include an evaluation by a health care professional familiar with concussions and the use of sideline assessment tools to rapidly evaluate athletes for removal from play. Before returning to play, athletes should have complete physical and cognitive rest until they are symptom-free. In addition, they should have a normal neurologic examination and normal imaging (if performed). Some programs employ neuropsychiatric testing, to evaluate for subtle deficits, in the evaluation of return to play. In general, emergency clinicians should stress to athletes being evaluated the serious nature of a concussion and not clear athletes to play from the ED but, rather, refer them through the appropriate protocols of their team.

Prognosis

Age is the most important prognostic factor in outcome. Younger children tend to do better than older children. It is still difficult to predict the outcome of any individual patient. Scalp lacerations, most skull fractures, and concussions are low-risk injuries. Intracranial hemorrhage, specific skull fractures, head injury secondary to nonaccidental trauma, and trauma accompanied by diffuse cerebral edema are high-risk injuries. If untreated, severe head injury may lead to death from herniation.

Other complications from severe head trauma are posttraumatic seizures, requiring lifelong treatment with anticonvulsants; hydrocephalus, necessitating placement of a ventriculoperitoneal shunt catheter; and persistent vegetative or severely impaired mental states. Penetrating head injuries can result in infections (eg, meningitis, abscess) and vascular injuries (eg, aneurysm, arteriovenous malformations). Sequelae such as postconcussion syndrome may result from less severe head trauma. Some of the characteristics of this syndrome include dizziness, headache, irritability, memory deficits, impaired behavior, and impaired cognitive development. These may persist for months after the head injury and can sometimes be permanent. These children may warrant formal neurobehavioral testing.

Prevention

Despite advancing medical knowledge and excellent critical care available to children with head trauma, little can be done to reduce the severity of primary brain injury once it has occurred. Therefore, pediatric health care professionals should make every attempt to educate patients and families about prevention strategies. Some of the most successful prevention strategies involve the required use of restraint devices such as seat belts and proper safety gear such as bicycle helmets. Anticipatory guidance and home safety recommendations provided to parents are also worthwhile. Finally, communities can contribute to injury prevention by providing playground resurfacing, reducing the height of playground equipment, and changing traffic laws. It is only through a combination of these prevention strategies that morbidity and mortality of pediatric head trauma will be truly reduced.

CASE RESOLUTION

The case scenario involves a young child with a significant mechanism of injury, brief loss of consciousness, and a depressed, altered mental status. Initial physical findings prompt suspicion of a depressed skull fracture and overlying soft tissue injury. Appropriate diagnostic tools after evaluation of airway, breathing, and circulation are a cranial computed tomography scan followed by admission for observation, monitoring, and serial neurologic examination. Operative repair of the skull fracture may be necessary.

Selected References

Atabaki SM, Stiell IG, Bazarian JJ, et al. A clinical decision rule for cranial computed tomography in minor pediatric head trauma. *Arch Pediatr Adolesc Med.* 2008;162(5):439–445

Bruce DA. Head trauma. In: Fleisher GR, Ludwig S, eds. *Textbook of Pediatric Emergency Medicine.* 5th ed. Baltimore, MD: Williams & Wilkins; 2005

Dunning J, Daly JP, Lomas JP, Lecky F, Batchelor J, Makway-Jones K. Derivation of the children's head injury algorithm for the prediction of important clinical events decision rule for head injury in children. *Arch Dis Child.* 2006;91(11): 885–891

Giza CC, Kutcher JS, Ashwal S, et al. Summary of evidence-based guideline update: evaluation and management of concussion in sports: report of the Guideline Development Subcommittee of the American Academy of Neurology. *Neurology.* 2013;80(24):2250–2257

Goldstein B, Powers KS. Head trauma in children. *Pediatr Rev.* 1994;15(6): 213–219

Halstead ME, Walter KD; American Academy of Pediatrics Council on Sports Medicine and Fitness. Sport-related concussion in children and adolescents. *Pediatrics.* 2010;126(3):597–615

Huh JW, Raghupathi R. New concepts in treatment of pediatric traumatic brain injury. *Anesthesiol Clin.* 2009;27(2):213–240

Hutchison JS, Ward RE, Lacroix J, et al. Hypothermia therapy after traumatic brain injury in children. *N Engl J Med.* 2008;358(23):2447–2456

Kirkwood MW, Yeates KO, Wilson PE. Pediatric sport-related concussion: a review of the clinical management of an oft-neglected population. *Pediatrics.* 2006;117(4):1359–1371

Kochanek P, Carney N, Adelson PD, et al. Guidelines for the acute medical management of severe traumatic brain injury in infants, children, and adolescents—second edition. *Pediatr Crit Care Med.* 2012;13(Suppl 1):S1–S82

Koestler J, Keshavarz R. Penetrating head injury in children: a case report and review of the literature. *J Emerg Med.* 2001;21(2):145–150

Kuppermann N, Holmes JF, Dayan PS, et al. Identification of children at very low risk of clinically-important brain injuries after head trauma: a prospective cohort study. *Lancet.* 2009;374(9696):1160–1170

McCrory P, Meeuwisse W, Johnston K, et al. Consensus statement on concussion in sport: the 3rd International Conference on Concussion in Sport held in Zurich, November 2008. *J Athl Train.* 2009;44(4):434–448

Michaud LJ, Duhaime AC, Batshaw ML. Traumatic brain injury in children. *Pediatr Clin North Am.* 1993;40(3):553–565

Osmond MH, Klassen TP, Wells GA, et al. CATCH: a clinical decision rule for the use of computed tomography in children with minor head injury. *CMAJ.* 2010;182(4):341–348

Palchak MJ, Holmes JF, Vance CW, et al. A decision rule for identifying children at low risk for brain injuries after blunt head trauma. *Ann Emerg Med.* 2003; 42(4):492–506

Palchak MJ, Holmes JF, Vance CW, et al. Does an isolated history of loss of consciousness or amnesia predict brain injuries in children after blunt head trauma? *Pediatrics.* 2004;113(6):e507–e513

Rivara FP. Epidemiology and prevention of pediatric traumatic brain injury. *Pediatr Ann.* 1994;23(1):12–17

Schutzman SA, Barnes P, Duhaime AC, et al. Evaluation and management of children younger than two years old with apparently minor head trauma: proposed guidelines. *Pediatrics.* 2001;107(5):983–993

Schutzman SA, Greenes DS. Pediatric minor head trauma. *Ann Emerg Med.* 2001;37(1):65–74

Sun BC, Hoffman JR, Mower WR. Evaluation of a modified prediction instrument to identify significant pediatric intracranial injury after blunt head trauma. *Ann Emerg Med.* 2007;49(3):325–332

Swaminathan A, Levy P, Legome E. Evaluation and management of moderate to severe pediatric head trauma. *J Emerg Med.* 2009;37(1):63–68

Tecklenburg FW, Wright MS. Minor head trauma in the pediatric patient. *Pediatr Emerg Care.* 1991;7(1):40–47

Zuckerman GB, Conway EE Jr. Accidental head injury. *Pediatr Ann.* 1997;26(10): 621–632

CHAPTER 68

Increased Intracranial Pressure

Kenneth R. Huff, MD

CASE STUDY

A 7-year-old boy has a 2-week history of recurrent vomiting. No fever, abdominal pain, or diarrhea has accompanied the vomiting; the vomiting has no particular relationship to meals; and the boy's appetite has decreased only slightly. The vomiting has gradually increased in frequency and is occurring every night. Yesterday there were 4 episodes. The boy's parents have noticed that their son is generally less active; he spends more time playing on the floor of his room and does not want to ride his bicycle or play with neighborhood friends. Some unsteadiness in the boy's gait has developed in the last few days. His parents attribute this to weakness from the vomiting.

The child's vital signs are normal except for a blood pressure of 130/80 mm Hg. Although the boy is somewhat pale and uncomfortable, he does not appear to be in acute distress. His abdominal examination is unremarkable. His speech is grammatically correct but sparse and hesitant, and he seems inattentive. On lateral and upward gaze the boy has coarse nystagmus, and upward gaze is somewhat limited. Dysconjugate left gaze is apparent, with slight failure of left eye abduction. The left eye does not blink as much as the right eye. Fundal examination discloses elevated disks with indistinct margins. No upper extremity weakness is evident. The right foot is slightly weaker than the left, ankle tone is bilaterally increased, and 3 to 4 beats of clonus on the right and bilateral positive Babinski reflexes are present. Some tremor occurs in both arms with finger-to-nose testing. The boy walks with shuffling, small steps; his gait has a slight lurching character; and he veers to the right.

Questions

1. What clinical situations are associated with increased intracranial pressure (ICP)?
2. What is the pathophysiological process leading to ICP?
3. What studies are used to evaluate children with ICP?
4. What measures are used to treat children with ICP?

The signs and symptoms of increased intracranial pressure (ICP) are often a signal of a serious intracranial process that may require surgical or intensive care intervention depending on the underlying cause. Although only a relatively small number of effective medical and surgical treatments for increased ICP are available, greater understanding is accumulating about when to initiate them. It is important to recognize signs and symptoms early and determine the underlying cause; treatment of the cause often resolves the secondarily increased ICP problem, particularly if deployed early in its course. In some cases, however, increased ICP is a potentially life-threatening critical care issue of itself where ongoing management, along with that of the underlying cause, is key for the child's survival.

Epidemiology

Head trauma is a leading cause of increased ICP. Infants may be victims of non-accidental trauma; older children may be stricken pedestrians or bicycle riders, occupants of crashed motor vehicles, or victims of falls or sports injuries; and children of any age may be victims of penetrating trauma such as gunshots. Such trauma is a major source of morbidity in children and requires careful monitoring and management of ICP.

Brain tumors are the most common solid neoplasms in children and frequently lead to increased ICP by direct mass effect or blockage of cerebrospinal fluid (CSF) flow. Ischemic brain damage resulting from a difficult delivery at birth, a submersion incident, or a major cerebral vessel thrombosis is also a cause of increased ICP. Cytotoxic causes of brain swelling, such as lead intoxication and liver failure in Reye syndrome, are less common etiologies.

Idiopathic intracranial hypertension (also called benign intracranial hypertension or pseudotumor cerebri) may also lead to increased ICP. This condition is associated most frequently with obese adolescent females but has also been seen with thrombosis of a venous sinus caused by a clotting diathesis or complicated otitis media or mastoiditis, following the use of high doses of vitamin A or tetracycline, or following withdrawal of steroid therapy.

Clinical Presentation

Children with increased ICP may present with a history of recurrent vomiting, lethargy, and new headaches of increasing frequency or severity (crescendo headaches) or that awaken them from sleep. A prior history of trauma, ischemia, meningitis, or having a CSF shunt, or a concomitant history of intoxication, such as with lead or metabolic aberration (ie, Reye syndrome or diabetic ketoacidosis), may also raise suspicions of increased ICP in the child with compatible examination findings. Neonates with intraventricular hemorrhage or meningomyelocele are prone to hydrocephalus. Children with cyanotic congenital heart disease are prone to abscesses, and children with sickle cell disease can present with strokes or hemorrhages causing increased ICP. In endemic areas of the world, cerebral malaria and intraventricular cysticercosis are frequent causes of increased ICP. Physical findings may include elevated optic disk, failure of upward gaze, hypertonicity of the extremities, and depressed alertness or inattention. Localized findings on neurologic examination may point to a lesion indicative of a space-occupying intracranial mass, which could contribute to increased ICP (D$_x$ Box).

Pathophysiology

The problem of increased ICP can be understood in terms of the Monro-Kellie doctrine, which applies to the rigid cranial compartment and pressure-volume relationships of the contents. This doctrine is conceptually useful even though not always quantitatively predictive because of the variable compliance of the child's skull and dural membranes, particularly in the first 2 years of life before most of the cranial sutures are fused. The skull and dura mater form a relatively rigid compartment; any increase in 1 of the 3 intracranial volume components—brain parenchyma, CSF, and blood—must occur at the expense of one or both of the other 2. Decreased volume leads to increased pressure in an inverse relationship; however, the rise becomes much steeper when initial compliance factors are overwhelmed. Irreversible damage to brain tissue occurs primarily as a result of pressure of the other components overtaking the arterial blood pressure and not allowing adequate tissue perfusion. In younger children, non-fused sutures allow more compliance if volume increases are relatively slow, but this factor is not as true for acute volume increases. In addition, pressure gradients exist across compartments or sites of CSF flow obstruction, or even around lesions within brain parenchyma, and this leads to focal findings in addition to those caused by global ICP or perfusion changes.

Changes in any of the 3 components making up the intracranial volume may result in increased ICP in several ways. First, the brain parenchyma component may be directly increased by mass lesions such as neoplasms, abscesses, or hemorrhages. Vasogenic edema may increase the brain parenchyma volume because of vascular leakage due to cytokines. Brain edema may also result from cytotoxic damage, cell death, and necrosis, producing increased interstitial oncotic pressure from released proteins and ions, and cellular inflammatory and repair processes. The immediate cause may be mediated by cellular insults including hypoxemia; intermediary

Dx Increased Intracranial Pressure

- Loss of appetite, nausea, vomiting, headache, or lethargy
- Inattention, decreased ability to arouse
- Papilledema, upward gaze paresis
- Increased tone, positive Babinski reflex
- Focal signs and history compatible with an intracranial mass
- Mass lesion, cerebral edema, or enlarged ventricles in an imaging study
- Elevated cerebrospinal fluid pressure measured manometrically in the intrathecal or intracranial space

metabolic toxins, including neuronal excitotoxins; and depletion of energy substrates which are consequential to major vessel thrombosis, contusional trauma or diffuse axonal injury, anoxia from cardiac arrest, hypertensive encephalopathy, encephalitic infection, or external metabolic poisoning. Edema with head trauma is worse in children than in adults and may be a combination of vasogenic and cytotoxic edema and related to neurogenic inflammatory release of substance P and calcitonin gene–related peptide at the molecular level.

Second, the pressure of the CSF volume component (ventricles or subarachnoid spaces) may increase in hydrocephalus. Hydrocephalus can result in 2 ways: from a discrepancy in the rate of formation of CSF relative to absorption and from an obstruction between the point of formation in the lateral ventricles and the sites of absorption at the arachnoid granulations. An obstruction can occur with a congenital malformation; a parenchymal or intraventricular mass such as a cyst or neoplasm; CSF inflammatory cells from meningitis, ventriculitis, or hemorrhage; subarachnoid protein or debris; displaced brain parenchyma from mass effect; or even overgrowth of dural tissue. The small passageways connecting the ventricular system, the foramen of Monro and the aqueduct of Sylvius; the exits of the ventricular system, the foramen of Magendie and foramen of Luschka; and the cisterns surrounding the brain stem are particularly vulnerable points of obstruction. Another type of brain edema, interstitial edema, is characterized by periventricular transudation of CSF into the adjacent white matter and is generally seen in patients with acute or subacute hydrocephalus.

Third, ICP may rise because the intravascular volume component may increase. One process that leads to this increase is venous outflow obstruction, such as with a dural sinus thrombosis. Many cases of idiopathic intracranial hypertension are associated with transverse sinus stenosis or thrombosis. Other processes that raise jugular venous pressure may also increase ICP. In addition, the intracranial arterial vascular volume is affected by carbon dioxide partial pressure. It not only increases with hypercapnia but also decreases with hypocapnia, which occurs with compensatory central neurogenic hyperventilation or iatrogenic lowering of ICP by mechanical hyperventilation.

Because the physiology is dynamic, it has proven useful to quantitate ICP for management purposes. Intracranial pressure is often measured as cm H_2O while blood pressure is noted as mm Hg; both types of units are noted here. Normal ICP levels are somewhat lower in the neonatal and infantile period at about 6 cm H_2O (5 mm Hg), but in adolescents, pressures above 25 cm H_2O (18 mm Hg) are abnormal and may produce symptoms. Although it is possible to have normal cognitive function at an ICP of 52 cm H_2O (40 mm Hg), this assumes an adequate perfusion pressure. The ICP becomes clinically significant when the perfusion pressure is compromised, which may occur when the ICP is 78 cm H_2O (60 mm Hg) below the mean arterial pressure, and it can become dangerous when the ICP is only 52 cm H_2O (40 mm Hg) below the mean arterial pressure. Decreased perfusion produces swollen, damaged tissue, which increases the brain parenchymal compartment volume and further exacerbates the pressure-volume problem in a snowballing fashion.

As ICP increases, brain perfusion pressure may be maintained transiently by a spontaneous increase in mean arterial pressure, a response referred to as the Cushing response (hypertension along with bradycardia and bradypnea). Although the relationship may not be universally reliable, when it is present with other suggestive clinical circumstances, the rise in systemic pressure can be a useful clinical sign of increased ICP. Normally, changes in arterial cerebrovascular resistance meet changes in perfusion pressure to maintain constant cerebral blood flow, a process called *autoregulation*. However, this process is frequently compromised after head trauma or asphyxia.

Acute or subacute changes in pressure within an intracranial compartment may produce a pressure gradient across compartments that may precipitate brain herniation syndrome (Figure 68-1). An ominous heralding sign of transtentorial herniation of the uncus of the temporal lobe is loss of the pupillary light reflex caused by entrapment of the third cranial nerve. This herniation often leads to irreversible brain stem damage as well as infarcts and additional secondary edema, which can end with brain death. Focally increased posterior fossa pressure may result in a pressure cone downward through the foramen magnum–compressing medullary centers, also leading to apnea and brain death. A marginally compensated system could be decompensated by an ill-advised lumbar puncture when the spinal compartment pressure is acutely lowered, increasing the pressure gradient across the foramen magnum and producing herniation.

Differential Diagnosis

Complicated migraine, seizures, and metabolic derangements are common problems that sometimes have a clinical presentation similar to increased ICP. A characteristic prodrome or the "pounding" nature of the pain may help separate migraine from increased ICP. At the initial headache presentation or when only a short headache history is present, the complicated migraine diagnosis may be one of exclusion. If children display focal neurologic signs with some of the general symptoms of increased ICP, an imaging study to rule out a space-occupying lesion and confirm the safety of a lumbar puncture, and a subsequent measurement of normal pressure by lumbar puncture manometry, may need to be performed as support for the diagnosis of migraine.

In children who are only partially responsive, the task of distinguishing a seizing or postictal state from a condition that may be producing increased ICP is sometimes difficult. Findings that suggest a seizure include rhythmic, clonic movements or sudden myoclonic jerks; rapid or variable changes of tone or posturing that are different from the decerebrate posturing that may accompany a process producing increased ICP; abrupt, fluctuating changes of autonomic function (eg, heart rate, blood pressure, pupillary size); saliva

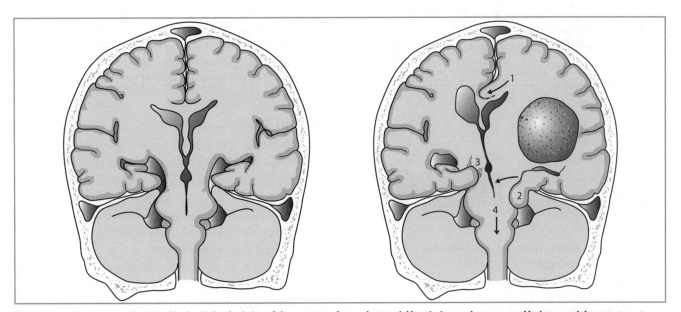

Figure 68-1. Left, depiction of a normal brain. Right, depiction of the anatomy of several potential herniation syndromes caused by intracranial compartment pressure gradients related to a mass (hematoma, neoplasm, or acutely necrotic brain tissue) in a cerebral hemisphere. 1, Trans-falcine herniation. 2, Uncal herniation. 3, Contralateral tentorial-midbrain damage. 4, Central herniation and foramen magnum pressure cone. These syndromes often lead to further brain ischemia and additional increases in intracranial pressure.

production without swallowing; and a history of prior seizures. Sometimes, however, only direct electroencephalogram (EEG) monitoring with ICP monitoring are able to distinguish ongoing electrographic "subclinical" seizure activity from increased ICP as the cause of the change in level of responsiveness.

In some cases, diffuse brain dysfunction from a toxic or metabolic etiology mimics increased ICP. Such toxic/metabolic causes include medication toxicity, electrolyte or blood chemistry imbalances, and systemic infections. With toxic/metabolic disorders, inattention is often accompanied by a confusional state with disorientation, incoherence, and sometimes agitation. In contrast, with subacutely increased ICP, inattention is frequently accompanied by slowness of thought, perseveration, decreased mental activity, and impaired gait.

Evaluation

History

A thorough neurologic history should be taken (Questions Box). Headache, nausea and vomiting, drowsiness, personality change, and changes in visual acuity are important historical factors. The headache history may crescendo in frequency or intensity and be of only a few days' or weeks' duration. The headache may be worsened by cough, micturition, defecation, or other Valsalva-like actions.

Physical Examination

Vital signs and head circumference should be noted. A careful neurologic examination is warranted whenever increased ICP is suspected. Particular attention should be paid to the components of the mental status and level of responsiveness and alertness of patients. The presence of papilledema and the cranial nerve functions should be assessed. Papilledema may not appear for a few days after ICP is increased. Retinal hemorrhages may raise the suspicion of non-accidental trauma. The sixth cranial nerve is particularly susceptible to increased ICP and an abnormality may be falsely localizing. Impaired upward gaze and lid retraction may be present. The head may be tilted to compensate for dysconjugate gaze. Specific muscle tone and strength as well as gait characteristics should be evaluated in children who are able to cooperate. Posturing responses to stimulation and the breathing pattern should be noted in comatose

Questions

Increased Intracranial Pressure

- How long has the child been vomiting and when does the vomiting occur?
- Do headaches awaken the child?
- Does the child have weakness or change in gait?
- Does the child have a recent history of trauma?
- Has there been a progressive decline in activity level or loss of developmental skills?

children to help ascertain brain stem localization of a lesion. In such children, findings should be reassessed at frequent intervals until stable to follow a potentially rapidly progressing devastating process, such as impending tentorial or brain stem herniation, which would necessitate immediate surgical intervention measures.

Useful quick-assessment instruments for initial, rapid evaluation and subsequent monitoring are the Glasgow Coma Scale (GCS) and Children's Coma Scale (for ages 4 years and younger) (see tables 67-1 and 67-2 in Chapter 67). These scales are a useful shorthand description for emergent triage purposes and perhaps for acute ventriculostomy decisions in trauma case but are not sufficient for all clinical decisions related to patients with increased ICP.

Newborns and infants may display a unique collection of signs—enlarged head circumference; bulging, raised fontanelle; frontal bone bossing with prominent venous distention; setting sun sign (inability to elevate the eyes and lid retraction from midbrain tectal pressure); hypertonicity; and hyperreflexia—that may be secondary to increased ICP from hydrocephalus. Papilledema is generally not present, perhaps related to greater compliance of the newborn/infant skull.

Chronic hydrocephalus as a cause of increased ICP may result in optic atrophy, depressed hypothalamic functions, spastic lower limbs, incontinence, and learning problems.

Laboratory Tests

If mental status changes suggest a toxic or metabolic aberration, appropriate laboratory screens should be performed, which may include electrolytes, toxicologic screen, liver function tests, and kidney function tests. If signs of meningeal irritation or infection are present without lateralized signs of altered tone or strength, evidencing an inter-compartmental pressure gradient, a CSF examination should be done. Otherwise the possibility of herniation after lumbar puncture might be clarified by a preceding imaging study. If there is lumbar tap danger, CSF analysis and pressure measurements can also be made from a ventriculostomy. If there are clinical signs of increased ICP and no focal clinical or imaging signs of a mass, a lumbar puncture can also be diagnostic and therapeutic for idiopathic intracranial hypertension.

Imaging Studies

A computed tomography (CT) scan should be performed whenever children's signs or symptoms indicate the possibility of increased ICP. Severe head trauma patients frequently have a particularly dynamic pathophysiology, and an additional early CT scan may be indicated for increasing hemorrhage, mass effect, or ventricular size along with ICP monitoring. Intravenous (IV) contrast should be given if a source of disruption in the blood-brain barrier (eg, infection, inflammation, neoplasia) is suspected. A magnetic resonance venogram can be obtained if there is a possibility of a venous sinus thrombosis. Computed tomography angiography or traditional intraluminal angiography with the option of intervention to prevent rebleeding may be the best studies in the case of an intracranial hemorrhage of unknown source.

Management

If idiopathic intracranial hypertension is diagnosed, the pressure can be monitored until stable with lumbar punctures. Increased ICP may respond to diuretics such as acetazolamide at high dose (20 mg/kg/d) or furosemide, as well as the removal of CSF during the lumbar puncture. The primary danger in this condition is an expanding blind spot and eventual blindness due to pressure at the optic nerve head. Visual fields should be monitored, and if medical therapy is not successful, lumbar or ventricular peritoneal shunt placement can be done surgically.

Encephalopathic children whose ICP is markedly elevated or likely to rise rapidly require treatment in an intensive care unit. When diagnostic imaging studies reveal an etiology for the increased ICP, such as a rapidly enlarging epidural hematoma, immediate **neurosurgical craniotomy** may be necessary. Other focal space-occupying lesions seen on scans may not require immediate craniotomy, depending on size and position of the lesion as well as the distortion of normal brain tissue and potential for imminent loss of perfusion; neoplastic lesions may require diagnostic biopsy or excisional biopsy within a few days if surgically accessible. **Mineralocorticoids (dexamethasone 0.25–0.5 mg/kg every 6 hours)** are useful in situations in which the pressure is produced by a component of vasogenic edema, such as that surrounding neoplasms. Measures should also be used to help prevent a stress ulcer. Hypotonic IV fluids should be avoided, and the patient should be monitored for the syndrome of inappropriate secretion of antidiuretic hormone with serum and urine osmolalities. Hypoglycemia and hyperglycemia should also be avoided. If acute danger of herniation due to a pressure gradient produced by CSF flow blockage is present, a temporary ventriculostomy may be indicated to relieve the CSF pressure. If an infectious process, including focal lesions, abscess, cerebritis, or encephalitis, is suspected, **antibiotics** or **antiviral** agents are indicated. Following directed specific treatment of the underlying lesion, the increased ICP may resolve spontaneously. If hydrocephalus due to CSF flow obstruction is still present after initial therapy is completed, **ventriculoperitoneal (VP) shunting of CSF** may be necessary. Endoscopic third ventriculotomy avoids long-term VP shunt hardware complications of obstruction and infection but is less often successful in relieving the pressure in younger children than older ones.

If there is no mass or other space-occupying lesion to be surgically removed, interventional therapies are directed toward maintaining perfusion of recovering brain tissue. In patients with head injury, a GCS score of 8 or less can be used as a guideline for ICP monitoring. Intracranial pressure can be monitored on an ongoing basis with commonly used neurosurgically placed devices, including the fiber-optic micro-transducer and intraventricular catheter or ventriculostomy. The former device can measure pressure in brain parenchyma as well as in fluid-filled spaces. A distinct advantage of the latter device is in allowing for therapeutic CSF drainage to relieve pressure, although it may be difficult to place if the ventricles are small or shifted and it carries a slight risk of hemorrhage or infection (increasing to a plateau at day 4 of 1%–2% per day).

Intracranial hypertension frequently peaks at 1 to 4 days after severe trauma. Intracranial pressure monitoring with devices and therapy based on the measurements, however, have not been helpful in most cases of severe ischemic damage, infection, or poisoning. This finding may be due to the widespread nature of the insult and brain involvement so that little normally responding tissue remains in which perfusion could be maintained.

Children with a decreased or fluctuating level of responsiveness may require EEG monitoring of cerebral electrical activity. Seizures may occur even in the presence of increased ICP. Anticonvulsant therapy is indicated if evidence of clinical or electrographic seizures is present. In addition, the EEG may be used to monitor barbiturate- or benzodiazepine-induced coma, used for severely increased ICP.

Respiratory physiology and ventilation are important in children with increased ICP because hypoxia and hypercapnia can contribute to vasodilation and increased pressure. Rapid sequence intubation and avoiding ketamine and succinylcholine help minimize elevations of ICP. Transmission of elevated intrathoracic pressure to intracranial vessels can be avoided by sedation and decreasing the inspiratory phase of the ventilator and avoiding high positive pressure and end-expiratory pressure. If acute lowering of pressure is necessary, hyperventilation to reduce the intracranial arterial blood volume is very effective, but on a chronic basis, carbon dioxide partial pressure should be kept at 32 to 38 mm Hg to avoid decreasing brain cell perfusion. Indomethacin is also a cerebral vasoconstrictor and carries the same risk to adequate perfusion. Elevating the head of the bed to about 30 degrees and avoiding flexion or turning of the neck to prevent jugular kinking are effective in reducing ICP. Pain, fever, shivering, and seizures must be treated aggressively. Because the goal is to ensure perfusion while lowering ICP, maintaining and even elevating systemic mean arterial pressure by appropriate use of fluid therapy and pressor agents are key therapeutic measures.

Diuretic agents such as mannitol (osmotherapy) (0.25–1 g/kg bolus) may also be useful through reducing brain volume by removing water, changing the rheologic characteristics of blood, and producing reflex vasoconstriction, but caution is advised. Mannitol, as a chronic infusion, can eventually cross the blood-brain barrier and draw more fluid into the brain. It is most effective where the blood-brain barrier is intact. Hypertonic saline (3%) (2–6 mL/kg bolus, then 0.1–1.0 mL/kg/h as a continuous infusion) may be an effective alternative. Serum osmolarity greater than 320 mOsm/kg can lead to renal failure. By giving diuretic agents at intervals as a bolus and titrating up to the ICP-lowering dose, such effects can generally be avoided. Sometimes these agents are used to counter ICP plateau waves or increased pressure with endotracheal suctioning or other procedures.

In children with severe refractory increased ICP, especially if secondary to an acute focal process, barbiturates such as pentobarbital or the benzodiazepine midazolam can be given as a continuous IV infusion with appropriate monitoring of brain electrical activity, serum levels, and systemic and brain perfusion pressures (Box 68-1). These agents may serve to reduce brain metabolism without impairing vascular autoregulation significantly. Their risk is in reducing

---

Box 68-1. Management Interventions in Increased Intracranial Pressure

- Keep head of bed elevated to 30 degrees.
- Maintain normal or elevated systemic blood pressure.
- Control hyperventilation to $Paco_2$ at 32–38 mm Hg and provide supplemental O_2 and PEEP as needed to keep Pao_2 >90 mm Hg
- If ICP progressively rises, pressure waves >20 mm Hg last longer than 5 minutes, or any pressure in first 24 hours is >30 mm Hg, give mannitol, 250–1,000 mg/kg IV. This may be repeated to maintain serum osmols at 300–320 mOsm.
- If mannitol needs repeating in <6 hours or osmolality is >320 mOsm
  —Give pentobarbital, 5 mg/kg IV, then 2 mg/kg/h IV monitoring to blood level of 25–35 mg/mL, burst-suppression pattern with 10 s between bursts on EEG, and cardiac index >2.7 L/min/m^2.
  or
  —Give midazolam by titrating the dose upward starting at 0.1 mg/kg/h IV to the same EEG criteria and limited by the same cardiac index criteria.

Particularly in trauma cases in which the cerebral lesion is primarily uni-hemispheric and pressure is rapidly Increasing, hemicraniectomy should be considered.

Abbreviations: EEG, electroencephalogram; ICP, intracranial pressure; IV, intravenous; $Paco_2$, carbon dioxide partial pressure; Pao_2, oxygen partial pressure; PEEP, positive end-expiratory pressure.

---

cardiac output and inducing associated infections, particularly pneumonia. Xenon CT measures multiple areas of local blood flow and may be a useful bedside technique to help specify targeted therapies. Decompressive craniotomy or craniectomy in early severe trauma in small series of patients has been associated with up to 50% good outcomes. Hypothermia to 93.2°F (34°C) for cardiac arrest and numerous "neuroprotective" agents continue to be studied as means to slow metabolism and the resulting excitotoxic glutamatergic damage and thereby reduce cytotoxic edema and spread of the volume of irreversibly damaged brain tissue into the surrounding penumbra of damaged but not dead brain.

Prognosis

Encephalopathic children with systemic hypotension, hyperglycemia, or disseminated intravascular coagulation have a worse prognosis. Some types of lesions generate increased ICP that may be too rapidly advancing for therapeutic measures to take effect or refractory to treatment, leading to irreversible brain tissue damage or death. However, children can recover from increased ICP if brain perfusion pressure is adequately maintained and the underlying brain lesion generating the increased pressure can be resolved.

CASE RESOLUTION

The boy in the case history has focal signs and symptoms referable to the posterior fossa brain stem and cerebellum as well as symptoms of increased intracranial pressure (ICP). An emergent computed tomography (CT) scan shows subacute hydrocephalus due to obstruction of cerebrospinal fluid flow produced by a large mass in the cerebellum and brain stem on the left side. He begins taking dexamethasone with some relief of increased ICP symptoms. Two days later a ventriculostomy is placed along with surgical removal of the mass, which is found to be a medulloblastoma. Because the ICP eventually subsides over the next few days and CT scans show decreasing ventriculomegaly, a ventriculoperitoneal shunt is not required and the ventricular drain is removed. The boy's recovery is otherwise uneventful, and he begins the staging evaluation for medulloblastoma radiotherapy and chemotherapy.

Selected References

Adelson PD, Wisniewski SR, Beca J, et al. Comparison of hypothermia and normothermia after severe traumatic brain injury in children (Cool Kids): a phase 3, randomised controlled trial. *Lancet Neurol*. 2013;12(6):546–553

Ball AK, Clarke CE. Idiopathic intracranial hypertension. *Lancet Neurol*. 2006;5(5):433–442

Christian CW, Block R; American Academy of Pediatrics Committee on Child Abuse and Neglect. Abusive head trauma in infants and children. *Pediatrics*. 2009;123(5):1409–1411

Del Bigio MR. Cellular damage and prevention in childhood hydrocephalus. *Brain Pathol*. 2004;14(3):317–324

Fishman RA. *Cerebrospinal Fluid in Diseases of the Nervous System*. 2nd ed. Philadelphia, PA: WB Saunders; 1992

Garton HJ, Piatt JH Jr. Hydrocephalus. *Pediatr Clin North Am*. 2004;51(2): 305–325

Huff K. Central nervous system failure. In: Osborn L, DeWitt T, First L, Zenel J, eds. *Pediatrics*. Philadelphia, PA: Elsevier; 2005

Kochanek PM, Carney N, Adelson PD, et al. Guidelines for the acute medical management of severe traumatic brain injury in infants, children, and adolescents—second edition. *Pediatr Crit Care Med*. 2012; 13(Suppl 1):S1–S82

Kotagal S. Increased intracranial pressure. In: Swaiman K, Ashwal S, Ferriero D, eds. *Pediatric Neurology Principles and Practice*. 4th ed. Philadelphia, PA: Mosby; 2006

Marcoux KK. Management of increased intracranial pressure in the critically ill child with an acute neurological injury. *AACN Clin Issues*. 2005;16(2):212–231

CHAPTER 69

Management of Dehydration in Children: Fluid and Electrolyte Therapy

Sudhir K. Anand, MD

CASE STUDY

A 2-year-old boy presents to your office after 2 days of vomiting and diarrhea. His siblings were both ill a few days ago with similar symptoms. Two weeks ago his weight was 12 kg at a well-child visit. Today his weight is 10.8 kg. He has a pulse of 130 beats/min, respiratory rate of 28 breaths/min, and blood pressure of 85/55. He is alert and responsive but appears tired. He has dry mucous membranes, no tears with crying, and slightly sunken-appearing eyeballs. His capillary refill is 2 seconds. He urinated a small amount about 6 hours ago. Despite his mother's best efforts in your office, the patient has vomited all of the oral rehydration therapy given to him. You draw serum electrolytes, blood urea nitrogen, and creatinine and initiate intravenous rehydration and give 2 boluses of 240-mL normal saline (0.9% sodium chloride solution) each.

Questions

1. How does one assess the magnitude of dehydration in children?
2. What are the different types of dehydration?
3. How does one determine the type and amount of fluid that a dehydrated child requires?
4. How does one assess renal status in a dehydrated child?
5. What is the role of electrolyte and acid-base laboratory studies in the evaluation of the dehydrated child?

Dehydration due to gastrointestinal (GI) and other disorders, especially diarrhea, is one of the most common medical problems encountered in children younger than 5 years. During the past 50 years or more, the usual therapy for children who are hospitalized with dehydration has been to administer intravenous (IV) fluids starting with 1 or 2 boluses of normal saline (NS) (0.9% sodium chloride [NaCl] solution at 20 mL/kg). This is followed by the administration of a sodium (Na$^+$) solution of variable concentration (usually 0.45% NaCl) mixed with 5% dextrose over next 24 to 48 hours until the child is able to take oral fluids. The exact amount of fluid and electrolytes is calculated using complicated formulas to provide maintenance fluids and correction of remaining deficit (deficit therapy). Holliday, who in the 1950s first recommended the calculation of maintenance therapy, more recently has suggested that dehydration management should focus on rapid restoration of extracellular fluids (ECF deficit) followed by oral rehydration therapy (ORT), and traditional calculations of fluid deficits should be abandoned. Alternatively, Moritz, along with other pediatric nephrologists and intensivists, has recommended that we forgo Na$^+$ calculations in hospitalized children and rely solely on isotonic NS (0.9% NaCl solution) for management. While this chapter incorporates these suggestions where appropriate, it continues the traditional approach to maintenance and deficit therapy because an understanding of the pathophysiology of dehydration helps in the management not only of dehydrated children but also of children with other types of fluid and electrolyte disorders.

Epidemiology

Over the past 25 years and associated with the advent of ORT, hospital admissions and mortality due to diarrhea and dehydration have decreased all over the world; nevertheless, diarrhea continues to be one of the leading medical problems in children younger than 5 years. In the United States an estimated 150,000 to 180,000 hospitalizations due to diarrhea occur each year in such children. In addition, diarrhea is responsible for 2 to 3 million outpatient visits.

Maintenance Fluid and Electrolyte Requirements

The body has a **maintenance fluid requirement** to replace daily normal losses that occur through the kidney, intestines, skin, and respiratory tract. Of the various methods used to determine fluid needs, the most common is the **caloric method,** also called the Holliday-Segar method, which is based on the linear relationship between metabolic rate and fluid needs. For every calorie expended in metabolism, a child requires about 1 mL of water. Metabolic rate in children is a function of body surface area. Infants, with higher relative surface areas per unit of body weight, have higher metabolic rates and, therefore, higher fluid requirements per unit weight. As children grow, their relative surface area decreases, as does their metabolic rate and fluid requirement per unit weight. Using this relationship, maintenance fluid needs can be calculated for the healthy child using the method outlined in Table 69-1. These calculations of fluid needs are often used to determine the amount of IV fluids provided to a hospitalized child or to calculate the approximate amount of fluid a healthy child requires orally to maintain hydration. However, **these calculations may not be appropriate for children who are critically ill, some of whom require fluid restriction and others of whom may have increased fluid needs.** Moreover, the caloric method makes no allowance for extra fluid needed for weight gain, growth, activity, or pathophysiological states that increase fluid needs (eg, fever). The fluid requirement derived from this method is valid to determine the daily fluid need for an essentially healthy child. Thriving infants normally drink more fluid than this method suggests. On average, growing infants may take 150 to 200 mL/kg/day of milk (human milk or infant formula) as desired to support the average weight gain of 30 g/day usually observed in the first few months of life.

Replacement of normal daily losses of electrolytes is considered when a child is not able to take adequate nutritional intake orally (as in the example in Box 69-1, in which the child receives nothing orally in preparation for surgery). Electrolyte quantities are usually expressed as milliequivalent (mEq) or millimole (mmol) amount per 100 mL of fluid required. Traditionally, the recommended Na^+ requirement for a healthy child is 3 mEq/100 mL fluid required (approximately 0.2% NaCl or ¼ NS), and the **potassium** (K^+) requirement is 2 to 2.5 mEq/100 mL of fluid (see Box 69-1, part B for sample calculation and IV order). As discussed in more detail

later in the chapter, K^+ should only be given to a patient after ensuring adequate renal function. These estimations of Na^+ and K^+ requirements are meant to replace normal daily losses and would not be adequate in the face of increased electrolyte losses that can occur in a number of pathologic conditions (eg, diarrhea). Moreover, there has recently been increasing focus on the risk of hyponatremia and related complications developing in hospitalized ill children.

Relatively healthy, well-nourished children receiving IV fluids for a brief period (ie, 1–2 days) while hospitalized do not routinely require supplementation with other electrolytes, such as calcium and magnesium. However, it is important to realize that standard IV fluids containing 5% dextrose, NaCl, and potassium chloride (KCl) provide only minimal caloric needs and do not adequately support weight gain or provide other necessary nutrients. Children who require prolonged IV therapy because of inadequate GI tract function should receive total parenteral nutrition to better meet their caloric and nutritional needs.

Alterations in Fluid Needs in Illness

A number of conditions alter fluid requirements. Conditions that increase a patient's metabolic rate (eg, fever) will also increase a patient's fluid requirement. A child's metabolic rate is increased 12%

Table 69-1. Caloric (Holliday-Segar) Method of Determining Maintenance Fluid Requirements in Healthy Children

Weight	Maintenance Fluid Requirement for 24 Hours
3[a]–10 kg	100 mL/kg/d[b] = 4 mL/kg/h
11–20 kg	50 mL/kg/d for each kg above 10 kg + 1,000 mL (fluid requirement for first 10 kg) = 40 + 2 mL/kg/h for each kg between 11–20 kg
>20 kg	20 mL/kg/d for each kg above 20 kg + 1,500 mL (fluid requirement for first 20 kg) = 60 + 1 mL/kg/h for each kg >20 kg

[a]Children weighing less than 3 kg may have altered fluid requirements owing to prematurity or other conditions.

[b]During the first 2 to 3 days of life, normal term newborns require less fluid (approximately 80 mL/kg) because they mobilize excess extracellular fluid.

Box 69-1. Example of Fluid Calculations[a]

Part A

Case: A 22-kg boy is given nothing orally in preparation for an elective abdominal surgery. How much IV fluid per hour should he receive as he awaits surgery?

- For first 10 kg: 100 mL/kg/d × 10 kg = 1,000 mL
- For next 10 kg (to get to 20 kg): 50 mL/kg/d × 10 kg = 500 mL
- For next 2 kg (to get to 22 kg): 20 mL/kg/d × 2 kg = 40 mL

1,000 mL + 500 mL + 40 mL = 1,540 mL/24 h

IV rate per hour = 64.2 mL/h (with a healthy child, round off to 65 mL/h for ease of administration)

Part B

Question: How much Na^+ and K^+ should this patient receive in his IV fluids?

Answer: 3 mEq Na^+/100 mL (1 dL) of fluid = 3 mEq × 15.4 dL = 46.2 mEq Na^+/d in 1,540 mL of water or 30 mEq NaCl/L

2.0 mEq K^+/100 mL (1 dL) of fluid = 2.0 × 15.4 = 30.8 mEq K^+/d in 1,540 mL of water or 20 mEq KCl/L

One possible way to write an IV order for this patient

D5 0.2% NaCl (or 0.25 NS) with 20 mEq KCl/L to run at 65 mL/h

---

Abbreviation: D5 = 5% dextrose water; IV, intravenous; K^+, potassium; Na^+, sodium; NS, normal saline.

[a]Normal saline contains 154 mEq NaCl/L and 0.2% NaCl contains 34 mEq NaCl. This solution is a widely available, premade IV solution that provides the approximate daily Na^+ requirement of the patient. Even though the calculations for sodium concentration are physiologic, at many institutions 0.5 NS in 5% dextrose is used preoperatively to prevent potential postoperative hyponatremia.

for every 1°C temperature elevation above normal. Most otherwise healthy children with free access to fluids will increase their own intake to account for increased needs when febrile. Other less common hypermetabolic states, such as thyrotoxicosis or salicylate poisoning, may have an even more dramatic effect, perhaps increasing metabolic rate by 25% to 50% over maintenance. In these cases and for children who are dependent on others to provide their fluids, clinicians must be aware of the magnitude of increased need and provide supplemental fluids to avoid dehydration.

Other conditions may decrease a child's fluid requirement. In hypometabolic states such as hypothyroidism, metabolic rate and fluid needs are decreased by 10% to 25%. Fluid requirements are decreased by 10% to 25% in high environmental humidity unless the ambient temperature is also high and results in visible sweating. In these situations, a healthy child with normal renal function given extra fluid beyond what is needed can, within limits, effectively excrete any excessive intake. Children with renal failure, however, pose a special challenge for the clinician in the management of fluid and electrolytes. When a child is unable to adequately excrete excessive fluid intake, this fluid can accumulate and lead to complications such as congestive heart failure and pulmonary edema. Without functioning kidneys, only **insensible fluid losses** need to be replaced. Insensible losses occur primarily through the skin and respiratory tract; they account for approximately 40% of maintenance fluid needs. However, fluid needs for patients with renal failure are usually estimated at 30% of the maintenance requirement, with additional fluids provided if needed. This is to avoid giving excessive fluids that may require dialysis for removal.

Fluid requirements may also be decreased under circumstances in which **arginine vasopressin** (AVP; also called antidiuretic hormone or ADH) is increased. In addition to hypovolemia or hypertonicity (hyperosmolality), AVP release is also stimulated by pain, nausea, surgery (postoperatively), central nervous system (CNS) infections such as meningitis and encephalitis, severe pneumonia or respirator use, and certain medications (including thiazide diuretics, chemotherapeutic agents, and selective serotonin reuptake inhibitors). Arginine vasopressin release in the absence of hypovolemia or hypertonicity results in hyponatremia, and is referred to as syndrome of inappropriate antidiuretic hormone **(SIADH)** secretion. In patients with SIADH, fluid restriction as well as administration of fluids with a higher Na^+ concentration may be indicated.

The most appropriate Na^+ concentration of IV fluids for hospitalized children admitted to a pediatric intensive care unit or in postoperative patients is an area of current controversy. Over the past 25 years, most such children have been maintained on a solution containing 5% dextrose water in half NS (D5 0.5 NS) or lower Na^+ concentrations (D5 0.25 NS). Studies suggest that these children, due to the kidney retaining free water in response to excessive AVP, are at risk for hyponatremia, hyponatremic encephalopathy, brain stem herniation, permanent brain damage, or death. Recently, some pediatric nephrologists and intensivists recommended forgoing Na^+ calculations in hospitalized very sick children and instead relying solely on isotonic fluids. Others have cautioned that we must make certain that the new recommendations to use isotonic fluids do not result in excessive congestive heart failure or hypernatremia before we abandon previous practices. Regardless of the approach that is taken, close attention to the type and quantity of fluids provided, quantity of body fluid output, weight change, and serial electrolyte assessments are important in the management of all sick children, and fluid and electrolytes must be individualized to prevent serious complications.

Pathophysiology

Dehydration is one of the most common pathophysiological alterations in fluid balance encountered in pediatrics. Although strictly speaking, *dehydration* means deficit of water only, most children with dehydration have lost water and electrolytes. Dehydration can result from diminished intake, excessive losses through the GI tract (eg, diarrhea, vomiting), excessive losses from the kidney or skin (eg, polyuria due to osmotic diuresis in uncontrolled diabetes), or a combination of these factors.

Children are at increased risk for episodes of dehydration for a number of reasons. Infants and young children have 2 to 4 times the body surface area per unit body weight compared with adults and so have relatively higher fluid needs. It is therefore much easier for children to become dehydrated in the face of decreased intake or increased losses that often accompany common childhood illnesses. For example, acute gastroenteritis, which is common in young children, often leads to anorexia, recurrent vomiting, and frequent or large-volume stools, with proportionately more severe fluid loss than in older children and adults. In addition, infants and young children are dependent beings who are unable to increase their own fluid intake in response to thirst and must rely on others to provide their fluid needs. If these fluid needs are not met or are underestimated, children can easily become dehydrated.

Dehydration is classified as **isotonic, hypotonic,** or **hypertonic.** When considering acute dehydration, these terms are often used interchangeably with **isonatremic, hyponatremic,** and **hypernatremic** dehydration, respectively, because it is the Na^+ content of the ECF that largely determines serum osmolality in otherwise healthy dehydrated children. In acute **isotonic** or isonatremic dehydration (serum Na^+ 135–145 mEq/L), the most common type of dehydration, there is net loss of isotonic fluid containing Na^+ and K^+ (Figure 69-1, top). Sodium, the primary ECF cation, is lost not only to the environment, but some also shifts to the intracellular fluid (ICF) to balance the loss of K^+ because K^+ losses from cells are generally not accompanied by intracellular anionic losses in acute dehydration. The Na^+ that has shifted into the ICF will return to the ECF compartment with rehydration. There is no net loss of fluid from the ICF in this process; the total water deficit in dehydration comes primarily from the ECF, although some have suggested, in the absence of valid data, that two-thirds of the losses come from ECF and one-third from ICF.

There are a variety of mechanisms by which **hyponatremia** (serum Na^+ <135 mEq/L) occurs in association with dehydration.

Figure 69-1. Pathophysiology of various types of dehydration. Abbreviations: ECF, extracellular fluid; ICF, intracellular fluid; Na$^+$, sodium; K$^+$, potassium; H$_2$O, water.

In **hypotonic** or hyponatremic **dehydration,** the ECF volume is compromised to a greater degree than in isotonic dehydration because of osmotic shifts of ECF into the cell, resulting in more severe signs of dehydration (Figure 69-l, middle). Hypotonic dehydration typically occurs in children with gastroenteritis when there are excessive Na$^+$ losses in stool along with a parent giving oral replacement with water or very low Na$^+$ beverages such as apple juice or tea. In hypotonic dehydration, the kidney often excretes a concentrated urine (ie, retains free water) despite hyponatremia because AVP is stimulated by the decreased effective circulating volume. Intravascular volume depletion seems to be a potent stimulus for AVP release, overriding the AVP suppressive effect of hypotonicity/hyponatremia. The result is that serum Na$^+$ levels are lowered due to dilution. Hypotonic dehydration may sometimes also occur due to excessive loss of Na$^+$ (relative to body water) in stool (eg, cholera) or in the urine (eg, adrenogenital syndrome, cerebral salt wasting, pseudohypoaldosteronism, other salt-wasting renal disorders).

Hypertonic or hypernatremic **dehydration** (serum Na$^+$ >145 mEq/L) occurs when net loss of water exceeds that of solute loss (Figure 69-1, bottom). It is usually seen in clinical conditions in which there is rapid loss of hypotonic fluid in stool, vomit, or urine accompanied by failure of adequate water intake due to anorexia or vomiting. Fever or hyperventilation, if present, may intensify the disproportionate loss of water. Occasionally, hypertonic dehydration may be due to excessive solute intake. Urinary excretion of excess solute obligates loss of large volumes of water, resulting in dehydration. The history may reveal that the child was accidentally fed a high Na$^+$ solution due to incorrect mixing of oral rehydration packets or concentrated formula. In hypertonic dehydration, there is shift of fluid from the ICF to the ECF to attain osmotic balance. As such, the ECF volume is somewhat spared at the expense of the ICF, and signs of dehydration may be delayed. However, fluid loss from the ICF results in intracellular dehydration, the most serious effect of which can occur in the brain. If hypernatremia occurs rapidly, there is not only a decrease in brain size but also a fall in cerebral spinal fluid (CSF) pressure owing to diffusion of water from CSF to the blood. As the brain shrinks, the bridging veins within the skull may stretch and even tear, resulting in subdural hemorrhage or other complications. If the hypertonic state develops more slowly, brain cell size may initially shrink minimally but will gradually return to normal size even in the face of continued hypernatremia. Preservation of the brain cell volume despite hypernatremia is thought to be due to the generation of idiogenic osmoles (myoinositol, trimethylamines, taurine, and other amino acids) that prevent water loss and attract water back into the cell and thus maintain cell volume. Rehydration of the patient with hypernatremia must occur slowly and cautiously to avoid brain cell swelling (Figure 69-2). The skin, on clinical examination, in hypertonic dehydration may sometimes feel "doughy" due to intracellular dehydration. This finding, however, is inconsistent even in the hands of experienced pediatricians and should not substitute for serum Na$^+$ measurements to diagnose hypernatremia.

Evaluation

History

In addition to signs and symptoms of the current illness, the history should focus on the cause of dehydration. Parents should be questioned on the type and amount of oral intake; the duration, quality, and frequency of vomiting or diarrhea; whether blood is present in the stool; the presence or absence of fever; frequency of urination; and whether a recent pre-illness weight is known for the child (Questions Box). When parents report change in mental status, it is of particular concern because this may occur because of significant electrolyte (eg, Na$^+$) disturbance, marked dehydration, or other serious infection or illness. The most accurate way to assess the degree of dehydration is to compare current weight with a recent pre-illness weight, although a prior weight is often unavailable. In acute dehydration, the loss of weight is primarily due to fluid loss. The difference between pre-illness and current weight can be used to determine the degree of the fluid deficit.

Physical Examination

An important goal of the physical examination of the dehydrated child is to assess the degree of dehydration. In the process, vital signs including blood pressure and a current weight should be obtained. Specific attention should be focused on the general appearance of the child and in particular whether he or she is ill-appearing, listless, or less reactive. In addition to the usual components of the

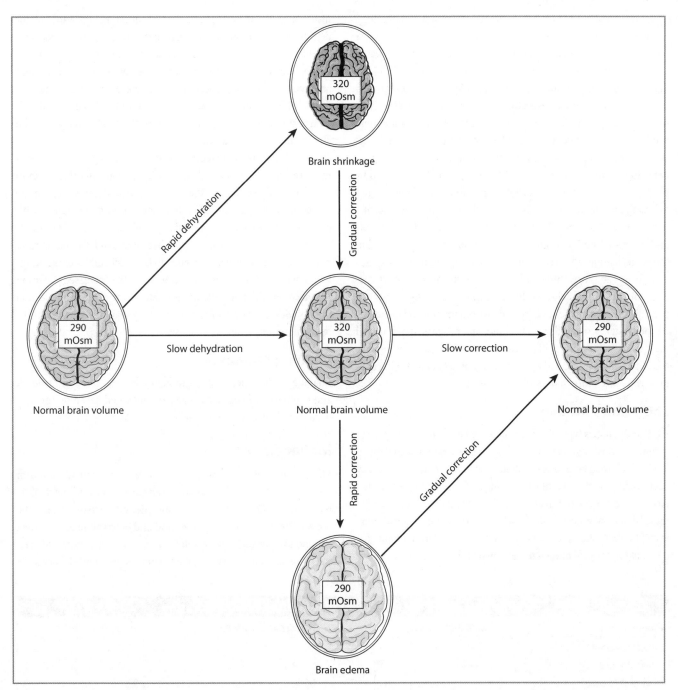

Figure 69-2. Hypertonic dehydration. Effects on brain volume of rapid versus slow development of hypernatremia and results of rapid versus slow correction of hypernatremia.

Questions

Dehydration

- Has the child had vomiting or diarrhea?
- Has the child had fever?
- What has the child been eating or drinking?
- Has the child been urinating? How many wet diapers did the child have?
- How much did the child weigh at the last visit to the physician?
- Has your child's behavior or level of alertness changed from normal?

physical examination, assessing for the following is important: whether the oral mucosal membranes appear tacky or dry, whether tears are present or absent, if tenting of the skin is present (abnormal when tenting remains after the skin is pinched between 2 fingers), and perfusion status of the extremities. In the process, it is important that the clinician recognize whether shock is present because this is a life-threatening condition that requires emergent treatment (see Chapter 63).

Because comparison to an accurate recent pre-illness weight usually is not possible, clinicians must rely on vital signs and clinical signs and symptoms to assess the degree of dehydration (Table 69-2). In infants and young children (<5 years), the estimated fluid loss for mild dehydration is less than or equal to 5% deficit of body water; moderate dehydration, 6 to 9%; and severe dehydration, 10 to 15%. The corresponding numbers for estimated fluid loss in older children are 3%, 6%, and 9%, respectively. A variety of clinical signs have been proposed to evaluate the degree of dehydration—some more valid and reliable than others. A 2004 systematic review found that assessment of capillary refill was the most useful single sign in detecting 5% or greater dehydration (capillary refill is assessed by placing brief pressure on the distal palmar aspect of a fingertip and assessing the amount of time for the blanched area to refill—normal is considered ≤2 seconds). Two other single signs found to be important in predicting 5% or greater dehydration were abnormal skin turgor (ie, tenting) and respiratory disturbance, in particular hyperpnea (deep, rapid breathing without other signs of respiratory distress) suggestive of acidosis. In general, the more signs that are present, the greater the severity of dehydration; however, a combination of delayed capillary refill time, absent tears, dry mucosal membranes, and general ill appearance may be equally as good as capillary refill, tenting, and hyperpnea combined in identifying children who have more than mild dehydration.

Laboratory Studies

Laboratory studies typically are not indicated in children who present with mild dehydration. Dehydrated children who are treated with IV fluids after having failed oral rehydration (at home or in the emergency department) should have initial assessment of their serum electrolytes, blood urea nitrogen, and creatinine. Initial and serial measurements of these laboratory studies should also be performed during rehydration in children with shock, severe dehydration, decreased urine output that does not improve after initial restoration of intravascular volume, or a history and clinical findings inconsistent with straightforward isotonic dehydration, or who are found to have dysnatremia (ie, serum Na^+ outside of the normal range [135–145], whether too low or too high). Dehydration in association with dysnatremia can have serious complications, and treatment requires special considerations. Hemolytic uremic syndrome, although uncommon, should be considered in any child with gastroenteritis, particularly with a history of grossly bloody stool, who also has decreased urine output.

Very ill children may require an arterial blood gas measurement to more accurately assess their acid-base status; in others, serum electrolytes are sufficient. The usual acid-base derangement in the moderately dehydrated child is a non-anion gap acidosis with decreased serum bicarbonate and hyperchloremia (due to bicarbonate losses in the stool). Severely dehydrated children, in addition, may have an anion gap acidosis due to lactic acid or ketone accumulation in the peripheral tissues secondary to the decreased perfusion that accompanies hypovolemia. An interesting exception is seen in infants with pyloric stenosis, who typically manifest a hypokalemic, hypochloremic metabolic alkalosis.

Imaging Studies

Imaging studies such as chest radiograph, abdominal ultrasound, and computed tomography scans are indicated based on the suspected etiology of the dehydration.

Management

Management of the dehydrated child involves consideration of 3 components: (1) normal **maintenance** fluid and electrolyte requirement, (2) fluid and electrolyte **deficit** incurred during the present illness, and (3) **ongoing fluid and electrolyte losses.** Most commonly, ongoing losses result from continued vomiting and diarrhea. Losses from diarrhea can be estimated at 10 mL/kg per stool

Table 69-2. Clinical Assessment of Magnitude of Dehydration			
Clinical Signs	*Mild Dehydration[a]*	*Moderate Dehydration*	*Severe Dehydration*

Loss of body weight
    Infant/young child
    Older child/adult
	
	≤5%
	3%
		
		6–9%
		6%
			
			≥10%
			9%

Skin turgor	Normal to slightly reduced	Decreased	Markedly decreased (tenting)
Skin color and temperature	Pale or normal	Ashen, cool	Mottled, cool
Dry mucous membranes	±	+	++
Absent tears	±	+	++
Sunken eyeballs	±	+	++
Increased pulse	±	+	++ (may be thready)
Blood pressure	Normal	Normal Postural decrease ±	Reduced (in late shock)
Urine output	Normal or reduced[b]	Oliguria[b]	Oliguria/anuria
Capillary refill time	Slightly prolonged	Prolonged	Prolonged

[a]In mild dehydration, only history of fluid loss in form of diarrhea, vomiting, or excessive urine output may be obtained, but no physical signs of dehydration described in this table may be present.
[b]Usually corrects with restoration of intravascular volume.

and from vomitus at 5 mL/kg per vomiting episode. Other forms of ongoing losses that occasionally must be considered and replaced include those associated with burns, gastric secretion suctioned via nasogastric tube, hyperventilation, or prolonged fever. The estimation of children's fluid and electrolyte needs and losses are almost always an approximation and require close follow-up, reassessment, and readjustment throughout treatment. At the very least, monitoring during treatment for dehydration requires regular assessment of vital signs, body weight, intake, and output.

Fluid given to dehydrated children may be provided **enterally** or **parenterally.** Whenever possible, **ORT** using oral rehydration solution (ORS) is preferred for children with mild dehydration and most children with moderate dehydration. Parenteral fluid therapy should be used in children with more severe dehydration, when oral therapy has failed despite an adequate trial (eg, due to intractable vomiting or lethargy), in children in shock or impending shock, or when an anatomic defect such as pyloric stenosis or ileus is suspected.

Parenteral Fluid Therapy

The parenteral management of moderate or severe dehydration can be divided into 2 phases: an initial phase (first 1–2 hours) and the main phase of rehydration. The aim of the initial phase is to restore intravascular volume, thus improving perfusion and renal function and reversing tissue hypoxia, metabolic acidosis, and increased AVP. Regardless of the type of dehydration (isotonic, hypertonic, or hypotonic), NS (0.9% NaCl) at 20 mL/kg/hour generally provides the most rapid and effective means to expand the intravascular volume at acute presentation. If shock is present or imminent, treatment is more aggressive (see Chapter 63). The child should in rapid succession receive 2 to 4 boluses of 20 mL/kg of NS given over 20 to 30 minutes each. After each bolus, the child should be reassessed, and if signs and symptoms of intravascular depletion persist, the next IV bolus of 20 mL/kg of NS should be given over 20 to 30 minutes and the child admitted to the hospital for further careful evaluation, including assessment for other causes of shock such as sepsis. **The rapid restoration of ECF volume with up to 4 boluses of NS is a change in recommendation for the management of dehydrated children when compared with the past.** Caution must be used not to give excessive fluids to a child with a compromised heart and thereby induce congestive heart failure. This approach will also decrease AVP/ADH levels and the chances of hyponatremia in subsequent therapy even if 0.45% NaCl (0.5 NS) solutions are used instead of NS to correct the remaining deficit and maintenance therapy. The validity of rapid restoration of ECF volume with up to 4 boluses of NS, however, has not been substantiated compared with the past standard rehydration therapy, when typically 1 or 2 boluses only were used (see Freedman et al). All ORT is based on the use of hypotonic fluids generally containing Na$^+$ concentration of 45 to 75 mEq/L.

During the second phase of rehydration, the remaining fluid and electrolyte deficits are replaced based on the magnitude of these losses. These replacements are in addition to the daily maintenance requirements as well as any ongoing losses, as discussed previously, but must take into consideration the NS boluses administered during the initial

phase, which may have already restored a substantial portion of the total fluid deficit. Each 20 mL/kg fluid bolus corrects 2% dehydration. Thus, a child who is moderately dehydrated and receives 3 boluses of 20 mL/kg of NS would correct 6% dehydration and may no longer have any remaining fluid deficit. Various protocols exist to restore fluid and electrolyte deficits; approaches to treatment of dehydration at different institutions will vary. Many of the differences in rehydration strategies lie in the composition of treatment fluid and the rate at which it is administered. Some clinicians prefer to administer half of the total fluid needs over the first 8 hours and the remainder over the next 16 hours; others replace the fluid at the same rate over the entire rehydration period. The latter method is presented in the case resolution at the end of the chapter. Usually the fluid deficit is replaced within 24 hours. There are noteworthy exceptions. Treating dehydration associated with **dysnatremia** (ie, abnormally low or high serum Na$^+$) should entail slower return (12 mEq serum Na$^+$ change per 24 hours or 0.5 mEq change per hour) to a normal range and may require 48 to 72 hours for correction.

Sodium replacement in the dehydrated child depends on the type of dehydration. In isotonic dehydration, some clinicians elect to replace the entire fluid deficit with NS, while others use a saline solution containing 110 mEq Na$^+$/L, and still others use 0.5 NS (77 mEq Na$^+$/L). We recommend NS (154 mEq Na$^+$/L) to replace the fluid deficit (see Case Resolution for example). This amount of Na$^+$ is somewhat more than the actual loss of Na$^+$ to the environment, which is closer to 110 mEq Na$^+$/L because during isotonic dehydration some Na$^+$, lost from the ECF, is shifted intracellularly to balance K$^+$ losses and thus will return to the ECF during rehydration. To calculate the ongoing losses, although the content of excreted body fluids can be analyzed for electrolyte content for more exact replacement, the diarrheal stools are commonly replaced with 0.5 NS at 10 mL/kg per stool. (This should be adequate in Na$^+$ content for most cases because diarrhea secondary to rotavirus contains approximately 30 to 40 mEq Na$^+$/L and enterotoxigenic *Escherichia coli,* 50 to 60 mEq/L; however, Na$^+$ stool losses in cholera are 90–120 mEq/L.)

Management of Dehydration With Dysnatremia

In hypertonic dehydration, the patient is considered to have a relative free water deficit but usually has lost not only body water but also some Na$^+$. The amount of free water a patient requires to restore serum Na$^+$ to normal (eg, 145 mEq/L is desired serum Na$^+$) is calculated as follows:

$$\text{[patient's weight in kilograms]} \times \text{[actual serum Na}^+ - 145] \times 4 \text{ mL/kg}$$

For serum Na$^+$ greater than 170 mEq/L, 3 mL/kg of free water is estimated to lower the Na$^+$ to the desired level (and thus the 4 mL/kg in the equation is changed to 3 mL/kg). The quantity of free water provided by this equation is only part of the patient's total needs. The remainder of the patient's fluid needs include isotonic losses that occurred during the dehydration process, ongoing losses, and maintenance fluids as well. Hypertonic dehydration is corrected slowly to avoid cerebral edema, which can lead to brain stem herniation and death. In hypernatremia, the various equations used for phase 2 of therapy often calculate the Na^+ concentration of the final solution at less than 30 mEq/L. Many clinicians, however, will initially provide 0.45% NaCl in 5% dextrose (a higher content Na^+ fluid than calculated by various equations) to ensure a slow rate of serum Na^+ decline and at a later stage decrease the Na^+ concentration to 0.2% NaCl. Serial monitoring of electrolytes is important to ensure that the serum Na^+ is decreasing at the expected slow rate and not so quickly as to lead to life-threatening brain complications.

Management of **hypotonic dehydration** also poses challenges. In addition to isotonic losses, additional Na^+ loss may have occurred. The amount of additional Na^+ (in mEq) to correct the serum Na^+ into a normal range (desired Na^+ level, eg, 135 mEq/L) has traditionally been calculated by the following equation (where 0.6 represents the body space affected by Na^+ changes):

$$[\text{patient's weight in kilograms}] \times [135 - \text{actual } Na^+ \text{ level}] \times 0.6$$

This amount of Na^+ represents an additional need beyond a patient's isotonic losses, ongoing losses, and maintenance requirements. Although precise calculations of Na^+ requirement to treat properly hypotonic dehydration may be desirable, in most patients with hyponatremia, treatment with NS (0.9% NaCl) in 5% dextrose is adequate to gradually correct their hyponatremia. The use of hypertonic saline (3% containing 513 mEq Na^+/L) is generally reserved for children with symptomatic hyponatremia (eg, a child who is seizing). Hypertonic saline is administered as 3.0 mL/kg of 3% saline given by IV over 15 to 30 minutes or until seizures stop. This volume of 3% saline will raise the serum Na^+ approximately 2.5 mEq/L and is usually sufficient to correct the serum Na^+ to a level at which serious signs and symptoms improve. This dose may be repeated once if there is no improvement in CNS-related symptoms. The remaining hyponatremia is corrected more slowly so as not to exceed 12 mEq/L per 24 hours because too rapid correction of serum Na^+, particularly when hyponatremia has been long-standing, can potentially cause pontine demyelination.

Hyponatremia in hospitalized children, as stated earlier (see Maintenance Fluid and Electrolyte Requirements on page 413), can result from other factors besides or in addition to Na^+ loss. Arginine vasopressin release in response to hypovolemia, hypertonicity, or other stimuli followed by free water retention can lead to dilutional hyponatremia (water intoxication). Hyponatremia in infants given excessively diluted baby formula (Special Supplemental Nutrition Program for Women, Infants, and Children syndrome) results from inadequate Na^+ intake and free water retention. There have been a number of recent reports of encephalopathy, brain stem herniation, and death occurring in hospitalized children with hyponatremia whose low Na^+ level was not appreciated or who received inappropriately low Na^+ content IV fluids or excessive volumes of IV fluids. The adverse effects of hyponatremia on the CNS seem to be accentuated in the setting of hypoxemia, thus further pointing to the importance of close monitoring of children with electrolyte disturbances. Moreover, with rehydration and provision of Na^+, the kidneys excrete relatively more dilute urine that can sometimes lead to rapid and unpredictable increases in serum Na^+ levels. As is the case with treatment of hypernatremia, close attention to type and quantity of fluids provided, quantity of body fluid output, weight change, and serial electrolyte assessment is important to prevent serious complications during therapy for low Na^+. When faced with such issues, consultation with a pediatric nephrologist or pediatric intensivist experienced in managing alterations in fluid and electrolyte balance is very important.

Potassium Replacement

Potassium deficits are more difficult to determine, and there is no specific method to calculate the exact amount of K^+ that a dehydrated child requires. Additionally, as the acidosis that commonly accompanies moderate and severe dehydration corrects, K^+ shifts intracellularly. What initially seems to be a normal serum K^+ may fall into the hypokalemic zone, potentially resulting in adverse effects on neuromuscular and cardiac function. Frequent reassessment of serum K^+ and adjustment of K^+ content of the IV fluids may be necessary. In general, once adequate urine output has been established, K^+ may be added to the IV fluids to provide 3 to 4 mEq/kg/24 hours. This need can usually be met by adding KCl 20 mEq/L to the IV fluids. Children who have decreased urine output or other indicators of renal impairment should not receive K^+ until normal urine output has been restored. Hyperkalemia, a serious and life-threatening condition, may occur if a child is unable to excrete excess K^+ via the kidney because of renal impairment.

Oral Rehydration

Oral rehydration therapy refers to specially prepared, balanced preparations of carbohydrates and electrolytes meant for oral consumption. Clinical trials have repeatedly shown that ORT is as efficacious as IV therapy in the treatment of the child with mild or moderate dehydration. Additional advantages of ORT over IV therapy are that it is less expensive and noninvasive and requires little technology. Oral rehydration therapy has been credited with the dramatic reduction in death associated with diarrhea in the developing world. In 2002, the World Health Organization and United Nations Children's Fund announced a new ORS with reduced osmolarity (proportionally lower Na^+ and glucose concentration) based on a number of clinical studies demonstrating less vomiting, lower stool output, and reduced need for IV fluids relative to the prior formulation.

In the United States, Pedialyte and generic equivalents are the most widely commercially available products. Flavored solutions and ice-pop versions of these solutions are available and often preferred by older children over the unflavored variety. Enfamil Enfalyte contains rice syrup solids as its carbohydrate source and is only available in unflavored, 6-oz, ready-to-use bottles. It is not necessary to change to ORT in a breastfed child who is tolerating human milk; these children can continue to receive human milk for rehydration, though they may require shorter, more frequent feedings.

The composition of various ORSs is presented in Table 69-3. The cost of commercially available ORS may be prohibitive for some

Table 69-3. Composition of Various Oral Rehydration Solutions

Solution	Carbo-hydrate (gm/L)	Sodium (mEq/L)	Potassium (mEq/L)	Base (mmol/L)	Osmolarity (mOsm/kg water)
Pedialyte	25	45	20	30	250
Enfalyte	30	50	25	33	160
World Health Organization–UNICEF oral rehydration solution (2002)	13.5	70	20	30	245

Box 69-2. Recipes for 2 Homemade Oral Rehydration Solutions[a]

Starch-Based Solution
- 1 qt clean water (4 cups or 32 oz)
- ½ teaspoon salt
- 1 cup dry baby rice cereal (about 2 oz in weight)

Sugar-Based Solution
- 1 qt clean water (4 cups or 32 oz)
- ½ teaspoon salt
- 6 teaspoons sugar

One teaspoon of flavored gelatin powder may be added to either recipe to improve palatability.

[a]The proportion of ingredients in these recipes is important. These recipes should only be given to families who have and know how to use measuring spoons and cups. (Courtesy of Kathi Kemper, MD, MPH.)

Table 69-4. Composition of Some Clear Liquids Not Appropriate for Rehydration

Liquid	Carbohydrate (g/L)	Sodium (mEq/L)	Potassium (mEq/L)	Base (mmol/L)	Osmolality
Cola	110	2	0	13	750
Apple juice	120	3	32	0	730
Chicken broth	0	250	8	0	500
Sport beverage	40	20	3	3	330

families. Given the simplicity of the ORS packet in the developing world and commercially available ORS in the developed world, these remain the first choice. However, homemade ORT, using the recipes in Box 69-2, can be effective as long as families have, and know how to use, measuring spoons and cups and have a clean source of water. Some solutions, such as fruit juices or chicken broth, do not contain the proper balance of Na^+ and carbohydrate to effectively rehydrate a dehydrated patient and should not be used (Table 69-4).

The amount of ORT fluid needed for rehydration can be calculated much the same way as is done when determining the parenteral fluid requirement for a dehydrated child. However, most children with mild dehydration can be rehydrated relatively quickly and then are likely to request, in response to thirst, the amount of fluid they need. Therefore, a simplified method of determining ORT

fluid requirements has been developed (Table 69-5). This quantity of fluid is given over a period of 3 to 4 hours. Children with ongoing losses should have these replaced. For the most part, it is not necessary to calculate the quantity of electrolytes that should be provided because these solutions are designed to adequately replace electrolytes in otherwise healthy children who are dehydrated.

Parents should receive guidance about the volume (converted into common household measures, eg, 5mL = 1 teaspoon and 15 mL = 1 tablespoon of water or ORS) and the frequency and duration of ORT to be given at home. Small volumes of 5 to 15 mL administered with a syringe or teaspoon every 2 to 5 minutes are much more likely to be retained by children who vomit larger volumes. Although this technique is labor intensive, it can be done by the parent and can deliver 150 to 300 mL/hour. As dehydration is corrected, vomiting often decreases and the child is then able to tolerate larger volumes. With ORT, the frequency and amount of stooling often increases during the initial period of treatment. Parents should be made aware that the primary purpose of ORT is to rehydrate and not to stop diarrhea, which will gradually decrease spontaneously. "Gut rest" is not appropriate in most cases, and early refeeding with a return to the usual formula or milk and solids, if appropriate, should be prioritized.

Prognosis

Children with mild or moderate dehydration as a consequence of a self-limited childhood illness are likely to recover completely when given timely and appropriate rehydration therapy. It is more difficult

Table 69-5. Treatment With Oral Rehydration Therapy

Degree	Dehydration ORT (Given Over 3–4 h)	Replacement of Losses	Dietary Therapy
Mild (5%) (older children = 3%)	50 mL/kg of ORS	10 mL/kg for each diarrheal stool 5 mL/kg for each vomitus	Return to formula or milk as soon as vomiting resolves. Children who eat solid food can continue their regular diet.
Moderate (10%) (older children = 6%)	100 mL/kg of ORS	10 mL/kg for each diarrheal stool 5 mL/kg for each vomitus	Return to formula or milk as soon as vomiting resolves. Children who eat solid food can continue their regular diet.

Abbreviations: ORS, oral rehydration solution; ORT, oral rehydration therapy.

to predict the prognosis of children with severe dehydration or significant aberrations in electrolyte balance. If managed appropriately, most of these children also completely recover; however, some, despite closely monitored care, may have permanent sequelae or poor outcomes.

CASE RESOLUTION

The opening vignette describes a child who is moderately dehydrated. Based on clinical assessment and weight change since his last clinic visit, he is approximately 10% dehydrated. He does not show evidence of shock. His laboratory studies show a sodium (Na$^+$) level of 140 mEq/L, potassium (K$^+$) of 3.7 mEq/L, chloride of 112 mEq/L, bicarbonate of 13 mEq/L, blood urea nitrogen (BUN) of 13 mg/dL, and creatinine of 0.4 mg/dL. His renal status is likely to be adequate because he is urinating, and BUN and creatinine are normal for patient age. The child's serum Na$^+$ is 140 mEq/L, which is in the isotonic range. The serum K$^+$ is 3.7 mEq/L, which is within normal range; however, this may not accurately reflect this patient's total body K$^+$ status. This level may decrease substantially as he is rehydrated and acidosis is corrected, indicating total body K$^+$ depletion. His serum bicarbonate is 13 mEq/L, and his anion gap is 15 [140 − (112 + 13)], which is mildly increased and probably related to ketosis or mild lactic acidosis.

A calculation of this child's fluid and electrolyte needs follows (his pre-illness weight was 12 kg):

Maintenance
Fluid needs: 1,000 mL for first 10 kg + 100 mL for next 2 kg = 1,100 mL
Sodium needs: 33 mEq Na$^+$ (3 mEq/100 mL of maintenance fluid requirement)

Deficit
Fluid: 10% of child's weight has been lost during this episode of dehydration = 1,200 mL deficit
Sodium: 185 mEq Na$^+$ (154 mEq/1,000 mL of isotonic losses: 154/1,000 × 1,200 = 185 mEq)

Ongoing Losses
Fluid: Estimate this child's ongoing losses at 10 mL/kg for each stool. He had one loose stool while in the office, so add 120 mL of additional fluid.
Sodium: The Na$^+$ content of diarrhea is variable; however, it is usually replaced with 0.5 normal saline (NS) or about 77 mEq/1,000/mL. We estimate about 9 mEq of Na$^+$ in his one loose stool.
Total fluid needs: 1,100 mL (maintenance) + 1,200 mL (deficit) + 120 mL (ongoing losses) = 2,420 mL/24 hours

Electrolyte Needs
Sodium: 33 mEq (maintenance) + 185 mEq (deficit) + 9 mEq (ongoing losses) = 227 mEq Na$^+$/24 hours
Potassium: Estimate his maintenance and replacement needs to be 20 mEq K$^+$/1,000 mL fluid provided.

Treatment
In the initial phase of therapy, provide 40 mL/kg/hour NS for about 2 hours. During this period, his heart rate normalizes and he urinates. The initial parenteral phase provides 480 mL fluid and 74 mEq Na$^+$. This amount of fluid and Na$^+$ is subtracted from the patient's total fluid needs. The remaining amount to be provided is 1,940 mL fluid and 153 mEq Na$^+$, or about 79 mEq Na$^+$/1,000 mL fluid. It is not necessary to prepare a special IV solution; 0.5 NS (77 mEq NaCl/L) with 5% dextrose ordered as **D5 0.5 NS with 20 mEq KCl/L to run at 80 mL/hour** is appropriate. As his gastrointestinal symptoms improve, intravenous therapy is discontinued and oral rehydration therapy (ORT) instituted. The patient tolerates the ORT well and is discharged home.

Selected References

Cheek DB. Changes in total chloride and acid-base balance in gastroenteritis following treatment with large and small loads of sodium chloride. *Pediatrics.* 1956;17(6):839–848

Denno D. Global child health. *Pediatr Rev.* 2011;32(2):e25–e38

Fischer TK, Viboud C, Parashar U, et al. Hospitalizations and deaths from diarrhea and rotavirus among children <5 years of age in the United States, 1993-2003. *J Infect Dis.* 2007;195(8):1117–1125

Freedman SB, Parkin PC, Willan AR, Schuh S. Rapid versus standard intravenous rehydration in pediatric gastroenteritis: pragmatic blinded randomised clinical trial. *BMJ.* 2011;343:d6976

Friedman AL. Pediatric hydration therapy: historical review and a new approach. *Kidney Int.* 2005;67(1):380–388

Holliday M. The evolution of therapy for dehydration: should deficit therapy be still taught? *Pediatrics.* 1996;98(2):171–177

Holliday MA, Ray PE, Friedman AL. Fluid therapy for children: facts, fashions and questions. *Arch Dis Child.* 2007;92(6):546–550

Holliday MA, Segar WE. The maintenance need for water in parenteral fluid therapy. *Pediatrics.* 1957;19(5):823–832

King CK, Glass R, Bresee JS, Duggan C; Centers for Disease Control and Prevention. Managing acute gastroenteritis among children: oral rehydration, maintenance, and nutritional therapy. *MMWR Recomm Rep.* 2003;52(RR-16):1–16

Moritz ML, Ayus JC. New aspects in the pathogenesis, prevention, and treatment of hyponatremic encephalopathy in children. *Pediatr Nephrol.* 2010;25(7):1225–1238

Moritz ML, Ayus JC. Prevention of hospital-acquired hyponatremia: do we have the answers? *Pediatrics.* 2011;128(5):980–983

Rose BD, Post TW. *Clinical Physiology of Acid-Base and Electrolyte Disorders.* 5th ed. New York, NY: McGraw Hill; 2001

Steiner MJ, DeWalt DA, Byerley JS. Is this child dehydrated? *JAMA.* 2004;291(22):2746–2754

Vega RM, Avner JR. A prospective study of the usefulness of clinical and laboratory parameters for predicting percentage of dehydration in children. *Pediatr Emerg Care.* 1997;13(3):179–182

Winters RW, ed. *The Body Fluids in Pediatrics.* Boston, MA: Little, Brown and Co; 1973

CHAPTER 70

Acute Kidney Injury

Gangadarshni Chandramohan, MD, MS, and Sudhir K. Anand, MD

CASE STUDY

A 10-month-old girl has a 2-day history of fever, vomiting, and watery diarrhea. The child has previously been healthy. Her diet has consisted of infant formula with iron, baby food, and some table food. Since the onset of her illness, she has not been drinking or eating well, and she has thrown up most of what she has eaten. Her mother has tried to give her Pedialyte and apple juice on several occasions but has had limited success. The child has had 8 to 10 watery stools without blood or mucus each day. Her temperature has varied between 98.6°F and 101.8°F (37.0°C and 38.8°C); the mother has given her daughter acetaminophen, which she has vomited. The girl's 4-year-old brother and her parents are doing well and have no vomiting or diarrhea.

The physical examination reveals a severely dehydrated (15%), listless infant. Her weight is 9.4 kg, her height is 74 cm, her temperature is 101.1°F (38.4°C), her heart rate is 168 beats/min, her respiratory rate is 30 breaths/min, and her blood pressure is 72/40 with an appropriately sized cuff. Capillary refill is 2 to 3 seconds. The skin appears dry, but no rash is present. Head and neck, chest, heart, and abdominal examinations are normal. Pending the results of her blood studies, an intravenous fluid bolus of 180 mL normal saline (20 mL/kg) over 20 to 30 minutes is administered. This is followed by 2 more boluses of 180 mL normal saline each. The girl is catheterized to obtain urine and determine the urine flow rate over the next several hours. A urinalysis is performed.

Questions

1. What are the 3 categories of acute kidney injury (AKI)?
2. What is the etiology of AKI?
3. How would one make an assessment of a patient with AKI?
4. What is the appropriate management for children with AKI?
5. What are the indications for renal replacement therapy?

Acute kidney injury (AKI) is encountered in outpatient and inpatient settings and is associated with high morbidity and mortality depending on the primary cause of the insult. There are more than 30 different definitions of AKI in the literature. For the past 50 to 60 years, a sudden decrease in kidney function, signified by the accumulation of nitrogenous waste products (ie, blood urea nitrogen [BUN] and various other metabolic products) has been called acute renal failure (ARF). With better understanding of the pathophysiology of acute deterioration in renal function, many nephrologists and intensivists have suggested that the term **AKI** be used instead of ARF. This is a better descriptive term than ARF in that it encompasses the full spectrum of renal dysfunction, from early and mild renal injury with only a small elevation in serum creatinine, to severe kidney injury requiring renal replacement therapy (dialysis) as a continuum.

To better delineate the progression of AKI, in 2004 the Acute Dialysis Quality Initiative work group set forth the RIFLE criteria, which is based on serum creatinine level and urine output. The acronym RIFLE defines 3 stages of progressively increasing severity of renal injury (*r*isk, *i*njury, and *f*ailure) followed by 2 outcome variables (*l*oss and *e*nd-stage renal disease). This criterion was recently modified for the pediatric population (pRIFLE), and the clinical use of it has been shown to improve outcomes in children (Figure 70-1). This classification is based in part on declining urine output; however, in

Figure 70-1. Modified pediatric RIFLE (pRIFLE) criteria. eGFR, estimated glomerular filtration route; ESRD, end-stage renal disease. (Adapted from Bellomo R, Ronco C, Kellum JA, Mehta RL, Palevsky P; Acute Dialysis Quality Initiative Workgroup. Acute renal failure—definition, outcome measures, animal models, fluid therapy and information technology needs: the Second International Consensus Conference of the Acute Dialysis Quality Initiative [ADQI] Group. *Crit Care*. 2004;8[4]:R204–R212.)

Risk	Urine output <0.5 mL/kg/h for 8h and/or eGFR is 75%
Injury	Urine output <0.5 mL/kg/h for 16h and/or eGFR is 50%
Failure	Urine output <0.3 mL/kg/h for 24h or anuric for 12h, and/or eGFR is 25%
Loss	Persistent failure for >4 weeks
ESRD	Persistent failure for >3 months

some children, urine output may remain normal or even increase, which is generally known as nonoliguric renal failure. The pRIFLE criteria, however, are not applicable in newborns during the first few days of life because newborns may be physiologically oliguric during the first 24 hours of life and their serum creatinine initially reflects maternal creatinine values.

The pRIFLE classification is intended to emphasize the reversible nature of the renal insult, which is often present in critically ill children admitted to pediatric intensive care units (PICUs). It is anticipated that this precise and universal definition of AKI will likely enable clinicians to rapidly recognize at-risk individuals and intervene promptly to improve immediate and long-term outcomes.

Epidemiology

Acute kidney injury occurs in children with a wide variety of medical or surgical conditions and especially in children who are critically ill. The exact incidence of AKI in children is unknown. Incidence of AKI has been increasing over the past few years because of the increasing number of cardiopulmonary bypass surgeries performed to treat congenital heart diseases, an increase in solid organ and bone marrow transplants, and usage of newly discovered nephrotoxic agents to treat a variety of disorders. Primary renal disease leading to AKI seems to be decreasing in incidence when compared with AKI caused by other systemic illnesses or their treatments. Acute kidney injury is often observed in patients in PICUs who are septic or have major trauma with severe bleeding and in the postoperative period following major heart surgery with a reported incidence of 20% to 40% (Fortenberry et al). The incidence of AKI is about 5% to 10% in neonatal intensive care units, and the most common cause is perinatal hypoxia and postnatal hypotension.

Clinical Presentation

Most children with AKI initially present with clinical findings of the primary condition that ultimately leads to the renal problem. In critically ill children, a small increase in serum creatinine may be the first indication of AKI. Other findings, such as decreased urine output, edema, and heart failure (following administration of excessive fluids), are specifically related to declining renal function (D_x Box). Additionally, hyperkalemia with cardiac arrhythmia, hyperventilation due to acidosis, and nausea and vomiting due to uremia may occur as renal failure progresses.

Dx Acute Renal Failure/Kidney Injury

- Decreased urine output
- Hypertension
- Hematuria
- Edema
- Elevated serum creatinine
- Blood urea nitrogen to creatinine ratio less than 20
- Elevated fractional excretion of sodium

Etiology and Pathophysiology

Because of the recent epidemiologic shift from renal to non-renal causes as common etiologic factors, primary care physicians and neonatal and pediatric intensivists should take an initiative to perform risk assessment using pRIFLE criteria in every child admitted to their unit and take necessary steps to prevent AKI before kidneys sustain serious injuries.

The causes of AKI are usually grouped into 3 categories: prerenal, postrenal, and intrinsic renal disorders (Box 70-1 and Figure 70-2). Although prerenal failure and acute tubular necrosis (intrinsic renal failure) may actually be on opposite ends of a continuum,

Box 70-1. Etiology of Acute Renal Failure/Kidney Injury in Children

Prerenal Disorders
- Decreased plasma volume
- Dehydration
- Hemorrhage
- Third spacing of plasma volume in burns, sepsis, bowel obstruction
- Other causes of renal hypoperfusion
- Shock
- Hypoxia
- Congestive heart failure
- Hepatorenal syndrome
- Bilateral renal artery stenosis
- Cardiac surgery

Postrenal Disorders
- Bilateral ureteropelvic or ureterovesical junction obstruction
- Posterior urethral valves
- Trauma to urethra
- Urethral stricture
- Neurogenic bladder
- Ureteropelvic or ureterovesical obstruction of a solitary kidney
- Obstruction due to kidney stone at the bladder neck

Intrinsic Renal Disorders
- Vascular: renal artery or vein thrombosis, disseminated intravascular coagulation.
- Glomerular: hemolytic uremic syndrome, severe (rapidly progressive) glomerulonephritis from any etiology.
- Interstitial: interstitial nephritis due to allergic reaction to drugs (eg, nonsteroidal anti-inflammatory drugs, oxacillin, methicillin), sepsis.
- Tubular (acute tubular necrosis): sepsis, post-cardiac surgery, ischemia due to prolonged hypoperfusion; all causes listed in prerenal category, if sufficiently prolonged, may lead to ATN.
- Nephrotoxins: aminoglycoside antibiotics, indomethacin, radiocontrast agents, ethylene glycol, methanol, heavy metals.
- Pigments: myoglobinuria, hemoglobinuria.
- Uric acid: hyperuricemia, tumor lysis syndrome.
- Congenital renal anomalies (especially in newborns and young infants).
- Bilateral cystic dysplastic kidneys, reflux nephropathy, polycystic kidneys, oligomeganephronia.

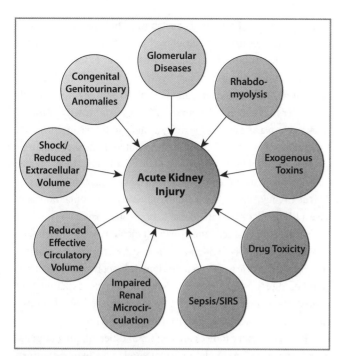

Figure 70-2. Common causes of acute kidney injury in children. SIRS, systemic inflammatory response syndrome.

rather than separate entities, this classification system still aids in the conceptualization of the underlying problem and formulation of the initial treatment plan. Correspondingly, it is important to note that postrenal failure could also inflict renal damage if intervention is not timely and ultimately can result in intrinsic renal failure.

Prerenal Disorders

Prerenal disorders are the most common cause of AKI in pediatrics and lead to a decrease in total or effective circulating blood volume. An absolute decrease in circulating volume can be caused by blood loss from acute hemorrhage secondary to trauma or fluid loss and dehydration secondary to gastroenteritis. Heart failure or redistribution of body fluids (third spacing) can lead to a decrease in effective circulating volume. In each of these situations, the resulting decrease in the glomerular filtration rate (GFR) can be readily reversed by improving renal perfusion in its early stages. If hypoperfusion is prolonged, however, ischemic damage to the kidney occurs and intrinsic renal failure develops.

Postrenal Disorders

In infancy and early childhood, urinary obstruction due to posterior or anterior urethral valves or other congenital lesions involving the urinary tract can lead to AKI. In older children, kidney stones or postoperative complications after pelvic surgeries or trauma could be the cause for postrenal failure.

Intrinsic Disorders

Intrinsic renal failure occurs because of injury to the vascular, glomerular, interstitial, or tubular components of the kidney (see Box 70-1). Intrinsic AKI can result from infection, ischemia, sepsis, or

toxins. Acute kidney injury resulting from renal tubular lesions is called acute tubular necrosis (ATN). Histologic changes that characterize ATN include loss of brush border microvilli in tubular cells, detachment of epithelial cells from basement membrane, and cast formation from cellular debris and protein.

Children with prolonged shock caused by sepsis, post-cardiac surgery, trauma (hemorrhage), or dehydration often develop ATN if effective circulating volume does not get reestablished. This is the most frequent type of intrinsic AKI observed in children. Nonsteroidal anti-inflammatory drugs are increasingly being recognized as a cause of AKI in children, especially when used in volume-depleted patients. In newborns and young infants, AKI may be superimposed on existing chronic congenital renal disease.

The pathogenesis of ATN in humans is controversial, and no single mechanism completely explains the sequence of events that lead to ATN. Ischemic and toxic ATN result from a complex interplay of hemodynamic, vascular, and tubulointerstitial changes, including decreased blood flow to glomerular and tubular capillaries, resulting in reduced GFR; injury to cortical and medullary tubules with their cellular debris, leading to tubular obstruction; and "back leak" of solute and water from the lumen to the interstitium with further decrease in GFR. Increased production of endothelin and reduced production of nitrous oxide in the microvascular smooth muscle cells lead to increased vasoconstriction and reduced perfusion, perpetuating the renal injury. Renal tubular cells respond to the injury in many different ways, including no or minimal damage, sublethal injury, apoptosis, or necrosis. In the tubules, at the cellular level, when there is decreased oxygen delivery, there is decreased production of adenosine triphosphate (ATP) that leads to damage to cell membranes and cell cytoskeletons. The cell damage alters the cell polarity, promotes entry of increased amounts of calcium into the cells, and increases intracellular free-radical formation that eventually results in altered cellular function, cellular swelling, and cell apoptosis/necrosis. On the other hand, low serum levels of bone morphogenetic protein 7, which is an antifibrotic, anti-inflammatory, and antiapoptotic factor that belongs to the transforming growth factor β superfamily of ligands, is thought to play a role in the pathogenesis of post-cardiac surgery-associated AKI. It is hoped that with better understanding of the pathophysiology of AKI, innovative, improved ways to prevent, diagnose, and treat the disease will be developed.

Differential Diagnosis

The diagnosis of AKI is established by the demonstration of a sudden increase in serum creatinine or BUN. Decreased urine output is also helpful. Identification of the clinical disorder that led to AKI is sometimes obvious, but at other times extensive evaluation to discover the etiology of the primary disorder may be necessary. It should also be determined whether children have chronic kidney disease or superimposition of AKI on a preexisting renal condition (Figure 70-2).

Evaluation

This is one of the few settings in which laboratory and radiologic tests are often more helpful diagnostically than history and physical examination.

History

The possibility of developing AKI should be anticipated in all children who are critically ill. A history of decreasing urine output, hematuria, dysuria, nausea, and vomiting should be sought in all patients. Prenatal and birth history may help to identify causes such as oligomeganephronia in children who were small for gestational age at birth or other complications that would have led to the current condition. The presence of previous genitourinary disorders, delayed growth, and anemia may point to preexisting kidney conditions (Questions Box). Also, family history of renal disorders can help in differential diagnoses.

Physical Examination

An evaluation of physical growth, hypotension or hypertension, arrhythmia, dehydration, and edema should be made. Examination of the flank area for renal enlargement or tenderness and of the bladder for distention is necessary to help determine the etiology of AKI.

Laboratory Tests

The following laboratory tests are recommended in all children with AKI: complete blood cell count, with red blood cell (RBC) morphology and platelet count; serum sodium, potassium, and bicarbonate; BUN; creatinine, uric acid, calcium, and phosphorus; glucose; total protein and albumin serum concentration; urinalysis and urine culture (if indicated); and spot urinary sodium and creatinine concentration and osmolality. If children are not voiding frequently, catheterization of the bladder is advisable temporarily (4–6 hours) to obtain urine for analysis. Residual volume should also be assessed, and the urinary flow rate (especially the response to initial fluid therapy) and presence of an outflow obstruction should be determined. All children with AKI and evidence of hyperkalemia should have an electrocardiogram (ECG).

Diagnosis of AKI can easily be established by laboratory tests and determination of urinary output over a specific time. *Oliguria* is defined as urine output less than 400 mL/m^2/day or less than 1 mL/kg/hour in infants younger than 1 year, less than 0.75 mL/kg/hour in children 2 to 6 years of age, and less than 0.5 mL/kg/hour in children older than 6 years. Urinalysis, urine-specific gravity or osmolality, urine-plasma creatinine ratio, urinary sodium concentration, and fractional excretion of sodium help differentiate prerenal from intrinsic AKI (Table 70-1). While a BUN-creatinine ratio of greater than 20:1 suggests prerenal azotemia in adults, this is not necessarily true in infants and young children because they often normally have a BUN-creatinine ratio equal to or greater than 20.

Tubular epithelial cells and brown-pigmented casts are often seen in patients with ATN. Evidence of hematuria or proteinuria signifies glomerular disease, especially glomerulonephritis. Presence of blood on dipstick but absence of RBCs on sediment examination suggests hemoglobinuria (eg, hemolytic uremic syndrome) or myoglobinuria (eg, rhabdomyolysis) as the basis of ATN.

Although urinary indices are helpful in differentiating prerenal from intrinsic AKI, a simple clinical method to distinguish between the 2 can be used. A therapeutic trial of volume expansion with 20 mL/kg of normal saline is administered intravenously over ½ to 1 hour (after the possibilities of congestive heart failure and urinary obstruction are excluded). If oliguria persists at the end of 1 hour, furosemide (2 mg/kg) can be given. If urinary output does not increase following furosemide administration, repeated administration of high-dose furosemide has few benefits and can cause toxicity, especially hearing loss, particularly in preterm newborns. Failure to respond to fluid and diuretic therapy suggests intrinsic AKI.

Many biomarkers have been investigated for the early diagnosis of AKI in adults and children (Al-Ismaili et al). The hope is that, one day, biomarkers found in the serum or urine will allow us to better

Questions

Acute Renal Failure/Kidney Injury

- How frequently is the child passing urine?
- Is the amount of daily urine decreased, increased, or unchanged?
- Does the child have hematuria or dysuria?
- Does the child have nausea or vomiting?
- Has the child had any previous urinary problems?
- (Older children) Does the child have a history of enuresis or nocturia?
- Is the child's physical development normal or delayed?
- Does the child have a history consistent with a primary condition that may have led to the acute renal failure/acute kidney injury?

Table 70-1. Diagnostic Indices in Acute Kidney Injury[a]

Test	Prerenal	Intrinsic Renal
Urinalysis	Normal, occasional granular casts	Renal epithelial cells; pigment casts
Urine osmolality (mOsm/kg H$_2$O)	>600	<400
Urine specific gravity	>1.020	<1.015
Urine sodium (mEq/L)	<15	>40
U-P creatinine	>40	<20
Fractional excretion of sodium (FE$_{Na}$)[b]	<1%	>2%

Abbreviation: U-P creatinine, urine-plasma creatinine ratio (mg/mg).

[a]Values in patients with nonoliguric AKI often overlap and fall between prerenal and renal values. In addition, values in newborns differ from those in children older than 1 year.

[b]FE$_{Na}$ = (UNa/UCr) × (PCr/PNa) × 100. UNa, urine sodium (mEq/L); FENa, fractional excretion of sodium; UCr, urine creatinine (mg/dL); PCr, plasma creatinine (mg/dL); PNa, plasma sodium (mEq/L).

detect early kidney injury, differentiate among multiple etiologies, and predict its severity. There are many promising urinary biomarkers, including IL-18, KIM-1, NGAL, β_2-microglobulin, and osteopontin, which have been recently identified by proteomic analysis, and all correlate with AKI to a variable degree. Both NGAL and β_2-microglobulin have been shown to correlate significantly with AKI in children seen in the emergency department with various forms of predisposing conditions. The concept of multiple biomarkers to determine changes in kidneys during the early phase of AKI has been recently entertained. Studies analyzing the value of this tool are still in progress. In parallel, studies looking at the value of renal angina index as a simplified alternative to already existing biomarkers are also in progress. Furthermore, more than one genetic polymorphism has been identified in adults known to be susceptible to AKI. Perhaps, in the future, this information can help physicians to recognize at-risk individuals and intervene early to prevent renal injury.

Imaging Studies

Renal ultrasonography is the most useful test for differentiating postrenal from other forms of AKI. Renal ultrasound can detect the presence or absence of kidneys, enlarged kidneys, dilated pyelocalyceal system, a distended bladder, and other congenital anomalies. Other investigative tests, such as voiding cystourethrography, renal scans, angiography, computed tomography, magnetic resonance imaging, or renal biopsy, may occasionally be necessary but are generally not indicated in children with AKI during the initial phase of the workup. Once a glomerular cause is suspected based on laboratory findings or radiologic evaluation, a biopsy is an appropriate next step. A chest radiograph may also be helpful in detecting cardiac enlargement or pulmonary edema caused by fluid overload.

Management

Prerenal azotemia is corrected by reestablishing adequate circulating volume, but unfortunately no current treatment leads to rapid recovery of renal function in humans with established intrinsic AKI. Although low-dose dopamine and furosemide are often used in the initial management of AKI, many studies have shown that these medications do not enhance recovery of renal function. Fenoldopam, a dopamine receptor agonist, has been used in critically ill, hemodynamically unstable patients with AKI to improve renal perfusion, with some benefit in selected patients. Certain drugs, such as ATP-magnesium chloride, thyroxine, atrial natriuretic hormone, and insulinlike growth factors (IGF-1) have been used in experimental animals and some human trials without much success. The goal of therapeutic management of intrinsic AKI is maintenance of normal body homeostasis while awaiting spontaneous improvement because proximal tubules can undergo repair and regeneration after damage.

After dehydration is corrected, **daily fluid intake** is limited to replacement of insensible water loss (about 30%–40% of daily recommended fluid intake for age), urinary losses, and fluid losses from non-renal sources (eg, nasogastric drainage). Hyperhydration should be avoided in patients with AKI because it can cause edema, congestive heart failure, hypertension, hyponatremia, encephalopathy, and seizures. Recent studies have shown that fluid overload in non-AKI patients in an intensive care unit setting can induce AKI, and in AKI patients, it can contribute to increased morbidity and mortality.

Patients with complete anuria require no sodium intake. **Sodium** losses should be replaced daily in patients with urinary output, however. Preferably, the amount of sodium required should be determined by measuring daily urinary sodium losses.

Once AKI is suspected, **potassium** intake from all sources should be restricted. Severe hyperkalemia can often be avoided early in the course of the disease with strict adherence to potassium restriction. The level of serum potassium as well as ECG changes should be closely monitored. Patients with mild hyperkalemia may be treated with ion exchange resins; sodium polystyrene sulfonate (Kayexalate) may be given orally every 4 to 6 hours or by retention enema every 1 to 2 hours. Sodium polystyrene sulfonate should be mixed in water and mixtures containing polysorbate avoided because the latter may lead to bowel perforation. Moderate hyperkalemia can be treated with insulin and glucose infusions or β-agonists, which will drive the potassium intracellularly. In patients who have ECG changes of hyperkalemia, such as tall T waves or widened QRS complexes, calcium gluconate should be given to stabilize the myocardium. If serum potassium continues to rise or there is evidence of cardiac instability despite conservative treatment, dialysis should be initiated to reduce the total burden on body potassium. Hypocalcemia and hyperphosphatemia are common in AKI, and small alterations in levels of **calcium** and **phosphorus** require no treatment. For serum phosphate greater than 8 mg/dL, phosphate binders such as calcium carbonate or calcium acetate may be used if the child can take nothing by mouth. If serum calcium is less than 8 mg/dL, intravenous (IV) or oral calcium should be administered to prevent tetany. If oral calcium supplements are given, the child will require 1,25 (OH) vitamin D (calcitriol by mouth or IV Calcijex) to enhance gastrointestinal absorption of calcium.

Mild metabolic acidosis is common in AKI and requires no treatment. If blood pH is less than 7.2 or serum bicarbonate is less than 12 mEq/L, sodium **bicarbonate** can be administered.

Adequate nutrition is important in AKI because it prevents excessive tissue breakdown. If renal failure is expected to be short in duration (3–4 days), most calories may be provided as carbohydrates. If AKI is expected to last longer, adequate calories in the form of carbohydrates along with daily protein intake of 1 g/kg should be provided.

Anemia should be identified and corrected if hemoglobin is less than 10 g/dL to improve oxygen and nutrient delivery to the tubules to facilitate regeneration of cells and establish their function. This can be achieved by maintaining an optimal hemoglobin level by transfusing packed RBCs and subcutaneous or IV administration of Epogen (recombinant erythropoietin) if renal failure is prolonged.

Many children with AKI can be managed by the conservative measures described previously. If renal failure lasts more than a few days or if complications develop, however, **dialysis** should be planned. The usual indications for dialysis include uncontrollable hyperkalemia or acidosis, volume overload with pulmonary edema or congestive heart failure unresponsive to diuretic treatment, progressive uremia with BUN greater than 100 mg/dL, or creatinine clearance less than 15 mL/min/1.73 m^2. In preemies and newborn babies, peritoneal dialysis is usually preferred over hemodialysis to avoid the major hemodynamic instability that is often seen with hemodialysis. In critically ill children with overwhelming sepsis or multisystem organ dysfunction, however, early continuous venovenous hemodiafiltration is indicated for more gradual fluid removal, avoiding significant fluctuations in the fluid balance and to optimize nutritional support.

Acute renal failure/AKI can often be prevented by anticipating its possible occurrence in children with high-risk conditions such as dehydration, trauma, sepsis, and shock, or after cardiac surgery. Prompt recognition of prerenal failure and its aggressive management with volume expansion may prevent the development of intrinsic AKI. Nephrotoxic agents such as gentamicin should be avoided in high-risk patients if possible. When these drugs are used, they should be monitored meticulously, with frequent measurement of blood levels.

Prognosis

The in-hospital complications and long-term complication in children with AKI can be associated with poor cardiovascular and renal prognosis. There are 3 scenarios in which a child with AKI can develop chronic kidney disease. First, the initial episode of AKI may cause permanent damage to the kidneys, resulting in end-stage renal disease (ESRD). Second, there may be an incomplete recovery from the initial episode, leading to relatively low renal function compared with baseline function and resulting in chronic kidney disease. Third, children who regain near-normal or normal renal function continue to have a higher risk of developing kidney failure years later, compared with those who did not have AKI.

The duration of oliguria in AKI may be short (1–2 days) or long (a few weeks). Recovery is usually first indicated by an increase in urinary output. Blood urea nitrogen and creatinine may rise during the first few days of diuresis before beginning to return to normal. During diuresis, large quantities of sodium and potassium may be lost in the urine. Serum electrolytes should be closely monitored, and adequate replacements should be made to prevent hyponatremia or hypokalemia.

In children with AKI, outcome largely depends on the primary condition, severity of damage to other organs, and physician expertise in managing AKI. Nonoliguric AKI is consistently associated with a shorter clinical course and better prognosis than oliguric AKI. Most children with ATN recover completely. However, children with more severe kidney involvement (cortical necrosis) may have residual renal impairment or chronic renal failure, and children who are critically ill have a 60% mortality rate. Early recognition of potential risk factors and prompt intervention will reduce long-term sequelae of AKI, particularly the development of ESRD years later.

CASE RESOLUTION

In the case scenario, a series of diagnostic studies are performed. The laboratory results are hemoglobin, 13.8 g/dL; hematocrit, 41%; white blood cell (WBC) count, 12,400/μL; neutrophils, 58%; band forms, 6%; lymphocytes, 32%; monocytes, 3%; and eosinophils, 1%. The platelet count is 277,500/μL. Serum sodium is 136 mEq/L; potassium, 5.1 mEq/L; chloride, 110 mEq/L; bicarbonate, 10 mEq/L; blood urea nitrogen, 84 mg/dL; creatinine, 2.8 mg/dL; and glucose, 68 mg/dL. The specific gravity is 1.015; the specimen shows protein trace, blood, WBC, and nitrite negative; and the sediment has many epithelial cells, 1 to 2 red blood cells, and many granular and pigmented casts. Spot urinary sodium is 65 mEq/L, creatinine is 39 mg/dL, and fractional excretion of sodium is 3.4%.

These results are most consistent with the diagnosis of intrinsic renal failure/acute kidney injury because the fractional excretion of sodium is increased. This began as prerenal failure, but later, prolonged hypovolemia contributed to ischemia of the kidneys resulting in intrinsic renal failure. Recovery may take a few days to a few weeks. The patient is admitted to the pediatric step-down unit where fluids are adjusted according to her urine output and electrolytes are monitored frequently.

Selected References

Akcan-Arikan A, Zappitelli M, Loftis LL, Washburn KK, Jefferson LS, Goldstein SL. Modified RIFLE criteria in critically ill children with acute kidney injury. *Kidney Int.* 2007;71(10):1028–1035

Al-Ismaili Z, Palijan A, Zappitelli M. Biomarkers of acute kidney injury in children: discovery, evaluation, and clinical application. *Pediatr Nephrol.* 2011;26(1):29–40

Askenazi DJ, Ambalavanan N, Goldstein SL. Acute kidney injury in critically ill newborns: what do we know? What do we need to learn? *Pediatr Nephrol.* 2009;24(2):265–274

Basu RK, Devarajan P, Wong H, Wheeler DS. An update and review of acute kidney injury in pediatrics. *Pediatr Crit Care Med.* 2011;12(3):339–347

Bellomo R, Ronco C, Kellum JA, Mehta RL, Palevsky P; Acute Dialysis Quality Initiative Workgroup. Acute renal failure—definition, outcome measures, animal models, fluid therapy and information technology needs: the Second International Consensus Conference of the Acute Dialysis Quality Initiative (ADQI) Group. *Crit Care.* 2004;8(4):R204–R212

Du Y, Zappitelli M, Mian A, et al. Urinary biomarkers to detect acute kidney injury in the pediatric emergency center. *Pediatr Nephrol.* 2011;26(2):267–274

Fortenberry JD, Paden ML, Goldstein SL. Acute kidney injury in children: an update on diagnosis and treatment. *Pediatr Clin North Am.* 2013;60(3):669–688

Goldstein SL, Jaber BL, Faubel S, Chawla LS; Acute Kidney Injury Advisory Group of the American Society of Nephrology. AKI transition of care: a potential opportunity to detect and prevent CKD. *Clin J Am Soc Nephrol.* 2013;8(3):476–483

Hsu CW, Symons JM. Acute kidney injury: can we improve prognosis? *Pediatr Nephrol.* 2010;25(12):2401–2412

Lameire N, Van Biesen W, Vanholder R. Acute renal failure. *Lancet.* 2005; 365(9457):417–430

Ringer SA. Acute renal failure in the neonate. *NeoReviews.* 2010;11(5):e243–e251

Schneider J, Khemani R, Grushkin C, Bart R. Serum creatinine as stratified in the RIFLE score for acute kidney injury is associated with mortality and length of stay for children in the pediatric intensive care unit. *Crit Care Med.* 2010;38(3): 933–939

Schrier RW, Wang W, Poole B, Mitra A. Acute renal failure: definitions, diagnosis, pathogenesis, and therapy. *J Clin Invest.* 2004;114(1):5–14

CHAPTER 71

Ingestions: Diagnosis and Management

Kelly D. Young, MD, MS

CASE STUDY

A 2-year-old girl is found by her mother with an open bottle of pills and pill fragments in her hands and mouth. She is rushed into the emergency department. She is sleepy but able to be aroused. The vital signs are temperature of 98.8°F (37.1°C), heart rate of 120 beats/min, respiratory rate of 12 breaths/min, and blood pressure of 85/42 mm Hg. Pupils are 2 mm and reactive. Skin color, temperature, and moisture are normal. She has no other medical problems.

Questions

1. What history questions should be asked to help identify the substance ingested?
2. What physical examination findings can give clues to the substance ingested and the seriousness of the ingestion?
3. What other diagnostic tests might be helpful in managing ingestion patients?
4. What are the management priorities?

Ingestions are a common problem faced by pediatric practitioners. Three scenarios frequently encountered are accidental ingestions by preschool-aged children, intentional suicide attempts by adolescents, and recreational drug use. This chapter discusses the general approach to the child who has ingested a potentially poisonous substance; ingestions of specific substances are beyond the scope of this chapter, as is toxicity occurring by dermal, ophthalmologic, or inhalational routes. However, the general approach to history, physical examination, laboratory tests and diagnostic studies, and management, especially decontamination, is useful for all ingestions.

Epidemiology

Most calls made to poison control centers involve pediatric patients. Poison control center data (2011) show that pediatric patients younger than 20 years accounted for 62% of exposures, and young children aged 0 to 5 years accounted for 49%. Boys were more commonly exposed in younger children, while girls predominated in adolescence. For children aged 0 to 12 years, 3% of exposures are intentional, while for adolescent 13- to 19-year-olds 24% are intentional, and for adults 72% are intentional.

The most common substances ingested overall are analgesics (including acetaminophen, nonsteroidal anti-inflammatory drugs, and narcotics) and cosmetics/personal care products. The most common fatal ingestion in children is narcotic analgesics (often not their own prescription). Also common pediatric fatal poisonings are stimulants and street drugs, cough and cold preparations, and carbon monoxide poisoning. A registry that included cases on which a medical toxicologist was consulted (presumably serious exposures) at 31 participating centers reported on the most common agents involved for infants and toddlers aged 2 years and younger: 16% cardiac drugs,

15% psychotropic drugs, 9% recreational drugs and controlled narcotics, 9% analgesics, 7% cleaning products, 5% scorpion stings, and 4% toxic alcohols.

Fatalities are uncommon overall and are more likely to be seen in intentional ingestions by older children. Poison control center data (2011) revealed 48 pediatric fatalities (0–12 years old) and 44 adolescent fatalities (13–19 years old). Children accounted for 4% of total toxicologic fatalities for the year, while adolescents accounted for 6% and adults for the remainder. Young children tend to ingest nontoxic substances or small quantities of toxic substances. Looking at trends over the last few years, there has been a decrease in overall calls but an increase in calls about serious exposures. Fatality rates have been stable.

An overall rise in adult prescription drug use has been associated with a rise in pediatric exposures, hence the predominance of analgesics (narcotics), cardiac drugs, and psychotropic drugs. Cough and cold medications have been an increasingly recognized source of toxicity in young children, and the US Food and Drug Administration (FDA) recommends against their use in children younger than 6 years. Another new source of serious toxic exposures in children is laundry and dishwasher detergent capsules, which can appear like candy. A rise in inadvertent pediatric marijuana exposures has been reported in states with legalized marijuana, with food sources playing a sizeable role.

Recreational drug use is another source of serious exposures in adolescents. Energy drinks with or without alcohol, synthetic cathinones ("bath salts"), synthetic cannabinoids ("K2," "Spice"), dextromethorphan, inhalants (especially computer cleaners), and the hallucinogenic herb salvia, which is legal in many states and also has opioid effects, are newer additions to still-popular narcotics, cocaine, amphetamines, and ecstasy.

Clinical Presentation

The clinical presentation varies considerably depending on the substance ingested. Some patients may not present with a clear history of a toxic ingestion. The clinician must maintain a high index of suspicion for poisoning as the cause of symptoms such as altered behavior, depressed level of consciousness, cardiac dysrhythmias, vomiting, seizures, and autonomic changes.

Pathophysiology

The pathophysiological picture depends on the substance. Some toxins act on a particular organ system (eg, acetaminophen on the liver, ethanol on the central nervous system), while others act diffusely at the cellular level (eg, cyanide). Generally, drugs are absorbed, distributed within the body, metabolized, then excreted. Drug levels obtained prior to completion of absorption and distribution may not reflect the peak level. Interventions focus on preventing absorption, sometimes on preventing metabolism into a more toxic by-product, and on enhancing excretion. Toxic effects may be delayed or prolonged when an extended-release form of a drug has been ingested, with drugs likely to form concretions (eg, iron, aspirin, theophylline), or when toxicity results from an active metabolite (eg, toxic alcohols, acetaminophen, acetonitrile, dapsone). Pharmacogenetics are increasingly recognized as playing an important role in individual responses to medications and toxins. Genetic variations in enzymatic activity in drug metabolism may result in toxicity through excessively rapid metabolism of a drug to its active metabolite, or through slow metabolism of a drug to its inactive metabolite. For example, a cytochrome P 450 CYP2D6 genotype has been linked to rapid metabolism of codeine to active morphine, resulting in toxicity and even fatality. The FDA has added a new boxed warning on codeine and a contraindication for its use after tonsillectomy or adenoidectomy in children.

Differential Diagnosis

The differential diagnosis of toxic ingestions is broad. If there is a history of ingestion, the differential is narrowed to substances available to the child. If no history of ingestion is given, practitioners should include ingestion in the differential when evaluating symptoms and signs such as altered mental status, altered behavior, metabolic derangements, cardiac dysrhythmias, hypotension and shock states, seizures, respiratory distress or apnea, cyanosis, vomiting, and diarrhea (Symptoms Box). In fact, almost any symptom complex may result from a toxic ingestion.

Evaluation

A detailed history of what and how much the patient ingested is key to the evaluation. Physical examination should focus on identifying symptoms and serious complications. Patients should be monitored and reassessed frequently. Laboratory and other diagnostic studies can be tailored to the specific ingestion.

History

The most important questions address the ingestion (Questions Box): What did the patient ingest? What is the maximum possible amount that was ingested? When did the ingestion occur? What symptoms are

---

Symptoms

Suspicious for Poisoning

- Bradycardia or tachycardia
- Hypothermia or hyperthermia
- Respiratory depression or hyperpnea
- Hypotension or hypertension
- Mydriasis or miosis
- Altered mental status or abnormal behavior
- Seizure
- Cardiac dysrhythmias
- Metabolic derangements
- Nausea, vomiting, diarrhea

---

occurring? History of previous medical conditions is also important to identify increased susceptibility to a particular toxin (eg, seizure disorder with ingestion of a substance that causes seizures); assess for factors that may have precipitated the ingestion, such as depression; and assess for medications that may interact with or exacerbate the toxic effects of the ingested substance (eg, acetaminophen ingestion in a patient taking a cytochrome P 450–inhibiting medication).

Parents should be encouraged to bring in the container and any remains of the substance ingested. The practitioner should try to obtain the exact formulation because generic and brand name drugs may differ. One must also be aware of possible combination products. Sleuthing methods such as calling or sending a family member to the home to identify the product, calling the pharmacy on a prescription label, or identifying a pill by comparing its picture and imprint to those in a pharmaceuticals reference may be necessary. Internet search engines may be used to search the imprint on a pill or to identify foreign medications.

Caregivers should be questioned about all available drugs or other toxic substances in the household. Sometimes caregivers must be encouraged to mention all substances in the household, even those they don't think the child could possibly have obtained. The practitioner must also ask about medications used by recent visitors (eg, grandparents) and the possibility of an exposure at a recently visited household or location. It is important not to overlook herbal preparations, vitamins, alternative medications, household products (including cleaning and personal care products), gardening products, chemicals used in hobbies or work, and alcohol or drugs of abuse belonging to an adult. Caregivers may initially overlook these as they concentrate only on recalling "medications." It may be

---

Questions

Poisonings

- What did the child take? (If unknown, what is available to the child?)
- How much did the child take? (If unknown, what is the maximum amount possible?)
- When did the child take it? (If unknown, how long was the child unattended or unobserved?)
- What symptoms have occurred, and when did the symptoms start relative to the time of ingestion?
- What other medical conditions does the child have? What medications does the child take regularly?

helpful to interview siblings or friends of an adolescent suspected of recreational drug use. Children may also be inadvertently exposed to parents' or other adults' recreational drugs. One must maintain a high index of suspicion for unreported co-ingestants, especially in adolescent suicide attempts.

Although often difficult, it is important to attempt to determine the quantity of drug that was available to the patient and how much is currently missing. One may need to count pills or measure liquid to determine this. For estimating liquids, the approximate volume of a swallow is 0.3 mL/kg. The practitioner should always assume the "worst case" (ie, the patient took all of the drug that is missing). History concerning the amount ingested may be inaccurate, especially when taken from adolescents with intentional ingestion.

The practitioner should try to determine approximately what time the ingestion occurred. Symptoms are usually expected within a defined time range. Recommended observation periods before discharge usually take into account expected symptoms based on the length of time since the ingestion. Timing may also be important in determining what substance was most likely ingested. For example, ingestion of mushrooms that cause a self-limited illness usually causes gastrointestinal (GI) upset within 4 to 6 hours, whereas *Amanita* mushrooms that may ultimately result in hepatic failure typically present with GI upset in 6 to 12 hours.

The practitioner should ask about current symptoms and when they started relative to the time of the ingestion. In a patient without a definite history of ingestion, certain combinations of symptoms may point toward a specific substance or class of substances. Whether the patient is symptomatic and what symptoms are present may guide the workup for an unknown ingestion, determine whether the patient needs to be hospitalized, or dictate therapy.

Physical Examination

If the substance ingested is known, the physical examination should be directed toward identifying expected symptoms of toxicity. A general physical examination should always be performed, however, because co-ingestion of another undisclosed substance must be considered. Particular attention should be paid to all 4 vital signs (ie, temperature, respiratory rate, heart rate, and blood pressure); pupillary size and reaction; breathing (eg, Kussmaul respiration seen in acidosis); mental status; distinctive breath odors; presence or absence of bowel sounds; and skin color, temperature, and moisture. The patient's weight should be measured because toxicity is often estimated based on milligrams of drug ingested per kilogram of body weight. Because symptoms may develop or worsen if peak levels of the toxic substance have not been reached at the time of initial evaluation, continual reassessment and cardiorespiratory monitoring are imperative. A recognizable set of symptoms suggestive of a certain class of medications or toxins is called a toxidrome. If a symptomatic patient is noted to have a typical toxidrome, therapy may be initiated based on the toxidrome without confirmation of the exact substance ingested. Some common toxidromes and their treatments are listed in Table 71-1.

Table 71-1. Toxidromes

Toxidrome	Toxins	Symptoms	Treatment
Narcotic or opiate	Oxycodone, hydrocodone, methadone, fentanyl, heroin, codeine, morphine	Nausea/vomiting, respiratory depression, miosis, altered mental status, or coma	Naloxone, respiratory support
Cholinergic (parasympathomimetic)	Organophosphate and carbamate pesticides	DUMBELLS mnemonic: *d*iarrhea, *u*rination, *m*iosis, *b*ronchorrhea and *b*ronchospasm, *e*mesis, *l*acrimation, *l*ethargy, *s*alivation	Atropine, pralidoxime (2-PAM)
Anticholinergic	Antihistamines, jimson weed, antipsychotics, some antidepressants, Parkinson medications	Flushing ("red as a beet"), dry skin and mucous membranes ("dry as a bone"), hyperthermia ("hot as a hare"), delirium ("mad as a hatter"), mydriasis ("blind as a bat"), also tachycardia, urinary retention, ileus/decreased bowel sounds	Supportive care
Sympathomimetic	Cocaine, amphetamines, ephedrine	Mydriasis, anxiety, tachycardia, hypertension, hyperthermia, diaphoresis	Quiet environment, benzodiazepines
Sympatholytic	Clonidine, β-blocker (eg, propranolol)	Bradycardia, hypotension, miosis, may have lethargy	Supportive care, fluids and pressors if needed for hypotension, atropine for symptomatic bradycardia
Tricyclic antidepressant	Imipramine, amitriptyline, many others	Seizures, tachycardia, prolonged QRS complex, altered level of consciousness, cardiac dysrhythmias	Sodium bicarbonate
Salicylate	Aspirin, methyl salicylate, oil of wintergreen	Hyperventilation, nausea/vomiting, tinnitus, hyperthermia, metabolic acidosis	Alkalinization with $NaHCO_3$ (confirm salicylate level)
Serotonin syndrome	Selective serotonin reuptake inhibitors, many other drugs	Altered mental status, neuromuscular rigidity, tremors, or hyperreflexia; autonomic instability: hyperthermia, mydriasis, tachycardia, hypertension or hypotension	Supportive care

Laboratory Tests (Box 71-1)

Qualitative drug screens (reporting only presence or absence of the drug) of urine or blood are often used when poisoning is part of a broader differential for symptoms such as altered mental status or acute behavioral changes. Such drug screens are rarely helpful acutely in the poisoned patient because results are often not rapidly reported, testing can only be done for a limited number of substances, and false-positives and false-negatives may occur. Given the frequency of narcotic ingestions, it is important to note that synthetic opioids (eg, fentanyl, methadone, oxycodone, hydrocodone) are not detected by typical hospital immunoassay "tox screens."

However, quantitative drug levels for specific drugs can be helpful to estimate severity of expected symptoms or to rule out ingestion of that drug. Examples include acetaminophen, salicylate, ethanol, methanol, ethylene glycol, iron, theophylline, lithium, anticonvulsants, and levels of carboxyhemoglobin or methemoglobin by blood gas analysis. Such levels should only be measured when suggested by history or physical examination, with the exception of acetaminophen and ethanol. Many experts in toxicology feel that because acetaminophen overdose produces few acute symptoms, may lead to fulminant hepatic failure, and is readily treatable with an antidote, and because acetaminophen is a frequent ingredient in combination products, all patients with a history of ingestion should have an acetaminophen level determined. In adolescents and adults, ethanol is a common co-ingestant, and ethanol levels are often routinely measured. Routine salicylate levels are likely to be low yield in the absence of suspicion by history or physical examination, although some practitioners also obtain them.

Serum chemistries and osmolarity may offer clues in ingestion of an unknown substance. The **anion gap** is calculated as [Na] − ([Cl] + [HCO$_3$]) and is normally 8 to 12 mEq/L. An elevated anion gap indicates presence of metabolic acidosis and is seen in ingestions and conditions identified by the **MUDPILES** mnemonic: *m*ethanol, *u*remia, *d*iabetic ketoacidosis, *p*araldehyde and *p*henformin,

---

Box 71-1. Laboratory Tests and Diagnostic Studies to Consider

- Specific drug levels as indicated
- Qualitative urine or blood toxicology screen
- Acetaminophen level; consider ethanol and salicylate levels
- Serum chemistries, calculated anion gap
- Serum osmolarity, calculated osmolar gap
- Liver function panel, renal function tests
- Rapid bedside glucose test
- Urine pregnancy test
- Pulse oximetry
- Electrocardiogram
- Arterial blood gas with carbon monoxide and methemoglobin levels
- Urinalysis
- Creatinine phosphokinase level
- Chest radiograph
- Abdominal film for radiopaque tablets

---

*i*ron and *i*soniazid, *l*actic acidosis, *e*thylene glycol and *e*thanol, and *s*alicylates and *s*olvents (eg, toluene). The **osmolar gap** is the difference between the measured serum osmolarity and the calculated osmolarity (given by the formula 2[Na] + [glucose]/18 + [BUN]/2.8). The normal osmolar gap is less than 10 mOsm. An elevated osmolar gap is seen with ingestion of alcohols such as ethanol, methanol, ethylene glycol, and isopropanol.

Depending on one's suspicion for acidosis, hypoxemia, or abnormal hemoglobins (carboxyhemoglobin and methemoglobin), arterial blood gas analysis may be indicated. Because hypoglycemia may be seen with some ingestions and is easily treated, a rapid bedside glucose test should be done on all patients. Urinalysis and creatinine phosphokinase–level tests may be performed to look for signs of rhabdomyolysis if the patient is deemed at risk. All females of childbearing age should have a urine pregnancy test. Assessment of liver and renal function is often important because many substances are metabolized by these routes.

Diagnostic Studies

Pulse oximetry and cardiorespiratory monitoring should be instituted for all serious ingestions. An electrocardiogram may be indicated if cardiac toxicity is expected. Other studies are tailored to the specific ingestion, such as endoscopy after ingestion of caustic acids or alkalis.

Imaging Studies

Specific imaging studies may be indicated for certain ingestions, such as chest radiography in hydrocarbon ingestion, to look for signs of aspiration. An abdominal film may be helpful in identifying ingestion of radiopaque substances and monitoring the effectiveness of GI decontamination procedures for removing such substances. The mnemonic **CHIPS** can be used for radiopaque medications: *c*hloral hydrate, *h*eavy metals, *i*ron, *p*henothiazines, and *s*low-release (enteric-coated) medications. In practice, abdominal radiography is primarily used in iron ingestion and suspected body-packing with illicit drugs.

Management

Management strategies are specific for the substance ingested. The regional poison control center should be consulted for advice on management and length of time to observe asymptomatic patients. A single number, 1-800-222-1222, automatically routes the caller to one of the appropriate 57 regional poison control centers in the nation. In general, the approach to management includes attention to the basic ABCs (airway, breathing, circulation) of resuscitation, decontamination methods, specific antidotes when available and indicated, and meticulous supportive care, often in an intensive care unit.

Decontamination

Decontamination techniques are strategies used to prevent or minimize absorption of the toxic substance and to enhance its elimination. They are a critical part of the management of acutely poisoned patients and should be used whenever a significant ingestion is suspected (Table 71-2).

Syrup of ipecac was commonly recommended in the past for home use to induce vomiting in the event of an accidental ingestion. **Gastric lavage,** in which a large nasogastric tube is placed and the stomach is washed with normal saline, is the hospital counterpart to syrup of ipecac. Both techniques theoretically remove toxic substance from the stomach, thus preventing absorption. However, at best (immediate performance after ingestion), less than one-third of gastric contents are removed by these methods. In addition, these techniques may interfere with the use of activated charcoal, usually a more effective therapy. Gastric lavage is technically difficult to perform in young children owing to the need to pass a large-bore tube. Gastric lavage also has a high rate of complications, such as aspiration and esophageal trauma. Neither syrup of ipecac nor gastric lavage is recommended for routine use. The American Academy of Pediatrics released a policy statement in 2003 stating that syrup of ipecac should no longer be kept in homes. Syrup of ipecac was administered in 0.01% of pediatric ingestions in 2011. The American Academy of Clinical Toxicology (AACT) reserves gastric lavage only for life-threatening ingestions presenting at fewer than 60 minutes since ingestion, with the caveat that there is no confirmed clinical benefit.

Activated charcoal is the mainstay in decontamination therapy of ingestion. Charcoal binds toxins, and because it is not absorbed in the GI tract, the charcoal-toxin complex passes through and is eliminated. Its efficacy decreases with increasing time since the ingestion, and ideally it should be started within an hour of the ingestion. The optimal dose of charcoal is 10 times the amount of substance ingested. Because the exact amount of toxin ingested is often unknown, activated charcoal is usually dosed at 1 to 2 g/kg. The amount of charcoal given is limited only by what the child is able to tolerate. Only a few substances are not absorbed by activated charcoal. The mnemonic **PHAILS** can be used to remember them: *p*esticides; *h*ydrocarbons and *h*eavy metals; *a*cids, *a*lkalis, and *a*lcohols; *i*ron; *l*ithium; and *s*olvents. The main complication of charcoal administration is aspiration pneumonitis, primarily seen in patients with altered level of consciousness and an unprotected airway. If charcoal is not voluntarily taken by the child, it may be administered via nasogastric tube. Endotracheal intubation (preferably with a cuffed tube) to protect the airway first may be necessary in the patient with altered mental status, as charcoal aspiration can result in severe chemical pneumonitis. It is imperative that nasogastric tube placement in the GI tract (as opposed to the respiratory tract) be confirmed prior to charcoal administration.

Cathartics (most commonly sorbitol) have been used to decrease transit time and improve elimination of the toxin through the GI tract and to counteract activated charcoal–induced constipation. The cathartic is often mixed with the activated charcoal and may serve to improve the palatability of the charcoal. A significant benefit from cathartic use has never been demonstrated, however, and there is a risk of dehydration and electrolyte disturbances, particularly in

Table 71-2. Summary of Gastric Decontamination Techniques

Technique	Dose	Contraindications
Syrup of ipecac	6 mo–1 y: 10 mL (use with caution) 1–12 y: 15 mL >12 y: 30 mL Follow with 8-oz water	**Not recommended for routine use** ALOC Caustics: acids and alkalis Hydrocarbons Expected ALOC (eg, tricyclic antidepressants)
Gastric lavage	15 mL/kg aliquots normal saline to maximum of 400 mL until lavage fluid is clear (may be several liters)	ALOC with unprotected airway Caustics: acids and alkalis Hydrocarbons Expected ALOC >1 h since ingestion
Activated charcoal	1–2 g/kg or <6 y: 25–50 g >6 y: 50–100 g	ALOC with unprotected airway Absent bowel sounds or bowel obstruction Substance not bound by charcoal
Cathartics	Magnesium citrate 4 mL/kg 70% sorbitol 1 g/kg	**Not recommended for routine use** Repeated doses can cause dehydration or electrolyte imbalances.
Whole-bowel irrigation	Toddler and preschool age: polyethylene glycol solution 500 mL/h 6–12 y: 1,000 mL/h Adolescent and adult: 1.5–2 L/h Continue until rectal effluent is clear	Bowel obstruction, ileus, perforation, or hemorrhage ALOC with unprotected airway
20% Intralipid	1.5 mL/kg initial bolus intravenous, then 0.25 mL/kg/min for 30–60 min	For lipophilic drug overdose with severe cardiotoxicity

Abbreviation: ALOC, altered level of consciousness.

young children. The AACT recommends *against* use of cathartics. Under no circumstances should repeated doses of cathartics be given.

Multiple-dose charcoal may remove drugs from the bloodstream by promoting diffusion back into the GI tract and subsequent binding to charcoal. It has been called "GI dialysis." Activated charcoal at the same dose previously used is repeated approximately every 4 hours. Cathartics should *not* be mixed with the charcoal for repeat doses. Multiple-dose charcoal is useful for a small number of drugs, such as phenobarbital, theophylline, carbamazepine, dapsone, and quinine. It should only be used if a potentially life-threatening amount has been ingested. It should not be used for drugs that can cause an ileus (eg, tricyclic antidepressants).

Whole-bowel irrigation involves infusion of a solution usually used for cleansing of the bowel prior to GI surgery (eg, polyethylene glycol). It is especially useful for slow-release medications, for tablets that dissolve slowly and may cause concretions (eg, iron), and in ingestions for which charcoal is not likely to be effective (eg, heavy metals). A nasogastric tube is used to infuse the solution at a rate of 500 mL/hour in young children and 1 to 2 L/hour in older children and adolescents. Clear rectal effluent is the end point; a bedpan may be necessary. Whole-bowel irrigation should not be used when there is bowel obstruction, ileus, perforation, or hemorrhage or altered mental status with an unprotected airway.

Hemodialysis may be used for serious ingestions of ethylene glycol, methanol, phenobarbital, lithium, salicylate, or theophylline. **Charcoal hemoperfusion,** in which blood goes through a charcoal cartridge instead of a dialysis machine, is used rarely for severe theophylline poisoning. **Urinary alkalinization** (by administration of sodium bicarbonate) can increase elimination of weak acids by keeping the drug in its ionic state, thus preventing reabsorption in the renal tubule. It is primarily used for significant salicylate, phenobarbital, and isoniazid poisonings.

Intralipid is becoming recognized as a potential treatment for lipophilic drug overdoses and has been used successfully for treating severe cardiotoxicity from bupivacaine, haloperidol, and verapamil overdoses. It is unclear by what method Intralipid works. Although ideal dosing and indications have not been established, one suggested treatment protocol to consider would be 1.5 mL/kg of 20% Intralipid initial bolus, followed by 0.25 mL/kg/min for 30 to 60 minutes. Boluses may be repeated for severe cardiotoxicity and dysrhythmias.

Supportive Care

Attention to the basic ABCs (airway, breathing, circulation) of resuscitation is always the first step in management. **Hypoglycemia** must be assessed and managed as soon as possible. Dextrose 0.5 to 1 g/kg intravenously is given; glucagon may be used if dextrose cannot be given. **Seizures** are generally treatable with benzodiazepines. Glucose and electrolyte levels should be normalized. With isoniazid ingestions, pyridoxine may be helpful. **Shock** requires aggressive fluid resuscitation. Fluid-resistant shock may require vasopressors, most commonly dopamine, epinephrine, or norepinephrine. Resistant shock in a β-blocker ingestion may respond to glucagon, and in a calcium channel blocker ingestion to insulin plus glucose.

Dysrhythmias should generally be treated by following pediatric advanced life support (PALS) protocols, although specific ingestions may respond to specific therapies. Sodium bicarbonate is the first-line treatment for dysrhythmias associated with ingestions of antihistamines, class 1 antiarrhythmics (ie, lidocaine, quinidine, procainamide), cocaine, and tricyclic antidepressants. β-blocker ingestions may respond to atropine and glucagon, while ingestions of calcium channel blockers are managed with calcium. Procainamide, found on PALS algorithms, should be avoided for dysrhythmias due to overdoses of antihistamines, quinidine and other class 1 antiarrhythmics, digoxin, quinine, and tricyclic antidepressants. Amiodarone, also found on PALS algorithms, should also be avoided in the treatment of antihistamine ingestions. Electrolyte imbalances should be assessed and corrected. **Suicidality** should be assessed, often in conjunction with a mental health professional.

Antidotes

Antidotes or medications that counteract the pathophysiological mechanisms of the toxin are available for only a few ingestions (Table 71-3). Important antidotes are N-acetylcysteine for acetaminophen, nalox-

Table 71-3. Antidotes	
Toxin	*Antidote*
Acetaminophen	N-acetylcysteine
Anticoagulants (Coumadin-like)	Vitamin K
Anticholinergic	Physostigmine
Benzodiazepine	Flumazenil
β-blocker	Glucagon
Calcium channel blocker	Calcium, insulin + glucose
Carbamate pesticide	Atropine
Carbon monoxide	Oxygen
Cyanide	Cyanide antidote kit
Digoxin	Digoxin immune Fab (ovine) (Digibind)
Ethylene glycol	Fomepizole, ethanol
Iron	Deferoxamine
Isoniazid	Pyridoxine
Lead	Dimercaprol (BAL), ethylene diamine tetra-acetic acid, DMSA
Mercury	BAL, DMSA
Methanol	Fomepizole, ethanol
Methemoglobinemia	Methylene blue
Narcotics	Naloxone
Organophosphate pesticide	Atropine, pralidoxime (2-PAM)
Rattlesnake bite	*Crotalidae* polyvalent immune Fab (ovine) (CroFab)
Sulfonylurea oral hypoglycemic	Dextrose, octreotide
Tricyclic antidepressant	Sodium bicarbonate

Abbreviations: BAL, British antilewisite; DMSA, dimercaptosuccinic acid.

Box 71-2. Substances Potentially Fatal in 1 to 2 Pills or Teaspoons

- Camphor (found in Vicks VapoRub, Campho-Phenique, Tiger Balm)
- Imidazoline decongestants (found in over-the-counter nasal drops and eyedrops)
- Acetonitrile nail glue remover
- Clonidine (available in transdermal patches also)
- Opiates (available in transdermal patches also)
- Methyl salicylate (oil of wintergreen, Bengay)
- Calcium channel blockers
- Toxic alcohols (methanol, ethylene glycol, ethanol, isopropanol)
- Tricyclic antidepressants
- Lomotil (opiate diphenoxylate + atropine)
- Sulfonylurea oral hypoglycemics
- Chloroquine and hydroxychloroquine antimalarial agents
- Hydrofluoric acid
- Selenious acid (gun bluing solution)
- Buffered saline solution
- Benzocaine-induced methemoglobinemia

pharmacies. Parents should not give activated charcoal without speaking to poison control center staff or medical personnel first.

Prognosis

Prognosis depends on the toxicity of the substance ingested. For a few substances, a small amount can be fatal (Box 71-2), whereas for others, even large ingestions are generally benign. Prognosis is generally excellent; fatalities in children are rare. Prognosis is worse for intentional ingestions, often because patients delay or fail to reveal that they attempted overdose.

CASE RESOLUTION

Because the respiratory rate of this 2-year-old is slow and there are symptoms of miosis and altered level of consciousness, narcotic ingestion is suspected and naloxone is administered. The child becomes more alert and respiratory rate increases to 24 breaths/min. The father is instructed to retrieve the bottle, and it turns out to be a prescription narcotic analgesic left in the house by a recent visitor. The child is given activated charcoal, observed overnight in the hospital, and discharged on the following day without sequelae.

one for narcotics, oxygen for carbon monoxide poisoning, bicarbonate for tricyclic antidepressant cardiotoxicity, digoxin immune Fab (ovine) (Digibind) for digoxin, and deferoxamine for iron. Antidotes are not without adverse effects themselves and should only be given in cases of symptomatic or potentially symptomatic (acetaminophen) ingestions of significant amounts. The poison control center staff can be very helpful in guiding practitioners in the use of antidotes.

Anticipatory Guidance and Prevention

Most ingestions are nontoxic and require only observation for a few hours. They do, however, provide an excellent opportunity to discuss poisoning prevention with parents and caregivers. Possible toxins, including prescription and over-the-counter medications, cleaning and household products, cosmetics and nail care products, toxic plants, gardening and hobby chemicals, and kitchen items such as alcohol should be kept out of reach of children. Visitors to the household should also be cautioned to keep medications out of reach of children. Substances should never be stored in unmarked containers, particularly in containers that typically hold beverages such as old soda bottles or cups. Medications should not be referred to as "candy" to entice youngsters to take them. Family members and visitors should be asked to store medications out of the child's reach and to dispose of leftover medications and used transdermal patches safely. Used transdermal patches may still contain up to 75% of the medication dose. Also, chewing on patches, as toddlers may do, releases the medication much faster. Parents should have the universal telephone number for the poison control center and telephone numbers for local emergency departments readily available. Carbon monoxide detectors should be placed near children's bedrooms. Activated charcoal for home use is controversial and not currently recommended, although it is available without prescription from many

Selected References

American Association of Poison Control Centers. http://www.aapcc.org. Accessed November 25, 2013

Bailey B. To decontaminate or not to decontaminate? The balance between potential risks and foreseeable benefits. *Clin Pediatr Emerg Med.* 2008;9:17–23

Bronstein AC, Spyker DA, Cantilena LR, Rumack BH, Dart RC. 2011 annual report of the American Association of Poison Control Centers' National Poison Data System (NPDS): 29th annual report. *Clin Toxicol (Phila).* 2012;50(10): 911–1164

Drugs.com. Pill identifier. http://www.drugs.com/pill_identification.html. Accessed November 25, 2013

Ferreirós N, Dresen S, Hermanns-Clausen M, et al. Fatal and severe codeine intoxication in 3-year-old twins—interpretation of drug and metabolite concentrations. *Int J Legal Med.* 2009;123(5):387–394

Finkelstein Y, Hutson JR, Wax PM, Brent J; Toxicology Investigators Consortium (ToxIC) Case Registry. Toxico-surveillance of infant and toddler poisonings in the United States. *J Med Toxicol.* 2012;8(3):263–266

Henry K, Harris CR. Deadly ingestions. *Pediatr Clin North Am.* 2006;53(2): 293–315

McGregor T, Parkar M, Rao S. Evaluation and management of common childhood poisonings. *Am Fam Physician.* 2009;79(5):397–403

Smith HS. Opioid metabolism. *Mayo Clin Proc.* 2009;84(7):613–624

US Food and Drug Administration. FDA drug safety communication: safety review update of codeine use in children; new Boxed Warning and Contraindication on use after tonsillectomy and/or adenoidectomy. http://www.fda.gov/Drugs/DrugSafety/ucm339112.htm. Accessed November 25, 2013

Weinberg G. LipidRescue resuscitation…for drug toxicity. http://lipidrescue.org. Accessed September 11, 2013

White ML, Liebelt EL. Update on antidotes for pediatric poisoning. *Pediatr Emerg Care.* 2006;22(11):740–749

Head, Neck, and Respiratory System

CHAPTER 72

Approach to the Dysmorphic Child

Julie E. Noble, MD

CASE STUDY

A 13-year-old boy presents to the office for the first time for an evaluation after moving to the area. Parents note that he has unexplained intellectual disability and has had problems with hyperactivity in school. The pregnancy was uncomplicated and the mother, who was a 32-year-old gravida 1, para 1 at the time of the child's birth, denies alcohol or drug use or exposure to any teratogens during pregnancy. Delivery was by cesarean birth secondary to cephalopelvic disproportion, but Apgar scores were 8 at 1 minute and 9 at 5 minutes. The newborn was noted to have macrocephaly and to be large for gestational age. He did well in the newborn period and had no feeding problems. Subsequently, he had no significant medical illnesses, including no seizures, but at 1 year of age was noted to be developmentally delayed. This delay continued, and he has been in special education classes throughout his school career. Family history is negative for any family members with disabilities.

On physical examination, the boy is greater than 90th percentile for height and weight. He is mildly prognathic with large ears. He has hyperextensible fingers. A complete examination reveals that his testicles appear large (6 cm) and his sexual maturity rating (Tanner stage) is 3. The rest of the examination is normal.

Questions

1. What history is important to elicit in evaluating a child with dysmorphic features?
2. What are the possible causes of errors in morphogenesis?
3. What clues on physical examination can aid in establishing a specific diagnosis?
4. What laboratory tests can confirm a diagnosis?
5. When is it appropriate to obtain a genetics consultation or refer a patient for genetic counseling?
6. What are the benefits of establishing a specific diagnosis?

Evaluation for structural anomalies is an essential part of all pediatric examinations. Visible errors in morphogenesis give the physician valuable information in evaluating a patient with abnormal symptoms, such as seizures. Additionally, major malformations frequently require treatment, and the presence of one anomaly suggests that others may also exist.

The study of these congenital defects was termed *dysmorphology* by David Smith in 1966. The anomalies fall into 2 categories: minor and major. Minor malformations are those of "no medical or cosmetic consequence to the patient." An example would be a supernumerary nipple that appears as a hyperpigmented papule along the nipple line. Identification of minor malformations is important because they may indicate the presence of a more generalized pattern of malformation. Major malformations are those that have "an adverse effect on either the function or social acceptability of the individual." A cleft lip and palate are major malformations that have functional as well as cosmetic relevance to the patient's health. Severe congenital malformations as defined by the Centers for Disease Control and Prevention are "defects that cause death, hospitalization or intellectual disability; necessitate significant surgical procedures; are disfiguring; or interfere with physical performance."

Epidemiology

Structural anomalies are common in the general population. Most are minor. In the first comprehensive analysis of minor structural anomalies, Marden in 1964 identified 7% to 14% of newborns with at least one minor anomaly on surface examination. Other studies identify up to 40% of newborns with one anomaly. Three or more minor malformations have predictive value in identifying a major malformation. Of newborns, 0.8% have 2 minor malformations, and 11% of these patients will have a major malformation. Three or more minor malformations occur in 0.5% of newborns, and 90% of these will have a major malformation. Data from the National Collaborative Perinatal Project revealed that 44.78% of these anomalies were craniofacial and 45.3% were skin. Males are affected with minor malformations more often than females. Autopsies of dead fetuses reveal an increased incidence of minor and major malformations. Frequencies of minor and major malformations vary along racial lines, depending on the specific malformations. For example, postaxial polydactyly is seen in 16 of 10,000 births in the white population and 140 of 10,000 births in the African American population. Hemangiomas are seen in 350 of 10,000 births in whites and only 100 of 10,000 births in African Americans.

Three percent of all pregnancies produce a child with a significant genetic disease or birth defect. These malformations account for a great proportion of morbidity and mortality in the pediatric population. Of all pediatric hospital admissions, one-third to one-half involve a child with a disease with a genetic component.

Clinical Presentation

With the advent of more prenatal tests and diagnostic modalities (see Chapter 22), the detection of anomalies may first occur in the prenatal period. Routine prenatal screening tests that are abnormal raise the possibility that the newborn will have an anomaly. For instance, an elevated maternal α-fetoprotein indicates the possibility of a spinal cord defect. Amniocentesis or chorionic villus biopsy may reveal abnormal chromosomes with associated structural defects. Prenatal ultrasound demonstrates structural defects in utero and a specific fetal ultrasound can further delineate those abnormalities.

Most structural anomalies develop during the first trimester of gestation and, if not detected prenatally, are noted at birth in the delivery room or newborn nursery. Many major congenital defects are obvious on a thorough physical examination. Some major defects, such as a tracheoesophageal fistula, will not be manifest on surface examination but will be readily apparent as the neonate adapts to extrauterine life and experiences symptoms when feeding begins. Minor anomalies may be overlooked on a neonate's initial examination. However, if that newborn manifests developmental delay at 6 months of age, the physician should thoroughly evaluate the infant for minor anomalies that may aid in identifying the cause of the developmental delay.

Sometimes dysmorphic features are not present at birth but become apparent later in life as the child grows and develops. These types of features are associated with dysplasias, defects in cellular metabolism that become manifest after birth. An example is a skeletal dysplasia that becomes more apparent as the bones grow.

Pathophysiology

The pathophysiology of structural defects can be separated into 4 different types of errors in morphogenesis: malformations, deformations, disruptions, and dysplasias (Box 72-1). All of these types of errors can result in a sequence of abnormalities.

Box 72-1. Pathophysiology of Structural Defects

Malformation
Chromosomal abnormality
Single gene disorder
Deformation
Disruption
Vascular compromise
Viral infection
Mechanical—amniotic bands
Teratogens—alcohol, drugs, irradiation
Dysplasia
Metabolic disorder

Previously, the term **malformation** was used descriptively to denote an anomaly, but it is also used to denote a specific pathogenic mechanism. Malformations are permanent defects in a structure caused by an intrinsic abnormality in the development of that structure. An example of a malformation is an endocardial cushion defect in a patient with Down syndrome. Malformations syndromes frequently are caused by chromosomal abnormalities and single-gene disorders that program for abnormal structure and environmental teratogens. Teratogens interfere with organ development during a critical period in embryogenesis and cause dysgenesis of fetal organs. Alcohol, specific drugs, irradiation, environmental exposures, and viral illnesses can all be teratogens. More than 30 drugs have been proven to be teratogenic.

Deformations occur in a newborn when external forces exert a mechanical pressure on the developing fetus. There is no intrinsic defect of the fetus. These deformations from intrauterine forces can be caused by uterine constraint, an abnormally shaped uterus, or multiparous pregnancy. A flexible talipes (clubfoot) is a deformation caused by uterine constraint. Postnatal deformations can also be caused by extrauterine forces such as plagiocephaly caused by an infant sleeping on his back. **Disruptions** occur when an agent outside a fetus causes cell death and a permanent defect in fetal development. These disruptive events result in tissue destruction. Disruptions can occur during development when there is tissue ischemia secondary to vascular compromise, when a viral infection disrupts development at a critical gestational age, or when a mechanical disruption interferes with normal development. An amniotic band is an example of a mechanical disruptive agent that can cause an amputation of a limb by constricting the extremity during development.

Dysplasias, often caused by a single-gene defect, are structural abnormalities that develop from abnormal cellular metabolism and organization. They can occur intrauterine and be apparent at birth, such as a skeletal dysplasia, or extrauterine. Mucopolysaccharidosis is a dysplasia that develops postnatally secondary to the absence of the lysosomal hydrolase of α-l-iduronidase. As a result, glycosaminoglycans accumulate in parenchymal and mesenchymal tissues. As affected children grow, they develop coarse facies, enlarged tongue, misshapen bones, and hepatosplenomegaly among other features.

Differential Diagnosis

In generating an appropriate differential diagnosis for a child who is dysmorphic, it is essential to identify all minor and major malformations. The differential will vary depending on the specific findings. A thorough history and physical examination will help greatly to establish the list of conditions to consider. If there are multiple anomalies, identifying the most specific and rarest anomaly can direct the practitioner to a narrower list of possible diagnoses. For example, nail hypoplasia, which is seen in fetal hydantoin syndrome, is much rarer than congenital cardiac disease, which is seen in multiple syndromes. A practitioner should be familiar with the prominent features of the more common syndromes but also should have readily available reference texts, such as *Smith's Recognizable*

Patterns of Human Malformation, to aid in establishing differential lists as well as finalizing diagnoses. In addition, the Internet has developed into a valuable tool through Web sites such as Online Mendelian Inheritance in Man (OMIM), PubMed, or Google, or those specifically developed for the delineation of syndromes and genetic disorders.

In evaluating a neonate or an infant with congenital anomalies, the practitioner should attempt to separate the findings into 1 of 5 categories: an isolated defect, a developmental field defect, a birth defect association, a sequence pattern, or a dysmorphic syndrome (Box 72-2). The first step is to determine whether the anomaly is **isolated.** If so, does it represent a failure in development in one location, such as a cleft lip? Most isolated anomalies are believed to have a multifactorial inheritance, representing the interaction between multiple genes and unknown external influences. They usually have a recurrence risk of 2% to 5%.

A **developmental field defect** is a pattern of anomalies that develops in structures that are together during embryologic development. These defects involve one limited region and are secondary to a disruptive event such as vascular compromise. They therefore have a low recurrence risk. An example would be hemifacial microsomia (oculoauriculovertebral defect), where the defects are secondary to disruption in vascular flow to the first and second branchial arches. This disruption results in hypoplasia of the malar, maxillary, and mandibular region on one side with associated microtia and vertebral defects.

Birth defect associations are diagnosed when the combination of anomalies occurs together frequently but the pattern does not fit a known field defect or syndrome. The etiology of association defects is unknown at this time, and recurrence risk is low. One of the more common associations is the VACTERL association (*v*ertebral anomalies, *a*nal atresia, *c*ardiac defects, *t*racheoesophageal fistula, *r*enal defects, and *l*imb defects). Emerging information in gene research may identify an etiology in the near future.

A **sequence pattern** of anomalies occurs when one malformation leads to multiple dysmorphic features. Potter oligohydramnios sequence results from renal agenesis. The renal malformation causes oligohydramnios with resultant fetal contractures, pulmonary hypoplasia, and a flattened face.

A **syndrome** is a pattern of anomalies that are pathologically related. Chromosomal abnormalities such as Down syndrome (trisomy 21), single-gene disorders, and teratogens fall into this category. Alcohol is the most common teratogen to which fetuses are exposed. Alcohol exposure in utero causes growth failure, developmental delay, microcephaly, a short nose, and small distal phalanges. Children with developmental delay and anomalies have a

higher likelihood of having a syndrome and should undergo a chromosome analysis.

Evaluation

History

A complete history is essential (Questions Box). The history begins prenatally with information from the mother on duration of pregnancy, possible teratogen exposure, fetal activity, diagnostic test results, and any complications of pregnancy. The delivery history should include type of delivery, newborn presentation, and size at birth, including growth percentiles. Neonatal adaptation and feeding patterns are important parameters to assess. The subsequent medical history should be obtained. The identification of associated intellectual disability is an essential part of the history.

A thorough family history is equally important, and a pedigree should be outlined. Specifically, the family should be questioned for parental age, possible consanguinity, and history of fetal loss or early infant deaths. Family history of birth defects or disabilities should be documented.

Physical Examination

The physical examination should be extremely thorough with all morphologic findings noted. As previously mentioned, the craniofacial area and skin are common sites for anomalies, but all organ systems should be extensively evaluated. Even minor anomalies, such as a supernumerary nipple or clinodactyly, may have significance. Objective measurements should be obtained when possible. Normal grids are available for evaluating, for example, inner canthus distance, palpebral fissure length, and ear length. Hair whorl patterns and dermatoglyphics should be evaluated. Physical data, including height, weight, and head circumference, should be plotted and the growth percentiles noted. A complete ophthalmologic evaluation may be indicated to detect abnormalities such as cataracts or cherry-red spots.

Box 72-2. Categories of Anomalies	
Isolated defect	Sequence pattern
Developmental field defect	Dysmorphic syndrome
Birth defect association	

Questions

The Dysmorphic Child

- How long was the pregnancy?
- Did the mother take any medications, smoke cigarettes, or use alcohol or any illicit drug?
- What was the fetal activity?
- Were there any complications of pregnancy?
- What was the type of delivery and presentation of the baby?
- What was the newborn's size at birth?
- How did the newborn feed?
- What is the subsequent medical and developmental history?
- Are the parents related?
- What are the parents' ages?
- Is there a history of fetal or infant deaths?
- Is there a history of birth defects in the family?
- Do any family members have disabilities?

Laboratory Tests

In assessments of children who appear dysmorphic, the physical examination is the most important part. Findings on physical examination direct which further studies will be of benefit. Additional studies may give added or confirmatory information about a suspected diagnosis. Prenatal screening tests may be used to detect a fetal abnormality, and specific prenatal tests are available to assess a fetus at risk for a given disease. Cytogenetic evaluation is essential in evaluating a child with a suspected syndrome and also in evaluating a child with malformations and developmental delay. Standard chromosomal analysis, G-banded karyotype, is the first-line laboratory test but may not detect many small chromosomal or gene defects. More sophisticated testing may be indicated. Small chromosomal aberrations can be detected by fluorescence in situ hybridization (FISH) analysis, in which labeled probes are applied to chromosomal preparations. These probes are specific for given disorders and should be used to confirm a suspected clinical syndrome. Prader-Willi and DiGeorge syndromes may be diagnosed by FISH analysis. Fluorescence in situ hybridization probes can now be applied to sub-telomeric regions of the chromosome, which are very gene rich. Whole chromosome painting is another technique in which FISH probes are used to paint the entire chromosome, thus identifying the origin of additional chromosomal material or cryptic translocations. Molecular testing is available for many single-gene disorders. Microarray-based comparative genomic hybridization (cgh) and single-nucleotide polymorphism (SNP) arrays are the cytogenetic methods for analysis of copy number changes in DNA. They are a supplement to a karyotype and the prime genome-wide screening method. These tests have revealed genetic etiologies of copy number variants in many previously unidentified patients with abnormalities.

Many dysplasias and some syndromes can be detected by metabolic testing. Serum amino acids and urine organic acids should be ordered if a diagnosis is suspected. Many states are now including an analysis for metabolic disorders in their expanded newborn screening protocols. There is a federal effort to standardize newborn screening guidelines statewide. Genomic sequencing may become part of newborn screening in the future.

Imaging Studies

Imaging studies are extremely useful in deriving information on internal malformations. Radiographs, including a skeletal survey, may detect skeletal anomalies. Echocardiogram, renal ultrasound, computed tomography scan, and magnetic resonance imaging (MRI) studies can all be used when appropriate. With the findings of anomalies and global developmental delay in a patient, the American Academy of Neurology recommends routine neuroimaging with an MRI.

Management

When children present with dysmorphic features, they should be evaluated to determine a specific diagnosis. Obtaining a diagnosis is of vital importance to the care of the patient and parental counseling. Knowing the diagnosis can direct subsequent testing for associated abnormalities. Treatment options may also be available for the condition, and a prognosis can be established. Defining the developmental prognosis for children is essential to establish appropriate school planning. If developmental delay is not associated with the diagnosis, such as with cleft lip and palate, parents should be reassured. Parents also need to know the recurrence risk for themselves and their children. Occasionally, further testing of parents may be necessary to determine the accurate recurrence risk. If one of the parents is a translocation carrier, the risk of subsequent children having the abnormality is increased.

Consultation with a geneticist can help the practitioner in establishing the correct diagnosis and provide the practitioner with the latest information on evaluation and possible treatment. New information in the field of genetic disease appears daily, and it is difficult for a primary care practitioner to stay abreast. A genetic consultation should also be obtained in patients with major malformations to confirm the diagnosis and help counsel parents.

Health supervision strategies have been established for specific disorders. For instance, published guidelines recommend hearing, ophthalmologic, and thyroid screening, among other tests, for patients with Down syndrome. A geneticist can also give guidance on revised recommendations.

If support groups are available for specific conditions, parents should be referred to these groups. Such groups can be invaluable in helping parents understand as well as adjust to the disorder. They can also advise parents about community and educational resources available for their child's care and help parents advocate for their child's unique needs.

A referral to a genetics counselor can provide parents with education about prenatal testing, recurrence risk, and alternatives for dealing with this recurrence risk. Counseling is extremely useful to help parents understand the inheritance pattern.

Prognosis

As with management, defining an accurate prognosis for each patient depends on recognition of the specific condition. Some conditions, such as trisomy 13, are lethal, while other conditions allow for a normal life span.

Malformations are permanent defects that generally have a recurrence risk. They may be correctable with surgery or treatment but frequently leave a residual disability.

Deformations usually resolve with treatment and have no recurrence risk unless the deformation is secondary to a uterine abnormality such as a bicornuate uterus.

A disruption may be treated with surgery or therapy to improve function, but as in malformations, a residual disability frequently remains. When the disruption is due to tissue ischemia or a mechanical agent, there is no recurrence risk. If it is due to a teratogen, the disruption will recur with the same teratogenic exposure.

Dysplasias tend to persist or worsen with time unless a specific treatment is available. Only a limited number of diseases have specific treatments available. Generally, there is a recurrence risk.

CASE RESOLUTION

The child in the case scenario has features that suggest a dysmorphic syndrome. The most specific finding on examination is macro-orchidism. This finding is associated with fragile X syndrome. The patient is referred to a genetic specialist for diagnosis and counseling. Specific DNA-based molecular analysis is performed and is positive for a fragile site on the X chromosome at Xq27.3.

Parents are counseled that this condition has an X-linked inheritance pattern. The child will have a normal life span but may need early intervention services and later a special education program, and may not be capable of independent living as an adult. The primary care physician will be notified of the diagnosis and coordinate further services. Parents are encouraged to attend a parents' support group and consult with experts to learn how their child's full potential may be realized.

Selected References

Aase JM. Dysmorphologic diagnosis for the pediatric practitioner. *Pediatr Clin North Am.* 1992;39(1):135–156

Brent RL. The role of the pediatrician in preventing congenital malformations. *Pediatr Rev.* 2011;32(10):411–422

Gropman AL, Batshaw ML. Epigenetics, copy number variation, and other molecular mechanisms underlying neurodevelopmental disabilities: new insights and diagnostic approaches. *J Dev Behav Pediatr.* 2010;31(7):582–591

Jones KL, Jones MC, Casanelles MD. *Smith's Recognizable Patterns of Human Malformation.* 7th ed. Philadelphia, PA: Elsevier Saunders; 2013

Mefford HC, Batshaw ML, Hoffman EP. Genomics, intellectual disability and autism. *N Engl J Med.* 2012;366(8):733–743

Moeschler JB, Shevell M; American Academy of Pediatrics Committee on Genetics. Clinical genetic evaluation of the child with mental retardation or developmental delays. *Pediatrics.* 2006;117(6):2304–2316

Poot M, Hochstenbach R. A three-step workflow procedure for the interpretation of array-based comparative genomic hybridization results in patients with idiopathic mental retardation and congenital anomalies. *Genet Med.* 2010;12(8): 478–485

Southard AE, Edelmann LJ, Gelb BD. Role of copy number variants in structural birth defects. *Pediatrics.* 2012;129(4):755–763

Toriello HV. Role of the dysmorphologic evaluation in the child with developmental delay. *Pediatr Clin North Am.* 2008; 55(5):1085–1098

Walker WO Jr, Johnson CP. Mental retardation: overview and diagnosis. *Pediatr Rev.* 2006;27(6):204–212

CHAPTER 73

Craniofacial Anomalies

Carol D. Berkowitz, MD

CASE STUDY

A 3,500-g boy is born by normal spontaneous vaginal delivery to a 28-year-old gravida 3, para 3 mother after an uncomplicated full-term gestation. Apgar scores are 9 and 10. On physical examination, the newborn is well but has an incomplete, left-sided unilateral cleft of the lip and palate.

No other family members have such a deformity, but the mother and father are distantly related. The mother had prenatal care. During the pregnancy she had no illnesses, took vitamins but no other medications, and did not smoke, drink alcohol, or use illicit drugs.

The mother is planning to feed the newborn with formula and wonders if she should do anything special. She is also wondering if her son's lip deformity can be repaired before she takes him home from the hospital. Except for the cleft, the physical examination is normal.

Questions

1. What craniofacial anomalies are common in children?
2. What are feeding considerations in newborns with cleft lip or palate?
3. What is the appropriate timing of surgery for the more common craniofacial anomalies?
4. What are the major medical problems that children with craniofacial anomalies, particularly clefts of the lip or palate, experience?
5. What is positional plagiocephaly? How is its prevalence related to the Back to Sleep campaign?

Neonates may be born with readily apparent craniofacial anomalies such as cleft lip, cleft palate, or microtia, or anomalies may emerge as an infant grows older. The latter includes conditions that may be genetically based but do not manifest until later, such as facial asymmetry (hemifacial microsomia) and premature closure of one or more sutures. Alternatively, these anomalies may be environmentally influenced, such as positional or deformational plagiocephaly. Deformational plagiocephaly is defined as a condition in which an infant's head and sometimes face are misshapen as a result of prenatal and, in recent years, postnatal external molding, which occur on the infant's malleable cranium.

Epidemiology

The overall incidence of cleft lip with or without cleft palate is 1 in 1,000 and that of isolated cleft palate is 1 in 2,500. Cleft lip with or without cleft palate is the fourth most common birth defect. There is racial, ethnic, and geographic variation in the incidence of clefts. For example, the incidence of clefts in parts of the Philippines is 1 in 200. Similarly, cleft lip with or without cleft palate is most common among Native Americans (1 in 230–1,000) and least common among African Americans (1 in 1,300–5,000). The gender distribution varies with the type of cleft. Isolated clefts of the palate occur twice as frequently in girls, but clefts of the lip with or without clefts of the palate appear twice as often in boys.

The type of cleft, the gender of the child, and whether parents or other siblings are similarly affected influence the risk for recurrence of clefts in subsequent offspring. In general, the risk for recurrence of clefts is 4% to 7% for cleft lip with or without cleft palate and 3% for isolated cleft palate.

Clefts may occur as isolated findings or as part of syndromes or sequences. In Van der Woude syndrome, clefts of the lip or palate are associated with lip pits. This condition is inherited in an autosomal-dominant manner. There are now more than 200 disorders associated with clefts, although only 10% to 15% of children with clefts fit a syndrome. Pierre Robin sequence includes micrognathia and glossoptosis (retrodeviated tongue) and a distinct u-shaped cleft. One theory relates the sequence to failure of the fetal neck to extend normally, leading to compression of the mandible on the chest, thereby restricting its growth and causing malposition of the tongue, thus preventing closure of the palate.

True craniosynostosis occurs in about 1 in 2,000 to 3,000 births, and this incidence is the same in all ethnic groups. There is gender variation among the different types of craniosynostosis. Mild deformational plagiocephaly is reported to be present in up to 13% of newborns, 16% of 6-week-olds, and nearly 20% of 4-month-olds. A study of 440 infants between 7 and 12 weeks of age reported an incidence of plagiocephaly of 46.6%; in 78.3%, it was mild. The term *plagiocephaly* comes from the Greek *plagio*, meaning oblique, twisted, or slanted, and *kephale* for head. Firstborn and male gender increase the risk of deformational plagiocephaly at birth. Most cases of deformational plagiocephaly resolve over time without specific medical intervention. When infants slept in the prone position, plagiocephaly occurred in 1 in 300. The prevalence of plagiocephaly increased to 1 in 60 following the recommendation for supine sleep position.

Microtia is less common and occurs in 1 in 6,000 to 8,000 births. Other ear malformations, such as auricular dystopia (ear located on the check) or total atresia of the external area, are less common and can be associated with other syndromes.

Clinical Presentation

Most craniofacial anomalies are readily apparent (D_x Box). Some anomalies, such as cleft lips or microtia, are noted immediately in the delivery room. Other anomalies, such as craniosynostosis, develop over time. Because the onset of craniosynostosis may be gradual, parents may fail to recognize the condition, which usually appears as asymmetry of the face or skull. Deformational plagiocephaly also evolves over time and is more often noted by the clinician rather than the parents.

Children with craniofacial anomalies may also have medical problems that occur secondary to the deformity. Newborns and infants with cleft palate may present with failure to thrive because of difficulty feeding. Older infants and children may experience recurrent otitis media, speech impairments, or psychosocial stress. Nasal regurgitation of liquids may occur in children with obvious palatal clefts or more subtle deformities, such as submucosal clefts of the soft palate.

Pathophysiology

Clefts of the lip and palate (Figure 73-1) are believed to develop as a result of an interruption in the merging of the middle and lateral portions of the face during the sixth to seventh week of gestation. The palate normally closes with an anterior to posterior progression. Any interference with this progression (eg, tumor or encephalocele in the roof of the mouth) leads to a cleft. A vascular disruption may also result in ischemia in the involved areas. Although the etiology of clefts is not fully determined, it is felt to be multifactorial. Studies establish a link between clefting and transforming growth factor–α (TGF-α). The locus for TGF-α is on the short arm of 2p13. As with other clinical conditions, genetic predisposition interacts with environmental factors to increase the risk of the emergence of a disorder. Newborns with the A2 form of the TGF-α gene are 8 times more likely to have facial clefts if their mothers smoke. Other environmental teratogens associated with clefts include hydantoin,

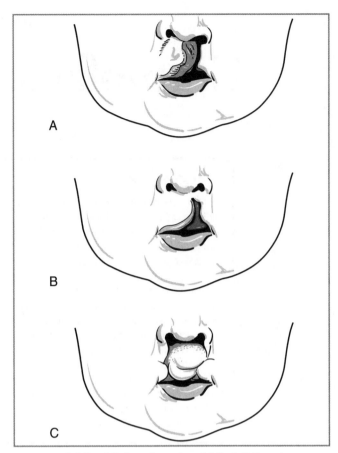

Figure 73-1. Cleft lips. A, Unilateral, complete cleft lip. **B,** Unilateral, incomplete cleft lip. **C,** Bilateral, complete cleft lip.

alcohol, warfarin, trimethadione, thalidomide, aminopterin, and topiramate.

The presence of a cleft palate affects normal oropharyngeal functioning, including sucking and speech. Children may exhibit hypernasal speech caused by the escape of air through the nose and have articulation problems. Recurrent otitis media seems to be related to dysfunction of the eustachian tube.

Microtia, a small atretic pinna of the ear, results from failure of development of the pinna and portions of the external auditory canal. It is most likely caused by a vascular accident during the 12th week of gestation. Similar anomalies have been created in laboratory animals by ligature of the stapedius artery. Microtia is considered in the spectrum of branchial arch defects.

Craniosynostosis refers to the premature closure of the sutures, which should remain open until 2 to 3 years of age. The newborn skull consists of membranous bones that meet at the suture lines. The newborn skull is therefore moldable, can change during the birthing process, and can expand in response to growth of the brain. Premature closure of the sutures is a pathologic process. What initiates this pathologic ossification is unclear. There is some evidence to suggest that skull compression, such as that which occurs in utero with breech presentation or twins, contributes to the process. When there are other associated anomalies, such as syndactyly, embryologic disturbances in fibrocartilaginous development are suspected.

Dx Craniofacial Anomalies

- Cleft of the lip or palate
- Small, atretic, or malformed ear
- Asymmetry of the face
- Misshapen skull
- Recurrent otitis media
- Speech impairment

Abnormalities in one region of chromosome 10 are implicated in syndromic synostosis. Genes associated with fibroblast growth factor receptor have been implicated in some genetic syndromes with craniosynostosis. Any or all of the sutures can be affected, and the closure may result in asymmetry of the skull or microcephaly. Single suture synostosis is classified as simple; multiple synostosis is classified as compound. When closure is related to pathology at the suture, the condition is primary. When there is underlying brain pathology, the disorder is secondary. Premature closure of all sutures is often associated with diseases of the central nervous system, with failure of the brain to grow.

Microcephaly may result from premature closure of some or all of the sutures as a primary event or from impairment of the brain and its growth related to some other problem, such as hypoxic encephalopathy or congenital infection. Other disorders involving head size include macrocephaly, in which the head circumference is greater than the 97th percentile. There are numerous causes of macrocephaly, including hydrocephalus, characterized by enlargement of the ventricular system, and macrencephaly, the latter of which may be due to enlargement of the brain from anatomic or metabolic conditions, including mucopolysaccharidoses. Children who have large heads and are neurologically normal have benign or idiopathic macrencephaly. Measuring parental head size is frequently a clue to the correct diagnosis.

Fusion of individual sutures prevents growth of the skull perpendicular to the suture, and skull expansion proceeds in an axis parallel to that of the suture (Figure 73-2). If the sagittal suture fuses prematurely, the head is long and narrow, a condition referred to as **scaphocephaly** (boat head). This is the most common type of craniosynostosis, occurring in about 54% to 58%. If the coronal sutures fuse too soon, the head is flattened; this condition is called **brachycephaly** and occurs in 18% to 29% of cases of craniosynostosis. The

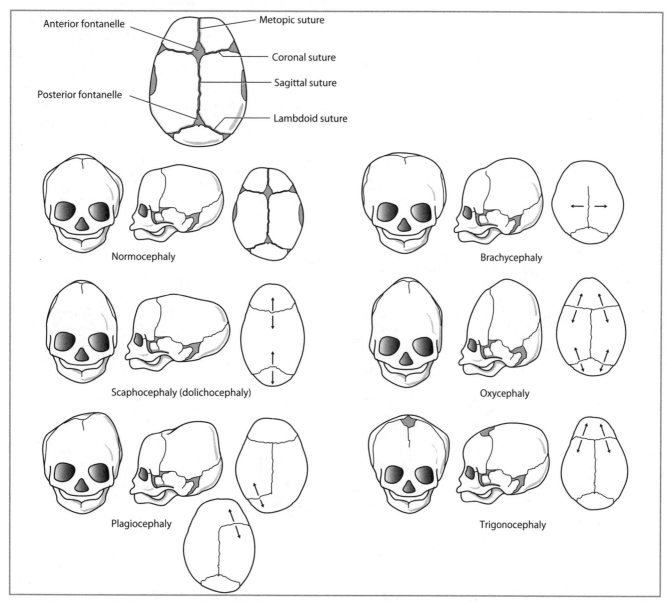

Figure 73-2. Changes in the shape of the skull when sutures fuse prematurely. Growth occurs parallel to the fused suture.

incidence is 1 in 10,000 live births. Unilateral fusion of a coronal suture produces facial asymmetry and a characteristic appearance of the orbit on the affected side, called a harlequin deformity, noted on facial radiograph. Premature closure of the metopic suture results in the triangular-shaped head characteristic of **trigonocephaly,** reported in 4% to 10%. Familial cases have been reported, as well as abnormalities of chromosomes 3, 9, and 11. *FGFR*3P25OR mutation has been reported in patients with nonsyndromic craniosynostosis, particularly with coronal or multi-suture synostoses.

Premature closure of the lambdoid sutures leads to **plagiocephaly** (oblique head) (Figure 73-3). Plagiocephaly may also result from malpositioning in utero or after birth, a condition referred to as nonsynostotic, deformational, or positional plagiocephaly. The skull has been likened to a parallelogram in appearance when there is also involvement of the facial structures. Torticollis, often related to injury to the sternocleidomastoid muscle at birth (see Chapter 110) and abnormal positioning after birth, may contribute to plagiocephaly. Plagiocephaly-torticollis sequence occurs in 1 in 300 live births. Malar and contralateral occipital flattening related to preferential positioning by infants are characteristically seen in affected infants. Some affected babies also have hip dislocation or positional talipes (clubfoot) from in utero constraint (see Chapter 104). Positional plagiocephaly may be seen without torticollis and has been attributed to supine sleeping.

Differential Diagnosis

In general, the differential diagnosis of clefts of the lip and palate presents few problems. However, submucosal clefts may be more difficult to diagnose. Children with such clefts may present with recurrent otitis media or hyper-nasal speech. Physical examination may reveal a bifid uvula and occasionally a notch at the junction of the hard and soft palates.

Determining whether any physical finding represents an isolated anomaly or is part of a genetic syndrome may be challenging. Any associated anomalies (eg, syndactyly, atrial septal defect) suggest the possibility of a genetic problem (boxes 73-1 and 73-2).

Microtia does not present a diagnostic dilemma. The anomaly usually appears sporadically as an isolated condition, although, like a cleft, it may be part of some other syndrome. Microtia is associated with midfacial hypoplasia and anti-Mongoloid slant to the eyes in Treacher Collins syndrome. Microtia may also occur in oculoauriculovertebral dysplasia (Goldenhar syndrome), which is characterized by several associated findings, including hemifacial microsomia (one side of the face smaller than the other), epibulbar dermoids, hemivertebrae, microphthalmos, and renal and cardiac anomalies.

Craniosynostosis may also be an isolated finding or associated with a condition such as Apert syndrome, in which clefts of the palate are also seen (Box 73-3). A careful neurodevelopmental assessment helps

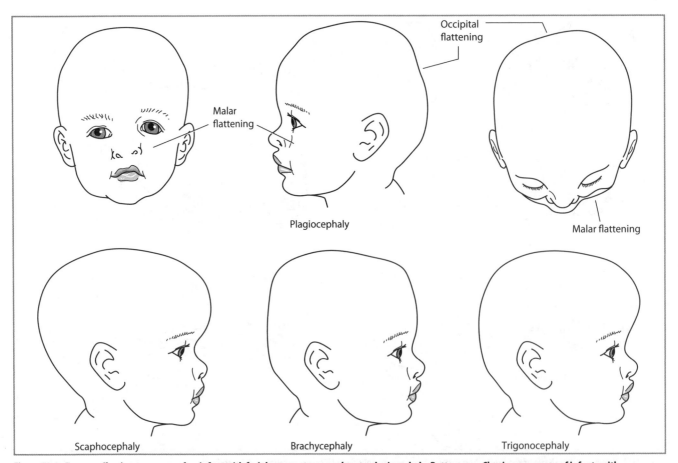

Figure 73-3. Top row, Classic appearance of an infant with facial asymmetry secondary to plagiocephaly. Bottom row, Classic appearance of infants with craniosynostosis.

Box 73-1. Genetic Syndromes Associated With Clefts	
Ankyloblepharon filiforme adnatum	Opitz
Apert	Oral-facial-digital (OFD1)
Ectrodactyly–ectodermal dysplasia–clefting	Popliteal web
Goldenhar (oculoauriculovertebral dysplasia)	Stickler (hereditary progressive arthro-ophthalmopathy)
	Treacher Collins
Meckel	Van der Woude

Box 73-2. Anomalies Associated With Cleft Lips and Palates	
Nasal glioma or encephalocele	Sacral agenesis
Persistent oropharyngeal membrane	Aniridia
Congenital neuroblastoma	Cleft larynx
Congenital heart disease	Polydactyly
Thoracopagus twins	Anencephaly
Congenital oral teratoma	Foot deformities
Forearm bone aplasia	Oral duplication
Lateral proboscis	Spina bifida
	Aplasia of trochlea
	Laryngeal web

Box 73-3. Genetic Disorders With Craniosynostosis	
Apert syndrome	Jackson syndrome
Crouzon syndrome	Pfeiffer syndrome

determine whether microcephaly is related to an underlying neuro-developmental disorder. Plagiocephaly may present a diagnostic dilemma: Is the condition related to unilateral craniosynostosis, torticollis, or supine sleeping? A careful assessment of the neck for masses or mobility helps determine the role of the neck musculature in cranial flattening and defines the management approach (eg, neck exercises).

Evaluation

Care must be taken to assess children and determine if the anomalies are isolated findings or components of a syndrome. This information is important in terms of patient care and genetic counseling for parents on the likelihood of having future offspring with similar anomalies.

History

A medical, family, and psychosocial history should be obtained (Questions Box). Whether the condition appeared at birth or some time later is particularly significant in lesions affecting the skull, such as craniosynostosis. Maternal use of certain medications, such as diazepam, phenytoin, and isotretinoin (Accutane), and alcohol is associated with

Questions

Craniofacial Anomalies

- Did the child suffer any injuries at birth?
- Was the child born in an abnormal position?
- What is the child's usual sleeping position?
- Have the findings been present since birth, or did they appear later?
- Has the anomaly led to any changes in the child's health, such as recurrent ear infections or speech difficulties?
- Does the child have any family history of craniofacial anomalies?
- Does the mother have a history of illness during pregnancy?
- Was the mother exposed to any medications, particularly teratogenic agents, during pregnancy?
- Did the mother use alcohol during pregnancy?
- Did the mother smoke during pregnancy?
- Is the child experiencing difficulties in school (eg, teasing)?
- How is the child performing in school?
- Is development progressing normally? What are the child's milestones?
- Is the child's speech understandable?
- Does the child have any trouble with eating or drinking? Are fluids expelled through the child's nose with swallowing?

an increased incidence of clefts of the lip and palate. Maternal smoking also increases the risk of clefting, especially in a genetically vulnerable population. Maternal smoking and high altitude are associated with an increased occurrence of craniosynostosis.

Physical Examination

Height, weight, and head circumference should be measured and plotted at each visit. Head circumference is especially important in children with craniosynostosis or facial asymmetry. The skull should be palpated to detect perisutural ridging. Inner canthal distance may reveal hypotelorism, a finding seen in trigonocephaly. The neck should be palpated for masses and the range of neck motion assessed. The growth of children with craniofacial anomalies must be carefully monitored. Problems with adequate weight gain are frequently experienced by newborns and infants with clefts.

The physical examination should focus on defining the extent of the anomaly and determining if associated abnormalities are present. Such abnormalities may involve the face or other parts of the body, including the skeleton. The pharynx should be carefully examined for mobility of the palate. While some children with nasal regurgitation have a structural deformity, such as a submucosal cleft, others, including infants with DiGeorge syndrome (22q11 deletion syndrome), have functional impairment with decreased palatal mobility. In children with microtia, the position of the ear should be noted. When the ear is displaced to the cheek, the condition is called *auricular malposition*. Cardiac murmurs may be noted in children with clefts, and these murmurs should be carefully evaluated.

Children with clefts should be carefully assessed for the presence of otitis media at each visit. Periodic hearing assessments should be carried out in children with clefts or microtia. Speech and development should also be evaluated.

Laboratory Tests

Routine laboratory tests are not indicated in most children with craniofacial anomalies. Chromosomal studies are indicated if a genetic disorder is suspected. Refined studies, including fluorescence in situ hybridization, may be needed to detect certain chromosomal abnormalities (see Chapter 72). Referral to a geneticist is warranted to ensure testing for the most recently identified gene associated with the condition and genetic counseling with the parents.

Imaging Studies

Radiographs and imaging studies may be indicated in children with facial asymmetry, microcephaly and macrocephaly, and craniosynostosis. A 3-dimensional computed tomography scan of the skull is particularly helpful in defining which, if any, sutures are fused but is not warranted in children with suspected positional plagiocephaly. Such studies are helpful in differentiating craniosynostosis and deformational disorders that will resolve on their own. Renal ultrasound may be indicated in children with microtia or other ear anomalies because of the association between ear and renal anomalies. Renal ultrasound is usually normal in children with isolated microtia but is abnormal in about 30% of children with auricular as well as other congenital anomalies, particularly when associated with certain syndromes.

Management

The management of children with craniofacial anomalies usually requires the expertise of a multidisciplinary team, including a pediatrician; plastic surgeon; ear, nose, and throat specialist; speech pathologist; social worker; psychologist; orthodontist; and prosthodontist. Primary care physicians who are not part of the team can receive information about appropriate patient care and follow-up. It is important for primary care physicians to be familiar with the appropriate nomenclature to be able to communicate with consultants. In brief, clefts of the lip are unilateral or bilateral and complete or incomplete. A complete cleft extends into the nares (see Figure 73-1). Clefts of the palate may involve the entire palate or be confined to the secondary or soft palate.

Routine **well-child care,** including monitoring of growth and administration of immunizations, is most important in the management of children with craniofacial anomalies. Some newborns and infants with clefts are slow feeders. Mothers should be told that although breastfeeding can be carried out, it may present unique challenges; however, the compliancy of the breast tissue creates a natural seal for the lip and palate. If difficulties are encountered, consultation with a lactation specialist may be especially helpful. Some formula-fed newborns and infants require the use of special adaptive nipples or feeders. A specific cleft palate feeder, which consists of a plastic bottle that allows for compression of the unit during feeding, is available. A soft, premature-type nipple can also be obtained. Long nipples, such as lamb's nipples, which are used to feed baby

lambs, are not routinely recommended because they cause newborns and infants to gag. Newborns and infants who gain weight slowly may need to be given concentrated formulas (see Chapter 133).

Hearing and speech should be monitored. Chronic prophylactic **antibiotics** or the insertion of **pressure equalization tubes** may be needed to manage recurrent otitis media (see Chapter 75). Speech problems require the expertise of a speech pathologist and placement of children in **speech therapy** in the community or school.

Surgical correction is indicated for many anomalies. Clefts are usually repaired as staged procedures during the first 2 years of life. Repair of the cleft lip, the first procedure, is traditionally scheduled when infants weigh 10 pounds and are 10 weeks of age and their hemoglobin is 10 (rule of 10s). Appropriate weight gain is therefore critical to ensure timely surgery. If skilled anesthesiologists and nurses are available, cleft lip repair can be carried out within the first 2 weeks of life. Early repair is recommended at some centers. Repair of the cleft palate, the second procedure, is usually undertaken when children are between 12 and 18 months of age. Better speech develops with earlier palatal repair. Surgical correction of clefts does not alter children's propensity to otitis media, although the incidence of otitis media appears to have decreased among children with clefts following the use of conjugated pneumococcal vaccine. The incidence of otitis media decreases as children get older, however. Refinement of the cosmetic results, including rhinoplasty, occurs throughout childhood. Orthodontia is frequently a key component to achieve a cosmetically acceptable result and appropriate occlusion of the dentition for speech and chewing. About 10% to 20% of children will develop velopharyngeal insufficiency following repair of a cleft palate. In these cases, the posterior soft palate fails to make a tight seal with the pharynx. Children may experience nasal regurgitation of food or hyper-nasal speech. Surgical correction of velopharyngeal insufficiency involves lengthening the shortened palate. Additional surgery may also be required by children who have significant jaw deformities. These may include the placement of bone grafts or maxillary advancement.

Children with isolated unilateral microtia often hear, and surgery is recommended to restore a normal anatomic appearance, even if hearing in the affected ear is not improved. Surgical correction of microtia is usually initiated when children are 5 years of age, before they start school. At this time, the ear has achieved 90% of its growth, and children are spared the potential embarrassment of their deformity in the school setting. Surgical reconstruction can involve the implantation of the child's costal cartilage or a porous polyethylene framework shaped like the pinnae. In either case, several surgical procedures are usually needed. If there are other facial anomalies, more extensive reconstructive surgery is indicated.

Craniosynostosis can be corrected surgically, although the procedure is major and has significant risks. Endoscopic craniosynostosis repair (endoscopic-assisted strip craniectomy) is less invasive and requires shorter operative time (average time: <1 hour) and a reduced length of hospital stay. Discharge can be as early as the first postoperative day. It is the preferred approach in many centers. The age of the infant and the site of the synostosis influence the complexity of the surgical procedure, although there is a move to do endoscopic surgery in infants younger than 16 weeks. Endoscopic strip craniectomy is usually followed by the use of a custom-made molding helmet for up to 7 months. A controversy about whether neurodevelopmental problems are related to craniosynostosis or whether they represent a preexisting condition has arisen. In developmentally normal children with evidence of closure of all sutures, surgical repair is believed to be warranted. In other cases, the procedure is thought to be reconstructive because it normalizes the appearance of children with a deformation.

In newborns and infants with plagiocephaly, when the deformation is believed to be related to torticollis, **passive stretching of the neck** 5 to 6 times a day (with each diaper change) is used to manage the condition. In addition, it is recommended that bright objects such as mobiles be placed over children's cribs to encourage head turning. Changing the crib position or the position of the newborn or infant in the crib may also encourage movement of the head. Studies have shown that 90% of newborns and infants with congenital torticollis improve with manual stretching. Infants who do not improve with stretching, who have a developmental delay in which they do not develop normal neck muscle strength or tone, or who have a deformity that is still present at 6 months of age may benefit from the use of a specially designed helmet or band, referred to as a *dynamic orthotic cranioplasty device*, that reshapes the skull. The device is not used prior to 6 months of age and is generally worn for a minimum of 4 months. In an effort to reverse the trend of increasing positional plagiocephaly related to supine sleeping, the American Academy of Pediatrics has recommended that parents rotate their infant's position when they are awake and allow for tummy time, which is time when infants are placed prone, sometimes with a rolled receiving blanket under their upper chest. Tummy time can be recommended with each diaper change. This promotes the development of the neck musculature and head control. Positional plagiocephaly secondary to supine sleeping usually resolves over time as the infant develops head control and spends less time in a supine position. Helmets can be used in refractory cases, but positional plagiocephaly does not require surgical intervention.

Psychologic counseling should be available to affected children and their families to help them adjust to anomalies and the reactions of society. Parents may be referred to community agencies such as the Cleft Palate Foundation (www.cleftline.org) to help them cope with the potential stress related to giving birth to children with this anomaly and to advise them about the medical and surgical interventions that are available. FACES: The National Craniofacial Association (www.faces-cranio.org) is a referral source for parents.

Prognosis

Some anomalies, such as deformational plagiocephaly, resolve spontaneously or with exercise and positioning. Most other anomalies can be surgically corrected, leaving little residual evidence of the deformity. School success and psychologic well-being may be more resistant to remediation and are highly dependent on the

supportiveness of the family and its emotional resources. Children who grow up in settings where the deformity is thought to be embarrassing have long-term problems with low self-esteem.

CASE RESOLUTION

The newborn in the case history has a cleft of the lip and palate. The mother is advised that her newborn can be given formula, and she is given a supply of special feeders. She is also given contact information for a parents' support group and meets other parents of children with similar anomalies. During her visit to the local craniofacial team, she views pictures of children who have undergone a repair and feels relieved.

The mother is advised about the timing of surgery and told that the surgery will be scheduled when the infant is approximately 10 weeks old. A follow-up appointment in about 2 weeks is arranged. Weight gain is monitored, and the adjustment between the mother and the newborn is assessed.

Selected References

Connolly JP, Gruss J, Seto ML, et al. Progressive postnatal craniosynostosis and increased intracranial pressure. *Plast Reconstr Surg.* 2004;113(5):1313–1323

Da Costa AC, Walters I, Savarirayan R, Anderson VA, Wrennall JA, Meara JG. Intellectual outcomes in children and adolescents with syndromic and nonsyndromic craniosynostosis. *Plast Reconstr Surg.* 2006;118(1):175–183

Damiano PC, Tyler MC, Romitti PA, et al. Health-related quality of life among pre-adolescent children with oral clefts: the mother's perspective. *Pediatrics.* 2007;120(2):e283–e290

Graham JM, Gomez M, Halberg A, et al. Management of deformational plagiocephaly: repositioning versus orthotic therapy. *J Pediatr.* 2005;146(2):258–262

Graham JM, Kreutzman J, Earl D, Halberg A, Samayoa C, Guo X. Deformational brachycephaly in supine-sleeping infants. *J Pediatr.* 2005;146(2):253–257

Harville EW, Wilcox AJ, Lie RT, Vindenes H, Abyholm F. Cleft lip and palate versus cleft lip only: are they distinct defects? *Am J Epidemiol.* 2005;162(5):448–453

Hunt O, Burden D, Hepper P, Stevenson M, Johnston C. Self-reports of psychosocial functioning among children and young adults with cleft lip and palate. *Cleft Palate Craniofac J.* 2006;43(5):598–605

Ishimoto S, Ito K, Karino S, Takegoshi H, Kaga K, Yamasoba T. Hearing levels in patients with microtia: correlation with temporal bone malformation. *Laryngoscope.* 2007;117(3):461–465

Jimenez DF, Barone CM, Cartwright CC, Baker L. Early management of craniosynostosis using endoscopic-assisted strip craniectomies and cranial orthotic molding therapy. *Pediatrics* 2002;110(1 Pt 1):97–104

Mawji A, Vollman AR, Hatfield J, McNeil DA, Sauvé R. The incidence of positional plagiocephaly: a cohort study. *Pediatrics.* 2013;132(2):298–304

Meng T, Shi B, Zheng Q, Wang Y, Li S. Clinical and epidemiologic studies of nonsyndromic cleft lip and palate in China: analysis of 4268 cases. *Ann Plast Surg.* 2006;57(3):264–269

Purugganan OH. Abnormalities in head size. *Pediatr Rev.* 2006;27(12):473–476

Samanich J. Cleft palate. *Pediatr Rev.* 2009;30(6):230–232

Schuster M, Maier A, Haderlein T, et al. Evaluation of speech intelligibility for children with cleft lip and palate by means of automatic speech recognition. *Int J Pediatr Otorhinolaryngol.* 2006;70(10):1741–1747

Shaw GM, Carmichael SL, Kaidarova Z, Harris JA. Epidemiologic characteristics of anotia and microtia in California, 1989–1997. *Birth Defects Res A Clin Mol Teratol.* 2004;70(7):472–475

van Vlimmeren LA, van der Graaf Y, Boere-Boonekamp MM, L'Hoir MP, Helders PJ, Engelbert RH. Risk factors for deformational plagiocephaly at birth and at 7 weeks of age: a prospective cohort study. *Pediatrics.* 2007;119(2):e408–e418

Wang RY, Earl DL, Ruder RO, Graham JM. Syndromic ear anomalies and renal ultrasound. *Pediatrics.* 2001;108(2):E32

Wilkie AO, Byren JC, Hurst JA, et al. Prevalence and complications of single-gene and chromosomal disorders in craniosynostosis. *Pediatrics.* 2010;126(2): e391–e400

Zarate YA, Martin LJ, Hopkin RJ, Bender PL, Zhang X, Saal HM. Evaluation of growth in patients with isolated cleft lip and/or cleft palate. *Pediatrics.* 2010; 125(3):e543–e549

CHAPTER 74

Common Oral Lesions

Charlotte W. Lewis, MD, MPH

CASE STUDY

A 7-year-old girl is brought to the office for evaluation of a swelling on the inside of her lower lip of 4 to 6 weeks' duration. Her mother reports that it increases and decreases in size. The girl says that the swelling is not painful, and she cannot remember hurting her lower lip. On examination, a raised, bluish, non-tender, 1 x 1 cm swelling is apparent along the mucosa of the lower lip.

Questions

1. What is the differential diagnosis of lip masses?
2. What laboratory or radiographic tests are useful in the evaluation of oral lesions?
3. What management strategies are used to treat cyst-like oral lesions?
4. When should children with oral lesions be referred to subspecialists?

Primary care physicians are often required to evaluate lesions in the oral cavity. Knowledge of common congenital, developmental, infectious, traumatic, and neoplastic conditions that affect the mouth and its structures can help physicians to recognize and manage these lesions appropriately. Although many oral lesions are benign or represent normal variants, others may require specific medical or surgical treatment. Some oral lesions offer clues to underlying syndromic diagnoses, indicate more serious systemic disease, or occur as side effects of certain medications.

Epidemiology

Oral pathology is common and covers a broad range of lesions. Benign oral lesions such as gingival cysts occur in about 75% of newborns. Approximately 20% of the population has at least a small **torus palatinus,** a benign bony overgrowth of the palate that usually begins in childhood. **Ankyloglossia,** commonly referred to as tongue-tie, affects approximately 5% of newborns. **Fissured tongue** affects approximately 2% of the population. Fissured tongue may be associated with **benign migratory glossitis** (geographic tongue), which occurs in approximately 1% to 2% of children. **Tobacco-associated keratosis** occurs at the site of habitual placement of snuff or chewing tobacco and is estimated to affect more than 300,000 US children. **Leukoplakia,** a premalignant condition associated with smokeless tobacco, occurs in approximately half of users. Although the resulting oral cancer is often diagnosed in the sixth or seventh decade of life, the habit of oral tobacco use typically starts in childhood—typically between 9 to 16 years of age. Among US high school students surveyed in 2011, 7.7% report current use of a smokeless tobacco product; use is significantly higher in boys than girls and in whites as well as American Indians/Alaska Natives relative to other racial/ethnic groups.

Aphthous ulcers (commonly known as canker sores) are one of the most common oral lesions seen in developed countries, with typical onset early in childhood. Approximately 20% to 25% of the US population experiences recurrent aphthous stomatitis (RAS). Oral lesions resulting from infections are also common. Approximately 35% of newborns and young infants will develop **oral candidiasis,** commonly known as thrush. Oral **herpes** lesions are also common and are caused by human herpesvirus, usually type 1. By young adulthood, more than half of US individuals will be seropositive for human herpesvirus 1. Approximately 20% to 40% of the population has experienced oral herpes at least one time.

Chronic ("ordinary") gingivitis usually has its onset in older children and will ultimately affect as many as 90% of adults.

Clinical Presentation

Oral lesions may come to the clinician's attention in any number of ways. Some may be obvious at birth, most notably a **congenital epulis,** which while benign in histology, typically presents as a mass protruding from a neonate's oral cavity and potentially interfering with breathing or eating. Oral lesions may be an incidental finding on physical examination. For example, in examining a newborn, the pediatrician may notice small (approximately 2–3 mm) yellow-white papules along the palatal midline and can then reassure the family that these are Epstein pearls, common lesions of no clinical significance. Most oral vascular malformations (1 of the 3 vessel types usually predominate: arterial, venous, or lymphatic) are present at birth, become more noticeable over time, and rarely regress. Microcystic lymphatic malformations often affect the tongue and surrounding soft tissue, can be friable, may interfere with eating and speaking, and can lead to overgrowth of adjacent bones. When these lesions become infected, they rapidly enlarge and can result in potential airway compromise.

The clinician or parent may be the first to notice thrush. The incidence of oral candidiasis peaks around the fourth week of life; thrush is uncommon in infants older than 6 to 9 months. Thrush can occur, however, at any age in predisposed patients (ie, immunosuppressed or deficient) and can affect the esophagus as well as the oropharynx. *Candida albicans* in combination with contact irritation has been implicated in **angular cheilitis,** which appear as crusty or scaling erythematous fissures at the corners of the mouth. Other benign oral lesions, such as benign migratory glossitis, are brought to the clinician's attention because parents are concerned that they represent pathology; however, reassurance is appropriate.

Concerns for ankyloglossia may arise when newborns have difficulty breastfeeding or as a cause of speech problems in older children, although these connections are controversial. Nevertheless, it can be difficult for children to use their tongue to clean food debris from around their teeth when the lingual frenulum is short. The maxillary labial frenulum can appear quite prominent in young children. It is common for parents to inquire whether this is contributing to what appears to be abnormal spacing between the upper central incisors (midline **diastema).** However, the prominent frenulum may be more a result of a diastema rather than a cause of it.

Clinicians may be the first to note swollen, friable, erythematous gingiva along with plaque buildup on and between the teeth representing the initial presentation of chronic gingivitis. Chronic gingivitis is the first stage of periodontal disease. Onset is typically in peri-pubertal children. Although young children experience gingivostomatitis from other causes, they do not usually harbor *Actinobacillus actinomycetemcomitans* or *Porphyromonas gingivalis* and thus do not commonly experience chronic gingivitis or periodontal disease. Thickening of the mucosa, usually in the labial vestibule, offers clues to smokeless tobacco use. The severity of tobacco-related oral lesions demonstrates a dose-response relationship with the amount, frequency, and duration of smokeless tobacco exposure. Tobacco-associated keratosis is a predictable lesion that manifests as an area of thickening at the site of habitual placement of snuff or chewing tobacco. Chronic exposure to smokeless tobacco can lead to the development of opaque-white to yellow-brown lesions with a wrinkled appearance, known as leukoplakia and considered to be a premalignant condition.

Other oral lesions may present in conjunction with systemic symptoms. **Primary herpetic gingivostomatitis** typically occurs in infants and young children with the initial human herpesvirus 1 infection and is characterized by multiple oral vesicular or ulcerative lesions, fever, malaise, cervical lymphadenopathy, and decreased oral intake. Reactivation of prior human herpesvirus 1 infection often affects the vermillion border of the lip, which is known as herpes labialis. Oral lesions may also indicate underlying serious systemic illness such as Crohn disease, systemic lupus erythematosus, or acute myelogenous leukemia. Some genetic syndromes are first detected because of oral lesions. For example, lip pits or mounds in conjunction with cleft lip/cleft palate are virtually pathognomonic of Van der Woude syndrome, an autosomal-dominant cause of orofacial cleft. Hyperpigmented lesions (brown or dark blue, similar to freckles) on the lips or buccal mucosa may provide a clue toward the diagnosis of Peutz-Jeghers syndrome, an autosomal-dominant condition of multiple intestinal hamartomas. Patients with Peutz-Jeghers syndrome may experience recurrent abdominal pain, intestinal obstruction, or bleeding, and have a 15-fold increased risk of intestinal cancer.

Pathophysiology

Neonatal and Other Developmental Lesions

Gingival cysts in the neonate include Epstein pearls, Bohn nodules, and dental lamina cysts and are caused by entrapment of tissues during embryologic development. Congenital epulis of the newborn is a rare, gingival tumor of unclear etiology that occurs more commonly in the maxilla than the mandible, with a marked female predilection (8:1), and may occur as a single or multiple tumors. The etiology of fissured tongue and geographic tongue are unknown. Fissured tongue tends to cluster in families, suggesting a genetic etiology, and can also be seen in Down syndrome. Benign migratory glossitis results from the loss of the tiny fingerlike projections, called papillae, on the tongue's surface, giving the tongue a maplike appearance. The inciting factors responsible for oral vascular malformations are not well understood.

Traumatic

Some of the most common oral lesions noted on physical examination result from minor accidental self-bites to the lip or buccal mucosa. Most of these resolve quickly, but recurrent trauma may lead to **pyogenic granuloma** or **fibroma** formation. A **mucocele** results from traumatic rupture of a minor salivary gland with subsequent cyst formation.

Infectious

Although an infectious etiology to aphthous ulcers has been proposed, their true etiology remains unclear. Oral herpes lesions are usually due to infection with human herpesvirus 1. **Herpangina** results from coxsackievirus A infection. *C albicans* causes oral candidiasis. Thrush occurs when normal host immunity is immature (as in neonates) or suppressed (eg, during steroid treatment) or when normal flora is disrupted (eg, while on antibiotics). Newborns may be colonized with *C albicans* during birth. Other sources of transmission to neonates include colonized skin (particularly around the breasts for breastfed newborns) or improperly cleaned bottle nipples.

Chronic gingivitis occurs after buildup of bacterial plaque on the teeth, adjacent gingiva, and pockets between teeth and gums. Bacteria within plaque (most common species involved are gram-negative anaerobic bacteria [*A actinomycetemcomitans* and *P gingivalis*]) release toxins that cause an inflammatory response.

Other

Drug-induced gingival hyperplasia can occur in patients taking corticosteroids, phenytoin (most common cause in children), cyclosporine A, and nifedipine. It results from fibrous tissue overgrowth but is exacerbated by poor oral hygiene and presence of plaque in much the same way as ordinary gingivitis is.

Differential Diagnosis

Age at onset, location and characteristics of the lesion, and accompanying signs and symptoms often help to narrow the differential diagnosis. The appearance of 1- to 3-mm cysts in the mouth of a neonate brings to mind (1) **Epstein pearls,** which are the most common and are usually present along the palatal midline; (2) **dental lamina cysts,** which are usually located bilaterally along the crest of the dental ridge about where the first molars usually will erupt; or (3) **Bohn nodules,** which are found on the buccal and lingual aspects of the ridge, away from the midline. A protuberant mass from the anterior maxillary ridge of a newborn should suggest a congenital epulis; however, examination by a pathologist after resection is important to confirm the diagnosis. A mucocele is a painless, clear or bluish, fluid-filled cyst that results from damage to the salivary duct leading to extravasation of mucus from the gland into the surrounding soft tissue.

White plaques involving the buccal, lingual, and palatal mucosa bring to mind oral candidiasis. Thrush can sometimes be confused with milk remaining in the child's mouth after feeding. Scraping the lesion to determine if the white substance is readily removed (as milk is) helps to differentiate this from oral candidiasis, where the white plaques do not easily scrape off, and after scraping, the base of the thrush lesion may be erythematous or bleed. Thrush involving the tongue may also be confused with the erythematous denuded areas of the tongue seen in benign migratory glossitis. In fissured tongue, grooves that vary in depth are noted along the dorsal and lateral aspects of the tongue.

Common oral ulcers include aphthous ulcers, herpes gingivostomatitis, or herpangina. Oral herpes may be characterized by multiple vesicular lesions, which after rupture appear as ulcers, involving the lips, skin around the mouth, tongue, and mucosal membranes, typically in the anterior portion of the mouth. The initial infection may occur between 1 to 3 years of age. Aphthous ulcers also involve the anterior mouth, typically along the wet vermillion, but they usually first appear at a somewhat older age (ie, in the preschool years or later) and with fewer lesions than oral herpes. Factors that may predispose to the development of RAS include familial tendency, trauma, hormonal factors, food or drug hypersensitivity, immunodeficiency, celiac disease, inflammatory bowel disease, and emotional stress. Herpangina may present similarly to herpes but it more typically involves the posterior pharynx and the palate. Similar lesions on the hands or foot, as in hand-foot-and-mouth disease, may lend support to coxsackievirus A as the etiology.

Trauma to the salivary duct may result in a mucocele. In contrast, a pyogenic granuloma is an erythematous, non-painful, smooth or lobulated mass that often bleeds easily when touched, while a fibroma is a moderately firm, smooth-surfaced, pink, sessile or pedunculated nodule, usually noted on the buccal mucosa in the occlusal plane.

Erythematous and friable gums often indicate the presence of chronic gingivitis. Typically plaque is seen on and between the teeth. In contrast with plaque-associated chronic gingivitis, which is usually painless, **acute necrotizing ulcerative gingivitis** is characterized by painful, edematous, bleeding gums with ulcers, necrosis, and pseudomembrane formation in affected areas. When this spreads to the oropharynx, it is referred to as **Vincent angina** (trench mouth), which can progress rapidly and interfere with speech and swallowing and obstruct the airway.

Evaluation

History

The history is very important in evaluating oral lesions and determining the need for further treatment or referral. Key factors to include in the history are age at onset, duration, inciting factors, other medical problems, medications, use of tobacco, family history, ill contacts, and associated or systemic symptoms such as fever (Questions Box).

Physical Examination

Physical examination of the oral structures should start with the lip (dry and wet vermillion) and surrounding skin (the "white lip"). The examination should then turn to the mucosa, gingiva, teeth, and palate; superior, lateral, and posterior aspect of the tongue; sublingual structures; frenums; and posterior pharynx. The clinician should note the number, size, location, and characteristics of the lesions because this information can be helpful in narrowing the differential diagnosis. Whether fever is present should be determined. The rest of the body should be examined with specific attention to the presence of other lesions, rashes, or arthritis.

Laboratory Tests

In otherwise healthy children who present with oral ulcerative lesions, supportive care is typically implemented without pursuing a definitive etiology. When there is need for specific diagnosis, human herpesvirus can be diagnosed via polymerase chain reaction techniques, immunofluorescence, or culture. Tzanck tests are no longer commonly performed to diagnose human herpesvirus because they require special skills and are not specific to human herpesvirus, and more specific tests are available. Likewise, oral candidiasis in an otherwise healthy infant is usually treated without diagnostic tests. However, a potassium hydroxide 10% microscopic slide preparation of scrapings from the lesion should demonstrate the characteristic

Questions

Common Oral Lesions

- How long has the child had the lesion?
- Is the lesion painful?
- Did the child recently injure the affected area?
- Has the child had any fever?
- Is the child eating as usual?
- Does the child have any other lesions?
- Is the child currently taking any medications? Has the child recently taken any medications?

spherical budding yeasts and pseudo-hyphae. An excisional biopsy or resection may be needed to determine histology and diagnosis of other oral lesions.

Laboratory tests, including a complete blood cell count, C-reactive protein, or erythrocyte sedimentation rate, may be helpful in the initial evaluation of the ill-appearing child with oral lesions or when serious infection, systemic illness, or inflammatory conditions are suspected.

Imaging Studies

Imaging studies are not indicated in the evaluation of most oral lesions unless the lesions are related to problems of dentition such as dental abscesses, in which case radiographs are obtained by the dentist rather than the pediatrician. Computed tomography is usually the best way to initially characterize oral vascular malformations.

Management

Many of the common oral lesions are developmental or normal variants or are self-limited, and their management entails observation to ensure the lesions follow their expected course. For example, gingival cysts in newborns typically regress spontaneously. Oral lesions such as torus palatinus or benign migratory glossitis do not require treatment. Although human herpesvirus 1 gingivostomatitis is self-limiting, primary infection can cause considerable pain and lead to decreased intake by mouth. Early (within 72 hours) antiviral therapy in the form of acyclovir 5 to 10 mg/kg/dose 5 times per day for 7 to 10 days has been shown to shorten duration of fever, lesions, and odynophagia. Other oral lesions respond well to supportive care. For example, a child with herpangina may benefit from regular ibuprofen or acetaminophen, topical application of a 1:1 mixture of attapulgite (Kaopectate) and diphenhydramine elixir (Benadryl) to form a protective coating over the lesion, avoidance of acidic beverages such as orange juice that may burn on contact with the ulcers, and close attention to fluid intake and signs/symptoms of dehydration. Amlexanox 5% oral paste or triamcinolone acetonide dental paste reduces pain, duration, and size of aphthous ulcers and is used in adults with RAS; however, safety of these treatments in children has not been established. Viscous lidocaine has been associated with systemic absorption and subsequent dysrhythmia or seizure; thus, substantial caution is warranted before prescribing. Over-the-counter topical anesthetic agents contain a high content of alcohol and should not be used in children.

Complicated vascular and lymphatic malformations of the oral cavity require specialty consultation with a team experienced in the care of these lesions. Unlike infantile hemangiomas, complicated vascular malformations do not involute. Treatment of choice for lymphatic malformations is usually surgical resection; however, microcystic lymphatic malformations are difficult to remove and may recur even after resection. Sclerosing therapy and laser treatment are sometimes options. Newer protocols for treatment of clinically significant hemangiomas include propranolol. Supportive care includes treatment with antibiotics when the lesion becomes infected and ongoing, aggressive preventive oral hygiene.

Other oral lesions require specific therapy. Thrush is typically treated with nystatin suspension (100,000 units/mL) as 1 mL swabbed to lesions 4 times per day until lesions are resolved. It is important to consider the possibility of an underlying immunodeficiency when thrush occurs outside of infancy or without a reasonable explanation. Angular cheilitis can be treated with nystatin cream or ointment and a low-potency hydrocortisone cream. Some oral lesions are best treated by resection; these would include congenital epulis, mucocele, pyogenic granuloma, and fibroma.

Treatment of gingivitis should start with ensuring that a child follows a regular home oral hygiene program, including twice-daily toothbrushing with fluoride toothpaste and flossing, and referral for professional dental care. Regular rinsing with alcohol-containing phenolic mouth rinse (eg, Listerine) or chlorhexidine gluconate oral preparation may also be beneficial. The goals of therapy for gingivitis are to reduce clinical signs of inflammation and gingival bleeding and arrest or reduce the risk of progression of the periodontal disease and maintain dentition. Drug-induced gingival hyperplasia requires similar therapy to ordinary gingivitis. In addition, if the causative medication cannot be discontinued or changed, patients can be referred for surgical removal of excess gingival tissue and fitting of a positive-pressure mouth guard to inhibit further tissue growth. Acute necrotizing ulcerative gingivitis should be treated with debridement, penicillin, or metronidazole.

Research evidence suggests that a frenotomy may improve breastfeeding ability in neonates born with ankyloglossia. Consultation with a lactation consultant is often helpful as a first step when questions arise about whether ankyloglossia is contributing to breastfeeding difficulty. Management of oral lesions may require consultation and collaboration with dental, oral surgery, head and neck surgery, or other subspecialty colleagues. If the etiology of a lesion is unclear or if an oral lesion does not follow its expected course, referral is essential to ensure appropriate diagnosis and treatment.

Prognosis

Most oral lesions in children respond to appropriate intervention without residual problems. However, oral lesions can signal the onset of or occur in association with serious systemic conditions. In addition, chronic gingivitis represents the first and only reversible stage of periodontal disease, which is the leading cause of tooth loss in adulthood. Because chronic gingivitis has its onset during childhood, physicians can play an important role in prevention of periodontal disease by promoting oral hygiene early in life. Once periodontal disease extends beyond the gums, it is no longer reversible and gradually destroys the bone and tissue that support the teeth, resulting in halitosis and tooth loss.

CASE RESOLUTION

The child described in the case history seems to have a mucocele. She should be referred to an oral or head and neck surgeon for surgical excision of the lesion.

Selected References

American Academy of Pediatric Dentistry Council on Clinical Affairs. Guideline on pediatric oral surgery. *Pediatr Dent.* 2005–2006;27(7 Suppl):158–164

Buckmiller LM, Richter GT, Suen JY. Diagnosis and management of hemangiomas and vascular malformations of the head and neck. *Oral Dis.* 2010;16(5): 405–418

Centers for Disease Control and Prevention. Youth risk behavior surveillance—United States, 2011. *MMWR Surveill Summ.* 2012;61(4):1–162

Ebbert JO, Carr AB, Dale LC. Smokeless tobacco: an emerging addiction. *Med Clin North Am.* 2004;88(6):1593–1605

Gibson AM, Sommerkamp SK. Evaluation and management of oral lesions in the emergency department. *Emerg Med Clin North Am.* 2013;31(2):455–463

Gonsalves WC, Chi AC, Neville BW. Common oral lesions: part I. Superficial mucosal lesions. *Am Fam Physician.* 2007;75(4):501–507

Gonsalves WC, Chi AC, Neville BW. Common oral lesions: part II. Masses and neoplasia. *Am Fam Physician.* 2007;75(4):509–512

Scully C. Clinical practice. Aphthous ulceration. *N Engl J Med.* 2006;355(2): 165–172

CHAPTER 75

Otitis Media

Nasser Redjal, MD

CASE STUDY

An 18-month-old boy is brought to your office with a 2-day history of fever and decreased food intake. He has had symptoms of an upper respiratory infection for the past 4 days but no vomiting or diarrhea. Otherwise, he is healthy.

The child appears tired but not toxic. On physical examination, the vital signs are normal except for a temperature of 101°F (38.3°C). The left tympanic membrane (TM) is erythematous and bulging, with yellow pus behind the membrane. The light reflex is splayed, and mobility is decreased. The right TM is gray and mobile, with a sharp light reflex. The neck is supple with shotty anterior cervical adenopathy, and the lungs are clear.

He has a 10- to 15-word vocabulary, and no one smokes in the household.

Questions

1. What are the differences between acute, persistent, and recurrent otitis media (OM)?
2. What factors predispose to the development of ear infections?
3. What are the most common presenting signs and symptoms of an ear infection in infants, older children, and adolescents?
4. How do the treatment considerations differ between acute, persistent, and recurrent ear infections?
5. What are some of the complications of OM?

Otitis media (OM) is the second most common reason after well-child care for a visit to the pediatrician and is the most common reason for which antibiotics are prescribed for children. It is estimated that approximately 30 million office visits per year are for the evaluation and treatment of OM and that billions of dollars are spent annually for OM care. Moreover, more than a quarter of all prescriptions written each year for oral antibiotics are for the treatment of middle-ear infections. In addition, many surgical procedures, such as **myringotomy** with **tympanostomy tube** placement or adenoidectomy, are performed on children for treatment of recurrent disease. Therefore, the primary care physician must have a good understanding of these very common pediatric conditions.

Otitis media can be classified into the following 5 categories: **acute OM (AOM), OM with effusion (OME), recurrent AOM, chronic OME,** and **chronic suppurative OM (CSOM).** It is important to distinguish between each of these entities because their presentation and management differ.

Acute OM (acute suppurative or purulent OM) is the sudden onset of inflammation of the middle ear, which is often accompanied by fever and ear pain (otalgia) (Box 75-1). In 2013, the American Academy of Pediatrics Subcommittee on the Management of Acute Otitis Media revised the definition of AOM to no longer include signs and symptoms of inflammation but stated that clinically, children with AOM may present with recent onset of ear pain and marked erythema of the tympanic membrane as the only findings on otoscopic examination. Otitis media with effusion is the presence of middle-ear fluid after antimicrobial treatment. Resolution

---

Box 75-1. Components of Acute Otitis Media

Definition

A diagnosis of acute otitis media (AOM) requires

1. A history of acute onset of signs and symptoms
2. The presence of middle-ear effusion (MEE)
3. Signs and symptoms of middle-ear inflammation

Elements of the definition of AOM are all of the following:

1. Recent, usually abrupt, onset of signs and symptoms of middle-ear inflammation and MEE
2. The presence of MEE that is indicated by any of the following:
   a. Bulging of the tympanic membrane (TM)
   b. Limited or absent mobility of the TM
   c. Air-fluid level behind the TM
   d. Otorrhea (not due to acute otitis externa)

Adapted with permission from Lieberthal AS, Carroll AE, Chonmaitree T, et al. The diagnosis and management of acute otitis media. *Pediatrics*. 2013;131(3):e964–e999.

---

of acute inflammatory signs has occurred, with persistence of a more serous, non-purulent effusion. Although the fluid may persist for 2 to 3 months, it resolves within 3 to 4 weeks in 60% of cases. Recurrent OM is defined as frequent episodes of AOM with complete clearing between each episode. A more specific definition is 3 new episodes of AOM requiring antibiotic treatment within a 6-month period or 4 documented infections in 1 year. This condition affects approximately 20% of children who are otitis prone; such children are usually infants who have their first infection at younger than 1 year. Chronic OME (serous OM, secretory OM, non-suppurative OM, mucoid OM, glue ear OM) is characterized by persistence of fluid in the middle ear for 3 months or longer. The tympanic membrane (TM) is retracted or concave with impaired mobility and without signs of acute inflammation. Affected children may be asymptomatic. These children are at greater risk for developing hearing deficits and speech delay. Chronic suppurative OM implies a non-intact TM (perforation or tympanostomy tube present) with 6 or more weeks of middle-ear drainage.

Epidemiology

The overall prevalence of OM is 15% to 20%, with the highest peak in children 6 to 36 months of age. An additional smaller peak occurs at about 4 to 6 years of age. Otitis media is relatively uncommon in older children and adolescents. The condition is more common in boys than girls.

Several epidemiologic risk factors for OM have been identified, including age younger than 2 years; first episode of AOM when younger than 6 months; familial predisposition; siblings in the household; low socioeconomic status; non-breastfed infant; altered host defenses (acquired or congenital immunodeficiencies); environmental factors, such as child care attendance; and the presence of an underlying condition, such as allergic disease of the upper airway, chronic sinusitis, a cleft palate, or other craniofacial anomalies. Children with Down, Goldenhar, and Treacher Collins syndromes and ciliary dysfunction also have an increased risk of OM. Race, bottle-feeding, use of pacifier, and exposure to cigarette smoke have not been identified consistently as risk factors for AOM. As one might expect, the highest rate of OM occurs during the winter months and in early spring, coinciding with peaks in the incidence of upper respiratory infections (URIs).

Worldwide OM leads to an estimated 50,000 deaths per year in children younger than 5 years because of the complications of CSOM. It is estimated to affect 65 million to 133 million people worldwide, 60% of whom suffer significant hearing loss. Chronic suppurative OM is a rare entity in developed countries where most OM is AOM or OME.

Etiology

In general, 50% to 90% of cases of AOM culture are bacterial, 20% to 50% are viruses, and 20% to 30% are no growth. Up until the widespread immunization of children with pneumococcal vaccine, the causative microorganisms for AOM were *Streptococcus pneumoniae* (25%–50%), *Haemophilus influenzae* (15%–30%; most strains not able to be typed), and *Moraxella catarrhalis* (3%–20%). Since vaccine licensure, there has been an overall decrease in the incidence of AOM, especially in children who are completely immunized. Group A streptococcus, *Staphylococcus aureus,* α-hemolytic *Streptococcus, Pseudomonas aeruginosa,* and anaerobic bacteria are other, less common causative organisms. Other uncommon organisms such as *Mycoplasma pneumoniae,* chlamydia, and *Mycobacterium tuberculosis* have been isolated. Bullous myringitis has shown a 97% bacterial-positive rate,

primarily with *S pneumoniae,* in contract with the previous belief that mycoplasma was the causative agent in this condition. Respiratory viruses such as respiratory syncytial virus, adenovirus, rhinovirus, parainfluenza, coronavirus, and influenza (A and B) also play a role. Respiratory syncytial virus, adenovirus, and coronavirus are associated with a higher rate of AOM, with 50% of children who have URIs caused by these viruses developing AOM, compared with only 33% of patients who have URIs caused by rhinovirus, influenza, parainfluenza, or enterovirus. The bacterial pathogens causing AOM in the first 6 weeks after birth are essentially the same as those in older children. However, 10.5% of neonates with AOM have gram-negative bacilli.

Currently, approximately 50% of *H influenzae* and 100% of *M catarrhalis* isolated from the upper respiratory tract are β-lactamase positive, and 15% to 50% (average 30%) of *S pneumoniae* are not susceptible to penicillin. The mechanism of penicillin resistance among isolates of *S pneumoniae* is not associated with β-lactamase production but to an alteration of penicillin-binding proteins. This effect varies widely by geographic location and results in resistance to penicillins and cephalosporins.

Clinical Presentation

Children with AOM often have a history of fever and ear pain. Associated symptoms include URI, cough, vomiting, diarrhea, and non-specific complaints such as decreased appetite, waking at night, generalized malaise, lethargy, or irritability. Purulent otorrhea with minimal ear pain and hearing loss may also occur. Fever occurs in approximately 30% to 50% of patients. Temperatures exceeding 104°F (40°C) are uncommon and suggest bacteremia or another complication. Older children may complain of tinnitus, vertigo, and hearing loss. Younger children are not able to express such complaints but may appear ataxic.

Pathophysiology

The most important factor in the pathogenesis of OM is abnormal function of the eustachian tube (Figure 75-1). Eustachian tube dysfunction occurs for 2 main reasons: abnormal patency and obstruction of the

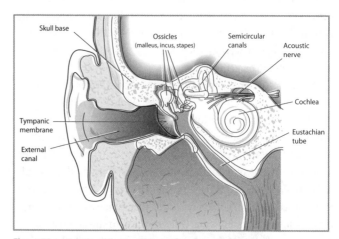

Figure 75-1. Relationship of middle ear to external and inner ears.

tube. Obstruction is functional (secondary to collapse of the tube), mechanical (from intrinsic or extrinsic causes), or both. Functional obstruction or collapse of the eustachian tube occurs commonly in infants and young children because the tube is less cartilaginous and therefore less stiff than in adults, as well as more horizontal and shorter. In addition, the tensor veli palatini muscle is less efficient in this age group. Extrinsically, the presence of lymphoid follicles (adenoidal enlargement) or tumors (rare) surrounding the opening of the tube contributes to reflux, aspiration, or insufflation of nasopharyngeal bacteria into the middle ear. Intrinsic mechanical obstruction of the eustachian tube occurs as the result of inflammation secondary to a URI or allergy in patients older than 5 years. In addition, viral infections may occur up to 6 to 12 times per year in children younger than 3 years. Subsequently, this causes eustachian tube dysfunction, leading to negative middle ear pressure, which occurs in 75% of children who have viral URIs. The presence of a viral URI enhances the ability of bacterial pathogens to adhere to and ascend from the nasopharynx to the middle ear via the eustachian tube. In addition, viruses can affect the local host immune response by impairing leukocyte function, exposing receptors for bacteria, and decreasing the effectiveness of the mucociliary escalator (see Figure 75-1).

Hematogenous spread of microorganisms also can lead to infection. Less often, primary mucosal disease of the middle ear from allergies or abnormal cilia contributes to OM.

Differential Diagnosis

The most common cause of otalgia, or ear pain, is AOM. Other causes include mastoiditis, which is almost always accompanied by OM; otitis externa; and referred pain from the oropharynx, teeth, adenoids, or posterior auricular lymph nodes. A foreign body in the canal can produce similar symptoms. In children with ear pain, a search for any of these other conditions must be undertaken if the TM appears completely normal.

Evaluation

History

The history should carefully delineate the symptoms of OM and differentiate from those indicating a more serious condition, such as meningitis (Questions Box).

For infants or children with a history of persistent or recurrent OM, it is important to find out when they had their last documented infection and what treatment they received. It is also critical to monitor development, particularly speech.

Physical Examination

To diagnose OM, the TM must be completely visualized and its mobility assessed. Occasionally, this may be difficult because of the presence of cerumen or otorrhea. Diagnosis is then made on the basis of the history, and treatment may be initiated without confirmation by physical assessment. In all other cases, the position, color, degree of translucency, and mobility of the TM are evaluated.

Otitis Media Questions

- Does the infant or child have fever, ear pain, hearing loss, or otorrhea?
- Is the infant or child inconsolable or lethargic?
- Has the infant or child had a previous ear infection? If so, when?
- Did the child complete the course of prescribed antibiotics?
- How many ear infections has the child had in the past year?
- Is the child taking any medication to prevent recurrent otitis media?
- Does the child attend child care?
- Is the child exposed to passive smoke?
- Is the infant breastfed?
- Does the child seem to hear?
- Is the child's speech development normal?

Classically, in AOM the TM is full, bulging, hyperemic, opaque, or has an air fluid level, with limited or no mobility. In addition, the light reflex is usually distorted or absent. In the case of persistent or chronic OM, signs of inflammation are usually absent and the TM may be retracted, with limited or no mobility.

Associated physical findings with an uncomplicated middle-ear infection may include posterior auricular and cervical adenopathy. Other significant findings on physical examination are pain on movement of the pinna, anterior ear displacement, posterior auricular pain, and, rarely, evidence of peripheral facial nerve (seventh cranial nerve) paralysis. The presence of these findings suggests other diagnoses such as an associated otitis externa or mastoiditis.

Positioning of infants or young children for examination of the ear is critical for an adequate examination. Several methods have been described, including allowing parents to hold the child in their arms or on their laps or restraining the child on the examination table (Figure 75-2). In addition, it may be difficult to visualize the TM in infants because the external auditory canal is slightly angulated. Lateral retraction of the pinna may help correct this problem.

Laboratory Tests

Although the diagnosis of OM is suspected on the basis of the history and then verified on physical examination, tympanometry may be helpful in distinguishing the normal ear from one with an effusion. In acute cases, audiometry is of limited diagnostic value, but it is helpful in evaluating the effects of a persistent, recurrent, or chronic middle-ear effusion (MEE) on hearing.

Figure 75-2. Three ways to position the infant or child for examination of the ear.

Tympanocentesis is the most definitive method of verifying the presence of middle-ear fluid and of recovering the organism responsible for the infection. Indications for tympanocentesis or myringotomy are listed in Box 75-2. Nasopharyngeal cultures are not helpful because they do not correlate with middle-ear fluid cultures.

Prevention

During infancy and early childhood, the incidence of respiratory tract infections and recurrent OM can be reduced by altering child care center attendance patterns.

Immunoprophylaxis with influenza vaccine and pneumococcal conjugate vaccine has proven effective in preventing OM. Avoiding supine bottle-feeding (bottle propping) and reducing or eliminating pacifier use in the second 6 months of life, as well as eliminating exposure to passive tobacco smoke, decreases the incidence of AOM.

Breastfeeding, which provides infants with immunologic protection against URIs, other viral and bacterial infections, and allergies, also has a protective effect. Facial musculature may mature differently in breastfed infants, thus influencing eustachian tube function and reducing the risk of aspiration of fluid into the middle ear. Positioning during breastfeeding also has some protective effect, although immune factors in human milk may serve as the most important mechanism for the reduced prevalence of OM.

Increased antibiotic resistance has eliminated the utility of routine antibiotic prophylaxis for recurrent AOM as a means of disease prevention.

Management

Current guidelines addressing the treatment of AOM consist of the use of antibiotics or observation without the use of antibacterial agents for children 6 months to 2 years with uncomplicated unilateral AOM with no otorrhea. Observation without antibiotics is also recommended for children older than 2 years with uncomplicated bilateral or unilateral AOM without otorrhea (Box 75-3). Antibacterial treatment is deferred in these children for 48 to 72 hours, and management is limited to symptomatic relief. In an era of conjugated

---

Box 75-2. Indications for Tympanocentesis or Myringotomy in Children With Otitis Media

- Otitis media in patients with severe ear pain, serious illness, or appearance of toxicity
- Onset of otitis media in children receiving appropriate and adequate antimicrobial therapy
- Otitis media associated with confirmed or potential suppurative complications, such as facial paralysis, mastoiditis, or meningitis
- Otitis media in newborns, sick neonates, or immunodeficient patients, in each of whom an unusual organism may be present
- Otitis media in patients with severe illness who have failed second-line antibiotic management
- Otitis media in patients with penicillin allergy who have failed first-line agent

---

Box 75-3. Indications for Antibiotics in the Treatment of Otitis Media

Criteria for antibacterial treatment or observation in children with non-severe illness

1. Younger than 6 months: antibacterial treatment
2. Six months to 2 years: antibacterial treatment with certain diagnosis or severe illness; observation with unilateral acute otitis media without otorrhea
3. Two years and older: antibacterial treatment with severe illness or observe with uncomplicated unilateral or bilateral acute otitis media

Observation is an appropriate option if

A. Caregiver is informed and agrees.
B. Caregiver is able to monitor the child and return should condition worsen.
C. Systems are in place for ready communication with the clinician, reevaluation, and obtaining medication, if necessary.

Adapted with permission from Lieberthal AS, Carroll AE, Chonmaitree T, et al. The diagnosis and management of acute otitis media. *Pediatrics.* 2013;131(3):e964–e999.

---

pneumococcal vaccine, the likelihood of bacteremia accompanying AOM is remote. Parents may be provided with a prescription to fill without recontacting the physician if the child remains symptomatic. Concern for serious infection among children younger than 6 months influences the decision for immediate antibacterial therapy in this age group. The recommended antibiotic therapy is noted in Table 75-1.

High-dose amoxicillin is recommended as the first-line treatment in most patients, although there are a number of medications that are clinically effective (see Table 75-1). The justification for the use of amoxicillin relates to its effectiveness against common AOM bacterial pathogens as well as its safety, low cost, acceptable taste, and narrow microbiological spectrum. In children who have taken amoxicillin in the previous 30 days, those with concurrent conjunctivitis, or those for whom coverage for β-lactamase-positive *H Influenzae* and *M catarrhalis* is desired, therapy should be initiated with high-dose amoxicillin-clavulanate (90 mg/kg/day of amoxicillin with 6.4 mg/kg/day of clavulanate in a ratio of amoxicillin to clavulanate of 14:1, given in 2 divided doses [less likely to cause diarrhea than other amoxicillin-clavulanate preparations]).

Alternative initial antibiotics include cefdinir (14 mg/kg/day in 1 or 2 doses), cefuroxime (30 mg/kg/day in 2 divided doses), cefpodoxime (10 mg/kg/day in 2 divided doses), or ceftriaxone (50 mg/kg, administered intramuscularly). It is important to note that alternative antibiotics vary in their efficacy against AOM pathogens. For example, recent US data on in vitro susceptibility of *S pneumoniae* to cefdinir and cefuroxime are only 70% to 80% compared with 84% to 92% amoxicillin efficacy. In vitro efficacy of cefdinir and cefuroxime against *H influenzae* is approximately 98%, compared with 58% efficacy of amoxicillin and nearly 100% efficacy of amoxicillin-clavulanate. A multicenter double tympanocentesis open-label study of cefdinir in recurrent AOM attributable to *H influenzae* showed eradication of the organism in 72% of patients.

Table 75-1. Recommended Antibiotics for (Initial or Delayed) Treatment and for Patients Who Have Failed Initial Antibiotic Treatment			
Initial Immediate or Delayed Antibiotic Treatment		**Antibiotic Treatment After 48–72 h of Failure of Initial Antibiotic Treatment**	
Recommended First-line Treatment	*Alternative Treatment (if Penicillin Allergy)*	*Recommended First-line Treatment*	*Alternative Treatment*
Amoxicillin (80–90 mg/kg per day in 2 divided doses)	Cefdinir (14 mg/kg per day in 1 or 2 doses)	Amoxicillin-clavulanate[a] (90 mg/kg per day of amoxicillin, with 6.4 mg/kg per day of clavulanate in 2 divided doses)	Ceftriaxone, 3 d Clindamycin (30–40 mg/kg per day in 3 divided doses), with or without third-generation cephalosporin
or	Cefuroxime (30 mg/kg per day in 2 divided doses)	or	Failure of second antibiotic
Amoxicillin-clavulanate[a] (90 mg/kg per day of amoxicillin, with 6.4 mg/kg per day of clavulanate [amoxicillin to clavulanate ratio, 14:1] in 2 divided doses)	Cefpodoxime (10 mg/kg per day in 2 divided doses)	Ceftriaxone (50 mg IM or IV for 3 d)	Clindamycin (30–40 mg/kg per day in 3 divided doses) plus third-generation cephalosporin
			Tympanocentesis[b]
	Ceftriaxone (50 mg IM or IV per day for 1 or 3 d)		Consult specialist[b]

Abbreviations: IM, intramuscular; IV, intravenous.

Note: Cefdinir, cefuroxime, cefpodoxime, and ceftriaxone are highly unlikely to be associated with cross-reactivity with penicillin allergy on the basis of their distinct chemical structures.

[a]May be considered in patients who have received amoxicillin in the previous 30 d or who have the otitis-conjunctivitis syndrome.

[b]Perform tympanocentesis/drainage if skilled in the procedure, or seek a consultation from an otolaryngologist for tympanocentesis/drainage. If the tympanocentesis reveals multidrug-resistant bacteria, seek an infectious disease specialist consultation.

Reproduced with permission from Lieberthal AS, Carroll AE, Chonmaitree T, et al. The diagnosis and management of acute otitis media. *Pediatrics.* 2013;131(3):e964–e999

For children allergic to penicillin, recent data suggest that cross-reactivity among penicillins and cephalosporins is lower than historically reported. Cross-reactivity is higher between penicillins and first-generation cephalosporins but is negligible with second- and third-generation cephalosporins. According to the Joint Council of Allergy, Asthma & Immunology, cephalosporin treatment of patients with a history of penicillin allergy, selecting out those with severe reaction histories, show a reaction rate of 0.1%. It recommends a cephalosporin in cases without severe or recent penicillin allergy reaction history when skin testing is not available.

Tympanocentesis is rarely performed nowadays prior to the initiation of antibiotics. Indications for tympanocentesis include severe ear pain (provides relief through decompression) or toxic appearance. Tympanocentesis is occasionally carried out in a child who has been receiving appropriate and adequate antimicrobial therapy but fails to improve; in the face of confirmed or potential suppurative complications, such as facial paralysis, mastoiditis, or meningitis; or in newborns, sick neonates, or immunodeficient patients in whom an unusual organism may be present (see Box 75-2).

Adjunctive medications such as topical analgesics and antipyretics are important therapeutic options and should be prescribed for children with significant pain or fever. Antihistamines, decongestants, or steroids play no documented role in the treatment of OME. Most resolving MEEs seen after AOM in otherwise healthy children do not need to be treated; the wait-and-watch approach is recommended.

Failure of antibiotic treatment and chronic effusions warrant a referral to an otolaryngologist for further evaluation for pressure equalization tubes, especially if effusion is present for more than 3 months and associated symptoms such as vestibular symptoms, school or behavioral problems, ear discomfort, or lowered quality of life are present. Clinicians may offer tympanostomy tubes for recurrent AOM (3 episodes in 6 months or 4 episodes in 1 year, with 1 episode in the preceding 6 months). Recurrent AOM has been defined as the occurrence of 3 or more episodes of AOM in a 12-month period that includes at least 1 episode in the preceding 6 months. These episodes should be well documented and separate acute infections. Other reasons for consultation include evidence of hearing loss; the presence of any anatomic abnormality, such as a defect of the TM (perforations, cholesteatomas) or intranasal problems (deviated septum, polyp); signs and symptoms of an OM but normal physical examination; and a predisposition to chronic recurrent OM (eg, children with a cleft palate or Down syndrome).

Duration of Therapy

For children younger than 2 years and children with severe symptoms, a standard 10-day course is recommended. A 7-day course of oral antibiotic appears to be equally effective in children 2 to 5 years of age with mild or moderate AOM. For children 6 years and older with mild to moderate symptoms, a 5- to 7-day course is adequate treatment.

Follow-up of the Patient With Acute Otitis Media

The physician may choose to reassess some children in 10 to 14 days, such as young children with severe symptoms or recurrent AOM or when specifically requested by the child's parent.

Persistent MEE is common and can be detected by pneumatic otoscopy (with or without verification by tympanometry) after resolution of acute symptoms. Two weeks after successful antibiotic treatment of AOM, 60% to 70% of children have MEE, decreasing to 40% at 1 month and 10% to 25% at 3 months after successful antibiotic treatment.

Complications

Complications associated with OM are much less common with appropriate antibiotic therapy and follow-up but occasionally occur. They can be divided into 2 categories: extracranial and intracranial. Extracranial complications include perforation of the TM, conductive and sensorineural hearing loss, cholesteatoma, mastoiditis, facial nerve (seventh cranial nerve) paralysis, osteomyelitis of the temporal bone, and Bezold abscess. Intracranial complications are meningitis, extradural as well as subdural abscesses, lateral venous sinus thrombosis, brain abscess, and hydrocephalus.

CASE RESOLUTION

In the case presented at the beginning of the chapter, the child displays the classic signs and symptoms of acute otitis media: fever, upper respiratory infection, decreased appetite, and an abnormal tympanic membrane on physical examination. Because of his age and fever and the certainty of diagnosis, he should be treated for 10 days with oral amoxicillin. The prognosis is good given his normal speech development.

Selected References

American Academy of Pediatrics. Antimicrobial stewardship: appropriate and judicious use of antimicrobial agents. In: Pickering LK, Baker CJ, Kimberlin DW, Long SS, eds. *Red Book: 2012 Report of the Committee on Infectious Diseases*. 29th ed. Elk Grove Village, IL: American Academy of Pediatrics; 2012:802–806

American Academy of Pediatrics Section on Breastfeeding. Breastfeeding and the use of human milk. *Pediatrics*. 2012;129(3):e827–e841

Arguedas A, Emparanza P, Schwartz RH, et al. A randomized, multicenter, double blind, double dummy trial of single dose azithromycin versus high dose amoxicillin for treatment of uncomplicated acute otitis media. *Pediatr Infect Dis J*. 2005;24(2):153–161

Berkun Y, Nir-Paz R, Ami AB, Klar A, Deutsch E, Hurvitz H. Acute otitis media in the first two months of life: characteristics and diagnosis difficulties. *Arch Dis Child*. 2008;93(8):690–694

Block SL, Heikkinen T, Toback SL, Zheng W, Ambrose CS. The efficacy of live attenuated influenza vaccine against influenza-associated acute otitis media in children. *Pediatr Infect Dis J*. 2011;30(3):203–207

Brunton S, Pichichero ME. Acute otitis media: influence of the PCV-7 vaccine on changes in the disease and its management. *J Fam Pract*. 2005;54(11):961–968

Casey JR, Pichichero ME. Changes in frequency and pathogens causing acute otitis media in 1995–2003. *Pediatr Infect Dis J*. 2004;23(9):824–828

Centers for Disease Control and Prevention. National, state, and urban area vaccination coverage among children aged 19–35 months—United States, 2005. *MMWR Morb Mortal Wkly Rep*. 2006;55(36):988–993

Coco A, Vernacchio L, Horst M, Anderson A. Management of acute otitis media after publication of the 2004 AAP and AAFP clinical practice guideline. *Pediatrics*. 2010;125(2):214–220

Coker TR, Chan LS, Newberry SJ, et al. Diagnosis, microbial epidemiology, and antibiotic treatment of acute otitis media in children: a systematic review. *JAMA*. 2010;304(19):2161–2169

Damoiseaux RA, van Balen FA, Hoes AW, Verheij TJ, de Melker RA. Primary care based randomised, double blind trial of amoxicillin versus placebo for acute otitis media in children aged under 2 years. *BMJ*. 2000;320(7231):350–354

DePestel DD, Benninger MS, Danziger L, et al. Cephalosporin use in treatment of patients with penicillin allergies. *J Am Pharm Assoc (2003)*. 2008;48(4):530–540

Gould JM, Matz PS. Otitis media. *Pediatr Rev*. 2010;31(3):102–116

Hoberman A, Paradise JL, Rockette HE, et al. Treatment of acute otitis media in children under 2 years of age. *N Engl J Med*. 2011;364(2):105–115

Joint Task Force on Practice Parameters; American Academy of Allergy, Asthma and Immunology; American College of Allergy, Asthma and Immunology; Joint Council of Allergy, Asthma and Immunology. Drug allergy: an updated practice parameter. *Ann Allergy Asthma Immunol*. 2010;105(4):259–273

Lieberthal AS, Carroll AE, Chonmaitree T, et al. The diagnosis and management of acute otitis media. *Pediatrics*. 2013;131(3):e964–e999

Ongkasuwan J, Valdez TA, Hulten KG, Mason EO, Kaplan SL. Pneumococcal mastoiditis in children and the emergence of multidrug-restraint serotype 19A isolates. *Pedatrics*. 2008;122(1):34–39

Piglansky L, Leibovitz E, Raiz S, et al. Bacteriologic and clinical efficacy of high dose amoxicillin for therapy of acute otitis media in children. *Pediatr Infect Dis J*. 2003;22(5):405–413

Rosenfeld RM. Diagnostic certainty for acute otitis media. *Int J Pediatr Otorhinolaryngol*. 2002;64(2):89–95

Siegel RM, Kiely M, Bien JP, et al. Treatment of otitis media with observation and a safety-net antibiotic prescription. *Pediatrics*. 2003;112(3 Pt 1):527–531

Spiro DM, Tay KY, Arnold DH, Dziura JD, Baker MD, Shapiro ED. Wait-and-see prescription for the treatment of acute otitis media: a randomized controlled trial. *JAMA*. 2006;296(10):1235–1241

Wald ER. Acute otitis media: more trouble with the evidence. *Pediatr Infect Dis J*. 2003;22(2):103–104

Whitney CG, Farley MM, Hadler J, et al. Decline in invasive pneumococcal disease after the introduction of protein-polysaccharide conjugate vaccine. *N Engl J Med*. 2003;348(18):1737–1746

CHAPTER 76

Hearing Impairments

Julie E. Noble, MD

CASE STUDY

A 15-month-old girl is brought to the office because her parents are concerned that she has not yet begun to speak. The child was the full-term product of an uncomplicated pregnancy. Her 25-year-old mother, who began to receive regular prenatal care during the second month of gestation, had no documented infections during the pregnancy, took no medications, and has denied using illicit drugs or alcohol. The child was delivered at home by a midwife and a newborn hearing screening was never done. The 27-year-old father is reportedly healthy. There is no family history of deafness, intellectual disability, or consanguinity.

The girl, who is otherwise healthy, has never been hospitalized, but she has had 3 documented ear infections. She rolled over at 4 to 5 months of age, sat at 7 months, and walked at 13 months. She is able to scribble. The parents report that their daughter smiles appropriately, laughs occasionally, and plays well with other children. As an infant, the girl cooed and babbled, but she now points and grunts to indicate her needs. She does not respond to loud noises by turning her head.

The child's growth parameters, including head circumference, are normal for age. The rest of the physical examination is unremarkable.

Questions

1. When should deafness be suspected in infants or children?
2. What is the relationship between hearing loss and language development?
3. What are the major causes of deafness in children?
4. What neonates are at risk for the development of hearing deficits?
5. What methods are currently available to evaluate hearing in infants and children?
6. What are the important issues to address with families who have infants or children with suspected hearing impairment?

Hearing loss, even a mild degree, is a significant childhood disability that can compromise speech and language development, academic performance, and psychosocial behavior. It is essential to identify hearing loss as soon as possible to implement early intervention, which has been shown to prevent many adverse consequences. Children may be born with a hearing deficit, termed *congenital deafness,* or may acquire the condition during childhood, termed *progressive* or *late-onset deafness.* A mild hearing deficit occurs with a 26 to 40 decibel (dB) loss. Severe hearing loss, on the other hand, is defined as 71 to 90 dB, and profound loss is 90 dB or greater. The most important period for speech and language development is from birth to 3 years of age. Reduced hearing acuity in both or even one ear during this time can significantly interfere with this important process (see Chapter 30). Therefore, primary care physicians must have a clear understanding of when to suspect impaired hearing in infancy and early childhood and must be familiar with the identification of, evaluation methods for, and treatment for hearing loss.

Epidemiology

The prevalence of congenital deafness in children is approximately 0.1%. In other words, 1 in 1,000 children is born severely to profoundly deaf. It has been estimated, however, that 3 to 5 in 1,000 children have mild to moderate hearing loss. The average age at diagnosis of most children who were born deaf was 2 to 3 years of age prior to the initiation of newborn hearing screening. Since its advent, the average age of diagnosis has dropped to 2 to 3 months of age. At this time in the United States, all 50 states have mandated universal newborn hearing screening programs and 95% of all newborns are screened. But as with any screening program, some newborns may get missed, especially with at-home births; as many as 40% of identified newborns may be lost to follow-up; and some forms of early-onset hearing loss are not apparent at birth. Therefore, careful assessment of hearing and language development by the pediatrician is essential at each patient encounter.

An estimated 20% to 30% of children who are hearing impaired develop the condition during childhood. Of these, 70% of children with acquired hearing loss are initially identified by parents rather than physicians. Any concern by parents that their child might have a hearing problem should be taken seriously by physicians and objective testing performed. Risk factors for acquired hearing loss in childhood include persistent otitis media with effusion, history of head trauma, bacterial meningitis, and identification of syndromes or neurologic disorders associated with hearing loss.

Graduates of the neonatal intensive care unit have a significantly increased risk of bilateral sensorineural hearing loss (SNHL) (1%–3%), termed *auditory neuropathy* or *dyssynchrony*. Associated factors such as prematurity (birth weight <1,500 g), hyperbilirubinemia, prolonged mechanical ventilation, extracorporeal membrane oxygenation treatment, perinatal asphyxia, exposure to ototoxic drugs, and neonatal sepsis increase this risk. Other factors associated with deafness in childhood include meningitis, parental consanguinity, craniofacial malformations, congenital viral infections, exposure to chemotherapy, and a family history of deafness.

Clinical Presentation

Newborns might present to their pediatrician having had an abnormal newborn hearing screening test. The initial newborn screen is mandated by 1 month of age, with definite testing by an audiologist for abnormal tests by 3 months of age. Therapy should begin by 6 months. If infants pass hearing testing but have positive risk factors, they should have communication skills assessed at every well-child visit and diagnostic audiologic assessment by 24 to 30 months of age.

Children with hearing impairments frequently present to physicians with delayed speech. Parents may be concerned that their toddler is indicating his or her needs by grunting and pointing rather than using words. Children also may display behavioral problems, such as inattention, temper tantrums, or aggressive play with other children (D$_x$ Box).

Hearing impairment can be more difficult to recognize in infants younger than 6 months because they may have no obvious symptoms of a hearing deficit. They may startle to moderately loud noises and begin to vocalize just like other infants (Figure 76-1). If the history is suggestive of a hearing deficit, audiologic testing should be performed.

Pathophysiology

Mechanism of Hearing

Sounds in the form of pressure waves are carried from the environment through the external auditory canal to the tympanic membrane (TM). These waves are converted to mechanical vibrations by the ossicles, and the mechanical vibrations are then transmitted from the TM to the inner ear, where they are transformed to fluid vibrations. Finally, these fluid vibrations are converted into nerve impulses

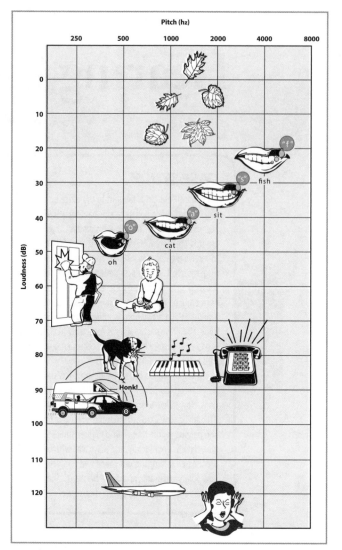

Figure 76-1. Loudness of everyday sounds.

by nerve endings within the organum spirale located in the cochlea in the inner ear. These impulses are conducted via the auditory nerve to the auditory cortex (Figure 76-2).

Hearing impairments can be classified according to the part of the auditory system affected or by the cause of the hearing loss.

Types of Hearing Loss

A **conductive hearing loss denotes an abnormality in the outer ear, TM, or middle-ear ossicles**. Cerumen impaction, otitis externa, serous otitis, recurrent otitis media, TM perforation, and ossicular discontinuity are examples of this type of hearing loss. Middle-ear effusions rarely cause more than a 20- to 30-dB loss.

The cochlea or inner ear or auditory nerve is affected in **SNHL.** Congenital infections, anomalies, and genetic disorders lead to this type of loss. The loss of cochlear function, usually from damage to sensory hair cells in the organum spirale, is the main cause of permanent childhood hearing loss. A **mixed disorder** has characteristics of conductive and sensorineural losses. In a **retrocochlear**

Dx **Hearing Impairment**

- Parental concern or suspicion of hearing loss
- Delayed speech and language development
- Associated risk factors including prematurity, exposure to ototoxic drugs, congenital or acquired central nervous system infections, family history of hearing loss, and craniofacial abnormalities
- History of behavioral problems or poor school performance
- Abnormal hearing test

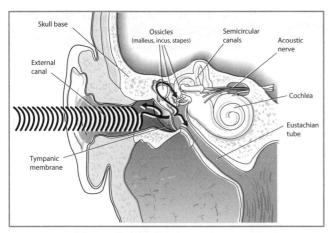

Figure 76-2. Sound waves passing through the external ear into the middle ear.

hearing loss, the auditory nerve, brain stem, or cortex is affected. This includes auditory neuropathy noted in neonates following neonatal intensive care unit stays.

Etiology of Hearing Impairment (Box 76-1)

Severe to profound hearing loss has 2 main causes: genetic and acquired environmental. Genetic causes account for approximately 68% of cases. There are more than 500 forms of syndromic hearing loss with associated clinical features. Autosomal-recessive Pendred syndrome with goiter is a more common example. Down (trisomy 21) syndrome and oculoauriculovertebral dysplasia (Goldenhar syndrome) have frequently associated hearing impairment. Alport syndrome with progressive SNHL and nephritis is also well recognized. But most cases of genetic hearing loss are nonsyndromic and result from a single gene defect encoding connexin 26 protein. This recessive disorder with mutations in the *GJB2* gene accounts for 30% to 50% of all cases in many populations. Genetic malformations of the ear pinnae or ossicles do occur but are the least common cause of hearing loss. Genetic mutations may result in different types of deafness with various presentations and outcomes; ie, hearing loss may be conductive, sensorineural, or mixed and may be static or progressive, with the initial presentation in infancy or later childhood.

Acquired environmental causes include prenatal, perinatal, or postnatal events and exposures such as congenital infections, bacterial meningitis, hyperbilirubinemia, complications of prematurity, and exposure to ototoxic medications. Cytomegalovirus (CMV) is probably the most frequently unrecognized congenital infection causing deafness. Ten percent of infants with congenital hearing loss are infected with CMV. However, toxoplasmosis, rubella, herpes simplex virus, HIV, and syphilis can also be implicated. Hearing loss associated with bacterial meningitis accounts for as many as 20% of cases, with *Streptococcus pneumoniae* as the prevalent responsible organism. The incidence of *S pneumoniae* and *Haemophilus influenzae* meningitis have decreased tremendously in young children following the advent of conjugate vaccine, and the prevalence of post-meningitic hearing loss has similarly declined. The role of steroids in the treatment of bacterial meningitis has also contributed to the decrease in SNHL in survivors.

With the recognition and treatment of hyperbilirubinemia in term newborns, hyperbilirubinemia as a cause of hearing loss is now rare in the United States and other developed countries. Prematurity as a cause of hearing loss is, however, not uncommon. Because of associated complications, premature newborns have higher rates of severe hearing loss than do full-term newborns. Some antibiotics, such as aminoglycosides, and other medications, like furosemide, can be irreversibly ototoxic; other drugs may cause only transient effects.

Any head injury causing significant middle-ear trauma may also cause deafness in children. Repeated acoustic trauma from continuous or significant exposure to loud noise can also cause irreversible hearing loss. With children's use of personal listening devices, this cause of hearing loss is increasing.

Differential Diagnosis

In addition to hearing loss, communication disorders should be considered in infants or children with delayed speech and language development. These include problems with speech perception, language comprehension, formulation of language output, and speech production. Unrecognized conditions such as intellectual disabilities or autism spectrum disorders can be responsible for some of these disorders. Other etiologies include specific central nervous system deficits as well as impairments of fine motor control of the oropharynx.

Box 76-1. Major Causes of Childhood Deafness	
Conductive Hearing Loss	**Sensorineural Hearing Loss**
Congenital • Microtia/atresia • Tympanic membrane abnormalities • Ossicular malformations	• Genetic disorders (syndromic, connexin 26, mitochondrial) • In utero infections (cytomegalovirus, measles, mumps, rubella, varicella, syphilis) • Anatomic abnormalities of the cochlea or temporal bone • Exposure to ototoxic drugs during pregnancy (alcohol, isotretinoin, cisplatin) • Hyperbilirubinemia
Acquired • Infection (acute otitis media, otitis externa, ossicular erosion) • Otitis media with effusion • Foreign body (including cerumen) • Cholesteatoma • Trauma (ossicular disruption, tympanic membrane perforation)	• Infections (bacterial meningitis, measles, mumps, rubella, Lyme disease) • Trauma (physical or acoustic) • Radiation therapy for head and neck tumors • Neurodegenerative or demyelinating disorders (Alport, Cogan syndromes)

Adapted from Gifford KA, Holmes MG, Bernstein HH. Hearing loss in children. *Pediatr Rev.* 2009;30(6):207–216.

Evaluation

Newborn Hearing Screening

In 1994, the Joint Committee on Infant Hearing (JCIH), composed of representatives from several professional organizations, endorsed universal newborn hearing screening. The goal was the early identification of hearing loss in newborns and infants before age 3 months and the implementation of intervention services by 6 months of age. As a result of these recommendations, states have implemented legislation mandating newborn hearing screening and intervention programs. A subsequent position statement was issued in 2000. The American Academy of Pediatrics endorsed this statement and promoted newborn hearing screening as well as periodic hearing assessment for every child. As a result, hearing screening has been established as an essential newborn evaluation, but there is a significant need to improve infrastructure to ensure that physicians receive and process screening results. The JCIH policy statement was most recently updated in 2007 and includes more specific guidelines for diagnostic audiologic evaluation, medical evaluation, and surveillance screening in the medical home. The policy notes that all infants and children, regardless of hearing screening results, should have ongoing assessment of communication skills beginning at 2 months of age. Any child with evidence of hearing loss in one or both ears should be offered early intervention.

History

Because the primary symptom of deafness is failure to learn to speak at the appropriate age, the most important aspect of the history in children with possible hearing loss is determining whether speech is developing normally. Even deaf infants may begin cooing and babbling in infancy, and these early attempts at verbalization are not useful milestones for assessment of hearing deficits. It helps to ask parents whether they are at all suspicious or concerned about their children's speech or hearing. Guidelines to assess language development are found in Table 76-1 (also see Chapter 30). An assessment of risk factors for deafness, such as a positive family history, infection during gestation, history of prematurity, hyperbilirubinemia, neonatal sepsis, and asphyxia, is also important (Questions Box).

Physical Examination

A complete physical examination should be performed on all children. In particular, any dysmorphic facial features that may suggest the presence of a syndrome with an associated hearing deficit should be noted. Other anomalies of the head and neck should be noted as well. Abnormal pigmentary conditions may be important clues. The eyes should be evaluated for heterochromia and hypertelorism findings seen in Waardenburg syndrome, which includes SNHL. The size and shape of the pinnae and external ear canals should be carefully inspected for abnormalities and patency, respectively. Preauricular pits or tags may be apparent. In addition, the TMs should be visualized and assessed for the presence of middle-ear effusion that may influence subsequent audiologic tests. Insufflation may be helpful to assess middle-ear effusion. The oropharynx should be examined for

Table 76-1. Expected Speech, Language, and Auditory Milestones		
Age	*Receptive Skills*	*Expressive Skills*
Birth	Turns to source of sound Shows preference for voices Shows interest in faces	Cries
2–4 mo		Coos Takes turns cooing
6 mo	Responds to name	
9 mo	Understands verbal routines (wave bye-bye)	Babbles Points Says mama, dada
12 mo	Follows a verbal command	Uses jargon Says first words
15 mo	Points to body parts by name	Learns words slowly
18–24 mo	Understands sentences	Learns words quickly Uses 2-word phrases
24–36 mo	Answers questions Follows 2-step commands	Phrases 50% intelligible Builds ≥3-word sentences Asks "what" questions
36–48 mo	Understands much of what is said	Asks "why" questions Sentences 75% intelligible Masters the early acquired speech sounds: m, b, y, n, w, d, p, and h
48–60 mo	Understands much of what is said, commensurate with cognitive level	Creates well-formed sentences Tells stories 100% intelligible
6 y		Pronounces most speech sounds correctly; may have difficulty with sh, th as in think, s, z, th as in the, l, r, and s in treasure
7 y		Pronounces speech sounds correctly, including consonant blends such as sp, tr, bl

Adapted from Feldman HM. Evaluation and management of language and speech disorders in preschool children. *Pediatr Rev.* 2005;26(4):131–142.

a cleft palate or bifid uvula, which may be associated with a submucosal cleft. The manner in which children communicate with parents should be noted, if possible, and the child assessed for response to sound.

Laboratory Tests

Tympanometry does not measure hearing but is useful in assessing the presence of middle-ear fluid and the mobility of the TM. Tympanometry can be particularly helpful with uncooperative, crying children in whom assessing the appearance of the TM and insufflation is difficult. Different types of hearing tests for evaluating infants

Hearing Impairment — Questions

- Does the child seem to respond to sounds?
- Does the child attempt to repeat sounds?
- How does the child indicate his or her desires or needs?
- How are the parents currently communicating with the child?
- Is there any evidence of a congenital infection, structural anomaly of the head and neck, or syndrome?
- Is there a history of prematurity or other prenatal or perinatal problem?
- Have there been any serious bacterial infections such as meningitis?
- Has the child had a history of repeated ear infections or exposure to ototoxic drugs?
- Aside from the hearing problem, is the child developmentally normal?
- Is there a family history of deafness, consanguinity, or multiple miscarriages or stillbirths?

and children for possible hearing deficits are available to general pediatricians (Box 76-2). **Automated auditory brain stem response (ABR)** and **brain stem auditory evoked response (BAER)** are electrophysiological measurements of activity in the auditory nerve and brain stem pathways. Electrodes are placed on the newborn, infant, or child's head to record brain wave activity while a specific auditory stimulus is presented through earphones to one ear at a time. Auditory thresholds can be estimated. The ABR is used for newborn hearing screening and only takes approximately 10 minutes, whereas the BAER is more comprehensive, requiring up to 90 minutes to perform. **Behavioral observation audiometry** measures a child's response to speech and frequency-specific stimuli presented through speakers in a soundproof room. This method of testing can only assess hearing in the better ear and cannot detect unilateral hearing loss. It is used with children at younger than 6 months' developmental age. **Evoked otoacoustic emissions** can be performed on children of all ages. It measures cochlear function in response to a specific stimulus via a small probe that contains a microphone that is placed in the ear canal. This test can be used for newborn hearing screening in low-risk newborns and can be performed in approximately 10 minutes. It has been implemented very successfully as the hearing screening test in primary care physician offices and has the advantage of being useful at all ages. **Conditioned play audiometry,** like **conventional audiometric testing,** measures auditory thresholds in response to frequency-specific stimuli presented

through earphones to one ear at a time. The patient is instructed to perform a particular task, such as putting a block in a container or raising his or her hand, when the stimulus is heard. Children as young as 3 years can be tested by conditioned play audiometry and 4 or 5 years of age via conventional audiometric testing. These are screening tests and, if abnormal results are obtained, should be used in conjunction with evaluations from audiologic and otolaryngologic consultations. In the case of high-risk infants, audiologic testing should be repeated at least every 6 months until 3 years of age and at appropriate intervals thereafter depending on the etiology of the suspected hearing loss and test results.

Diagnostic tests to consider in evaluating the cause of deafness include titers for congenital infections such as CMV, toxoplasmosis, HIV, and rubella and fluorescent treponemal antibody absorption tests for syphilis. In the newborn period, a CMV culture may be helpful. Testing for the *GJB2* gene, the mitochondrial A1555G mutation that predisposes one to ototoxicity from drugs, and the *SLC26A4* gene for Pendred syndrome, along with CMV testing, would reveal an etiology for 40% of congenital hearing loss and 60% of late-onset hearing loss. Thyroid function tests are necessary if Pendred syndrome is suspected, especially in school-aged children with goiters. Proteinuria and hematuria should also be ruled out by urine dipstick, especially in boys with a positive family history of deafness and renal failure, findings suggestive of Alport syndrome. An electrocardiogram is recommended to detect conduction defects such as QT prolongation in Jervell and Lange-Nielsen syndrome.

Imaging Studies

Occasionally, a computed tomography scan or magnetic resonance imaging of the temporal bone may be used to view the anatomy of the middle and inner ear, particularly in cases of a suspected cochlear or vestibular malformation or fistula. Necessity for such studies should be determined by an audiologist or otolaryngologist.

Management

Studies have shown that the earlier the hearing deficit is detected and remediation begun in an otherwise normal newborn, the greater the likelihood the child will have language development close to that of a hearing child. Initiation of intervention prior to 6 months of age produces infants who are able to develop language as well as social and emotional skills appropriate for their age. School performance and communication skills have been shown to be better in those identified at a younger age. There is a critical period for hearing and speech development that appears to be from birth to 3 years of age. All newborns, infants, and children identified with a hearing deficit should be referred to an otolaryngologist and audiologist for immediate assessment and recommendation for assistive devices.

If a child is diagnosed with bilateral otitis media with effusion, recent guidelines indicate that if the effusion lasts for 3 months or longer, a hearing test should be done. If a hearing loss is identified, tympanostomy tubes should be inserted.

Additional assessment for children with identified hearing loss includes an ophthalmologic evaluation and referral to a geneticist.

Box 76-2. Tests to Evaluate Hearing

- Automated auditory brain stem response: used for newborn hearing screening
- Behavioral observation audiometry
- Brain stem auditory evoked response
- Evoked otoacoustic emissions: newer type of newborn hearing screening
- Conditioned play audiometry
- Conventional audiometric testing

Once infants or children are found to have a hearing impairment, careful follow-up is necessary so that any further reduction in hearing is promptly identified. The role of primary care physicians thus becomes even more crucial. Coordination of care with speech and language specialists as well as educators who have experience working with deaf children is essential. Parents and other family members may initially be devastated by the diagnosis of a hearing impairment, especially if the deficit is severe to profound. They often have multiple questions about children's medical prognosis and educational future. The possibility of further speech and language development may also be a foremost concern in their minds. In addition to providing patients with comprehensive care, all of the parents' questions and concerns must be addressed and anticipated.

Future Audiologic Evaluations

In newly diagnosed patients with SNHL, **audiology testing** should be repeated every 3 months in the first year, then every 6 months when children are in preschool, and at least annually after children have begun school. Continued monitoring is essential to detect any progression of the hearing deficit.

Assistive Devices

Although **hearing aids** may not restore normal hearing, all children with conductive hearing loss as well as SNHL benefit from amplification. Several different types of hearing aids are available for children; these devices should be fitted appropriately and adjusted regularly. In addition, it is also recommended that all patients receive bilateral hearing aids to improve auditory localization and training, particularly in the context of different learning situations.

An **FM system** is an additional assistive listening device that can be used in a classroom. A speaker uses a microphone to transmit to a receiver the child wears to improve reception. **Closed-caption television** (signed or subtitled) is another method of auditory training. In addition, **teletype telephone systems** are available for children who can read.

Cochlear implants may be surgically placed in the cochlea to improve hearing. Implants were first approved by the US Food and Drug Administration for use in children in 1990. The implant consists of an electrode array placed in the cochlea with a receiver-stimulator under the skin and a processor worn over the ear that transmits by radio waves an impulse that produces an electrical discharge within the cochlea. These electrical pulses effectively stimulate the auditory system. The implant can be used in children at 12 months or older with severe to profound SNHL. Its use is now considered to be standard of care for patients with SNHL and is being used in infants as young as 6 months. Speech, language, and special education resources should be provided. Most patients with implants show significant improvement in communication skills. Children with cochlear implants are at increased risk for meningitis; therefore, pneumococcal and routine *H influenzae* type b vaccines are recommended.

Education and Communication

Much controversy exists regarding the optimal method of communication for deaf children. **Oral communication (lipreading)** and **sign language** each have their advantages as well as disadvantages depending on children's age, type of deafness, and whether the deficit is congenital or acquired. Whether the children already know a language is also important to consider. The preferred methods seem to vary from region to region; therefore, schools, other institutions, and resource groups often use the most popular communication method in a particular area. In general, some authors recommend that children with minimal hearing loss may do better with lipreading than those with greater hearing loss, who will most likely benefit more from sign language. Early intervention and education programs can be home-based or in a group setting, but it is recommended that educators be familiar with working with children who are hearing impaired.

Whether to mainstream children with severe hearing loss in a regular classroom with an interpreter or place them in a school for deaf children is another controversial issue. Parents should be encouraged to explore the possibilities of each option and to make a decision based on the individual needs of their children and not current trends. The expertise of an educator who is knowledgeable in this field can be helpful when making this decision.

Outside Resources and Referrals

As previously mentioned, it takes a team to properly evaluate a child with hearing loss. Newly diagnosed children should be evaluated by **otolaryngologists** with pediatric expertise, **audiologists,** pediatric **ophthalmologists,** and medical **geneticists.** Any refractory error should be treated and followed closely because children with severe hearing difficulties are more dependent on vision. A genetics evaluation is important for diagnostic reasons as well as for providing families with information and counseling about the risk of recurrence.

Speech assessment and therapy are an essential part of long-term management, as are special education resources. Support groups and referrals to national organizations for hearing-impaired individuals can be valuable for parents and families. Resources for financial support should also be explored. Agencies with multidisciplinary teams are particularly important for newborns, infants, and children with other associated disabilities.

Prognosis

The goals of early recognition and treatment of newborns, infants, and children with hearing deficits are to minimize possible long-term sequelae of persistent speech and language problems and maximize cognitive development. An additional goal is to prevent the development of learning disabilities with subsequent educational failure. The earlier the intervention, the more likely children are to succeed and maximize their potential. With appropriate treatment, children should be able to lead a normal life.

CASE RESOLUTION

In the case study at the beginning of the chapter, the child has a history that is classically positive for a hearing deficit. She does not turn to loud noises, she has not developed any specific words, and she indicates her needs nonverbally. Although there are no obvious historical risk factors for hearing loss, a behavioral audiogram or brain stem auditory evoked response should be performed by an audiologist. The physician's suspicion should be discussed with the family, and a follow-up visit should be arranged to review hearing test results as soon as possible.

Selected References

Feldman HM. Evaluation and management of language and speech disorders in preschool children. *Pediatr Rev.* 2005;26(4):131–141

Foust T, Eiserman W, Shisler L, Geroso A. Using otoacoustic emissions to screen young children for hearing loss in primary care settings. *Pediatrics.* 2013;132(1): 118–123

Gifford KA, Holmes MG, Bernstein HH. Hearing loss in children. *Pediatr Rev.* 2009;30(6):207–216

Harlor ADB, Bower C; American Academy of Pediatrics Committee on Practice and Ambulatory Medicine and Section on Otolaryngology–Head and Neck Surgery. Hearing assessment in infants and children: recommendations beyond neonatal screening. *Pediatrics.* 2009;124(4):1252–1263

Joint Committee on Infant Hearing. Year 2007 position statement: principles and guidelines for early hearing detection and intervention programs. *Pediatrics.* 2007;120(4):898–921

Kennedy CR, McCann DC, Campbell MJ, et al. Language ability after early detection of permanent childhood hearing impairment. *N Engl J Med.* 2006;354(20): 2131–2141

Kral A, O'Donoghue GM. Profound deafness in childhood. *N Engl J Med.* 2010;363(15):1438–1450

Morton CC, Nance WE. Newborn hearing screening—a silent revolution. *N Engl J Med.* 2006;354(20):2151–2164

Papsin BC, Gordon KA. Cochlear implants for children with severe-to-profound hearing loss. *N Engl J Med.* 2007;357(23):2380–2387

Rosenfeld RM, Schwartz SR, Pynnonen MA, et al. Clinical practice guideline: tympanostomy tubes in children. *Otolaryngol Head Neck Surg.* 2013;149 (1 Suppl):S1–S35

Ross DS, Visser SN. Pediatric primary care physicians' practices regarding newborn hearing screening. *J Prim Care Community Health.* 2012;3(4):256–263

Russell JL, Pine HS, Young DL. Pediatric cochlear implantation: expanding applications and outcomes. *Pediatr Clin North Am.* 2013;60(4):841–863

Smith RJ, Bale JF, White KR. Sensorineural hearing loss in children. *Lancet.* 2005;365(9462):879–890

Weichbold V, Nekahm-Heis D, Welzl-Mueller K. Universal newborn hearing screening and postnatal hearing loss. *Pediatrics.* 2006;117(4):e631–e636

CHAPTER 77

Sore Throat

Stanley H. Inkelis, MD, and Casey Buitenhuys, MD

CASE STUDY

An 8-year-old girl has had a sore throat and fever for 2 days. She also has pain on swallowing, a headache, and a feeling of general malaise but no stridor, drooling, breathing difficulty, or rash. Other than the current illness, the girl is in good health. Although she has had sore throats in the past, she has never had one this severe. One week ago, her mother and father had sore throats and fever that resolved after 5 days with no medication.

The child has a temperature of 102.2°F (39.0°C). The physical examination is normal except for red tonsils with exudate bilaterally, palatal petechiae, and tender cervical lymphadenopathy.

Questions

1. What are the causes of sore throat in children?
2. What is the appropriate evaluation of children with sore throat? What laboratory tests are necessary?
3. What is the appropriate management for children with sore throat?
4. When should otolaryngologic consultation be obtained?

Sore throat, one of the most common illnesses seen by the primary care physician, is a painful inflammation of the pharynx, tonsils, or surrounding areas. In most cases, children with sore throat have mild symptoms that require little or no treatment. However, sore throat may be the presenting complaint of a severe illness such as epiglottitis or retropharyngeal abscess. Young children may not able to define their complaints very well, which makes a careful history from parents or other caregivers and a good physical examination essential for correct diagnosis. Optimal management of sore throat, especially if group A beta-hemolytic streptococcus (GABHS; *Streptococcus pyogenes*) is suspected, is still very controversial.

Epidemiology

Sore throat accounts for approximately 15 million outpatient physician visits each year, and approximately 5% of all pediatric emergency department visits are for pharyngitis. Sore throats are most common in children between 5 and 15 years of age. They are uncommon in infants younger than 1 year. Like other respiratory infections, sore throats occur most often in the late fall and winter months. Approximately 11% of all school-aged children receive medical care for pharyngitis. Twenty percent to 30% or more of cases of pharyngitis in these children are caused by GABHS. The estimated medical and nonmedical costs for GABHS pharyngitis are $205 per visit or approximately $224 million to $539 million per year, with much of the indirect costs related to parental loss of time from work.

The organisms that cause bacterial and viral pharyngitis are present in saliva and nasal secretions and are almost always transmitted by close contact. Spread between children in school is the common mode of transmission.

Clinical Presentation

The clinical presentation of sore throat is variable and often depends on etiology (D_x Box; also see Differential Diagnosis on page 474). Most children with sore throat present with sudden onset of pain and fever. The height of the fever is variable and is typically higher in younger children. In older children, especially if the sore throat is associated with a common cold, fever is minimal or absent. The throat or tonsils are red, and the breath may be malodorous. Headache, nausea, vomiting, and abdominal pain may occur, especially

---

Dx — Sore Throat

Viral
- Pain in throat
- Fever (variable)[a]
- Rhinorrhea (common)
- Cough (common)
- Erythema of pharynx or tonsils
- Follicular, ulcerative, exudative lesions of pharynx or tonsils[a]
- Conjunctivitis
- Non-scarlatiniform rash
- Occipital or posterior cervical adenopathy

Bacterial
- Pain in throat, usually sudden onset
- Fever
- Marked erythema of pharynx, tonsils, or uvula
- Headache, nausea, vomiting, abdominal pain
- Tonsillar and posterior pharyngeal wall exudate
- Tender, swollen cervical lymphadenopathy
- Scarlatiniform rash
- Absence of rhinorrhea or cough
- Positive rapid antigen test or throat culture result
- Distortion of natural anatomy

[a]Dependent on etiology (see Differential Diagnosis).

if children are febrile. Appetite may be decreased and children may be less active than usual.

In children with the common cold, rhinorrhea and postnasal discharge are present. A pharyngeal and tonsillar exudate is not typical. Although the cervical lymph nodes may be enlarged, they are usually not very tender. In contrast, children with streptococcal pharyngitis typically have high fever, pharyngeal and tonsillar exudate, and tender cervical lymph nodes.

Pathophysiology

Various bacteria and viruses produce sore throat symptoms by causing inflammation in the ring of posterior pharyngeal lymphoid tissue that consists of the tonsils, adenoid, and surrounding lymphoid tissue. This ring of tissue, called Waldeyer tonsillar ring, drains the oral and pharyngeal cavity and defends against infection of the mouth and throat. Other host defenses that protect against infection include the sneeze, gag, and cough reflexes; secretory immunoglobulin A; and a rich blood supply.

Viral sore throats may be acquired by inhalation or self-inoculation from the nasal mucosa or conjunctiva. The local respiratory epithelium becomes infected with the virus, and inflammation occurs. In some instances, inflammatory mediators may be responsible for the pain of sore throat. Group A streptococcus and other bacterial organisms directly invade the mucous membranes. Enzymes produced by this organism, streptolysin O and hyaluronidase, aid in the spread of infection.

Differential Diagnosis

Although most children who present with sore throat have common viral or bacterial pharyngitis, other, less common disorders such as infectious mononucleosis, acute HIV seroconversion syndrome, epiglottitis, retropharyngeal abscess, or peritonsillar abscess should be considered.

Viral Infection

Viral infection, the most common cause of sore throat in children, is most often associated with an upper respiratory infection caused by a rhinovirus. Cough and rhinorrhea associated with a sore throat suggest this etiology. Influenza virus infections may present with sudden onset of high fever, headache, cough, sore throat, and myalgia.

Adenovirus often leads to exudative pharyngitis, frequently in children younger than 3 years. Pharyngoconjunctival fever, caused by adenovirus 3, is characterized by a high fever (temperature >102.2°F [39.0°C]) for several days, conjunctivitis, and exudative tonsillitis.

Coxsackievirus and echovirus (enteroviruses) are the usual cause of herpangina. Vesicles and ulcers are generally apparent on the anterior tonsillar pillars and soft palate. They may also be found on the tonsils, pharynx, or posterior buccal mucosa. Children may have a high fever (temperature >102.2°F [39.0°C]), be irritable, and refuse to eat or drink; dehydration may result. Coxsackievirus A16, A6, and enterovirus 71 cause hand-foot-and-mouth disease, which is characterized by ulcerative oral lesions on the tongue and buccal mucosa and, less frequently, on the palate and anterior tonsillar pillars. Vesicular and papulovesicular lesions are evident on the hands and feet and occasionally on other parts of the body, most commonly the knees and buttocks. It usually occurs in children younger than 5 years but can occur in older children as well. A more severe form of hand-foot-and-mouth disease is associated with coxsackievirus A6, a virus new to the United States in 2012. Enterovirus 71 is sometimes associated with severe central nervous system disease. Enteroviral infections typically occur in the late spring, summer, and early fall.

Human herpesvirus may lead to pharyngotonsillitis but can be distinguished from most of the enteroviral infections because human herpesvirus almost always involves the anterior portion of the mouth and lips and is associated with gingivitis (herpes gingivostomatitis). The lesions often appear as whitish-yellow plaques with an erythematous base and are sometimes ulcerative. This illness is characterized by a high fever (temperature >102.2°F [39.0°C]) for up to 7 to 10 days and frequent refusal to eat or drink because of the painful lesions. Dehydration may occur.

Epstein-Barr virus (EBV) may cause exudative pharyngotonsillitis alone or as part of the infectious mononucleosis syndrome that includes fever, malaise, lymphadenopathy, palatal petechiae, and hepatosplenomegaly. Fatigue, malaise, eyelid edema, organomegaly, and a maculopapular rash without the other characteristics of a scarlet fever rash help distinguish between infectious mononucleosis and GABHS infection.

Cytomegalovirus may cause an infectious mononucleosis syndrome similar to EBV but is not as commonly associated with pharyngitis and splenomegaly.

HIV seroconversion syndrome may present with low-grade fevers, myalgia, nonexudative pharyngitis, diffuse adenopathy, anorexia, and weight loss. Generally, onset of symptoms is about 1 week after exposure but may be within the first month after exposure.

Bacterial Infection

Group A beta-hemolytic streptococcus is the most common cause of bacterial sore throat in children older than 3 years. The pharynx is typically very red and sometimes edematous, and the tonsils are red, enlarged, and covered with exudate. Occasionally, the uvula is very inflamed as well. Children may also have dysphagia, fever, vomiting, headache, malaise, and abdominal pain. Swollen anterior cervical lymphadenopathy and petechiae on the soft palate and uvula are usually apparent. In addition, the occurrence of a scarlatiniform rash, strawberry tongue, and Pastia lines (petechiae in the flexor skin creases of joints) indicates scarlet fever, which is diagnostic of group A streptococcal infection (see Chapter 126). Sore throat from GABHS typically occurs in the winter and early spring. Rheumatic fever and glomerulonephritis are nonsuppurative complications of group A streptococcal infection.

Peritonsillar abscess or cellulitis and cervical lymphadenitis are suppurative complications of GABHS. Children with peritonsillar abscess often experience trismus and drooling and speak with a "hot potato" voice. The abscess in the affected tonsil causes a bulge in the posterior soft palate and pushes the uvula away from the midline to the unaffected side of the pharynx. On palpation, the abscess may feel fluctuant. Peritonsillar cellulitis typically produces a bulge in the soft palate but does not cause deviation of the uvula.

Parapharyngeal and retropharyngeal abscesses that typically occur in children younger than 6 years are additional life-threatening complications of GABHS. Sore throat is associated with these conditions, but dysphagia is usually more evident when the child swallows. Children with a retropharyngeal or parapharyngeal abscess are toxic-appearing, also complain of trismus, have a fever, have dysphonia, refuse to swallow, and drool. In addition, the child may have meningism and may be short of breath. A fluctuant mass may be palpated deep to the tonsils. The patient may have pain when the trachea is manipulated in a lateral direction. The neck may be stiff and the patient may resist passive neck movements. Stridor may be present but usually is an ominous sign of impending airway compromise.

Group B, C, and G beta-hemolytic streptococci (non-GABHS) have all been isolated from children with pharyngitis. *Streptococcus pneumoniae* and *Arcanobacterium haemolyticum* infrequently cause pharyngitis in children. The latter organism is associated with a scarlatiniform rash in some patients and is most common in adolescents and young adults. In contrast with scarlet fever, palatal petechiae and strawberry tongue are not present with the pharyngitis caused by this bacterium. Although *Corynebacterium diphtheriae* (diphtheria) rarely causes sore throat in immunized children, this organism should be considered in non-immunized children or children from developing countries who have exudative pharyngotonsillitis and a grayish pseudomembrane that bleeds when removal is attempted.

Chlamydia trachomatis may lead to pharyngitis and tonsillitis in adolescents and young adults through sexual transmission. The role of *Chlamydia pneumoniae* as a cause of sore throat in children remains unclear. *Mycoplasma pneumoniae* does not usually produce sore throat in children unless they have lower respiratory tract disease. *Neisseria gonorrhoeae* may lead to sore throat in sexually active adolescents. Its occurrence in prepubertal children is often secondary to sexual abuse. The appearance of the throat is not characteristic, and diagnosis is made by cultures when the degree of suspicion is high. **Tularemia** is a rare cause of exudative pharyngitis in children but should be suspected if contact with wild animals has occurred.

Fusobacterium necrophorum is a gram-negative anaerobe that may cause an exudative pharyngitis, tender adenopathy, and fever. Untreated, it may progress to Lemierre syndrome or septic thrombosis of the internal jugular vein. Direct extension of the bacterial pharyngitis leads to perivenular inflammation and septic thrombosis of the internal jugular vein. Patients may present with fever, severe lateral neck pain, torticollis, and prominent internal and external jugular veins with erythema and induration. Patients may also present with additional signs and symptoms if septic emboli propagate, including acute neurologic signs (central nervous system retrograde propagation) and shortness of breath and multilobar pneumonia with or without cavitation (pulmonary propagation). Paradoxical septic emboli may cause other symptoms if a right-to-left cardiac shunt is present.

Other Causes

Candida albicans may be responsible for sore throat in infants and children who are immunocompromised or taking antibiotics. Children with oral candidiasis usually present with whitish plaques on the labial or buccal mucosa that do not wipe off easily. When the pharynx and tonsils are involved, some discomfort or dysphagia, but usually not significant pain, may occur.

Epiglottitis (supraglottitis) may present as sore throat. Prior to the *Haemophilus influenzae* type B (Hib) conjugate vaccine, epiglottitis typically affected children 2 to 7 years of age who would present with signs of toxicity, stridor, difficulty swallowing, and drooling. In relatively well-appearing children with sore throat but no stridor, neither epiglottitis nor retropharyngeal abscess is a likely cause of sore throat. In the past, epiglottitis was almost always caused by Hib. With the widespread use of the Hib conjugate vaccine, this organism is now rarely the etiology, thus diminishing the prevalence of epiglottitis and making this entity an uncommon cause of sore throat in children. Although rare in adolescents, epiglottitis may present with severe sore throat out of proportion to clinical findings. Other signs and symptoms include dysphagia, odynophagia, a muffled voice, and pain on palpation of the anterior neck around the hyoid bone. *Streptococcus pneumoniae, Staphylococcus aureus,* and group A, B, and C beta-hemolytic streptococci are unusual but reported causative agents of epiglottitis.

Children with croup may have sore throat and stridor, but they do not usually appear toxic and do not have difficulty swallowing. Affected children are usually between 6 months and 3 years of age (see Chapter 60).

Odontogenic infections may cause localized infection, inflammation, and swelling of the submental and submandibular space. Significant infection of this space may present with Ludwig angina, which is characterized by difficulty with secretions, dyspnea, airway compromise, and elevated position of the tongue and "woody" induration and tenderness of the sublingual space.

Trauma from penetrating objects, burns, or exposure to caustic materials may cause sore throat in children. Household smoking may also lead to pharyngeal irritation. In addition, allergic rhinitis with postnasal drip may result in sore throat. Tumor rarely causes sore throat in children but should be considered if a mass is present or pharyngeal inflammation persists. Persistent sore throat may also be a symptom of Kawasaki disease.

Evaluation

History

A thorough history often reveals the etiology of the sore throat (Questions Box). Questions about duration, fever, headache, vomiting, pain on swallowing, rash, oral lesions, abdominal pain, and history of

Sore Throat

- How long has the child had a sore throat?
- Does the child have fever, headache, or vomiting?
- How rapid was the onset of fever?
- Does the child have pain on swallowing?
- Are there any voice changes?
- Does the child have a rash or oral lesions?
- Does the child have abdominal pain?
- Does the child have any ill contacts?
- Are the child's immunizations up-to-date?
- Is the child having any difficulty breathing?
- Does the child have a history of allergies?
- Has the child suffered any trauma to the throat or neck?
- Has the child been exposed to environmental smoke?
- For sexually active adolescents or children with a history of sexual abuse with non-responding sore throats, has there been any oral sexual activity? Any other risk-taking behavior?

contact with other family members or classmates with similar symptoms suggest the most common causes of sore throat (infections with viruses and GABHS). A history of rapid onset of fever, toxicity, difficulty swallowing, drooling, and respiratory distress suggest epiglottitis and retropharyngeal abscess. Voice changes suggest peritonsillar abscess or tonsillar hypertrophy associated with infectious mononucleosis (EBV). Immunization history or history of immigration from a developing country helps assess the risk of diphtheria. Oral sexual activity suggests the possibility of a sexually transmitted infection. A history of allergies, trauma, and environmental smoke may help diagnose other causes of sore throat. Red eye or pinkeye with a rash, persistent fever (>5 days), and sore throat suggest Kawasaki disease. A teenager with at-risk behavior and an influenza-like illness may be presenting with HIV seroconversion syndrome.

Physical Examination

A general physical examination should be performed. It is important to note whether children appear toxic. The skin should be examined for a scarlatiniform, sandpaper-like rash; a vesicular rash involving the hands and feet; or a generalized maculopapular rash. The eyes should be evaluated for conjunctivitis and the nose for rhinorrhea (serous or purulent). The mouth, pharynx, and tonsils should be examined for vesicular lesions, ulcers, and gingivitis. The pharynx should be checked for redness, exudate, vesicles, edema, and foreign bodies. The tonsils and uvula should be examined for these same findings as well as asymmetry, and the neck should be checked for nuchal rigidity. The lymph nodes should be evaluated for enlargement (adenopathy) and inflammation (adenitis). The abdomen should be examined for hepatosplenomegaly.

Laboratory Tests

Although many signs and symptoms may suggest streptococcal pharyngitis, diagnosis can be confirmed only with laboratory tests. The

throat culture is the gold standard for diagnosis. When done correctly, throat culture has a sensitivity of 90% to 95% in detecting pharyngeal GABHS. Specimens should be obtained from the surfaces of both tonsils and posterior pharynx without touching other parts of the pharynx or mouth. The main disadvantage of throat culture is that the results are not available for a day or more after the specimen is obtained. Nevertheless, throat culture is the most reliable way to confirm streptococcal infection.

Rapid antigen detection tests (RADTs) are available for on-the-spot diagnosis. False-positive results are uncommon (specificity ≥95%), but false-negative results for most RADTs occur commonly (sensitivity 80%–90%). Because a negative test may not exclude a streptococcal infection, it is currently recommended by many authors and guidelines that this result should be confirmed by throat culture. Because RADTs are highly specific, it is not necessary to confirm a positive test result with a throat culture.

Newer RADTs using optical immunoassay (OIA) and chemiluminescent DNA probes boast sensitivities of greater than 99%. Recent data suggest that a negative OIA RADT may not always need routine confirmation with a throat culture, especially if physicians confirm in their practice setting that the newer RADT has a sensitivity comparable to the sensitivity of throat culture. In addition, it has been suggested in several studies that the recommendation to obtain a backup throat culture in all patients with a negative RADT is not a cost-effective approach. However, a negative backup throat culture may offer more assurance that the cause of the pharyngitis in the child or adolescent is not from GABHS infection.

Rapid and sensitive OIA RADTs reduce antibiotic prescription rates by 50% in pediatric emergency care visits related to sore throat. An antistreptolysin-O titer and an anti-deoxyribonuclease-B titer are not useful for the acute diagnosis of GABHS infection because these titers do not increase until 1 to 2 weeks after the onset of pharyngitis and peak at 3 to 4 weeks. However, measurement of these titers may help confirm a prior streptococcal infection if the throat culture is negative, particularly in children in whom there is a high suspicion of acute rheumatic fever or acute poststreptococcal glomerulonephritis. Diagnostic studies are typically not necessary for children younger than 3 years because GABHS pharyngitis is uncommon and the risk of developing acute rheumatic fever and suppurative complications is low. However, if a child is younger than 3 years and there is a school-aged household contact with GABHS infection, an RADT or throat culture should be ordered if the child is symptomatic.

Differentiating between viral and bacterial pharyngitis is often difficult, and the rapid streptococcal antigen tests and throat cultures should be reserved for patients who have signs and symptoms common for both illnesses. There are some children whose clinical findings are not consistent with bacterial pharyngitis. For example, afebrile children with a sore throat, runny nose, and cough who have slight pharyngeal erythema almost certainly have viral pharyngitis and do not need further workup. However, children with a constellation of signs and symptoms suggesting bacterial pharyngitis, such as sudden onset of sore throat, fever, headache, swollen and erythematous tonsils, tonsillar or posterior pharyngeal wall exudate, uvulitis, tender and enlarged cervical lymphadenopathy, absence of runny nose or cough, or exposure to an individual with streptococcal pharyngitis, may need further testing with RADT or throat culture to confirm group A streptococcal pharyngitis because an accurate diagnosis cannot be made on clinical grounds alone. Approximately 20% of all children are asymptomatic carriers of GABHS in the pharynx, especially during winter and spring. If tested, these children will be positive for GABHS even though they may have a viral illness and will be unnecessarily treated with antibiotics. Guidelines for clinical prediction have been evaluated and have suggested different approaches to the need for RADT or throat culture and antibiotic management. The Centor criteria were derived and validated in adult patients and overestimate the likelihood of GABHS pharyngitis in children. A modified McIsaac score predicts better in children but is still not sensitive or specific enough to rely on alone. In a meta-analysis of signs and symptoms predicting GABHS, presence of a tonsillar exudate, pharyngeal exudate, or exposure to strep infection in the previous 2 weeks (positive likelihood ratios 3.4, 2.1, and 1.9, respectively) and the absence of tender anterior cervical nodes, tonsillar enlargement, or exudate (negative likelihood ratios of 0.6, 0.63, and 0.74), were most predictive. Guidelines that recommend identifying patients who are likely to have group A streptococcal pharyngitis based on clinical or epidemiological findings and providing antibiotics for only those confirmed by RADT or throat culture decrease the unnecessary overuse of antibiotics.

Viral throat cultures and acute and convalescent titers to determine viral pharyngitis are rarely indicated unless systemic infection occurs (eg, herpes encephalitis). Epstein-Barr virus infection can be determined by specific serologic antibody assays, but nonspecific tests for heterophil antibody (eg, mononucleosis spot [monospot] test) are most available and are usually the tests of choice for diagnosing infectious mononucleosis. However, it may be negative in children younger than 4 years or early in the course of the infection. Only 75% of infected children between 2 and 4 years of age and fewer than 30% of children younger than 2 years are identified by this test. The monospot test, a rapid slide test for heterophil antibodies, may remain positive for months after the infection and incorrectly may suggest the diagnosis of infectious mononucleosis in children who do not have this disorder. A complete blood cell count with more than 50% to 60% lymphocytes or more than 10% atypical lymphocytes is suggestive of mononucleosis. When these tests are inconclusive, the specific serologic antibody tests for EBV infection are helpful in establishing the diagnosis. Cytomegalovirus-specific antibody tests should be considered in the patient with a mononucleosis syndrome and negative laboratory test results for EBV. Culture or fluorescent antibody evaluation of the pseudomembrane may be used to diagnose diphtheria. Culture or presence of serum agglutinins confirms tularemia. Thayer-Martin culture plates should be used to diagnose suspected gonorrheal sore throat. HIV antibody tests are of little use in the evaluation of acute seroconversion syndrome because antibody titers take 4 to 6 weeks to become detectable. If acute seroconversion is suspected, quantitative RNA polymerase chain reaction should be ordered.

Imaging Studies

If epiglottitis or retropharyngeal abscess is suspected but not clinically apparent, a lateral neck radiograph may be obtained. The radiograph should be performed with a physician in attendance who is capable of performing endotracheal intubation in case the child has respiratory failure (see Chapter 60). Computed tomography of the neck is indicated in the stable patient with suspected deep parapharyngeal or retropharyngeal infection. Emergency bedside ultrasound is an effective and sensitive tool for differentiating between peritonsillar cellulitis and a peritonsillar abscess.

Management

Management of children with sore throat is based on the etiology of the condition. The early recognition of potentially serious conditions based on history and physical examination is essential to providing optimal care. **Otolaryngologic consultation** should be obtained in children with peritonsillar abscess, retropharyngeal abscess, parapharyngeal abscess, submental abscess, epiglottitis, significant pharyngeal trauma, or pharyngeal tumor. Recurrent tonsillitis, especially in children who miss school, may be a reason for referral to an otolaryngologist.

Outpatient Treatment

For most children with sore throat, the physician must differentiate between viral and streptococcal pharyngitis. Viral sore throat can be managed symptomatically. Treatment with **analgesics such as acetaminophen or ibuprofen to relieve pain and maintaining hydration** are the mainstays of therapy for young children with viral or bacterial sore throat. Gargling with warm water and sucking on hard candy may provide additional symptomatic relief for older children. The use of steroids for reducing pain for pharyngitis is controversial. A recent systematic review demonstrated a relatively small reduction in time to significant pain relief of 4.5 hours and a negligible reduction in pain in 24 hours when a single dose of dexamethasone (0.6 mg/kg, maximum 10 mg) is given. The decision to administer steroids should be made on a case-by-case basis.

The pain from lesions of herpes stomatitis often responds to acetaminophen or ibuprofen. For those children with persistent pain, acetaminophen with hydrocodone may be helpful. **Anesthetics** such as lidocaine may also decrease the pain. A convenient way of delivering lidocaine is in a mixture (1 part each) of lidocaine, diphenhydramine (Benadryl), and a liquid antacid. This mixture, called "magic mouthwash," may be used in older children. However, there is little evidence supporting a benefit. If used, it may be inserted into each side of the mouth, gargled, or placed on a gloved finger or cotton swab and applied directly on the oral lesions of the tongue and labial and buccal mucosa. It is best used about 30 minutes before feeding or drinking, especially in children who refuse to drink. Lidocaine should be used cautiously because it can suppress the gag reflex. The dose should never exceed 3 mg/kg. Too much lidocaine may result in seizures. Magic mouthwash can also be prepared without lidocaine, especially for younger children. Parents should be given instruction on how to monitor fluid intake and the signs of dehydration.

In children without clear-cut evidence of streptococcal pharyngitis, a positive rapid streptococcal antigen test helps direct antibiotic treatment. A negative test in the presence of positive symptoms should be accompanied by a throat culture. However, the OIA rapid test may preclude the need for culture confirmation. Patients can await the results of culture before beginning antibiotic therapy. **Antibiotics** without confirmation from rapid streptococcal tests or cultures are indicated in children who appear toxic, who have scarlet fever or peritonsillar cellulitis/abscess, or who have a history of rheumatic fever. Most evidence suggests that early treatment results in more rapid clinical improvement, although this is controversial. Rheumatic fever can be prevented if treatment is started within 9 days of sore throat symptom development. Glomerulonephritis probably is not affected by antibiotic therapy.

Evidence suggests that children with streptococcal pharyngitis should be treated with antibiotics to relieve symptoms, shorten the course of their illness, and prevent disease dissemination, suppurative complications, and rheumatic fever. Penicillin is the antibiotic of choice. It may be administered orally as penicillin V (phenoxymethyl penicillin) in a dose of 250 mg 2 to 3 times a day for 10 days for children and 500 mg 2 to 3 times a day for adolescents and adults. Most patients will feel better after 2 to 3 days, but it is important to stress to parents that their children need to complete the full 10-day course. Amoxicillin, given once a day (50mg/kg, maximum 1,000 mg) for 10 days is as effective as penicillin V given 2 to 3 times a day for 10 days, making compliance more likely. In addition, amoxicillin is more acceptable to young children because the oral suspension is better tasting. (See Table 77-1 for dosages.)

If the risk of noncompliance is high or if the risk of complication is great (eg, children have a history of rheumatic fever), penicillin should be administered intramuscularly. Intramuscular penicillin has 2 disadvantages: pain associated with the injection and increased incidence of a potentially more severe allergic reaction. The dose of benzathine penicillin for children weighing less than 27 kg (60 lb) is 600,000 U. The dose for larger children and adults is 1.2 million U. Bicillin CR, which contains 900,000 U of benzathine penicillin and 300,000 U of procaine penicillin, is a satisfactory alternative form of delivering penicillin intramuscularly in children and may be preferable because it causes less pain and less severe local reaction. This preparation has not been determined to be effective in heavier patients (adolescents and adults); therefore, the benzathine preparation noted previously is recommended for this group. The injection of benzathine penicillin is less painful if it is given after it reaches room temperature. (See Table 77-1 for dosage information.) A first-generation oral cephalosporin, such as cephalexin, is recommended for most penicillin-allergic children but should not be used in children with an immediate or type 1 hypersensitivity to penicillin. Clindamycin may also be used for patients allergic to penicillin; however, the liquid preparation is not palatable and compliance may be poor. Azalides and macrolides such as azithromycin or

Table 77-1. Antibiotics Used in the Management of Sore Throat in Children	
Drug *(for Streptococcal Pharyngitis)*	**Dosage**
Penicillin V	250 mg 2–3 times/d for children and 500 mg 2–3 times/d for adolescents orally for 10 d
Amoxicillin	50 mg/kg once daily orally for 10 d (maximum 1,000 mg)
Cephalexin	25–50 mg/kg/d every 12 h orally for 10 d (maximum 500 mg every 12 h)
Clindamycin	20 mg/kg/d in 3 divided doses (maximum 1.8 g/d) orally for 10 d (for chronic streptococcal carriers or suspected *Fusobacterium necrophorum*)
Azithromycin	12 mg/kg once daily orally for 5 d (maximum 500 mg)
Clarithromycin	15 mg/kg/d every 12 h orally for 10 d
Benzathine penicillin	600,000 U (<27 kg or 60 lb); 1.2 million U (>27 kg or 60 lb) as single intramuscular injection
Bicillin CR	900,000 U benzathine penicillin and 300,000 U procaine penicillin for children as single intramuscular injection
Rifampin	10 mg/kg/dose orally every 12 h for 4 d (given last 4 d of treatment with penicillin V or benzathine penicillin for chronic streptococcal carriers)
Drug *(for Gonococcal Pharyngitis)*	**Dosage**
Ceftriaxone **Plus**	125 mg intramuscularly in a single dose if <45 kg, 250 mg intramuscularly in a single dose if >45 kg
Azithromycin **or**	20 mg/kg (maximum 1 g) orally in a single dose
Erythromycin **or (if ≥9 y)**	50 mg/kg/d (maximum 2 g/d) orally every 6 h for 14 d
Doxycycline	100 mg orally 2 times/d for 7 d

clarithromycin may be substituted in children who are allergic to penicillin. They are preferred to erythromycin because they are associated with fewer gastrointestinal side effects. Azithromycin has the added advantage of once-a-day dosing and a shortened course of therapy of only 5 days. Additionally, shorter-duration alternatives to penicillin were superior in time to symptom improvement as well as duration of fever. Macrolide resistance, however, is 5% to 8% in most areas of the United States. Tetracyclines; sulfonamides, including trimethoprim-sulfamethoxazole; and fluoroquinolones are not recommended for the treatment of streptococcal pharyngitis.

If children continue to be symptomatic and have a persistently positive throat culture after completing a course of therapy, they may be re-treated with the same antibiotic, given another oral antibiotic (as noted previously and in Table 77-1), or given an intramuscular dose of penicillin, especially if compliance is in question.

As noted previously, approximately 20% of children are asymptomatic carriers of group A streptococci. In general, these children do well, and eradication of the bacteria is not necessary. Cultures after treatment are generally not recommended, except for children with recurring or persistent symptoms or those with a previous history of rheumatic fever. In selected cases of children whose throat cultures remain positive, eradication of the pharyngeal carriage should be strongly considered. These indications are as follows: if there is an outbreak of acute rheumatic fever or poststreptococcal glomerulonephritis, if there is an outbreak of group A streptococcal pharyngitis in a closed or semi-closed community, if there is a family history of rheumatic fever, or if repeated episodes of documented symptomatic group A streptococcal pharyngitis recur within a family over several weeks despite appropriate therapy. If cultures remain positive, these children may be treated with benzathine penicillin and oral rifampin for 4 days in an attempt to eradicate the organism. (See Table 77-1 for dosages.) Clindamycin is reportedly more effective in eradication of the organism from symptom-free carriers. (See Table 77-1 for dosages.)

Mycoplasma pneumoniae pharyngitis is usually associated with a generalized infection. Because it is often a self-limited illness, it does not require antibiotic therapy unless symptoms persist. Treatment with any of the macrolide antibiotics may be helpful. However, clarithromycin and azithromycin have fewer side effects and are likely to produce better compliance. Macrolides are also the drugs of choice for children with *A haemolyticum* pharyngitis.

Diphtheria, seen almost exclusively in less-advantaged countries, is a life-threatening infection that requires prompt diagnosis and treatment. Penicillin G or erythromycin must be given to kill *C diphtheriae*; in addition, equine antitoxin must be administered to neutralize the exotoxin. Tularemia pharyngitis is unusual, but if suspected, it is treated with gentamicin.

For gonococcal pharyngitis caused by *N gonorrhoeae*, intramuscular ceftriaxone is the drug of choice. (See Table 77-1 for dosages.) Additional antibiotic coverage for associated *C trachomatis* infection should be administered. Oral azithromycin or doxycycline should also be given to children 9 years or older. (See Table 77-1 for dosages.) Azithromycin or erythromycin may be used for younger children. Children should be examined and cultured for sexually transmitted infections in other sites and should have a serological test for syphilis at the first visit and have a repeat test 6 to 8 weeks later. They should also be evaluated for concurrent hepatitis B and HIV infection. Sexual abuse should be considered in all cases of gonococcal pharyngitis, particularly in prepubertal children (see chapters 101 and 132).

Children with croup usually respond to steroids. Oral nystatin can be used in children with oral candidiasis. Adolescents with uncomplicated peritonsillar abscess may be managed as outpatients in selected cases with needle aspiration and oral antibiotics.

Inpatient Treatment

Children with sore throat should be admitted to the hospital if they have airway obstruction or need intavenous (IV) hydration or antibiotics. Children with retropharyngeal abscess and epiglottitis require IV antibiotics and should be managed in consultation with an otolaryngologist. Preadolescent children or adolescents with complicated peritonsillar abscess also require IV antibiotics. Surgical intervention is indicated if the abscess is fluctuant, the child is toxic or has severe trismus or airway compromise, or there is no resolution within 24 hours. Needle aspiration may be acceptable in selected cases. Intravenous hydration is occasionally needed for patients with severe herpes stomatitis who will not drink because of pain and who become dehydrated.

Patients with Lemierre syndrome should be admitted and started on IV antibiotics covering a polymicrobial infection, including anaerobic organisms. If simple *F necrophorum* pharyngitis is suspected, antibiotics covering anaerobes are indicated, such as clindamycin.

Suspected deep space infection of the pharynx other than an uncomplicated peritonsillar abscess requires inpatient admission and treatment. Retropharyngeal and parapharyngeal abscesses usually require incision and drainage during or after antibiotics have been initiated. Ludwig angina requires IV antibiotics for an uncomplicated cellulitis or an incision and drainage procedure in the operating room. Meticulous monitoring of the patient's airway is required if it is not secured preoperatively.

The role of tonsillectomy or adenotonsillectomy for children with recurrent sore throat is still controversial. However, the American Academy of Otolaryngology–Head and Neck Surgery convened a panel of clinicians from various disciplines to develop evidence-based guidelines to identify children who are most likely to benefit from tonsillectomy. These guidelines, containing content based on previous work done by Paradise et al about children with recurrent sore throats, have been recently published. Most children with sore throat improve on their own, and recommendations are therefore for watchful waiting if there are fewer than 7 documented sore throat episodes in the past year, fewer than 5 per year over the past 2 years, and fewer than 3 per year over the past 3 years. Parental report does not qualify as documentation. If the number of documented sore throats meets or exceeds these numbers and there are associated findings (eg, temperature >101°F [38.3°C], cervical lymphadenopathy, tonsillar exudate, positive test for GABHS), the clinician may recommend tonsillectomy. Consultation with an otolaryngologist and a period of watchful waiting should be considered. If a child with recurrent sore throat does not meet these criteria, the child should be assessed for other factors that may favor tonsillectomy over observation, including, but not limited to, multiple antibiotic allergy or intolerance, PFAPA syndrome (*p*eriodic *f*ever, *a*phthous stomatitis, *p*haryngitis, and *a*denitis), or a history of peritonsillar abscess. Although these guidelines are evidence-based and the recommendations are better defined than before, each case should be individualized. As with all clinical decisions, there is a role for shared decision-making with the child's caregiver and primary care physician about the need for tonsillectomy.

Education

Patients and families should receive general education about sore throats. Medication for pain with drugs such as acetaminophen or ibuprofen is useful, especially if children are having difficulty swallowing. Gargling with warm salt water or sucking on hard candy may soothe the pain of sore throat. For children with herpes gingivostomatitis, avoidance of acidic or spicy food products may prevent pain during eating. Children with bacterial pharyngitis may return to school after 24 hours of antibiotic therapy and the disappearance of fever. It should be recommended that symptomatic family members see a physician. Parents should call or return to the physician if their children have respiratory or swallowing difficulties, drooling, severe pain, or fever (temperature >101°F [38.3°C]) for more than 48 hours after the initiation of appropriate antibiotics.

Prognosis

The prognosis for children with viral sore throat is excellent because of its self-limited nature. The outlook for children with streptococcal sore throat is also excellent. If the infection is not diagnosed and treated appropriately, however, suppurative (eg, peritonsillar abscess) and non-suppurative complications (eg, rheumatic fever, acute glomerulonephritis) may occur. With early diagnosis and prompt treatment, the prognosis for unusual, life-threatening causes of sore throat is also very good. Research in the development of a polyvalent synthetic oligosaccharide vaccine for GABHS is underway. The cross-immunogenicity of GABHS presents a unique and challenging case for vaccine development.

CASE RESOLUTION

In the case presented, the child has palatal petechiae and tonsillar exudate, which are signs and symptoms consistent with streptococcal pharyngitis. A streptococcal rapid antigen detection test is performed and is positive. The child is treated with oral penicillin. Neither of her parents has sore throat symptoms.

Selected References

Altamimi S, Khalil A, Khalaiwi KA, Milner RA, Pusic MV, Al Othman MA. Short-term late-generation antibiotics versus longer term penicillin for acute streptococcal pharyngitis in children. *Cochrane Database Syst Rev.* 2012;8:CD004872

American Academy of Pediatrics. Group A streptococcal infections. In: Pickering LK, Baker CJ, Kimberlin DW, Long SS, eds. *Red Book: 2012 Report of the Committee on Infectious Diseases.* 29th ed. Elk Grove Village, IL: American Academy of Pediatrics; 2012:668–680

Ayanruoh S, Waseem M, Quee F, Humphrey A, Reynolds T. Impact of rapid streptococcal test on antibiotic use in a pediatric emergency department. *Pediatr Emerg Care.* 2009;25(11):748–750

Baltimore RS. Re-evaluation of antibiotic treatment of streptococcal pharyngitis. *Curr Opin Pediatr.* 2010;22(1):77–82

Baugh RF, Archer SM, Mitchell RB, et al. Clinical practice guideline: tonsillectomy in children. *Otolaryngol Head Neck Surg.* 2011;144(1 Suppl):S1–S30

Bisno AL, Gerber MA, Gwaltney JM Jr, Kaplan EL, Schwartz RH; Infectious Diseases Society of America. Practice guidelines for the diagnosis and management of group A streptococcal pharyngitis. *Clin Infect Dis.* 2002;35(2):113–125

Bulloch B, Kabani A, Tenenbein M. Oral dexamethasone for the treatment of pain in children with acute pharyngitis: a randomized, double-blind, placebo-controlled trial. *Ann Emerg Med.* 2003;41(5):601–608

Cherry JD. Pharyngitis (pharyngitis, tonsillitis, tonsillopharyngitis, and nasopharyngitis). In: Feigen RD, Cherry JD, Demler-Harrison GJ, Kaplan SL, eds. *Textbook of Pediatric Infectious Diseases.* 6th ed. Philadelphia, PA: Saunders; 2009:161–170

Clegg HW, Ryan AG, Dallas SD, et al. Treatment of streptococcal pharyngitis with once-daily compared with twice-daily amoxicillin: a noninferiority trial. *Pediatr Infect Dis J.* 2006;25(9):761–767

Dale JB, Fischetti VA, Carapetis JR, et al. Group A streptococcal vaccines: paving a path for accelerated development. *Vaccine.* 2013;31(Suppl 2):B216–B222

Edmonson MB, Farwell KR. Relationship between the clinical likelihood of group A streptococcal pharyngitis and the sensitivity of a rapid antigen-detection test in a pediatric practice. *Pediatrics.* 2005;115(2):280–285

Fine AM, Nizet V, Mandl KD. Large-scale validation of the Centor and McIsaac scores to predict group A streptococcal pharyngitis. *Arch Intern Med.* 2012; 172(11):847–852

Fleisher GR. Sore throat. In: Fleisher GR, Ludwig S, eds. *Textbook of Pediatric Emergency Medicine.* 6th ed. Philadelphia, PA: Lippincott; 2010:579–583

Gerber MA. Diagnosis and treatment of pharyngitis in children. *Pediatr Clin North Am.* 2005;52(3):729–747

Gerber MA, Baltimore RS, Eaton CB, et al. Prevention of rheumatic fever and diagnosis and treatment of acute streptococcal pharyngitis: a scientific statement from the American Heart Association Rheumatic Fever, Endocarditis, and Kawasaki Disease Committee of the Council on Cardiovascular Disease in the Young, the Interdisciplinary Council on Functional Genomics and Translational Biology, and the Interdisciplinary Council on Quality of Care and Outcomes Research: endorsed by the American Academy of Pediatrics. *Circulation.* 2009; 119(11):1541–1551

Gieseker KE, Roe MH, MacKenzie T, Todd JK. Evaluating the American Academy of Pediatrics diagnostic standard for *Streptococcus pyogenes* pharyngitis: backup culture versus repeat rapid antigen testing. *Pediatrics.* 2003;111(6 Pt 1):e666–e670

Jaggi P, Shulman ST. Group A streptococcal infections. *Pediatr Rev.* 2006;27(3): 99–105

Joachim L, Campos D Jr, Smeesters PR. Pragmatic scoring system for pharyngitis in low-resource settings. *Pediatrics.* 2010;126(3):e608–e614

Linder JA, Bates DW, Lee GM, Finkelstein JA. Antibiotic treatment of children with sore throat. *JAMA.* 2005;294(18):2315–2322

Linder JA, Chan JC, Bates DW. Evaluation and treatment of pharyngitis in primary care practice: the difference between guidelines is largely academic. *Arch Intern Med.* 2006;166(13):1374–1379

Martin JM, Green M, Barbadora KA, Wald ER. Group A streptococci among school-aged children: clinical characteristics and the carrier state. *Pediatrics.* 2004;114(5):1212–1219

McIsaac WJ, Kellner JD, Aufricht P, Vanjaka A, Low DE. Empirical validation of guidelines for the management of pharyngitis in children and adults. *JAMA.* 2004;291(13):1587–1595

Millar KR, Johnson DW, Drummond D, Kellner JD. Suspected peritonsillar abscess in children. *Pediatr Emerg Care.* 2007;23(7):431–438

Paradise JL, Bluestone CD, Colborn DK, Bernard BS, Rockette HE, Kurs-Lasky M. Tonsillectomy and adenotonsillectomy for recurrent throat infection in moderately affected children. *Pediatrics.* 2002;110(1):7–15

Park SY, Gerber MA, Tanz RR, et al. Clinicians' management of children and adolescents with acute pharyngitis. *Pediatrics.* 2006;117(6):1871–1878

Pfoh E, Wessels MR, Goldmann D, Lee GM. Burden and economic cost of group A streptococcal pharyngitis. *Pediatrics.* 2008;121(2):229–234

Rafei K, Lichenstein R. Airway infectious disease emergencies. *Pediatr Clin North Am.* 2006;53(2):215–242

Ramirez-Schrempp D, Dorfman DH, Baker WE, Liteplo AS. Ultrasound soft tissue applications in the pediatric emergency department: to drain or not to drain? *Pediatr Emerg Care.* 2009;25(1):44–48

Shaikh N, Leonard E, Martin JM. Prevalence of streptococcal pharyngitis and streptococcal carriage in children: a meta-analysis. *Pediatrics.* 2010;126(3): e557–e564

Shulman ST, Bisno AL, Clegg HW, et al. Clinical practice guideline for the diagnosis and management of group A streptococcal pharyngitis: 2012 update by the Infectious Diseases Society of America. *Clin Infect Dis.* 2012;55(10):e86–e102

Van Howe RS, Kusnier LP 2nd. Diagnosis and management of pharyngitis in a pediatric population based on cost-effectiveness and projected health outcomes. *Pediatrics.* 2006;117(3):609–619

Webb KH. Does culture confirmation of high-sensitivity rapid streptococcal tests make sense? A medical decision analysis. *Pediatrics.* 1998;101(2):E2

Webb KH, Needham CA, Kurtz SR. Use of a high-sensitivity rapid strep test without culture confirmation of negative results: 2 years' experience. *J Fam Pract.* 2000;49(1):34–38

Wessels MR. Clinical practice. Streptococcal pharyngitis. *N Engl J Med.* 2011; 364(7):648–655

Wing A, Villa-Roel C, Yeh B, Eskin B, Buckingham J, Rowe BH. Effectiveness of corticosteroid treatment in acute pharyngitis: a systematic review of the literature. *Acad Emerg Med.* 2010;17(5):476–483

CHAPTER 78

Nosebleeds

Katherine E. Remick, MD, and Stanley H. Inkelis, MD

CASE STUDY

A 3-year-old boy is brought to the office one winter day. He has had 4 nosebleeds in the past week as well as a cold with a runny nose and cough, which began the day before the first nosebleed. The nosebleeds occurred at night or during sleep and stopped spontaneously or with gentle pressure. Other than the cold and nosebleeds, the boy is in good health. He is active, with bruises over both tibias but none elsewhere. The many cuts and scrapes he has had in the past resulted in minimal bleeding. His family has no history of a bleeding disorder or easy bruising.

The child's physical examination is entirely normal except for a small amount of blood in the left anterior naris.

Questions

1. What are the common causes of nosebleeds in children?
2. What systemic diseases are associated with nosebleeds?
3. How should nosebleeds be evaluated in children?
4. How should minor and severe nosebleeds be managed in children?

Nosebleed, or epistaxis, occurs commonly in children, especially in those between the ages of 2 and 10 years. In most cases, nosebleeds are secondary to local trauma and can be cared for by primary care physicians. In rare instances, however, a nosebleed may be difficult to control or a manifestation of a serious systemic illness. Referral to an otolaryngologist or a hematologist/oncologist is usually not required except in these situations, and hospitalization is generally unnecessary. Parents and children are often frightened by nosebleeds and frequently overestimate the amount of blood lost. Providing reassurance and a basic understanding of the most common causes are important in allaying anxiety.

Epidemiology

Thirty percent of children have one nosebleed by the time they are 5 years of age. In children between the ages of 6 and 10 years, the frequency increases to 56%. Nosebleeds are rare in infancy and infrequent after puberty. They occur much more frequently in the late fall and winter months, when upper respiratory infections (URIs) are common, environmental humidity is relatively low, and the use of heating systems results in dryness. Nosebleeds are also more common in children who live in dry climates, especially in the presence of a concomitant URI or chronic allergic rhinitis.

Clinical Presentation

Most children with nosebleeds have a history of bleeding at home and have minimal or no bleeding at the time of presentation (D$_x$ Box). However, children with underlying clotting disorders (eg, hemophilia) may have recurrent nosebleeds and a history of prolonged bleeding, easy bruising, or multiple bruises in uncommon locations such as the gingivae or joints. Less commonly, nosebleeds

---

Dx Nosebleeds

- Blood in anterior nares, nasopharynx, or mouth
- History of any of the following:
  — Frequent digital manipulation (nose picking)
  — Upper respiratory infection (recent)
  — Allergic rhinitis
  — Dry climate
  — Foreign body in nose
  — Trauma to nose
  — Prolonged or difficult-to-stop bleeding or easy bruising
- Physical examination consistent with any of the following:
  — Rhinorrhea
  — Dry, cracked nasal mucosa
  — Foreign body in nose
  — Trauma to nose
  — Multiple bruises

---

are one of the first manifestations of an undiagnosed malignancy or other systemic illness. In unusual situations, children with gastrointestinal or respiratory tract bleeding may present with blood exiting through the nose. Alternatively, some children with nosebleeds may present with hematemesis, hemoptysis, melena, or anemia. In these cases, a nasal source should be considered.

Nosebleeds are generally categorized by anatomic location as anterior or posterior. With anterior nosebleeds, vessels from the anterior portion of the nose rupture, resulting in readily visible blood loss through the nares. With posterior nosebleeds, most of the blood runs into the nasopharynx and mouth, although some blood may exit through the nose as well. Posterior nosebleeds tend to be heavier and more difficult to control, and though uncommon, children have a propensity to become hemodynamically unstable.

Pathophysiology

Most nosebleeds in children (>90%) are anterior and easily controlled. Anterior bleeding originates approximately 0.5 cm from the tip of the nose, known as the Kiesselbach area. This area is a confluence of small vessels supplied by the anterior and posterior ethmoid arteries, the sphenopalatine artery, and the septal branches of the superior labial artery (Figure 78-1). The mucosa covering the Kiesselbach area is thin and friable, thereby providing little structural support to the small vessels supplying the nasal mucous membrane.

Congestion of vessels located in the Kiesselbach area due to URIs or drying of the mucosa secondary to low environmental humidity makes this area susceptible to bleeding. Viral respiratory infections, such as infectious mononucleosis and influenza, may predispose children to nosebleeds because of their local inflammatory effect. Nosebleeds in children with these infections are more common in areas of low environmental humidity. However, even in the absence of URI-like symptoms, children may suffer from nosebleeds in such environments, especially in the winter, when inhaling dry, hot air from heating systems causes desiccation of the nasal mucosa (rhinitis sicca). Nosebleeds also occur more commonly in children who have nasal colonization with *Staphylococcus aureus*. It is postulated that *S aureus* replaces existing flora and leads to inflammation and new vessel formation.

Posterior nosebleeds are unusual in children and most commonly associated with trauma. If bleeding is vigorous or poorly controlled with anterior nasal packing or involves both nares, a posterior source is likely to be identified. Posterior nosebleeds generally arise from the turbinate or nasal wall. Significant bleeding, usually from a branch of the sphenopalatine artery, may occur. Because of the posterior location, children often present with symptoms other than frank epistaxis (eg, hematemesis, hemoptysis, melena, anemia).

Differential Diagnosis

Trauma from nose picking and **inflammation** of the nasal mucosa from a URI are by far the most common causes of nosebleeds in children. Repetitive, habitual nose picking results in the formation of friable granulation tissue that bleeds when congested blood vessels are traumatized (epistaxis digitorum). As the nasal mucosa dries, it may lead to crust formation and cracking. Bleeding may occur spontaneously or from nose rubbing, but more often it results from forceful nose blowing and sneezing that increases venous pressure in the more vascularized nasal septum.

Foreign bodies may cause direct trauma or pressure necrosis to the vessels of the nasal mucosa. Toddler-aged children may place small toys, beads, pebbles, or food items into the nares. Button batteries are particularly troublesome and should be removed immediately to avoid septal perforation. Children with unilateral epistaxis with purulent or foul-smelling nasal drainage should be evaluated for a foreign body. **External trauma**, secondary to falls or blunt force, can cause tears to the nasal mucosa or nasal fractures. If bleeding from mucosal vessels occurs but the mucosa remains intact, a septal hematoma may develop. The nasal septum must, therefore, be carefully examined. Abscess formation or septal perforation may occur if the septal hematoma is not drained. **Non-accidental** trauma should be considered in any infant or child younger than 2 years with a nosebleed.

Allergic rhinitis with inflammation and subsequent drying may also lead to nosebleeds. Airborne environmental pollutants have been associated with increased inflammation of the nasal mucosa. Children with allergic rhinitis who take decongestants or use topical nasal decongestants or topical nasal steroid sprays may be more likely to suffer from nosebleeds. In addition, the dispenser tip of these sprays may traumatize the already dry and friable mucosa, causing the nose to bleed.

Although nosebleeds are usually benign conditions, they may be one of the first signs of serious illness. Persistent or recurrent nosebleeds with no obvious cause should raise the suspicion of **bleeding disorders.** Thrombocytopenia is the most common coagulation defect causing nosebleeds. Idiopathic thrombocytopenic purpura is the most frequent thrombocytopenic disorder associated with nosebleeds. Leukemia, aplastic anemia, and HIV infection should also be considered and ruled out in children with nosebleeds and thrombocytopenia. Finally, platelet aggregation disorders may be a cause of recurrent nosebleeds.

The most commonly inherited bleeding disorder associated with nosebleeds is von Willebrand disease, an autosomal-dominant bleeding disorder characterized by varying degrees of factor VIII deficiency and platelet dysfunction (decreased platelet adhesiveness). Hemophilia (factor VIII, IX, or XI) deficiency, factor VII deficiency,

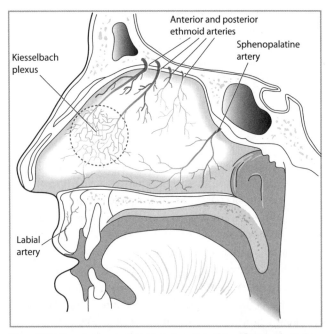

Figure 78-1. Vascular supply of nasal septum. Note the confluence of vessels that forms the Kiesselbach area (plexus).

Labels in figure:
Anterior and posterior ethmoid arteries
Sphenopalatine artery
Kiesselbach plexus
Labial artery

Glanzmann thrombasthenia, and Bernard-Soulier syndrome are other inherited bleeding disorders that may lead to nosebleeds. Hepatic disease, severe vitamin K deficiency, or malabsorption syndrome is associated with an acquired coagulopathy, which may present with nosebleed. Valproic acid administration has been associated with acquired von Willebrand disease and nosebleeds.

Nosebleeds may be a manifestation of hereditary or acquired **blood vessel disorders**. Hereditary hemorrhagic telangiectasia (Osler-Weber-Rendu disease) is an inherited autosomal-dominant disease with multiple mucosal telangiectasias, especially in the nose. Because telangiectasias are deficient in muscular and connective tissue, these telangiectasias may rupture spontaneously and bleed profusely. An association between migraine headaches and recurrent nosebleeds has also been reported.

Neoplasms, particularly malignancies, are uncommon causes of nosebleeds in children. Though generally benign, **nasal polyps** are usually present in association with cystic fibrosis or allergies. Capillary, cavernous, and mixed hemangiomas may occur in the nose and be a source of bleeding. Juvenile nasopharyngeal angiofibroma occurs almost exclusively in adolescent males who present with nasal obstruction and bleeding. Rhabdomyosarcomas, lymphomas, and squamous cell carcinomas of the nose, sinuses, or nasopharynx are rare causes of nosebleeds.

Drugs such as aspirin and nonsteroidal anti-inflammatory drugs, which interfere with platelet function, and warfarin and heparin, which inhibit clotting factors, increase the risk of nasal hemorrhage with minor trauma, infection, or inflammation. Accidental ingestion of these medications should be suspected if they are available. Cocaine or heroin snorting may cause nasal septal perforation and nosebleeds.

Hypertension is rarely associated with nosebleeds in children. Wegener granulomatosis and lethal midline granuloma are rare idiopathic inflammatory diseases in children that lead to nasal tissue destruction and bleeding. Nosebleeds during menstruation, known as vicarious menstruation, may be secondary to hormonal changes causing vascular congestion of the nasal mucosa.

Evaluation

History

A thorough history often reveals the etiology of the nosebleed (Questions Box). Information concerning the side of the nose from which the bleeding occurred, amount of bleeding, measures used to stop the bleeding, and time required to stop the bleeding may be helpful to quickly assess the severity of the nosebleed.

Physical Examination

A general physical examination should be performed. In children with significant blood loss, particular attention should be directed toward the mental status and vital signs to determine hemodynamic stability. If vital signs are normal, these children should also be evaluated for orthostatic changes. If blood pressure is elevated, it should

---

Questions

Nosebleeds

- Does the child pick his or her nose?
- Has the child suffered any trauma recently?
- Is there suspicion of non-accidental trauma?
- Has the child recently had an upper respiratory infection?
- Has the child recently had any systemic viral or bacterial illness?
- Does the child have any allergies?
- Is the child exposed to dry conditions (eg, dry climate, dry heat, dehumidified air)?
- Has the child put or tried to put foreign objects in his or her nose?
- Is there a history of easy bruising or prolonged, difficult-to-stop bleeding in the child or family?
- Does the child or anyone in the family use any aspirin, aspirin-containing medications, nonsteroidal anti-inflammatory drugs, or warfarin?
- Which side of the nose was bleeding?
- How extensive was the bleeding?
- Did the child spit out or swallow blood? Was there blood in the mouth?
- What measures were used to stop the bleeding? How long did it take to stop the bleeding?
- Was this the first nosebleed? If nosebleeds are recurrent, how often do they occur and how long do they last?

---

be reassessed at a time when the anxiety related to the nosebleed has dissipated.

In addition, the skin and mucous membranes should be checked carefully for petechiae, purpura, and ecchymoses, which are signs of easy bruising. The abdomen should be examined for hepatosplenomegaly, and the child should be evaluated for lymphadenopathy. Telangiectasias in the oropharynx or mucous membranes suggest hereditary hemorrhagic telangiectasia (Osler-Weber-Rendu disease). The oropharynx and nasopharynx should be examined for masses and blood dripping downward from a posterior bleed. The nose should then be inspected for the site of bleeding, with special attention directed toward the Kiesselbach area in the anterior septum. In children younger than 2 years with nosebleeds, suspicion of non-accidental trauma should be considered, especially if nosebleeds are recurrent, the event is not witnessed, or the story given by the caregiver changes.

Diagnostic Studies

Laboratory tests are rarely indicated in most children with nosebleeds. A hematocrit/hemoglobin should be obtained if the nosebleeds are severe or recur frequently. Blood for type and crossmatch should be sent in children who have signs or symptoms of hypovolemia (ie, increased pulse; cool, clammy skin; increased capillary refill; decreased blood pressure) or a marked drop in hematocrit. If the history or physical examination suggests that a coagulopathy may be present, a complete blood cell count with platelet count, prothrombin time, and partial thromboplastin time should be obtained and screening for von Willebrand disease considered if the other laboratory tests are negative.

Radiographs and other imaging studies are rarely necessary in children with nosebleeds. However, if a mass is visualized, further imaging may be necessary to evaluate the mass. The most commonly used modalities include magnetic resonance imaging and contrast-enhanced computed tomography. Rarely, pseudoaneurysm of the internal carotid artery has been associated with epistaxis and may require angiography for further evaluation.

Management

Children who present to primary care physicians with a history of a nosebleed or nosebleeds that have resolved spontaneously or with application of pressure to the nose need no further treatment in the office or emergency department setting, provided that the history and physical examination are consistent with a benign cause. These children or their parents should be instructed to apply a lubricant such as **petroleum jelly** or an antibiotic ointment inside the septal portion of the involved naris twice a day for 3 to 5 days with a cotton-tipped swab or little finger. Often the child's little finger is used because it is non-threatening and it "knows where to go." Further nose picking should be discouraged, and fingernails should be trimmed to minimize trauma. In addition, a bedside **humidifier** helps to moisturize the air, especially in dry climates or during the winter when forced hot-air heat is used. Children whose nares moisten from rhinorrhea and then dry and crack also benefit from humidified air. Buffered saline nasal spray may also be helpful in humidifying the nose. Those children who are prone to recurrent nosebleeds in whom serious causes have been ruled out may benefit from regular use of some of the mentioned measures when they have URIs or allergic manifestations or are in a dry season or environment. In addition, for children with *S aureus* nasal colonization, eradication should be considered.

Children or parents should be given advice about how to care for nosebleeds at home. These instructions can also be given to parents who seek advice over the telephone about how to stop children's nosebleeds. Practitioners should reassure parents and children that most nosebleeds are easily controlled. Children should sit upright and lean forward slightly while **direct pressure** is applied to the nose. External compression of the nares between 2 fingers for 5 to 10 minutes should be sufficient. Pressure applied to the anterior and mid-portion of the nose rather than at the base is more effective in stopping the bleeding because most nosebleeds originate here.

Children who are actively bleeding through the nose when seen by primary care physicians should be positioned sitting upright and leaning forward slightly, and they should be given a basin and facial tissue. Direct pressure should be applied by a nurse or physician to the anterior and mid-portion of the nose while following universal precautions. A cotton dental roll may be placed under the upper lip to compress the labial artery in older children in whom concern about displacement and possible aspiration of the cotton is minimal. If the bleeding continues after external compression, children should be instructed to blow their noses to remove as much clot as possible. Fresh blood should be removed with suction. Cotton pledgets moistened with a few drops of a topical **vasoconstrictor,** such as 0.05% oxymetazoline (Afrin), 0.25%

phenylephrine (Neo-Synephrine) or epinephrine (1:1,000) mixed with 4% lidocaine for local anesthesia, or topical thrombin, should be inserted into the side of the nose involved. Pressure should then be applied for an additional 10 minutes.

If the bleeding persists, **cauterization** of the bleeding site with a silver nitrate stick is indicated. If not already applied, topical anesthesia with 2% to 4% lidocaine should be applied before cauterization. Continued bleeding is slowed by first cauterizing a small ring around the bleeding point to interrupt flow from surrounding vessels and then rolling the tip of the applicator onto the bleeding site for 5 seconds or less. Cauterization is often difficult in children, and consultation with an otolaryngologist is advisable. Cauterization should not be performed in children with a bleeding diathesis. In addition, cauterization should only be done unilaterally. Cauterizing both sides of the nasal septum can result in septal ischemia and possible necrosis and ultimately septal perforation.

If the bleeding continues or as a modality to attempt prior to cauterization, an absorbable **nasal sponge** made from oxidized cellulose (OxiCell, Surgicel) or gelatin (Gelfoam) may be directly applied to the bleeding site to form an artificial clot. Hemostatic seals (Floseal, Avitene) may also be used and are composed of collagen or thrombin derivatives to support platelet aggregation and clot formation when applied to the bleeding site. Alternatively, though less well tolerated, a **nasal tampon** (Merocel, Rhino Rocket), made from a dehydrated material that expands when it becomes moist, may be inserted to tamponade the area of bleeding. Applying antibiotic ointment, preferably mupirocin or chlorhexidine-neomycin, to the tampon allows for easier insertion and removal as well as potentially preventing *S aureus* colonization and infection. Alternatively, an inflatable balloon (Rapid Rhino) coated with a platelet aggregator can be inserted to stop the bleeding. Continued uncontrolled bleeding requires anterior **nasal packing** with antibiotic-impregnated, preferably mupirocin, 1-inch petrolatum gauze strips, which should remain in place for approximately 2 to 3 days. Prophylactic **antibiotics** should be started because sinusitis is a complication of anterior nasal packing. Antibiotics providing coverage for staphylococcal organisms, in particular methicillin-resistant *S aureus*, and sinusitis should be strongly considered.

Posterior nosebleeds, which are more difficult to control, should be suspected if the measures described previously are ineffective, bleeding is vigorous and the cause cannot be identified, or most of the bleeding is into the nasopharynx and mouth. A posterior nasal pack can be created using rolled gauze or a nasal tampon. Alternatively, a Foley catheter or an Epi-Stat inflatable nasal balloon catheter may be used to control posterior nosebleeds. Posterior packs should never be used without the presence of a concurrent anterior nasal pack. Thus, double-balloon catheters are now available (eg, Gottschalk Nasostat, Xomed Epi-Stat) such that 2 separate packing mechanisms can be avoided. Posterior packing can result in significant discomfort for the patient, and appropriate analgesia should be provided. However, significant pain with balloon inflation should not occur and overinflation may result in ischemia if the balloon is not slightly deflated. Posterior packing should be left in place for 2 to 3 days and antibiotics initiated to prevent sinusitis. In addition, posterior packing can result in hypoventilation and hypoxia. Therefore, all patients with posterior packing should be admitted and placed on a cardiorespiratory monitor. This also allows for monitoring of potential complications, namely aspiration due to accidental dislodgment; septal ischemia secondary to packing; and development of hypotension, bradycardia, or apnea secondary to a pronounced nasal-vagal response.

The need for **otolaryngologic consultation** depends on the experience of the individual physician and availability of consultation. Prompt consultation, if available, should be obtained for children with severe nosebleeds who need volume replacement, with nosebleeds that do not stop or that recur after the mentioned measures have been taken, who may need anterior or posterior nasal packing, and with recurrent, difficult-to-stop nosebleeds. Surgical consultation should be sought in patients with suspected nasal fractures prior to the placement of nasal packing. In some cases, obtaining consultation before cauterization with silver nitrate is advisable, particularly in those patients with known bleeding disorders. Children with septal hematomas, tumors, polyps, telangiectasias, and intractable bleeding should be referred to an otolaryngologist for further care and possible surgical intervention. Children with a documented or suspected bleeding disorder should be referred to a hematologist. Selective angiographic embolization by an interventional radiologist or sphenopalatine artery ligation may be indicated for patients with persistent, intractable nosebleeds. Intranasal laser surgery may be indicated in patients with recurrent nosebleeds from abnormal vascular malformations such as hereditary hemorrhagic telangiectasia (Osler-Weber-Rendu disease).

Children with severe nosebleeds should have an intravenous line started early, blood sent for type and crossmatch, and fluids replaced, depending on the amount of blood loss and physical evidence of hypovolemia. In children who are frightened or in whom certain procedures (eg, cauterization of bleeding site, drainage of septal hematoma) are performed, procedural sedation should be strongly considered. Intravenous pain medication should be used in children who need anterior or posterior packing. If procedures that cause undue pain or discomfort are necessary, general anesthesia in an operating room setting may be indicated.

Hospitalization is rarely necessary for children with nosebleeds. However, children who are hemodynamically unstable on presentation usually require inpatient treatment. As mentioned previously, children who need placement of a posterior nasal pack should be admitted to the hospital for close airway observation. Hospitalization may be necessary for children with difficult-to-stop bleeds who need an anterior nasal pack or who have a bleeding disorder or underlying chronic illness such as leukemia, aplastic anemia, or HIV infection.

Prognosis

The prognosis for nosebleeds in children is excellent. Almost all nosebleeds are easily controlled with a minimal amount of home care or medical management. Surgery is rarely indicated. Complications associated with significant nosebleeds include hypovolemia from blood loss and sinusitis and toxic shock syndrome from *S aureus* associated with anterior or posterior nasal packing. Even for rare causes of nosebleeds, the prognosis is very good with prompt diagnosis and treatment.

CASE RESOLUTION

In the case presented, the boy has experienced several nosebleeds of short duration associated with an upper respiratory infection and winter dryness. His history and physical examination are unremarkable for a bleeding disorder or chronic illness. The small amount of blood in his nose is consistent with an anterior nosebleed originating from the Kiesselbach area with inflammation and drying of the nasal mucosa. Laboratory tests are not indicated. The parents should be instructed to apply petroleum jelly to the septal portion of the left side of the child's nose twice a day for 3 to 5 days and to humidify the child's bedroom. They should also be reassured that their child has a common condition that he will outgrow.

Selected References

Bernius M, Perlin D. Pediatric ear, nose, and throat emergencies. *Pediatr Clin North Am.* 2006;53(2):195–214

Briskin, KB. Epistaxis. In: Baren JM, Rothrock SG, Brennan JA, Brown L, eds. *Pediatric Emergency Medicine.* Philadelphia, PA: Saunders; 2008:402–404

Douglas R, Wormald PJ. Update on epistaxis. *Curr Opin Otolaryngol Head Neck Surg.* 2007;15(3):180–183

Gifford TO, Orlandi RR. Epistaxis. *Otolaryngol Clin North Am.* 2008;41(3):525–536

Kasperek ZA, Pollock GF. Epistaxis: an overview. *Emerg Med Clin North Am.* 2013;31(2):443–454

Manning SC, Culbertson MC Jr. Epistaxis. In: Bluestone CD, Stool SE, Alper CM, et al, eds. *Pediatric Otolaryngology.* 4th ed. Philadelphia, PA: Saunders; 2003:925–931

McIntosh N, Mok JY, Margerison A. Epidemiology of oronasal hemorrhage in the first 2 years of life: implications for child protection. *Pediatrics.* 2007;120(5):1074–1078

Nadel F, Henretig FM. Epistaxis. In: Fleischer GR, Ludwig S, eds. *Textbook of Pediatric Emergency Medicine.* 6th ed. Philadelphia, PA: Lippincott Williams and Wilkins; 2010:236–239

Patel PB, Kost SI. Management of epistaxis. In: King C, Henretig FM, eds. *Textbook of Pediatric Emergency Procedures.* 2nd ed. Philadelphia, PA: Lippincott Williams and Wilkins; 2008:603–614

Riviello RJ, Brown NA. Otolaryngologic procedures. In: Roberts JR, Hedges JR, eds. *Clinical Procedures in Emergency Medicine.* 5th ed. Philadelphia, PA: Saunders Elsevier, 2010:1178–1216

Sandoval C, Dong S, Visintainer P, Ozkaynak MF, Jayabose S. Clinical and laboratory features of 178 children with recurrent epistaxis. *J Pediatr Hematol Oncol.* 2002;24(1):47–49

Whymark AD, Crampsey DP, Fraser L, Moore P, Williams C, Kubba H. Childhood epistaxis and nasal colonization with *Staphylococcus aureus. Otolaryngol Head Neck Surg.* 2008;138(3):307–310

CHAPTER 79

Strabismus

Teresa Rosales, MD

CASE STUDY

The mother of an 8-month-old complains that every time her son looks to either side, his eyes seem crossed. Otherwise, he is growing and developing normally. A symmetric pupillary light reflex, bilateral red reflex, and normal extraocular eye movements in all directions are noted on physical examination of the eyes.

Questions

1. What is strabismus?
2. What conditions make infants' eyes appear crossed? What is the differential diagnosis?
3. What tests are used in the office evaluation of children suspected of having strabismus?
4. Which infants with crossed eyes require referral for further evaluation and treatment?

Strabismus refers to any abnormality in ocular alignment, whether the eyes go in or out or one eye is higher than the other. It is one of the most common eye problems observed in infants and children. The pediatrician plays an important role in the early detection and prompt referral of children with suspected ocular alignment abnormalities.

Epidemiology

Strabismus affects approximately 3% of the population, and the condition is seen most commonly in children younger than 6 years. About 50% of all affected children have a positive family history of strabismus, although the exact genetic mode of inheritance is unclear. Up to 75% of normal newborns and infants have transient intermittent strabismus during the first 3 months of life.

Clinical Presentation

Children with ocular misalignment have an asymmetric corneal light reflex test. Eye movement is noted with cover testing. Children with paralytic strabismus may present with torticollis or head tilting in an effort to avoid diplopia (D$_x$ Box).

Strabismus

- Head tilt
- Double vision (diplopia)
- Squint
- Asymmetric corneal light reflex
- Eye movement with cover testing

Pathophysiology

Normal binocular vision is the result of the fusion of images from both eyes working synchronously across the visual field. Six extraocular muscles control all eye movements. Orthophoria is proper alignment of the eyes, and strabismus results from an imbalance in muscle movements.

Strabismus

The classification of strabismus is complex. Based on etiology, it may be considered nonparalytic (comitant) or paralytic (noncomitant). Strabismus may also be classified as congenital or acquired, intermittent or constant, and alternating or unilateral. In **nonparalytic strabismus,** the extraocular muscles and nerves that control them are normal. The degree of deviation is constant or nearly constant in all directions of gaze. Nonparalytic strabismus is the most common type of strabismus seen in children, and congenital or infantile esotropia is usually of this kind. Ocular or visual defects such as cataracts or high refractive errors occasionally cause nonparalytic strabismus.

In **paralytic strabismus,** paralysis or paresis of one or more of the extraocular muscles produces a muscle imbalance. The deviation is asymmetric, and characteristically the degree of deviation is worse when gazing in the direction of the affected muscle. Paralytic strabismus may be congenital or acquired. **Congenital paralytic strabismus** may result from birth trauma, muscle anomalies, abnormal development of the cranial nerve nuclei, or congenital infections affecting the eyes. Congenital strabismus may be seen in association with neurodevelopmental disorders such as cerebral palsy. **Acquired paralytic strabismus** due to extraocular muscle palsies usually indicates the presence of a serious underlying condition, such as an intracranial tumor, a demyelinating or neurodegenerative disease, myasthenia gravis, a progressive myopathy, or a central nervous system (CNS) infection. Children may present with a complaint of double vision or a compensatory torticollis (head tilt) to avoid double vision (diplopia).

Intermittent (latent) misalignment of the eyes is referred to as a **phoria.** Under normal conditions, the fusional mechanisms of the CNS maintain eye alignment. Eye deviation is appreciated only under certain conditions, such as illness, fatigue, or stress, or when fusion is interrupted by occluding one eye (eg, during cover testing). Some degree of phoria may be found in almost all individuals and is usually asymptomatic. Larger degrees of phoria may give rise to troublesome symptoms such as headaches, transient diplopia, or asthenopia (eyestrain).

Constant misalignment of the eyes is referred to as **heterotropia.** This condition occurs because normal fusional mechanisms are unable to control eye deviation; children are unable to use both eyes together to fixate on an object. In alternating heterotropias, both eyes appear to deviate equally, and vision generally develops normally in each eye because children have no preference for fixation. If strabismus affects only one eye, the other eye is always used for fixation, and there is a danger of developing amblyopia or loss of vision in the deviating eye.

Convergent deviation, a turning in or crossing of the eyes, is called an esodeviation (eg, esotropia or esophoria). Divergent deviation, a turning out of the eyes, is an exodeviation. Hypertropia is used for upward vertical deviations. Esodeviations are the most common types of ocular misalignment, accounting for 50% to 75% of all cases of strabismus. Vertical deviations represent less than 5% of all cases of strabismus.

Amblyopia

Amblyopia is a potential complication if strabismus is not corrected in a timely manner. It refers to poor vision in one eye or, rarely, both despite correction of any refractive errors. If children have no significant refractive error and the visual acuity of one eye is worse than the other, they have amblyopia. To be considered amblyopia, visual acuity, as measured by reading an eye chart, should differ by at least 2 lines (eg, 20/20 in one eye and 20/40 in the other). It is the leading cause of preventable visual loss in children.

Amblyopia may be classified into 3 major categories. **Deprivational amblyopia** generally results when a unilateral lesion or developmental defect in one of the structures of the eye or its visual pathways obstructs vision. Causes of deprivational amblyopia include congenital cataract, ptosis, corneal opacity, retinal detachment, retinoblastoma, colobomas, optic nerve defects (eg, optic nerve hypoplasia), or orbital tumors. These conditions cause a lack of formation of a retinal image or a blurred retinal image, usually in one eye. **Refractive amblyopia** refers to a blurring of the retinal image due to large or asymmetric refractive errors. Amblyopia is usually considered a unilateral abnormality but may be bilateral in cases of large refractive errors (usually astigmatism or hyperopia). In **strabismic amblyopia,** the immature or developing brain suppresses images from the deviating eye to prevent diplopia. Strabismic amblyopia is most commonly associated with strabismus that develops in children younger

than 4 years. If the condition leading to amblyopia is not corrected while the brain's visual pathways are still malleable (eg, before approximately 6–7 years of age), children may have some degree of permanent visual loss.

Differential Diagnosis

The differential diagnosis of strabismus may be divided into 3 categories: transient neonatal strabismus, congenital or infantile strabismus, and acquired strabismus. True strabismus must be differentiated from the illusion of deviation created by facial asymmetry or anatomic variations (ie, pseudostrabismus).

Transient Neonatal Strabismus

Eye alignment in normal newborns and infants during the first 2 to 3 months of life may vary from normal to intermittent esotropia or exotropia. These deviations are believed to result from CNS immaturity and resolve spontaneously in most infants by 4 months of age. If such deviations are constant or persist beyond this age, children should be referred to an ophthalmologist for further evaluation.

Congenital or Infantile Strabismus

This type of strabismus is defined as a deviation that occurs during the first 6 months of life. Because the deviation may not always be present at birth, the term *infantile* may be more accurate. The differential diagnosis of infantile strabismus is presented in Box 79-1. **Pseudo-esotropia** is an illusion or apparent deviation and not a true deviation. In many infants, the broad, flat nasal bridge and prominent epicanthal folds may obscure a portion of the sclera near the nose and create the appearance of esotropia (Figure 79-1). This illusion resolves as children mature. Symmetric corneal light reflexes or normal cover tests differentiate pseudo-esotropia from true esotropia.

Esotropia is one of the more common types of childhood strabismus. The constant deviation of infantile esotropia is usually readily apparent because of the large angle of deviation. Affected children usually have good bilateral vision because of the alternation of fixation from one eye to the other. Cross-fixation, in which children look to the left with the adducted right eye and to the right with the adducted left eye, may be evident because of the large angle of deviation. Rarely, esotropia may be caused by abducens palsy (ie, palsy of the sixth cranial nerve) in isolation or association with other cranial nerve palsies (eg, Möbius syndrome).

Infantile exotropia is less common than esotropia. Like esotropia, exotropia develops within the first 6 months of life and is characterized by a large angle of deviation. Other causes of infantile exotropia include trochlear palsy (ie, congenital third nerve palsy) (paralytic strabismus) and abnormalities of the bones of the orbit (eg, Crouzon syndrome).

Acquired Strabismus

Acquired strabismus may result from a variety of causes (Box 79-1). Accommodative esotropia and intermittent exotropia are the 2 most common types of acquired strabismus. **Accommodative esotropia**

Box 79-1. Differential Diagnosis of Strabismus

Congenital or Infantile Strabismus

Esophoria/Esotropia

Infantile esotropia

Pseudo-esotropia

Möbius syndrome

Abducens palsy (congenital sixth nerve palsy)

Duane syndrome

Exophoria/Exotropia

Congenital exotropia

Trochlear palsy (congenital third nerve palsy)

Abnormalities of the bony orbit (Crouzon syndrome)

Esophoria/Esotropia and Exophoria/Exotropia

Duane syndrome (esotropia more common than exotropia)

Acquired Strabismus

Esophoria/Esotropia

Accommodative esotropia

Abducens palsy (benign sixth nerve palsy)

Exophoria/Exotropia

Intermittent exotropia

Overcorrection after surgery for esotropia

Esophoria/Esotropia and Exophoria/Exotropia

Poor vision

Orbital trauma causing entrapment of extraocular muscles

Intracranial tumors or tumors involving the orbit (eg, retinoblastoma)

Myasthenia gravis

Central nervous system infection (eg, meningitis)

Central nervous system tumor

Orbital cellulitis

Figure 79-1. Child with pseudo-esotropia. Note the wide nasal bridge and prominent epicanthal folds.

typically develops in children between 2 to 4 years of age but may appear as early as 6 months or as late as 8 years. Children with hyperopia use accommodation (attempts to focus) to see clearly. The accommodative reflex is closely linked to convergence; when accommodation occurs, so does convergence. If children have severe hyperopia (farsightedness), the amount of convergence that occurs with accommodation may be severe and lead to the development of esotropia. Such esotropia is usually intermittent initially and only gradually becomes constant. The deviating eye frequently becomes amblyopic.

Intermittent exotropia, the most common form of exodeviation seen in children, develops between birth and 4 years of age. Although it begins as an intermittent condition in which children's eyes appear to deviate outward, especially when they are tired, ill, or fixating at a distance, the exotropia can become constant with time. Children may also close one eye in bright sunlight, presumably in an effort to prevent diplopia.

Evaluation

History

Evaluation of infants or children suspected of having strabismus should begin with a thorough family history because strabismus often runs in families (Questions Box). Parental description of the ocular deviation is useful because misalignments, especially intermittent deviations that may only become manifest when children are tired, may not always be evident during the office visit. A history of head or orbital trauma may help in the evaluation of acquired strabismus.

Physical Examination

On physical examination, the presence of any dysmorphic features and structural abnormalities of the face or neck (eg, torticollis) should be noted. Children with paralytic strabismus (eg, trochlear palsy [fourth nerve palsy], superior oblique palsy) may compensate for their paretic lesion by tilting their head to avoid diplopia. It is important that visual screening of children begin during the neonatal period. Newborn screening should emphasize the presence of a bilateral red reflex. An abnormal red reflex or a white reflex may indicate the presence of a cataract or retinoblastoma. These require immediate referral to an ophthalmologist. Evaluation for ocular alignment should begin at the 4-month health maintenance visit.

Questions

Strabismus

- Does the infant or child have a family history of strabismus?
- Does the infant or child constantly tilt the head toward one side?
- Does the infant or child squint?
- Has the infant or child complained of blurred or double vision?
- Does the infant or child close one eye in bright sunlight?
- Has the infant or child had any recent trauma to the eyes or head?

Intermittent misalignment of the eyes is often seen in normal infants younger than 4 months. However, constant misalignment requires immediate attention at any age.

Vision Testing

Testing visual acuity is essential in the evaluation of children with suspected strabismus. Such testing may be performed as early as 3 years of age if children are cooperative. Charts with symbols, figures, or letters can be used. The traditional Snellen eye chart with letters can generally be used in children 4 years of age. Decreased vision in one eye may be indicative of ocular abnormalities, including ocular deviations.

The 2 basic tests for strabismus that can be easily performed in the office are the corneal light reflex test, or Hirschberg method, and the cover test. The pediatrician should be comfortable performing both tests.

The **corneal light reflex test** is the simplest and quickest test for the evaluation of strabismus. In this test, a penlight is projected simultaneously onto the corneas of both eyes as the child looks straight ahead. The examiner compares the placement of the corneal light reflex in each eye with respect to the center of the pupil. If the eyes are straight, the reflection appears symmetrically in the center of both pupils or on the same point on each cornea. If the light reflex appears off center in one eye compared with the other, an ocular deviation or heterotropia is present. Nasal deviation of the light reflex on the cornea indicates exotropia on that side, temporal deviation signifies esotropia, and inferior deviation indicates hypertropia.

Unlike the corneal light reflex test, which may be performed even in uncooperative children, **cover tests** require a child's cooperation and ability to fixate on a specified object. These tests are used to detect heterophoria. Two types of cover tests, alternate cover and cover-uncover, are used. Only the alternate cover test detects both heterophorias and heterotropias. This test may be preferred by the primary care physician as a screening tool. The cover-uncover test detects only manifest deviations or heterotropias. In the alternate cover test, one eye and then the other is covered as the child fixates on an object at a distance. If neither eye moves as the cover is moved rapidly between the eyes, the eyes are in alignment or orthophoric. With heterotropia, the deviating eye moves when the fixating eye is occluded; in heterophoria, the deviating eye moves when it is uncovered (Figure 79-2).

The alternate cover test may be illustrated with the following example: A child presents with constant esotropia of the left eye. When the right or fixating eye is occluded, the left eye is forced to fixate so that the child can see, and the left eye moves outward as the right eye is occluded. In the case of a child with an esophoria or latent deviation of the left eye, the eye deviates inward when it is occluded because it is not being forced to fixate. As the cover is moved from the left eye to the right, the left eye moves outward and returns to a position of fixation.

The alternate cover test may be more difficult to interpret in children with bilateral or alternating strabismus who use both eyes in turn for fixation. It is not necessary for the pediatrician to identify exactly what type of strabismus is present; abnormal movement should be noted and children should be referred for further evaluation. An ophthalmologist is able to perform a more detailed examination.

Management

The goals of management are the attainment of the best possible vision in each eye, straight eyes cosmetically, and fusion. The sooner deviations are corrected, the better the child's chances for equal bilateral vision. Treatment includes correction of any underlying refractive error with **corrective lenses.** Such lenses, which remedy the refractive error and minimize the need for accommodation, are used to treat accommodative esotropia. Glasses are also used in anisome-

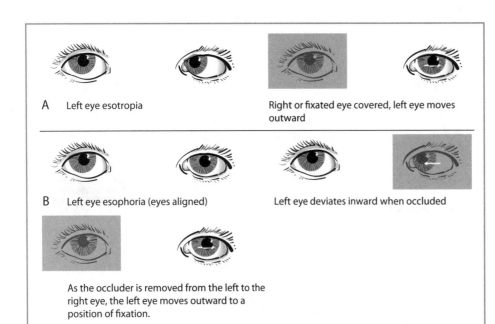

A Left eye esotropia

Right or fixated eye covered, left eye moves outward

B Left eye esophoria (eyes aligned)

Left eye deviates inward when occluded

As the occluder is removed from the left to the right eye, the left eye moves outward to a position of fixation.

Figure 79-2. Alternate cover test in the detection of strabismus. Normally, both eyes appear to be aligned and centrally fixed. A, Detection of esotropia. The right eye is fixating and a left esotropia is present. When the right or fixating eye is covered, the left eye moves outward (away from the nose). B, Detection of esophoria. The eyes are aligned with a left esophoria. When the left eye is covered, it deviates inward. As the cover is moved from the left eye to the right eye, the left eye moves outward to a position of fixation.

tropic amblyopia in which one eye has a significantly different refractive error than the other.

Children who do not see equally well from both eyes may be at risk for amblyopia if they preferentially fixate with only one eye. If detected, amblyopia should be corrected with occlusion therapy of the fixating "good" eye. **Occlusion therapy** forces children to use the amblyopic eye. This treatment is best accomplished by constantly patching the eye with better vision during waking hours or penalization with dilating drops in the better-seeing eye. Children require repeat evaluations and close monitoring during this therapy.

If nonsurgical methods fail to align the eyes, surgical correction may be necessary. **Surgery** may be used to achieve the best possible ocular alignment and is usually required for treatment of infantile esotropia. It is generally performed in infants between 6 months and 1 year of age, while the visual system is still pliable enough to allow for development of postsurgical binocular vision. Surgery also may be needed in children with intermittent exotropia if the frequency of deviation is increasing.

Prognosis

Certain conditions, such as pseudo-esotropia or infrequent intermittent exotropia, may resolve as children mature. Others, such as infantile esotropia, require early detection and treatment to achieve the best binocular vision. Amblyopia and permanent vision loss may result if correction of strabismus is delayed.

CASE RESOLUTION

The infant in the case history has pseudo-esotropia. Although the boy's eyes appear to deviate, the corneal light reflex and cover tests are normal. Physical examination reveals prominent epicanthal folds and a broad, flat nasal bridge.

Selected References

Campos EC. Why do the eyes cross? A review and discussion of the nature and origin of essential infantile esotropia, microstrabismus, accommodative esotropia and acute comitant esotropia. *J AAPOS*. 2008;12(4):326–331

Ekdawi NS, Nusz KJ, Diehl NN, Mohney BG. Postoperative outcomes in children with intermittent exotropia from a population-based cohort. *J AAPOS*. 2009;13(1):4–7

Greenberg AE, Mohney BG, Diehl NN, Burke JP. Incidence and types of childhood esotropia: a population-based study. *Ophthalmology*. 2007;114(1):170–174

Keech R. Practical management of amblyopia. In: Wright K, ed. *Focal Points: Clinical Modules for Ophthalmologists*. Vol. XVIII, No. 2. San Francisco, CA: American Academy of Ophthalmology; 2000:1–3

Louwagie CR, Diehl NN, Greenberg AE, Mohney BG. Long term follow-up of congenital esotropia in a population-based cohort. *J AAPOS*. 2009;13(1):8–12

Ludwig IH, Clark RA, Stager DR Sr. New strabismus surgical techniques. *J AAPOS*. 2013;17(1):79–88

Olitsky SE, Hug D, Plummer LS, Stass-Isern M. Disorders of eye movement and alignment. In: Kliegman RM, Behrman RE, Jenson HB, Stanton BF, eds. *Nelson Textbook of Pediatrics*. 19th ed. Philadelphia, PA: Saunders Elsevier; 2011:2157–2162

Parks MM. Binocular vision. In: Tasman W, Jaeger EA, eds. *Duane's Ophthalmology*. 15th ed. Philadelphia, PA: Lippincott Williams & Wilkins; 2009

Simon J, ed. *Pediatric Ophthalmology and Strabismus*. San Francisco, CA: American Academy of Ophthalmology; 2006–2007:9–12, 67–118

Wallace DK, Chandler DL, Beck RW, et al. Treatment of bilateral refractive amblyopia in children three to less than 10 years of age. *Am J Ophthalmol*. 2007;144(4):487–496

CHAPTER 80

Infections of the Eye

Teresa Rosales, MD

CASE STUDY

A 10-day-old has a 1-day history of red, watery eyes and nonproductive cough with no fever. The girl is breastfed and continues to eat well. She was the 7-lb, 2-oz (3,238-g) product of a term gestation, born via normal spontaneous vaginal delivery without complications to a 26-year-old woman. The pregnancy was also uncomplicated. No one at home is ill.

On examination, the infant is afebrile with normal vital signs. Examination of the eyes reveals bilateral conjunctival injection with only a mild amount of purulent discharge. Bilateral red reflexes are present. The rest of the physical examination is within normal limits.

Questions

1. What is the differential diagnosis of conjunctivitis during and following the neonatal period?
2. What laboratory tests, if any, should be performed?
3. When is a chest radiograph indicated in the evaluation of neonates with conjunctivitis?
4. What are management strategies for eye infections?

Infections of the eye and surrounding structures are commonly seen by pediatricians. Such infections range in severity from common problems such as blepharitis and conjunctivitis, which lack serious sequelae, to severe and less common infections such as periorbital and orbital cellulitis. The presenting complaint in many children with eye infections is a red-appearing eye. Familiarity with the common causes of a red eye makes prompt diagnosis and treatment possible.

Epidemiology

Conjunctivitis, which affects children of all ages, is perhaps the most common eye infection of childhood. The incidence of conjunctivitis in the newborn period is estimated to range from 1.6% to 12%. The incidence of chlamydial conjunctivitis is about 8 in 1,000 live births. About two-thirds of acute childhood conjunctivitis has a bacterial etiology, and one-third is viral. *Haemophilus influenzae* and *Streptococcus pneumoniae* are the most common bacterial agents and account for about 40% and 10% of culture-proven cases, respectively. The incidence of *H influenzae* is decreasing with the advent of the *H influenzae* type b vaccine. The incidence of community-associated methicillin-resistant *Staphylococcus aureus* (CA MRSA) is increasing. *S aureus* is isolated from the conjunctivas of children with acute conjunctivitis, but it is found with about the same frequency in the eyes of children without conjunctivitis. Adenovirus is the most common viral isolate. Most cases of acute conjunctivitis in young adults have a viral etiology. Serious eye infections such as periorbital and orbital cellulitis occur far less often.

Clinical Presentation

Red eyes and discharge are the common presenting signs of infections of the eyelids and conjunctivas. Eyelid edema and erythema surrounding the eye characterize periorbital and orbital cellulitis. Proptosis, abnormal extraocular movement, or loss of visual acuity may signal spread of the infection beyond the orbital septum (orbital cellulitis) (D_x Box).

Pathophysiology

Eye infections may be divided into 2 types: those affecting the structures surrounding the orbit and those involving the orbital contents themselves (Figure 80-1). Although all structures surrounding the eye may potentially become inflamed or infected, the eyelids, nasolacrimal drainage system (dacryocystitis; see Chapter 81), conjunctiva, and cornea are most commonly involved. Orbital cellulitis is defined as an infection of the orbital structures posterior to the orbital septum. The orbital septum, an extension of the periosteum of the bones of the orbit, extends to the margins of the upper and lower eyelids and provides an anatomic barrier to the spread of most infectious and inflammatory processes. Preseptal or periorbital cellulitis is localized to structures superficial to the orbital septum, whereas post-septal or orbital cellulitis implies that the disease process involves orbital structures extending beyond the septum.

Differential Diagnosis

Infections of the eye are included in the differential diagnosis of conditions presenting with red eye (Box 80-1). Also included in the differential diagnosis are congenital, inflammatory, traumatic, and

Eye Infections

Eyelid Infections
- Redness
- Itching (blepharitis)
- Burning (blepharitis)
- Scales at the base of the lashes (seborrheic blepharitis)
- Swelling (hordeolum or chalazion)
- Pain (hordeolum)

Conjunctivitis
- Conjunctival injection and edema
- Excessive tearing
- Discharge or crusting
- Itching (allergic conjunctivitis)

Uveitis
- Conjunctival injection
- Pain
- Blurred vision
- Photophobia
- Headache

Periorbital Cellulitis
- Unilateral eyelid edema
- Erythema surrounding the eye
- Pain
- Fever

Orbital Cellulitis
- Eyelid edema
- Proptosis
- Decreased extraocular movements
- Loss of visual acuity
- Fever
- Ill appearance
- Associated sinusitis

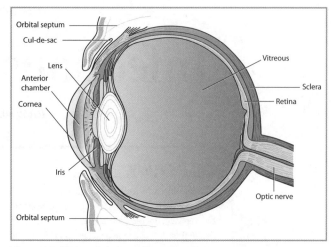

Figure 80-1. The eye and surrounding structures.

Box 80-1. Differential Diagnosis of Red Eye

Congenital Anomalies
- Nasolacrimal duct obstruction
- Congenital glaucoma

Infection
- Keratitis
- Conjunctivitis
- Dacryocystitis
- Corneal ulcer
- Periorbital and orbital cellulitis

Inflammation
- Blepharitis
- Hordeolum
- Chalazion

Trauma
- Corneal abrasion
- Foreign body
- Blunt trauma: hyphema
- Perforating injuries
- Exposure to chemicals or other noxious substances

Systemic Illnesses
- Kawasaki disease
- Varicella
- Measles
- Lyme disease
- Stevens-Johnson syndrome
- Ataxia-telangiectasia
- Juvenile rheumatoid arthritis

systemic processes. Although infection and irritation are by far the most common causes of an acute onset of red eye, other possibilities, including trauma, glaucoma, or underlying systemic disease, must be considered.

Eyelid Infections

Common conditions affecting the eyelid and its related structures are blepharitis, hordeolum, and chalazion.

Blepharitis is an inflammation of the lid margins. This condition, which is often bilateral, may be chronic or recurrent. The 2 most common causes of blepharitis are staphylococcal infection and seborrheic dermatitis. Children with staphylococcal blepharitis often present with scales at the base of the lashes, ulceration of the lid margin, and loss of lashes. The infection may spread to the conjunctiva or cornea, producing conjunctivitis or keratitis. In contrast, seborrheic blepharitis is characterized by greasy, yellow scales attached to the base of the lashes. In addition, associated seborrhea of the scalp or eyebrows may be present. Mixed staphylococcal-seborrheic infections, which occur as staphylococcal superinfection, may complicate seborrheic blepharitis. Less commonly seen forms of blepharitis are parasitic blepharitis, which results from infestation of the lids by the head louse, *Pediculus humanus capitis,* or crab louse, *Phthirus pubis,* and primary or recurrent human herpesvirus 1 infections that may manifest as clusters of vesicles on the eyelids. Rosacea may rarely occur in childhood and can present very similarly to chronic blepharitis.

The glands of the eyelid can also be infected. *Staphylococcus aureus* is the most common organism. A **hordeolum,** or common sty, results from an infection of the meibomian glands located along the lid margins. The glands become obstructed and an abscess can form. Affected children present with a well-circumscribed, painful swelling that may be at the lid margin or deeper in the lid tissue. These generally rupture or resolve without complications when treated aggressively with hot compresses.

A chalazion is a hordeolum that has not resolved over weeks to months. It is no longer an infectious process but has become a chronic granulomatous inflammation of the meibomian glands. The resulting firm, non-tender, slow-growing mass within the upper or lower eyelid may be painful if secondary infection is present.

Infections of the Conjunctiva

Conjunctivitis refers to any inflammation of the conjunctiva. The condition may be allergic, chemical, viral, or bacterial in etiology. In addition, it may be a sign of systemic disease such as Kawasaki disease or Stevens-Johnson syndrome.

Acute conjunctivitis, or pinkeye, is common during childhood and can be extremely contagious. The usual signs are conjunctival injection, tearing, discharge, crusting of the lashes, and conjunctival edema (chemosis). Pain and decreased vision are uncommon symptoms and may signal corneal involvement.

In general, it is difficult to distinguish bacterial conjunctivitis from viral conjunctivitis on clinical features alone. Certain clinical characteristics may guide the diagnosis. The average age of children affected with **bacterial conjunctivitis** tends to be younger than the age of those with viral conjunctivitis, which occurs more frequently in adolescents; however, considerable overlap occurs. Children with bacterial conjunctivitis typically present with an acute onset of unilateral or bilateral injection and edema of the palpebral and bulbar conjunctiva, minimal to copious purulent discharge, and crusting of the eyelashes. Children may have difficulty opening their eyes on awaking in the morning because of the exudate. An association between conjunctivitis and concomitant otitis media has been well described. *Haemophilus influenzae,* which is often resistant to ampicillin, is the pathogen most commonly isolated from affected children.

The diagnosis of **viral conjunctivitis** is considered if signs of viral upper respiratory infection (eg, low-grade fever, cough, rhinorrhea) are evident. Viral infection is associated with conjunctival injection, watery or thin mucoid discharge, and only mild lid edema and erythema. Adenoviral infection is usually bilateral, with significant conjunctival injection and chemosis of the conjunctiva, and is often accompanied by a tender preauricular lymph node. Epidemic keratoconjunctivitis is a highly contagious form of adenoviral conjunctivitis. Affected children often complain of foreign body sensation beneath the lids or photophobia due to corneal involvement. Pharyngeal conjunctival fever, another presentation of adenoviral conjunctivitis, usually manifests as conjunctivitis in association with pharyngitis and fever.

Infants who suffer from **chronic or recurrent conjunctival discharge** may have an obstruction of the nasolacrimal duct, whereas older children with chronic conjunctivitis may have allergic diseases, recurrent blepharitis, or chlamydial infections. Blepharitis is the most common cause of chronic conjunctivitis in older children. *Staphylococcus aureus* is frequently implicated in these infections.

Itching, tearing, and conjunctival edema are the hallmarks of **allergic conjunctivitis,** a noninfectious form of conjunctival inflammation often seen in children with other allergic disorders such as asthma or hay fever. Conjunctival injection tends to be mild, bilateral, and seasonal. The etiology is most often a hypersensitivity to pollens, dust, or animal dander. Vernal conjunctivitis is a bilateral, severe form of allergic conjunctivitis seen primarily during childhood. Most cases occur during the spring and summer. Severe itching and tearing are the most frequent complaints. The palpebral conjunctiva may have a cobblestone appearance due to the accumulation of inflammatory cells, or there may be small, elevated lesions of the bulbar conjunctiva at the corneal limbus. The pathogenesis is unclear, but atopy seems to play a role.

Chlamydial conjunctivitis frequently affects neonates and adolescents. Inclusion conjunctivitis is an acute infection of the eyes caused by sexually transmitted *Chlamydia trachomatis* (usually serotypes D–K). This condition may be seen in neonates or sexually active adolescents. Trachoma, the most common cause of impaired vision and preventable blindness worldwide, is a chronic conjunctivitis usually caused by *C trachomatis* serotypes A, B, and C. Although this disease is rarely seen in North America, it is endemic among certain populations, especially Native Americans. Inclusion conjunctivitis and endemic trachoma are characterized initially by conjunctivitis with small lymphoid follicles in the conjunctiva.

Neonatal conjunctivitis, or ophthalmia neonatorum, occurs during the first month of life. The major causes of neonatal conjunctivitis are chemical, chlamydial, and bacterial (in decreasing order of frequency). Ophthalmia neonatorum may be produced by the same bacteria that cause childhood conjunctivitis but also results from organisms such as *C trachomatis* or *Neisseria gonorrhoeae.* Newborns may acquire these latter pathogens following premature rupture of membranes or passage through an infected or colonized birth canal. *Chlamydia trachomatis* is the organism most commonly identified. It has been isolated from 17% to 40% of neonates with conjunctivitis. Neonates born to mothers with active cervical chlamydial infection have a 20% to 50% chance of developing chlamydial conjunctivitis. Viruses are uncommon causes of neonatal ocular infections. Human herpesvirus is the primary viral agent involved in neonatal conjunctivitis. The presence of characteristic vesicular skin lesions or corneal dendritic lesions helps in the diagnosis.

Time of onset of symptoms is related to the etiologic agent. Inflammation secondary to the **silver nitrate** drops instilled at birth to prevent gonococcal infection presents as mild conjunctivitis 12 to 24 hours after birth in 10% to 100% of treated newborns. This condition usually resolves spontaneously in 24 to 48 hours. This is more of historic interest because erythromycin ointment 0.5% has replaced silver nitrate in most hospitals. (Silver nitrate was ineffective against *C trachomatis*.) Conjunctivitis due to *N gonorrhoeae* appears 2 to 5 days after birth and is associated with copious purulent discharge. Conjunctivitis due to *C trachomatis* occurs at 5 to 14 days, a result of a longer incubation period. Time of onset and severity of symptoms of these 2 conditions may overlap, however. The presentation of gonococcal infection may be delayed for 5 days or more because of the partial suppression of the infection by the prophylactic drops instilled at birth. Chlamydial infection can vary in severity from mild erythema of the eyelids to severe inflammation and copious purulent discharge. Chlamydial infection is primarily localized to the palpebral conjunctiva and only rarely affects the cornea. Gonococcal conjunctivitis is considered a medical emergency because the gonococcus can penetrate the cornea, resulting in corneal ulceration and perforation of the globe within 24 hours if untreated.

Concomitant nasopharyngeal chlamydial infection is commonly seen. Spread of the organism from the nasopharynx to the lungs is a sequela of colonization. Ten percent to 20% of newborns and infants with conjunctivitis have chlamydial pneumonia. It may occur simultaneously with the conjunctivitis or up to 4 to 6 weeks later. Affected newborns and infants are usually afebrile and present with symptoms of increasing tachypnea and cough.

Anterior uveitis may be confused with conjunctivitis. The uvea consists of the iris, ciliary body, retina, and choroid. Inflammation of the iris or ciliary body may produce conjunctival injection, which may be associated with decreased visual acuity, pain, headache, and photophobia. Systemic conditions associated with uveitis include Kawasaki disease, juvenile rheumatoid arthritis, Lyme disease, tuberculosis, sarcoidosis, *Toxocara* infection, toxoplasmosis, and spondyloarthropathies.

Infections of the Eye and Surrounding Tissues

Preseptal cellulitis and **orbital cellulitis** are 2 serious infections of the eyelids and surrounding structures. Although these infections are not as frequent as those that are limited to the eye, they have serious sequelae. The preseptal space is defined by the skin of the eyelid on one side and the orbital septum on the other. Children with preseptal cellulitis, or **periorbital cellulitis,** usually present with acute onset, unilateral upper and lower eyelid edema, erythema, and pain. The condition is often associated with systemic signs and symptoms such as ill appearance, fever, and leukocytosis. The eye itself usually appears normal. Infection may follow hematogenous seeding of the preseptal space, most often with *H influenzae* type b or *S pneumoniae*, or after traumatic breaks in the skin that usually lead to *S aureus* infection.

Orbital cellulitis is an infection of the contents of the orbit posterior to the orbital septum. Usually an insidious onset of eyelid edema, proptosis, decreased extraocular movements, and loss of visual acuity occur. As with periorbital cellulitis, children are often febrile and ill-appearing. Contiguous spread of infection from adjacent sinusitis (most often ethmoid) is the most common cause. The organisms most often involved are the same

as those in acute sinusitis *(S aureus, S pneumoniae,* and nontypeable *H influenzae)*. Untreated, the infection may progress to orbital abscess formation or progress posteriorly in the orbit to the cavernous sinus and brain.

Primary Human herpesvirus infection can affect the skin surrounding the eyes as well as the eye itself. Most of these infections are caused by human herpesvirus 1, although human herpesvirus 2 infections may be seen in newborns. Children with **herpetic infections of the eye** usually present with unilateral skin vesicles and a mild conjunctivitis or keratitis. Herpetic keratoconjunctivitis can recur following fever, exposure to sunlight, or mild trauma. The characteristic corneal lesion of herpetic keratitis is the dendritic corneal ulcer, which appears as a tree branch pattern on fluorescein staining of the cornea. Although this lesion may be seen with primary infection, it is more common in recurrent infections. Skin vesicles may not appear with a recurrence, which makes it difficult to distinguish herpetic infection from other causes of conjunctivitis. Steroids may lead to progression of the herpetic infection and permanent corneal scarring as well as cataracts and glaucoma. Empiric topical steroid treatment for presumed viral conjunctivitis should be avoided for this reason. Neonatal herpetic infections of the eye primarily result from human herpesvirus 2. Infections may be isolated to the eye, or the eye may be infected secondarily due to central nervous system (CNS) or disseminated disease. Proper diagnosis is important because disseminated herpetic disease has a mortality of about 85%, and CNS disease has a mortality of 50%. Isolated herpetic eye disease is actually quite rare in neonates.

Evaluation

History

A careful history taken from the parent or primary caregiver as well as the child can guide the diagnosis (Questions Box). It is important to exclude the possibility of ocular trauma or exposure to noxious chemicals when evaluating children with red, irritated eyes.

Questions

Eye Infections

- How long has the child had symptoms?
- Is the child having any difficulty seeing clearly?
- Is the child complaining of light sensitivity?
- Has the child had fever, cold symptoms, or purulent nasal discharge (eg, green, yellow)?
- Are the eyes pruritic (itchy) or painful?
- Does the child have difficulty opening the affected eye on awaking in the morning or after naps?
- Have the parents noticed any discharge from the eyes or crusting around the eyelids?
- Is the child complaining of earache or sore throat?
- Does the child have allergies, asthma, or hay fever?
- Has there been any trauma or bug bites?

Physical Examination

A thorough examination of the eyes should be performed. The eyelids, conjunctiva, and cornea should be inspected for evidence of inflammation or foreign bodies. The presence of any discharge or crusting of the eyelids as well as light sensitivity or pain should be noted. Extraocular movements should be checked, and their symmetry should be noted. Visual acuity should be determined, and an ophthalmoscopic examination of the retina should be performed whenever possible. A slit-lamp examination of the eye is indicated if uveitis is suspected. In addition, it is important to perform a thorough head and neck examination, noting the presence of associated sinusitis, otitis media, pharyngitis, or preauricular nodes.

Laboratory Tests

Laboratory assessment is guided by the history and physical examination. Although clinical differentiation between a bacterial and viral etiology is difficult, cultures are usually not required because acute conjunctivitis in children is a self-limited disease. In neonatal conjunctivitis, however, the time of onset of illness and clinical findings overlap and Gram stain and cultures are essential. Gonococcal infection is assessed by Gram stain and culture. Treatment may be initiated on the basis of Gram stain alone because of the serious potential for corneal involvement and subsequent loss of visual acuity.

If human herpesvirus is suspected, viral cultures should be obtained. If chlamydial infection is suspected, a nasopharyngeal culture should be sent in addition to conjunctival scraping. Purulent material may be examined for gonococci, but conjunctival scrapings are required for chlamydia because chlamydia is an obligate intracellular organism. Laboratory assessment of periorbital cellulitis includes a complete blood cell count (CBC), blood culture, and a lumbar puncture in young infants or children with signs of meningeal irritation. The reported prevalence of meningitis is 1% in children with periorbital cellulitis and 10% in children with bacteremia and periorbital cellulitis. As with periorbital cellulitis, laboratory assessment of orbital cellulitis includes a CBC and blood culture.

Imaging Studies

Imaging studies are required infrequently in the assessment of eye infections. A chest radiograph to detect pneumonia should be taken if infants with neonatal conjunctivitis have respiratory symptoms. Characteristic features on chest radiograph include hyperinflation and diffuse or patchy interstitial infiltrates. In orbital cellulitis, a computed tomography scan of the orbit and sinuses may be useful for assessing the degree of involvement.

Management

Most common eye infections resolve spontaneously or respond readily to **hygiene** and **topical antibiotics.** Treatment of staphylococcal and seborrheic blepharitis consists of daily lid hygiene (usually at bedtime), including application of a warm compress and removal of the scales and crusts with a moistened, warm washcloth. The eyelashes and lid margins may also be scrubbed with a washcloth soaked in a 50:50 mixture of baby shampoo and water. When staphylococcal blepharitis is present, an ointment containing an antistaphylococcal antibiotic agent, such as erythromycin, may be applied to the eyelids after cleansing. Treatment of parasitic blepharitis consists of application of petrolatum ophthalmic ointment (to smother the nits) several times a day for 1 week, followed by removal of the remaining parasites and their ova with tweezers or forceps.

Treatment for hordeola consists of application of hot compresses several times a day. This usually causes the abscess to come to a point and drain. Occasionally, surgical excision and drainage may be required if the abscess does not resolve. Unlike the hordeolum, a chalazion generally requires surgical excision because spontaneous resolution is uncommon.

Most cases of acute childhood conjunctivitis can be managed successfully by primary care physicians. Acute conjunctivitis in childhood is generally a self-limited disease. However, antibiotic treatment of bacterial conjunctivitis hastens recovery and may help prevent secondary cases by eradicating the bacterial pathogen. It is helpful to determine clinically whether the infection is bacterial and initiate empiric treatment with topical antibiotic preparations. Trimethoprim and polymyxin B sulfate (Polytrim), sodium sulfacetamide (Bleph-10), gentamicin (Garamycin), tobramycin (Tobrex), and moxifloxacin (Vigamox) are some of the commonly prescribed antibiotics. Trimethoprim/polymyxin B sulfate and gentamicin are still highly effective against MRSA. Avoid neomycin-containing products because sensitivity to neomycin occurs frequently. Antibiotic ointments may be easier to instill in infants and young children. Antibiotic drops should be used in older children during the day because the ointments can blur the vision; ointments may be used at bedtime. Systemic therapy can be considered for concomitant conjunctivitis and otitis media. Good hygiene with special attention to hand washing is important to prevent the spread of the infection to the other eye and family and friends. Children should not go to school until the discharge and drainage have resolved (even if on antibiotic drops). If symptoms persist for more than 7 to 10 days or if the diagnosis is in question, appropriate cultures should be taken. Complicated cases such as suspected herpetic, gonococcal or MRSA infection; foreign bodies that cannot be removed easily; loss of visual acuity; presence of significant pain; those involving children with a history of recent penetrating ocular trauma or surgery; and those involving children who use contact lenses should be referred to an ophthalmologist immediately. Contact lens wearers with red eyes are at high risk for corneal ulcers. They should be instructed to leave their lenses out until seen by the ophthalmologist.

Allergic conjunctivitis can be managed with cool compresses. Topical decongestant drops may provide symptomatic relief if treatment is indicated. Vernal conjunctivitis may be treated with topical cromolyn sodium drops or medications designed to relieve redness and itching and stabilize mast cells, such as olopatadine (Patanol) or ketorolac (Acular). Caution should be used when prescribing corticosteroid preparations for the eye because they may lead to progression of an undiagnosed herpetic eye infection. Chronic use of topical steroids can cause cataracts and glaucoma.

Treatment of neonatal conjunctivitis depends on the diagnosis. If **gonococcal infection** is suspected and Gram stain result is positive for gram-negative diplococci, immediate parenteral therapy with ceftriaxone should be initiated. **Chlamydial conjunctivitis** should be managed with systemic rather than topical treatment to prevent systemic disease. Oral erythromycin is the drug of choice. Although oral treatment provides adequate local antibiotic levels, topical erythromycin ointment may be used in conjunction with systemic therapy to provide more prompt relief of ophthalmic symptoms. The parents should also be treated.

Empiric parenteral antibiotic therapy (eg, cefuroxime) should be initiated for **periorbital cellulitis.** Repeat evaluations for signs of progression should be performed frequently during the initial 24 to 48 hours. If **orbital cellulitis** is suspected, an ophthalmologist should be consulted, and hospitalization and systemic antibiotics should be instituted. Surgical drainage of the sinuses or an orbital abscess is sometimes necessary.

Children with suspected **herpetic infection** should be referred to an ophthalmologist. Intravenous acyclovir is often recommended for the treatment of isolated herpetic eye infections in neonates.

Prognosis

Most common eye infections such as blepharitis, hordeolum, and acute childhood conjunctivitis resolve without sequelae. Recurrence is common for hordeola, and periorbital cellulitis may be a potential complication in rare or untreated cases. Unlike acute conjunctivitis, chronic conjunctivitis may not be self-limited. Appropriate diagnosis and management are extremely important to prevent serious sequelae in some children. For example, endemic trachoma may progress to produce conjunctival scarring, pannus formation, and even blindness if not appropriately treated with systemic erythromycin or tetracycline. (In general, systemic tetracycline should not be used in children younger than 8 years to avoid discoloration of the teeth.)

Periorbital cellulitis generally resolves without sequelae if treated promptly with systemic antibiotics. Orbital cellulitis should be considered a true ophthalmologic emergency because the potential for complications is high. The optic nerve may become involved, resulting in loss of vision or spread of the infection into the cranial cavity. This spreading may lead to meningitis, cavernous sinus thrombosis, or brain abscess.

CASE RESOLUTION

The newborn presented in the case history has neonatal conjunctivitis. A Gram stain of the purulent discharge should be examined, and cultures should be taken from the eye and nasopharynx. If the Gram stain result is negative for gonococci, empiric treatment may begin with oral erythromycin.

Selected References

Amato M, Pershing S, Walvick M, Tanaka S. Trends in ophthalmic manifestations of methicillin-resistant Staphylococcus aureus (MRSA) in a northern California pediatric population. *J AAPOS.* 2013;17(3):243–247

Gold RS. Treatment of bacterial conjunctivitis in children. *Pediatr Ann.* 2011;40(2):95–105

Golde KT, Gardiner MF. Bacterial conjunctivitis in children: a current review of pathogens and treatment. *Int Ophthalmol Clin.* 2011;51(4):85–92

Liesegang T, Skuta G, Cantor L. Infectious and allergic ocular diseases. *J Pediatr Ophthalmol Strabismus.* 2006;17:215–238

Liu S, Pavan-Langston D, Colby KA. Pediatric herpes simplex of the anterior segment: characteristics, treatment, and outcomes. *Ophthalmology.* 2012;119(10):2003–2008

Nageswaran S, Woods CR, Benjamin DK Jr, Givner LB, Shetty AK. Orbital cellulitis in children. *Pediatr Infect Dis J.* 2006;25(8):695–699

O'Hara MA. Ophthalmia neonatorum. *Pediatr Clin North Am.* 1993;40(4):715–725

Ohnsman CM. Exclusion of students with conjunctivitis from school: policies of state departments of health. *J Pediatr Ophthalmol Strabismus.* 2007;44(2):101–105

Patel PB, Diaz MC, Bennett JE, Attia MW. Clinical features of bacterial conjunctivitis in children. *Acad Emerg Med.* 2007;14(1):1–5

Pichichero ME. Bacterial conjunctivitis in children: antibacterial treatment options in an era of increasing drug resistance. *Clin Pediatr (Phila).* 2011;50(1):7–13

Rimon A, Hoffer V, Prais D, Harel L, Amir J. Periorbital cellulitis in the era of Haemophilus influenzae type B vaccine: predisposing factors and etiologic agents in hospitalized children. *J Pediatr Ophthalmol Strabismus.* 2008;45(5):300–304

Wagner RS. The differential diagnosis of the red eye. *Contemp Pediatr.* 1991;8:26–4

CHAPTER 81

Excessive Tearing

Teresa Rosales, MD

CASE STUDY

A 4-week-old girl has had a persistent watery discharge from both eyes since birth. Her mother has noticed white, crusty material on her daughter's eyelids for the past few days. The infant's birth and medical history are unremarkable. Examination of the eyes, including bilateral red reflexes and symmetric extraocular movements, is normal, except that the left eye appears "wetter" than the right.

Questions

1. What is the differential diagnosis of excessive tearing in infancy?
2. How do physical findings such as corneal enlargement and haziness influence the differential diagnosis?
3. How should infants with excessive tearing be managed?
4. When should a child with excessive tearing be referred to an ophthalmologist?

Infants or young children with excessive tearing or epiphora in one or both eyes are a common pediatric ophthalmologic concern. The pediatrician must be capable of differentiating benign causes of this common childhood condition from more serious illnesses, such as glaucoma, that potentially threaten vision.

NASOLACRIMAL DUCT OBSTRUCTION

Epidemiology

Congenital obstruction of the nasolacrimal duct or dacryostenosis, which occurs in 1% to 6% of newborns and infants, is the most common cause of excessive tearing in infancy. Eighty percent will resolve spontaneously by 6 months of age.

Clinical Presentation

Infants with dacryostenosis usually present with a history of a mucoid discharge and crusting along the eyelid margins. The affected eye appears "wetter" than the normal eye, and a small pool of tears may be noted along the lower eyelid. Frequent tearing is reported. Commonly, the patient has repeated episodes of infection with purulent discharge (D_x Box).

Pathophysiology

The lacrimal system (Figure 81-1) produces and drains tears away from the eyes and into the nose. Reflex tearing is usually present shortly after birth but may be delayed for several weeks to months until the lacrimal gland begins to function. Tears drain away from the eyes through the superior and inferior puncta into the superior and inferior canaliculi and finally into the nasolacrimal duct, which drains beneath the inferior turbinate into the nose.

Dx Excessive Tearing

- Conjunctival edema or injection
- Crusting of the eyelids
- Rhinorrhea
- Photophobia
- Corneal haziness
- Reflux of tears with gentle pressure on medial canthus
- Wetness of eye

Outflow obstruction, most often due to obstruction of the nasolacrimal duct or dacryostenosis, is the most common cause of excessive tearing in infancy. The obstruction is usually bilateral and occurs during fetal development. Most commonly, a persistent, thin membrane (Hasner membrane) obstructs the opening of the sac in the nose. The membrane is usually located in the distal or nasal segment of the duct rather than the proximal portion. The term *dacryocystitis* is used if acute infection or inflammation is associated with the obstruction. If the canaliculi and nasolacrimal duct are obstructed, a mucocele over the nasolacrimal sac may be noted at birth. This sac appears as a bluish, firm mass located over the lacrimal sac. Atresia of some portion of the drainage system may also occur, but this is extremely rare.

Differential Diagnosis

Box 81-1 outlines the differential diagnosis of excessive tearing in infancy. Although obstruction of the nasolacrimal duct is the most common cause of excessive tearing in newborns and infants, it is important to consider and rule out glaucoma when evaluating neonates and infants with this complaint. Infantile glaucoma may be unilateral or bilateral.

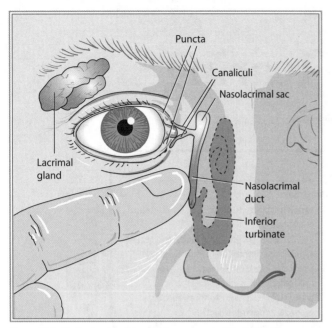

Figure 81-1. The lacrimal system, showing massage of the lacrimal sac.

Box 81-1. Differential Diagnosis of Excessive Tearing in Newborns and Infants

Increased Production
- Infantile glaucoma
- Allergy
- Conjunctivitis
- Corneal abrasion
- Foreign body under the eyelid

Outflow Obstruction
- Nasolacrimal duct obstruction (dacryostenosis)
- Anomalies of the lacrimal drainage system
- Mucocele of the lacrimal sac
- Atresia of the lacrimal punctum or canaliculus
- Nasal congestion
- Craniofacial anomalies involving the midface

Acute onset of excessive tearing in older children is usually due to ocular irritation. Any irritation of the conjunctiva, cornea, or eyelids may produce tearing. Conjunctivitis and corneal abrasion, usually secondary to a retained foreign body or human herpesvirus keratoconjunctivitis, are the 2 most common causes. Eye infections are discussed in Chapter 80.

Evaluation

History

Evaluation of excessive tearing should begin with a thorough history. The nature of any discharge (eg, watery, mucoid, purulent) should be noted. Parents or other caregivers should be questioned about the appearance of the infant's eyes (Questions Box). The excessive mucoid discharge in the medial canthal region and on the

Questions

Excessive Tearing

- How old was the infant when the excessive tearing appeared?
- Are one or both eyes affected?
- How does the eye appear? How has its appearance changed?
- Is there a family history of infantile glaucoma?
- Is the infant photophobic or light sensitive (eg, closes eyes in bright sunlight)?
- Has the infant had any persistent, watery discharge?
- Does the infant have difficulty opening the affected eye on awaking in the morning or after a nap?

eyelashes is noticeable to the family, as is the increased tearing. Crusting along the eyelashes caused by drying of the mucoid material is usually noted when infants awake in the morning or after a nap. Mucopurulent discharge may be noted if an associated acute infection is present (dacryocystitis).

Physical Examination

A careful examination of the eyes in infants includes inspection, evaluation of extraocular movements, and funduscopic examination. Funduscopic examination may be difficult in this age group, but bilateral red reflexes should at least be elicited. Signs of **dacryostenosis,** which usually appear days to weeks after birth, include tearing, mucoid discharge, and crusting of the eyelids. Tearing may be as mild as an increased wetness of the affected eye; this is best evaluated prior to disturbing the infant. Visible overflow of tears from the affected eye is not unusual and is typically seen when the eye is irritated (eg, due to cold or wind). If dacryostenosis is present, there may be associated erythema and edema of the eyelids. Dacryocystitis may also spread to the surrounding tissues, producing a periorbital cellulitis; systemic signs of infection such as fever may be noted. Gentle pressure along the medial canthal region over the lacrimal sac may produce a reflux of tears or mucoid discharge onto the surface of the eye, thus confirming the diagnosis of obstruction.

Laboratory Tests

Routine laboratory assessment is generally not necessary.

Management

Spontaneous resolution of dacryostenosis is common by 6 to 8 months of age. The primary medical treatment of uncomplicated nasolacrimal duct obstruction consists of **local massage** and **cleansing,** beginning when symptoms are noted. Parents are instructed to massage the nasolacrimal duct several times a day by applying firm, downward pressure over the medial canthal region with a finger and sliding the finger down toward the mouth (Crigler maneuver) (Figure 81-1). This maneuver attempts to move fluid trapped within the nasolacrimal sac down through the duct to break the obstruction with hydrostatic pressure. Parents may be asked to cleanse the eyes with warm water before performing this maneuver. Antibiotic ointments and drops should be prescribed only if the discharge is purulent or associated conjunctivitis is evident.

Controversy exists regarding when probing of the nasolacrimal duct should be performed. Some ophthalmologists prefer probing the duct before infants are 6 months of age because prior to this time, the procedure may be performed in the office without general anesthesia. Others state that more than 80% of obstructions resolve with conservative medical management by 6 months of age and prefer to delay probing until the age of 9 to 12 months. At this age, the procedure needs to be performed under general anesthesia. Deciding when to proceed with the probing depends on the standard of practice within the community, severity of symptoms, response to medical management, and level of parental concern.

Ophthalmologic referral is necessary for affected infants by 6 months of age if the obstruction has not resolved. Referral should be made sooner if symptoms are severe or infections recur.

Prognosis

Most cases of dacryostenosis resolve spontaneously during the first year of life without further sequelae. If tear duct probing is necessary, it is 90% to 95% successful if performed before 13 months of age. The success rate drops to 70% between 13 to 15 months and 50% over 18 months.

CONGENITAL GLAUCOMA

Epidemiology

Congenital or infantile glaucoma, a serious cause of excessive tearing, is quite rare; the incidence is about 1 in 10,000 live births. Although glaucoma may be present at birth, onset during the first few weeks to months of life is more common. Approximately 25% of cases are diagnosed at birth and 80% by 1 year of age. The severity of the disease is worse with earlier onset. Most affected infants are male; the male-female ratio in older infants is 2:1. Infantile glaucoma seems to have a multifactorial inheritance pattern, but most cases are sporadic. In families with one affected infant or a parental history of infantile glaucoma, the chance of having an infant with glaucoma is about 5%. Although glaucoma may be unilateral or bilateral, most infants (75%–90%) who present before 3 months of age have bilateral glaucoma.

Clinical Presentation

In addition to excessive tearing, other clinical signs of infantile glaucoma include blepharospasm (spasmodic blinking of the eyelids), photophobia, corneal enlargement and corneal haziness due to corneal edema, progressive enlargement of the eye (buphthalmos), and cupping and atrophy of the optic nerve (D_x Box).

Pathophysiology

Glaucoma is the most serious and potentially sight-threatening etiology for excessive production of tears. Glaucoma refers to an increase in intraocular pressure that is severe enough to damage the eye and alter vision. In infants and children, glaucoma is usually a result of a developmental abnormality of the iridocorneal angle, interfering with drainage of aqueous humor from the anterior chamber. Young infants differ from adults in that the globe in infants' eyes is distensible; the increased intraocular pressure not only produces corneal enlargement and edema but also expands the globe itself. Breakdown of the corneal epithelium and resultant irritation of the eyes produce reflex tearing and photophobia. Untreated glaucoma may lead to optic nerve damage with resultant loss of visual acuity, decreased visual field, and even blindness. Glaucoma in children younger than 3 years is referred to broadly as infantile glaucoma, and glaucoma that occurs in children between 3 and 20 years of age is called juvenile glaucoma. Infantile glaucoma is further classified as being primary or secondary. Primary glaucoma refers to isolated abnormalities of the iridocorneal angle, whereas secondary glaucoma may be associated with other ocular or systemic diseases. Juvenile glaucoma is a form of open-angle glaucoma.

Differential Diagnosis

Excessive tearing may be caused by increased production or obstruction to outflow (see Box 81-1). Infants with increased production of tears will demonstrate rhinorrhea in association with epiphora, a finding that distinguishes glaucoma from dacryostenosis. Rhinorrhea is not associated with dacryostenosis because the nasolacrimal duct is obstructed and no tears drain out of the nose. Ocular irritation, which occurs with conjunctivitis, corneal abrasion, or a foreign body under the eyelid, can also produce excessive tearing, especially in older children. In addition, allergies are associated with excessive tearing due to overproduction.

Disorders associated with outflow obstruction include dacryostenosis, anomalies of the lacrimal drainage system (mucocele of the lacrimal sac and atresia of the lacrimal punctum or canaliculus), nasal congestion, and craniofacial anomalies involving the midface.

Evaluation

A corneal diameter greater than 12 mm in infants is suggestive of infantile glaucoma. Corneal edema is more common in newborns and younger infants (younger than 3 months) and may cause the red reflex to appear dull in the affected eye. The optic cup may be enlarged. A cup-to-disk ratio greater than 0.3 or an asymmetry of the ratio between the eyes may indicate glaucoma.

As in adults, loss of visual fields occurs in children with glaucoma. Visual fields are difficult to evaluate in infants and young children because of their inability to cooperate with the examination.

Management

Suspected cases of glaucoma should be referred to an ophthalmologist immediately for further evaluation, including measurement of intraocular pressure. Pressures greater than 20 mm Hg are suggestive of glaucoma (normal pressures are 10–20 mm Hg in infants and young children as well as in adults).

Surgery is the primary treatment. The goal is to normalize intraocular pressure and minimize irreversible corneal and optic nerve damage.

Prognosis

Infantile glaucoma, if left untreated, may progress to blindness. The visual prognosis depends on several factors, including the age at onset of glaucoma (the earlier the onset, the worse the prognosis), the amount of optic nerve damage, and the degree of myopia caused by the enlargement of the eye. In addition, amblyopia, secondary to deprivation due to corneal opacities or unequal refractive errors, is often seen (see Chapter 79).

CASE RESOLUTION

The infant in the case history has dacryostenosis. This can be managed with medical treatment such as local massage and cleansing at this stage. If her symptoms persist beyond the age of 6 months, consultation with an ophthalmologist is recommended.

Selected References

Al-Faky YH, Al-Sobaie N, Mousa A, et al. Evaluation of treatment modalities and prognostic factors in children with congenital nasolacrimal duct obstruction. *J AAPOS*. 2012;16(1):53–57

Becker BB. The treatment of congenital dacryocystocele. *Am J Ophthalmol*. 2006;142(5):835–838

Guez A, Dureau P. Diagnosis and treatment of tearing in infancy. *Arch Pediatr*. 2009;16(5):496–499

Kushner BJ. The management of nasolacrimal duct obstruction in children between 18 months and 4 years old. *J AAPOS*. 1998;2(1):57–60

Olitsky S, Medow N, Rogers G. Diagnosis and treatment of congenital nasolacrimal duct obstruction. *J Pediatr Ophthalmol Strabismus*. 2007;44(2):80–83

Pediatric Eye Disease Investigator Group. Resolution of congenital nasolacrimal duct obstruction with nonsurgical management. *Arch Ophthalmol*. 2012;130(6):730–734

Pediatric Eye Disease Investigator Group; Repka MX, Chandler DL, Beck RW, et al. Primary treatment of nasolacrimal duct obstruction with probing in children younger than 4 years. *Ophthalmology*. 2008;115(3):577–584

Robb R. Nasolacrimal duct obstruction in children. In: *Focal Points: Clinical Modules for Ophthalmologists*. Module 8. San Francisco, CA: American Academy of Ophthalmology; 2004:XXII, 1–10

Stamper RL, Lieberman MF, Drake MV. *Becker-Shaffer's Diagnosis and Therapy of the Glaucomas*. 7th ed. St Louis, MO: Mosby; 1999

Walton DS, Katsavounidou G. Newborn primary congenital glaucoma: 2005 update. *J Pediatr Ophthalmol Strabismus*. 2005;42(6):333–341

CHAPTER 82

Neck Masses

Casey Buitenhuys, MD, and Stanley H. Inkelis, MD

CASE STUDY

A 2-year-old boy is brought to the office with a 1-day history of an enlarging red, tender "bump" beneath his right mandible. He has a fever (temperature 101.6°F [38.5°C]) and sores around his nose, upper lip, and cheek. These sores have been present for 3 days and have not responded to an over-the-counter antibiotic ointment. He had an upper respiratory tract infection 1 week ago, which has almost entirely resolved. He is otherwise in good health. The family has no history of tuberculosis or recent travel, and the child has not been playing with cats or other animals.

The physical examination is completely normal except for fever, mild rhinorrhea, honey-crusted lesions on the nares and upper lip, and a 4 × 5-cm, right submandibular neck mass that is erythematous, warm, and tender to palpation.

Questions

1. What are the common causes of neck masses in children?
2. What steps are involved in the evaluation of children with neck masses?
3. What clinical findings suggest that neck masses are neoplasms? When should neck masses be biopsied or removed?
4. What is involved in the treatment of the different types of neck masses in children?
5. When should children with neck masses be referred for further consultation?

Neck masses are any swellings or enlargements of the structures in the area between the inferior mandible and the clavicle. Normal variants, such as the angle of the mandible or tip of the mastoid, may occasionally appear as swellings, and parents sometimes confuse these with neck masses. If the swelling is not a normal structure, a well-directed history and physical examination usually determine the etiology.

Lymphadenopathy from viral or bacterial throat infections is the most common cause of neck **masses** in children. Therefore, neck masses are common because children frequently have sore throats. Most parents know about swollen lymph glands, and they usually do not seek medical advice unless the glands become very large or do not recede in a few days. Neck masses in children may have many other causes besides lymphadenopathy. Most of these masses may be categorized as inflammatory, neoplastic, traumatic, or congenital in origin. A well-described mnemonic in the adult literature, KITTENS, can summate many of the causes of neck masses in children as well (Table 82-1).

Epidemiology

Most neck masses are benign. Almost 50% of all 2-year-olds and up to 90% of children between 4 and 8 years of age have palpable cervical lymph nodes. Although more than 25% of malignant tumors in children are found in the head and neck region (this is the primary site in only 5%), less than 2% of suspicious head and neck masses are malignant.

The epidemiology of neck masses of infectious origin depends on the infectious agent itself, geographic location of the child, and the child's immediate environment. Neck masses of viral origin may be related to focal infection of the oropharynx or respiratory tract but are often associated with generalized adenopathy. Neck masses of bacterial origin typically occur from normal bacterial flora of the nose, mouth, pharynx, and skin that secondarily spreads to lymph nodes. These organisms are not usually transmitted from person to person. Pathologic flora such as group A streptococcus and *Mycobacterium tuberculosis* that result in neck masses can spread by human-to-human contact, however. Additionally, cat-scratch disease is caused by *Bartonella henselae*, a vector-borne pathogen.

Clinical Presentation

Children with neck masses present in a variety of ways depending on the etiology of the mass. Typically, a swelling or enlargement in the neck, which parents often notice more than children, is evident. Associated signs and symptoms include fever, upper respiratory tract infection, sore throat, ear pain, pain or tenderness over the mass, changes in skin color over the mass, skin lesions of the head or neck, and dental caries or infections (D_x Box). Malignant tumors are usually slow-growing, firm, fixed, non-tender masses. Congenital neck masses and benign tumors, which have frequently been present since birth or early infancy, are soft, smooth, and cyst-like and may be recurrent. Neck masses associated with trauma are often rapidly evolving and may lead to airway obstruction. Temporal development of neck masses is a helpful predictor of mass etiology. The Skandalakis rule of 7s may be applied and adapted to pediatric neck masses (Table 82-2).

Table 82-1. KITTENS Mnemonic for Neck Masses	
K	**Congenital/Developmental Anomalies** • Thyroglossal duct cyst • Branchial cleft cyst • Dermoid cyst • Vascular malformation
I	**Infectious/Inflammatory** • Lymphadenitis/cervical adenopathy • Viral adenitis (multiple causes) • Bacterial adenitis (multiple causes) • Retropharyngeal/parapharyngeal abscesses
T	**Trauma** • Hematoma • Pseudoaneurysm • Laryngocele
T	**Toxic** • Thyroid toxicosis • Medications (eg, carbamazepine)
E	**Endocrine** • Thyroid neoplasms • Parathyroid neoplasms • Thyroiditis • Goiter
N	**Neoplasms** • Hemangioma • Lipoma • Salivary gland • Parapharyngeal space • Lymphoma
S	**Systemic Disease** • Sarcoidosis • Sjögren syndrome • Kimura disease • Histiocytic necrotizing lymphadenitis (Kikuchi disease) • Castleman disease • Kawasaki disease • AIDS

Table 82-2. Rule of 7s	
Mass duration	*Likely mass etiology*
7 min	Trauma
7 d	Inflammation/infection
7 mo	Neoplastic
7 y	Congenital

Adapted from Skandalakis LJ, Skandalakis JE, Skandalakis PN, eds. *Surgical Anatomy and Technique.* New York, NY: Springer; 2009.

Neck Masses

Inflammatory/Infectious
- Swelling or enlargement in the neck
- Fever
- Sore throat, dental infection, skin infection of head or neck
- Pain or tenderness over the mass (usually)

Neoplastic
- Slowly enlarging mass
- Unilateral, discrete
- Firm or rubbery
- Fixed to tissue
- Deep within the fascia
- Non-tender (usually)

Traumatic
- Rapidly enlarging mass
- Hematoma
- Acute airway obstruction

Congenital
- Enlargement in neck (usually present since birth or soon after)
- Soft, smooth, cyst-like
- Non-tender (unless infected)
- Recurrent

Pathophysiology

The pathophysiology of neck masses in children is dependent on etiology. Most neck masses are related to inflammation or infection of lymph nodes. Enlargement of lymph nodes usually results from proliferation of intrinsic lymphocytes or macrophages already present in the lymph node (eg, lymphadenopathy caused by a viral infection) or from infiltration of extrinsic cells (eg, lymphadenitis, metastatic tumor). Neck masses from trauma occur from leakage of fluid into the neck, and congenital anatomic abnormalities become apparent because of fluid collection or infection of the defect. The parotid gland may be enlarged from inflammation (eg, blocked salivary gland duct), infection (eg, mumps), or tumor (eg, pleomorphic adenoma), but the swelling primarily involves the face rather than the neck and obscures the angle of the jaw. Other salivary glands may be infected or obstructed and may cause submandibular swelling, erythema, and tenderness.

Differential Diagnosis

Neck masses in children are usually the result of inflammation or infection of lymph nodes, tumors of lymph nodes and other neck structures, trauma, and congenital lesions. The location of the mass is often a clue to its etiology (Figure 82-1).

Lymphadenopathy/Lymphadenitis

Lymphadenopathy is lymph node enlargement or hyperplasia secondary to localized infection or antigenic stimulation proximal to the involved node or nodes. Because lymphoid tissue steadily

Figure 82-1. Differential diagnosis of neck mass by location. 1, Parotid—cystic hygroma, hemangioma, lymphadenitis, parotitis, Sjögren syndrome, infantile cortical hyperostosis (Caffey-Silverman syndrome), lymphoma. 2, Postauricular—lymphadenitis, branchial cleft cyst (first), squamous epithelial cyst. 3, Submental—lymphadenitis, cystic hygroma, thyroglossal duct cyst, dermoid, sialadenitis. 4, Submandibular—lymphadenitis, cystic hygroma, sialadenitis, tumor, cystic fibrosis. 5, Jugulodigastric— lymphadenitis, squamous epithelial cyst, branchial cleft cyst (first), parotid tumor, normal-transverse process C2, styloid process. 6, Midline neck— lymphadenitis, thyroglossal duct cyst, dermoid, laryngocele, normal hyoid, thyroid. 7, Sternomastoid (anterior)—lymphadenitis, branchial cleft cyst (second, third) pilomatricoma, rare tumors. 8, Spinal accessory— lymphadenitis, lymphoma, metastasis from nasopharynx. 9, Paratracheal— thyroid, parathyroid, esophageal diverticulum. 10, Supraclavicular—cystic hygroma, lipoma, lymphoma, metastasis, normal fat pad, pneumatocele of upper lobe. 11, Suprasternal—thyroid, lipoma, dermoid, thymus, mediastinal mass. (From May M. Neck masses in children: diagnosis and treatment. *Pediatr Ann*. 1976;5[8]:517–535, with permission from SLACK Inc.)

increases until puberty, palpable lymph nodes, including those in the cervical area, are a common, normal finding in children. Palpable cervical lymph nodes are present in up to 90% of children between 4 and 8 years of age. Any lymph node in the neck larger than 10 mm qualifies as cervical lymphadenopathy.

The most common cause of cervical lymphadenopathy is a viral infection of the upper respiratory tract. Lymphadenopathy usually begins and resolves with the acute infection. Occasionally, the swelling remains for several days or months, however, and children present because of parental concern. Bacterial pharyngitis, usually from infection with group A beta-hemolytic streptococcus (GABHS), is often associated with cervical lymphadenopathy. Cervical as well as generalized lymphadenopathy may be seen in children with systemic illness (eg, Kawasaki disease, sarcoid, HIV, mononucleosis). Cat-scratch disease, toxoplasmosis, fungal infection, and mycobacterial and atypical mycobacterial infections may be associated with lymphadenopathy that may later progress to lymphadenitis. Viral illnesses, including Epstein-Barr virus (EBV) (mononucleosis), adenovirus, enterovirus, human herpesvirus 1 and 2, human herpesvirus 6

(HHV-6), and cytomegalovirus (CMV) commonly cause lymphadenopathy and lymphadenitis.

Lymphadenitis is infection or inflammation of the lymph node that occurs when microorganisms and neutrophils infiltrate the node, leading to necrosis and abscess formation. This condition is usually associated with proximal bacterial infection that drains to the affected nodes by connecting afferent lymphatic channels. Lymphadenitis is often a progression of disease, resulting in enlarged nodes that measure 2 to 6 cm. These nodes, which are typical of bacterial disease, are often termed "hot nodes," and they are erythematous, warm, tender, and sometimes fluctuant. Subacute or chronic inflammation of lymph nodes typical in illnesses such as cat-scratch disease, mycobacterial infection, or toxoplasmosis are not warm to the touch and are usually not as tender. They are typically not suppurative and may be difficult to distinguish from nodes that are simply enlarged (Figure 82-2).

Staphylococcus aureus and group A streptococcus are responsible for 50% to 90% of cases of acute unilateral cervical lymphadenitis. These organisms spread from a primary site to the lymph nodes, draining those sites. Common primary sites of infection are the throat, teeth and gums, and skin (lesions), particularly on the scalp or ears. Infections at these sites may result from trauma, such as scratches or scabs, or from primary infection, such as impetigo. Anaerobic oral flora constitute a small portion of causes for bacterial cervical adenitis, especially in older children with poor dentition. *Staphylococcus aureus* or group B streptococcus usually causes cervical lymphadenitis in neonates or very young infants. Such staphylococcal infections, which are often nosocomially spread from contact in the newborn nursery, present as discrete masses. Group B streptococcus causes the "cellulitis-adenitis" syndrome, which presents as cervical adenitis associated with a facial cellulitis. *Pseudomonas aeruginosa* is an unusual cause of cervical adenitis in newborns.

Mycobacterial disease must always be considered in children of all ages who present with cervical adenitis particularly involving posterior cervical nodes. The child with *M tuberculosis* cervical adenitis

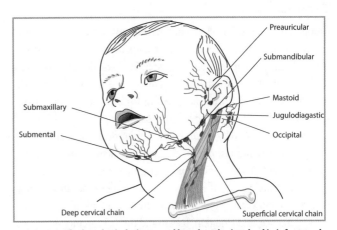

Figure 82-2. The lymphatic drainage and lymph nodes involved in infants and children with cervical lymphadenitis. (Reproduced with permission from Feigin RD, Cherry JD, eds. *Textbook of Pediatric Infectious Diseases*. 5th ed. Philadelphia, PA: Saunders; 2004:186.)

often has multiple nodes, sometimes bilateral, usually non-tender, and usually not erythematous or warm. These children are typically older, commonly reside in an urban setting, have a history of tuberculosis exposure, and often have an abnormal chest radiograph. Intradermal placement of a purified protein derivative (PPD) often produces more than 15 mm of induration in most children with typical mycobacterial infection. A reaction of 5 to 14 mm may be caused by tuberculous or nontuberculous mycobacterial infection. Atypical mycobacterial infection usually occurs in children between 1 and 6 years of age with unilateral rather than bilateral lymph node enlargement and a normal chest radiograph.

Cat-scratch disease should be considered in children who have cats or kittens or who play with them. The infection may result from a cat scratch or from a cat licking a child's broken skin. If the inoculum is near the head and neck area, cervical adenitis develops. Contact with the hand may result in axillary lymphadenitis. Occasionally, generalized lymphadenopathy is present. An associated non-painful papule or papules where the cat scratch or lick occurred may be apparent. *Bartonella henselae* has been identified as the organism causing cat-scratch disease.

Toxoplasmosis may be accompanied by adenitis, usually in the posterior cervical area. Nodes are painless and may fluctuate in size, and children are often asymptomatic. Multiple lymph nodes are involved in about one-third to half of cases.

Children presenting with recurrent cervical adenitis and recurrent fevers may have PFAPA syndrome (*p*eriodic *f*ever, *a*phthous stomatitis, *p*haryngitis, and cervical *a*denitis). This entity usually occurs in children younger than 5 years and can be aborted with steroids.

Kikuchi disease, or histiocytic necrotizing lymphadenitis, has an Asian and female predilection and is characterized by fever, leukopenia, and cervical lymphadenopathy. The illness is self-limited, and follow-up is recommended because of a possible association with systemic lupus erythematosus.

Less common bacterial, viral, and fungal causes of cervical adenitis are listed in Box 82-1.

Tumors

Compared with other neck masses, **malignant neck tumors** occur rarely; nevertheless, they should be considered in any children with enlarging or persistent neck masses. Hodgkin disease and non-Hodgkin lymphoma are the most frequent cause of head and neck malignancies in children, accounting for almost 60% of cases. Rhabdomyosarcomas are the next most frequent head and neck malignancy, followed by thyroid tumors, neuroblastoma, and nasopharyngeal carcinomas. Age is an important factor in determining the likelihood of specific tumors. Neuroblastoma, leukemia, and rhabdomyosarcoma are the most common tumor types in children younger than 6 years. Non-Hodgkin lymphoma typically occurs in preadolescence, and Hodgkin disease and thyroid carcinoma are the most common malignancies in adolescents.

Benign neck tumors, with the exception of those mentioned later in the discussion of congenital lesions, are uncommon. They include epidermoid inclusion cysts, lipomas, fibromas, neurofibromas, pilomatricomas (benign skin neoplasms of hair follicle origin), keloids, goiters, and ranulas (intraoral mucocele) and plunging ranula (an extension of the oral ranula into the neck).

Trauma

Trauma to the neck may be associated with bleeding and edema. Large hematomas that affect vital structures are potentially life-threatening. Significant trauma and structural injury usually accompany expanding neck hematomas. Neurologic deficits and stroke after neck trauma should alert the clinician to consider cervical arterial dissection. In children with mild injuries and neck hematomas, bleeding disorders are a possible cause of the hematoma. Twisting injuries to the neck may lead to muscle spasm of the sternocleidomastoid muscle (torticollis) and an apparent mass that is the contracted muscle. Additionally, intramuscular hematoma or bleeding from vaginal delivery may cause torticollis in the neonatal period. The neck is bent toward the side of the affected sternocleidomastoid muscle. Child abuse should also be considered in children who have neck injuries that are not consistent with their histories.

A foreign body in the neck may present as a mass because of the foreign body itself (eg, piece of glass or metal, bullet) or surrounding inflammation. A crepitant neck mass following trauma to the neck or chest suggests subcutaneous emphysema from tracheal injury or a pneumomediastinum. Crepitant neck masses may also be seen secondary to pneumomediastinum in children with obstructive lung diseases such as asthma or cystic fibrosis.

Congenital Lesions

Children with congenital neck lesions can present with a neck mass in early infancy or later in childhood. Some congenital lesions are not discovered until adulthood. The most common of these benign lesions are thyroglossal duct cysts, branchial cleft cysts, lymphatic malformations (cystic hygromas/lymphangiomas), and hemangiomas (Figure 82-3).

Thyroglossal duct cysts are almost always midline in the neck and inferior to the hyoid bone. They usually move upward with tongue protrusion or swallowing. Most branchial cleft cysts occur anterior to the middle third of the sternocleidomastoid muscle. Less commonly, branchial cleft cysts may appear in the posterior triangle of the neck and the preauricular area. Branchial cleft sinus tracts appear as slit-like openings anterior to the lower third of the sternocleidomastoid muscle and may present as neck masses if they become infected. Thyroglossal duct cysts and branchial cleft cysts may also present for the first time as infected neck masses.

Cystic hygromas are usually large, soft, easily compressible masses found in the posterior triangle behind the sternocleidomastoid muscle in the supraclavicular fossa. They transilluminate well. Two-thirds of cystic hygromas are present at birth, and 80% to 90% are identified before 3 years of age. They are more common on the left side of the neck. Cystic hygromas occasionally become secondarily infected, with findings of erythema, warmth, and tenderness.

Box 82-1. Differential Diagnosis of Neck Masses

Cervical Lymphadenopathy/Lymphadenitis	**Tumor**	**Immunologic Disorders**

Cervical Lymphadenopathy/Lymphadenitis

Bacterial origin

Staphylococcus aureus (methicillin sensitive)

Staphylococcus aureus (methicillin resistant)

Group A beta-hemolytic streptococcus

Mycobacterium tuberculosis

Atypical mycobacteria

Cat-scratch disease *(Bartonella henselae)*

Anaerobes

Gram-negative enteric bacteria

Haemophilus influenzae

Plague

Actinomycosis

Diphtheria

Tularemia

Brucellosis

Syphilis

Group B streptococcus (neonates)

Viral origin

Epstein-Barr virus (infectious mononucleosis)

Adenovirus

Cytomegalovirus

Human herpesvirus types 1 and 2

Enterovirus

HIV

Measles

Rubella

Human herpesvirus 6

Influenza virus

Fungal origin

Histoplasmosis

Coccidioidomycosis

Aspergillosis

Candidiasis

Sporotrichosis

Cryptococcosis

Parasitic origin

Toxoplasmosis

Leishmaniasis

Tumor

Malignant

Hodgkin disease

Non-Hodgkin lymphoma

Lymphosarcoma

Rhabdomyosarcoma

Neuroblastoma

Leukemia

Langerhans cell histiocytosis

Thyroid tumors

Nasopharyngeal squamous cell carcinoma

Salivary gland carcinoma

Benign

Epidermoid cyst

Lipoma

Fibroma

Neurofibroma

Pilomatricoma

Keloid

Goiter

Osteochondroma

Teratoma (may be malignant)

Ranula

Congenital Disorders

Hemangioma

Cystic hygroma (lymphangioma)

Branchial cleft cyst

Thyroglossal duct cyst

Laryngocele

Dermoid cyst

Cervical rib

Sternocleidomastoid tumor

Trauma

Hematoma (acute or organized)

Subcutaneous emphysema

Foreign body

Arteriovenous malformation

Immunologic Disorders

Local hypersensitivity reaction (sting or bite)

Pseudolymphoma (from phenytoin)

Serum sickness

Sarcoidosis

Infantile cortical hyperostosis (Caffey-Silverman syndrome)

Kawasaki disease

Systemic lupus erythematosus

Juvenile rheumatoid arthritis

Kikuchi disease (necrotizing lymphadenitis)

Kimura disease

Miscellaneous

Sialadenitis

Parotitis

Storage disorders

   Niemann-Pick disease

   Gaucher disease

Obstructive airway disease (asthma, cystic fibrosis)

Hemangiomas are usually not present at birth but appear in early infancy and may enlarge rapidly. In most cases, they recede spontaneously by 9 years of age. They are usually much smaller than cystic hygromas, do not transilluminate, and may be recognized by their reddish color (capillary or strawberry hemangioma) or by a bluish hue of the overlying skin (cavernous hemangioma).

Small infants who present with torticollis should be examined for a sternocleidomastoid mass ("tumor"), which represents fibrosis and contracture of that sternocleidomastoid muscle so that the head tilts toward the affected side with the chin rotating to the opposite side. Contusion of the sternocleidomastoid muscle from traumatic extraction of the head during delivery with subsequent hemorrhage and healing has been implicated as the cause of the fibrotic mass. However, it is more likely that this mass occurs prior to birth because it contains mature fibrous tissue. In addition, the mass may be present following cesarean delivery and is associated with hip dysplasia and other congenital lesions, suggesting that the condition is related to abnormal positioning in utero. Venous occlusion of the sternocleidomastoid muscle in utero or at the time of delivery has also been proposed as a cause.

Figure 82-3. Head and neck congenital lesions seen in children in frontal and lateral views. The shaded areas denote the distribution in which a given lesion may be found. A, Dermoid cyst. B, Thyroglossal duct cyst. C, Second branchial cleft appendage. D, Second branchial cleft sinus. E, Second branchial cleft cyst. F, First branchial pouch defect. G, Preauricular sinus or appendage. (Reproduced with permission from Fleisher GR, Ludwig S, eds. *Textbook of Pediatric Emergency Medicine.* 5th ed. Philadelphia, PA: Lippincott Williams & Wilkins; 2006:1594.)

Evaluation

History

A thorough history is important in establishing the etiology of the neck mass (Questions Box).

Physical Examination

A general physical examination should be performed. The neck mass should be examined for anatomic location, color, size, shape, consistency, tenderness, fluctuation, and mobility. The mass should also be measured. A mass that has an audible bruit or palpable thrill is suggestive of a vascular malformation or traumatic injury. The head, neck, and face should be examined for lesions, most often infections that drain into neck lymph nodes. Lesions can frequently be found on the scalp, neck, face, ears, mouth, teeth, tongue, gums, and throat. Hairstyles such as tight braids can sometimes provide ports of entry for bacteria. Occasionally, sinus tracts or fistulas may be the entry point of infection. In addition, other lymph node groups should be examined to determine if the lymphadenopathy is local or generalized. Particular attention should be paid to the supraclavicular area because enlarged supraclavicular nodes are more frequently associated with malignant pathology such as Hodgkin disease. The chest should be examined for use of accessory muscles, equality of breath sounds, and wheezing. The abdomen should be examined for hepatosplenomegaly.

Neck Masses   **Questions**

- How old is the child?
- How long has the neck mass been present?
- What signs and symptoms are associated with the neck mass?
- Has the child been exposed to tuberculosis?
- Has the child ever drunk any unpasteurized cow's milk?
- Has the child been in contact with any cats or kittens? Rabbits? Other animals?
- Has the child traveled to areas where endemic diseases such as histoplasmosis or coccidioidomycosis are prevalent?
- Has the child suffered any trauma recently?
- Does the child have any allergies?
- Does the child have any risk factors for HIV?

Laboratory Tests

Laboratory tests are rarely indicated in children with cervical lymphadenopathy or lymphadenitis of acute onset. Although a rapid streptococcal antigen detection test or throat culture is helpful in children with suspected streptococcal sore throat, it may be unnecessary if antibiotic therapy is empirically prescribed for lymphadenitis. If the adenitis is fluctuant, aspiration and culture may be helpful in determining the specific bacteriologic diagnosis. Fine-needle aspiration cytology and polymerase chain reaction assays may help differentiate between tuberculous and nontuberculous mycobacterial disease. Superficial cervical nodes or axillary nodes, if enlarged, are appropriate first-line aspiration sites because of their superficial nature. In addition, a PPD test should be applied to all children who present with lymphadenitis.

If the adenitis does not resolve or improve after 2 to 3 days of observation or therapy, laboratory tests directed by the history and physical examination should be considered. A complete blood cell count (CBC) with differential and a monospot or serologic antibody tests for EBV may be helpful in the diagnosis of infectious mononucleosis. If the mass in the neck is a hematoma and a bleeding disorder is suspected, a CBC with platelet count, prothrombin time, and partial thromboplastin time should be obtained. Possible additional tests include an erythrocyte sedimentation rate, C-reactive protein, and, if indicated, serologic tests for toxoplasmosis, CMV, HHV-6, coccidioidomycosis, histoplasmosis, tularemia, *B henselae,* and syphilis should be performed. Skin tests for fungi should be considered in those patients coming from endemic areas. These tests should be placed after serologic tests are performed so that false-positive serologic test results are not obtained.

Similar laboratory tests should be considered for children who present for the first time with enlarged or enlarging lymph nodes of long duration or those who do not respond after 2 weeks of antibiotic therapy. The physician may choose to do more of these laboratory tests at the initial evaluation or after a therapeutic trial because the likelihood of viral lymphadenopathy decreases and the possibility of a more unusual etiology increases. HIV testing should also be considered.

Thyroid function tests should be considered in children with a thyroid mass or suspected thyroglossal duct cyst. An ultrasound or a thyroid scan should be considered for the child with a thyroid mass.

Unless cat-scratch disease is very likely, immediate lymph node biopsy is indicated for enlarged supraclavicular nodes or lymph nodes in the lower half of the neck, rapidly progressive and enlarging nodes, fixed nodes, nodes deep within the fascia, or firm or hard nodes. Children who have a persistent fever or weight loss should have a biopsy at 1 week if a diagnosis has not been established. Asymptomatic children without an established diagnosis should have a biopsy at 2 weeks if the node increases in size, at 4 to 6 weeks if the node is not increased in size but is persistent, and at 8 to 12 weeks if the node has not regressed to a normal size. In some cases, the initial biopsy is non-diagnostic, but on subsequent biopsy, a specific diagnosis may be made. Consequently, children with persistent adenopathy should be followed closely and be biopsied again if indicated. Fine-needle aspiration biopsy in children is controversial but has some demonstrated benefits. It is being used more often to differentiate between benign and malignant disease and to potentially decrease the need for open biopsy. However, if malignancy is a consideration, consultation with an oncologist is advisable to determine the biopsy method of choice.

Imaging Studies

A chest radiograph should be obtained in all children with suspected tuberculosis or tumor (eg, enlarged supraclavicular nodes) as well as in children with crepitant neck masses or in whom the diagnosis of the adenitis remains uncertain. If a foreign body in the neck is suspected, anteroposterior and lateral neck radiographs should be obtained.

Almost all neck masses can be evaluated by ultrasonography, computed tomography (CT), or magnetic resonance imaging (MRI). Because there is no ionizing radiation associated with ultrasonography, it is quickly available, is noninvasive, and does not need sedation; it is the initial imaging study of choice, particularly for thyroid masses, thyroglossal duct cysts, branchial cleft cysts, and parotid masses. If malignancy is suspected or the mass cannot be delineated in the field of view, MRI or CT may be more definitive studies. Ultrasonography with color Doppler is helpful in differentiating cystic from solid masses and determining if the mass is vascular. In addition, demonstration of a normal thyroid gland by ultrasound in patients with a thyroglossal duct cyst confirms a source of thyroid hormone. Consequently, a thyroid scan is not necessary.

Computed tomography and MRI scans provide better definition and extent of the mass. Computed tomography scan with contrast is the preferred method of imaging for deep neck abscesses that present with a neck mass and for enlarged salivary glands. Magnetic resonance imaging provides the best anatomic detail, and it is the preferred imaging study for children with vascular and lymphatic malformations and neoplasms; however, it is not as available as CT and often requires a greater degree of sedation.

Management

Neck masses are rarely acutely life-threatening. If neck masses impinge on the airway, children may experience stridor, hoarseness, drooling, increased effort of breathing, unequal breath sounds, or evidence of shock. Resuscitation and stabilization should be initiated immediately. The algorithm in Figure 82-4 outlines the management of cervical lymphadenitis.

Children with lymphadenitis who do not appear toxic and have no evidence of sepsis may be treated empirically with **oral antibiotics** that cover *S aureus*, particularly methicillin-resistant *S aureus* (MRSA), and GABHS. Clindamycin or a combination of cephalexin (administered until the culture from the lymph node, if available, for group A streptococcus is negative) and trimethoprim-sulfamethoxazole may be used to provide coverage for these organisms. If methicillin-susceptible *S aureus* (MSSA) is cultured and sensitivities are deter-

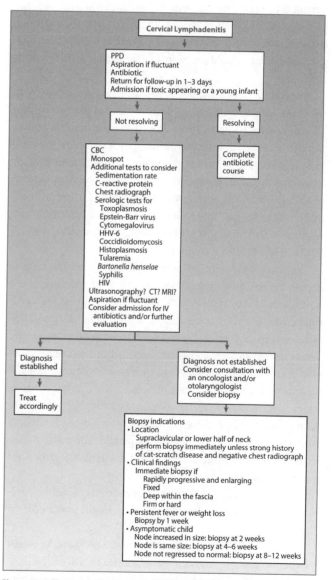

Figure 82-4. **Management of cervical lymphadenitis. Abbreviations: CBC, complete blood cell count; CT, computed tomography; HHV-6, human herpesvirus 6; HIV, human immunodeficiency virus; IV, intravenous; MRI, magnetic resonance imaging; PPD, purified protein derivative.**

mined, a first-generation cephalosporin such as cephalexin (50 mg/kg/day), dicloxacillin (50 mg/kg/day), or amoxicillin/clavulanic acid (40 mg/kg/day [amoxicillin]) may provide satisfactory coverage. Treatment should be continued for a minimum of 10 days but for no less than 5 days after resolution of acute signs and symptoms. Lack of clinical improvement after 36 to 48 hours suggests that the diagnosis and proposed therapy need to be reevaluated.

Infants and small children, as well as those older children who do not respond to oral antibiotic therapy, may require admission for **intravenous antibiotics,** such as clindamycin or vancomycin (especially for a potentially life-threatening infection) until culture results are available. If MSSA is cultured and sensitivities are determined, oxacillin or a cephalosporin may be satisfactory alternatives. Incision and drainage of large, fluctuant nodes that are clearly from bacterial disease should be done in consultation with an otolaryngologist or surgeon to promote resolution of the lymphadenitis. Alternatively, treatment by needle aspiration instead of incision and drainage has been advocated by some physicians. If *M tuberculosis,* atypical mycobacterial infection, or infection with *B henselae* is suspected, incision and drainage should not be done because persistent sinus tracts may result.

Atypical mycobacterial infection is generally unresponsive to treatment with antituberculous medications. **Surgical excision** of all visibly affected nodes, deep as well as superficial, is recommended. However, in cases in which surgery is refused or is incomplete or disease is recurrent, macrolide or azalide monotherapy (clarithromycin or azithromycin) or a macrolide in combination with ethambutol, rifampin, or rifabutin has been helpful in treating nontuberculous adenitis. Tuberculous mycobacterial adenitis usually responds to short-course medical therapy. Antituberculous medication for 6 to 9 months is recommended.

Lymphadenitis from cat-scratch disease usually resolves spontaneously in 2 to 4 months. Azithromycin may shorten the course and is recommended by some experts. Antibiotic therapy is indicated if children are severely ill or appear toxic with systemic cat-scratch disease, have hepatic or splenic involvement, are immunocompromised, develop meningoencephalitis, or are admitted for a suppurative adenitis. Treatment with oral antibiotics such as azithromycin, rifampin, trimethoprim-sulfamethoxazole, or ciprofloxacin may be beneficial. If there is no improvement, the addition of parenteral gentamicin to the regimen may be considered. **Aspiration** is indicated to relieve symptoms in patients with fluctuant or painful suppurative nodes. Incision and drainage should not be done. Total removal of the node is sometimes necessary to effect a cure.

There is no specific therapy for lymphadenitis caused by *Toxoplasma gondii*. Excision of the affected node may be indicated if the diagnosis is questionable.

If a tumor is suspected, consultation with a pediatric oncologist is recommended. The mass should be biopsied for a definitive diagnosis. If it is malignant, a treatment plan should be generated with the appropriate consultants.

Congenital torticollis from fibrosis of the sternocleidomastoid muscle is best treated with nonoperative intervention. Repetitive passive range-of-motion exercises over several weeks usually result in loosening the tight muscle and increasing the range of motion.

Fifty percent of hemangiomas will usually resolve by the time children are 5 years of age, 70% by age 7, and 90% by age 9. Surgical intervention is rarely indicated. Recent literature has demonstrated a profound benefit with oral propranolol therapy in the management of hemangiomas. Oral propranolol therapy demonstrates a considerable flattening and effacement of cutaneous and mucous membrane hemangiomas within 24 hours and marked improvement after weeks of propranolol therapy. While studies are small and underpowered, recent evidence suggests excellent efficacy with oral propranolol for the treatment of life-threatening, vital-organ–impairing (eg, vision loss), refractory, or disfiguring hemangiomas. Dosing is titrated up to 2 mg/kg/day and continued for weeks until resolution of the hemangioma. Patients should be closely monitored for hypoglycemia, bradycardia, hypotension, and congestive heart failure during institution of therapy for adverse effects usually requiring consultation with a cardiologist and a short hospitalization. Propranolol initiation is increasingly performed in the outpatient setting. Corticosteroids, previously the mainline treatment modality for hemangiomas, are now considered an adjunctive treatment with propranolol. Additional therapies include interferon alfa-2a and various cytotoxic medications. Interferon alfa-2a has been associated with transient or permanent neurologic disabilities, so it is important to balance the benefits and risks of this medication. High-potency topical corticosteroids such as clobetasol or topical beta blockers such as timolol may be used in selected cases.

Surgical excision is usually indicated for cystic hygromas (lymphangiomas), branchial cleft cysts, and thyroglossal duct cysts. A thyroid ultrasound should be performed before removal of a thyroglossal duct cyst to confirm that other thyroid tissue is not present. Endocrinologic consultation is recommended in these cases. Thyroid nodules in children may be cancerous, especially in children who have had irradiation to the head and neck region. Consultation with an endocrinologist and surgeon should be obtained. Goiters in children should be evaluated by an endocrinologist.

Prognosis

The prognosis for children with neck masses is generally excellent but differs depending on the cause. Children with an infectious etiology do very well if diagnosed and treated with appropriate antimicrobials. Mycobacterial lymphadenitis may result in sinus tract formation or disseminated disease. Surgical excision usually cures atypical mycobacterial infection. Cat-scratch disease is usually benign and self-limited. Encephalopathy is a rare complication of this disorder.

The prognosis for benign tumors of the neck is excellent. The outlook for children with malignant neck tumors depends on etiology of the tumor and spread of the malignancy to other organs. Early diagnosis and treatment are clearly important in improving outcome.

Children with neck masses from trauma usually have had significant injury. The outcome often depends on establishment of an airway, provision of ventilatory support, and management of hemodynamic instability. Availability of surgical support is often essential to a good outcome.

Children with congenital lesions of the neck usually have an excellent prognosis. Some lesions resolve spontaneously, while others require simple surgical excision. Cystic hygromas may require multiple operations for complete removal because of their diffuse nature.

CASE RESOLUTION

In the case presented, the boy has signs and symptoms consistent with submandibular bacterial cervical lymphadenitis. The location of the neck mass in relation to the honey-crusted lesions (nonbullous impetigo) implicates spread of bacteria from the primary site of infection to the lymph nodes. Laboratory tests are unnecessary because the child does not appear septic. Culture of the impetigo may be helpful in determining if the organism causing the infection is methicillin-resistant *Staphylococcus aureus* (MRSA). If the affected lymph node is fluctuant, aspiration of fluid for culture is indicated and incision and drainage should be considered. The child should be treated as an outpatient with an oral antibiotic directed against MRSA and group A beta-hemolytic streptococcus, such as clindamycin or a combination of cephalexin and trimethoprim-sulfamethoxazole, as well as an analgesic for pain as needed. If methicillin-susceptible *S aureus* is cultured and sensitivities are determined, cephalexin, amoxicillin-clavulanic acid, or dicloxacillin may be administered. If the child appears toxic or if there is marked lymph node enlargement, the child should be admitted for intravenous antibiotics. A purified protein derivative skin test should be placed. The child should be followed up in 1 to 3 days for clinical improvement depending on the severity of the infection.

Selected References

Acierno SP, Waldhausen JH. Congenital cervical cysts, sinuses and fistulae. *Otolaryngol Clin North Am.* 2007;40(1):161–176

Bauer PW, Lusk RP. Neck masses. In: Bluestone CD, Stool SE, Alper CM, et al, eds. *Pediatric Otolaryngology.* 4th ed. Philadelphia, PA: Saunders; 2003:1629–1647

Chadha NK, Forte V. Pediatric head and neck malignancies. *Curr Opin Otolaryngol Head Neck Surg.* 2009;17(6):471–476

Frieden IJ, Drolet BA. Propranolol for infantile hemangiomas: promise, peril, pathogenesis. *Pediatr Dermatol.* 2009;26(5):642–644

Goff CJ, Allred C, Glade RS. Current management of congenital branchial cleft cysts, sinuses, and fistulae. *Curr Opin Otolaryngol Head Neck Surg.* 2012;20(6):533–539

Gross E, Sichel JY. Congenital neck lesions. *Surg Clin North Am.* 2006;86(2):383–392

Holmes WJ, Mishra A, Gorst C, Liew SH. Propranolol as first-line treatment for rapidly proliferating infantile haemangiomas. *J Plast Reconstr Aesthet Surg.* 2011;64(4):445–451

Knight PJ, Mulne AF, Vassy LE. When is lymph node biopsy indicated in children with enlarged peripheral nodes? *Pediatrics.* 1982;69(4):391–396

Lawley LP, Siegfried E, Todd JL. Propranolol treatment for hemangioma of infancy: risks and recommendations. *Pediatr Dermatol.* 2009;26(5):610–614

Léauté-Labrèze C, Dumas de la Roque E, Hubiche T, Boralevi F, Thambo JB, Taïeb A. Propranolol for severe hemangiomas of infancy. *N Engl J Med.* 2008;358(24):2649–2651

Malley R. Lymphadenopathy. In: Fleisher GR, Ludwig S, eds. *Textbook of Pediatric Emergency Medicine.* 5th ed. Philadelphia, PA: Lippincott; 2006:421–428

Pasha R. *Otolaryngology: Head and Neck Surgery Clinical Reference Guide.* 2nd ed. San Diego, CA: Plural Publishing, Inc; 2006:79, 207

Pruden CM, McAneney CM. Neck mass. In: Fleisher GR, Ludwig S, eds. *Textbook of Pediatric Emergency Medicine.* 6th ed. Philadelphia, PA: Lippincott Williams and Wilkins; 2010:385–391

Rajasekaran K, Krakovitz P. Enlarged neck lymph nodes in children. *Pediatr Clin North Am.* 2013;60(4):923–936

Sans V, de la Roque ED, Berge J, et al. Propranolol for severe infantile hemangiomas: follow-up report. *Pediatrics.* 2009;124(3):e423–e431

Skandalakis JE. Neck. In: Skandalakis LJ, Skandalakis JE, Skandalakis PN, eds. *Surgical Anatomy and Technique.* 3rd ed. New York, NY: Springer; 2009:2

Tanphaichitr A, Bhushan B, Maddalozzo J, Schroeder JW Jr. Ultrasonography in the treatment of a pediatric midline neck mass. *Arch Otolaryngol Head Neck Surg.* 2012;138(9):823–827

CHAPTER 83

Allergic Disease

Kenny Yat-Choi Kwong, MD, and Nasser Redjal, MD

CASE STUDY

A 3-year-old girl is rushed to the office by her mother after her daughter developed a pruritic rash, facial swelling, and hoarseness shortly after eating a peanut butter sandwich. She had eaten peanut butter once before and her parents noticed a few small hives on her cheek, which self-resolved. Previously, she has been well except for recurrent nasal congestion every spring that has responded to antihistamines. She has also had an intermittent skin rash that has been treated with topical steroid creams. She has never had an acute reaction before and has no history of asthma. Her father had asthma as a child.

Physical examination reveals a well-developed, 3-year-old girl with marked facial swelling and a **generalized rash** who is in mild respiratory distress. Vital signs, including blood pressure, are normal. The girl has a diffuse,

blotchy, erythematous rash with central wheals; a hoarse voice; and a mild expiratory wheeze on auscultation of her chest. The remainder of the examination is normal.

Questions

1. What are the various symptoms of allergic disease?
2. What is the appropriate evaluation of children with manifestations of allergic disease?
3. What allergens are common triggers for allergic symptoms?
4. What management is helpful in the treatment of children with manifestations of allergic disease?
5. Can allergic disease be prevented?

Allergic disease, which occurs frequently in the general population, is manifested in many ways. Asthma, atopic dermatitis, allergic rhinitis, allergic conjunctivitis, urticaria, angioedema, anaphylaxis, and food, insect, and drug allergies are all types of allergic diseases. Allergic symptoms result from the production of specific immunoglobulin E (IgE) antibody following exposure to a foreign antigen. The process has 2 steps. The first step is the sensitization or antibody induction stage. The individual develops IgE antibody against an inhaled, ingested, or injected substance. The process usually takes a period of time ranging from several days or weeks for medications and foods to months or years for inhalant allergens like pollens. Newly formed antigen-specific IgE antibody adheres to IgE receptors on circulating blood basophils or to tissue mast cells. On reexposure, the allergen then binds to several specific IgE antibodies on the surface of these cells and triggers degranulation of preformed and rapidly formed mediators such as histamine and leukotrienes, resulting in the early phase of the reaction. Clinically, this is manifested by sneezing, rhinorrhea, and pruritus in allergic rhinitis; wheal/flare in urticaria/angioedema, and shock in anaphylaxis. Mast cell degranulation also releases peptides that attract inflammatory peptides such as IL-4 and IL-5, which release mediators that result in chronic inflammation. This is called the late phase of inflammation and is responsible for congestion and hyperreactive mucosa in allergic rhinitis and delayed reactions in anaphylaxis (see chapters 84 and 125). This chapter focuses on the remaining manifestations of allergies, including allergic rhinitis, conjunctivitis, food allergies, and anaphylaxis.

Epidemiology

Allergic disease or some form of allergic symptom is found in 12% to 20% of the general population. The prevalence of symptoms varies depending on the population being investigated. Factors such as age, genetic background, and place of residence are significant. Allergic rhinitis occurs in 10% of children, as does asthma. Up to 6% of children younger than 3 years develop food allergies. Urticaria occurs at some time in about 10% to 20% of the population.

It is generally accepted that if neither parent is atopic (ie, has the allergic tendency to manufacture IgE on antigen exposure), the chance that children will develop allergic symptoms is less than 1 in 5. If one parent is atopic, the risk doubles. If both parents are atopic, the chance is better than 3 in 5.

Pathophysiology and Clinical Presentation

Allergic rhinitis, like all allergic manifestations, is caused primarily by an antigen-antibody reaction involving IgE. Antigen-specific IgE is produced by the B lymphocytes of allergic patients on exposure to a particular antigen, which attaches to immune cell receptors located on basophils in the circulation and mast cells in the tissue. On reexposure, the antigen reacts with this specific IgE on the mast cells, releasing vasoactive mediators including histamine, leukotrienes, kinins, and prostaglandins. These mediators produce vasodilation and edema, and they also stimulate neural reflexes to produce mucous hypersecretion and sneezing. Eosinophils, basophils, and other inflammatory cells induced by chemotactic factors enter the affected organ, releasing mediators, thereby worsening the inflammation and damaging tissues. Secretions and released tissue proteins exacerbate existing edema. Other immunologic mechanisms can also be involved.

Children with allergic rhinitis often present with rhinorrhea, sneezing, nasal pruritus, and congestion. Allergic eye symptoms (allergic rhinitis and conjunctivitis) may accompany nasal rhinitis with ocular pruritus, injection of the conjunctiva, and clear tearing.

Urticaria, the clinical rash produced by capillary leak vasodilation and edema of the skin, occurs when histamine and other vasoactive peptides such as prostaglandins and leukotrienes are released from the epidermal mast cells. Mast cell degranulation occurs commonly in sensitized patients on reexposure to antigens found in food, medications, supplements, and insect venom when antigen-specific IgE found on mast cells are triggered by these allergens. The mast cell, however, can also be activated and release mediators by a wide number of stimuli independent of IgE mechanisms, including viral, bacteria, parasitic, and fungal infections; collagen vascular disease; malignancy; and endocrine disease. Some patients also experience urticaria to physical factors such as heat, cold, pressure, sun, and vibration.

An urticarial rash appears as erythematous lesions of various sizes with pale, papular centers. Lesions may coalesce, the rash blanches on pressure, and the skin is intact. Usually, lesions last less than 24 hours at a single location, although they may recur in the same place often.

Angioedema is the extension of the urticarial process deeper into the dermis of the skin, producing swelling. The mucous membranes may be affected. Pathophysiology is similar to that for urticaria. A hereditary type of angioedema, which is not allergy related, is caused by an inherited deficiency of the C1 esterase inhibitor, resulting in unopposed production of the potent vasoactive amine bradykinin. Unlike urticaria, there is no distinct rash and the skin is not pruritic. Capillary leak and edema of the dermis results in tissue swelling, a sense of tightness, and possibly pain. Involvement of the abdominal viscera may produce colicky abdominal pain.

Chronic urticaria and angioedema are considered chronic when they persist beyond 6 weeks. More than 90% of chronic urticaria and angioedema in an otherwise healthy patient is idiopathic and termed chronic idiopathic urticaria. Up to half of patients with chronic idiopathic urticaria have a circulating mast cell anti-IgE receptor antibody (IgG) that chronically causes cutaneous mast cell to degranulate in these patients.

Anaphylaxis is an acute, systemic allergic reaction resulting from antigen-specific IgE on mast cells and basophils. Pathophysiology is similar to allergic rhinitis, but the reaction occurs in mast cells in many locations simultaneously, and prior sensitization to an allergen is essential. Anaphylactic reactions may be life-threatening. Massive vasoactive mediator release results in large reductions in peripheral resistance due to capillary leak and vasodilation. This eventually overwhelms compensatory increases in cardiac output (blood pressure = cardiac output × total peripheral resistance), leading to hypotension

and shock. Pooling of blood in the periphery also reduces venous return, resulting in diminished preload and cardiac output. Reactions can occur in seconds or as late as 1 hour after exposure. Up to 20% of adult patients may experience a late or biphasic phase hours after the first reaction due to late recruitment and activation of basophils and other inflammatory cells. Children with anaphylaxis have a lower risk of late phase reaction, likely around 3% to 5%. Common causes of anaphylaxis include food, medications and biologic agents, and stinging insect venom. The drug most frequently implicated in anaphylaxis is penicillin. Patients initially experience tightness and intense itching of the skin. Nausea, vomiting, and abdominal pain may ensue. Subsequently, the full spectrum of anaphylaxis appears. Certain agents such as radiocontrast media and blood products may cause massive mast cell degranulation via an IgE-independent mechanism. This results in clinical symptoms that are indistinguishable from anaphylaxis. These reactions, termed anaphylactoid reactions, are generally less severe.

There is confusion among less experienced clinicians as to what combination of symptoms constitutes anaphylaxis, which may lead to overdiagnosis and underdiagnosis. In general, anaphylaxis is highly likely when there are cutaneous findings plus respiratory or hemodynamic compromise; involvement of 2 or more of the skin, respiratory, and gastrointestinal (GI) organ systems; and hemodynamic compromise (Box 83-1).

A **food allergy** may produce IgE-mediated reactions and diseases, including acute urticaria or angioedema, anaphylaxis, acute rhinitis, and atopic dermatitis. The localization of IgE-sensitized mast cells to that specific antigen determines the symptoms produced by an allergy. The antigen enters through the GI mucosal barrier. Intact food proteins may enter the circulation, stimulating the production of antigen-specific IgE. In addition, food allergens may result in some non–IgE-mediated diseases, including eosinophilic esophagitis, food protein–induced enterocolitis syndrome (FPIES), allergic proctocolitis, and Heiner syndrome, a rare reaction

---

Box 83-1. Practical Definition of Anaphylaxis

One of the following criteria is fulfilled:

1. Acute onset of mucosa or cutaneous findings such as hives, pruritus, lip swelling, AND one of the following:
   - Respiratory compromise
   - Cardiovascular compromise such as hypotension or end-organ dysfunction such as syncope

2. TWO of the following after likely exposure to allergen:
   - Respiratory compromise
   - Mucocutaneous symptoms
   - Hypotension
   - Persistent gastrointestinal symptoms

3. Reduced blood pressure appropriate for age

Adapted from Sampson HA, Muñoz-Furlong A, Campbell RL, et al. Second symposium on the definition and management of anaphylaxis: summary report—second National Institute of Allergy and Infectious Disease/Food Allergy and Anaphylaxis Network symposium *Ann Emerg Med.* 2006;47(4):373–380, with permission.

to cow's milk protein. Finally, many patients have nonimmune-mediated reactions to foods termed *food intolerances* (eg, lactose intolerance).

In young children, the most common food allergens are milk, egg, soy, wheat, peanuts, and tree nuts, while adults and older children are allergic to peanuts, shellfish, and fish. Adults and older children with atopic predisposition and allergic rhinitis or asthma often become sensitized to tree and weed pollens via the respiratory tract. They exhibit cross-reactivity between common elements of these inhalant tree or weed pollen peptides and similar peptides found in fruits and vegetables, resulting in local (oral) IgE symptoms of tingling and mild swelling when ingesting these foods. These mild reactions are called pollen food allergy syndrome (PFAS).

Patients with IgE-mediated food allergy may experience urticaria or angioedema, eczematoid rash, vomiting, wheezing, and, in severe cases, anaphylaxis. Eosinophilic esophagitis presents with nonspecific symptoms, including vomiting, reflux, dyspepsia, poor appetite, and failure to thrive. Infants with FPIES present with severe vomiting and bloody stools, generalized edema, and, in some cases, shock on initial ingestion of cow's milk, although soy and other foods have, in rare cases, been implicated. Allergic proctocolitis presents in infants on first exposure to cow's milk protein, including via human milk, but symptoms are mild and only involve blood-streaked stools. Heiner syndrome is a rare IgG-mediated reaction to cow's milk protein that results in anemia, wheezing, hemoptysis, melena, and pulmonary infiltrates. Older patients experiencing PFAS to fruits and vegetables experience lip and oral mucosa, tongue tingling, and minimal swelling. These are local and mild and rarely progress to anaphylaxis.

Differential Diagnosis

Most patients with **allergic rhinitis** have clear-cut signs and symptoms consistent with a history of exposure; however, other etiologies should be considered, especially when there is poor response to treatment. Children experience many upper viral respiratory infections a year that can mimic allergic rhinitis. There are many types of nonallergic rhinitis and mechanisms responsible are unclear, although cholinergic pathways are likely involved. Vasomotor and cholinergic rhinitis often result in copious amounts of clear rhinorrhea in response to cholinergic stimuli such as cold air (skier nose) or spicy foods (gustatory rhinitis). Medications such as angiotensin-converting enzyme inhibitors and nonsteroidal anti-inflammatory drugs may cause rhinitis but usually in adults and older children. Similarly, hormone surges, such as during ovulation, may result in nasal symptoms. Overuse of topical decongestants containing α-agonists results in rebound rhinitis (rhinitis medicamentosa). In children, foreign bodies produce unilateral nasal obstruction and often malodorous purulent discharge. Finally, patients a with history of basilar skull fractures with cerebrospinal fluid leak may present with clear rhinorrhea.

Urticaria and angioedema have a distinct clinical presentation that is usually easy to distinguish from other skin conditions. As mentioned previously, the challenge is to determine the cause of urticaria and angioedema given the numerous possible etiologies. Urticaria and angioedema may last for weeks; however, individual lesions should persist for less than 24 hours, though they can recur at one area. Urticarial vasculitis is a distinct form of urticaria that results from the persistence of antigens arising from collagen vascular disease, serum sickness, and neoplasia. The rash from urticarial vasculitis lasts for more than 24 hours, has a burning sensation, causes less pruritus, and leaves an area of hyperpigmentation on resolution. Other rashes that mimic urticaria include insect bites, erythema multiforme, mastocytosis, and contact dermatitis. Anaphylaxis is usually associated with cutaneous, respiratory, cardiovascular, and systemic symptoms such as skin rash, edema, wheezing, arrythmia, occasionally fever, and shock. A history of an acute exposure is more likely to be seen with anaphylaxis.

Signs and symptoms of **food allergies** vary. It is important to determine whether there is actual immune-mediated disease or if the patient has food intolerance. Food may contain toxic peptides, such as in scombroid fish poisoning, in which bacteria in unrefrigerated fish convert amino acids into histamine, which results in allergy-like symptoms when ingested. Patients with enzyme deficiencies such as lactose intolerance will experience GI symptoms when eating dairy products. Finally, food may have pharmacologic properties such as those found in caffeinated drinks.

Non–IgE-mediated food allergies may produce signs and symptoms similar to other disorders, which can be life-threatening (eg, FPIES, often indistinguishable from sepsis; Heiner syndrome, which shares similarities with serious diseases such as pulmonary hemosiderosis and Wegner granulomatosis). These conditions must be ruled out during the evaluation of these forms of food allergies.

Lastly, the majority of patients with symptoms associated with foods do not have an immune-mediated reaction but have food intolerances. Some manifestations have well-defined mechanisms, such as in lactase deficiency or galactosemia, while others, such as gustatory rhinitis, are less clear.

Evaluation

History and Physical Examination

Allergic Rhinitis and Conjunctivitis

Children with possible allergic rhinitis have a history of sneezing, itching, nasal discharge, and nasal blockage. The eyes, ears, palate, and throat may itch. They may also have a history of mouth breathing and snoring at night, sleep disturbances, and daytime fatigue from nasal obstruction. Other signs include sinusitis, postnasal drip, halitosis, cough, and morning sore throat. Symptoms may be seasonal or associated with a specific stimulus. In addition, systemic symptoms of fatigue, headache, anorexia, and irritability may be present.

The history should also include a search for other manifestations of allergies (eg, wheezing, atopic dermatitis) as well as a family history of atopy. An environmental history of allergen exposure, including pets and tobacco smoke, is also important to obtain.

The physical examination should be thorough. The skin should be inspected for atopic dermatitis and the lungs for evidence of asthma. The nasal mucosa should be examined with an otoscope. In children with allergic rhinitis, the nasal mucosa is swollen, pale, and sometimes cyanotic with copious clear discharge. Nasal polyps, if present, should be noted. Although polyps are most often present on an allergic basis, they may occur with cystic fibrosis. A transverse crease across the nose ("allergic creases") can occur from repeatedly using the palm of the hand in an upward thrust on the nares to relieve itching and open the nasal airway ("allergic salute"). Dark circles under the eyes ("allergic shiners") may be present from chronic periorbital edema and venous stasis. Morgan fold (also called Dennie sign), a wrinkle just beneath the lower eyelids, is present from early infancy and is associated with atopic dermatitis and allergic rhinitis. Allergic gape or adenoid facies is secondary to chronic mouth breathing during the first several years of life and results in a characteristic pattern of maldevelopment of facial bones, causing a high-arched palate, flat maxilla, and angulated mandible with a recessed chin and dental malocclusion (Figure 83-1). If affected, the conjunctivae are erythematous with a clear discharge and may have a follicular appearance. The mouth may reveal a high-arched palate from chronic mouth breathing, and hypertrophic lymphoid follicles in the oropharynx often can be seen.

Classification of allergic rhinitis, while not as stringent as that of asthma, is important because it guides the choice of optimal therapy. According to the World Health Organization Allergic Rhinitis and Its Impact on Asthma guidelines, allergic rhinitis is considered to be intermittent if symptoms occur fewer than 4 days a week or fewer than 4 weeks in duration, while persistent rhinitis is defined as symptoms occurring more than 4 days a week or more than 4 weeks in duration. Further, mild allergic rhinitis is defined as having no sleep disturbances; normal daily activities, sports, and leisure; normal school or work; and no troublesome symptoms. One or more of these symptoms results in classification of moderate/severe persistent allergic rhinitis (Box 83-2). Thus, allergic rhinitis may be classified as mild intermittent, moderate/severe intermittent, mild persistent, and moderate/severe persistent.

Complications of chronic allergic rhinitis may be evident on examination, including chronic serous otitis, recurrent otitis media, hearing loss secondary to otitis, sinusitis, nasal polyps, sleep apnea, or dental malocclusion.

Urticaria and Angioedema

Because the most common causes of urticaria and angioedema in children are foods, medications, supplements, and viral infections, questions should focus on recent exposures to drugs, dietary changes, new soaps or detergents, environmental agents, and recent viral illnesses. Consideration should also be given to other serious conditions such as collagen vascular disease and neoplasm. Laboratory tests are usually not required unless the history and physical examination suggests a potential etiology (eg, a patient with urticaria, joint swelling, pallor, and fatigue requires testing for evidence of systemic lupus erythematosus and malignancy).

Anaphylaxis

The focus of the history in a patient with anaphylaxis is an acute exposure to a foreign antigen (eg, medication, food, venom). Although most patients react within minutes to hours after exposure to the causative agent, there are reports of anaphylactic reactions many hours to days after exposure. Therefore, the history must be inclusive of this time frame.

Hemodynamically, patients have reduced peripheral resistance resulting from vasodilation and capillary leak. This results in warm skin and flushing. Compensatory increases in cardiac output result in tachycardia and bounding pulses. Patients often feel a sense of doom. Hypotension ensues if shock is untreated. Respiratory

Figure 83-1. Characteristic facial features in children with allergic diseases. A, Allergic shiner. B, Allergic salute. C, Adenoid facies.

Box 83-2. Classification of Allergic Rhinitis		
Frequency	**Severity**	
	Mild No sleep disturbances No impairment of activities, sports, leisure Normal school and work No troublesome symptoms	**Moderate/severe** One or more of • Sleep disturbance • Impairment of activities, sports, leisure • Abnormal school and work • Troublesome symptoms
Intermittent <4 d/wk <4 wk	**Mild intermittent**	**Moderate/severe intermittent**
Persistent >4 d/wk >4 wk	**Mild persistent**	**Moderate/severe persistent**

Adapted from Adkinson NF Jr, Bochner BS, Busse WW, et al, eds. *Middleton's Allergy: Principles and Practice.* 7th ed. St. Louis, MO: Mosby; 2009.

Box 83-3. Specific Food Immunoglobulin E Levels and Likelihood of Clinical Reactivity			
Food	IgE (kU/L)	PPV	NPV
Egg	7	98	36
Egg (<2 y)	2	95	
Milk	15	95	53
Milk (<1 y)	5	95	
Peanut	14	99	36
Soy	30	73	82
Fish	20	99	89
Wheat	26	74	87

Abbreviations: IgE, immunoglobulin E; NPV, negative predictive value; PPV, positive predictive value.

Adapted from Adkinson NF Jr, Bochner BS, Busse WW, et al, eds. *Middleton's Allergy: Principles and Practice.* 7th ed. St. Louis, MO: Mosby; 2009.

symptoms include airway edema with upper airway obstruction and stridor, and smooth muscle constriction results in wheezing and respiratory distress. Some patients will have GI symptoms including vomiting, abdominal discomfort or pain, and diarrhea. The majority of patients with anaphylaxis will have skin manifestations, usually urticaria.

The most common cause of death from anaphylaxis is respiratory compromise followed by hemodynamic collapse.

Food Allergies

Diagnosing food allergy is not difficult if there is a clear association of a reaction after ingestion of a specific food. Timing of the reaction is usually minutes to a few hours after ingestion. This is obviously less clear after a meal with multiple ingredients. An accurate diet diary will help narrow down the list of potential reactive foods. Negative food allergy test results via skin or in vitro serum IgE are reliable in ruling out a food; however, positive test results have limited predictive value unless values are high (Box 83-3). Therefore, positive test results suggest a food is responsible for a reaction, and confirmation should be pursued via an elimination period followed by food challenge. The double-blind, placebo-controlled food challenge is the gold standard; however, it is impractical in most community clinical settings. National food allergy guidelines recommend using open food challenges to confirm a diagnosis. An absolute exception is when there is serious systemic reaction, such as anaphylaxis, in which case a strong history and a positive skin or serum test result will suffice for diagnosis.

Laboratory Tests

The diagnosis of an allergic disease can be made with a thorough history and physical examination and empiric therapy with no further investigations. Additional tests are performed when the diagnosis is in question, to provide optimal avoidance strategies, and if allergen immunotherapy is needed. Testing may be needed for the diagnosis of food allergy and further evaluation of urticaria and angioedema.

History of exposure followed by symptoms can suggest causative agents, but the combination of **allergy testing** with history will improve the positive predictive value of a specific antigen causing the symptoms. For example, a patient with year-round indoor symptoms of rhinorrhea and nasal pruritus may be allergic to dust mites, cats, dogs, cockroaches, or mold. Subsequent allergen testing will thus elucidate which single allergen or combination of allergens is responsible. This results in a more focused and effective approach to environmental control. Allergen testing is also necessary if allergen immunotherapy is being considered.

Allergy testing may be achieved with in vivo skin-prick testing or in vitro specific IgE testing. Skin tests are sensitive and accurate. Positive test results indicate the presence of an antigen-specific IgE. Although skin testing may be less reliable in infants because their skin is less reactive, these tests have been performed in infants as young as 4 months. Fewer allergens are usually tested in children younger than 2 years because these patients have not been sensitized to a wide range of antigens. Currently, skin-prick testing is the recommended method for skin tests. Intradermal testing involving injection of allergen under the skin is used for testing of stinging insect allergy and various medication hypersensitivity and rarely required for the diagnosis of inhalant or food allergen sensitization. When evaluating food allergy, intradermal testing should not be performed because of the risk of precipitating a systemic reaction.

In vitro allergen-specific IgE concentrations (ImmunoCap/ radioallergosorbent tests) in sera, which are also available for the laboratory assessment of allergies, provide a measure of the amount of IgE specific for individual allergens. In general, in vitro tests have similar sensitivity and specificity as skin testing but are more expensive. In vitro tests have an advantage in that they can be performed on patients who are using medications that affect skin-testing reactivity, such as antihistamines and tricyclic antidepressants. In addition, they are preferred tests in patients who have poor skin reactivity, such as the very young and very old, those who do not have skin findings, such as atopic dermatitis and dermographism, and who may have anaphylaxis to the allergens being tested.

For inhalant allergens, in vivo and in vitro tests have good negative and positive predictive values. Both tests have good negative predictive value for food allergy but positive predictive value of approximately 50%. For certain foods, very high levels of specific IgE have good positive predictive values (see Box 83-3).

Other screening tests may include a nasal smear for eosinophils. More than 10% eosinophils is consistent with allergic rhinitis. Although serum IgE levels are elevated in 60% of patients with allergic rhinitis and asthma, they are not sensitive or specific and have limited value. Rhinoscopy in adults and older children provides a painless method to detect pathology not visible by anterior inspection via the nares. These include identification of nasal polyps, deviated nasal septum, adenoidal hypertrophy extending into the nares, sinusitis, vocal cord edema, and polyps and potential masses. Computed tomography (CT) scans are clinically very useful because they reveal structural abnormalities and mucosal disease, including findings within sinus cavities. The need for such information has to be weighed against the high doses of radiation associated with CT scans. Plain sinus radiographs are rarely indicated due to their limited ability to detail nasal anatomy and high rates of false negatives for sinusitis along with exposure to radiation.

Management

General Principles

Avoidance of allergen triggers is a natural way to control allergy symptoms without medication and should be encouraged in all patients with allergic disease. It is currently the only option available to patients with food allergy and anaphylaxis.

For patients with allergic rhinitis, conjunctivitis, and asthma, allergic triggers consist of perennial and seasonal allergens. Perennial allergens usually include house dust mites, warm-blooded animals with fur (eg, cats, dogs, rodents), cockroaches, and indoor pollens (usually molds). Seasonal allergens include pollen from trees, grasses, weeds, and outdoor molds. Effective environmental controls for these are outlined in Box 83-4. In addition to allergic triggers, nonallergic irritant triggers such as tobacco smoke, automobile exhaust, smog, and perfumes should be avoided.

While environmental controls are safe and effective, they may be labor intensive, expensive, and, in rare cases, psychologically detrimental. For instance, removal of carpeting is difficult and expensive, especially in rented housing. Dust mite–proof coverings are expensive and cumbersome to wash in hot water weekly. Removal of family pets may lead to psychologic issues if children have become attached. Patients are more likely to institute environmental controls if there is evidence of allergic sensitization via skin-prick or blood tests.

Currently, there is no therapy to treat patients with food allergies except avoidance of the triggering food. Food avoidance should be undertaken only after a careful history, allergy testing, and a trial of food elimination and challenge to correctly identify the culprit. A poor history and false-positive testing result in many foods being

Box 83-4. Environmental Control Strategies	
Dust mites	• Cover mite reservoirs with mite-proof covers (eg, mattress, pillows, box springs, comforter). • Wash linen in hot water once a week. • Remove mite reservoirs such as carpets and, if possible, stuffed toys. • Use HEPA filter in conjunction with mite reduction strategies. • Use vacuum cleaner that has HEPA filtration.
Pets (eg, dogs, cats)	• Do not get a warm-blooded furry pet (even if initially not allergic to cats or dogs) because children may sensitize to them later, at which time it will be difficult to remove the pet from the home. • Bathing the pet once a week will reduce allergen load. • Have child's room pet free or, if possible, have outside cat or dog. • Use of HEPA filter may help • Re-home pet, if possible. (Note: Cat dander may linger for many months, and continuous house cleaning is required even after removal of pet.)
Cockroaches/ rodents	• Use of boric acid for cockroach control is a pesticide-free strategy. • Rodents and cockroach often require professional extermination.
Mold	• Repair water damage. • Reduce humidity.
Pollens	• Use HEPA filter. • Close windows at night (plants usually pollinate in early morning).

Abbreviation: HEPA, high-efficiency particulate air.

implicated, a draconian elimination diet, and undernutrition. Patients truly allergic to multiple foods benefit from consultation with a registered nutritionist or dietitian. Additionally, patients should be taught to read food labels to avoid offending foods.

Children generally lose sensitivity to milk, soy, egg, and wheat by school age. For instance, one large study noted that 85% of milk-allergic and 66% of egg-allergic children lost their sensitivity by 5 years of age. Only about 20% of peanut-allergic patients will lose their sensitivity, and even less become tolerant of fish and shellfish. Understanding the natural history of food allergies allows the clinician to liberalize the diet if retesting shows negative or reduced reactivity and a supervised food challenge is negative. The decision to challenge depends on the nutritional and social importance of a particular food.

Many patients with FPIES, allergic proctocolitis, and Heiner syndrome also outgrow their food hypersensitivities. The natural history of eosinophilic esophagitis is less clear. Rechallenge to more severe diseases like FPIES must be performed in a monitored settings with staff competent at resuscitation.

Anaphylaxis is a **medical emergency.** Rapid reversal of cardiovascular or respiratory compromise is essential. Epinephrine is the first agent given to increase systemic vascular resistance, reverse bronchospasm, and lessen airway edema. A 0.01 mL/kg per dose of 1:1,000 aqueous solution is given intramuscularly in the lateral thigh. This route achieves high serum concentrations in the shortest time compared with other routes. Subcutaneous injection is no longer recommended. If symptoms progress or do not improve, epinephrine may be repeated in 5 to 10 minutes. Refractory symptoms have been treated with intravenous (IV) epinephrine diluted to 1:10,000. However, because of the significant cardiac effects of IV epinephrine, cardiac monitoring must be instituted. Because vasoactive mediators result in capillary leak of fluids into the peripheral tissue, rapid volume expansion with normal saline or similar colloids should be instituted early, especially if there is poor response to epinephrine. Administration of epinephrine must not be delayed; the majority of deaths from anaphylaxis have been associated with delayed epinephrine administration.

Oxygen therapy should be instituted and bronchodilator drugs, such as albuterol, given for bronchospasm and wheezing concomitant with epinephrine. H_1- and H_2-receptor antagonists, such as diphenhydramine and ranitidine, are usually given as well as systemic corticosteroids such as methylprednisolone. Intravenous administration of these drugs ensures systemic delivery, especially if there is vomiting. However, antihistamines and corticosteroids are rapidly absorbed orally, and absorption of diphenhydramine is also good intramuscularly. These routes should considered if IV access cannot be established in a timely fashion.

Due to the risk of a late-phase reaction or a biphasic reaction, patients with anaphylaxis must be observed for a period, usually 4 to 8 hours. Administration of systemic corticosteroids and antihistamines does not adequately reduce the risk of late-phase reactions. Patients must be discharged with an epinephrine auto-injector and taught how to use it (0.15 mg for patients up to 66 lb; 0.3 mg for patients ≥66 lb). Inpatient observation is appropriate for patients experiencing severe reactions or who need prolonged resuscitation, when triggers are unclear, if there is difficulty getting an epinephrine auto-injector, and if parents are not capable of recognizing anaphylactic symptoms or administering treatment. Medical alert bracelets should be issued if the offending agent is known.

The management of **urticaria and angioedema** should begin with the identification of the causal agent and its elimination. Offending foods or medications should be avoided, underlying infections should be treated, and more serious etiologies, such as collagen vascular disease and malignancy, should be worked up and managed. Medications are required to treat bothersome symptoms and include H_1- and H_2-receptor antagonists and, in severe or persistent cases, corticosteroids. Tricyclic antidepressants are also used in adults and older children because of their potent antihistamine effects.

Medications

Avoidance of allergens and triggers is sufficient in mild disease, but often, addition of medications is usually required when symptoms persist or are more severe.

Antihistamines or H_1-receptor antagonists have been used extensively in the treatment of allergic diseases and are effective in reducing symptoms of pruritus, rhinorrhea, and sneezing. They are less effective in relieving nasal congestion, although many patients report that their nasal congestion improves with these agents. These agents are also effective in reducing hives, swelling, and pruritus in urticaria and angioedema. First-generation antihistamines include diphenhydramine, chlorpheniramine, and brompheniramine, which, though effective, have significant sedating side effects. Even when administered at bedtime, patients show diminished concentration and attention the next day; sedating antihistamines can impair learning in schoolchildren. Newer H_1-receptor antagonists, such as loratadine, cetirizine, and fexofenadine, are less sedating and should be used as first-line agents in children. Some patients report lower efficacy of these less-sedating antihistamines compared with older ones. Newer intranasal antihistamines, such as desmethyl azelastine, have a rapid onset of action, are effective, and are very safe but are also sedating.

Anti-inflammatory agents include intranasal corticosteroids, intranasal cromolyn sodium, and systemic corticosteroids. Intranasal corticosteroids have become the mainstay in treatment of allergic rhinitis because of their powerful, broad anti-inflammatory properties and excellent safety profile. They are effective in reducing pruritus, rhinorrhea, sneezing, and congestion when used on a chronic preventive basis. Topical intranasal therapy has minimal to no effects on the hypothalamic-pituitary-adrenal axis when newer corticosteroids such as fluticasone and mometasone are used. Older agents such as beclomethasone have more bioavailability, and children may experience very small but significant growth delays. Cromolyn sodium is a mast-cell stabilizer and has virtually no side effects. Clinical efficacy is, however, poor, and it is now used infrequently. Although most patients with allergic rhinitis do not require systemic corticosteroids, some patients refractory to treatment may benefit from a short course of oral corticosteroids, such as prednisone. Systemic steroids are usually used to control urticaria and angioedema and are mandatory in the management of anaphylaxis.

Alpha-adrenergic agents are used systemically as well as topically to treat rhinitis. Oral agents such as pseudoephedrine and phenylephrine are effective but cause alpha-adrenergic side effects, such as tachycardia and jitteriness. Topical agents, such as oxymetazoline, are potent vasoconstrictors and can dramatically improve nasal obstruction, but routine use for more than 3 to 5 days results in rebound congestion with persistent and worse symptoms (rhinitis medicamentosa).

Leukotrienes have biological effects similar to histamine and also recruit inflammatory cells into tissue. Therefore, the leukotriene-receptor antagonist, montelukast, can be used as monotherapy for the treatment of allergic rhinitis. Intranasal corticosteroids have better efficacy than montelukast, but the latter is an oral agent that promotes better compliance. Additionally, allergic rhinitis is often comorbid with asthma, and montelukast has the advantage of treating both conditions.

Normal saline washes provide a medication-free adjunctive treatment of allergic rhinitis, and their use has increased in popularity among patients.

Immunotherapy is very effective for the long-term treatment of allergic rhinitis, allergic conjunctivitis, and stinging insect venom hypersensitivity and is also recommended for asthma and atopic dermatitis when avoidance strategies and medications are not controlling symptoms. This treatment is effective for symptoms caused by dust mites, pollens, animal dander, molds, and insect venom. Immunotherapy involves a series of injections with extracts of allergens specific for individual patients, producing tolerance to particular antigens. The mechanism of action of immunotherapy is related to the development of allergen-specific blocking antibody (IgG), increased allergen-specific T regulatory cells, decreased lymphocyte cytokine response to an allergen, and decreased basophil histamine release in response to an allergen. The results of skin testing dictate which allergens to use. Initially, injections are given weekly with increasing doses until maintenance concentrations are achieved, at which point they are spaced out to every 4 weeks. Immunotherapy is given in a supervised setting with an observation period of approximately 20 minutes because there is a small possibility of anaphylaxis.

In Europe, immunotherapy using sublingual delivery of antigens has been used effectively for many years without the need for injections. Commercial extracts of sublingual immunotherapy antigens were beginning to be approved in the United States at the time of publication.

Caveats About Treatment

Because patients with **allergic rhinitis** are repeatedly exposed to allergens, they may require use of anti-inflammatory agents such as intranasal corticosteroids as first-line therapy. Current national guidelines recommend anti-inflammatory agents as first-line therapy for moderate/severe persistent disease and can be considered for mild persistent and moderate/severe intermittent disease. Patients may require long-term use of anti-inflammatory agents in combination with antihistamines (Figure 83-2).

Allergic conjunctivitis often coexists with allergic rhinitis. Control of nasal symptoms may result in improvement of eye symptoms, but ocular medications may also be required. Available medications include antihistamines, mast-cell stabilizers, vasoconstrictors, and combination agents. The sight-threatening allergic ocular conditions of vernal conjunctivitis and atopic keratoconjunctivitis (caused by corneal ulcerations) require prompt referral to an ophthalmologist.

In mild and sporadic cases of **urticaria and angioedema,** the needed use of antihistamines is sufficient. With frequent and persistent eruptions, routine use of H_1 blockers with the addition of H_2 blockers may be required. In more severe and refractory cases, older first-generation antihistamines are needed, with dosage pushed to maximal recommendations. In adults and older children, tricyclic antidepressants such as doxepin can be added when high doses of H_1- and H_2-receptor antagonists do not provide relief. Systemic steroids are very effective in controlling symptoms of urticaria and angioedema; however, symptoms may recur after stopping, and patients may become dependent on them for relief.

Chronic urticaria and angioedema may last months to years, some in waxing and waning fashion. Patients with chronic idiopathic urticaria and angioedema must be counseled that the disease is not caused by an external agent. The aforementioned medications need to be used long term to allow these patients to lead symptom-free lives until the pathology self-extinguishes.

Prevention

The cost of medical care, lost school days and workdays, disability from complications, and actual lives lost from allergic disease take a great toll on the population. Prevention will significantly reduce the health burden.

Evidence currently suggests that sensitization to foods can occur in the first 6 to 12 months of life and even in utero. Strategies to avoid allergic foods during the third trimester and first year of life have not diminished the prevalence of food allergies. Rather than avoiding

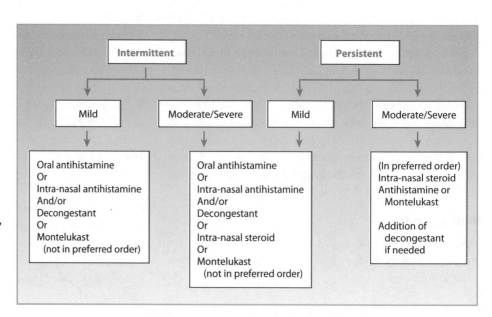

Figure 83-2. Allergic rhinitis treatment. (Adapted from Bousquet J, Schünemann HJ, Samolinski B, et al. Allergic Rhinitis and Its Impact on Asthma (ARIA): achievements in 10 years and the future. *J Allergy Clin Immunol.* 2012;130[5]:1049–1062, with permission.)

certain highly allergenic foods, small but well-designed studies have shown that introduction of allergic foods such as peanuts early on is associated with a lower incidence of food allergies. Large prospective studies are being conducted in the United States to confirm this.

Strategies to prevent development of inhalant allergies have not been universally effective. For patients at risk for development of allergic rhinitis and asthma, early avoidance of allergens is reasonable; however, this may merely delay sensitization until patients are older. Strategies include removal of dust mite reservoirs such as carpets, covering of mattresses and pillows with mite-proof covers, not having a warm-blooded furry pet, and repair of water damage to reduce mold growth. Prevention of tobacco smoke exposure is essential.

Recently, the hygiene hypothesis has received attention. In this paradigm, exposure to bacterial components like endotoxin results in a natural shift of lymphocytes from IgE-facilitating Th_2 to Th_1. Global shifts away from endotoxin-exposing agrarian societies to more sterile urban societies reduces this shift and may result in the increase of atopy worldwide. There is, however, the misconception that children exposed to a dirty environment with multiple pets, respiratory infections, and dirt will be protected against atopy. Unfortunately, the endotoxin-facilitated shift of Th_2 to Th_1 is likely to occur in a narrow window in utero and during the first year of life. Thus, exposure of older children to a dirty environment is unlikely to protect against atopy, and exposure of children with allergic disease exacerbates symptoms.

The method to prevent progression of allergic disease (allergic march) is immunotherapy. Immunotherapy against inhalant allergens in children with allergic rhinitis significantly decreases the risk of asthma. The need for weekly, then monthly injections reduces the acceptance of this method, but the approval of sublingual immunotherapy may improve patient compliance.

Prognosis

Prognosis for children with allergic disease is good. Some patients lose their allergy naturally or following immunotherapy. For others, allergic rhinitis, urticaria, and anaphylactic reactions persist throughout life on exposure to antigens. However, with appropriate management, children can thrive and live a normal life. Methods to prevent development of inhalant and food allergies is less understood; however, ongoing research will elucidate these mechanisms and allow effective prevention strategies in the future.

CASE RESOLUTION

In the case presented at the beginning of the chapter, the girl's symptoms of rash, swelling, and wheezing after exposure to an antigen suggest an anaphylactic reaction. Treatment with epinephrine, antihistamines, and systemic corticosteroids is clearly indicated. She should be observed for the occurrence of late-onset reactions. The child and family should be counseled to avoid any foods that contain peanuts. Parents should read all food labels and carry an epinephrine autoinjector (EpiPen) at all times for emergency use. A medical alert bracelet indicating peanut allergy should be ordered. The patient should be referred to an allergist for further evaluation.

Selected References

Adkinson N, Yunginger J, Busse W, et al, eds. *Middleton's Allergy: Principles and Practice.* 7th ed. St. Louis, MO: Mosby; 2009

Barnes ML, Menzies D, Fardon TC, Burns P, Wilson AM, Lipworth BJ. Combined mediator blockade or topical steroid for treating the unified allergic airway. *Allergy.* 2007;62(1):73–80

Berger W, Hampel F Jr, Bernstein J, Shah S, Sacks H, Meltzer EO. Impact of azelastine nasal spray on symptoms and quality of life compared with cetirizine oral tablets in patients with seasonal allergic rhinitis. *Ann Allergy Asthma Immunol.* 2006;97(3):375–381

Berkowitz RB, McCafferty F, Lutz C, et al. Onset of action of fexofenadine hydrochloride 60 mg/pseudoephedrine hydrochloride 120 mg in subjects aged 12 years with moderate to severe seasonal allergic rhinitis: a pooled analysis of two single-dose, randomized, double-blind, placebo-controlled allergen exposure unit studies. *Clin Ther.* 2006;28(10):1658–1669

Bodtger U, Linneberg A. Remission of allergic rhinitis: an 8-year observational study. *J Allergy Clin Immunol.* 2004;114(6):1384–1388

Bousquet J, Schünemann HJ, Samolinski B, et al. Allergy Rhinitis and Its Impact on Asthma (ARIA): achievements in 10 years and the future. *J Allergy Clin Immunol.* 2012;130(5):1049–1062

Brozek JL, Bousquet J, Baena-Cagnani CE, et al. Allergy Rhinitis and Its Impact on Asthma (ARIA) guidelines: 2010 revision. *J Allergy Clin Immunol.* 2010;126(3):466–476

Craig TJ, Ferguson BJ, Krouse JH. Sleep impairment in allergic rhinitis, rhinosinusitis, and nasal polyposis. *Am J Otolaryngol.* 2008;29(3):209–217

Cutler DL, Banfield C, Affrime MB. Safety of mometasone furoate nasal spray in children with allergic rhinitis as young as 2 years of age: a randomized controlled trial. *Pediatr Asthma Allergy Immunol.* 2006;19:146

Ellis AK, Day JH. Incidence and characteristics of biphasic anaphylaxis: a prospective evaluation of 103 patients. *Ann Allergy Asthma Immunol.* 2007;98(1):64–69

Fleischer DM, Spergel JM, Assa'ad AH, Pongracic JA. Primary prevention of allergic disease through nutritional interventions. *J Allergy Clin Immunol Pract.* 2013;1(1):29–36

Food Allergy Research & Education. http://www.foodallergy.org. Accessed March 6, 2014

Joint Task Force on Practice Parameters; American Academy of Allergy, Asthma, and Immunology; American College of Allergy, Asthma and Immunology; Joint Council of Allergy, Asthma and Immunology. The diagnosis and management of anaphylaxis: an updated practice parameter. *J Allergy Clin Immunol.* 2005;115(3 Suppl 2):S483–S523

Kim KT, Rabinovitch N, Uryniak T, Simpson B, O'Dowd L, Casty F. Effect of budesonide aqueous nasal spray on hypothalamic-pituitary-adrenal axis function in children with allergic rhinitis. *Ann Allergy Asthma Immunol.* 2004;93(1):61–67

Kwong KY, Leibel S. Update on immunotherapy for treatment of allergic disease. *Adv Pediatr.* 2013;60(1):141–165

Meltzer EO. Allergic rhinitis: managing the pediatric spectrum. *Allergy Asthma Proc.* 2006;27(1):2–8

Meltzer EO, Blaiss MS, Derebery MJ, et al. Burden of allergic rhinitis: results from the Pediatric Allergies in America survey. *J Allergy Clin Immunol.* 2009;124(3 Suppl):S43–S70

Norman PS. Immunotherapy: 1999–2004. *J Allergy Clin Immunol.* 2004;113(6):1013–1024

Patel P, Philip G, Yang W, et al. Randomized, double-blind, placebo-controlled study of montelukast for treating perennial allergic rhinitis. *Ann Allergy Asthma Immunol.* 2005;95(6):551–557

Pitsios C, Papadopoulos D, Kompoti E, et al. Efficacy and safety of mometasone furoate vs nedocromil sodium as prophylactic treatment for moderate/severe seasonal allergic rhinitis. *Ann Allergy Asthma Immunol.* 2006;96(5):673–678

Platts-Mills TA. Allergen avoidance. *J Allergy Clin Immunol.* 2004;113(3): 388–391

Pratt EL, Craig TJ. Assessing outcomes from the sleep disturbances associated with rhinitis. *Curr Opin Allergy Clin Immunol.* 2007;7(3):249–256

Ramey JT, Bailen E, Lockey RF. Rhinitis medicamentosa. *J Investig Allergol Clin Immunol.* 2006;16(3):148–155

Rudders SA, Banerji A, Vassallo MF, Clark S, Camargo CA Jr. Trends in pediatric emergency department visits for food-induced anaphylaxis. *J Allergy Clin Immunol.* 2010;126(2):385–388

Sampson HA, Muñoz-Furlong A, Campbell RL, et al. Second symposium on the definition and management of anaphylaxis: summary report—second National Institute of Allergy and Infectious Disease/Food Allergy and Anaphylaxis Network symposium. *Ann Emerg Med.* 2006;47(4):373–380

Wallace DV, Dykewicz MS, Bernstein DI, et al. The diagnosis and management of rhinitis: an updated practice parameter. *J Allergy Clin Immunol.* 2008;122(2 Suppl):S1–S84

Wander AA, Bernstein IL, Goodman DL, et al. The diagnosis and management of urticaria: a practice parameter. *Ann Allergy Immunol.* 2005;85:525–544

Wang J, Sampson HA. Food anaphylaxis. *Clin Exp Allergy.* 2007;37(5):651–660

Wu CC, Kuo HC, Yu HR, Wang L, Yang KD. Association of acute urticaria with *Mycoplasma pneumoniae* infection in hospitalized children. *Ann Allergy Asthma Immunol.* 2009;103(2):134–139

Zuraw BL, Christiansen SC. Pathogenesis and laboratory diagnosis of hereditary angioedema. *Allergy Asthma Proc.* 2009;30(5):487–492

CHAPTER 84

Wheezing and Asthma

Nasser Redjal, MD, and Kenny Yat-Choi Kwong, MD

CASE STUDY

A 7-year-old boy is referred to the office after being seen in the emergency department (ED) for wheezing. He has been treated in the ED for wheezing 4 times in the past month and was once hospitalized for 3 days. The boy's father and paternal grandmother both have asthma.

The child's physical examination is remarkable for end-expiratory wheezing on forced expiration.

Questions

1. What are the most common causes of wheezing in infants and children?
2. What are the causes of reversible bronchospasm?
3. What is the pathophysiology of reversible bronchospasm?
4. How should children with asthma be managed?

Recurrent wheezing is a frequent symptom of obstructive airway disease in children that may be caused by intrinsic or extrinsic compression of the airway, bronchospasm, inflammation, or defective clearance of secretions. Ten percent to 15% of infants wheeze during their first year of life, and as many as 25% of children younger than 5 years present to their clinicians with wheezing during a respiratory illness. Most infants and young children with recurrent wheezing have asthma; however, a wide variety of congenital and acquired conditions can cause narrowing of the extrathoracic or intrathoracic airways and may present with wheezing. Reactive airway disease is the most common cause of wheezing in childhood. Childhood asthma typically falls into 1 of 3 categories. **Transient wheezing** occurs in infants who are born with smaller caliber airway and wheeze with viral lower respiratory tract infections and bronchiolitis. They do not have atopy and usually have no more wheezing by 3 years of age. The majority of patients with no atopic predisposition who wheeze in the early years of life fall into this category. **Late transient wheezing** occurs in children who usually have a history of serious lung insult, such as severe respiratory syncytial virus (RSV) infections, and persistent wheezing beyond 3 years of age. They also have no atopy, and symptoms usually slowly resolve over time. **Atopic wheezing** occurs in children who have a strong atopic predisposition. They are most likely to develop asthma that persists throughout the school-age years.

Wheezes can originate from airways of any size, from the large extrathoracic upper airway to the intrathoracic small airways. In addition to narrowing or compression of the airway, wheezing requires sufficient airflow to generate airway oscillation and produce sound. Thus, the absence of wheezing in a patient who presents with acute asthma may be an ominous finding, suggesting impending respiratory failure. The audible musical or squeaking sounds noted with obstruction are caused by turbulence of the air as it is forced through a narrowed airway. Infants and young children are more prone to wheezing when they have airway obstruction because air forced through smaller airways is more turbulent than air forced through the larger airways of older children and adults. Infection-induced wheezing in children younger than 2 years is associated with RSV, especially in infants with passive exposure to smoke, and with rhinovirus in children older than 2 years. The most common causes of wheezing in infants and children are asthma, bronchiolitis, and pneumonia. Less common causes include congenital structural anomalies, gastroesophageal reflux and aspiration, cardiac failure, cystic fibrosis, foreign bodies, and vocal cord dysfunction (Box 84-1).

The modified Asthma Predictive Index (mAPI) is a clinical instrument to predict persistence of asthma. Predictive factors include wheezing before 3 years of age and the presence of one major risk factor (parental history of asthma, personal history of atopic dermatitis, or patient sensitized to aeroallergen) or 2 of 3 minor risk factors (patient sensitized to food, wheezing apart from colds, or eosinophilia). The mAPI has a positive predictive value of 76% and a negative predictive value of 95%. More than 80% of infants who have a history of wheezing in the first postnatal years do not wheeze after 3 years of age.

Asthma is a common chronic disorder of the airways characterized by variable and recurring symptoms, airflow obstruction, bronchial hyperreactivity, and underlying inflammation. Bronchospasm is reversible spontaneously or with treatment. In some patients, permanent alterations in the airway structure, referred to as **airway remodeling,** develop and are not prevented by or fully responsive to currently available treatment. Clinically, asthma is characterized by recurrent episodes of cough, chest tightness, dyspnea, prolonged expiration, wheezing, hyperinflation of the chest (air trappings), use of accessory chest muscles (retractions), and, in severe cases, cyanosis.

Epidemiology

Asthma is the most common chronic childhood illness. In 2007, the National Health Interview Survey noted that 9% of children 0 to 17 years of age (6.7 million) had asthma. Asthma is the leading cause

---

Box 84-1. Causes of Wheezing

Infection
- Bronchiolitis
- Pneumonia
- Bronchitis
- Laryngotracheobronchitis
- Bacterial tracheitis
- Toxocariasis
- Ascariasis

Reactive Airway Disease
- Asthma
- Exercise-induced asthma
- Anaphylaxis
- Nighttime cough asthma
- Toxic exposure (smoke, organophosphate poisoning)
- Allergic aspergillosis

Laryngeal Dysfunction

Congenital Structural Anomalies
- Vascular rings
- Bronchiectasis
- Lung cysts
- Laryngotracheoesophageal cleft
- Tracheobronchomalacia

Defective Secretion Clearance
- Cystic fibrosis
- Immotile cilia syndrome

Tumor
- Mediastinal tumors (lymphoma, teratoma, neuroblastoma, thymoma)

Chronic Aspiration
- Gastroesophageal reflux
- Bulbar palsy
- Tracheoesophageal fistula

Other Causes
- Bronchopulmonary dysplasia
- α_1-Antitrypsin deficiency
- Pulmonary hemosiderosis
- Sarcoidosis

Foreign Body

Cardiac Disease

Immunodeficiency

---

of emergency department (ED) visits, hospital admissions, and school absenteeism. Over the last several decades, the prevalence of asthma has increased worldwide, an increase that varies from 40% in some areas of the United Kingdom and Australia to 3% in Indonesia, China, and India. Asthma prevalence, mortality, and hospitalization rates are higher in blacks than in whites. One-third of patients initially experience symptoms in the first year of life, and 80% are diagnosed by the time they reach school age. In the United States, asthma is a leading diagnosis for children admitted to children's hospitals. Hospitalization rates have remained relatively stable, with lower rates in some age groups but higher rates in children

0 to 4 years of age. In addition, asthma is a major cause of school absence; 23% of school days missed can be attributed to asthma. The male-female ratio is 2:1 until age 10 years and is equal from ages 10 to 14 years; after puberty, asthma incidence is greater in girls and women.

In recent years, the incidence of more serious disease in younger children and adolescents has increased. Low socioeconomic status is associated with an increase in asthma prevalence, morbidity, and mortality. Inner-city African Americans are most at risk, but studies suggest that socioeconomic class and health care disparities only partially account for these differences.

Clinical Presentation

Children with asthma may present with acute symptoms of cough, shortness of breath, prolonged expiration, use of accessory muscles of respiration, wheezing, complaints of chest tightness or congestion, hyperinflation of the chest, cyanosis, exercise intolerance, tachycardia, and abdominal pain.

Wheezing may be audible and detected by the parent or may not be appreciated until the child is examined by a physician. There may be no wheezing in children with severe bronchoconstriction because the flow of air is impeded, but wheezing may appear after bronchodilator treatment, owing to partial opening of the airway.

Some children have cough, which may be nocturnal or recurrent as a predominant symptom. Some pediatric patients have symptoms such as cough or wheezing that are precipitated or exacerbated by exercise (D_x Box).

Abdominal pain and vomiting also are common in younger children and may be followed by temporary relief of respiratory symptoms. During an acute asthma attack, a low-grade fever, profuse sweating, and fatigue from the hard work of breathing may be apparent.

Pathophysiology

Asthma is a chronic inflammatory disorder of the airways. The immunohistopathologic features of asthma include alteration and denudation of the airway epithelium, thickening of the basement membrane, fibrotic changes in the subbasement membrane, bronchial smooth muscle hypertrophy, edema and angiogenesis, mast cell activation, and inflammatory cell infiltration (neutrophils, lymphocytes, eosinophils),

Asthma

- Recurrent wheezing
- Shortness of breath
- Exercise intolerance
- History of allergies
- History of atopic dermatitis
- Nasal polyps
- History of nighttime cough

which release mediators such as histamine, prostaglandin, leukotriene, and major basic proteins. These changes lead to airway hyperreactivity, airflow limitation, respiratory symptoms, and disease chronicity. The limitation to the flow of air results from acute bronchoconstriction, airway edema, mucus plug formation, and airway wall remodeling. The unique anatomy and physiology of the lung in infants compared with adults predisposes infants to obstructive airway disease. These anatomic differences include reduced number and size of the alveolar pores and Lambert canals, causing deficient collateral ventilation and a predisposition to atelectasis distal to obstructed airway. Mucous gland hyperplasia favors increased intraluminal mucus production. Decreased smooth muscle in the peripheral airway results in less support and narrower airways. Decreased number of fatigue-resistant skeletal muscle fibers in the diaphragm, its horizontal insertion to the rib cage (versus oblique in adult), and a highly compliant rib cage increase the work of breathing in children. Decreased static elastic recoil predisposes to early airway closure during tidal breathing, resulting in mismatching of ventilation and perfusion and hypoxemia.

Atopy, the genetic predisposition to the development of immunoglobulin (Ig) E–mediated response to common aeroallergens, is a predisposing factor for developing asthma. There are at least 50 genes that influence susceptibility to asthma and its clinical expression. Sites located on chromosomes 6p, 12q, 5q, 11q, and 16p are known to be associated with allergic diseases and encoding for major histocompatibility complex, IgE, interferon, and cytokine.

Environmental changes such as wind, temperature fluctuations, and increased exposure to allergens or air pollutants, such as tobacco smoke, ozone, sulfur dioxide, and nitrogen dioxide, and particulate matter, such as diesel exhaust and biologic residues (eg, endotoxin), may precipitate clinical attacks. Inhalant allergens, particularly indoors, play an important role. The most important allergens are house dust mite feces (Der p1 and Der p2), cat dander (Feld l), and cockroach saliva (Bla g2, Bla g4, and Bla g5). Other inhalant allergens such as dog dander, outdoor fungus (ie, *Alternaria*), and some pollens, also play a role. Infections, particularly respiratory ones, are implicated, influencing not only asthma's exacerbation but also its inception and persistence. Viral infections, such as RSV, parainfluenza, and rhinovirus, are the most frequent precipitants of asthma exacerbations in infancy. The frequency of lower tract respiratory infection during early childhood with these viruses is a strong independent factor in development of asthma. *Mycoplasma* and *Chlamydia* infections can cause wheezing and persistence of asthma. Emotional stress may also play a role in the exacerbation of asthma.

The physiological changes involved in asthma occur in 2 phases. An immediate response (early phase) to the offending agent causes edema and bronchial smooth muscle constriction that lead to narrowing of the airway and plugging with secretions. Air is trapped behind the narrowed airways, resulting in altered gas exchange, increased respiratory rate, decreased tidal volume, and increased work of breathing. The late response, which occurs 4 to 12 hours after the initial symptoms, primarily involves infiltration of the airways with inflammatory cells. The end pathway in the disease process is obstruction to airflow. The pathophysiology of asthma is reviewed in Figure 84-1.

Differential Diagnosis

An extensive differential diagnosis is listed in Box 84-1. Most conditions are differentiated from asthma by the presence of associated symptoms or the child's response to bronchodilators.

Evaluation

History

A thorough history, including how the child and family are coping with the asthma, should be obtained (Questions Box). If acute respiratory distress is present, an abbreviated history focusing on potential precipitating factors and medication use should be obtained first and the more detailed history gotten at a later time.

Physical Examination

Vital signs including pulse oximetry should be obtained. Objective determination of pulmonary function involves measuring the peak expiratory effort. Paradoxical pulse, the difference between systolic arterial blood pressure during inspiration and expiration, is usually under 10 mm Hg. This difference may be increased during an acute asthma exacerbation, but the measurement is difficult in young children. Breath sounds, work of breathing, the inspiratory-expiratory ratio, use of accessory muscles, presence of retractions, quality of breath sounds (whether decreased), presence of prolonged expiration, and quality of wheezing should be carefully assessed (Table 84-1). Polyphonic wheezing (many different pitches, starting and stopping at varying points in the respiratory cycle) and cough are highly suggestive of asthma. Monophonic wheezing (a single, distinct noise of one pitch and starting and stopping at one discrete time) and cough should always raise suspicion of large airway obstruction caused by foreign body aspiration, vascular ring, or tracheomalacia. The nose and associated nasal passages should be examined for secretions, edema, pallor, and polyps. The skin should be assessed for eczema and other rashes. The chest should be carefully checked for increased anteroposterior diameter of the chest wall, a sign of air trapping. Fingers should be examined for signs of digital clubbing, which suggests a diagnosis other than asthma.

Laboratory Tests

Laboratory assessment of wheezing children is indicated if the diagnosis is unclear or to eliminate disorders that mimic asthma. Pulmonary function tests are noninvasive, objective, and cost-effective in the diagnosis and follow-up of patients with asthma. These tests can be performed in children older than 5 years with appropriate coaching. After the administration of an aerosolized bronchodilator, dynamic tests of airflow increase or return to normal. An improvement in forced expiratory volume in 1 second (FEV_1) greater than 12% is virtually diagnostic, but lack of improvement in FEV_1 does not preclude asthma. Exercise tolerance tests using a treadmill

Figure 84-1. Proposed pathways in the pathogenesis of bronchial inflammation and airway hyperreactivity. (Reproduced from the National Heart, Lung, and Blood Institute. *National Asthma Education Program Expert Panel Report: Guidelines for Diagnosis and Management of Asthma.* **Bethesda, MD: National Institutes of Health; National Heart, Lung, and Blood Institute; 1991. NIH Publication No. 91-3042.)**

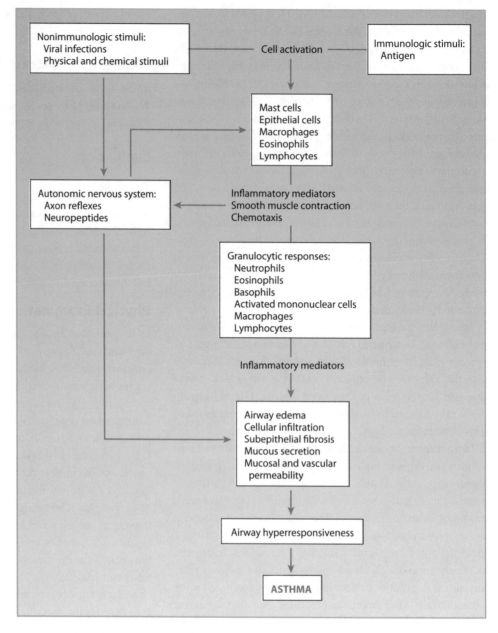

or free running followed by pulmonary function tests can be performed; a decrease greater than 12% in FEV_1 or 30% in forced expiratory flow is diagnostic of exercise-induced asthma. Peak flow meters, which measure forced peak expiratory flow (PEF), are useful in the office and at home to monitor expiratory flow rate. A decrease in PEF may predict the onset of an exacerbation and suggests the need for early intervention, using additional drug therapy. A complete blood cell count with a differential count may suggest infection or allergies. Peripheral eosinophil counts may be elevated in asthma. Pulse oximetry assesses the degree of oxygen saturation.

Sputum smear, stained with eosin-methylene blue, may show numerous eosinophils and granules from disrupted white blood cells, eosinophils, and epithelial cells. The presence of more than 5% to 10% eosinophils suggests allergic inflammatory disease. Other findings in the sputum include Curschmann spirals, which are threads

of glycoprotein; Creola bodies, which are clusters of epithelial cells; and Charcot-Leyden crystals, which are derived from eosinophils.

Total serum IgE is not as helpful as antigen-specific IgE and is elevated in 80% of children with allergen-induced asthma. Allergy skin testing or serologic testing, such as radioallergosorbent testing, is indicated to identify potentially important environmental allergens. Allergens may play a significant role in asthma, and 85% of asthma patients have a positive skin test reaction to common aeroallergens. Extensive laboratory testing should be reserved for children with severe disease who may benefit from consultation with an allergy specialist.

Imaging Studies

Children suspected of having asthma rarely require a chest radiograph unless there is concern about other pathology. Radiograph findings may range from normal to hyperinflation, increased

Questions

Asthma

- What symptoms (eg, wheezing, exercise intolerance) does the child experience?
- Does the child experience any nocturnal awaking or cough?
- What time of day and year do the symptoms occur?
- When did the symptoms begin? How old was the child?
- Are the symptoms associated with any particular activity? Does anything seem to trigger the symptoms?
- Are the child's activities limited in any way?
- How often do asthma attacks occur?
- What is the child's living situation? Are there pets in the home?
- Does anyone smoke in the home?
- Do asthma attacks cause the child to be absent from school?
- Does the child manage the condition at home with any particular treatments or medications?
- Has the child visited any urgent care or emergency departments for treatment for asthma or related episodes in the past? Has the child had any hospitalizations?
- Does the child have a history of allergies?

Table 84-1. Parameters Used to Estimate the Severity of Acute Asthma

Sign/Symptom	Mild	Moderate	Severe
Respiratory rate	Normal	Increased	Increased >2 SD
Breath sounds	Normal (some end-expiratory wheezes)	Wheezing in inspiration and expiration	Decreased ±wheezing
Shortness of breath	None (can speak in sentences)	Can speak in phrases	Speaks only single words
Skin color	Normal (pink)	Pale	Pale to cyanotic
Work of breathing	Normal	Moderate retractions; some use of accessory muscles	Severe retractions, nasal flaring, use of accessory muscles
Pulse	Normal	Normal or increased	Increased
Level of consciousness	Normal	Normal	Diminished; may be lethargic or combative
Paradoxical pulse	<10 mm Hg	10–20 mm Hg	20–40 mm Hg
Oxygen saturation	>95%	90%–95%	<92%
Pulmonary function	80% of predicted	50%–70% of predicted	<50% of predicted

Abbreviation: SD, standard deviation.

bronchial marking, and atelectasis, especially during acute exacerbation. Infiltration, pneumothorax, pneumomediastinum, and pneumonia are less common findings.

Management

The long-term goals of asthma therapy are as follows:

- Prevent chronic and disabling symptoms (eg, coughing, sleep disturbances, exercise intolerance, shortness of breath).
- Maintain normal or near-normal pulmonary function.
- Maintain normal activity levels.
- Prevent recurrent exacerbations and minimize the need for ED visits and admission to the hospital.
- Provide drug therapy that is effective with minimal side effects.
- Meet the expectations of the child and family for the care of asthma.
- Encourage self-management of asthma.

Assessment measures for asthma should include monitoring of the following: signs and symptoms, pulmonary function through peak flow or respirometry, quality of life or functional status, acute disease exacerbations, pharmacologic therapy, and satisfaction of the child and family with the asthma care.

Selecting the appropriate therapy for an asthma patient depends on the age, disease severity, and developmental level of the child; tolerance for a specific pharmacologic agent; and routes of administration. The pharmacologic treatment for symptom control and reduction of inflammation is predicated on the severity of the asthma, as categorized according to National Heart, Lung, and Blood Institute (NHLBI) guidelines. Box 84-2 contains an overview of these medications. Quick-relief medications ("rescue meds") are used for acute exacerbations; the long-term control medications are used for chronic therapy. Non-pharmacologic measures aim at prevention and serve as an adjunct to drug therapy.

Short-term Management

Acute attacks can be managed in the office if the staff is prepared to deal with children in respiratory distress. Otherwise, children can be referred to the ED. Equipment and supplies for resuscitation of infants and children must be available in offices that care for children with asthma.

The goal of therapy is to relieve airflow obstruction and prevent respiratory failure. All children with moderate or severe asthma should be placed in a position of comfort and given oxygen by nasal prongs or mask as tolerated. Assessment of work of breathing and the use of pulse oximetry help guide oxygen therapy. Nebulized β_2-agonists such as albuterol are used until symptoms subside. Children may require drug therapy every 20 to 30 minutes. Not only are nebulized β_2-adrenergic agonists more effective than oral medications, they are associated with fewer side effects. Ipratropium bromide used in conjunction with a β-agonist in the urgent care setting has been shown to reduce risk of hospitalization. Systemic corticosteroids, which help reduce the inflammation associated with clinical attacks, are indicated in most moderate and severe cases. Response to therapy is determined by clinical assessment of work of breathing, respiratory rate, objective

Box 84-2. Pharmacologic Therapy: An Overview of Medications Used to Treat Asthma

Long-term Control Medications (Controller Class)

Corticosteroids

Most potent and effective anti-inflammatory medication currently available. Inhaled form is used in the long-term control of asthma. Systemic corticosteroids are often used to gain prompt control of the disease when initiating long-term therapy.

Cromolyn Sodium and Nedocromil

Mild anti-inflammatory medication. May be used as monotherapy in mild persistent asthma. Can also be used as preventive treatment prior to exercise or unavoidable exposure to known allergens.

Long-Acting β₂-Agonists

Long-acting bronchodilator used concomitantly with anti-inflammatory medications for long-term control of symptoms, especially nocturnal symptoms. Includes salmeterol and formoterol.

Methylxanthines

Sustained-release theophylline is a mild-to-moderate bronchodilator used principally as adjuvant to inhaled corticosteroids for prevention of nocturnal asthma symptoms. May have mild anti-inflammatory effect.

Leukotriene Modifiers

Montelukast, a leukotriene receptor antagonist, or zileuton, a 5-lipoxygenase inhibitor, may be considered an alternative therapy to low doses of inhaled corticosteroids, or cromolyn or nedocromil, in mild persistent asthma.

Systemic Corticosteroids

- Used for moderate-to-severe exacerbations to speed recovery and prevent recurrence of exacerbations.
- **Omalizumab** (anti-IgE), a recombinant DNA–derived humanized monoclonal antibody of the Fc portion of the IgE antibody, binds to that portion, thereby preventing IgE binding to its high-affinity receptor (fcER1) on mast cells and basophils, leading to a decrease in the release of mediators in response to allergen exposure.

Quick-Relief Medications (Reliever Class)

Short-Acting β₂-Agonists

Albuterol and levalbuterol are therapy of choice for relief of acute symptoms and prevention of exercise-induced bronchoconstriction.

Anticholinergics

Ipratropium bromide provides additive benefit to inhaled β₂-agonists in acute exacerbations. May be an alternative bronchodilator for patients who do not tolerate inhaled β₂-agonists.

Box 84-3. Therapeutic Goals for Children With Chronic Asthma

- Maintain a normal, age-appropriate activity level.
- Maintain near-normal pulmonary function.
- Prevent symptoms such as exercise intolerance, chronic cough, and shortness of breath.
- Prevent acute exacerbations of the disease that require acute therapy.
- Minimize adverse effects of the drugs used to treat the disease.
- Promote self-esteem and a sense of well-being.

changes in pulmonary function, and pulse oximetry. Children with incomplete responses to initial therapy may require several hours of treatment or hospitalization.

Long-term Management

The goals of long-term management are shown in Box 84-3.

Continuous and longitudinal primary care of children with asthma can profoundly affect the course of their disease. Primary care practitioners, children, and their families must work together to achieve good control of symptoms. Prevention of exacerbations may be accomplished by removal of offending allergens. Minimization of exposure to known allergens and irritants has been shown to decrease symptoms and exacerbation. The most commonly implicated irritants are tobacco smoke; fumes from gas, oil, and kerosene stoves and wood-burning appliances; and sprays and strong odors. House dust mites are microscopic insects that feed on human scales, require humidity greater than 50%, and are found in stuffed furniture, carpets, and mattresses. House dust mite infestation can be reduced by encasing mattresses, blankets, and pillows in mite-proof covers; removing carpeting; and decreasing humidity to less than 50%.

Allergen immunotherapy may be considered for asthma patients when there is evidence of a clear relationship between symptom and exposure to an allergen, and symptoms are poorly controlled with pharmacologic management (eg, medication ineffective, multiple medications are required, patient does not accept or tolerate medication). Adherence with appropriate medications and in home peak-flow measurement helps in prevention and control of asthma. Periodic assessment ensures appropriate therapy and compliance with treatment. Practitioners should make sure that families can afford the necessary medications. During routine visits, home monitoring and therapy as well as any diaries and records should be reviewed, children's and families' expectations about the course of the disease should be discussed, and all parties should be allowed to express their concerns about the development of a treatment plan. Other factors, such as rhinitis, sinusitis, and gastroesophageal reflux, which may influence the severity of asthma or a child's quality of life, should be assessed and treated appropriately.

Family members and children should be given a written action plan based on patients' personal best peak flow (Figure 84-2) and instructed in the use of peak flow meters to indicate when medical treatment is necessary. Some meters have 3 color zones: a green zone, which indicates good airflow; a yellow zone, which signals the need for treatment; and a red zone, which suggests that a visit to the ED may be indicated.

Pharmacologic Therapy

The 2007 NHLBI guidelines for asthma management are based on age group: children 0 to 4 years of age (Table 84-2), children 5 to 11 years of age (Table 84-3), and children 12 years and older (Table 84-4).

Asthma severity is categorized by *impairment* and *risk.* Impairment considers the frequency and severity of daytime and nighttime

For: _____ Doctor: _____ Date: _____

Doctor's Phone Number: _____ Hospital/Emergency Department Phone Number: _____

GREEN ZONE

Doing Well   Take these long-term control medicines each day (include an anti-inflammatory).

| No cough, wheeze, chest | **Medicine** | **How much to take** | **When to take it** |

No cough, wheeze, chest

tightness, or shortness of _____ → _____ → _____

breath during the day or night _____ → _____ → _____

Can do usual activities

And, if a peak flow meter is used,   **Identify and avoid and control the things that make your asthma worse, like (list here):**

Peak Flow: more than _____ _____

(80% or more of my best peak flow) _____ _____.

My best peak flow is: _____

     Before exercise, if prescribed, take: ☐ 2 or ☐ 4 puffs _____

                 5–60 minutes before exercise

YELLOW ZONE

Asthma Is Getting Worse → First Add: quick-relief medicine and keep taking your GREEN ZONE medicine.

       _____ ☐ 2 or ☐ 4 puffs, every 20 minutes for up to 1 hour

       (short-acting β_2-agonist) ☐ Nebulizer once

Cough, wheeze, chest tightness, or shortness of breath,   **If applicable, remove yourself from the thing that made your asthma worse.**

      or   → **Second, if your symptoms (and peak flow, if used) return to GREEN ZONE after**

Waking at night due to asthma, or   **1 hour of treatment:**

Can do some but not all usual activities   ☐ Continue monitoring to be sure you stay in the green zone.

– Or –   **If your symptoms (and peak flow, if used) do not return to GREEN ZONE after**

Peak flow: _____   **1 hour of treatment:**

       (50%–79% of my best peak flow)   ☐ Take: _____ ☐ 2 or ☐ 4 puffs or ☐ nebulizer

                                (short-acting β_2-agonist).

                                ☐ Add: _____ mg per day for _____ (3–10 days)

                                (oral corticosteroid).

                                ☐ Call the doctor _ ☐ before/☐ within ___ hours after taking oral corticosteroid.

RED ZONE

Medical Alert!   **Take this medicine:**

Very short of breath, or   ☐ _____ ☐ 4 or ☐ 6 puffs or ☐ nebulizer

Quick-relief medicines have not helped, or   (short-acting β_2-agonist)

Cannot do usual activities, or   ☐ _____ mg

Symptoms are same or get worse   (oral corticosteroid)

After 24 hours in Yellow Zone   **Then call your doctor NOW.** Go to the hospital or call an ambulance

                                if:

– Or –   ☐ You are still in the Red Zone after 15 minutes AND

Peak flow: less than _____   You have not reached your doctor.

       (50% of my best peak flow)

DANGER SIGNS

Trouble walking and talking due to shortness of breath

Lips or fingernails are blue

Take ☐ 4 or ☐ 6 puffs of your quick-relief medicine AND

Go to the hospital or call for an ambulance _____

Figure 84–2. Asthma action/medicine plan. (Source: National Heart, Lung, and Blood Institute, National Institutes of Health, US Department of Health and Human Services. NIH Publication No 075251, October 2006.)

Table 84-2. Classifying Asthma Severity: Ages 0 to 4 Years

Components of Severity		Classifying of Asthma Severity and Initiating Treatment (0–4 y)			
			Persistent		
		Intermittent	Mild	Moderate	Severe
Impairment	Symptoms	≤2 d/wk	>2 d/wk but not daily	Daily	Throughout the day
	Nighttime awakenings	0	1–2x/mo	3–4x/mo	>1x/wk
	Short-acting β$_2$-agonist use for symptom control (not prevention of EIB)	≤2 d/wk	>2 d/wk but not daily	Daily	Several times per day
	Interference with normal activity	None	More limitation	Some limitation	Extremely limited
Risk	Exacerbation requiring oral systemic corticosteroids	0–1/y	≥2 exacerbations in 6 mo requiring oral systemic corticosteroids, or ≥4 wheezing episodes/1 y lasting >1 d AND risk factors for persistent asthma		
		Consider severity and interval since last exacerbation. Frequency and severity may fluctuate over time. Exacerbations of any severity may occur in patients in any severity category.			
Recommended Step for Initiating Therapy (See Table 84-5 for treatment steps.)		Step 1: SABA PRN	Step 2: Low-dose ICS	Step 3: Medium-dose ICS and consider short course of OCS	
		In 2–6 wk, depending on severity, evaluate level of asthma control that is achieved. If no clear benefit is observed in 4–6 wk, consider adjusting therapy or alternative diagnoses.			

Abbreviations: EIB, exercise-induced bronchoconstriction; ICS, inhaled corticosteroids; OCS, oral corticosteroids; PRN, as needed; SABA, short-acting β$_2$-agonist.

Adapted from the National Asthma Education and Prevention Program. *Expert Panel Report 3: Guidelines for the Diagnosis and Management of Asthma, 2007.* Bethesda, MD: National Heart, Lung, and Blood Institute; 2007. NIH Publication No. 07-4052.

Table 84-3. Classifying Asthma Severity: Ages 5 to 11 Years

Components of Severity		Classifying of Asthma Severity and Initiating treatment (5–11 y)			
			Persistent		
		Intermittent	Mild	Moderate	Severe
Impairment	Symptoms	≤2 d/wk	>2 d/wk but not daily	Daily	Throughout the day
	Nighttime awakenings	≤2x/mo	3–4x/mo	>1x/wk but not nightly	Often 7x/wk
	Short-acting β$_2$-agonist use for symptom control (not prevention of EIB)	≤2 d/wk	>2 d/wk but not daily	Daily	Several times per day
	Interference with normal activity	None	More limitation	Some limitation	Extremely limited
	Lung function	Normal FEV$_1$ between exacerbations FEV$_1$ >80% predicted FEV$_1$/FVC >85%	FEV$_1$ ≥80% predicted FEV$_1$/FVC >80%	FEV$_1$ = 60%–80% predicted FEV$_1$/FVC = 75%–80%	FEV$_1$ <60% predicted FEV$_1$/FVC <75%
Risk	Exacerbation requiring oral systemic corticosteroids	0–1/y (See note.)	≥2/y (See note.)		
		Consider severity and interval since last exacerbation. Frequency and severity may fluctuate over time.			
		Relative annual risk of exacerbations may be related to FEV$_1$.			
Recommended Step for Initiating Therapy (See Table 84-5 for treatment steps.)		Step 1: SABA PRN	Step 2: Low-dose ICS	Step 3: Medium-dose ICS option	Step 3, Medium-dose ICS option or step 4
				Consider short course of OCS.	
		In 2–6 wk, evaluate level of asthma control that is achieved and adjusting therapy accordingly.			

Abbreviations: EIB, exercise-induced bronchoconstriction; FEV$_1$, forced expiratory volume in 1 second; FVC, forced vital capacity; ICS, inhaled corticosteroids; OCS, oral corticosteroids; PRN, as needed; SABA, short-acting β$_2$-agonist.

Adapted from the National Asthma Education and Prevention Program. *Expert Panel Report 3: Guidelines for the Diagnosis and Management of Asthma, 2007.* Bethesda, MD: National Heart, Lung, and Blood Institute; 2007. NIH Publication No. 07-4052.

Table 84-4. Classifying Asthma Severity: 12 Years and Older

Component of Severity		Classifying of Asthma Severity and Initiating Treatment (≥12 y)			
				Persistent	
		Intermittent	Mild	Moderate	Severe
Impairment	Symptoms	≤2 d/wk	>2 d/wk but not daily	Daily	Throughout the day
	Nighttime awakenings	≤2x/mo	3–4x/mo	>1x wk, but not nightly	Often 7x/wk
	Short-acting β₂-agonist use for symptom control (not prevention of EIB)	≤2 d/wk	>2 d/wk but not daily and more than 1x on any day	Daily	Several times per day
	Interference with normal activity	None	More limitation	Some limitation	Extremely limited
	Lung function	Normal FEV₁ between exacerbations FEV₁ >80% predicted FEV₁/FVC >85%	FEV₁ ≥80% predicted FEV₁/FVC normal	FEV₁ >60, but <80% predicted FEV₁/FVC = reduced 5%	FEV₁ <60% predicted FEV₁/FVC reduced <5%
Risk	Exacerbation requiring oral systemic corticosteroids	0–1/y	≥2 y		
		Consider severity and interval since last exacerbation. Frequency and severity may fluctuate over time. Exacerbations of any severity may occur in patients in any severity category.			
Recommended Step for Initiating Therapy (See Table 84-5 for treatment steps.)		Step 1: SABA PRN	Step 2: Low-dose ICS	Step 3: Low-dose ICS + LABA	Step 4/5: Medium/High-dose ICS + LABA
				Consider short course of OCS.	
		In 2–6 wk, depending on severity, evaluate level of asthma control that is achieved. If no clear benefit is observed in 4–6 wk, consider adjusting therapy or alternative diagnoses.			

Abbreviations: EIB, exercise-induced bronchoconstriction; FEV_1, forced expiratory volume in 1 second; FVC, forced vital capacity; ICS, inhaled corticosteroids; LABA, long-acting β₂-agonist; OCS, oral corticosteroids; PRN, as needed; SABA, short-acting β₂-agonist.

Adapted from the National Asthma Education and Prevention Program. *Expert Panel Report 3: Guidelines for the Diagnosis and Management of Asthma, 2007.* Bethesda, MD: National Heart, Lung, and Blood Institute; 2007. NIH Publication No. 07-4052.

asthma symptoms, use of short-acting β₂-agonist for other than exercise-associated symptoms, effect on activities, and pulmonary function testing. Risk assesses the frequency of asthma exacerbations requiring the use of oral corticosteroids. The most severe level of symptoms, medication use, and other factors defines the level of severity, which determines the long-term approach to management. Patients with intermittent asthma may respond to short-acting bronchodilator as needed, whereas children with persistent asthma require a controller medication such as inhaled corticosteroids (ICS) to reduce inflammation. Treatment of asthma is based on its severity and control. For **intermittent asthma only,** short-acting β₂-agonists are required on an as-needed basis to treat symptoms. Prophylactic use of β₂-agonists, cromolyn, or nedocromil may be used for exercise-induced asthma before the onset of activity. For **mild persistent asthma,** daily anti-inflammatory medications (controllers) are required with low-dose ICS as recommended therapy or alternative monotherapy with cromolyn, nedocromil, or leukotriene modifier agents, such as montelukast. Use short-acting β₂-agonists for acute exacerbations. For **moderate persistent asthma,** medium-dose ICS or low-dose ICS plus a second agent is

recommended, depending on the age group. Second agents include long-acting β₂-agonists, leukotriene modifiers, and theophylline. For **severe persistent asthma,** usually high-dose ICS plus a second agent is required. Systemic corticosteroids may be required to gain asthma control in patients with moderate to severe persistent asthma. In patients with difficult-to-control asthma, especially those experiencing severe exacerbations despite optimal controller therapy, omalizumab has been shown to decrease risk of asthma attacks. Patients of all asthma severities require short-acting β₂-agonists for quick relief of symptoms and prevention of exercise-induced asthma.

Inhaled corticosteroids act topically on lung epithelium, inhibiting cell migration and activation and reducing airway hyperreactivity. Inhaled corticosteroids are the most effective anti-inflammatory medication for asthma. Inhaled corticosteroids reduce asthma symptoms, improve lung function, reduce acute exacerbations of asthma, and reduce the risk of death from asthma. Recent data show that ICS are well-tolerated, safe medications at the recommended dosages.

Leukotriene modifiers interfere with the action of leukotrienes, inflammatory mediators released from mast cells, eosinophils, and basophils. Long-acting β₂-agonists provide at least 12 hours of

				Table 84-5. Stepwise Approach for Managing Asthma By Age Group[a]		
Age	Step 1	Step 2[b]	Step 3[b]	Step 4[b]	Step 5[c]	Step 6[c]
0–4 y	SABA PRN	Low-dose ICS alternative: cromolyn or montelukast	Medium-dose ICS	Medium-dose ICS + either LABA or montelukast	High-dose ICS + either LABA or montelukast	High-dose ICS + OCS + either LABA or montelukast
5–11 y	SABA PRN	Low-dose ICS alternative: cromolyn, LTRA, or theophylline	Low-dose ICS + either LABA, LTRA, or theophylline OR medium-dose ICS	Medium-dose ICS + LABA alternative: medium-dose ICS + either LTRA OR theophylline	High-dose ICS + LABA alternative: high-dose ICS + either LTRA OR theophylline	High-dose ICS + LABA + OCS alternative: high-dose ICS + either LTRA OR theophylline + OCS
12 y–adult	SABA PRN	Low-dose ICS alternative: cromolyn, LTRA, or theophylline	Low-dose ICS + LABA OR medium-dose ICS alternative: low-dose ICS + either LTRA OR theophylline or zileuton	Medium-dose ICS + LABA alternative: medium-dose ICS + either LTRA OR theophylline or zileuton	High-dose ICS + LABA AND Consider omalizumab for patients who have allergies.	High-dose ICS + LABA + OCS AND Consider omalizumab for patients who have allergies.

Abbreviations: ICS, inhaled corticosteroid; LABA, long-acting β₂-agonist; LTRA, leukotriene receptor antagonist; OCS, oral corticosteroids; PRN, as needed; SABA, short-acting β₂-agonist.

[a]All patients need quick-relief medication (SABA).

Each step: Patient education, environmental control, and management of comorbidities.

[b]Steps 2–4 (5 y–adult): Consider subcutaneous allergen immunotherapy for patients who have persistent, allergic asthma.

[c]Steps 5–6 (12 y–adult): Consider omalizumab for patients who have allergies.

Adapted from the National Asthma Education and Prevention Program. *Expert Panel Report 3: Guidelines for the Diagnosis and Management of Asthma, 2007.* Bethesda, MD: National Heart, Lung, and Blood Institute; 2007. NIH Publication No. 07-4051.

bronchodilation by stimulating β₂ receptors in the airway, which increases the concentration of cyclic adenosine monophosphate, causing relaxation of airway smooth muscle. Long-acting β₂-agonists should never be used alone without concomitant use with ICS in treatment of asthma.

Patients may be started at a higher level of medications at the onset, to establish prompt control, and then step-down reduction should be implemented to reach the minimum medication necessary to maintain control (Table 84-5).

Prognosis

Asthma can result in significant morbidity and mortality if children are not managed appropriately. Children without longitudinal primary care generally require expensive therapy in EDs or inpatient settings. A significant number of individuals with asthma have fatal outcomes because of lack of timely and appropriate care. Virtually all of these deaths are preventable.

CASE RESOLUTION

The 7-year-old boy in the case study who visits the office for asthma requires not only medication but also education and longitudinal primary care. It is particularly important to assess possible environmental factors (eg, pets), exposure to smoke, and poor compliance with previous recommendations, which have contributed to his recurrent symptoms.

Selected References

Abadoğlu O, Mungan D, Paşaoglu G, Celík G, Misirligil Z. Influenza vaccination in patients with asthma: effect on the frequency of upper respiratory tract infections and exacerbations. *J Asthma.* 2004;41(3):279–283

Adkinson N, Yunginger J, Busse W, et al, eds. *Middleton's Allergy: Principles and Practice.* 7th ed. St. Louis: Mosby; 2009

Akinbami L; Centers for Disease Control and Prevention National Center for Health Statistics. The state of childhood asthma, United States, 1980–2005. *Adv Data.* 2006;(381):1–24. http://www.cdc.gov/nchs/data/ad/ad381.pdf. Accessed March 6, 2014

Apter AJ, Szefler SJ. Advances in adult and pediatric asthma. *J Allergy Clin Immunol.* 2006;117(3):512–518

Bacharier LB, Strunk RC, Mauger D, White D, Lemanske RF Jr, Sorkness CA. Classifying asthma severity in children: mismatch between symptoms, medication use, and lung function. *Am J Respir Crit Care Med.* 2004;170(4):426–432

Bisgaard H, Hermansen MN, Loland L, Halkjaer LB, Buchvald F. Intermittent inhaled corticosteroids in infants with episodic wheezing. *N Engl J Med.* 2006;354(19):1998–2005

Bloom B, Cohen RA, Freeman G. Summary health statistics for U.S. children: National Health Interview Survey, 2007. *Vital Health Stat.* 2009;(239):1–80

Boushey HA, Sorkness CA, King TS, et al. Daily versus as-needed corticosteroids for mild persistent asthma. *N Engl J Med.* 2005;352(15):1519–1528

Bousquet J, Wenzel S, Holgate S, Lumry W, Freeman P, Fox H. Predicting response to omalizumab, an anti-IgE antibody, in patients with allergic asthma. *Chest.* 2004;125(4):1378–1386

Brussee JE, Smit HA, van Strien RT, et al. Allergen exposure in infancy and the development of sensitization, wheeze, and asthma at 4 years. *J Allergy Clin Immunol.* 2005;115(5):946–952

Bueving HJ, Bernsen RM, de Jongste JC, et al. Influenza vaccination in children with asthma: randomized double-blind placebo-controlled trial. *Am J Respir Crit Care Med.* 2004;169(4):488–493

Busse W, Corren J, Lanier BQ, et al. Omalizumab, anti IgE recombinant humanized monoclonal antibody, for the treatment of severe allergic asthma. *J Allergy Clin Immunol.* 2001;108(2):184–190

Castro-Rodríguez JA, Holberg CJ, Wright AL, Martinez FD. A clinical index to define risk of asthma in young children with recurrent wheezing. *Am J Respir Crit Care Med.* 2000;162(4 pt 1):1403–1406

Covar RA, Spahn JD, Murphy JR, Szefler SJ; Childhood Asthma Management Program Research Group. Progression of asthma measured by lung function in the childhood asthma management program. *Am J Respir Crit Care Med.* 2004; 170(3):234–241

Eder W, Ege MJ, von Mutius E. The asthma epidemic. *N Engl J Med.* 2006;355(21): 2226–2235

Friedman H, Wilcox T, Reardon G, Crespi S, Yawn BP. A retrospective study of the use of fluticasone propionate/salmeterol combination as initial asthma controller therapy in a commercially insured population. *Clin Ther.* 2008;30(10): 1908–1917

Greenstone IR, Ni Chroinin MN, Masse V, et al. Combination of inhaled long-acting beta2-agonists and inhaled steroids versus higher dose of inhaled steroids in children and adults with persistent asthma. *Cochrane Database Syst Rev.* 2005;(4):CD005533

Griffiths B, Ducharme FM. Combined inhaled anticholinergics and short-acting beta2-agonists for initial treatment of acute asthma in children. *Cochrane Database Syst Rev.* 2013;8:CD000060

Guilbert TW, Morgan WJ, Zeiger RS, et al. Long-term inhaled corticosteroids in preschool children at high risk for asthma. *N Engl J Med.* 2006;354(19): 1985–1997

Huynh PN, Scott LG, Kwong KY. Long-term maintenance of pediatric asthma: focus on budesonide/formoterol inhalation aerosol. *Ther Clin Risk Manag.* 2010;6:65–75

Jenkins CR, Thien FC, Wheatley JR, Reddel HK. Traditional and patient-centred outcomes with three classes of asthma medication. *Eur Respir J.* 2005;26(1): 36–44

Kwong KY, Huynh P. Treatment of pediatric asthma. In: Martin CR, Preedy VR, eds. *Scientific Basis of Health Care. Asthma.* Enfield, NH: Science Publishers; 2012:205–238

Masoli M, Weatherall M, Holt S, Beasley R. Moderate dose inhaled corticosteroids plus salmeterol versus higher doses of inhaled corticosteroids in symptomatic asthma. *Thorax.* 2005;60(9):730–734

Morgan WJ, Crain EF, Gruchalla RS, et al. Results of a home-based environmental intervention among urban children with asthma. *N Engl J Med.* 2004;351(11): 1068–1080

National Asthma Education and Prevention Program. *Guidelines the Diagnosis and Management of Asthma: Expert Panel Report 3.* Bethesda, MD: National Institutes of Health, National Heart, Lung and Blood Institute; 2007

National Heart, Lung, and Blood Institute. *National Asthma Education and Prevention Program Expert Panel Executive Summary Report: Guidelines for the Diagnosis and Management of Asthma—Update on Selected Topics 2002.* Bethesda, MD: National Institutes of Health; National Heart, Lung, and Blood Institute; 2002. NIH Publication No. 02-5075

Nelson KA, Zorc JJ. Asthma update. *Pediatr Clin North Am.* 2013;60(5): 1035–1048

Ng D, Salvio F, Hicks G. Anti-leukotriene agents compared to inhaled corticosteroids in the management of recurrent and/or chronic asthma in adults and children. *Cochrane Database Syst Rev.* 2004;(2):CD002314

Paull K, Covar R, Jain N, Gelfand EW, Spahn JD. Do NHLBI lung function criteria apply to children? A cross-sectional evaluation of childhood asthma at National Jewish Medical and Research Center, 1999–2002. *Pediatr Pulmonol.* 2005;39(4):311–317

Salpeter SR, Buckley NS, Ormiston TM, Salpeter EE. Meta-analysis: effect of long-acting beta-agonists on severe asthma exacerbations and asthma-related deaths. *Ann Intern Med.* 2006;144(12):904–912

Sigurs N, Gustafsson PM, Bjarnason R, et al. Severe respiratory syncytial virus bronchiolitis in infancy and asthma and allergy at age 13. *Am J Respir Crit Care Med.* 2005;171(2):137–141

Verbanck S, Schuermans D, Paiva M, Vincken W. The functional benefit of anti-inflammatory aerosols in the lung periphery. *J Allergy Clin Immunol.* 2006;118(2): 340–346

Wood PR, Hill VL. Practical management of asthma. *Pediatr Rev.* 2009;30(10): 375–385

Zeiger RS, Hay JW, Contreras R, et al. Asthma costs and utilization in a managed care organization. *J Allergy Clin Immunol.* 2008;121(4):885–892

CHAPTER 85

Cough

Nasser Redjal, MD, and Kenny Yat-Choi Kwong, MD

CASE STUDY

A 3-year-old boy presents with a cough that he has had for 4 weeks. In the past, he has had coughs with colds, but this cough is persistent and deeper in quality. The cough seemed to develop suddenly when he was playing at a friend's house. It occurs all day and disrupts his sleep at night. The boy has had no nasal congestion, fever, or sore throat. No one at home is coughing, and the boy has not traveled recently. Neither the boy nor his family has a history of allergies or asthma. Over-the-counter cough preparations have not helped relieve his symptoms. On examination, growth parameters are normal. The child has a persistent cough with no respiratory distress. Chest examination reveals a normal respiratory rate, no retractions, and no use of accessory muscles, but diffuse expiratory wheezing is noted in the right lower lobe. The remainder of the examination is normal.

Questions

1. What are common parental concerns about cough?
2. What diagnoses in children with persistent cough should be considered?
3. What historical factors and physical findings are important to determine the etiology of cough?
4. What diagnostic workup is appropriate?
5. How should children with chronic cough be managed?

Cough is an essential protective reflex that allows for clearance of secretions and particulates from the airways. Its persistence can be distressing to the patient and often causes parental anxiety because of uncertainty of its etiology. Cough may be acute, subacute, or chronic. Acute cough lasts less than 2 weeks and is often associated with respiratory tract infections in children. Cough lasting 2 to 4 weeks is subacute, and when cough lasts more than 4 weeks, it is persistent or chronic. In children older than 15 years and adults, *chronic* is usually defined as persistent cough lasting more than 8 weeks. Parental sensitivity as well as accessibility to medical care influence when in the course of disease children present with this problem. Most cough resolves in children without treatment, but some may be caused by underlying conditions such as asthma or, rarely, foreign body aspirations or bronchiectasis.

Epidemiology

Cough is a very common complaint initiating pediatric office visits. In the National Ambulatory Medical Care Survey, 6.7% of pediatric office visits involved children who presented with cough. Typically, preschool children have up to 8 upper respiratory infections with associated cough in a winter season. Persistent cough is also very common, with an estimated prevalence of 5% to 7% in preschoolers and 12% to 15% in older children. Cough is more common among boys than girls up to 11 years of age and may be less common in developing countries than in affluent countries.

Clinical Presentation

Presentation varies greatly depending on the etiology of the cough. Most children have no evidence of respiratory compromise, but on occasion, some will present with respiratory distress. Depending on the underlying etiology, they may manifest other symptoms of chronic lung disease such as clubbing and failure to thrive, although the majority are found to be in good health.

Pathophysiology

Coughing is a protective reflex that is automatically triggered by cough receptors found throughout the human airway, including the nose, paranasal sinuses, posterior pharynx, larynx, trachea, bronchi, and pleura. They can also be found outside of the respiratory tract in the ear canal, stomach, pericardium, and diaphragm (Figure 85-1).

Proximal airways (larynx and trachea) are more sensitive to mechanical stimulation and distal airways are more sensitive to chemical stimulation. Lung parenchymal (bronchiolar and alveolar) tissue contains no cough receptors, so pneumonia may not produce a cough. Stimulation of any of these receptors by an irritant, whether mechanical, chemical, thermal, or inflammatory, can initiate the cough reflex. Impulses from stimulated cough receptors traverse afferent nerves (vagus, glossopharyngeal, trigeminal, or phrenic) to a "cough center" in the medulla, which itself is under some control by higher cortical centers. The cough center generates an efferent signal that travels down the vagus, phrenic, and spinal motor nerves to expiratory musculature, thereby producing the cough. The cough center can be voluntarily stimulated or suppressed. Once initiated, the cough reflex propels excess mucus up the airways at the pressures of up to 300 mm Hg and at flows of up to 5 to 6 L/sec.

The actual cough experienced by patients may be broken down into 4 phases. First, the glottis opens with an inspiratory gasp. Second,

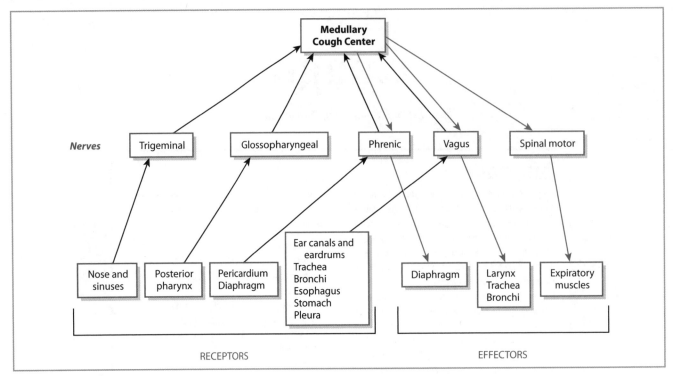

Figure 85-1. The cough reflex.

the glottis closes with forceful contraction of the chest wall, diaphragm, and abdominal muscles. Third, the glottis again opens with release of airway pressure in an expiratory phase. Fourth, the chest wall and abdominal muscles relax. This process expels mucus or irritants from the airways, helping maintain lung health. Children who do not cough effectively may be at risk for atelectasis, recurrent pneumonia, and chronic airway disease from aspiration or retention of secretions.

Differential Diagnosis

Any pathology present along the airway from the nose to the alveoli can elicit a cough response; therefore, the list of differential diagnoses of cough is long (Box 85-1). Narrowing the list of causes can be accomplished by paying attention to several factors (D_x Box).

As with any pediatric symptom, the child's **age** influences the diagnostic possibilities and management of the cough. Congenital anomalies, which are most likely to present in the first few months of life, include tracheoesophageal fistula, laryngeal cleft, vocal cord

paralysis, and tracheobronchomalacia. Congenital heart disease can produce a cough from heart failure and pulmonary edema. Congenital mediastinal tumors cause infants to cough if the tumor presses on the bronchial tree. Many children with asthma experience cough or wheezing in infancy, often precipitated by episodes of respiratory viral infection with respiratory syncytial virus (RSV), rhinovirus, or metapneumovirus.

The **duration of the cough** also suggests its possible cause. Most acute coughs are infectious in origin. Upper respiratory infections can initiate an acute cough through stimulation of the cough receptors in the nose and posterior pharynx. If nasal congestion and cough persist, a diagnosis of allergic rhinitis or sinusitis should be considered. Serous otitis media can also cause a persistent cough and may occur in children with chronic congestion.

Respiratory infections with viral pathogens are the most likely cause of cough in children. Adenovirus, RSV, rhinovirus, and human metapneumonic virus occur in infants and younger children, and influenza and parainfluenza may produce cough in children of all ages. Cough that persists may be due to *Bordetella pertussis*, mycoplasma, and chlamydia. Cough can occur in patients with pneumonia, and pneumococcus is the most probable agent. Other infections, such as tuberculosis and coccidioidomycosis, should also be considered in endemic areas or high-risk populations. Chronic infectious coughs, such as those associated with influenza and pertussis, can last many months. Host factors that may predispose to chronic cough should also be investigated. Children with cystic fibrosis, bronchopulmonary dysplasia, HIV, and other immunodeficiency syndromes as well as congenital pulmonary malformations may present with chronic, recurrent cough.

Cough

- Quality: dry, productive, brassy, honking
- Duration: acute, subacute, chronic, recurrent
- Timing: during day, at night, on awakening, with exercise
- Fever or upper respiratory infection associated with infectious origin
- Allergic findings of rhinorrhea, sneezing, wheezing, atopic dermatitis associated with asthma or allergic rhinitis
- Failure to thrive (indicates chronic disease)

Box 85-1. Causes of Cough

Congenital Anomalies	**Bacterial**	**Chronic Disease**
Tracheoesophageal fistula	Pertussis	Cystic fibrosis
Laryngeal cleft	Pneumococcal	HIV infection
Vocal cord paralysis	Staphylococcal	Immunodeficiency syndrome
Mediastinal masses	Tuberculosis	Dyskinetic cilia
Pulmonary malformations	**Fungal**	*Allergic Conditions*
Tracheobronchomalacia	Coccidioidomycosis	Allergic rhinitis
Congenital heart disease	**Parasitic**	Asthma
Infections (eg, upper respiratory,	Paragonimiasis	Serous otitis media
sinusitis, pneumonia)	Echinococcosis	*Mediastinal Tumors*
Viral	**Other**	*Foreign Body Aspiration*
Adenovirus	Chlamydial	*Gastroesophageal Reflux*
Influenza	Mycoplasmosis	*Environmental Irritants*
Parainfluenza	*Cardiac Disease*	*Psychogenic Cough*
Respiratory syncytial virus	Congestive heart failure	*Drug-Induced Conditions*
Rhinovirus	Pulmonary hypertension	*Sarcoidosis*
Human metapneumovirus		*Tourette Syndrome (tics)*

Children who have cough independent of respiratory infections often have postnasal drip caused by rhinitis (allergic and nonallergic) and sinusitis (acute and chronic). Asthma may present as solely cough without wheezing or dyspnea in children and adults (cough variant asthma). Stomach acid from gastroesophageal reflux disease (GERD) may activate receptors in the larynx, resulting in cough even if there is no aspiration into the airways.

An unexplained persistent cough, primarily in toddlers, may be the result of foreign body aspiration if the initial aspiration was not observed. In some studies, a history of choking episodes is absent in approximately 50% and chest radiograph examination produces normal results in approximately 20% to 40% of children who have foreign bodies present on bronchoscopy. The foreign object acts as a chronic airway irritant that stimulates coughing, and it may be the cause of recurrent infections. Other irritants that initiate cough include dust, allergens, wood- and gas-burning stoves, chemicals, and passive or active exposure to smoke from tobacco, marijuana, cocaine, or other substances. In older children and adults, drugs such as β-adrenergic receptor antagonists and angiotensin-converting enzyme (ACE) inhibitors can also induce a chronic cough, probably by increasing the sensitivity of the cough reflex. Patients previously treated with cytotoxic drugs or thoracic radiation are at risk of interstitial lung disease. Cough along with symptoms of pancreatic insufficiency, recurrent bacterial pneumonia, or failure to thrive should raise suspicion of cystic fibrosis. Cough with a history of dyspnea or hemoptysis should trigger a search for organic lung disease. Hemoptysis should also raise concerns of bronchiectasis, cavitary lung disease (tuberculosis or bacterial abscesses), congestive heart failure, hemosiderosis, neoplasm, foreign bodies, vascular lesions, endobronchial lesions, menstrual (ectopic endometrial tissue) bleeding, and clotting disorders.

Etiologies for chronic cough are similar to those for acute cough except the stimuli persist for longer periods. Generally, viral infections self-resolve before the threshold of 4 to 8 weeks required to define chronic cough in children and adults, respectively, although cough from some rare viruses may linger for many months. In children 15 years and older and adults with normal history, physical examination, and chest radiograph, postnasal drip, asthma, and GERD are the most likely causes of chronic cough, followed by medications such as ACE inhibitors and smoking. These patients often have more than one etiology contributing to persistent symptoms. Recent studies, however, have found that the aforementioned etiologies result in chronic cough in only 10% of children with cough lasting more than 4 weeks. Therefore, in children 15 years and younger, a broader differential should be considered, especially with regard to more serious causes such as foreign body aspiration and bronchiectasis.

Evaluation

History

A complete history should be obtained when children present with cough (Questions Box). All symptoms should be noted. Vomiting with cough can indicate phlegm production and accumulation of mucus in the stomach, with resultant delayed gastric emptying. In some children with a chief complaint of vomiting, it is actually the cough that precipitates the vomiting. Post-tussive vomiting is characteristic of, though not specific for, pertussis.

The presence of a nighttime cough can be important. Pathologic coughs, including those caused by sinusitis with postnasal drip, gastroesophageal reflux, and asthma, are more likely to occur at night.

Physical Examination

A complete physical examination should be performed on all children who present with cough. Growth parameters and vital signs

Cough

Questions

- How old is the child?
- How long has the child had the cough?
- How frequently does the child cough?
- Does the cough occur at night?
- Does exercise make the cough worse?
- Do any factors, such as environmental irritants, seem to precipitate the cough?
- Does the child have any related infectious symptoms, including fever and nasal congestion?
- Does the child have any other symptoms?
- Has the child had any previous episodes of coughing or associated symptoms?
- Has the child lost weight recently?
- What is the child's birth history?
- Has the child had any pulmonary injuries?
- What is the child's immunization status?
- Does the child have a history of recent travel?
- Has a family member had similar symptoms?
- Does the family have a history of pulmonary disease or allergies?
- Has the child been treated with any medications for the cough? Have they helped?
- Is the child taking any other medications?

should be assessed. Skin should be examined for evidence of cyanosis or atopy. Facial petechiae or subconjunctival hemorrhage indicates particularly forceful coughing. Extremities should be evaluated for fingernail clubbing, which is a sign of chronic pulmonary disease. The nose should be assessed for evidence of congestion. Allergic disease produces pale, edematous mucosa, whereas infection results in more inflammatory mucosa. Tympanic membranes should be examined and mobility tested; halitosis, tonsillar hypertrophy, pharyngeal cobblestone, and tenderness on the sinus area suggest sinus disease.

The **character** of the cough is another factor to consider in assessment because certain etiologies may be associated with a very specific type of cough. A barking cough is consistent with laryngeal edema and croup. A cough with stridor may be seen with proximal airway disease, such as laryngomalacia or tracheomalacia, laryngotracheobronchitis, or a foreign body. An inspiratory whoop is characteristic of pertussis or parapertussis. Staccato cough in infants can be the result of infection with *Chlamydia trachomatis*. The psychogenic or habitual cough is a strange, honking sound (Canadian goose-like); disappears at night; and is typically at its worst and most disruptive during school classes. Chronic paroxysmal cough triggered by exercise, cold air, sleep, or allergens is often seen in patients with asthma. In contrast, a chronic productive (or "wet") cough suggests a suppurative process and may require further investigation to exclude bronchiectasis, cystic fibrosis, active infection, immune deficiency, or congenital malformation.

Respiratory effort, including the use of accessory muscles, should also be noted. Careful attention should be paid to breath sounds; whether abnormal sounds are in the inspiratory or expiratory phase

of respiration should be determined. Stridor is classically an inspiratory sound (see Chapter 60), whereas wheezing is usually an expiratory sound. Chronic cough and wheeze are often noted in combination. Even in the absence of a history of wheeze, clinicians should listen carefully for this finding during the physical examination. Wheezing that is characterized by many different pitches and starting and stopping at varying points in the respiratory cycle is termed *polyphonic* and in association with cough is highly suggestive of asthma. Other causes of polyphonic wheezing include viral bronchiolitis, obliterative bronchiolitis, bronchiectasis, bronchopulmonary dysplasia, congestive heart failure, immunodeficiency, bronchomalacia, and aspiration syndromes.

Monophonic wheezing (a single, distinct, one pitch that starts and stops at one discrete time) and cough should always raise suspicion of large airway obstruction caused by foreign body or by tracheomalacia. Extrinsic airway compression as occurs with vascular rings, lymphadenopathy, and mediastinal tumors is also associated with monophonic wheezing. Tuberculosis should be considered in a child with a monophonic wheeze, particularly in areas where the disease is prevalent.

Prolongation of the expiratory phase is associated with wheezing and also indicates airway obstruction. Abnormal breath sounds should be localized, if possible. Because the character of the cough can establish the diagnosis, listening to the cough is probably the most important part of the physical examination. A parental description of the cough may be less diagnostic.

Laboratory Tests

Laboratory investigations are usually not necessary in management of cough. Studies should be directed at proving or disproving the most likely diagnosis in a specific patient and guided by the history and physical examination.

If, after the history, physical examination, and chest radiograph, an infectious etiology for cough is suspected, a complete blood cell count with differential and a purified protein derivative skin test for tuberculosis maybe ordered. Appropriate cultures should be sent, if possible. Most children swallow their phlegm, so sputum cultures may be difficult to obtain. Gastric aspirates can sometimes yield a reasonable sputum specimen for culture, although this is uncomfortable and only used when absolutely necessary, such as in management of tuberculosis. Nasopharyngeal cultures and rapid antigen detecting assays are useful for diagnosing pertussis and respiratory viruses.

If a specific diagnosis is suspected, laboratory tests (Table 85-1) should be directed toward that diagnosis (eg, sweat chloride to rule out cystic fibrosis; quantitative immunoglobulins to rule out immunodeficiency). Allergy skin testing or specific allergen IgE serum (radioallergosorbent test type) testing may be indicated to exclude inhalant allergy.

Imaging Studies

The chest radiograph (anteroposterior and lateral views) remains the mainstay of the diagnostic evaluation of cough and should be

Table 85-1. Tests to Consider for Evaluation of Chronic Cough

Allergy	Allergy skin test or blood-specific immunoglobulin E test
Asthma	Pulmonary function test (PFT), bronchial hyperreactivity test such as methacholine challenge test, exhaled nitric oxide, trial of asthma treatments
Ciliary dyskinesia	Ciliary function tests
Congenital anomalies	Bronchoscopy, chest radiograph, computed tomography (CT)/magnetic resonance imaging, angiography
Fungal infections	Coccidioidomycosis: antibody assay (precipitin, complement fixation) Histoplasmosis: antibody assay (complement fixation, immunoprecipitating) Serum and urine antigen detection
Cystic fibrosis	Sweat chloride test, genetic test
Idiopathic pulmonary fibrosis, autoimmune disease	PFT and diffusion CT, autoantibodies
Foreign body	Chest radiograph, bronchoscopy
Gastroesophageal reflux	Barium swallow, 24-hour pH recording, and bronchoalveolar lavage (BAL)
Pertussis, chlamydia, or other infectious etiologies	Cultures, serology, polymerase chain reaction testing
Purulent infection	Cultures (sputum, BAL), chest radiograph, CT, microbiology immunology, sweat test
Sinusitis	Imaging of sinuses with radiograph or CT scan
Tuberculosis	Mantoux testing

ordered when there are definitive signs on physical examination and when the cough has been chronic. A lateral decubitus film can provide additional information about pleural fluid or air trapping. Inspiratory and expiratory films can be obtained if a foreign body is suspected. An area of inflation that fails to deflate on exhalation or remains present in the decubitus position is suggestive of a foreign body. Congenital lobar emphysema and unilateral emphysema (Swyer-James syndrome) are rare causes of focal or unilateral hyperinflation. If a nodular pulmonary lesion is found on radiograph, bronchoscopy may be the next step to further define the lesion. Bronchiectasis is a characteristic of cystic fibrosis, immune deficiency, primary ciliary dyskinesia, chronic aspiration, and previous history of severe infection (most commonly adenovirus and pertussis). If sinusitis is suspected, computed tomography scan of the sinuses can be performed, though radiation exposure must be considered. An upper gastrointestinal series of radiographs or a pH probe study would help to define gastroesophageal reflux if the cough is associated with meals or episodes of vomiting or at night.

In children with asthma, the chest radiograph may be totally normal. Further diagnostic testing with pulmonary function tests in cooperative children can be done to demonstrate restriction or obstruction of the airway. The most helpful test to diagnose asthma may be response to inhaled corticosteroids and bronchodilator.

Management

Cough should not be treated until the cause has been identified by a thorough consideration of the differential diagnoses. Therapy should then be directed toward treating that etiology. However, many children do not have any evidence of chronic disease based on a detailed history, physical examination, radiography, and pulmonary function testing. When the initial evaluation outlined previously is unrevealing, cough variant asthma, post-viral cough, increased cough receptor sensitivity, and functional disorders (including habit cough and tic disorders) should be considered. Empiric courses of therapy for asthma, rhinitis, sinusitis, or gastroesophageal reflux can be considered if suggestive findings exist. The external ear is innervated by the vagus nerve, and removal of irritants from the external auditory canal may reduce the coughing. Airflow obstruction may be apparent at the first visit, and a trial of asthma therapy is warranted, particularly if other signs of allergic disease are present or if the child's cough is precipitated by typical asthma triggers. A cough of an infectious etiology should be treated with appropriate antibiotics. Expectorants and mucolytic agents in cough syrups have little effect on relieving coughs. Most over-the-counter children's cough medications are marginally effective, provide no greater benefit compared with placebo, and may be associated with adverse or paradoxical reactions.

Caveat in Management of Chronic Cough

Chronic cough often causes frustration and anxiety among patients and their parents. Clinicians may be unable to provide a definitive etiology and timely relief of symptoms, resulting in patients seeking answers from multiple clinicians and trying many ineffective over-the-counter products. Key to effective management of these patients is good communication. Patients and parents need to be informed that irritation of the airways resulting in chronic cough often takes time to resolve, and improvement of cough symptoms should be measured in weeks, not a few days.

In children 15 years and older and adults with a normal history and physical examination (and preferably a normal chest radiograph), treatment for rhinitis, asthma, and GERD should be initiated if there are suggestive signs such as postnasal drip, rhinorrhea, and heartburn. However, many adult practitioners initiate empiric treatment even in absence of findings. Because symptoms may be the result of a combination of etiologies, treatment of one pathology may only result in partial improvement; treatment of the other causes is needed for full resolution. For instance, therapy with intranasal steroid and antihistamines for 2 weeks may result in partial improvement of symptoms, while the addition of a proton pump inhibitor would result in full resolution. Medications that may provoke chronic cough, such as ACE inhibitors, should be changed and exposure to tobacco smoke eliminated.

In the past, management of chronic cough in children younger than 15 years was done in a similar fashion as with adults—using empiric trials of medications. The American College of Chest Physicians, however, changed this recommendation in 2006 after it was found that predominant causes of chronic cough in adults were only present in approximately 10% of children with similar symptoms. Cough and cold preparations used to empirically treat allergic conditions in adults have been found to have unacceptable side effects in children. Other serious causes of cough should be considered in children with persistent cough and worked up if there is no disease resolution. For instance, children with cough that was preceded by choking should be evaluated for foreign body aspiration; progressive cough with weight loss and fevers requires workup for tuberculosis; wet cough, sinusitis, and history of pneumonia may need immunodeficiency workup; and cough with seasonal sneezing and rhinorrhea may need treatment for allergic rhinitis and postnasal drip. Fortunately, viral infections are the predominant cause of chronic cough in children, and reassurance may be the only management needed until resolution of symptoms. Most children do not require treatment, but benign agents such as warm liquids with honey (>1 year) often suffice.

The exception to the rule of not using empiric treatment for children in diagnosis and treatment of chronic cough is asthma, which can present in a cough-variant form without wheezing or respiratory distress. Empiric trial of inhaled corticosteroids or bronchodilators is recommended for a period of a few weeks, after which response is assessed. Pretreatment and posttreatment spirometry, if available, will provide an additional objective measure for asthma diagnosis.

Prognosis

With thoughtful evaluation, it is usually possible to identify the causes of acute and chronic cough. Most symptoms resolve with appropriate therapy. If the cough persists with treatment, alternate diagnoses should be considered.

CASE RESOLUTION

In the case presented at the beginning of this chapter, the child's cough began acutely and developed into a chronic cough. The boy has no history of allergies or symptoms consistent with an infectious process. Physical examination reveals localized wheezing. A chest radiograph is ordered, which reveals hyperinflation of the right lung. His symptoms and presentation are most consistent with foreign body aspiration, and he is admitted to the hospital for bronchoscopy.

Selected References

Adkinson N, Yunginger J, Busse W, et al, eds. *Middleton's Allergy: Principles and Practice.* 7th ed. St. Louis, MO: Mosby; 2008

Bucca CB, Bugiani M, Culla B, et al. Chronic cough and irritable larynx, *J Allergy Clin Immunol.* 2011;127(2):412–419

Carr BC. Efficacy, abuse, and toxicity of over-the-counter cough and cold medicines in the pediatric population. *Curr Opin Pediatr.* 2006;18(2):184–188

Chang AB, Glomb WB. Guidelines for evaluating chronic cough in pediatrics: ACCP evidence-based clinical practice guidelines. *Chest.* 2006;129(1 Suppl):260S–283S

Chung KF, Chang AB. Therapy for cough: active agents. *Pulm Pharmacol Ther.* 2002;15(3):335–338

Chung KF, Pavord ID. Prevalence, pathogenesis, and causes of chronic cough. *Lancet.* 2008;371(9621):1364–1374

de Jongste JC, Shields MD. Cough. 2: chronic cough in children. *Thorax.* 2003; 58(11):998–1003

Eysink PE, Bottema BJ, ter Riet G, Aalberse RC, Stapel SO, Bindels PJ. Coughing in pre-school children in general practice: when are RASTs for inhalation allergy indicated? *Pediatr Allergy Immunol.* 2004;15(5):394–400

Irwin RS, Baumann MH, Bolser DC, et al. Diagnosis and management of cough executive summary: ACCP evidence-based clinical practice guidelines. *Chest.* 2006;129(1 Suppl):1S–23S

Kelkar P, Weldon D. Approach to the patient with chronic cough. In: Adkinson NF, Bochner BS, et al. *Middleton's Allergy Principle and Practice.* 7th ed. Mayland Heights, MO: Elsevier; 2009:1395–1404

Morice AH, Fontana GA, Belvisi MG, et al. ERS guidelines on the assessment of cough. *Eur Respir J.* 2007;29(6):1256–1276

Morice AH, Fontana GA, Sovijarvi AR, et al. The diagnosis and management of chronic cough. *Eur Respir J.* 2004;24(3):481–492

Morice AH, Geppetti P. Cough. 5: the type 1 vanilloid receptor: a sensory receptor for cough. *Thorax.* 2004;59(3):257–258

Ramanuja S, Kelkar P. Habit cough. *Ann Allergy Asthma Immunol.* 2009;102(2): 91–97

Ramanuja S, Kelkar PS. The approach to pediatric cough. *Ann Allergy Asthma Immunol.* 2010;105(1):3–11

Santamaria F, Montella S, Camera L, Palumbo C, Greco L, Boner AL. Lung structure abnormalities, but normal lung function in pediatric bronchiectasis. *Chest.* 2006;130(2):480–486

Schwartz J. Air pollution and children's health. *Pediatrics.* 2004;113(4 Suppl):1037–1043

Tan H, Büyükavci M, Arik A. Tourette's syndrome manifests as chronic persistent cough. *Yonsei Med J.* 2004;45(1):145–149

Hematologic Disorders

CHAPTER 86

Anemia

Joseph L. Lasky III, MD, and Eduard H. Panosyan, MD

CASE STUDY

An 18-month-old girl is brought to the office with a 3-day history of cough, rhinorrhea, low-grade fever, mild scleral icterus, and pallor. During her first week of life, the girl had hyperbilirubinemia of unknown etiology that required phototherapy. Her family history is significant for mild anemia in her father; the cause of his condition is unknown. A paternal aunt and grandfather had cholecystectomies while in their 30s.

On physical examination, the girl is tachycardic and tachypneic (no respiratory distress) with scleral icterus and pallor. Her spleen is palpable 3 cm below the midcostal margin. The remainder of her examination is normal.

Questions

1. What hemoglobin/hematocrit values are associated with anemia?
2. What is the appropriate initial evaluation of children with anemia?
3. What emergency situations in children who present with anemia should be recognized by the primary pediatrician?
4. When should a child with anemia be referred to a hematologist?
5. How is the family history relevant in the evaluation of anemia?

Anemia occurs when there is a reduction in hemoglobin concentration or red blood cell (RBC) number, leading to decreased oxygen-carrying capacity of blood. Anemia is defined as a hemoglobin or hematocrit value that is less than 2 SDs below the mean for age and gender. With this statistical definition, 2.5% of the healthy population will be categorized as having anemia. These values vary throughout infancy and childhood as hematopoiesis evolves from fetal to adult type, and it is important to reference normal age- and gender-related values when interpreting a hemoglobin or hematocrit result (Table 86-1). In addition, there is racial variation with African American children having lower average hemoglobin values when compared with white children. Cardiopulmonary status should also be considered because children with cyanotic heart disease or chronic respiratory insufficiency typically have hemoglobin values that are higher than the normal range and may be functionally anemic when the hemoglobin value falls, even if it is within the lower range of normal.

Epidemiology

Iron deficiency is the most common cause of anemia in childhood, occurring most frequently during late infancy through the first few years of life and again during adolescence. This prevalence pattern corresponds to periods of rapid growth, and when combined with poor dietary intake can predispose to iron deficiency. Other contributing factors to iron deficiency include prematurity, blood loss (most commonly menstrual or gastrointestinal), and GI conditions associated with decreased iron absorption.

Table 86-1. Values (Mean and Lower Limits of Normal) for Hemoglobin, Hematocrit, and Mean Corpuscular Volume Determinations

Age, y	Hemoglobin (g/dL)		Hematocrit (%)		MCV (μ^3)	
	Mean	Lower Limit	Mean	Lower Limit	Mean	Lower Limit
0.5–1.9	12.5	11.0	37	33	77	70
2–4	12.5	11.0	38	34	79	73
5–7	13.0	11.5	39	35	81	75
8–11	13.5	12.0	40	36	83	76
12–14						
Female	13.5	12.0	41	36	85	78
Male	14.0	12.5	43	37	84	77
15–17						
Female	14.0	12.0	41	36	87	79
Male	15.0	13.0	46	38	86	78
18–49						
Female	14.0	12.0	42	37	90	80
Male	16.0	14.0	47	40	90	80

Abbreviation: MCV, mean corpuscular volume.

From Brugnara C, Oski FA, Nathan DG. Diagnostic approach to the anemic patient. In: Orkin SH, Nathan DG, Ginsburg D, Look AT, Fisher DE, Lux SE, eds. *Nathan and Oski's Hematology of Infancy and Childhood*. 7th ed. Philadelphia, PA: Saunders Elsevier; 2009:456, with permission.

Other epidemiologic factors that contribute to anemia are presented in Box 86-1. Anemias that have a genetic etiology, including hemoglobinopathies (eg, sickle cell disease, thalassemias), RBC enzyme deficiencies (eg, glucose-6-phosphate dehydrogenase, pyruvate kinase), and RBC membrane disorders (eg, hereditary spherocytosis), are commonly diagnosed in childhood. The highest incidence of sickle cell disease, thalassemia, and G6PD deficiency is in individuals of African, Mediterranean, and Southeast Asian descent within the "malaria belt" near the equator, likely reflecting an evolutionary advantage against malaria. Dietary factors can cause impaired hematopoiesis as in iron, folate, or vitamin B_{12} deficiency. Ingestion of oxidants (eg, fava beans, medications) can trigger hemolysis in G6PD deficiency. Ingestion of toxins such as lead can also result in impaired hematopoiesis. Lead poisoning occurs more commonly in children who live in cities and older housing. In an otherwise healthy child, viral infections can cause a pure red cell aplasia (transient erythroblastopenia of childhood), an autoimmune hemolytic anemia, or an aplastic anemia. Children with congenital hemolytic anemias are at risk for hemolytic and aplastic crises associated with infectious illnesses.

Clinical Presentation

The clinical presentation of anemia depends on the age of the child, severity and cause of the anemia, and rapidity of onset (D_x Box). Most often, anemia is detected on a routine screen or as part of an evaluation for an acute illness and the child is asymptomatic with no significant physical findings. Children who have developed anemia gradually may be relatively asymptomatic because time has afforded compensatory mechanisms such as plasma volume expansion and increased cardiac contractility. With severe anemia, easy fatigability and exercise intolerance can develop and pallor, fatigue, headache, dizziness, and irritability may occur. On examination, pallor, tachycardia, tachypnea, edema, and in severe cases, outright congestive heart failure (CHF) may be present. Children with an abrupt drop in hemoglobin from blood loss or hemolysis will present more acutely with signs of tachycardia, tachypnea, and possible hypotension and shock. If the anemia is caused by acute hemolysis, accompanying jaundice, icterus, and dark urine may be seen.

Pathophysiology

Erythrocytes develop from pluripotent stem cells within the bone marrow under the influence of various hematopoietic growth factors. Erythropoietin is the primary growth factor regulating RBC production and is produced primarily by renal interstitial peritubular cells. The primary function of the erythrocyte is the delivery of oxygen to tissues for aerobic metabolism. To this end, hemoglobin is the main intracellular protein of the erythrocyte. Hemoglobin consists of 4 polypeptide subunits, each containing an active heme group that is capable of binding to an oxygen molecule. A normal erythrocyte has a life span of approximately 120 days and is subsequently removed from circulation as it passes through the reticuloendothelial system. Under steady state conditions, the daily 1% loss of aged

---

Box 86-1. Epidemiologic Factors Related to Anemia

Genetic
- Autosomal-dominant: hereditary spherocytosis
- Autosomal-recessive: most Embden-Meyerhof pathway enzyme deficiencies (pyruvate kinase deficiency), most hemoglobinopathies (sickle cell disease, β-thalassemia)
- X-linked: G6PD deficiency

Ethnicity
- Northern European: hereditary spherocytosis, pyruvate kinase deficiency
- Mediterranean (Italian, Greek, North African): β-thalassemia, G6PD deficiency
- African: sickle cell disease, hemoglobin C, hemoglobin D, G6PD deficiency, α-thalassemia trait, hereditary elliptocytosis
- Southeast Asian: α-thalassemia, hemoglobin E, G6PD deficiency

Dietary
Poor dietary intake (iron, folate, or vitamin B_{12} deficiency)
- Iron (excessive cow's milk intake)
- Folate (excessive goat's milk intake)
- Vitamin B_{12} (vegan diet)

Poor gastrointestinal absorption
- Iron, absorbed in duodenum (small bowel disease)
- Folate, absorbed in duodenum and jejunum (small bowel disease)
- Vitamin B_{12}, absorbed in terminal ileum (surgical resection, pernicious anemia, small bowel disease)

Ingestion of oxidants (medications such as sulfa drugs, fava beans in G6PD deficiency)

Toxins (lead)

Socioeconomic
- Living near highways: increased incidence of lead poisoning
- Poverty: associated with pica and lead poisoning

Infectious
- Malaria: heterozygous form of sickle cell disease, thalassemia, G6PD-deficiency confer protection
- Viral infections: transient erythroblastopenia of childhood, autoimmune hemolytic anemias, hemolytic crisis in patients with congenital hemolytic anemias
- Parvovirus: aplastic crisis in patients with hemolytic anemias
- Viral hepatitis: aplastic anemia

Abbreviation: G6PD, glocuse-6-phosphate dehydrogenase.

Dx Anemia

- Pallor, fatigue
- Scleral icterus
- Hepatosplenomegaly
- Lymphadenopathy
- Weight loss
- Congestive heart failure

erythrocytes is compensated by a normal active erythropoiesis. Also of note, red cell loss is greater (1.5%) and life span is shorter (90 days) during the late fetal and early neonatal period. Anemia occurs when there is an imbalance between erythrocyte production and destruction. It can arise from conditions leading to **decreased production, increased destruction** (ie, hemolysis), or **blood loss.** Deficient production may be due to nutrient deficiency (iron, folate, vitamin B_{12}), bone marrow failure (acquired or inherited), or bone marrow infiltration (eg, malignancy). Increased destruction of erythrocytes can occur as a consequence of disorders intrinsic to the erythrocyte (eg, hemoglobinopathies, enzymopathies, membranopathies) or extrinsic factors (immune or nonimmune etiologies).

Differential Diagnosis

The differential diagnosis of anemia can be determined by considering the underlying mechanism of anemia (decreased production/increased destruction/blood loss) and the size of the erythrocyte (mean corpuscular volume). The differential diagnosis of anemia based on pathophysiology and erythrocyte size can be found in Table 86-2 and Box 86-2. In determining the cause of anemia, the reticulocyte count is the most useful test in ascertaining whether the anemia is caused by decreased production or increased destruction. A reduced reticulocyte count indicates decreased marrow production, whereas an elevated reticulocyte count is highly suggestive of hemolysis. Anemia based on erythrocyte size can be classified as microcytic (low MCV), normocytic (normal MCV), or macrocytic (high MCV). Microcytic anemias reflect a defect in hemoglobin synthesis and are most commonly due to iron deficiency, thalassemia, lead poisoning, and chronic disease. Macrocytic anemias reflect a relative decrease in DNA synthesis during impaired erythropoiesis and are usually of nutritional origin (vitamin B_{12} or folate deficiency). The many other causes of anemia commonly fall into the normocytic category and can be further divided based on the reticulocyte count. Etiology and erythrocyte size, the 2 systems for classification of anemia, are not mutually exclusive—simultaneous application of these systems will enable the pediatrician to make a primary diagnosis of anemia and determine its probable causes.

Microcytic Anemias

Iron deficiency is the most frequent cause of microcytic anemia in childhood and occurs as a result of inadequate intake, increased requirements due to growth, blood loss, and malabsorption of iron. As iron deficiency evolves, depletion of iron stores occurs first, then iron-deficient erythropoiesis without anemia, and finally, iron deficiency anemia. The combination of rapid growth and inadequate iron intake is responsible for the common occurrence of iron deficiency anemia in toddlers and adolescents. Many young newborns and infants are spared because of adequate iron stores acquired in utero and the ingestion of iron-fortified formulas. Exclusively breastfed newborns and infants may require supplemental iron before 6 months of age and should be evaluated for anemia. Premature newborns are the exception, as they have lower baseline iron stores (much of the iron stores are acquired by the fetus in the third

trimester). As iron stores become depleted during late infancy and cow's milk is introduced into the diet, the ever-growing older infant/toddler becomes at risk for iron deficiency. Excessive cow's milk intake during the first few years of life predisposes to iron deficiency because cow's milk has minimal bioavailable iron (<1 mg/L). Large intake of cow's milk results in early satiety and prevents adequate intake of other iron-containing foods. Iron deficiency is often further compounded by trace amounts of GI blood loss due to GI mucosal damage or cow's milk allergy enteropathy. Adolescents, particularly menstruating females, are also prone to iron deficiency because of the pubertal growth spurt and suboptimal dietary habits. In young infants and children older than 3 years, purely dietary iron deficiency is uncommon, and an evaluation for blood loss or malabsorption is warranted. Blood loss can occur as hematochezia or melena (inflammatory bowel disease, diarrhea, Meckel diverticulum, polyp, ulcer), menorrhagia, epistaxis, hematuria (intravascular hemolysis), or rarely as pulmonary bleeding (pulmonary hemosiderosis). Iron is absorbed primarily in the duodenum, and a number of dietary factors (eg, coffee, tea) as well as primary intestinal disorders can impair absorption (ie, celiac disease).

The **thalassemias** are a heterogeneous group of inherited anemias that are characterized by impaired or absent synthesis of the α or β chains that make up the normal adult hemoglobin tetramer. The **β-thalassemias** are caused by a decrease in the production of β-globin chains. Anemia observed in the severe forms of β-thalassemia occurs as a result of ineffective erythropoiesis. This is because of the instability of excess α chains, which precipitate and cause oxidative damage to the cell membrane, leading to premature destruction of the erythrocyte within the bone marrow. Erythrocytes that do survive in circulation have a shortened life span because of increased hemolysis. Severe forms (compound heterozygous or homozygous state) are classified as **β-thalassemia intermedia** or **β-thalassemia major** depending on the clinical presentation and degree of anemia. Individuals with β-thalassemia major develop a severe anemia during the first year of life because decreasing levels of fetal hemoglobin ($\alpha_2\gamma_2$) cannot be replaced by normal adult hemoglobin ($\alpha_2\beta_2$). Hemoglobin values fall in the range of 3 to 4 g/dL and regular transfusions are required. Individuals with β-thalassemia intermedia usually present later in life and do not require early intervention with blood transfusions. Hemoglobin values are in the 7 to 8 g/dL range, and individuals may be intermittently transfusion-dependent. Individuals with **β-thalassemia trait** (β-thalassemia minor), the heterozygous form, have a mild microcytic anemia with a hemoglobin that is approximately 2 g/dL below the normal mean for age. Clinically it is an asymptomatic anemia; however, it is of diagnostic relevance in that it must be distinguished from iron deficiency anemia, which may be a concomitant problem.

The **α-thalassemias** are caused by a decrease in the production of α chains and are generally milder than β-thalassemias. This reflects the fact that the excess of β chains that occurs in α-thalassemia is more stable, resulting in less membrane damage and intramedullary erythrocyte destruction. In humans, there are

Table 86-2. Differential Diagnosis of Anemia Based on Pathophysiology

Pathophysiological Mechanism	General Diagnostic Features	Specific Diagnostic Features
Decreased Production of RBCs	**Evidence of decreased production:** ↓ reticulocytes	

Marrow infiltration
  Secondary to tumor infiltration
  Secondary to infiltration with nonmalignant cells
    Lipidoses
    X-linked lymphoproliferative disorder
Osteopetrosis
Decreased production of hematopoietic elements (bone marrow failure)
  Decreased RBC production only
    Constitutional: Congenital hypoplastic anemia
    Acquired
      Acquired pure red cell aplasia
Transient erythropenia of childhood
  Decreased RBC and WBC production
    Constitutional
      Fanconi syndrome
      Shwachman syndrome
  Decreased production of RBCs, WBCs, and platelets (aplastic anemia)
    Constitutional
      Fanconi syndrome
      Shwachman syndrome
    Acquired: aplastic anemia
Dietary deficiency
  Iron deficiency
  Folic acid deficiency
  Vitamin B$_{12}$ deficiency
  Vitamin C deficiency
  Protein deficiency
  Hypothyroidism
		Pancytopenia due to bone marrow infiltration with leukemia, neuroblastoma, etc
		
		Lipid-filled macrophages
		Hepatosplenomegaly
		Poor growth and bony encroachment on cranial nerve foramina
		
		Multiple physical deformities
		
		Associated with thymoma
		Associated with parvovirus infection
		
		Multiple physical deformities
		Pancreatic insufficiency
		
		Multiple physical deformities
		Pancreatic insufficiency
		History of hepatitis B, toxin exposure, idiopathic
		
		↓ MCV, ↓ MCH, ↑ RDW, ↓ serum iron, ↓ serum ferritin, excessive milk intake
		↑ MCV, ↑ RDW, megaloblastic marrow, low serum and RBC folate
		↑ MCV, ↑ RDW, megaloblastic marrow, low serum B$_{12}$ levels, Schilling test
		Clinical scurvy
		Kwashiorkor
		Low T4, elevated TSH

Increased Production (Hemolysis)	**Evidence of hemolysis:** ↑ reticulocytes	

Intrinsic RBC defects
  RBC membrane defects (spherocytosis, elliptocytosis)
  RBC enzyme defects (G6PD deficiency, pyruvate kinase)
  Hemoglobin defects
    1. Qualitative defects (sickle cell anemia, HbC, HbE)
    2. Quantitative defects (thalassemia)
	Hyperbilirubinemia
	LDH (RBC)
	MCV may be increased if reticulocytes high.
	
	MCV low with thalassemia
		+ Osmotic fragility, spectrin deficiency (HS)
		+ Enzyme assays
		
		Hb electrophoresis
		HbA$_2$ (β-thalassemia), targets cells

Extrinsic RBC disorders
  Immune
    Isoimmune hemolytic anemia (eg, ABO, Rh incompatibility)
    Autoimmune hemolytic anemia
    Idiopathic
    Secondary: post-viral, autoimmune disorders, Evans syndrome
 	
  Nonimmune (eg, DIC, HUS)
		+ Antiglobulin test
		
		+ Antiglobulin test
		+ ANA
		Concomitant thrombocytopenia or neutropenia
		Concomitant renal disease (HUS)

Blood Loss	**Reticulocytes normal (acute loss),** ↑↓ *(chronic)*	
Overt (eg, splenic sequestration, gastrointestinal, nasal bleeding) Occult (eg, bleeding Meckel diverticulum, pulmonary hemosiderosis)	↑ Reticulocytes (chronic loss, not iron deficient) ↓ Reticulocytes (chronic loss, iron deficient); may have rapidly falling hematocrit	Sickle cell anemia (splenic sequestration) Pulmonary infiltrates iron deficiency (pulmonary hemosiderosis)

Abbreviations: ANA, antinuclear antibodies; DIC, disseminated intravascular coagulation; G6PD, glucose-6-phosphate dehydrogenase; Hb, hemoglobin; HS, hereditary spherocytosis; HUS, hemolytic uremic syndrome; LDH, lactate dehydrogenase; MCH, mean corpuscular hemoglobin; MCV, mean corpuscular volume; RBC, red blood cell; RDW, red cell distribution width; TSH, thyroid-stimulating hormone; WBC, white blood cell.

Adapted from Lanzkowsky P. *Manual of Pediatric Hematology-Oncology*. New York, NY: Churchill Livingstone; 1989:2–3.

Box 86-2. Differential Diagnosis of Childhood Anemias Based on Red Blood Cell Size

Hypochromic, Microcytic Anemia (Low MCV)
- Iron deficiency anemia
- Thalassemias
- Lead poisoning
- Anemia of inflammation or chronic disease

Normochromic, Normocytic Anemia (Normal MCV)
- High reticulocyte count
  —Intrinsic red cell disorders
- Hemoglobinopathies (hemoglobin SS disease)
- Enzymopathies (G6PD, PK)
- Membranopathies (HS)
  —Extrinsic red cell disorders
- Immune-mediated
- Nonimmune (thrombotic thrombocytopenic purpura [eg, hemolytic uremic syndrome])
- Low reticulocyte count
  —Pure red cell aplasia (congenital hypoplastic anemia, TEC)
  —Pancytopenia (marrow failure or infiltration)

Macrocytic Anemia (Increased MCV)
- Folate deficiency
- Vitamin B_{12} deficiency
- Congenital hypoplastic anemia
- Myelodysplastic syndromes
- Chemotherapy agents

Abbreviations: G6PD, glucose-6-phosphate dehydrogenase; HS, hereditary spherocytosis; MCV, mean corpuscular volume; PK, pyruvate kinase; SS, 2 sickle β-globin genes; TEC, transient erythroblastopenia of childhood.

4 α-globin genes. Individuals with a deletion of one α-globin gene are **silent carriers** and are asymptomatic with a normal hemoglobin value and MCV. Individuals with 2-gene deletions have **α-thalassemia trait** and have a very mild microcytic anemia that is asymptomatic. Three α-globin gene deletions causes **hemoglobin H disease,** a moderate chronic hemolytic anemia that may be intermittently transfusion-dependent. This occurs primarily in individuals of Southeast Asian descent. Four-gene deletion causes **hydrops fetalis,** an almost universally fatal condition essentially resulting in fetal CHF and intrauterine demise.

Although **lead** inhibits heme synthesis and red cell function on many levels, microcytic anemia is a late finding of lead intoxication. Iron deficiency and lead poisoning often occur together with a complex relationship. Pica is a risk factor for lead ingestion. In the presence of lead, iron uptake by the erythrocyte is diminished and iron deficiency increases lead retention and toxicity. Intestinal absorption and uptake of lead by red cells is decreased in the presence of iron. In addition, iron deficiency and lead poisoning tend to occur in the same lower socioeconomic population, and both are exacerbated by concomitant nutritional deficiencies.

Anemia of inflammation or chronic disease can be seen in children with chronic infections, generalized inflammatory disorders (rheumatoid arthritis), and some cancers. It is characterized by a decrease in serum iron and iron binding capacity, an increase in ferritin, and the presence of iron in bone marrow macrophages indicating impaired iron mobilization from storage sites. Increased synthesis of hepcidin, an iron regulatory hormone, under the influence of inflammatory cytokines seems to be responsible for the hypoferremia observed in anemia of inflammation. In general, anemia of inflammation is mild and may be microcytic or normocytic.

Macrocytic Anemias

Folate and **vitamin B_{12} deficiency** cause a macrocytic anemia as a consequence of defective erythroid precursor nuclear maturation and megaloblastic changes in the bone marrow. Folate is absorbed in the duodenum and jejunum and is widely available in meats, green leafy vegetables, and cereals. Because of the ubiquity of folate, dietary deficiency is uncommon; however, newborns and infants fed exclusively goat's milk are at risk because of the exceedingly low levels of folate in goat's milk. Individuals with chronic hemolytic anemias may also become folate-deficient because of high bone marrow activity and increased demand.

Vitamin B_{12} is available from animal sources and is actively absorbed in the terminal ileum in association with intrinsic factor. Vitamin B_{12} deficiency can occur in individuals with a strict vegan diet (or in exclusively breastfed newborns and infants of women following a strict vegan diet); however, it usually occurs as a consequence of malabsorption. Decreased absorption can occur in the setting of pernicious anemia (decreased intrinsic factor), surgical resection (ie, following necrotizing enterocolitis), or GI disease.

Other causes of macrocytic anemias include congenital hypoplastic anemias (eg, congenital hypoplastic anemia), myelodysplastic syndromes, chemotherapeutic agents (eg, methotrexate), and hypothyroidism.

Normocytic Anemias

Normocytic anemias can be classified as hemolytic (associated with a reticulocytosis) and hypoplastic (reticulocytopenia). **Hemolytic anemias** can be further divided into disorders that are intrinsic or extrinsic to the RBC. Intrinsic RBC disorders include hemoglobinopathies, enzymopathies, and membranopathies.

Sickle cell disease is the most common hemoglobinopathy worldwide and is concentrated in individuals of African or mixed African descent. Inheritance of 2 sickle β-globin genes (hemoglobin SS) is the most common form; however, other significant sickle syndromes include hemoglobin SC, Sβ$^+$ thalassemia, and Sβ° thalassemia. Hemolytic anemia and painful vasoocclusive episodes are the hallmarks of sickle cell disease. The anemia is generally well tolerated with hemoglobin values in the 6.5 to 8.5 g/dL range with an associated reticulocytosis (5%–15%). The 2 most common hematologic complications in sickle cell disease are aplastic crises and splenic sequestration—both of which can cause an acute drop in hemoglobin. Aplastic crises are generally the result of infection with parvovirus, which temporarily causes the complete cessation of red cell production. Splenic sequestration occurs most commonly in infants and young children with sickle cell disease, often in association with a viral illness. Large amounts of blood can be quickly trapped in the spleen, causing hypovolemia, shock, and massive splenomegaly. See Selected References for further information on and excellent reviews of this multisystem disorder.

Glucose-6-phosphate dehydrogenase deficiency, the most common RBC enzyme deficiency, is an X-linked recessive hereditary disease that renders the red cell susceptible to oxidant stress and hemolysis. A number of variants have been defined; however, the most common variants are those associated with acute intermittent hemolytic anemias with exposure to oxidant stresses (fava beans, medications). Variants associated with chronic hemolytic anemias are very rare.

Pyruvate kinase deficiency is the most common red cell enzyme defect, causing a chronic congenital hemolytic anemia. The degree of hemolysis is variable, ranging from a mild, fully compensated hemolytic process without anemia to a transfusion-dependent anemia. Individuals with severe hemolysis may be chronically jaundiced and may develop the clinical complications of chronic hemolytic states (gall stones, transient aplastic crises in association with infections, folate deficiency, and infrequently, skin ulcers.) **Hereditary spherocytosis** is the most common red cell membranopathy and is characterized by the presence of spherical-shaped erythrocytes on the peripheral blood smear. Increased membrane fragility due to defects in proteins of the red cell membrane (spectrin, ankyrin, band 3, protein 4.2) leads to membrane vesiculation and membrane loss and the assumption of a spheroidal shape. Hemolysis occurs as these spherocytes are then trapped within the spleen. Clinically, the degree of hemolysis varies from mild anemia to severe transfusion dependence. Complications of a chronic hemolytic state such as gallstones, aplastic crises, and folate deficiency can also be observed.

Hemolytic anemias that are due to factors extrinsic to the red cell can be further classified as immune-mediated or nonimmune. **Immune-mediated anemias** may be due to alloantibodies that occur in the setting of neonatal Rh or ABO incompatibility or transfusion reactions. Autoantibodies may occur in association with infection, autoimmune disorders, malignancy, or drugs. In children, autoantibodies (warm immunoglobulin G, cold immunoglobulin M) are often seen in association with a viral illness or mycoplasma infection. **Nonimmune hemolytic anemias** include thrombotic thrombocytopenic purpura and macroangiopathy anemias caused by a myriad of etiologies, including infections, drugs, toxins, burns, and artificial heart valves.

Reticulocytopenic anemias can be congenital or acquired and can occur in isolation or in the setting of pancytopenia. **Congenital hypoplastic (Diamond-Blackfan) anemia** is a ribosomal disorder that causes a congenital pure red cell aplasia that presents early in infancy. The bone marrow typically shows red cell aplasia with a paucity of red cell precursors, and the red cells may be normocytic or macrocytic. Associated congenital anomalies, such as craniofacial anomalies, radial abnormalities, and renal and cardiac defects, are seen in approximately 25% of affected individuals. **Transient erythroblastopenia of childhood** is an acquired reticulocytopenic anemia that typically occurs following a viral illness. Usual age of presentation is between 2 to 3 years in an otherwise healthy child, and complete recovery is the natural course. Aplastic processes such as idiopathic aplastic anemia and hereditary Fanconi syndrome usually present with neutropenia or thrombocytopenia in addition to anemia.

Evaluation

History

When evaluating an infant or child with anemia, the age, rapidity of symptom onset, MCV, and suspected underlying mechanism of anemia will direct the history (Questions Box). In most instances, it is important to inquire about dietary habits, with particular attention to the type and amount of milk ingested per day (number of bottles/ounces). Ingestion of more than 24 oz of cow's milk should raise suspicion of iron deficiency anemia. Medication use, potential toxin ingestion (lead), or a history of pica should be determined as well. In addition, inquiries to potential sources of blood loss (hematochezia, melena, menorrhagia, hematuria, epistaxis, pulmonary) should be addressed. Acute onset of jaundice, icterus, or dark urine is suggestive of hemolysis and should elicit questions about possible triggers (fava beans, medications, illnesses). A personal history of neonatal hyperbilirubinemia or a family history of anemia, gallstones, cholecystectomy, or splenectomy is highly suggestive of a congenital hemolytic anemia. Acute onset of hemolysis with a viral illness is consistent with an autoimmune hemolytic anemia. Marrow failure syndromes often present with a prolonged history of increased fatigue and pallor, with occasional history of previous red cell transfusions prior to diagnosis. In acquired marrow failure states such as aplastic anemia, the history is occasionally consistent with antecedent hepatitis, a viral syndrome, or, rarely, exposure to toxins such as benzene and toluene-containing compounds or oral chloramphenicol use (commonly available over the counter in Latin America).

Questions

Anemia

- Does the child eat meat?
- Does the child drink too much milk (>24 oz/day)?
- Has the child had any bleeding recently?
- Has the child had a recent illness?
- Is the child taking any medications?
- Have the child's eyes appeared yellow?
- Does the child have a family history of anemia, jaundice, gallstones, or splenectomy?
- Did the child or siblings have jaundice at birth requiring phototherapy or exchange transfusion?
- Was the child born premature, and if so, how early?

Physical Examination

Most children who present with anemia will have a normal physical examination. Depending on the degree of anemia, pallor, tachycardia, or tachypnea may be present. In severe cases of anemia (hemoglobin <3 g/dL) with chronic onset and moderate anemia (hemoglobin of 3–7 g/dL) with acute onset (blood loss), CHF can occur. Other physical findings are unique to certain red cell disorders. Infants with sickle cell disease may present with dactylitis, a form of painful crisis that manifests as swelling of the digits associated with pain and sometimes fever. Splenomegaly can be seen in sickle cell disease (in younger children prior to autosplenectomy), β-thalassemia major and intermedia, and red cell membrane disorders, most commonly hereditary spherocytosis. In children with severe chronic hemolysis, regardless of etiology, classic facies (often called thalassemic facies) can develop, with frontal bossing and flattened nasal bridge, due to thinning of the facial bones from brisk intramedullary hematopoiesis. Children with congenital hypoplastic anemia or Fanconi syndrome may have physical anomalies, such as thumb or radial abnormalities, short stature, cardiac or renal anomalies, and developmental delay. Aplastic anemia or malignant infiltration of the bone marrow may present with concomitant neutropenia and thrombocytopenia. If neutropenic (absolute neutrophil count <1,000/mL), signs of fever or infection may be present. If thrombocytopenic, bruises, petechiae, and mucosal bleeding from the mouth, nose, and GI tract may also be present. With malignancy, such as leukemia, lymphadenopathy and hepatosplenomegaly may also be observed. Severe Vitamin B_{12} deficiency can result in neurologic findings such as ataxia, impaired vibratory sensation, or even psychiatric symptoms.

Laboratory Tests

Complete blood cell count (CBC) and peripheral blood smear provide a wealth of information and should be evaluated closely to narrow the differential diagnosis. The first step is to determine if the child is truly anemic by referencing the normal **hemoglobin/hematocrit** values for the child's age and gender. The second step is to evaluate the red cell indices. The **MCV** is a direct measure of red cell size and allows for classification of the anemia as microcytic, normocytic, or macrocytic (Figure 86-1). The mean corpuscular hemoglobin **(MCH)** is a calculated value that typically parallels the MCV. The **MCH concentration** is a measure of the red cell hydration status and is useful when elevated, as this reflects the presence of spherocytes. The red cell volume distribution width (RDW) reflects the variation in red cell size (usually normal with thalassemia trait and elevated in iron deficiency). The RBC count can be useful because it is typically elevated (>5 million/mL) in a child with thalassemia trait and decreased in iron deficiency anemia. Review of the **white blood cell and platelet count** will provide information

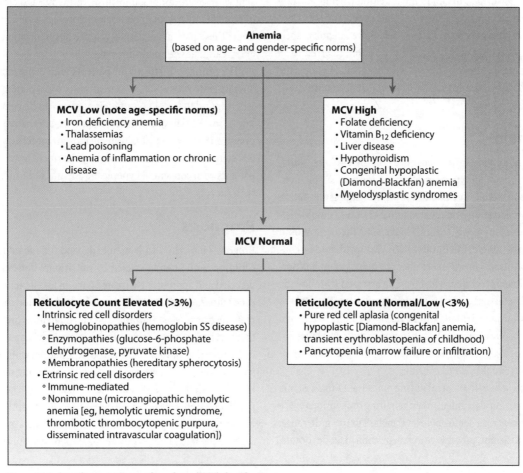

Figure 86-1. Anemia mean corpuscular volume (MCV) classifications.

as to whether other cell lines are affected. The **peripheral blood smear** provides information on RBC morphology characteristic of different red cell disorders (sickle cells, spherocytes, elliptocytes, schistocytes, bite cells). The presence of polychromasia is suggestive of a hemolytic process. White blood cell morphology can also suggest the etiology of the anemia (hyper-segmented neutrophils in folate or vitamin B_{12} deficiency, or basophilic stippling in lead poisoning). The **reticulocyte count** provides clues to the underlying mechanism of anemia. An elevated reticulocyte count is consistent with a hemolytic or blood loss picture, whereas a reduced or normal reticulocyte count in the face of anemia suggests a production problem. If hemolysis is evident, a **direct antiglobulin test (Coombs test)** should be performed to determine if this is an immune-mediated process. Hemoglobin analysis (using isoelectric focusing or high-pressure liquid chromatography) will diagnose sickle cell disease and related disorders and can help distinguish between α- and β-thalassemia traits.

With the CBC, peripheral blood smear, and reticulocyte count, a focused differential diagnosis can be generated and more specific testing can be performed. Further studies specific for individual hemolytic diseases or particular diseases secondary to marrow failure are summarized in Table 86-2.

Imaging Studies

Few children routinely need imaging studies in the evaluation of their anemia. If performed in children with chronic hemolytic disorders, radiographs may reveal "hair-on-end" appearance of bones due to increased hematopoiesis. Patients who have anemia associated with lead poisoning may have lead deposition, referred to as **lead lines,** in their long bones. Patients with congenital hypoplastic anemia or Fanconi syndrome may have skeletal abnormalities visible on plain radiographs.

Management

The treatment of anemia varies depending on the etiology. Nutritional anemias require dietary counseling and nutrient supplementation. With **iron deficiency anemia,** oral iron supplementation (3–6 mg/kg/day elemental iron divided into 2–3 doses) should generate a brisk reticulocytosis within 7 days, and the hemoglobin should increase by 1.0 g/dL/week thereafter. Therapy should be continued for an additional 6 to 8 weeks after the hemoglobin has normalized to replete iron stores, which can be assessed by following ferritin levels. Dietary education is key to ensure that milk intake is reduced and that iron-rich foods are encouraged. Failure to respond to iron therapy is most commonly due to noncompliance; however, alternative diagnoses (thalassemia trait), ongoing blood loss, or malabsorption states should also be considered.

Patients with severe thalassemia syndromes (ie, β-thalassemia major) are transfusion-dependent, often requiring transfusions every 3 to 4 weeks to maintain a hemoglobin level in the 9 to 10.5 g/dL range. With transfusion therapy, progressive iron deposition in tissues occurs, leading to cardiac, hepatic, and endocrinologic complications, which can be fatal if not prevented. Iron chelation with deferoxamine or deferasirox has improved survival; however, compliance remains an issue. Hematopoietic stem cell transplantation has been performed in patients with severe thalassemias and sickle cell disease.

Depending on the degree of hemolysis and compensation, individuals with congenital hemolytic anemias may require no transfusions, intermittent transfusions (due to aplastic crises), or regular transfusions. Individuals may require folate supplementation and should be monitored for potential complications such as gallstones and aplastic crises. The more severely affected individuals may benefit from splenectomy. Individuals with G6PD deficiency should be counseled on the avoidance of potential triggers of hemolysis.

Two anemia-related conditions constitute emergencies. Prompt recognition of these conditions is vital if proper treatment is to be initiated. **Splenic sequestration** occurs in infants and young children with sickle cell disease who sequester large volumes of blood within the spleen over a period of hours. This results in a rapidly dropping hemoglobin, clinically resembling anemia due to massive blood loss. The blood pooled in the spleen is not available to the circulation, and affected children are subject to fatal splenic rupture. Early recognition is essential and treatment involves emergency volume repletion followed by transfusion or exchange transfusion. **Severe autoimmune hemolytic anemia** is the second anemia-related emergency. Children with this disorder can occasionally present with severe antiglobulin-positive anemia and clinical evidence of rapid hemolysis; their hemoglobin may fall as much as 1 g/dL per hour. These patients generally require hospitalization, transfusion, and treatment with high-dose steroids.

The primary treatment for patients with congenital hypoplastic anemia is steroids and RBC transfusions. Most patients (50%–75%) will respond to steroids, and their anemia can be controlled at very low doses. For steroid-refractory patients, alternative immunosuppressive therapy and RBC transfusions are necessary. Hematopoietic stem cell transplantation can be performed in steroid-refractory patients with congenital hypoplastic anemia and Fanconi syndrome with success.

Prognosis

Prognosis for a child with anemia depends on the underlying cause. Children with anemia caused by nutritional deficiencies that are detected and appropriately treated have an excellent prognosis. Children with transient erythroblastopenia of childhood can expect complete recovery. Most immune-mediated anemias are responsive to therapy; however, if associated with an underlying autoimmune disorder, they may have a relapsing course. Children with chronic hemolytic disorders will have varying courses depending on the degree of hemolysis. Early diagnosis and intervention through newborn screening for children with sickle cell disease has significantly reduced early mortality for this disease. Children with β-thalassemia major or severe congenital hemolytic anemias will be transfusion-dependent and subject to the complications of iron overload, which can be addressed with chelation therapy. Some children with transfusion-dependent congenital hemolytic anemias may be candidates for splenectomy, with normalization of their hemoglobin values post-splenectomy. Prognosis for children with congenital hypoplastic anemia depends on their responsiveness to steroid therapy and need for transfusions. These individuals, along with children with Fanconi syndrome, are also at risk for certain malignancies (eg, acute myeloid leukemia).

When to Refer

Children with anemia caused by chronic inherited or acquired red cell disorders are at risk for complications during the course of their disease and are best served at a center that offers pediatric hematology expertise. Sickle cell disease and severe thalassemias are usually diagnosed by newborn screening programs and are automatically referred to subspecialists. Any anemia that is complicated by thrombocytopenia or neutropenia also warrants immediate referral to a hematologist.

CASE RESOLUTION

The girl described in the case history has hereditary spherocytosis. Her history is highly suggestive of a hereditary hemolytic disorder, and the combination of spherocytes in the peripheral smear, a negative antiglobulin test, and a positive, incubated, osmotic fragility test are diagnostic of the condition. At the age of 9 years, she undergoes a splenectomy and has no more hemolytic episodes that require transfusions.

Selected References

Baker RD, Greer FR; American Academy of Pediatrics Committee on Nutrition. Diagnosis and prevention of iron deficiency and iron-deficiency anemia in infants and young children (0–3 years of age). *Pediatrics.* 2010;126(5):1040–1050

Brugnara C, Oski FA, Nathan DG. Diagnostic approach to the anemic patient. In: Orkin SH, Nathan DG, Ginsburg D, Look AT, Fisher DE, Lux SE, eds. *Nathan and Oski's Hematology of Infancy and Childhood.* 7th ed. Philadelphia, PA: Saunders Elsevier; 2009:455–466

Charache S, Lubin B, Reid CD, eds. *Management and Therapy of Sickle Cell Disease.* Bethesda, MD: National Institutes of Health; 1995. NIH Publication No. 96–2117

Cherrick I, Karayalcin G, Lanzkowsky P. Transient erythroblastopenia of childhood. Prospective study of fifty patients. *Am J Pediatr Hematol Oncol.* 1994;16(4):320–324

Fixler J, Styles L. Sickle cell disease. *Pediatr Clin North Am.* 2002;49(6):1193–1210

Gazda HT, Sieff CA. Recent insights into the pathogenesis of Diamond-Blackfan anaemia. *Br J Haematol.* 2006;135(2):149–157

Hermiston ML, Mentzer WC. A practical approach to the evaluation of the anemic child. *Pediatr Clin North Am.* 2002;49(5):877–891

Lo L, Singer ST. Thalassemia: current approach to an old disease. *Pediatr Clin North Am.* 2002;49(6):1165–1191

McCavit TL. Sickle cell disease. *Pediatr Rev.* 2012;33(5):195–206

Robins EB, Blum S. Hematologic reference values for African American children and adolescents. *Am J Hematol.* 2007;82(7):611–614

CHAPTER 87

Bleeding Disorders

Joseph L. Lasky III, MD, and Eduard H. Panosyan, MD

CASE STUDY

A 6-year-old girl presents with a several-month history of recurrent epistaxis. Episodes occur every 2 to 3 weeks and last 15 to 20 minutes at a time. Both nares are affected. Her mother also notes that the girl has always bruised easily. On physical examination, several 2- to 3-cm ecchymoses are noted on her lower extremities. Initial laboratory evaluation includes a complete blood cell count, which is normal (platelet count 300,000/μL); a normal partial thromboplastin time of 30 seconds; and a normal prothrombin time of 12.5 seconds, with international normalized ratio 1:1.

Questions

1. What conditions should be considered when easy bruising is the chief complaint?
2. What is the appropriate laboratory evaluation for children with clinical signs of bleeding?
3. What management is appropriate for the most common pediatric bleeding disorders?
4. What are the common medical complications that children with bleeding disorders face?
5. When is consultation with a hematologist appropriate in a child who easily bruises?

When evaluating a child with bruising or bleeding symptoms, the major challenge facing the pediatrician is to ascertain whether the degree of bleeding is appropriate for the hemostatic stress or whether further evaluation for a potential bleeding disorder is warranted. Bruising and bleeding are common childhood complaints and usually follow minor injury or trauma. However, in the child with an underlying hemostatic disorder, non-accidental trauma, or both, the bruising or bleeding may be more extensive than expected. A thorough medical history and physical examination and an understanding of hemostasis will aid in focusing the laboratory evaluation and elucidating the underlying etiology.

Epidemiology

Bleeding disorders can be inherited or acquired. Of the inherited bleeding disorders, von Willebrand disease is the most common, with a reported incidence ranging between 1 in 100 and 1 in 1,000. Von Willebrand disease is autosomally inherited, affecting males and females equally; however, more females are diagnosed because of the inherent hemostatic challenges that females face (menses, childbirth). Hemophilia is the most common severe bleeding disorder, affecting about 1 in 5,000 males. Approximately 80% of cases are hemophilia A (factor VIII deficiency) and 20% are hemophilia B (factor IX deficiency). Hemophilia is inherited in an X-linked fashion, but one-third of newly diagnosed males have no previous family history and represent new mutations. Other inherited coagulation and platelet disorders are rare and are listed in Table 87-1.

Acquired abnormalities of coagulation or platelets are much more common. These can occur in the setting of liver disease, vitamin K deficiency, renal disease, disseminated intravascular coagulation (DIC), infection, medications, malignancy, massive transfusion, post-surgery, and autoimmunity or alloimmunity. Immune thrombocytopenic purpura (ITP) is a common acquired childhood bleeding disorder with an incidence of 4 to 8 per 100,000 children per year. Neonatal alloimmune thrombocytopenia occurs in approximately 1 in 1,800 live births. Common acquired bleeding disorders are also listed in Table 87-1.

Clinical Presentation

Bleeding disorders can present in various ways depending on the etiology. Inherited bleeding disorders will often present during infancy or early childhood; mild disorders, however, may go undiagnosed until later in life. In general, disorders of primary hemostasis (ie, von Willebrand disease, platelet disorders, collagen vascular disorders) will present with superficial, immediate, mucocutaneous-type bleeding. Characteristic bleeding symptoms include easy bruising, epistaxis, gum bleeding, menorrhagia, postpartum bleeding, and bleeding with dental extractions or surgeries. Disorders of secondary hemostasis, such as hemophilia A or B, will often present with deep, delayed bleeding, such as hemarthroses or muscular hematomas.

Acquired bleeding disorders typically present with an acute onset and often involve abnormalities of primary and secondary hemostasis. Acute onset of bleeding symptoms in a toxic or ill-appearing child suggests a systemic process such as sepsis, DIC, malignancy, or hepatic or renal dysfunction. A well-appearing child with acute bleeding symptoms suggests ITP, an acquired inhibitor, or a medication-related cause.

Pathophysiology

Following vascular injury, hemostasis is initiated by exposure of flowing blood to subendothelial collagen and tissue factor. The primary phase of hemostasis leads to the production of a platelet plug. Von

Table 87-1. Inherited Versus Acquired Bleeding Disorders

Disorder	Inherited	Acquired

Coagulation	• von Willebrand disease
	• Hemophilia A (FVIII)
	• Hemophilia B (FIX)
	• Hemophilia C (FXI)
	• FII, FV, FVII, FX, or FXIII deficiency
	• Disorders of fibrinogen
	  —Dysfibrinogenemia, hypofibrinogenemia, or afibrinogenemia
	• Disorders of fibrinolysis
	  —α_2-antiplasmin
	• PAI-1 deficiency
		• Vitamin K deficiency
		• Liver disease
		• DIC
		• Massive transfusion syndrome
		• Disorders of fibrinogen (dysfibrinogenemia or hypofibrinogenemia)
		  —Liver disease
		  —Renal disease
		  —Medication
		• Disorders associated with malignancy and therapy (ie, asparaginase)
		• Coagulation inhibitors

Platelet	• Quantitative
	  —TAR syndrome
	  —Megakaryocytic thrombocytopenia
	  —Fanconi syndrome
	• Qualitative
	  —Glanzmann thrombasthenia
	  —Storage pool disorders
	  —Release defects
	• Quantitative/qualitative
	  —Bernard-Soulier syndrome
	  —Wiskott-Aldrich syndrome
	  —Gray platelet syndrome
		• Quantitative
		  —Increased destruction
		    ~Nonimmune-mediated
		      • HUS
		      • TTP
		      • DIC
		    ~Immune-mediated
		      • ITP
		      • Evans syndrome
		      • NAIT
		      • Medications
		  —Decreased production
		    ~Aplastic anemia
		    ~Malignancy infiltrating bone marrow
		    ~Medications
		• Qualitative
		  —Medication
		  —Liver disease
		  —Uremia
		  —Post-cardiopulmonary bypass surgery

Abbreviations: DIC, disseminated intravascular coagulation; F, factor; HUS, hemolytic uremic syndrome; ITP, immune thrombocytopenic purpura; NAIT, neonatal alloimmune thrombocytopenic purpura; PAI, plasminogen activator inhibitor; TAR, thrombocytopenia–absent radius; TTP, thrombotic thrombocytopenic purpura.

Willebrand factor (vWF), a multimeric glycoprotein of varying size, attaches to exposed subendothelial collagen and binds platelets via the platelet glycoprotein Ib/IX receptors. Von Willebrand factor also serves as a carrier protein for FVIII, thereby localizing FVIII to areas of endothelial disruption. Once platelets adhere to vWF, they become activated and release their granular contents, produce thromboxane A$_2$, and express the fibrinogen receptor glycoprotein IIb/IIIa (GPIIb/IIIa). The release of thromboxane A$_2$ and other granular contents leads to local vasoconstriction and activation of additional platelets and their respective GPIIb/IIIa receptors, allowing for platelet aggregation. Fibrinogen binds to all of the exposed activated GPIIb/IIIa sites, clumping the platelets together to form a platelet plug. The platelet plug stops local bleeding and provides a phospholipid surface for the coagulation reactions of secondary hemostasis to occur to form a definitive fibrin plug.

Secondary hemostasis is also initiated at the time of endothelial disruption with exposure of tissue factor to circulating blood. Tissue factor binds to FVIIa, and this complex serves as the key initiator of in vivo hemostasis by activating other tissue factor FVII (TF:FVII) complexes, as well as FIX, and factor X (FX). Once activated (by FIXa or TF:FVIIa), FXa, along with its cofactor, factor Va, activates prothrombin (FII) to thrombin (FIIa). Thrombin cleaves circulating fibrinogen to fibrin monomers that self-polymerize. Factor XIII then stabilizes the fibrin clot by forming cross-links within the clump of fibrin polymers. These coagulation reactions occur on the surface of the platelet plug and, with the generation of cross-linked fibrin, the primary platelet plug is converted into a definitive fibrin plug that prevents further bleeding. An overview of hemostasis is depicted in figures 87-1 and 87-2. Deficiencies or impairments in any of these elements can lead to abnormal test results or inadequate hemostasis and excessive hemorrhage.

The delicate balance of hemostasis and thrombosis is maintained by inhibitors (protein C, protein S, antithrombin, tissue factor pathway inhibitor) at each step of the coagulation cascade. These natural

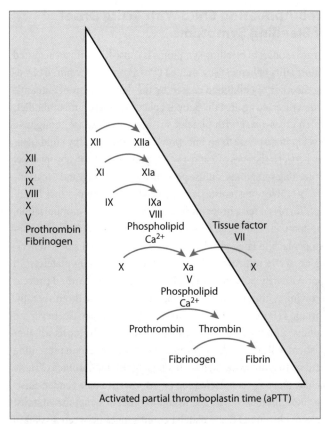

Figure 87-1. Intrinsic pathway reflected by activated partial thromboplastin time.

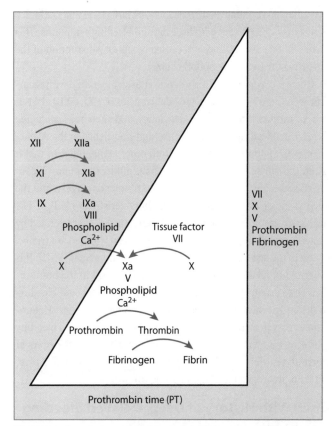

Figure 87-2. Coagulation pathway. Extrinsic pathway reflected by prothrombin time.

anticoagulants serve to prevent excessive thrombus formation. Fibrinolysis is mediated by plasmin, which cleaves fibrinogen and fibrin within a thrombus, allowing for restoration of vessel patency following hemostasis. Plasmin is activated by tissue plasminogen activator (tPA) and urokinase. Fibrinolysis is kept in check by plasminogen activator inhibitor (PAI-1), which inactivates tPA, and α_2-antiplasmin, which inactivates plasmin. Any defects in the fibrinolytic system that leads to an increase in fibrinolysis can result in excessive bleeding.

Differential Diagnosis

In developing the differential diagnosis for a child with bleeding symptoms, it is important to obtain a thorough bleeding history and physical examination. The age, bleeding pattern, duration of symptoms, family history, and overall clinical status of the child will help to narrow the spectrum of possibilities.

Child With Chronic History of Mucocutaneous Bleeding

In a child who presents with a history of easy bruising, epistaxis, or menorrhagia, the primary differential diagnosis includes von Willebrand disease, platelet disorders, and collagen vascular disorders (disorders of primary hemostasis). **Von Willebrand disease** is caused by a quantitative or qualitative defect of vWF. Von Willebrand factor plays an important role in primary hemostasis (mediates platelet adhesion at sites of vascular injury) and secondary hemostasis (stabilizes FVIII in plasma). Von Willebrand disease is autosomally inherited and

classified into 3 different types. Type 1 refers to a partial quantitative deficiency of vWF. Type 2 refers to qualitative abnormalities of vWF with a number of subtypes that fall within this classification. Type 3, the most severe form, refers to a complete deficiency of vWF, which is caused by homozygous or compound heterozygous mutation and is inherited in autosomal-recessive fashion. Type 1 is the most common form, accounting for 70% to 80% of cases. Bleeding symptoms tend to be mild and are characterized by easy bruising, epistaxis, menorrhagia, and prolonged oozing after minor or major surgeries. Only the most severely affected patients (type 3), with very low FVIII levels, will have soft tissue bleeding and hemarthroses similar to an individual with moderate or severe hemophilia.

Qualitative platelet disorders also present with mucocutaneous bleeding, often during infancy. In **Bernard-Soulier syndrome,** platelets lack a functional glycoprotein Ib/IX receptor complex on the platelet surface, resulting in defective platelet adhesion to vWF at sites of vascular injury. It is an autosomal-recessive disorder and is usually seen in consanguineous families. The platelets tend to be large on peripheral smear, and there may be a degree of thrombocytopenia. **Glanzmann thrombasthenia** is characterized by an absence or defect in the platelet membrane GPIIb/IIIa receptor, the main fibrinogen receptor on the platelet surface that allows for platelet aggregation. It is autosomal-recessively inherited and is more common in the presence of consanguinity. Other qualitative platelet disorders such as **storage pool disorders** and **platelet release defects** can also present in a similar manner.

Collagen-vascular disorders, such as Marfan and Ehlers-Danlos syndromes, can present with bruising and bleeding symptoms. This increased bleeding diathesis is caused by an easy disruption of the integrity of the vascular endothelium.

Other rare coagulation disorders to consider in a child with recurrent bleeding symptoms include deficiencies of FXI, FXIII, PAI-1, and α_2-antiplasmin. **Factor XI deficiency,** also known as *hemophilia C,* is a rare bleeding disorder with a high prevalence in the Ashkenazi Jewish population. It differs from other hemophilias in that it is autosomally inherited and tends to have milder symptoms. Bleeding episodes are typically in response to trauma or surgery, and the deep tissue or intra-articular bleeds characteristic of FVIII or FIX deficiency are not seen. **Factor XIII deficiency** is characterized by delayed or prolonged bleeding because the clots formed are friable, owing to the lack of cross-linkage of fibrin monomers by FXIII. It is inherited in an autosomal-dominant pattern, and in the homozygous state usually presents in infancy with umbilical cord bleeding or delayed separation, as well as intracranial hemorrhage. Heterozygotes may present later in life with delayed or prolonged bleeding following trauma or surgery and poor wound healing. **Disorders of fibrinolysis** (deficiency of PAI-1 or α_2-antiplasmin) can also present with prolonged bleeding following trauma.

Child With History of Deep, Delayed Bleeding

Deep tissue and intra-articular bleeding is the hallmark bleeding pattern of **hemophilia.** Differential diagnosis for a child who presents with this type of bleeding is hemophilia A (FVIII deficiency) or B (FIX deficiency), FVII deficiency, and type 3 von Willebrand disease. Clinically, hemophilia is classified according to the factor level, with less than 1% factor activity as severe, 1% to 5% as moderate, and greater than 5% as mild. The factor level correlates with the bleeding tendency. Males with severe hemophilia can have "spontaneous" bleeds or bleeding with minimal trauma. Males with moderate or mild hemophilia will bleed with more significant trauma. The bleeding pattern of hemophilia varies as the child grows. Infants may present with a cephalhematoma or intracranial hemorrhage, particularly if the delivery was complicated with the use of forceps or vacuum extraction. Bleeding with circumcision, heel sticks, or blood draws may also occur. As the infant starts crawling, bruises and soft tissue hematomas on the lower extremities become common. As the toddler becomes upright, the first hemarthroses can occur, typically involving the ankle. The older child has hemarthroses primarily involving the knees and elbows.

Factor VII deficiency is very rare; however, it can present with a bleeding pattern similar to hemophilia A or B. Type 3 von Willebrand disease, which is characterized by an absence of vWF (the carrier protein for FVIII), can have FVIII levels as low as an individual with severe or moderate hemophilia A. In addition to the characteristic mucocutaneous bleeding seen with von Willebrand disease, these individuals can also have deep tissue and intra-articular bleeding.

Well-Appearing Child With Acute Onset of Bleeding Symptoms

An acute onset of bleeding symptoms is consistent with an acquired abnormality of hemostasis. Acute **ITP** is a common acquired bleeding disorder of childhood caused by the development of autoantibodies directed against the patient's platelets. These autoantibodies, which cross-react with platelet surface antigens, are thought to develop in response to an infection. Typically, a healthy child (usually between the ages of 2 and 4 years) presents with an abrupt onset of bleeding symptoms, diffuse petechiae and bruising, and occasionally, "wet" bleeding (epistaxis, gum bleeding, gastrointestinal bleeding). There is often a history of a viral illness or recent immunization. The complete blood cell count (CBC) reveals an isolated thrombocytopenia, and large platelets are seen on peripheral smear reflecting an active marrow with the production of young platelets. In approximately 80% of cases, ITP is an acute, self-limited process resolving within 6 months of diagnosis with or without therapy. Chronic ITP exists when the thrombocytopenia persists beyond 6 months. Although it is not possible to predict at diagnosis whether a patient will go on to have chronic ITP, there are certain presenting features that are associated with a higher risk for chronicity. These include older age at presentation (>10 years), female gender, existing autoimmune disease, and insidious onset of symptoms. In most cases of chronic ITP, the platelet count ranges between 40,000 to 80,000, and bleeding symptoms are minimal.

Acquired coagulation inhibitors are rare in children without an underlying coagulation disorder; however, they can occur in the setting of malignancy, infection, or post-surgery. Acquired FVIII deficiency due to FVIII inhibitor occurs primarily in the adult population but has been previously reported in children. Acute onset of severe bleeding symptoms is the common presentation. Antiphospholipid antibodies can cause a prolongation of the partial thromboplastin time (PTT) or prothrombin time (PT); however, these antibodies are not associated with bleeding and are typically transient following a viral illness. The exception is if the antiphospholipid antibody is directed against prothrombin, resulting in low levels of prothrombin. In this situation, bleeding may be associated but is usually mild and intervention unnecessary.

Acquired abnormalities of coagulation or platelet function can also occur in association with **medications.** Aspirin and nonsteroidal anti-inflammatory drugs are common medications that affect the function of platelets. Warfarin, a vitamin K antagonist, is commonly used as an anticoagulant. One percent to 3% of patients on therapeutic warfarin can experience bleeding complications. Chronic antibiotic use can result in vitamin K deficiency and a depletion of the vitamin K–dependent factors (II, VII, IX, X).

Ill-Appearing Child With Acute Onset of Bleeding Symptoms

Acute onset of bleeding in an ill-appearing child suggests an acquired systemic process. **Disseminated intravascular coagulation** is a consumptive coagulopathy that can occur secondary to a number of disorders, including sepsis, trauma, or malignancy. Disseminated intravascular coagulation occurs as a result of endothelial disruption and initiation of abnormal coagulation, fibrin deposition, and depletion of multiple clotting factors, inhibitor proteins, and platelets.

Because the liver is the primary site of synthesis for most of the coagulation factors, **liver dysfunction** caused by any illness can result in an imbalance in the hemostatic system. In addition, thrombocytopenia may be present with chronic liver disease because of portal hypertension and associated splenomegaly with sequestration. Causes of the depletion of vitamin K–dependent factors, such as obstructive jaundice, malabsorptive states (cystic fibrosis), parenchymal liver disease, and chronic antibiotic use, can also predispose to bleeding.

Renal disease with uremia impairs platelet function and can present with bleeding symptoms as well. A **malignancy** infiltrating the bone marrow, such as leukemia, lymphoma, or neuroblastoma, can cause thrombocytopenia and resultant platelet bleeding. Acquired von Willebrand disease can occur with Wilms tumor and present with mucocutaneous bleeding. **Bone marrow failure syndromes** such as aplastic anemia and Fanconi syndrome can also present with thrombocytopenia and associated bleeding.

Newborn/Infant With Bleeding Symptoms

A newborn or an infant who presents with bleeding symptoms may have a congenital bleeding disorder or an acquired condition. **Inherited coagulation deficiencies** (VII, VIII, IX, XI, XIII, type 3 von Willebrand disease) and qualitative platelet disorders may present in the newborn period with intracranial hemorrhage or cephalhematoma, bleeding with heel sticks or blood draws, umbilical cord bleeding, and bleeding with circumcision. **Congenital thrombocytopenias** usually present within the first year of life and are associated with other syndromic features. Thrombocytopenia–absent radius (TAR) syndrome is an autosomal-recessive condition, typically recognized in the newborn period, characterized by thrombocytopenia, skeletal anomalies (most commonly radial agenesis), and renal and cardiac abnormalities. Other congenital thrombocytopenias include megakaryocytic thrombocytopenia, Fanconi syndrome (also with associated skeletal anomalies), and Wiskott-Aldrich syndrome (eczema, frequent infections, small platelets).

Neonatal alloimmune thrombocytopenia (NAIT) is a rare condition in which a newborn inherits platelet antigens from the father that are different from the mother. The mother becomes alloimmunized to the newborn's platelet antigens during pregnancy, similar to erythrocyte alloimmunization from Rh incompatibility. The maternal immunoglobulin G alloantibodies cross the placenta and destroy the newborn's platelets, resulting in a transient but severe thrombocytopenia in the newborn. Antibodies against the human platelet antigen-1a (HPA-1a) are responsible for 80% of NAIT cases in the white population. Thrombocytopenia in the newborn or infant can last several weeks until the maternal antibody is cleared. Unlike Rh alloimmunization, NAIT can occur in the first pregnancy. The risk of intracranial hemorrhage is significant, with a reported incidence of up to 20% in some series, and can occur in utero. Neonatal

thrombocytopenia can also occur as a consequence of **maternal ITP** with maternal transfer of antibody. Bleeding tends to be mild in this setting and intracranial hemorrhage is rare. The thrombocytopenia resolves after several weeks. An acquired thrombocytopenia most often occurs in the setting of an ill newborn or infant with sepsis, congenital viral infection (*Toxoplasma,* rubella, cytomegalovirus, HIV), necrotizing enterocolitis, respiratory distress syndrome, asphyxia, or congenital heart disease. Drug-associated thrombocytopenia can also occur in the hospitalized newborn or infant.

Vitamin K deficiency in the neonate has 3 different presentations. **Classic hemorrhagic disease of the newborn** presents between days 2 to 7 of life and is due to immature neonatal liver and impaired clotting factor synthesis, inadequate vitamin K intake, and sterile neonatal gut. With the advent of vitamin K prophylaxis at birth, this form of vitamin K deficiency is rarely seen. **Early hemorrhagic disease of the newborn** presents in the first 24 hours of life and is due to maternal medications that affect vitamin K metabolism (anticonvulsants). **Late vitamin K deficiency** occurs after the first week of life and is associated with a number of conditions in which vitamin K stores may be low, such as inadequate intake in breastfed neonates and infants, impaired absorption in neonates and infants with chronic diarrhea, antibiotic use, cystic fibrosis, and other GI disorders. Bleeding symptoms associated with vitamin K deficiency can be quite severe with a significant incidence of GI, deep tissue, and intracranial hemorrhage.

Exposures to superwarfarin vitamin K antagonists (found in rat poisons) are relatively common in children but are usually asymptomatic because a large quantity of ingested rat poison is necessary to induce significant coagulopathy. However, this intoxication should be considered in patients presenting with extreme coagulopathy and unexplained elevation of PT and activated PTT (aPTT) secondary to depletion of vitamin K–dependent factors.

Evaluation

History

A thorough bleeding history and physical examination should enable the pediatrician to determine the likelihood of an underlying bleeding disorder. The pattern of bleeding, timing of the symptoms (acute vs chronic), overall health of the child, and family history are important in helping to determine the underlying etiology. The Questions Box lists the pertinent questions to ask when obtaining a bleeding history.

Bruises are a common childhood complaint. Normal bruising that occurs in an active child must be differentiated from pathologic bruising owing to a possible bleeding disorder or non-accidental trauma. Bruises over exposed bony prominences such as the anterior tibial region or the knees are common. Bruises of a size inconsistent with the degree of reported trauma, and bruises in nonexposed or unusual areas (back, chest, shoulders, or upper arms), should alert the pediatrician to a possible bleeding disorder or non-accidental trauma. Linear or geometric bruises are concerning for non-accidental trauma. Epistaxis, another common complaint, is most often due to digital trauma or allergic rhinitis. However, epistaxis unrelieved by

Bleeding History

- Is bleeding history positive or child presents for incidentally discovered abnormal tests (eg, prolonged prothrombin time/activated partial thromboplastin time)?
- Is the bleeding acute or chronic?
  —For acute onset bleeding
    ~What type of bleeding is the child experiencing?
    ~Is the child well-appearing or toxic?
    ~Is there a history of recent illness?
    ~Is the child taking any medications?
    ~Does the child have any medical problems?
  —For chronic history of bleeding
    ~What type of bleeding is the child experiencing?
    - Bruising (location, size, palpable hematoma)
    - Epistaxis (duration of bleeding, history of packing, cauterization, or transfusion)
    - Bleeding with vaccinations, injections, minor cuts
    - Bleeding with dental extractions/surgeries
    - Menses (total number of days of bleeding, leaking, alteration of activities during menses, diagnosis of iron deficiency, use of oral contraceptives, history of transfusion)
    ~Medications
    ~Family history (obstetric and gynecologic history of female relatives)

15 minutes of appropriately applied pressure or epistaxis requiring packing, cautery, or transfusions is highly suggestive of a bleeding disorder. Menorrhagia, defined as menstrual flow greater than 7 days, and a history of frequently stained clothes or iron deficiency anemia in an adolescent female are concerning. Persistent or recurrent bleeding with dental extractions (beyond the day of the procedure) or with surgeries also merits a closer evaluation. However, if a child has undergone previous dental extractions or surgeries without bleeding complications, an underlying bleeding disorder is unlikely. Finally, a history of deep muscle bleeding or unexplained hemarthroses would suggest an inherited factor deficiency.

Physical Examination

Depending on the underlying bleeding disorder and the time of presentation, the physical examination may be completely normal. If there is active bleeding, physical signs may include petechiae, ecchymoses, mucosal bleeding (nasal, oral, vaginal), hematuria, swollen joints (hemarthrosis), or limited range of motion. Children with bleeding associated with an acquired disorder such as infection, malignancy, autoimmunity, or liver or renal dysfunction may have physical signs specific to the underlying illness. Children with bleeding associated with a genetic disorder may have a normal examination or congenital anomalies associated with a particular syndrome.

Laboratory Tests

The extent of laboratory evaluation is dependent on the bleeding history and clinical presentation. Initial laboratory studies for a potential bleeding disorder should include a CBC with a peripheral smear, a PT, and an aPTT.

The **CBC** is useful in providing a platelet count to identify suspected thrombocytopenia. In addition, abnormalities in the white blood cell count or red cell indices can provide clues to the underlying process. A microcytic anemia consistent with iron deficiency would suggest chronic blood loss and raise suspicion of an underlying bleeding disorder. Pancytopenia would suggest an underlying bone marrow failure syndrome or a possible malignancy such as leukemia. Review of the **peripheral smear** can confirm the presence of true thrombocytopenia and allow for an assessment of platelet, white blood cell, and red blood cell morphology.

The **PT** reflects the extrinsic and common pathway; the **aPTT** reflects the intrinsic and common pathway. A prolonged PT or PTT should be followed up with a 1:1 mixing study to determine whether the prolongation is caused by a factor deficiency or the presence of an inhibitor. **Bleeding time** is a reflection of primary hemostasis (platelets, vWF, vascular integrity) but is rarely performed in pediatrics because of the unreliability and difficulty of performing this test in children. **Platelet function assay** is a screening test of platelet function, measuring platelet adhesion and aggregation (primary hemostasis).

A stepwise approach to more specific testing is dictated by the clinical presentation and screening test results and is best performed with the consultation of a pediatric hematologist. When an abnormality of primary hemostasis is suspected, the initial evaluation should focus on von Willebrand disease because it is the most common disorder. A **vWF panel,** which includes vWF antigen, ristocetin cofactor activity (functional measure of vWF), FVIII activity, and a vWF multimer analysis, should be performed. Many factors may transiently increase vWF levels (stress, inflammation, hormones, exercise, oral contraceptives), and normal results are frequently encountered in patients with type 1 von Willebrand disease. Repeat testing is often necessary to make the diagnosis and should be pursued if suspicion is high. For hemophilia or any other suspected factor deficiency, a specific **coagulation factor assay** must be performed. For patients with suspected qualitative platelet disorder, **platelet aggregation studies** (measuring the degree and pattern of platelet aggregation to various agonists) or **flow cytometry** (measuring the platelet surface GP expression) can be performed. On a case-by-case basis, additional studies such as fibrinogen, D dimer, fibrin split products, thrombin time, factor inhibitor assay, autoimmune studies, liver function tests, creatinine, or blood urea nitrogen may be indicated. Table 87-2 lists the major screening tests for hemostasis.

Imaging Studies

In general, imaging studies are not indicated. Bone films may be taken of the upper extremities in patients with thrombocytopenia to rule out Fanconi and TAR syndromes. Computed tomography may be considered for evaluating the extend of highly suspected intracranial hemorrhage or iliopsoas bleeding in patients with hemophilia (appropriate factor replacement is a priority).

Table 87-2. Laboratory Evaluation for Hemostasis

Laboratory Test	Measured Hemostatic Function
CBC	Platelet count
Peripheral blood smear	Platelet morphology
aPTT	Factors I, II, V, VIII, IX, XI, XII (intrinsic and common pathway)
PT	Factors I, II, V, VII, X (extrinsic and common pathway)
aPTT and PT mixing studies	Performed when aPTT/PT is prolonged; patient plasma and normal plasma is mixed 1:1, then aPTT/PT repeated. If aPTT/PT corrects, there is a factor deficiency; if not, there is an inhibitor.
Bleeding time (not recommended)	Primary hemostasis (platelets, vWF, endothelial integrity)
PFA-100 screen	Primary hemostasis (platelets, vWF)
Thrombin time	Fibrinogen
vWF panel	vWF antigen (amount of vWF) Ristocetin cofactor activity (function of vWF) Factor VIII activity vWF multimer analysis (distribution of multimers)
Coagulation factor assays	Specific factor activity
Platelet aggregation studies	Platelet function; patient platelets are exposed to agonists and the degree of aggregation and pattern of the response is unique for various qualitative platelet disorders.

Abbreviations: aPTT, activated partial thromboplastin time; CBC, complete blood cell count; PFA, platelet function assay; PT, prothrombin time; vWF, von Willebrand factor.

Management

The management of bleeding disorders is dependent on the underlying abnormality. However, general supportive measures, such as local pressure for bleeding, avoidance of blood draws, and avoidance of medications that affect the function of platelets or hemostasis, can be applied to most clinical scenarios of bleeding.

Treatment of **von Willebrand disease** is dependent on the subtype and severity of bleeding symptoms. For mild bleeding symptoms, supportive measures alone may be all that is necessary—applying appropriate pressure for epistaxis, ice pack for bruises, and avoidance of antiplatelet medications. For type 1 von Willebrand disease, DDAVP (synthetic vasopressin) can be used and is available as a concentrated nasal spray or intravenously. DDAVP stimulates endothelial release of vWF and can increase levels 2- to 3-fold. For type 3 and most cases of type 2 von Willebrand disease, replacement therapy with FVIII concentrates that contain vWF is necessary for significant bleeding episodes. Antifibrinolytic agents such as aminocaproic acid are very effective for mucosal bleeding and can be used alone for mild cases or in conjunction with DDAVP or FVIII/vWF concentrates in more severe episodes of bleeding. For

females with menorrhagia, a trial of oral contraceptives is reasonable because estrogen can increase vWF levels. This response is variable, however, and if not effective, aminocaproic acid and nasal DDAVP may be necessary.

Treatment for most **qualitative platelet disorders** is supportive. Mild bleeding episodes can be treated nonspecifically with antifibrinolytic agents or DDAVP. Platelet transfusions should be reserved for life-threatening bleeds and otherwise avoided because of the risk for developing antibodies.

The management for **acute ITP** consists of family education, supportive measures, and in selected cases, pharmacologic therapies. The use of pharmacologic therapies in acute ITP remains controversial. The natural course of acute ITP is for the platelet count to rise within 1 to 3 weeks of presentation. The impetus to treat is the theoretical prevention of intracranial hemorrhage; however, incidence of this complication is less than 0.5%, and there are no data to confirm that any of the currently available therapies actually prevent this complication. Pharmacologic intervention will increase the platelet count more rapidly and may prevent a significant bleeding complication. In those at risk, the use of pharmacologic intervention will not reduce the likelihood of developing chronic ITP. The decision to treat must be individualized, taking into consideration the child's age, bleeding symptoms, child's activity level, and parental anxiety level. Treatment options include observation without medical therapy, corticosteroids, intravenous (IV) gamma globulin, and anti-D immunoglobulin. Anti-D immunoglobulin can only be used in patients who are Rh positive. In all cases, parents should be instructed to avoid the use of aspirin, ibuprofen, and other antiplatelet medications; avoid intramuscular injections; and postpone immunizations and allergic desensitization injections that may exacerbate the degree of thrombocytopenia. Physical activity should be limited with specific instruction to avoid activities that may cause head injury. Parents should also be educated to the signs and symptoms of an intracranial hemorrhage and given instructions as to what to do in the event of an emergency. Therapeutic options for **chronic ITP** include observation without therapy, corticosteroids, regular infusions of IV immune globulin (IVIG) or anti-D immunoglobulin (for Rh+ patients), immunosuppressive agents, rituximab, and laparoscopic splenectomy. Rituximab is a chimeric monoclonal antibody directed against CD20 (found primarily on the surface of B cells) and has been shown to be effective in chronic ITP and other autoimmune conditions. Treatment for acute bleeding in **neonatal alloimmune thrombocytopenia** includes transfusion of **maternal washed** platelets and IVIG. If maternal **washed** platelets are not available, random platelets, preferably crossmatched or HPA-1a negative, can be used along with IVIG.

Prevention and early treatment of bleeding episodes, family education, and good well-child care are important in providing comprehensive **hemophilia** care. The current standard of care for patients with severe hemophilia is prophylaxis, IV factor replacement therapy on a regular schedule (every other day, 3 times a week, or twice a week depending on the type of hemophilia) to prevent bleeding episodes. Prophylaxis is usually initiated during the first few years of life. A subcutaneous central venous catheter is inserted for this purpose and, as the child grows, the parents, and eventually the child, are taught how to administer factor by peripheral infusion. For acute bleeds, prompt treatment is essential to prevent long-term complications. In 30% of patients with hemophilia A and 2% to 3% of patients with hemophilia B, an inhibitor to the respective factor can develop. In the presence of an inhibitor, acute bleeds must be treated with bypassing agents such as prothrombin concentrates or recombinant FVIIa. In the long term, immune tolerance is attempted by exposing the child to high doses of factor on a daily basis in an attempt to eradicate the inhibitor. A number of immune tolerance regimens have been in use with varying success.

Acquired causes of coagulation or platelet abnormalities can be treated supportively or by replacing the deficiency or removing the offending causative agent. Children with **DIC** may be given fresh frozen plasma, cryoprecipitate, and platelets as needed while the underlying etiology of the DIC is treated. In children in whom **vitamin K deficiency** is suspected as the cause of bleeding, one dose of vitamin K should correct the coagulopathy within 12 to 36 hours. Depending on the underlying cause of vitamin K deficiency, regular replacement may be required, as during prolonged antibiotic therapy. Clinically important bleeding in children with superwarfarin rodenticide ingestions may necessitate GI decontamination in addition to administrations of fresh frozen plasma and high-dose vitamin K.

Prognosis

Most patients with inherited bleeding disorders will have an excellent prognosis if the diagnosis is made in a timely fashion and appropriate intervention is initiated.

Patients with **von Willebrand disease** usually have mild bleeding symptoms and, with appropriate education and intervention, the prognosis is excellent. Patients with **hemophilia** will also have an excellent prognosis assuming early diagnosis, family education, prophylaxis, and early treatment of bleeds. With the advent of prophylaxis, the severe hemophilic arthropathy that plagued older generations of males with hemophilia has been largely averted or minimized. In addition, the use of recombinant factor products and highly purified plasma-derived products in the pediatric population has largely eliminated the risk for viral transmission. **Acute ITP** resolves spontaneously by 6 months in 80% of cases, regardless of pharmacologic intervention, and the risk for significant hemorrhage is exceedingly low. For individuals with **chronic ITP,** most cases will also resolve with time, and individuals do not usually have significant bleeding complications.

When to Refer

Most cases of elevated PT/PTT are due to nonspecific inhibitors that are transient and do not cause bleeding. These generally do not require subspecialty referral. Routine ITP can often be managed by a primary pediatrician; however, if there are any questions as to the diagnosis, a hematologist should be consulted. Patients with hemophilia and other severe bleeding disorders are usually diagnosed in infancy and require close follow-up with a pediatric hematologist in the setting of a comprehensive hemophilia treatment center.

CASE RESOLUTION

A van Willebrand factor (vWF) panel was performed and revealed a vWF antigen of 20%, ristocetin cofactor activity of 30%, factor VIII activity of 40%, and a normal multimer analysis. The girl was diagnosed with type 1 von Willebrand disease. A DDAVP challenge was performed in clinic, and she was found to have an excellent response. She was prescribed nasal DDAVP (Stimate) and aminocaproic acid for significant bleeding episodes.

Selected References

Allen GA, Glader B. Approach to the bleeding child. *Pediatr Clin North Am.* 2002;49(6):1239–1256

Andrew M, Vegh P, Johnston M, Bowker J, Ofosu F, Mitchell L. Maturation of the hemostatic system during childhood. *Blood.* 1992;80(8):1998–2005

Astermark J, Petrini P, Tengborn L, Schulman S, Ljung R, Berntorp E. Primary prophylaxis in severe haemophilia should be started at an early age but can be individualized. *Br J Haematol.* 1999;105(4):1109–1113

Cherrick I, Karayalcin G, Lanzkowsky P. Transient erythroblastopenia of childhood. Prospective study of fifty patients. *Am J Pediatr Hematol Oncol.* 1994;16(4): 320–324

Cines DB, Blanchette VS. Immune thrombocytopenic purpura. *N Engl J Med.* 2002;346(13):995–1008

Gazda HT, Sieff CA. Recent insights into the pathogenesis of Diamond-Blackfan anaemia. *Br J Haematol.* 2006;135(2):149–157

Ingels M, Lai C, Tai W, et al. A prospective study of acute, unintentional, pediatric superwarfarin ingestions managed without decontamination. *Ann Emerg Med.* 2002;40(1):73–78

Manco-Johnson MJ, Abshire TC, Shapiro AD, et al. Prophylaxis versus episodic treatment to prevent joint disease in boys with severe hemophilia. *N Engl J Med.* 2007;357(6):535–544

Neunert C, Lim W, Crowther M, et al. The American Society of Hematology 2011 evidence-based practice guideline for immune thrombocytopenia. *Blood.* 2011; 117(16):4190–4207

Nichols WL, Hultin MB, James AH, et al. Von Willebrand disease (VWD): evidence-based diagnosis and management guidelines, the National Heart, Lung, and Blood Institute (NHLBI) Expert Panel report (USA). *Haemophilia.* 2008; 14(2):171–232

Raipurkar M, Lusher JM. Clinical and laboratory approach to the patient with bleeding. In: Orkin SH, Nathan DG, Ginsburg D, Look AT, Fisher DE, Lux SE, eds. *Nathan and Oski's Hematology of Infancy and Childhood.* 7th ed. Philadelphia, PA: Saunders Elsevier; 2009:1449–1461

Tarantino MD, Buchanan GR. The pros and cons of drug therapy for immune thrombocytopenic purpura in children. *Hematol Oncol Clin North Am.* 2004; 18(6):1301–1314

CHAPTER 88

Lymphadenopathy

Eduard H. Panosyan, MD, and Joseph L. Lasky III, MD

CASE STUDY

A 12-year-old girl is brought to the office with swelling of the anterior cervical nodes, which she has had for 2 weeks. Intermittent fever with temperatures as high as 101°F (38.3°C) and decreased appetite have been associated with the condition. On examination, her temperature is 100.4°F (38.0°C) and her other vital signs are normal. Three to 4 non-tender nodes 1 to 2 cm in diameter are present bilaterally. The remainder of the examination is normal.

Questions

1. When is lymphadenopathy of medical concern?
2. What are the clinical features of childhood diseases that present as cervical lymphadenopathy?
3. What are the diagnostic approaches to the evaluation of children with lymphadenopathy?
4. What is an appropriate therapeutic approach to cervical lymphadenopathy in children?

Lymphadenopathy is one of the most common clinical problems encountered in pediatrics. Palpable lymph nodes are a source of anxiety for parents, often prompting a pediatrician visit for evaluation. While most cases are caused by a benign, self-limited infectious process, lymphadenopathy may also signal a serious underlying systemic illness. It is important for the pediatrician to make this distinction so that appropriate diagnostic and therapeutic measures can be initiated when necessary.

Epidemiology

Lymphadenopathy occurs frequently in childhood, and even healthy children may have palpable lymph nodes in the anterior cervical, inguinal, and axillary regions. Localized lymphadenopathy is largely caused by an infectious etiology, whereas generalized lymphadenopathy occurs with systemic illnesses, such as systemic infections (viral, bacterial, protozoal, fungal), autoimmune disorders, storage disorders, and malignancies.

Clinical Presentation

Lymphadenopathy may be localized or generalized on presentation. **Localized** or **regional** lymphadenopathy refers to enlargement of lymph nodes within contiguous regions, whereas **generalized** lymphadenopathy involves more than 2 noncontiguous lymph node groups (D_x Box). Infection is the most frequent cause of localized lymphadenopathy in children. The anterior cervical lymph node region is the most commonly involved area reflecting the high frequency of upper respiratory infections (URIs). Bilateral cervical lymphadenopathy is often seen with viral and bacterial URIs, and the nodes tend to be soft, mobile, and non-tender. Viruses such as Epstein-Barr virus (EBV) or cytomegalovirus (CMV) can present with prominent posterior cervical lymphadenopathy as well as generalized adenopathy and occasionally hepatosplenomegaly. Direct

 Dx

Lymphadenopathy

- Enlarged lymph nodes
- Fever
- Tenderness or warmth over the lymph nodes (lymphadenitis)
- Antecedent infection (eg, pharyngitis, upper respiratory infection, otitis media, skin and soft tissue infections)
- Pallor
- Weight loss
- Bone pain
- Night sweats

bacterial invasion of lymph nodes produces lymphadenitis, which is typically unilateral, tender, erythematous, and fluctuant. Subacute or chronic lymphadenopathy may be caused by atypical mycobacterial infections, tuberculosis, cat-scratch disease, EBV, CMV, toxoplasmosis, coccidioidomycosis, or HIV. Generalized lymphadenopathy is concerning for an underlying systemic illness (infection, autoimmune process, storage disease, or malignancy). Lymphadenopathy due to malignancy is typically characterized by fixed, firm, non-tender lymph nodes in the setting of other signs and symptoms, such as fever, pallor, night sweats, and weight loss.

Pathophysiology

Lymph nodes are an integral part of the immune system in which phagocytic cells filter microorganisms and particulate matter, and antigens are presented provoking a cellular or humoral mediated lymphocyte response. Lymph nodes are distributed in groups throughout the body and drain specific regions (head, neck, axilla, mediastinum, abdomen, extremities) (Table 88-1). Enlargement of

Table 88-1. Lymph Node Drainage Patterns	
Group	*Drainage Pattern*
Occipital	Posterior scalp
Preauricular	Superficial orbital and periorbital tissue, temporal scalp
Submental/ submandibular	Mouth
Cervical	Mouth, pharynx, ear, parotid gland, deep structures of neck (thyroid, larynx, trachea, upper esophagus)
Supraclavicular	Head, neck, arms, lungs, mediastinum, and abdomen
Mediastinal	Lungs, heart, thymus, esophagus
Axillary	Chest wall, breast, upper extremity
Abdominal	Abdominal organs, pelvis, lower extremities
Iliac and inguinal	Lower extremities, genitalia, buttocks, pelvis

a lymph node may be caused by proliferation of lymphocytes intrinsic to the lymph node (as a physiological immune response or a malignant transformation) or infiltration by pathogens or extrinsic inflammatory or metastatic malignant cells.

Differential Diagnosis

The duration and extent of lymphadenopathy (localized vs generalized), characteristics of the lymph nodes, and presence of associated symptoms will help to focus the differential diagnosis. A list of common causes of lymphadenopathy in children is provided in Table 88-2.

Localized lymphadenopathy is most often caused by an infectious etiology. Acute bilateral cervical lymphadenopathy is most frequently caused by viral URIs (respiratory syncytial virus, adenovirus, parainfluenza and influenza viruses) or EBV and CMV, which can also cause generalized adenopathy. Bacterial pharyngitis (most commonly *Streptococcus* species) and oral infections or dental abscesses can present with cervical adenopathy. Unilateral lymphadenitis is most often caused by *Staphylococcus aureus,* followed by *Streptococcus pyogenes,* anaerobes, and other species. When the condition appears subacute, cat-scratch disease, tuberculosis (scrofula), atypical mycobacteria, toxoplasmosis, tularemia, and, less commonly, histoplasmosis, brucellosis, and syphilis should be considered. Cervical lymphadenopathy can also occur with Kawasaki disease, with high fever (5 days); redness, swelling, and desquamation of extremities; conjunctivitis; rash; and swollen lips and tongue.

Generalized lymphadenopathy may be caused by systemic infections (eg, EBV, CMV, HIV, toxoplasmosis), autoimmune disorders (eg, juvenile idiopathic arthritis, systemic lupus erythematosus), storage disorders (eg, Niemann disease, Gaucher disease), histiocytic disorders (eg, Langerhans cell histiocytosis, hemophagocytic lymphohistiocytosis), drug reactions (eg, phenytoin), or malignancies. Malignancies include leukemia and lymphoma (Hodgkin and non-Hodgkin) as well as solid tumors that can metastasize to lymph nodes (eg, neuroblastoma, rhabdomyosarcoma). With neoplastic infiltration, enlarged nodes are generally non-tender, firm, rubbery,

and immobile. In Hodgkin disease, the nodes enlarge sequentially, with involvement spreading from one chain to the next. Supraclavicular or epitrochlear adenopathy is highly suggestive of malignancy.

A number of head and neck lesions that occur in the pediatric population are often confused with cervical lymphadenopathy. These lesions include cystic hygromas, branchial cleft cysts, thyroglossal duct cysts, and epidermoid cysts. These are congenital malformations that often present as a neck mass in the young child and can easily be mistaken for a lymph node, particularly if infected (see Chapter 82).

Evaluation

History

A thorough history and review of symptoms is essential in determining the underlying etiology of lymphadenopathy in children. Inquiries should be made about the duration of the lymphadenopathy, rate of nodal enlargement, and occurrence of associated fever and other constitutional symptoms, such as bone pain, weight loss, fever, and night sweats. Recent illnesses or infections, insect or animal bites, and local trauma should be determined. A history of distant travel, recent emigration from countries with endemic tuberculosis (eg, Mexico, Central America, Southeast Asia), recent travel to areas with endemic histoplasmosis (southeastern United States) or coccidioidomycosis (San Joaquin Valley, CA), a detailed history of pet contact (cats/kittens, which can transmit toxoplasmosis and cat-scratch disease), and exposure to ill contacts, particularly individuals known to have tuberculosis, are also important (Questions Box). In addition, it is important to obtain a history of chemical exposure and steroid use.

Physical Examination

When evaluating a child with lymphadenopathy, the enlarged nodes should be examined and measured at their widest diameter and evaluated for evidence of erythema, tenderness, and warmth, all of which are suggestive of infection. The characteristics of the enlarged lymph node should be noted (eg, soft, firm, rubbery, mobile, matted, tender, discrete). The surrounding skin and soft tissue region that is drained by the involved lymph node should be examined for signs of inflammation or skin breakdown. The extent of the lymphadenopathy should be determined, as well as the presence or absence of hepatosplenomegaly.

Laboratory Tests

In most cases, a thorough history and physical examination can establish the likely diagnosis without any laboratory testing. If studies are deemed necessary, a complete blood cell count, peripheral blood smear, tests of renal and hepatic function, and tumor lysis laboratory tests are useful to screen for an underlying systemic illness that may be associated with lymphadenopathy. Lymphocytosis with atypical lymphocytes on peripheral blood smear is consistent with a viral etiology such as EBV or CMV. Leukocytosis with a left shift

Table 88-2. Differential Diagnosis of Lymphadenopathy			
Diagnostic Category	Clinical Features	Epidemiologic Features	Laboratory Features, Initial Radiologic Studies
Infections			
Viral (EBV, CMV, rubella, HIV)	Usually generalized, not purulent or tender; may have hepatosplenomegaly		EBV/CMV with atypical lymphocytes on peripheral blood smear, viral titers, and PCRs
Mycobacterial (TB, atypical mycobacteria)	Usually localized; often tender, red, flocculent		PPD, chest radiograph, QuantiFERON-TB Gold
Bacterial (staphylococcal and streptococcal infections, cat-scratch disease, tularemia, plague, diphtheria)	Usually localized; often tender, red, flocculent		Titers (cat scratch), Gram stain/culture
Protozoal (toxoplasmosis)	Generalized		Titers
Spirochete (syphilis)			Titers
Fungal (histoplasmosis, coccidioidomycosis)	May be generalized	Suspicion should be raised based on regional incidence	Titers
Neoplastic Conditions			
Hodgkin lymphoma	Often associated with "B" symptoms (eg, fever, weight loss, night sweats), pruritus	Common among higher socioeconomic groups, adolescents	ESR (can be >100), LDH, elevated eosinophils, anergy, elevated ferritin, chest radiograph
Non-Hodgkin lymphoma	See Hodgkin lymphoma.		Abdominal ultrasound
Leukemia	Generalized lymphadenopathy, hepato-splenomegaly, petechiae, purpura, pallor		Cytopenias (leukopenia, neutropenia, thrombocytopenia, or anemia). Lymphocy-tosis and blasts on peripheral blood smear (may be absent), hyperuricemia, hyperkale-mia, hyperphosphatemia, elevated LDH
Solid tumors (eg, rhabdomyo-sarcoma, neuroblastoma)	Depends on location and character of underlying malignancy		
Langerhans cell histiocytosis	Eczema, failure to thrive, bony lesions, diabetes insipidus, proptosis, hepatospleno-megaly, and early teeth eruption all possible		Characteristic pathology with Birbeck granules and CD1a+
Sinus histiocytosis with massive lymphadenopathy			
Autoimmune Disorders			
JIA	Generalized lymphadenopathy seen in systemic form (Still disease) (eg, fever, hepatosplenomegaly, evanescent rash, arthritis)	Equal incidence in males and females	ESR, anemia, negative ANA, and rheumatoid arthritis in JRA (Still disease)
Lupus	Arthritis, butterfly facial rash, effusions (lung, joint, cardiac), CNS, nephrotic syndrome	Increased incidence in girls	ESR; positive ANA; anti-dsDNA; C3, C4, or CH50; anemia; low platelets; proteinuria
Other			
Storage disorders (eg, Niemann disease, Gaucher disease)	Generalized lymphadenopathy, hepatosplenomegaly		
Drugs (eg, phenytoin)	Generalized lymphadenopathy		
Sarcoidosis	Bilateral hilar lymphadenopathy, noncaseating granulomas (lung, liver)	In African Americans and those of Irish heritage	Serum angiotensin-1–converting enzyme, serum lysozyme

Abbreviations: ANA, antinuclear antibody; CMV, cytomegalovirus; CNS, central nervous system; EBV, Epstein-Barr virus; ESR, erythrocyte sedimentation rate; HIV, human immunodeficiency virus; JIA, juvenile idiopathic arthritis; JRA, juvenile rheumatoid arthritis; LDH, lactate dehydrogenase; PCR, polymerase chain reaction; PPD, purified protein derivative; TB, tuberculosis.

Lymphadenopathy — **Questions**

- How long have the nodes been enlarged?
- Was the child sick before the swelling began?
- Does the child have any symptoms now, such as fever, weight loss, pallor, night sweats, or anorexia?
- Does the child come in contact with any animals, particularly cats?
- Has the child traveled anywhere?
- Is the child taking any medications?
- Has the child been in contact with anyone who is ill?

suggests a bacterial etiology. Cytopenias or blasts on peripheral blood smear are concerning for leukemia. Uric acid, phosphorus, and lactate dehydrogenase are typically elevated in the setting of leukemia or lymphoma. An erythrocyte sedimentation rate is nonspecific but may be helpful. Depending on the clinical scenario, serum antibody studies and viral polymerase chain reactions for various infections may be warranted (ie, EBV, CMV, HIV, *Bartonella henselae* for cat-scratch disease, *Bartonella quintana* for trench fever). In addition, a purified protein derivative (PPD) skin test for tuberculosis or serologic tests for fungal disease should be considered. Certain populations may also benefit from new T-cell–based assays for tuberculosis (eg, QuantiFERON-TB Gold). In lupus and juvenile idiopathic arthritis, an antinuclear antibody may be positive and complement levels may be reduced.

If infectious lymphadenitis is suspected, an aspirate for a Gram stain and culture may be helpful, particularly if the infection has been unresponsive to empiric antibiotics. However, if there is *any* concern for malignancy, a fine needle aspiration is *not* the preferred method for diagnosis. An excisional biopsy should be performed so that the entire lymph node and its architecture can be visualized and adequate samples for testing will be available. See Figure 88-1 for the suggested approach to generalized lymphadenopathy in children.

Imaging Studies

A chest radiograph should be performed in any child with significant lymphadenopathy if there is suspicion of an underlying systemic process. If leukemia or lymphoma is suspected, a chest radiograph is obtained to evaluate for an anterior mediastinal mass. Other imaging studies are not routinely performed; however, if the nature of an enlarged lymph node requires further definition, an ultrasound can be done. Massive lymphadenopathy in the head and neck region may warrant evaluation with computed tomography or magnetic resonance imaging. In the setting of malignancy, additional radiographic studies are performed for staging purposes.

Management

Management is dictated by the underlying cause of lymphadenopathy (see Figure 88-1). Cervical lymphadenopathy associated with URIs will typically resolve without intervention. Bacterial lymphadenitis can be treated with a trial of **antibiotics** with antistaphylococcal and antistreptococcal coverage. Underlying fungal and mycobacterial diseases should be treated with appropriate **antifungal or antibacterial agents,** with the exception of cervical adenopathy due to atypical mycobacteria, which requires **surgical removal.** Malignancies may require **multimodal therapy** with surgery, chemotherapy, or targeted therapy or radiation, depending on the specific diagnosis and stage (see Chapter 145).

Prognosis

The outcome of lymphadenopathy depends entirely on the underlying etiology. In most cases, the cause is infectious and the lymphadenopathy is self-limited or resolves with the use of appropriate antibiotics. Lymphadenopathy associated with an underlying systemic illness may have a more chronic or relapsing course, depending on the disease.

CASE RESOLUTION

In the case study, the bilateral nature of the swelling and lack of tenderness of the nodes are very worrisome and suggest a systemic involvement. The girl had a throat culture, an intermediate purified protein derivative, and a chest radiograph, the results of all of which were negative. A complete blood cell count revealed leukocytosis with 28,000 white blood cells per deciliter (60% lymphocytes) with a normal hemoglobin and platelet count. A heterophile test result for infectious mononucleosis was positive. Supportive measures were recommended, and the child made a complete recovery in 3 weeks.

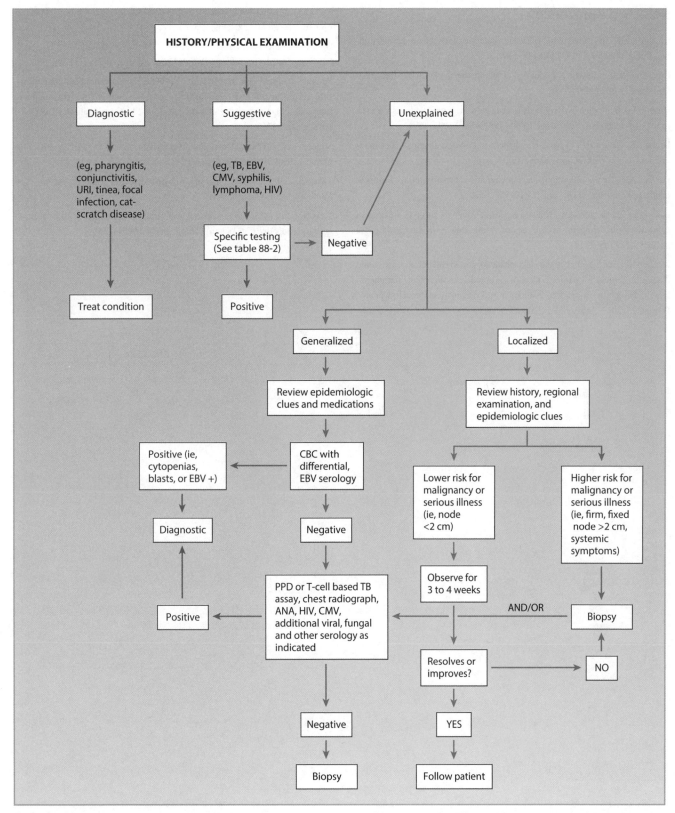

Figure 88-1. Approach to the management of lymphadenopathy. (Modified from Ferrer R. Lymphadenopathy: differential diagnosis and evaluation. *Am Fam Physician*. 1998;58[6]:1313–1320, with permission.)

Selected References

Ginsburg AM. The tuberculosis epidemic: scientific challenges and opportunities. *Public Health Rep.* 1998;113:128–136

Grossman M, Shiramizu B. Evaluation of lymphadenopathy in children. *Curr Opin Pediatr.* 1994;6(1):68–76

Larsson LO, Bentzon MW, Berg Kelly K, et al. Palpable lymph nodes of the neck in Swedish schoolchildren. *Acta Paediatr.* 1994;83(10):1091–1094

Leung AK, Davies HD. Cervical lymphadenitis: etiology, diagnosis, and management. *Curr Infect Dis Rep.* 2009;11(3):183–189

Loeffler AM. Treatment options for nontuberculous mycobacterial adenitis in children. *Pediatr Infect Dis.* 2004;23(10):957–958

Ludwig BJ, Wang J, Nadgir RN, Saito N, Castro-Aragon I, Sakai O. Imaging of cervical lymphadenopathy in children and young adults. *AJR Am J Roentgenol.* 2012;199(5):1105–1113

McClain KL, Fletcher RH. Peripheral lymphadenopathy in children: evaluation and diagnostic approach. UpToDate. http://www.uptodate.com/contents/peripheral-lymphadenopathy-in-children-evaluation-and-diagnostic-approach. Updated February 5, 2014. Accessed February 28, 2014

Nield LS, Kamat D. Lymphadenopathy in children: when and how to evaluate. *Clin Pediatr (Phila).* 2004;43(1):25–33

Oguz A, Karadeniz C, Temel EA, Citak EC, Okur FV. Evaluation of peripheral lymphadenopathy in children. *Pediatr Hematol Oncol.* 2006;23(7):549–561

Painter JA, Graviss EA, Hai HH, et al. Tuberculosis screening by tuberculosis skin test or QuantiFERON-TB Gold in-tube assay among an immigrant population with a high prevalence of tuberculosis and BCG vaccination. *PLoS ONE.* 2013;8(12):e82727

Stutchfield CJ, Tyrrell J. Evaluation of lymphadenopathy in children. *Paediatr Child Health.* 2012;22(3):98–102

Twist CJ, Link MP. Assessment of lymphadenopathy in children. *Pediatr Clin North Am.* 2002;49(5):1009–1025

Yaris N, Cakir M, Sözen E, Cobanoglu U. Analysis of children with peripheral lymphadenopathy. *Clin Pediatr (Phila).* 2006;45(6):544–549

SECTION VI

Cardiovascular System

CHAPTER 89

Heart Murmurs

Robin Winkler Doroshow, MD, MMS, MEd

CASE STUDY

A 6-year-old girl is brought to the office for a physical examination for school. Her medical history is unremarkable, and her growth and development have been normal. She is asymptomatic. Her physical examination is normal except for a grade 2/6 low-pitched vibratory systolic ejection murmur that is loudest at the left lower sternal border, with radiation to the apex and upper sternal border. The murmur increases to 3/6 in the supine position.

Questions

1. What is the significance of a heart murmur in asymptomatic children?
   How reassuring are a negative history and the absence of other physical findings?
2. What workup should be done by primary care physicians?
3. What are the costs of excessive tests and unnecessary consultation?
   What are the costs of an inadequate workup?
4. When should physicians refer children to specialists for consultation?

Asymptomatic children with heart murmurs are commonly encountered by physicians. A murmur is a finding rather than a medical sign or symptom because it is detected incidentally at an examination conducted for another purpose.

Correct assessment of the significance of a heart murmur is important to ensure appropriate management of children with heart disease. Complications of undiagnosed cardiac disease in children include progressive hemodynamic impairment, endocarditis, and even sudden death.

The misinterpretation of an innocent murmur as organic in nature can also take its toll, primarily as parental anxiety. Unnecessary restriction of activities may result, which can have a negative effect on children's school and social lives as well as self-image. As adults they may be denied life insurance and certain types of employment. In addition, misdiagnosis costs money and uses limited resources, with unnecessary tests and doctor visits, as this "non-disease" is evaluated and followed.

Epidemiology

An estimated 50% of healthy children have heart murmurs. The overall incidence of congenital heart disease (CHD), including symptomatic cases, is just under 1%, most of which are identified prenatally or in the newborn period. Some children with CHD have no murmur. Therefore, about 98 out of 100 murmurs noted during childhood are "innocent" (ie, have no organic basis).

Clinical Presentation

Heart murmurs are usually detected on routine examination for well-child care or on evaluation for an unrelated problem. Innocent murmurs are not associated with signs or symptoms because they are normal findings. Most of the symptoms sometimes associated with organic murmurs (ie, murmurs of heart disease) are related to the presence of congestive heart failure (CHF) (see Chapter 92) and usually appear during infancy. Some children with murmurs come to medical attention with complaints of exercise intolerance or chest pain. It is necessary to determine whether these problems are actually referable to the heart, which is uncommon (see Chapter 93).

The noting of a murmur in a child for the first time may be viewed as a "new murmur," which in the adult can be serious finding heralding new onset of acquired heart disease such as mitral insufficiency due to poor ventricular function or aortic insufficiency due to infective endocarditis. In the pediatric patient, these are rare. Much more commonly, a murmur not previously noted may be heard for the first time for benign reasons. Innocent murmurs have characteristic ages at which they appear. Previously very soft murmurs may be more pronounced under different conditions such as fever or anxiety. Murmurs that are predominantly audible in the supine position may not have been noted when the child was examined only in the upright position or vice versa. The lower heart rate and better level of cooperation of the child, compared with the infant, may allow the examiner to identify a murmur not heard on previous examinations.

Pathophysiology

A murmur is a sustained sound that can be detected with a stethoscope placed on the chest. This sound is produced by turbulence of blood flow in the heart or great vessels. This turbulence may be the result of structural abnormalities (eg, aortic valve stenosis), benign or normal flow patterns, or exaggeration of normal flow patterns (seen in high output states such as fever, exercise, anxiety, or anemia and sometimes termed *functional*).

Not all significant heart disease in children is heralded by a murmur. Structural heart disease may be silent and indicated by other findings. For example, transposition of the great arteries results in cyanosis, anomalous pulmonary venous return in pulmonary edema and hypoxia, and anomalous origin of the left coronary artery from the pulmonary artery in CHF. Acquired heart disease, such as Kawasaki disease, myocarditis, or cardiomyopathy, often produces no murmur.

Common innocent murmurs are better recognized than understood. Because they occur in normal, healthy individuals, there are few hemodynamic or anatomic data to correlate with the murmur, and pathophysiology is in some cases conjectural. **Still murmur,** which was once thought to be caused by easily appreciated aortic valve flow, is now believed to result from vibration of normal fibrous bands ("false tendons") that cross the left ventricle. This murmur may also be heard in children who have undergone spontaneous closure of a membranous ventricular septal defect, with a small residual aneurysm in the septum. The **pulmonary flow murmur** seems to be caused by normal flow across the pulmonary valve, perhaps made more apparent because of high cardiac output, close proximity to the chest wall, and (in adolescent females) mild anemia. The **venous hum** is attributed to turbulence at the confluence of the innominate veins, which is exacerbated in the upright position by gravity.

The **physiologic peripheral pulmonic stenosis (PPPS) murmur** in newborns is produced by turbulence at the origins of the left and right pulmonary arteries. Because less than 10% of the combined ventricular output of the fetus goes to these branches, they are small and arise at a sharp angle from the main pulmonary artery. When postnatal circulation abruptly requires the entire cardiac output to enter these vessels, a relative stenosis is encountered. This physiologic stenosis resolves gradually with remodeling of the pulmonary artery tree by 2 to 3 months of age.

Differential Diagnosis

In healthy children, the differential diagnosis of a heart murmur includes innocent murmurs and murmurs resulting from structural lesions, most of which are congenital. The specific features of a particular murmur usually provide most if not all necessary clues to the diagnosis. It is therefore important to develop and maintain auscultatory skills. No written or visual material is a good substitute for practice with recordings and actual patients. A good quality stethoscope, with diaphragm and bell correctly sized for the patient and snugly fitting but comfortable earpieces, is essential. Conditions should be optimized: The patient should be kept comfortable and, if necessary, distracted, and extraneous environmental noise should be minimized.

Some features may alert examiners to the organic nature of a murmur. Although very loud murmurs (grades 4–6; ie, with associated precordial thrill) are usually not innocent, some innocent murmurs may be as loud as grade 3, particularly with high cardiac output (eg, fever, anxiety, anemia). Diastolic murmurs and continuous murmurs, other than the easily recognizable venous hum, are usually pathologic, as are high-pitched and harsh murmurs, which are better heard with the diaphragm of the stethoscope. Murmurs that change strikingly with body position are rarely due to CHD.

The common innocent murmurs of childhood are recognizable on auscultatory examination. **Still murmur,** or the **innocent vibratory murmur,** is a low-pitched, vibratory, or musical murmur that sounds like a groan. Because of its low frequency, the murmur is better heard with the bell. It is loudest at the left lower sternal border but is often distributed widely over the precordium. This murmur is often quite loud, particularly in the supine position, and is extremely common in school-aged children, but may also be heard in the infant. The characteristics of the murmur are diagnostic, although the absence of other findings is supportive.

The **pulmonary flow murmur,** usually heard in older children, is a short, blowing systolic ejection (ie, crescendo-decrescendo) murmur localized to the left upper sternal border. It may be louder in the supine position.

The **venous hum** is a soft continuous murmur, similar to the sound heard in a seashell. Because of its constancy, it is often overlooked. This murmur is very commonly heard in preschool- and school-aged children. Loudest in the right subclavian area, it may also be heard on the left. This murmur is highly variable with head and neck position and compression of the neck veins, which may increase or diminish it. It usually disappears in the supine position.

The **PPPS** murmur is an innocent murmur found in newborns. Best heard at the upper left sternal border, this blowing systolic ejection murmur radiates strikingly over the lung fields into the back and both axillae. It usually disappears by 3 months of age, whereas the murmur of true stenosis of the pulmonary arteries will persist.

Evaluation

History

The history may be helpful in assessment of the child with a murmur. If a thorough history shows that the child has no symptoms, this suggests the absence of severe heart disease and helps exclude many major or complex defects as well as CHF. The absence of symptoms does not, however, exclude several common defects that may require intervention (Table 89-1).

Table 89-1. Common Organic Murmurs in Asymptomatic Children	
Lesion	*Other Clues*
Atrial septal defect	Fixed split S_2
Ventricular septal defect (small to moderate)	Loud heart sounds
Patent ductus arteriosus (small to moderate)	Full or bounding pulses
Pulmonic stenosis	SEC
Aortic stenosis	SEC; suprasternal thrill
Coarctation of the aorta	Weak or absent femoral pulses

Abbreviation: SEC, systolic ejection click.

The most common cardiac symptom reported by children or their parents is easy fatigability (Questions Box). This is difficult to quantitate. Determining exercise intolerance on the basis of history is very subjective; it may be due, of course, to noncardiac causes and unrelated to the murmur. Easy fatigability during infancy may be reported as slow or poor feeding. Chest pain, a common symptom in adults with heart disease, is rarely cardiac in origin in children (see Chapter 93). A history of rapid breathing, excessive sweating, and other complaints referable to CHF suggests organic heart disease. Central cyanosis (ie, involving the oral mucosa rather than the perioral area or fingers) may be reported occasionally by parents of children with cyanotic CHD but is often not recognized.

Physical Examination

The physical examination often gives strong clues to the cardiac diagnosis beyond the murmur itself. Even in children with known CHD, the non-auscultatory portions of the examination are critical in assessing the cardiac status (ie, how the patient is tolerating the defect). **Vital signs,** preferably obtained with the child at rest or sleeping, yield information about cardiac status more than specific diagnosis. Tachypnea and tachycardia are present in CHF. A normal resting respiratory rate (ie, <60 breaths/min in infants) argues strongly against CHF. Blood pressure is normal in most patients with CHD. It may be useful to measure blood pressure in the legs, especially if coarctation of the aorta is suspected because of diminished pulses in the lower extremities or a pulse oximetry difference between upper and lower extremities.

The **growth pattern** may reflect the presence of any chronic illness, including hemodynamically significant CHD. Affected patients, particularly infants and children with large left-to-right shunts (with or without CHF), gain weight poorly. Height and head circumference are usually normal, although in more severe or prolonged situations height may also be affected.

A complete **cardiac examination** should be performed. Is the chest asymmetric, a sign of long-standing cardiomegaly? Is the precordial impulse hyperdynamic? Are extra sounds (eg, clicks, rubs, gallops) heard? Is the second sound normal in intensity and in width and motion of splitting (ie, variation with respiration)?

Additional pertinent findings include lethargy, dysmorphic features suggestive of a genetic syndrome, noncardiac anomalies commonly associated with CHD, central cyanosis, and clubbing. Hepatomegaly is found in children with CHF. The peripheral pulses should be normal in volume, neither diminished (eg, pedal pulses in coarctation) nor bounding (eg, in patent ductus arteriosus), and equal in all extremities. The temperature and capillary refill of the extremities in children who are not chilled reflect adequacy of peripheral circulation.

Diagnostic Studies

Routine laboratory studies are not warranted in the evaluation of most murmurs. An **electrocardiogram (ECG)** is indicated when heart disease is known or strongly suspected, but a normal ECG may not rule out significant CHD, particularly in the infant. A **chest radiograph**

Heart Murmurs

- Is the child easily tired? Is his sleeping/napping pattern normal for his or her age?
- Does the child keep up with others of his or her age?
- If the child is having a good time—for example, at a park or a party—how is the child's endurance?
- Does the child have a family history of congenital heart disease?
- Was the child exposed antenatally to possible teratogens such as maternal diabetes?
- Does the child ever complain of chest pain? At rest or with activity?
- Does the child ever appear blue?
- Does the child perspire excessively?

may be helpful in this setting, but its potential benefits are usually outweighed by the risks of discomfort and radiation exposure. In the case of some tests, such as **echocardiography** or **magnetic resonance imaging**, the manner in which the examination is carried out will vary depending on the suspected diagnosis; direct input from a cardiologist may be necessary to maximize the yield from these studies. Such tests are not suitable for screening purposes and should be obtained only after consultation with a pediatric cardiologist.

Management

If a heart murmur is suspected of being organic in origin because of its features or associated findings, referral to a pediatric cardiologist is indicated. For the young infant (particularly the newborn), the level of concern is high because of the serious risks inherent in ductus-dependent defects (see Chapter 91), which may present with a simple murmur. However, those cases that are critical will usually be identified prior to newborn discharge from the hospital, particularly in areas in which routine pulse oximetry screening is performed. Thus, a newborn with a murmur who "passes" the oximetry screen and has an otherwise normal examination (including femoral pulses) does not require echocardiography or cardiology consultation on an emergent basis.

In the case of a child who is asymptomatic there is no urgency, but parental and physician anxiety can best be allayed by proceeding to consultation promptly (ie, within weeks). In some cases, a repeat examination may be useful before deciding whether to consult a specialist, particularly if the murmur is initially heard under nonphysiological conditions such as fever. Tests are usually best used if selected and ordered by specialists. Not all cardiologists perform all tests on all patients. Because pediatric cardiologists are particularly skilled and experienced in cardiac auscultation, an examination by a confident specialist may be all that is indicated. Innovative methods are under development to enable long-distance auscultation via telemedicine using digital recordings obtained by the primary physician, and even automatic computerized murmur assessment. These approaches may be particularly helpful in overcoming geographic challenges in underserved or widely spread populations.

Management of organic heart disease in infants or children is also best handled by specialists. Treatment may include **medications, interventional catheterization,** or **cardiac surgery.** Communication between the primary care physician and cardiologist, however, is essential to delivery of optimal patient care.

If the murmur is innocent, physicians must complete the following steps:

1. Children and their families must be informed about the presence of the murmur. Even if the murmur is benign, patients have a right to know that it was heard. In addition, they are likely to be examined by other practitioners who will report it, which may lead to the erroneous suspicion of a new murmur or negligence on the part of the first examiner.

2. The diagnosis must be clearly explained to parents and children (depending on the age). It is essential that they understand that this is a normal finding rather than a minor abnormality. In some cases, notification of teachers or athletic coaches may be appropriate to prevent misunderstanding. Physicians must stress that no further evaluation is needed and no restrictions are indicated. Printed brochures that explain innocent murmurs are available from organizations such as the American Heart Association.

3. The description of the murmur and the diagnosis itself must be documented in the medical record. A murmur that is clearly and unequivocally innocent, with no evidence of heart disease, should not affect, for example, the child's access to insurance or participation in sports. Medical documentation also helps protect patients from unnecessary reevaluations in the future.

4. Medical professionals should proceed no further. No laboratory studies or consultations need be performed. If the evaluation has been completed by a specialist because of suspicion of CHD by the referring physician, no follow-up with the specialist is indicated. The child is referred back to the primary practitioner.

Prognosis

The prognosis for children with heart murmurs depends on the cause of the murmur. Children with an innocent murmur, who by definition have normal hearts, have a normal prognosis—with one exception. If parents mistakenly believe their children to have heart disease, parents may treat the children inappropriately (eg, unnecessary testing, restriction of activities). As a result, children may develop sedentary habits and inferior self-image.

With appropriate medical attention, the prognosis is normal or near normal in most cases of CHD. Children with minor defects not requiring intervention (eg, small ventricular septal defect, mild pulmonic stenosis) need only infrequent cardiology follow-up visits. With the development of refined cardiac surgery and interventional catheterization, even children with the most complex cardiac

anomalies now have a good outlook with respect to quality of life and life expectancy.

CASE RESOLUTION

In the case presented, a healthy girl with no history of cardiovascular symptoms has a heart murmur and an otherwise unremarkable physical examination. The murmur is a typical Still (innocent vibratory) murmur, which is identifiable by its low-pitched, vibratory quality. No further evaluation is necessary. The diagnosis is explained, the girl and her parents are reassured, and the murmur and diagnosis are noted in the medical record.

Selected References

Bergman AB, Stamm SJ. The morbidity of cardiac nondisease in schoolchildren. *N Engl J Med.* 1967;276(18):1008–1013

Danford DA, Nasir A, Gumbiner C. Cost assessment of the evaluation of heart murmurs in children. *Pediatrics.* 1993;91(2):365–368

Gaskin PR, Owens SE, Talner NS, Sanders SP, Li JS. Clinical auscultation skills in pediatric residents. *Pediatrics.* 2000;105(6):1184–1187

Geggel RL, Horowitz LM, Brown EA, Parsons M, Wang PS, Fulton DR. Parental anxiety associated with referral of a child to a pediatric cardiologist for evaluation of a Still's murmur. *J Pediatr.* 2002;140(6):747–752

Haney I, Ipp M, Feldman W, McCrindle BW. Accuracy of clinical assessment of heart murmurs by office based (general practice) paediatricians. *Arch Dis Child.* 1999;81(5):409–412

Hohn AR. Congenital heart disease—the first test. *West J Med.* 1992;156(4): 435–436

Mahnke CB, Mulreany MP, Inafuku J, Abbas M, Feingold B, Paolillo JA. Utility of store-and-forward pediatric telecardiology evaluation in distinguishing normal from pathologic pediatric heart sounds. *Clin Pediatr (Phila).* 2008;47(9): 919–925

Mangione S, Nieman LZ. Cardiac auscultatory skills of internal medicine and family practice trainees. A comparison of diagnostic proficiency. *JAMA.* 1997; 278(9):717–722

Moss AJ. Clues in diagnosing congenital heart disease. *West J Med.* 1992;156(4): 392–398

Newburger JW, Rosenthal A, Williams RG, Fellows K, Miettinen OS. Noninvasive tests in the initial evaluation of heart murmurs in children. *N Engl J Med.* 1983;308(2):61–64

Smythe JF, Teixeira OH, Vlad P, Demers PP, Feldman W. Initial evaluation of heart murmurs: are laboratory tests necessary? *Pediatrics.* 1990;86(4):497–500

Vukanovic-Criley JM, Criley S, Warde CM, et al. Competency in cardiac examination skills in medical students, trainees, physicians, and faculty: a multicenter study. *Arch Intern Med.* 2006;166(6):610–616

Zühlke L, Myer L, Mayosi BM. The promise of computer-assisted auscultation in screening for structural heart disease and clinical teaching. *Cardiovasc J Afr.* 2012; 23(7):405–408

CHAPTER 90

Palpitations

Robin Winkler Doroshow, MD, MMS, MEd, and Nefthi Sandeep, MD

CASE STUDY

A previously healthy 10-year-old girl comes to the office complaining of an episode of "racing heart." This occurred about a week ago while she was watching TV. Her heart suddenly started pounding hard, and the sensation stopped just as suddenly about 30 minutes later. During the episode, the child's mother felt the girl's chest and noted her heart was beating extremely fast and hard; the child looked scared but was in no respiratory distress and was alert. Her parents drove her to the local emergency department (ED), but the symptoms stopped en route. On arrival in the ED, she was fine and had normal vital signs and physical examination and a normal electrocardiogram. In retrospect, she has had brief such episodes in the past.

Questions

1. What is the significance of palpitations in an otherwise well child?
2. How likely is this symptom to be cardiac in origin, and if so, how likely to be life-threatening?
3. How can transient cardiac events be documented?
4. What does the primary care physician need to do and know prior to referring the child to a cardiologist?

The term *palpitations* is currently used more by medical personnel than by patients. It refers to a sensation of increased awareness of the heart beating faster, harder, or less evenly than expected. Frequently used lay terms for this perception are racing, fluttering, or pounding of the heart. Some patients simply report a sudden unexplainable feeling of being afraid, or they may interpret the symptom as pain or other indescribable discomfort in the chest.

Epidemiology

The incidence of this complaint is not reported. It is a fairly common reason for referral of pediatric patients to cardiologists, although significantly less common than murmurs or chest pain. Because articulating this complaint requires significant verbal skills as well as bodily awareness, it is not usually reported before age 3 or 4 years; beyond this threshold, it may occur at any age. It should be noted that cardiac arrhythmias, the most likely significant cause of this symptom, occur at any age and even in utero, but the presenting complaint in younger patients will usually reflect secondary or tertiary physiological changes such as altered mental status, color change, syncope, or respiratory distress.

Clinical Presentation

As in chest pain, patients' descriptions of these symptoms are quite variable. They are almost always episodic, with a sudden sensation of the heartbeat taking the child by surprise. Because this feeling may be alarming or at least disconcerting (even to adults), the patient may not have been a good observer, and thus the report of the episode(s) may be lacking in clarity or detail. The sense of alarm may stem from the unexpected nature of its appearance, interpretation (in an older child or an adult observer) that a dangerous cardiac event such as a heart attack is occurring, or misinterpretation of a rapid heartbeat as a reflection of fear. It is also not unusual to see a child entirely unconcerned about this symptom accompanied to the visit by an extremely concerned parent.

The vast majority of patients with this complaint report its occurrence in the absence of other medical issues, as in the Case Study at the beginning of this chapter.

Pathophysiology

Palpitations are a subjective symptom and may reflect a cardiac issue (most commonly arrhythmia), anxiety, or simply increased somatic awareness. Only the first of these has a significant component of abnormal physiology.

The degree to which cardiac function may be compromised in cases of arrhythmia will depend on the nature of the rhythm, rate, duration of the episode, and presence or absence of underlying cardiac disorders, congenital or acquired. In ventricular tachycardia (VT), the rate is usually in the range of 150 to 180 beats per minute, and filling is not seriously impaired; however, loss of atrioventricular synchrony and inefficient ventricular *emptying* result in poor cardiac output in most cases. In addition, this rhythm can deteriorate to ventricular fibrillation, with essentially no functional cardiac output, a life-threatening situation. Supraventricular tachycardia (SVT) is by far the most frequently diagnosed arrhythmia in the pediatric population. Its rate is substantially higher, often greater than 250 beats per minute, with relatively less time in diastole and more in systole. This leads to compromise of ventricular *filling* and secondarily the cardiac output, as well as an unfavorable myocardial supply-demand ratio, which may cause angina-like chest pain. Atrioventricular block is uncommon in otherwise healthy children and is more likely to produce pre-syncope or syncope than palpitations, but the latter may also occur. This rhythm impairs cardiac output by a decrease in ventricular rate and loss of atrioventricular synchrony.

Some patients report erratic, very brief pounding sensations caused by single premature ventricular contractions (PVCs), while others are unaware of this common arrhythmia (Figure 90-1). Those who do perceive them are sensing the increased cardiac output of the immediate post-PVC beat as a "thump" and rarely experience associated symptoms. Premature atrial contractions are very common but rarely perceived by the patient.

Palpitations related to anxiety disorders will often be associated with other catecholamine-induced symptoms such as dyspnea or tremor; these somatic symptoms may dominate over psychiatric symptoms and divert the clinician's attention away from the pursuit of a psychologic cause.

Differential Diagnosis

The differential diagnosis of palpitations has been alluded to herein and is summarized in Box 90-1. In cases of sudden onset of isolated rapid pounding of the heart, SVT, which includes reentrant SVT (Figure 90-2), junctional tachycardia, ectopic atrial tachycardia, and atrial flutter, dominates the cardiac causes in frequency. Saarel et al found that of 238 consecutive children who transmitted their rhythms trans-telephonically during palpitations, 35 had SVT; no other significant arrhythmias were found in the remainder. Other tachyarrhythmias and bradyarrhythmias must be considered, despite their rarity, however, because of the poorer prognosis and importance of instituting therapy.

Sinus tachycardia in the absence of anxiety may be experienced by those with decreased stroke volume, such as patients with myocarditis or cardiomyopathy, either of which may present with palpitations. Children receiving stimulant therapy for attention-deficit/hyperactivity disorder experience palpitations with surprising infrequency, perhaps because their slight overall increase in heart rate is chronic rather than episodic. Cardiac arrhythmias in this setting are no more common than in the general pediatric population. However, stimulants in the form of so-called energy drinks are becoming increasingly popular in the adolescent and preadolescent population and may lead to inappropriate sinus tachycardia. Caffeine is the main active ingredient in most energy drinks. However,

Box 90-1. Differential Diagnosis of Palpitations in Children and Adolescents

Cardiac Arrhythmias
- Atrioventricular block (rare cause)
- Premature atrial contractions (uncommon cause)
- Premature ventricular contractions (common cause)
- Sinus tachycardia
  - —Caused by high-output states (eg, hyperthyroidism, anemia) (uncommon cause)
  - —Caused by low cardiac output (eg, in myocarditis or cardiomyopathy) (rare cause)
  - —Caused by stimulants (eg, amphetamines, beta agonists, caffeine) (common cause)
- Supraventricular tachycardia (common cause)
- Ventricular tachycardia (rare cause)

Psychogenic
- Hypochondria (common cause)
- Panic attacks and other anxiety disorders (uncommon cause)
- School phobia (common cause)

Other
- Somatic hyperawareness (common cause)

there are often additional caffeine-containing plant-based substances, such as guarana, that have inotropic and chronotropic properties. Of course, abuse of drugs such as amphetamines may also lead to this rhythm, but patients rarely report this as a complaint. Hyperthyroidism, similarly to chronic use of stimulant medication, leads to sustained sinus tachycardia, which is rarely reported by the patient, but can also occasionally lead to significant cardiac arrhythmias.

Psychogenic palpitations are quite common in childhood, reported by Ginsburg et al in almost 50% of pediatric patients with anxiety disorders and panic disorder. This complaint may be the presenting symptom and should not be dismissed by the clinician as unimportant. On the other hand, in those cases in which these disorders are ruled out, simple somatic hyperawareness, such as is often

Figure 90-2. Supraventricular tachycardia at 257 beats/min. Note ST depression (arrow) caused by relative myocardial ischemia.

Figure 90-1. Premature ventricular contractions (arrows).

seen in healthy adolescents ("My heart speeds up when I take a test"), may lead to the same complaint but respond to reassurance.

Evaluation

The keystones for evaluation of children with palpitations are the history and documentation of cardiac rhythm. The first of these guides the clinician in determining which direction to pursue and, in particular, how extensive an arrhythmia workup is appropriate. When arrhythmia is suspected, documentation ("capturing" the arrhythmia) is essential prior to intervention.

History

It is important to obtain as much descriptive information as possible from the child himself or herself and any witnesses (Questions Box). If the child reports a rapid heart rate, a witness may have taken the child's pulse rate, or the patient himself or herself may be able to "tap out" a representation of the rate on his or her chest or a table. A rough idea of the pulse rate will aid the physician in formulating a differential diagnosis; language such as "very fast" may be interpreted differently by different people and, thus, is not helpful. A witness can also report whether the patient had a change in color, respiratory pattern, or mental status.

Palpitations of abrupt onset and offset are more likely to reflect paroxysmal cardiac arrhythmias, while sinus tachycardia due to stimulants or anxiety is more likely to have a gradual onset and resolution. Some arrhythmias may be triggered by certain events or actions, such as exertion, emergence from anesthesia, or exposure to stimulants such as beta agonists. If the palpitations resolve in response to an action such as Valsalva maneuver or vomiting, conversion of an arrhythmia may have taken place.

The presence or absence of associated symptoms may give a clue as to the seriousness of a cardiac event. Ventricular arrhythmias such as sustained VT often cause an abrupt fall in cardiac output, resulting

in loss of consciousness or even sudden death. Brief episodes of SVT may not be associated with any complaints other than the palpitations themselves but, if sustained, may be associated with fatigue, breathlessness, chest pain, nausea, or dizziness.

Most children reporting palpitations have no relevant **past medical history.** However, patients with past history of congenital heart disease (particularly if treated surgically), inflammatory heart disease such as myocarditis, or exposure to cardiotoxins such as anthracycline chemotherapeutic agents, are more likely to have experienced a significant arrhythmia than others and are less likely to tolerate arrhythmia well. In these settings, prompt and thorough evaluation is essential. As mentioned previously, if the patient becomes alarmed, he or she may also experience symptoms reflective of increased catecholamine output, such as breathlessness or pallor, complicating the assessment. These additional symptoms may respond to reassurance even when the palpitations persist.

The history must include a search for a **family history** of heritable rhythm disorders, such as long QT syndrome, or events, such as unexpected sudden death, that may reflect one of these disorders, which may have been inherited by the patient.

Physical Examination

The physical examination of the patient presenting with isolated episodic palpitations is rarely contributory. Certainly the cardiac rhythm and rate should be noted, but they will rarely give a direct clue as to the diagnosis. Findings such as a heart murmur or gallop may point toward an underlying cardiac disorder not previously identified.

Synthesis

Having completed the history and physical examination, the pediatrician will have established a level of concern about the likelihood of cardiac causes for the palpitations, which will in turn guide him or her to recommend elective referral to a cardiologist, emergent referral to an emergency department (ED) or hospital, elective referral to a psychologist or psychiatrist, or, alternatively, to manage the problem without further referral.

Laboratory Studies

In the primary care setting, laboratory studies are not often needed to make the determination of whether to refer the patient; the history and examination will usually suffice. If there is significant suspicion of arrhythmia, the cardiology consultant will consider various studies (Table 90-1), focusing on documenting the rhythm during symptoms and seeking evidence of underlying causes of arrhythmia.

Electrocardiogram

Electrocardiogram (ECG) is a readily available test that is often diagnostic if obtained during palpitations. Parents should be instructed to take the child to an urgent care center or ED promptly if the child experiences a prolonged episode (eg, lasting an hour) and request that an ECG be done immediately on arrival. In the absence of symptoms at the time of the visit, the ECG will not often shed light on the

---

Questions

Palpitations

- What does it feel like? If the heartbeat is fast, how fast?
- What symptoms are associated with the palpitations?
- Do the symptoms start gradually or abruptly? How do they end? Can the patient cause them to end?
- How frequent are the episodes, and how long do they last?
- Are they precipitated by certain events?
- How disruptive are these symptoms to activities of daily living?
- Does the child have a history of cardiac problems such as congenital heart disease or other symptoms that point to an underlying defect?
- Did the onset of these episodes correlate with other life or medical events?
- Is the child taking or using stimulant medication or beverages that might be contributing to these symptoms?
- Is there a family history suggestive of cardiac arrhythmia, such as sudden unexpected death or long QT syndrome?

Table 90-1. Laboratory Tests Used in the Evaluation of Palpitations in Children	
Test	**Information**
ECG	Diagnostic if obtained during symptoms Underlying predisposition such as WPW or LQTS
Holter monitor (ambulatory ECG)	Captures rhythm during symptoms during a 24-hour recording period
Event detector	Captures rhythm during symptoms over an extended period (eg, 30 days)
Implantable monitor	Captures rhythm during symptoms over an extended period (up to several months)
Exercise test	Provocation of symptoms or arrhythmia in patients who have symptoms induced by exercise
EPS	Provokes arrhythmias Identifies additional conducting pathways that support arrhythmias Opportunity to intervene (eg, ablation)
Echocardiogram	Identifies underlying structural or functional cardiac disorder
Cardiac magnetic resonance imaging	Assesses cardiac anatomy in complex congenital heart disease Evaluates for arrhythmogenic right ventricular cardiomyopathy
Hematocrit	Identifies underlying anemia
Thyroid function tests	Identifies underlying hyperthyroidism
Toxicology screen	Identifies drug exposure

Abbreviations: ECG, electrocardiogram; EPS, electrophysiology study; LQTS, long QT syndrome; WPW, Wolff-Parkinson-White syndrome.

Figure 90-3. Wolff-Parkinson-White syndrome. Note the short PR interval (left arrow) and the delta wave (right arrow) created by preexcitation.

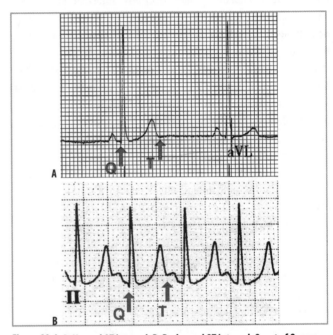

Figure 90-4. A, Normal QT interval. B, Prolonged QT interval. Onset of Q wave and end of T wave indicated by arrows.

diagnosis. It is important, however, to look for predisposition to arrhythmia, such as Wolff-Parkinson-White syndrome (Figure 90-3) predisposing to SVT, and long QT syndrome (Figure 90-4) predisposing to VT (and in particular to torsades de pointes). Either of these conditions may be only intermittently apparent on a surface ECG, so their absence on a single tracing does not exclude them.

Documentation of Cardiac Rhythm During Symptoms

This is indeed the key to making a diagnosis of arrhythmia and, more often, to ruling out arrhythmia as a cause of palpitations. Multiple techniques are available, each with advantages and disadvantages. The **Holter monitor** is a well-established, sensitive, high-quality random 24-hour tracing. Only in cases with very frequent (ie, almost daily) palpitations is it likely to capture the symptomatic rhythm itself, but in some cases subclinical arrhythmias such as brief bouts of SVT may go unnoticed by the patient but will be seen on the Holter. The test is readily available but not well tolerated by very young children; it is not monitored by clinicians or technologists in real time; and its value is substantially undermined in cases in which the patient or his parents fail to provide an accompanying symptom

diary. Similar to ECGs, Holter monitors have excellent specificity (ie, low rate of false-positive results) but poor sensitivity (ie, high rate of false-negative results); hence, a negative Holter result does not definitively rule out an arrhythmia.

Less frequent episodic palpitations are more frequently captured on **event detectors,** also known as **trans-telephonic monitors (TTMs).** These are small devices that can be taken home with the patient for several weeks and can be used to capture the ECG in the event of symptoms, then convert that signal into an audio code which can be transmitted over the telephone to a doctor's office or monitoring service. The quality of its output is poorer than that of a Holter monitor. Most TTMs are **post-event monitors,** which require the patient to actively produce the recording. This requires patient cooperation and symptoms that last long enough to elicit patient-initiated recording, usually over 3 to 4 minutes. This method fails to capture the onset of the arrhythmia. These obstacles may be overcome with a **loop-type event recorder,** which continuously records and erases a short loop of

ECG. The patient depresses a button when experiencing the symptoms and the device will save the previous 2 to 3 minutes, thus enabling capture of the onset of the arrhythmia or even an arrhythmia that has ceased by the time the patient activates the device. Some of these devices may also be programmed to automatically record in certain situations, such as when the heart rate exceeds a selected threshold. Loop recorders require that stick-on leads must be worn more or less continuously, and patient tolerance for them is therefore not high.

As technology continues to improve, the range of diagnostic monitor options and quality of their output increase. Some patients will benefit from a small **implantable monitor,** such as the Reveal, which can automatically record the ECG when certain parameters are met and also be activated by the patient. In addition to higher cost, these devices have the disadvantage of requiring minor surgery for implantation (usually in the left pre-pectoral pocket) and removal and require the patient to report to a cardiac center for downloading.

Stress Testing

In selected cases in which physical exercise consistently triggers palpitations, a treadmill or bicycle exercise test may occasionally be used to provoke the symptom.

Electrophysiology Study

If there is a high enough suspicion of a serious arrhythmia that cannot be captured by one of the previously described methods in a reasonable period, invasive electrophysiology testing may yield information as to provokable arrhythmias (eg, VT) or abnormal conducting pathways not manifest on the surface ECG. These complex studies are not without risk and are only performed by experienced cardiac electrophysiologists. They have the advantage of offering the opportunity to intervene during the same procedure and also provide the opportunity to perform a highly detailed arrhythmia evaluation in a controlled setting.

Echocardiogram

In the absence of past history, symptoms, or physical findings suggesting underlying heart disease, the echocardiogram is unlikely to be abnormal. If the patient does have one of these risk factors, it may be helpful. Particular emphasis is placed on evaluation of ventricular function. Abnormal contractility may lead to arrhythmia, and the converse is also true if the arrhythmia is persistent rather than transient.

Cardiac Magnetic Resonance Imaging

In patients with ventricular arrhythmias of unknown etiology, cardiac magnetic resonance imaging may be diagnostic for arrhythmogenic right ventricular cardiomyopathy (ARVC). Echocardiography is not sensitive for this diagnosis.

Blood Tests

Many cardiologists screen for thyroid dysfunction in patients with isolated tachyarrhythmias. This is rarely productive, particularly in the absence of physical findings such as resting sinus tachycardia, tremor, or sweating. Because anemia of at least moderate degree may cause sinus tachycardia or pounding sensation due to high stroke volume, a complete blood cell count may be considered in some cases.

Toxicology Screen

Patients experiencing tachyarrhythmias in an acute setting should be evaluated for possible drug abuse as an underlying cause.

Management

The most common outcome of this type of evaluation is that cardiac arrhythmia is ruled out. When one of the methods of documentation described previously demonstrates normal sinus rhythm during the symptoms, reassurance is all that is needed.

If sinus tachycardia is documented during symptoms, consideration must be given to the possibility of a psychosomatic disorder, anxiety disorder, drug effect, hyperthyroidism, and other causes of sinus tachycardia. For management of these disorders, the reader is referred to other chapters.

Minor, clinically insignificant cardiac arrhythmias such as isolated low-grade **PVCs** usually do not require treatment; the patient and parents are reassured.

If a clinically significant cardiac dysrhythmia is diagnosed, there are multiple management options from which to choose, depending on the nature of the rhythm and its risk to the patient. Serious **ventricular arrhythmias** such as VT may require aggressive treatment such as antiarrhythmic medication, beta blockers, or, in some cases, insertion of an implantable cardioverter-defibrillator (ICD). This decision and these interventions are usually accomplished by a cardiac electrophysiologist.

Supraventricular tachycardia is the most frequently diagnosed arrhythmia that is clinically significant in children. Beyond the newborn period and in the absence of underlying heart disease, these rhythms are not life-threatening unless sustained for very long periods (eg, days), which is uncommon. They may, however, be very unpleasant and highly disruptive. When this is not the case, but the child only experiences infrequent fleeting episodes of well-tolerated SVT, no intervention may be required. For more troublesome cases, pharmacologic management is usually well tolerated and highly efficacious in prevention of recurrences. In the current era, results of interventional catheterization, such as cryoablation or radiofrequency ablation of accessory pathways, are excellent and attained at low risk. This option may enable the child to be free not only of the arrhythmia but also of the need to take daily medications.

Prognosis

For those patients in whom the concern for heart disease is low, and for those in whom it is excluded or found not to be clinically significant, the prognosis is, of course, the same as for other children. Those found to have paroxysmal SVT usually respond well to pharmacologic management, although some experimentation may be needed to find the best-tolerated and most effective treatment. Ablative procedures, in the absence of the rare complication of complete heart block, yield an excellent prognosis and are, in fact, often curative.

Prognosis is less certain for children with serious ventricular arrhythmias, particularly in the setting of ARVC or LQTS. However, the evolution of ICDs suitable for children has already led to improvement in quantity and quality of life.

CASE RESOLUTION

The child wore a Holter monitor, during which time she did not have symptoms. She was then issued an event detector and 2 weeks later successfully recorded and transmitted her electrocardiogram during an episode of palpitations. It demonstrated SVT at a rate of 250 beats per minute that terminated spontaneously after 20 minutes. Her parents elected to have her undergo electrophysiology study, which demonstrated an aberrant pathway, which was successfully ablated without complication. At her 1-year follow-up visit, she was free of palpitations, on no medications, and participating actively in age-appropriate activities.

Selected References

Babikar A, Hynes B, Ward N, Oslizok P, Walsh K, Keane D. A retrospective study of the clinical experience of the implantable loop recorder in a paediatric setting. *Int J Clin Pract.* 2008;62(10):1520–1525

Cooper WO, Habel LA, Sox CM, et al. ADHD drugs and serious cardiovascular events in children and young adults. *N Engl J Med.* 2011;365(20):1896–1904

Ginsburg GS, Riddle MA, Davies M. Somatic symptoms in children and adolescents with anxiety disorders. *J Am Acad Child Adolesc Psychiatry.* 2006;45(10):1179–1187

Hegazy RA, Lotfy WN. The value of Holter monitoring in the assessment of pediatric patients. *Indian Pacing Electrophysiol J.* 2007;7(4):204–214

Ko JK, Deal BJ, Strasburger JF, Benson DW Jr. Supraventricular tachycardia mechanisms and their age distribution in pediatric patients. *Am J Cardiol.* 1992;69(12):1028–1032

Olfson M, Huang C, Gerhard T, et al. Stimulants and cardiovascular events in youth with attention-deficit/hyperactivity disorder. *J Am Acad Child Adolesc Psychiatry.* 2012;51(2):147–156

Rajagopalan K, Potts JE, Sanatani S. Minimally invasive approach to the child with palpitations. *Expert Rev Cardiovasc Ther.* 2006;4(5):681–693

Saarel EV, Stefanelli CB, Fischbach PS, Serwer GA, Rosenthal A, Dick M. Transtelephonic electrocardiographic monitors for evaluation of children and adolescents with suspected arrhythmias. *Pediatrics.* 2004;113(2):248–251

Scalvini S, Zanelli E, Martinelli G, Baratti D, Giordano A, Glisenti F. Cardiac event recording yields more diagnoses than 24-hour Holter monitoring in patients with palpitations. *J Telemed Telecare.* 2005;11(Suppl 1):14–16

Seifert SM, Schaechter JL, Hershorin ER, Lipshultz SE. Health effects of energy drinks on children, adolescents, and young adults. *Pediatrics.* 2011;127(3):511–528

CHAPTER 91

Cyanosis in the Newborn

Robin Winkler Doroshow, MD, MMS, MEd

CASE STUDY

A 3,500-g term male neonate born to a 29-year-old, gravida 2, para 2, healthy mother by spontaneous vaginal delivery is well until 24 hours of age, when a nurse notes that he is cyanotic. On examination, he appears blue but in no distress. The vital signs are temperature (axillary) 37°C (98.6°F), pulse 130 beats/min, respirations 40 breaths/min, and blood pressure 80/60 mm Hg in the right arm. His general appearance is normal except for the cyanosis. His heart sounds are normal, and no murmur is heard. His liver is not palpable, and the peripheral pulses are normal and equal in all extremities. Capillary refill is normal. Oxygen saturation is 65% by pulse oximetry.

Questions

1. What are the causes of cyanosis in newborns?
2. What is the appropriate evaluation of cyanosis in newborns?
3. How urgent is the assessment? What are the risks and benefits of further evaluation?
4. Which aspects of management should be initiated by a primary physician at a community hospital?
5. Which types of treatment should be undertaken by the consulting pediatric cardiologist at the referral center?

Cyanosis is a bluish appearance of the skin resulting from the presence of reduced hemoglobin in the tissues. Central cyanosis, which is detected initially in the oral mucosa and nail beds but is generalized when severe, indicates at least 4 to 5 g of reduced hemoglobin per 100 mL blood. Hypoxemia is usually the cause. This condition is frequently present in neonates with pulmonary pathology but is also one of the most common presentations of severe congenital heart disease (CHD).

Because cyanotic CHD in newborns may be life-threatening, it must not go undiagnosed. Most diagnostic studies have minimal risk. Even the risk of cardiac catheterization, rarely indicated, is relatively low in this setting. Most of the lesions that cause cyanotic CHD can be palliated or corrected, and the prognosis is good.

Epidemiology

Cyanotic CHD occurs in about 2 to 3 of every 1,000 live-born neonates. Approximately 80% to 90% of these cases, usually the most severe ones, are detected prenatally or in the first 30 days of life. However, failure to diagnose major CHD *before newborn discharge* occurs in at least 10% of cases, leading to unnecessary morbidity and mortality. Newborns with low pulmonary blood flow or lesions causing poor mixing most often present with obvious cyanosis, although initially they otherwise appear well and comfortable. Those with high pulmonary flow are less blue and often present first with congestive heart failure (CHF) or a murmur but may be detected earlier using screening pulse oximetry.

Most cyanotic CHD is not diagnosed before birth. The antenatal history, gestational age, birth weight, and delivery room examination are unremarkable. Failure to identify CHD in the setting of a routine obstetric ultrasound study does not rule it out;

the sensitivity of such scans in the general population is very low. Congenital heart disease is more likely in some situations that can be anticipated prenatally (Box 91-1). In these settings, increased suspicion may lead to antenatal detection using specialized echocardiography.

Clinical Presentation

Neonates with cyanotic CHD often present within the first week of life with cyanosis of the oral mucosa. In more severe cases, generalized cyanosis occurs. The abnormal color may be more apparent with effort (eg, feeding, passing stool) or crying. Respiratory distress, heralded by grunting, nasal flaring, and retractions, is minor or absent in many newborns with cyanotic CHD, in striking contrast with those who have respiratory disease such as respiratory distress syndrome or aspiration pneumonia. In cases of severe hypoxia, metabolic acidosis leads to poor perfusion and compensatory tachypnea with hyperpnea, a sign of critical heart disease. Additional findings depend on the nature of the causal lesion (D_x Box). It is important to note that the absence of associated physical findings does not exclude cyanotic CHD.

Box 91-1. Settings With Increased Risk of Congenital Heart Disease

- Genetic syndromes (eg, trisomies, DiGeorge syndrome)
- Certain extracardiac anomalies (eg, omphalocele, forearm anomalies)
- High incidence of congenital heart disease in the family
- Maternal diabetes if poorly controlled during first trimester
- Fetal exposure to cardiac teratogen (eg, lithium, isotretinoin)
- Fetal or neonatal arrhythmia other than premature atrial beats

---

Dx Cyanosis in the Newborn: Possible Associated Findings

- Low oxygen saturation
- No improvement with oxygen
- Heart murmur
- Tachypnea
- Increased perspiration
- Abnormal cardiac silhouette on radiograph
- Abnormal electrocardiogram
- Abnormal echocardiogram

Pathophysiology (Box 91-2)

Cardiac cyanosis is due to **right-to-left shunting** so that systemic venous blood bypasses the pulmonary circulation and enters the systemic circulation. Two conditions are usually necessary to produce this type of shunting: a communication, such as a septal defect, for the blood to shunt across and a cause, such as pulmonic stenosis, for the blood to be shunted away from the lungs. The most notable exception is simple transposition of the great arteries (TGA), where the fundamental connections are abnormal and all systemic venous blood is directed to the systemic arterial circulation. Lesions associated with cyanosis may be divided into 3 groups.

1. The *low pulmonary blood flow (LPBF) group* consists of tetralogy of Fallot, pulmonary atresia with intact ventricular septum, and virtually any combination of defects that includes pulmonary atresia or severe pulmonic stenosis. Pulmonary flow is diminished and may derive entirely from the ductus arteriosus while it remains patent. Aside from obvious cyanosis (and associated oxygen saturation below 80%), neonates often appear well.

2. The *high pulmonary blood flow (HPBF) group* includes truncus arteriosus, single ventricle, and combinations of defects that involve mixing of oxygenated and unoxygenated blood and little or no obstruction to pulmonary flow. Although a right-to-left shunt is present, the left-to-right shunt is even greater. Pulmonary venous return is therefore voluminous and contributes disproportionately to systemic output. Cyanosis is less apparent;

saturation is greater than 80% and may be as high as 95%. Pulmonary flow increases over the first days and weeks of life as the pulmonary vascular resistance falls, and CHF develops, as in patients with isolated shunt lesions (eg, ventricular septal defect). Some neonates with HPBF lesions also have obstruction to systemic blood flow (eg, coarctation of the aorta, hypoplastic left heart syndrome) and may depend on the ductus arteriosus to carry some or all of this flow.

3. The *poor mixing group* is limited to TGA and its variants. The right and left circuits are in parallel rather than in series, and survival depends on interchange of oxygenated and unoxygenated blood between them. Most newborns with poor mixing present with marked cyanosis (saturation <80%), like patients in the LPBF group.

Severe hypoxemia (oxygen partial pressure [P_{O_2}] <35 mm Hg for the average newborn) is not compatible with prolonged survival. Neonates experience tissue hypoxia, anaerobic glycolysis, and metabolic acidosis. Respiratory compensation may occur at first. Even with a normal pH, however, the presence of metabolic acidosis (large base deficit) indicates life-threatening hypoxia, necessitating immediate intervention, without which death ensues in a matter of hours.

Differential Diagnosis

The major causes of cyanosis are cardiac (Box 91-2) and respiratory (Box 91-3). Diagnoses in the latter group include problems of the lung, chest, airway, or respiratory drive.

The syndrome of **persistent fetal circulation** is perhaps most often confused with cyanotic CHD. It is also known as **persistent pulmonary hypertension of the newborn.** In this syndrome the heart and great vessels are structurally normal, but high pulmonary vascular resistance, which is often seen in post-term newborns with perinatal distress or pulmonary disease, causes blood to shunt away from the lungs at the foramen ovale and ductus arteriosus. Profound cyanosis that is unresponsive to supplemental oxygen, particularly in post-ductal sites such as the lower extremities, may be the only abnormal finding, and echocardiography is required to exclude CHD.

Pulmonary cyanosis may be due to **infection** (eg, group B streptococcal pneumonia); **aspiration** (eg, meconium, tracheoesophageal fistula); **pulmonary hypoplasia** (eg, oligohydramnios sequence, diaphragmatic hernia); **respiratory distress syndrome** (eg, prematurity); or a host of other problems of the lung, chest, or airway. Neurologic depression may produce hypoventilation with resultant hypoxia.

Box 91-2. Cyanotic Congenital Heart Defects

- Low pulmonary blood-flow lesions
  - Tetralogy of Fallot
  - Pulmonary atresia with intact ventricular septum
  - Complex lesions with severe pulmonary stenosis or atresia
  - Obstructed total anomalous pulmonary venous return
- High pulmonary blood-flow lesions with mixing
  - Truncus arteriosus communis
  - Tricuspid atresia
  - Transposition with ventricular septal defect
- Poor mixing
  - Transposition of the great arteries

Box 91-3. Noncardiac Causes of Neonatal Cyanosis

- Persistent fetal circulation
- Upper airway obstruction (eg, choanal atresia)
- Pulmonary infection (eg, group B streptococcal infection)
- Aspiration (eg, meconium aspiration syndrome, tracheoesophageal fistula)
- Pulmonary hypoplasia (eg, Potter syndrome , diaphragmatic hernia)
- Respiratory distress syndrome (eg, in prematurity)
- Thoracic hypoplasia (eg, thanatophoric dwarfism)
- Hypoventilation (eg, neurologic depression)

Evaluation

Evaluation of the cyanotic newborn must be expeditious so that management is not delayed. In some cases, therapy may be initiated before the evaluation is complete. All available data, including the statistical likelihood of CHD and the risk-benefit ratio of the treatment, must be taken into account.

History

Review of the history may be helpful, particularly in certain situations, such as in newborns with pulmonary disease (Questions Box). It is important to note that a negative response to any or all of the questions does not render cyanotic CHD unlikely; in fact, negative responses are noted in most cases.

Physical Examination

Cyanosis may be the only abnormal physical finding in cardiac patients, but a careful, thorough examination often yields information about the underlying cardiac defect and overall circulatory status. External anomalies or abnormal phenotypic appearance may indicate a genetic disorder with associated cardiac anomalies. Dyspnea (grunting, nasal flaring, intercostal retractions) is more often seen with lung disease, but tachypnea (rapid respiration) is common with severe heart disease and pulmonary problems. Tachypnea results from CHF in HPBF lesions and hyperpnea (deep breathing) from metabolic acidosis in severe hypoxia or impaired perfusion. Poor perfusion is also manifested by abnormal color (a gray or ashen appearance if combined with cyanosis), cool extremities, delayed capillary refill, and diminished pulses.

The peripheral pulses must be palpated in all extremities. Abnormalities or discrepancies between extremities should be confirmed by measuring blood pressures. Weak pulses may be found in cardiogenic shock, and bounding pulses may be noted with diastolic runoff lesions such as patent ductus arteriosus or aortic insufficiency. Pulse quality and blood pressure may differ between extremities if an aortic arch abnormality such as coarctation is present. The abdominal examination may reveal hepatomegaly (in CHF) or abnormal situs (as in Ivemark syndrome, usually associated with complex cyanotic CHD).

The cardiac examination may disclose a loud murmur if an obstruction such as pulmonary stenosis is present. The examiner should note, however, that atresia, being a total obstruction, produces no murmur. Heart sounds may be loud and the precordium hyperdynamic, particularly in newborns with HPBF. Splitting of the second sound confirms that 2 patent semilunar valves are present, but this finding is often difficult to appreciate even in normal newborns.

Laboratory Tests

A number of laboratory studies are available (see Chapter 92, Table 92-1). As in CHF, it is initially more important to determine whether patients have heart disease than to obtain a precise, complete diagnosis. In cyanotic CHD, sophisticated studies such as echocardiography, magnetic resonance imaging, and catheterization are usually needed to make a detailed diagnosis.

The suspicion of arterial hypoxemia should be confirmed by **pulse oximetry,** an indirect measurement. It is readily available and noninvasive but has shortcomings. Perfusion must be adequate to obtain a reading. Accuracy is diminished at saturations below 75%, although the presence of profound hypoxia can still be confirmed. Cyanotic CHD cannot be ruled out by pulse oximetry, however, because readings of 100% saturation may reflect Po_2 values that range anywhere between 75 and 250 mm Hg (Figure 91-1). **Arterial blood gases** are more accurate and give important additional information about ventilation and acid-base status. Arterialized capillary gases may suffice if perfusion is adequate.

Oxygenation may differ between the extremities in newborns with certain lesions (eg, coarctation). The site of sampling should be noted. If possible, the saturation should be measured at sites proximal and distal to the ductus arteriosus (ie, the right arm and either leg).

A **shunt study,** also known as a hyperoxia challenge, may be performed to determine whether a right-to-left cardiac shunt is present, particularly if echocardiography is not readily available. Pure

Figure 91-1. Comparison between oxygen partial pressure (Po₂) by arterial blood gas measurement and oxygen saturation by pulse oximetry. (Reproduced with permission from Niehoff J, DelGuercio C, LaMorte W, et al. Efficacy of pulse oximetry and capnometry in postoperative ventilatory weaning. *Crit Care Med.* 1988;16[7]:701–705.)

Cyanosis in the Newborn

Questions

- Has the neonate been in any distress?
- Has the neonate had difficulty feeding?
- Was the neonate suspected of having a heart problem prior to birth (eg, fetal arrhythmia, abnormal heart on ultrasound)?
- Is the mother diabetic?
- Did the mother take any drugs (prescribed or not) during the pregnancy?
- Was the mother ill during the first trimester?
- Is there a positive family history of congenital heart disease or other birth defects?
- Did any perinatal problems (eg, passage of meconium in utero) occur?

oxygen (fraction of inspired oxygen in gas [FIO₂] = 1.00) is given for 5 to 10 minutes by hood. In patients with LPBF or TGA, increasing the inspired oxygen does not affect the oxygenation of the blood because the blood is unable to enter the lungs; this is a positive result. In patients with pulmonary disease or hypoventilation, oxygenation increases strikingly, often to a Po₂ exceeding 200 mm Hg; this negative result rules out cyanotic CHD.

A blunted shunt study, characterized by a rise in Po₂ but rarely to levels above 150 mm Hg, is seen in patients with severe pulmonary disease and in those with HPBF lesions. With such lesions the pulmonary venous blood is high in volume, and the rise in its saturation causes a definite rise in arterial oxygenation. This effect is exaggerated by the further increase in pulmonary flow due to the vasodilating effect of oxygen.

A positive shunt study may be identified with pulse oximetry. It is difficult or impossible, however, to distinguish between a blunted study and a negative one with this tool. The oxyhemoglobin dissociation curve is flattened at the upper end, and the saturation changes very little over a wide range of Po₂ (Figure 91-2). Capillary gases may be equally inaccurate in this range, but directly measured arterial blood gases are highly reliable. In addition, they may reveal hypercapnia, with or without respiratory acidosis, suggesting a pulmonary cause for the hypoxia.

Electrocardiogram (ECG), a fairly inexpensive test, is readily available and noninvasive. However, it does not often help distinguish cyanotic CHD from other causes of cyanosis, particularly for those practitioners who lack experience with neonatal ECGs. The normal range is large in neonates, with much overlap between normal and CHD. Care must be taken in placing the leads correctly and minimizing artifacts; incorrect technique may lead to a false-positive result.

Imaging Studies

The **chest radiograph,** a relatively inexpensive and readily available test, is often extremely helpful in differentiating between cardiac and noncardiac disease. Pulmonary disease is often readily apparent on

Figure 91-2. Oxyhemoglobin dissociation curve. Note that the position of the curve itself may vary with temperature, pH, oxygen partial pressure (Po₂), and 2,3-diphosphoglycerate.

chest radiograph. This test also helps define the cardiac diagnosis broadly but not precisely. Patients with LPBF lesions have small hearts and diminished pulmonary blood flow. In contrast, patients with HPBF lesions have large hearts and increased flow, such as is seen in neonates with simple left-to-right shunts. With many cyanotic lesions, the cardiac silhouette is abnormal in configuration (eg, boot-shaped heart in tetralogy of Fallot) or position (eg, dextrocardia in patients with heterotaxy syndromes), but this finding may be obscured by the generous thymus in the newborn. Transposition of the great arteries may be more misleading; pulmonary flow may be increased despite the severe cyanosis, and the heart size may be normal. An apparently normal radiograph does not exclude TGA.

Under optimal conditions, **echocardiography** enables the physician not only to recognize CHD but to identify details of anatomy and physiology. Conversely, a properly performed, complete, negative echocardiogram rules out CHD. The performance of a high-quality study requires the appropriate equipment (with high-resolution imaging), an experienced sonographer, and an experienced cardiologist for interpretation. In the absence of these elements, preliminary echocardiography may be used cautiously as a screening device as part of the initial assessment to confirm the presence of heart disease prior to referral to a specialist. Recently, availability of telemedicine for echocardiography has helped to fill this gap in some hospitals and avoid some unnecessary transports. When there is significant suspicion of cyanotic CHD, referral should not be delayed until echocardiography can be performed.

Management

Initial management prior to cardiac consultation (often with transfer to another institution) includes surveillance, assistance, direct medical management, and supportive care.

Close **surveillance,** including transfer to the highest level of neonatal care available, use of a cardiopulmonary monitor and continuous pulse oximetry, frequent monitoring of vital signs, and repeat physical examinations, is begun as soon as cyanotic CHD is identified. Even if the newborn is feeding well, it is best to suspend feedings because of the likelihood of invasive procedures or spontaneous deterioration in the near future. An orogastric tube is placed to decompress the stomach, reducing the work of breathing as well as the risk of aspiration. At least one secure intravenous (IV) line should be placed for administration of fluids, glucose, and medications. If umbilical arterial catheterization can be expeditiously established, it will allow close monitoring of arterial blood gases and blood pressure. The latter may be difficult to measure by cuff in the compromised newborn.

While undertaking these measures, the physician should make every effort to seek **assistance** from a pediatric cardiologist. A neonatologist may be consulted if a pediatric cardiologist is not immediately available. Much advice may be obtained over the telephone. In addition, plans for immediate consultation or transfer of patients may be discussed in this way.

The need for **supportive care** depends on the case. In the absence of metabolic acidosis or impaired perfusion, no special measures are indicated in this category. In some cases, IV fluid boluses, inotropic agents, and other treatments may be needed as part of early management. Mechanical ventilation should be used in patients with metabolic acidosis, whether compensated or uncompensated, because of the increased oxygen requirement produced by hyperventilation and the tendency for tiring, leading to superimposed respiratory acidosis.

The temptation to give supplemental oxygen for more than the few minutes necessary to perform a shunt study is great but must be resisted. Oxygen is rarely helpful and may be harmful in this setting. In neonates with TGA or LPBF lesions, oxygenation is not affected. In newborns with HPBF lesions, oxygenation is usually adequate in room air (saturation >80%), and an increase in F_{IO_2} may exacerbate CHF. Patients at greatest risk for deterioration due to administration of oxygen are those with total anomalous pulmonary venous return with obstruction, in whom pulmonary arteriolar vasodilation precipitates severe pulmonary edema and secondary right heart failure. Oxygen may also directly constrict the ductus arteriosus on which the cyanotic newborn may depend.

The possibility of ductal dependency should prompt consideration of administering the ductus dilator, **prostaglandin E₁ (PGE₁).** The definitive diagnosis of cyanotic CHD need not be made prior to institution of this lifesaving treatment. In newborns who remain adequately oxygenated (no acidosis) and perfused, the drug can be prepared but administration deferred pending consultation. The benefits of giving PGE_1 to severely hypoxic neonates or neonates with compromised perfusion far outweigh the risks, which include apnea and fever. A dramatic improvement is often seen within seconds to minutes, supporting the diagnosis of a ductal-dependent lesion, and enabling the physician to stabilize the patient until more definitive evaluation and intervention can take place.

Prognosis

If untreated, LPBF lesions and TGA are usually fatal during infancy, most often during the neonatal period, because of severe hypoxia. Untreated HPBF lesions may lead to death in infancy from CHF or complications such as pneumonia. If the systemic blood flow is ductus dependent (eg, interruption of the aortic arch), death occurs shortly after ductal closure, usually during the first week of life. Delayed diagnosis, even when not fatal, may result in a suboptimal outcome, including end-organ injury such as renal dysfunction or neurologic sequelae.

With early recognition and intervention, however, the prognosis for newborns with cyanotic CHD is surprisingly good in the absence of a genetic syndrome (eg, trisomy 18) or a major complicating extracardiac malformation (eg, neural tube defect). If diagnosed before the onset of severe circulatory compromise, neonates can be stabilized and evaluated promptly, and palliative or corrective procedures can be performed in the operating suite or catheterization laboratory. Most of these patients can survive well into adulthood with a good quality of life. Newborns with lesions in which all 4 chambers are adequate in size (eg, tetralogy of Fallot) have a better lifetime prognosis than those with a hypoplastic chamber (eg, tricuspid atresia). Even neonates with abnormalities such as Ivemark syndrome (asplenia syndrome) or hypoplastic left heart syndrome now have a reasonable outlook with complex staged reconstructive surgery or heart transplantation.

CASE RESOLUTION

In the case presented at the beginning of the chapter, marked hypoxia is present in the absence of other cardiac findings, such as a heart murmur. The oxygen saturation does not rise after the newborn breathes 100% oxygen for 10 minutes. The chest radiograph shows a small, boot-shaped heart and diminished pulmonary blood flow, and the electrocardiogram is normal. Transport is arranged. Because of the marked cyanosis, infusion of prostaglandin E₁ is begun, and saturation increases to 80%, with the oxygen partial pressure rising from 33 to a safer 48 mm Hg. The neonate is transferred to a tertiary care center, where consultation is obtained. An echocardiogram is also performed, which demonstrates tetralogy of Fallot with pulmonary atresia. A modified Blalock-Taussig shunt is placed in the newborn period, and complete repair using a pulmonary artery homograft is performed at 1 year of age.

Selected References

Brown KL, Ridout DA, Hoskote A, Verhulst L, Ricci M, Bull C. Delayed diagnosis of congenital heart disease worsens preoperative condition and outcome of surgery in neonates. *Heart.* 2006;92(9):1298–1302

de-Wahl Granelli A, Wennergren M, Sandberg K, et al. Impact of pulse oximetry screening on the detection of duct dependent congenital heart disease: a Swedish prospective screening study in 39,821 newborns. *BMJ.* 2009;338:a3037

Freed MD, Heymann MA, Lewis AB, Roehl SL, Kensey RC. Prostaglandin E1 infants with ductus arteriosus-dependent congenital heart disease. *Circulation.* 1981;64(5):899–905

Jones RW, Baumer JH, Joseph MC, Shinebourne EA. Arterial oxygen tension and response to oxygen breathing in differential diagnosis of congenital heart disease in infancy. *Arch Dis Child.* 1976;51(9):667–673

Niehoff J, DelGuercio C, LaMorte W, et al. Efficacy of pulse oximetry and capnometry in postoperative ventilatory weaning. *Crit Care Med.* 1988;16(7):701–705

Oster ME, Lee KA, Honein MA, Riehle-Colarusso T, Shin M, Correa A. Temporal trends in survival among infants with critical congenital heart defects. *Pediatrics.* 2013;131(5):e1502–e1508

Pfammatter JP, Stocker FP. Delayed recognition of haemodynamically relevant congenital heart disease. *Eur J Pediatr.* 2001;160(4):231–234

Sable CA, Cummings SD, Pearson GD, et al. Impact of telemedicine on the practice of pediatric cardiology in community hospitals. *Pediatrics.* 2002;109(1):e3

Sasidharan P. An approach to diagnosis and management of cyanosis and tachypnea in term infants. *Pediatr Clin North Am.* 2004;51(4):999–1021

Thangaratinam S, Brown K, Zamora J, Khan KS, Ewer AK. Pulse oximetry screening for critical congenital heart defects in asymptomatic newborn babies: a systematic review and meta-analysis. *Lancet.* 2012;379(9835):2459–2464

Victorica BE. Cyanotic newborns. In: Gessner IH, Victorica BE, eds. *Pediatric Cardiology: A Problem Oriented Approach.* Philadelphia, PA: W. B. Saunders; 1993

CHAPTER 92

Congestive Heart Failure

Robin Winkler Doroshow, MD, MMS, MEd

CASE STUDY

A 2-month-old boy is brought to the office by his mother, who complains that her son has been eating poorly and breathing oddly for the past few days. The perinatal history is unremarkable. A heart murmur was noted at the 1-month checkup.

The infant is scrawny and irritable. Physical examination shows that the baby's weight, which was at the 50th percentile at birth, is now at the fifth percentile; his height, which was at the 50th percentile, is now at the 25th percentile. He is afebrile, and his heart rate is 165 beats/min, with respirations 70 breaths/min and shallow but without respiratory distress. The skin is pale and diaphoretic, and the mucous membranes are pink. Examination of the head and neck is normal; no jugular distention is present. The lungs are clear. The precordium is hyperdynamic, and the heart sounds are loud; a prominent systolic murmur is audible at the left lower sternal border.

The liver edge is palpable 4 cm below the right costal margin in the right midclavicular line, and the spleen is not palpable. The extremities are thin, with normal pulses and no edema. Capillary refill is slightly delayed.

Questions

1. What are acute and chronic signs of cardiac disease in children?
2. What are the signs of congestive heart failure (CHF) in children? How do these signs in children differ from those in adults?
3. What underlying disorders can cause CHF in young infants?
4. What is the appropriate emergent management for infants with CHF? What are the risks of treatment if the diagnosis is incorrect?

Congestive heart failure (CHF) is the most common presentation of serious heart disease in infants. Although this condition also occurs in older children, an estimated 90% of cases of CHF in the pediatric population begin in the first year of life. In children CHF is most often caused by structural congenital heart disease (CHD). Compensatory mechanisms are fewer and less successful in small infants. Other causes of CHF are included in Box 92-1.

Epidemiology

The precise incidence of CHF in children is unknown; it is approximately 0.1%. Most cases result from CHD, which occurs in 0.8% of live births. The incidence of CHD varies little with geography, ethnic group, or gender, but it is far more common in children with recognizable genetic syndromes (eg, Down syndrome, Turner syndrome).

Clinical Presentation

Most commonly, complaints about CHF take the form of concerns about an infant's feeding. Comments are often vague (eg, "My baby is not a good eater") but may be more precise (eg, "He is taking less formula with each feeding"; "He is taking longer to nurse"). Parents may also describe rapid breathing, excessive sweating, or decreased activity, but usually only on specific questioning.

Box 92-1. Causes of Congestive Heart Failure in Children

Volume Overload
- Left-to-right shunts (eg, ventricular septal defect)
- Bidirectional shunts (eg, truncus arteriosus)
- Valvular insufficiency (eg, mitral regurgitation)
- Extracardiac conditions (eg, anemia, arteriovenous malformation)

Pressure Overload
- Outflow obstruction (eg, coarctation of the aorta)
- Inflow obstruction (eg, obstructed anomalous pulmonary veins)
- Vascular resistance (eg, hypertension, chronic pulmonary disease)

Myocardial Dysfunction
- Intrinsic conditions (eg, cardiomyopathy, anthracycline toxicity)
- Inflammatory conditions (eg, viral myocarditis, rheumatic fever)
- Coronary insufficiency (eg, anomalous left coronary artery)

Arrhythmias
- Tachyarrhythmia (eg, paroxysmal supraventricular tachycardia)
- Bradyarrhythmia (eg, third-degree atrioventricular block)

Congestive heart failure may also be detected on examination during routine infant checkups or for unrelated complaints. Careful assessment of the physical findings, including vital signs, reveals **tachypnea, tachycardia,** and **hepatomegaly** and frequently signs of underlying structural heart defects, such as a murmur (D_x Box).

Congestive Heart Failure

- Tachycardia
- Tachypnea
- Hepatomegaly
- Sweating
- Decreased feeding
- Irritability
- Easy fatigability

Pathophysiology

High cardiac output may lead to CHF in infants with large left-to-right shunts. Myocardial contractility is relatively normal, and children remain on the "normal" line of the Starling curve, which relates cardiac output to diastolic volume (also called *preload*) or pressure (Figure 92-1). The shunt requires a very large volume of output, primarily to the pulmonary bed. Although the heart may be able to meet this demand, preload is high, leading to "congestive" signs and symptoms (eg, tachypnea, hepatomegaly). In more severe cases, systemic output may be compromised, resulting in hypotension, renal failure, and metabolic acidosis.

Left-sided failure caused by elevated pulmonary venous pressure produces increased lung water. Initially, this fluid is interstitial,

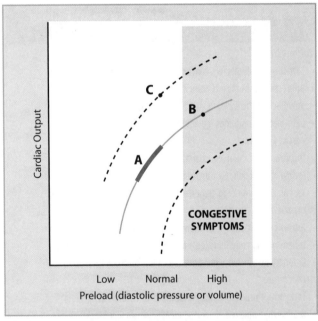

Figure 92-1. Relationship of cardiac output to preload. The solid curve represents normal myocardial contractility, and the dotted curves represent impaired function (shifted downward) and the positive inotropic state (shifted upward). A, Normal range (no heart disease). B, Left-to-right shunt with congestive heart failure (CHF). Note that overall output is high, but most of it is shunted. C, Same situation as B but after treatment for CHF. Cardiac output is the same or better, but preload is now out of the range that results in congestive symptoms.

and it does not interfere with gas exchange but does trigger reflex tachypnea. Minute volume is kept normal by decreasing tidal (breath-to-breath) volume, leading to shallow as well as rapid breathing (sometimes called "happy tachypnea" because of the absence of dyspnea). Only when the ability of the pulmonary lymphatics to drain this fluid is overcome by large volume does fluid accumulate in the alveoli; rales and respiratory distress, or dyspnea, result and gas exchange may be compromised.

Right-sided failure caused by an elevated systemic venous load usually produces more volume than pressure load on this system, possibly as a result of the greater venous compliance in infants compared with adults. The liver becomes very distended and is easily palpated. As long as the liver can absorb the increased venous volume, the portal pressure does not rise, and splenomegaly does not occur. Because the venous pressure rises very little, jugular distention, which is difficult to detect in young infants in any case, is rarely seen, and edema is also rare.

The left and right (systemic and pulmonary) circulations are more interdependent in infants and younger children than they are in older children or adults. As a result, **bilateral heart failure** is much more common than right-sided or left-sided failure alone. Although this means that recognition of CHF may be easier, determination of the underlying condition may be more difficult because the clues are less specific. For example, in an adult with left-sided failure, the differential diagnosis includes mitral, but not tricuspid, valve disease.

Differential Diagnosis

When tachycardia, tachypnea without dyspnea, and hepatomegaly are present, the diagnosis of CHF is straightforward. Congestive heart failure is most commonly confused with major respiratory infections such as bronchiolitis or pneumonia. Pulmonary infections are frequently associated with dyspnea as well as tachypnea, impaired gas exchange, and other respiratory findings. Rhinorrhea, cough, fever, or wheezing may also be present. Rales may accompany pneumonia but are rare in CHF in infancy or early childhood. Hyperinflation due to lung disease may lead to a false impression of hepatomegaly. In some children, CHD, CHF, and respiratory infections coexist and compound one another to increase morbidity and mortality, as is seen with respiratory syncytial virus.

Clues to the presence of structural heart disease, such as a murmur or absent femoral pulses, may support the diagnosis of CHF. Severe CHF, with low cardiac output or even shock, has a broader differential diagnosis. In addition to cardiac causes, sepsis, hypovolemia, and disorders associated with inborn errors of metabolism should be considered.

Evaluation

History

The history should include specific questions about feeding and growth (Questions Box). Poor feeding, often a nonspecific complaint in infants who are chronically or subacutely ill, results from tachypnea and

Congestive Heart Failure

Questions

- How has the infant been feeding? Does he or she get out of breath or appear exhausted?
- Has the infant's growth pattern changed recently?
- Does the infant tire easily? With eating? With playing?
- Does the infant perspire excessively, especially with efforts such as feeding?
- Does the infant breathe rapidly, even at rest?

Table 92-1. Laboratory Tests Used in the Evaluation of Heart Disease in Children	
Test	**Information**
Chest radiograph	Presence and direction of shunt. Hints concerning specific diagnosis (and possible pulmonary disease ruled out)
Serum BNP and NT-proBNP	Presence and severity of congestive heart failure
ECG	Cardiac rhythm and conduction. Chamber overload. Coronary insufficiency
Ambulatory ECG (24-hour ECG)	Subacute rhythm assessment. Correlation of symptoms with rhythm
Oximetry	Presence and degree of hypoxemia
Arterial blood gases	Hypoxemia. Acid-base status
Hematocrit	Anemia. Polycythemia
Exercise test	Quantitation of exercise tolerance. Provocation of symptoms or arrhythmia
Echocardiogram	Specific structural diagnosis and hemodynamics. Chamber enlargement and function. Presence of pericardial effusion
Cardiac magnetic resonance imaging or computed tomography	Specific structural diagnosis and hemodynamics. Chamber enlargement and function
Cardiac catheterization	Specific structural diagnosis and hemodynamics. Cardiac electrophysiology
Tilt test	Autonomic function

Abbreviations: BNP, brain natriuretic peptide; ECG, electrocardiogram.

fatigability in infants with heart disease. Growth failure may result from poor feeding and increased cardiopulmonary work. The physician should specifically query parents about possible excessive sweating or rapid breathing in infants because parents may not volunteer this information (see Chapter 63).

Physical Examination

The diagnosis of CHF is primarily based on clinical findings, and physical examination is essential. The resting respiratory rate must be precisely counted because infants in CHF most often have tachypnea without dyspnea. The liver edge is palpable more than 1 cm below the right costal margin in the midclavicular line, and the degree of enlargement mirrors the severity of the CHF.

The physical examination may also give clues as to the underlying cause of CHF, such as a heart murmur or gallop, or pulses weaker in the lower extremities than the upper extremities.

In the older child or adolescent, physical findings are more similar to those of the adult with CHF. Additional findings that may be present in this age group include jugular venous distension, basilar rales, and peripheral pitting edema.

In severe CHF, where cardiac output is declining, flow to end organs is compromised. The skin will be cool and pale or ashen, and capillary refill will be delayed; the peripheral pulses will be diminished. Mental status may be affected, resulting in lethargy or even unresponsiveness.

Laboratory Tests

Many laboratory tests can be performed to assess infants' hearts (Table 92-1), including electrocardiogram (ECG) and echocardiogram. However, some procedures are very costly, and some are invasive and therefore carry risk. The value of most of these tests depends on the expertise of the individuals who perform and interpret them. It is important to remember that although test results and consultation with a pediatric cardiologist may be invaluable in the identification of the underlying lesion, *these procedures are not usually required to make a diagnosis of CHF.*

Pressure or volume overload of the ventricles causes them to release a neurohumoral peptide, brain natriuretic peptide (BNP), which acts as a natural natriuretic, diuretic, and vasodilator. Studies in adults have demonstrated that blood levels of **BNP** and its precursor, N-terminal proBNP (**NT-proBNP**) are elevated in CHF, and

the degree of elevation closely reflects severity of CHF. This test, which may be performed at the bedside on very small samples of blood, may be used to distinguish between CHF and other similar disorders such as acute pulmonary disease. Because it closely parallels changes in severity of CHF, it may also be used to track response to treatment. Recent studies in children suggest that it may be similarly useful in the pediatric population; BNP levels may be very effective in distinguishing between cardiac and noncardiac causes of CHF in children (Figure 92-2).

Imaging Studies

Because elucidation of the structure and function of the heart is central to assessment of the underlying cause of CHF in the pediatric population, imaging studies play a key role (see Table 92-1) in evaluation of these patients. Moreover, these tests (particularly **echocardiography**) may be used as a means of tracking response to

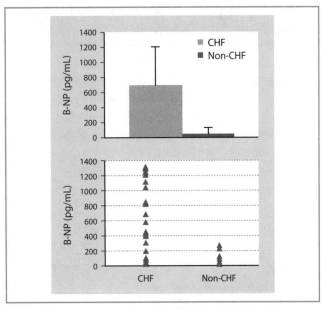

Figure 92-2. Utility of brain natriuretic peptide (BNP) in differentiating congestive heart failure (CHF) from lung disease in pediatric patients with respiratory distress. (From Koulouri S, Acherman RJ, Wong PC, Chan LS, Lewis AB. Utility of B-type natriuretic peptide in differentiating congestive heart failure from lung disease in pediatric patients with respiratory distress. *Pediatr Cardiol.* 2004;25[4]:341–346, with permission from Springer Science + Business Media.)

Table 92-2. Therapy for Pediatric Congestive Heart Failure

Category	Example
Chronic (Ambulatory)	
Cardiac glycosides	Digoxin
Diuretics	Furosemide, spironolactone
Angiotensin-converting enzyme inhibitors	Enalapril, captopril
Angiotensin receptor blockers	Losartan
Selective β-blockers	Carvedilol, metoprolol
Acute (Inpatient)	
Diuretics	Furosemide, bumetanide
β-agonists	Dobutamine, dopamine
Phosphodiesterase inhibitors	Milrinone, inamrinone
Vasodilators	Nitroprusside, oxygen, inhaled nitric oxide
Severe, Refractory	
Mechanical support	Extracorporeal membrane oxygenation, ventricular assist
Cardiac or cardiopulmonary transplantation	
Exogenous brain natriuretic peptide	Nesiritide

treatment. The **ECG** may provide clues as to underlying pathology but does not aid in the diagnosis of CHF per se.

Chest radiograph, preferably in anteroposterior and lateral projections, may be very useful as a *supportive* study. It may show cardiomegaly, pulmonary venous congestion, and hyperinflation. Cardiomegaly is most commonly due not to myocardial dysfunction but to volume overload from the shunt. In the absence of cardiac enlargement, the diagnosis of CHF must be seriously questioned. (However, CHF may occur in the absence of cardiomegaly in total anomalous pulmonary venous return with obstruction, which usually presents in the first week of life in association with hypoxia.) Pulmonary venous congestion occurs in left-sided heart failure, but increased pulmonary arterial flow from a left-to-right shunt often obscures the congestion. Hyperinflation resulting from peribronchial edema is also a common finding.

In children with severe CHF, further studies are indicated. **Arterial blood gases** show evidence of metabolic acidosis due to tissue anoxia, with respiratory compensation in early stages and superimposed respiratory acidosis in later stages. A **complete blood cell count** shows leukocytosis due to stress. It may not differentiate between heart disease and sepsis.

Management

All infants and children with CHF should be under the care of a pediatric cardiologist, often in concert with a pediatrician, intensivist, or neonatologist. Prompt referral to a cardiologist will aid not only in management of the CHF but also in assessment and management of the underlying disorder.

The numerous pharmacologic treatments for pediatric CHF fall into a small number of categories based on mechanism of action (Table 92-2). Preload can be optimized by the administration of diuretics and vasodilators and afterload by the use of arteriolar dilators, some of which also have inotropic effects. Contractility is enhanced by inotropic agents, and antiarrhythmics control tachycardia and bradycardia to optimize heart rate. The most effective control of CHF is attained when more than one mechanism is used.

Inotropes and **diuretics** are used in the initial management of CHF in children. Inotropic support results in a shift to a higher Starling curve (see Figure 92-1), which allows affected patients to maintain the high volume output necessitated by the underlying CHD at lower diastolic pressures, thus alleviating congestive symptoms. **Digoxin,** a form of digitalis, is the drug of choice in such cases in which cardiac output is not severely impaired and is therefore often used in outpatients. This agent is readily available, easily absorbed, safe in the therapeutic range, and easy to administer (elixir for oral administration). If digoxin is initially given at the maintenance dose (10 μg/kg/d), therapeutic levels are not attained for about a week; therefore, loading is preferable (Table 92-3) but may require hospitalization. Digoxin is well tolerated and rarely causes side effects. Because of the safety and reliability of absorption, blood levels need not be checked unless overdose is suspected (eg, history of overadministration, toxic ingestion, unexplained vomiting, second- or third-degree heart block). In the neonate, blood levels may be

Table 92-3. Digoxin: Total Oral Loading Dose in Children[a]	
Age	*Dose (μg/kg)*
Preterm newborns	20–30
Term newborns and infants	25–35
1–5 y	30–40
5–10 y[b]	20–30
10 y to adult[b]	10–15

[a]Intravenous loading dose = 75%–89% of oral dose. Usually given ½, followed 8 hours later by ¼, followed 8 hours later by ¼, followed 12 hours later by initiation of maintenance dose. Assumes normal renal function; the maintenance dose must be adjusted downward for renal failure.

[b]In children older than 5 years, loading dose is more often based on surface area (0.5–1.0 mg/m²).

difficult to interpret because of the presence of natural digoxin-like immunoreactive substance in the blood.

The elevated diastolic preload of CHF is the result of neurohumorally mediated sodium and water retention. **Diuretics** reverse this phenomenon. **Furosemide,** a potent loop diuretic that is available in an oral suspension and is fairly well absorbed, is the most frequent drug of choice for the outpatient. The starting dose is 1 mg/kg once or twice daily. Initially, furosemide may be given intravenously or intramuscularly rather than orally, which reduces the time to onset of action and is more effective. Such treatment also supports the patient while digoxin loading is in progress. **Spironolactone,** a less potent diuretic, may be used in combination with furosemide for its potassium-sparing effects and may also reduce the deleterious histopathologic and structural changes known as *myocardial remodeling* that can accompany CHF.

Fluid and sodium restriction, often used in adults with CHF, is difficult to achieve with infants because their diet is predominantly or exclusively liquid. High-calorie diets using concentrated formulas, complex carbohydrate additives, or medium-chain triglyceride oils may reduce the intake of free water and the effort of feeding without compromising caloric intake. Human milk and most proprietary formulas have a low sodium load. In older infants and children with CHF, salt intake is more easily modified and should be minimized.

Certain pediatric patients with chronic CHF may benefit from the addition of **angiotensin-converting enzyme inhibitors** or **angiotensin receptor blockers** (ARBs) to their regimen. These arteriolar dilators help control afterload and have been shown to be effective in children with dilated cardiomyopathy and those with large left-to-right shunts, such as ventricular septal defects (VSDs). Recent observations suggest that third-generation **β-blockers** such as carvedilol may be useful to control chronic CHF in children with dilated cardiomyopathy. Randomized, controlled clinical trials in adults with similar pathology have been very encouraging, despite poor understanding of the mechanism involved; similar trials in children have thus far been disappointing.

Children with acute, severe, or refractory cases of CHF may require additional medications or interventions, necessitating hospitalization, often in an intensive care unit. These therapies include

β-agonists and **phosphodiesterase inhibitors** for inotropic support and **vasodilators** for afterload reduction, **correction of anemia** (eg, transfusion), **treatment of fever** (eg, antipyretics), and **reduction of metabolic demands** (eg, ventilatory support, bed rest, sedation). **Diuretics,** usually given intravenously, provide effective control of congestive symptoms. Because of the importance of fluid balance and nutrition in the child hospitalized with CHF, close and accurate monitoring of fluid intake and output, measurement of daily weight, and measurements of serum electrolytes are essential data in the management of CHF. Feeding is often problematic because of its increased workload, conflict with the increased work of breathing, and diminished circulation to the gut. In some cases, tube feedings may be an option; in others, all enteric feedings must be discontinued and hydration and nutrition maintained intravenously.

In a minority of cases, CHF is refractory to all of these measures. This may be seen in very severe acute myocarditis, long-standing cardiomyopathy of various causes, and during the postoperative period after complex CHD surgery. Additional options include **resynchronization therapy** in which an artificial pacemaker alters the sequence of ventricular depolarization and contraction, and **mechanical support** such as extracorporeal membrane oxygenation and ventricular assist devices. **Exogenous recombinant BNP** (nesiritide), which has shown some promise in the setting of adult CHF, may be helpful. In some cases, replacement of the ailing heart or heart-lung unit by **transplantation** may be the only remaining alternative.

Ultimately, the best management for CHF is **treatment of the underlying disorder.** In many cases, failure to treat the underlying disorder will result in limited or no success of other treatment modalities. The degree of urgency depends on the nature of the disorder and the severity of the CHF. For example, in neonates with ductus-dependent lesions such as hypoplastic left heart syndrome, maintenance of ductal patency with prostaglandin E₁ is crucial to initial management. In infants with CHF caused by supraventricular tachycardia, prompt conversion to normal sinus rhythm is often the only treatment necessary. Congestive heart failure caused by severe anemia responds dramatically to correction of hemoglobin levels, often using exchange transfusion to avoid additional acute volume overload. Cor pulmonale, often seen in children with severe chronic lung disease, is most responsive to measures directed at improving the lung disease or decreasing pulmonary vascular resistance, such as supplemental oxygen or inhaled nitric oxide. When CHF is caused by structural CHD (the most common situation), surgery or interventional catheterization to palliate the problem (eg, pulmonary artery banding in certain cases with large net left-to-right shunts) or correct the defect (eg, repair of VSD) usually reverses the CHF. Fortunately, it is rarely necessary to "tolerate" prolonged, uncontrolled CHF in children or to treat the condition aggressively at the expense of a major change in lifestyle.

Family counseling, which should begin when CHF is identified, is essential. Several important points should be included, in addition to a general description of the cardiac defect and CHF. The term *heart failure,* which is commonly thought by nonmedical professionals to refer to a sudden deterioration of heart function or even cardiac arrest, must be clarified. It is also important to stress that affected infants should be treated as normally as possible, with the exception of administration of medicines and keeping medical appointments. Contrary to popular belief, most infants with cardiac conditions are not fragile. Addressing quality-of-life issues such as parental concern, assuaging guilt, and normalizing existence are key responsibilities of the medical professional.

Prognosis

In most young infants and children with CHF, the prognosis is excellent. Congestive heart failure responds well to treatment, and the underlying defect can usually be corrected or at least palliated. Without cardiac surgery for CHD, CHF often remits spontaneously over months or years as a result of maturation of compensatory mechanisms, spontaneous improvement in the defect (eg, decrease in the size of a VSD), or increase in pulmonary vascular resistance because of long-standing high pulmonary artery pressure and flow (Eisenmenger syndrome). "Catch-up" growth occurs with remission of CHF, and children have the potential to reach their genetically determined height and weight.

CASE RESOLUTION

The case presented at the beginning of the chapter is typical of an otherwise normal infant with a large ventricular septal defect (VSD) who becomes symptomatic with the development of congestive heart failure (CHF). The baby's growth failure can be attributed to the chronicity of his illness.

The loud murmur and presentation in infancy strongly suggest the existence of underlying structural congenital heart disease as the cause of CHF. The time of onset of CHF also suggests a specific mechanism. When the onset is slightly delayed after birth, a lesion with changing postnatal hemodynamics, such as left-to-right shunt, which has increased as pulmonary resistance has fallen, is suggested. (Note that a ductus-dependent defect would have presented more acutely and severely in the first week of life.)

This infant responded fairly well to oral diuretics and digoxin but continued to grow slowly and tire easily, and the VSD showed no signs of spontaneous decrease in size. He underwent surgical repair of the VSD at 5 months of age with an excellent result and no longer has symptoms or requires medication. His growth parameters are now within normal limits, and his prognosis is excellent.

Selected References

Bruns LA, Chrisant MK, Lamour JM, et al. Carvedilol as therapy in pediatric heart failure: an initial multicenter experience. *J Pediatr.* 2001;138(4):505–511

Costello JM, Goodman DM, Green TP. A review of the natriuretic hormone system's diagnostic and therapeutic potential in critically ill children. *Pediatr Crit Care Med.* 2006;7(4):308–318

Hsu DT, Pearson GD. Heart failure in children: part I: history, etiology, and pathology. *Circ Heart Fail.* 2009;2(1):63–70

Hsu DT, Pearson GD. Heart failure in children: part II: diagnosis, treatment and future directions. *Circ Heart Fail.* 2009;2(5):490–498

Koulouri S, Acherman RJ, Wong PC, Chan LS, Lewis AB. Utility of B-type natriuretic peptide in differentiating congestive heart failure from lung disease in pediatric patients with respiratory distress. *Pediatr Cardiol.* 2004;25(4):341–346

Mahle WT, Cuadrado AR, Kirshbom PM, Kanter KR, Simsic JM. Nesiritide in infants and children with congestive heart failure. *Pediatr Crit Care Med.* 2005;6(5):543–546

Maisel AS, Krishnaswamy P, Nowak RM, et al. Rapid measurement of B-type natriuretic peptide in the emergency diagnosis of heart failure. *N Engl J Med.* 2002;347(3):161–167

Medoff-Cooper B, Naim M, Torowicz D, Mott A. Feeding, growth, and nutrition in children with congenitally malformed hearts. *Cardiol Young.* 2010;20(Suppl 3):149–153

O'Connor MJ, Rosenthal DN, Shaddy RE. Outpatient management of pediatric heart failure. *Heart Fail Clin.* 2010;6(4):515–529

Price JF, Thomas AK, Grenier M, et al. B-type natriuretic peptide predicts adverse cardiovascular events in pediatric outpatients with chronic left ventricular systolic dysfunction. *Circulation.* 2006;114(10):1063–1069

Rosenthal D, Chrisant MR, Edens E, et al. International Society for Heart and Lung Transplantation: practice guidelines for management of heart failure in children. *J Heart Lung Transplant.* 2004;23(12):1313–1333

Simpson KE, Canter CE. Can adult heart failure regimens be applied to children: what works and what does not? *Curr Opin Cardiol.* 2012;27(2):98–107

CHAPTER 93

Chest Pain

Robin Winkler Doroshow, MD, MMS, MEd

CASE STUDY

A previously healthy 13-year-old boy comes to the office complaining of recurrent chest pain occurring approximately once a week over the past 2 months. The pain is stabbing in nature, located at the mid-sternum, and not associated with any other symptoms, and occurs randomly, at rest and with exercise. It lasts for 2 to 3 minutes, is ranked as 4 on a severity scale of 10, and subsides spontaneously. The patient does not appear very concerned about the pain, but his mother is quite anxious to have it checked out. His teacher has sent him home from school twice because of the pain, and the soccer coach will not let him play until he is cleared by a doctor. His physical examination is unremarkable.

Questions

1. What is the significance of chest pain in an otherwise healthy child?
2. How likely is serious heart disease to be heralded by chest pain?
3. How much testing, and what type, is appropriate in working up chest pain?
4. Which patients with chest pain should be referred to a cardiologist? To other specialists?

Chest pain in children is one of the most common reasons for referral to a pediatric cardiologist, second only to heart murmurs. It is, however, one of the least common presenting complaints of cardiac disease. In fact, from an etiologic standpoint, it would be more suitable for this chapter to be located in the section on gastrointestinal disorders, respiratory problems, psychological and psychogenic disorders, or hematology, rather than cardiology.

Why, then, approach it in the cardiology section, along with discussions of heart murmurs, cyanosis, and congestive heart failure? Perhaps the strongest reason is that it is the greatest fear of the patient, parent, and physician that chest pain could herald a serious—even lethal—heart problem in an otherwise healthy youngster. This fear is exacerbated by 2 social phenomena in our culture: the widespread press given to cases of sudden unexpected death in young, apparently healthy athletes (who had not, in fact, experienced chest pain in most cases), and the appropriately high level of concern over the underdiagnosis of ischemic heart disease in the adult population. Public information targeting the adult with chest pain may, unfortunately, be misinterpreted as applying also to the child. It is this apprehension, and the associated medicolegal defensive posture, that can so often drive the patient and his referring primary care physician to seek cardiology consultation and testing.

Epidemiology

The epidemiology of pediatric chest pain is not well studied. Published series have looked retrospectively at patients seen in an emergency department (ED), with a rate of about 0.25%; in an outpatient clinic at about 0.3%; or, as mentioned previously, at a high rate in a pediatric cardiology clinic. In the primary care office setting, chest pain is the third most frequent pain complaint, after abdominal pain and headache, leading to more than 600,000 office visits per year in the United States. The most common age range is 8 to 18 years, peaking between 11 and 13 years of age. There is no gender or racial predilection, although the etiologic distribution may vary by gender.

Cardiac causes of chest pain are very uncommon for 2 reasons. Such pain is either a rare symptom in a common cardiac disorder (eg, aortic stenosis) or caused by a rare condition (eg, anomalous origin of coronary artery [AOCA]).

Clinical Presentation

There is substantial variability in the complaint of chest pain in children (Questions Box). Some youngsters experience a single, protracted, severe episode that brings them to the ED. In that setting, the patient may have other signs or symptoms of an acute medical problem, such as fever, shortness of breath, or hypotension, raising the level of suspicion for a serious organic cause.

More frequently, children report repeated episodes occurring sporadically over a period of months or even years. The pain may be induced or exacerbated by exercise, deep breathing, lying down, or eating. It can begin and end abruptly or gradually. It may be accompanied by other symptoms, which can give major clues to the diagnosis. In cases in which the pain occurs on exercise, is this a consistent, predictable experience, or is it unpredictable?

Most (up to 97%) children seen for chest pain have no serious medical history, and most have an unremarkable physical examination.

Chest Pain

Questions

- What is the pain like? Where is it located? Does it radiate? How severe is it?
- How long has the child been having pain? Did it begin after trauma? How often does the pain occur? How long does it last? Does it start and end suddenly?
- What brings the pain on? Is it related to exercise and, if so, is it consistent?
- Does the child have associated symptoms with the pain, such as syncope, shortness of breath, palpitations, fever, nausea, sour taste, wheezing, or cough?
- Does the child at other times have cardiac symptoms, such as easy fatigability, cyanosis, exertional dyspnea, edema, or syncope?
- Does the child's medical history include potentially pertinent disorders such as asthma, gastroesophageal reflux disease, psychiatric problems, heart disease, or sickle cell disease?
- How much impact is the pain having on the child's life? Is he or she missing school or sports?
- Is there a family history of sudden unexpected death, recurrent syncope, or known genetic syndrome?

Pathophysiology

The pathophysiology varies with the underlying cause of the pain, for which there is a broad differential diagnosis (Box 93-1). It is important for the patient, parent, and physician to understand that thoracic or abdominal pain, and particularly visceral pain, is poorly localized. This makes it difficult to distinguish between, for example, esophagitis and cardiac ischemia; hence, the term *heartburn* for the former. Thus, precordial pain may originate from any intrathoracic organ or from the chest wall itself, and the patient cannot identify the source of her discomfort, which in itself is a cause of distress.

Cardiac causes are a heterogeneous category, which can best be viewed as ischemic and non-ischemic in origin (Box 93-2). None of these causes is common. Ischemic chest pain, or angina, is caused by a drop, often sudden, in the myocardial oxygen supply to demand ratio, causing pain or, in rare cases, sudden death. This may occur because of diseased coronary arteries as in adults, due to accelerated coronary atherosclerosis, which is very rare in the pediatric population. It may be seen in progeria, mucopolysaccharidosis, posttransplant coronary disease, and severe familial hypercholesterolemia. It may occur as a result of previous inflammation (as in Kawasaki disease with coronary aneurysms) leading to coronary artery stenosis. A congenital AOCA from the opposite sinus aortae (Figure 93-1) or from the pulmonary artery may result in ischemia due to compression of the anomalous vessel between the great arteries, obstruction from a slit-like orifice at the origin, or in the case of the pulmonary artery, low pressure and low saturation in the perfusing blood.

The chest pain seen in a small minority of patients with left ventricular outflow obstruction (aortic valve stenosis and hypertrophic obstructive cardiomyopathy) is likely also due to ischemia. The

Box 93-1. Differential Diagnosis of Chest Pain in Children and Adolescents

Chest Wall
- c Trauma
- c Overuse
- c Inadequate breast support
- c Chronic cough
- u Costochondritis
- u Precordial catch syndrome
- r Slipping rib syndrome

Gastrointestinal
- c Gastroesophageal reflux disease
- u Esophagitis due to repeated vomiting
- r Esophageal stricture
- r Foreign body

Pulmonary
- c Exercise-induced asthma
- c Pneumonia
- u Pleurodynia, pleurisy
- r Pneumothorax/pneumomediastinum
- r Pulmonary embolism

Psychological
- c Anxiety disorder
- c Depression
- u Conversion reaction
- r Munchausen syndrome
- r Bulimia nervosa

Miscellaneous
- c Idiopathic
- u Acute chest syndrome (sickle cell disease)
- r Thoracic tumors
- r Herpes zoster

Cardiac
See Box 93-2.

Abbreviations: c, common cause of chest pain; r, rare cause of chest pain; u, uncommon cause of chest pain.

already diminished supply to demand ratio due to hypertrophy and hypertension of the left ventricle falls further with strenuous exercise, causing pain or arrhythmia.

In abuse of drugs such as cocaine, chest pain may be attributable to arrhythmia, myocardial hypoperfusion, or a combination of the two; this may present as chest pain or overt collapse, in some cases with cardiac arrest.

Although many children with cardiac arrhythmias are asymptomatic or present with palpitations, dizzy spells, or syncope, some do complain of chest pain. In the case of the younger child, this may reflect an inability to express the discomfort of palpitations as other than "hurting." In addition, ischemia does occur in some individuals with tachyarrhythmia, such as paroxysmal supraventricular tachycardia (SVT), due to high myocardial oxygen consumption and shortened diastole, compromising perfusion. In these patients, ST

Box 93-2. Cardiac Causes of Chest Pain in Children

Ischemic

u   Tachyarrhythmia (supraventricular tachycardia, ventricular tachycardia)

u   Cocaine abuse

r   Aortic stenosis

r   Hypertrophic obstructive cardiomyopathy

r   Anomalous origin of a coronary artery

r   Accelerated coronary atherosclerosis (eg, progeria, hyperlipidemia, cardiac transplantation)

r   Coronary artery stenosis secondary to Kawasaki disease

Non-ischemic

u   Pericarditis (viral, bacterial, autoimmune, postoperative)

u   Mitral valve prolapse

r   Myocarditis

r   Aortic root dissection (eg, in Marfan syndrome)

Abbreviations: r, rare cause of chest pain; u, uncommon cause of chest pain.

Figure 93-1. Schematic diagram of the 2 forms of anomalous origin of a coronary from the wrong sinus that are associated with myocardial ischemia. A, Anomalous origin of the left main coronary artery (LMA) from the right sinus aortae. B, Anomalous origin of the right coronary artery (RCA) from the left sinus aortae. In each case, the anomalous coronary artery can be seen coursing between the aorta and pulmonary artery (PA). L, left aortic sinus; LAD, left anterior descending; LCx, left circumflex; R, right aortic sinus.

segment depression may be seen on the electrocardiogram (ECG) during the arrhythmia and may persist for several minutes after the arrhythmia is terminated.

Non-ischemic cardiac causes of chest pain include pericarditis and, less commonly, myocarditis, aortic dissection, and mitral prolapse. The most common form of inflammatory heart disease is acute viral infection; acute bacterial pericarditis is more severe and associated with greater systemic toxicity. Connective tissue disease, such as lupus erythematosus or juvenile rheumatoid arthritis, is frequently associated with immune-mediated pericarditis, as is the postpericardiotomy syndrome seen shortly after cardiac surgery. In these disorders the pain is caused by inflammation of the pericardium and epicardium, directly stimulating the many sensory nerve endings in this area.

Aortic dissection also results in direct stimulation of pain fibers, in this case in the aortic wall. It is very rare in the normal pediatric population but may occur in the setting of Marfan syndrome and related disorders. Chest pain is also seen in patients with mitral valve prolapse, but it is often difficult to establish a clear causal relationship in this setting. Interestingly, gastroesophageal reflux disease (GERD) can be demonstrated in a high percentage of these patients.

Differential Diagnosis

The differential diagnosis of pediatric chest pain is presented in Box 93-1, and cardiac causes are listed in Box 93-2. The relative frequencies of these causes vary in reported series, but all report higher frequencies of respiratory, idiopathic, traumatic, and psychogenic etiologies and low frequencies of cardiac etiologies, usually in the range of 1% to 5% in patients with no previous cardiac history. These data must be viewed as approximations because the ultimate etiologic classification of cases in these series is not usually based on a definitive result but rather an attribution by the physician involved. Therefore, cultural factors and individual preferences may lead to higher reported rates of "idiopathic" chest pain in some centers, "chest wall pain" in others, and "anxiety disorder" in still others. Some studies report a higher incidence of cardiac etiologies because they classify any patient with chest pain with a cardiac finding (eg, premature beats, abnormal ECG), regardless of whether it may explain the pain. Among children referred to a cardiologist for evaluation of chest pain, almost half have psychiatric diagnoses of at least moderate severity; in 29% of referred children, it is of marked severity. Anxiety disorders predominate in this subpopulation, but depression is also seen more commonly than in the general population.

Evaluation

The keystones to the evaluation of the child with chest pain are a thorough, methodical history and careful physical examination; indeed, in many cases these will suffice to arrive at a diagnosis and formulate a management plan.

History

The major questions to be addressed are outlined in the Questions Box. Because there are many pertinent details to be included in the **history of present illness,** and they are often provided in a variable sequence, some physicians find it helpful to use a printed format as a guide. Some offer a questionnaire for the patient or parent to complete. Witnesses to the episodes may provide additional helpful information, especially if the patient is not verbally expressive. The witness may estimate a pain score based on observation, which may differ substantially from the score assigned by the patient himself.

Pain that occurs repeatedly over time is less likely the result of an organic cause of a serious nature, particularly if it is not reproducible. A severe, protracted episode (eg, lasting hours) is more likely to be organic in origin. The location of the pain has not been a strong predictor of diagnosis in reported series. Its timing and association with other symptoms, however, may provide major clues. Reflux esophagitis may occur after eating, more often when supine or very active, and may be accompanied by a sour taste; it may be relieved by eating or use of an antacid. Associated symptoms that may raise a red flag for a cardiac cause include syncope, palpitations, sweating, and nausea; reproducible pain at a given level of exertion is also more likely anginal. Because pain and accompanying anxiety may cause sinus tachycardia, which can be interpreted by the patient as palpitations, it is important to get a sense of the heart rate experienced by patients with that complaint. The child can be asked to tap his chest or clap his hands as fast as his heart was racing during the palpitations; serious tachyarrhythmia, such as supraventricular tachycardia and ventricular tachycardia, are usually very rapid.

Recent fever and malaise are often present in pneumonia, pleurisy, or pericarditis. Exercise-induced asthma (EIA), in addition to being related to exertion, is sometimes accompanied by cough or wheezing. Shortness of breath is very frequently reported by patients in association with their pain; this may reflect anxiety or sensitivity to movement rather than pulmonary pathology.

In youngsters with psychogenic pain, other symptoms of anxiety or depression may be reported, although not necessarily simultaneously with the chest pain and often preceding it in onset. A history of recent stressors may be uncovered. These patients may also report other recurrent somatic complaints.

The nature, severity, and abruptness of the pain may also yield diagnostic clues. Exercise-induced asthma is often described as a chest "tightness," is usually gradual in onset, and lasts beyond the exertion itself. The precordial catch syndrome, a poorly understood disorder also known as *Texidor twinge,* is a sudden, sharp, localized pain that is exacerbated by deep breathing, and lasts only seconds or minutes. In contrast, slipping rib syndrome, in which the cartilaginous tips of the eighth, ninth, and 10th ribs become transiently subluxated, produces pain at the costal margin, is very sensitive to movement, and is often associated with a "popping" or "slipping" sensation in the affected area. Gastroesophageal reflux disease pain is usually described as "burning" and may awaken the patient from sleep. In contrast, the pain of angina is reported as "crushing" and may radiate to the left arm or the neck. The diffuse pain of pericarditis is often ameliorated by sitting forward. Aortic dissection results in an acute, tearing sensation.

A history of recent chest trauma will naturally suggest chest wall injury as the cause, but the fall or sports mishap may be forgotten if the onset of the pain is not temporally associated with the event. Chest wall pain may also result from overuse, as seen in weight lifters, or from inadequate breast support, as seen in female runners. Drug abuse, particularly with cocaine, may be disclosed if the patient is questioned in private. In some cases this may have occurred several days before the onset of pain.

The patient's **medical history,** if positive, may lead the clinician toward the underlying diagnosis. In children with sickle cell disease, acute chest syndrome must be considered early in the assessment. A history of respiratory disease may point to an acute respiratory infection or EIA. Children with known heart disease, who may experience benign chest pain, are more likely to have a cardiac etiology than their peers, depending on the cardiac diagnosis. Most congenital heart defects, for example, do not cause pain but may raise the level of anxiety in the family and lead to the perception or exaggeration of chest pain. Of greater concern is a history of heart disease that may affect myocardial perfusion, such as Kawasaki disease or cardiac surgery involving the coronary arteries (eg, arterial switch operation for transposition of the great arteries).

The **family history** must not be overlooked. Although most pediatric chest pain is not due to hereditary disorders, some of the more severe causes may be hereditary, such as hypertrophic cardiomyopathy, some arrhythmias, asthma, sickle cell disease, and aortic dissection in Marfan syndrome. It is also noted that in children with nonorganic chest pain, such as psychogenic pain, there is often a history of a close relative having had recent heart surgery or a heart attack, bringing attention to this area during a time of emotional stress.

A complete **review of systems** is essential in the assessment of children with chest pain because of the wide range of differential diagnoses.

Physical Examination

A careful physical examination is imperative; in children with no history of serious illness, this should be focused on, but not be limited to, the chest. General inspection will immediately aid in distinguishing between the acutely ill child and the otherwise well child with chest pain. Abnormal vital signs, such as fever, tachycardia, or tachypnea, are associated with acute etiologies such as infection or inflammation. The child's pain level should be quantified with the aid of a pain scale. If the patient is dyspneic, pulse oximetry should be measured.

The chest wall should be examined for signs of trauma and for tenderness. Care must be taken with the latter because it is easy to obtain a false-positive examination for costochondritis, for example, because the costochondral junctions have some degree of normal tenderness, as do the female breasts. Asymmetry of tenderness, and a report that the pain produced is similar to that experienced, suggests chest wall injury. In patients with rib injury, the pain can be elicited not only on direct palpation but also indirectly by compression of the thoracic cage from another location. In girls with inadequate breast support, the breast ligaments may be symmetrically tender.

Auscultation of the lungs and heart will, of course, yield useful clues to diagnosis, especially in children with acute inflammatory processes (rales, rub) and in those with left ventricular outflow obstruction, such as aortic stenosis (murmur). It must be remembered, however, that many of the organic causes of chest pain, such as GERD, EIA, intermittent arrhythmias, and AOCA, will have a normal examination if the patient is not experiencing the pain at the time of the visit.

Other portions of the physical examination may also aid in the evaluation of the child with chest pain. Jugular distention, hepatomegaly, and peripheral edema suggest congestive heart failure or pericardial effusion with tamponade. The child's behavior pattern and interaction with his parents may suggest a psychological disorder such as anxiety or depression. Poor dentition and halitosis in an adolescent with weight loss may be a sign of bulimia as a source of esophagitis. Excessive signs of trauma such as multiple ecchymoses may indicate a coagulopathy and also raise the possibility of non-accidental trauma.

Laboratory Studies

A wide variety of diagnostic studies is available to help in arriving at a diagnosis; it is incumbent on the physician to select those appropriate to the individual patient, guided by the findings of the history and physical examination.

In the patient presenting with **acute chest pain,** often to the ED, there is a greater need for tests because the differential diagnosis more often includes serious, even life-threatening, disorders than in the child with chronic recurrent pain. Reported series show the chest radiograph to have a reasonably high yield of positive findings; a negative radiograph is reassuring in ruling out pathology such as pleural effusion, pneumonia, pneumothorax, pneumomediastinum, and thoracic tumor but cannot be used to exclude most cardiac etiologies. More detailed imaging such as magnetic resonance imaging may be needed when major chest trauma is reported or aortic dissection suspected. Dyspnea or hypoxemia, particularly in the setting of recent immobilization or in an adolescent female taking oral contraceptives, should lead one to suspect pulmonary embolism, for which a spiral computed tomography or nuclear perfusion scan is indicated.

Although ECG is routinely performed as part of the evaluation for acute chest pain in children, it is rarely helpful in establishing a diagnosis other than arrhythmia, which may be suspected from the history or examination. ST segment changes may reflect pericardial irritation or myocardial ischemia if the ECG is done at the time of the pain. If ongoing myocardial ischemia is suspected, myocardial enzymes (creatine kinase MB fraction, troponin I) should be measured and a toxicology screen performed. If signs of acute infection such as fever are noted, a complete blood cell count, sedimentation rate or C-reactive protein, and appropriate cultures are indicated. Echocardiography is highly sensitive and specific for pericardial effusion and should be performed early in the evaluation of the patient with chest pain and jugular distention, a friction rub, fever, or ST segment elevation on ECG.

In patients presenting with **chronic recurrent chest pain,** the likelihood of serious pathology is very low. When the examination is normal and the history reassuring, the yield of "screening" tests such as chest radiograph and ECG is extremely poor, and the cost in dollars and anxiety not justifiable. In most cases the history and physical examination are adequate to lead to a focused selection of diagnostic tests, if any are needed. A description of pain suggestive of esophagitis, for example, may lead to endoscopy or upper gastrointestinal series. When EIA is suspected, pulmonary function testing is appropriate, in some cases with an exercise challenge. Strong suspicion of psychogenic causes should prompt further psychological evaluation at the initial encounter, including querying the patient about suicide; further testing or consultation may be indicated.

The finding of a murmur of left ventricular outflow tract obstruction is an indication for echocardiography, which will confirm the diagnosis and yield further details that will guide management. A history of palpitations or syncope raises the possibility of arrhythmia; an ECG may give clues such as Wolff-Parkinson-White syndrome as a substrate for SVT, but a normal ECG does not rule out arrhythmia if the patient is asymptomatic at the time. Here an ambulatory ECG (Holter) monitor or trans-telephonic event detector may enable the clinician to document the rhythm during an episode of pain. Consistent exertional pain merits evaluation for ischemia, using resting ECG and often exercise stress testing. These study results, unfortunately, can be negative between episodes in patients with AOCA. This diagnosis can, however, be identified by echocardiography, but only if the study is deliberately directed toward that diagnosis; therefore, the study should be done in a pediatric echocardiography laboratory, and the sonographer must be aware of the diagnosis in question.

Management

The management of pediatric chest pain depends on the underlying diagnosis or lack thereof. For management of GERD, acute chest syndrome, pneumonia, pericarditis, connective tissue disorders, thoracic tumors, anxiety disorder, pneumothorax, cocaine abuse, and chest wall trauma, as well as other serious disorders discussed under differential diagnosis, the reader is directed to other sources within and beyond this text.

When there is a strong suspicion of cardiac pathology, on the basis of history and physical examination or of subsequent testing as described previously, prompt referral to a pediatric cardiologist is indicated. Management may include surgery (eg, for AOCA), antibiotics, anti-inflammatories, pericardiocentesis (eg, for pericarditis), antiarrhythmics, interventional catheterization (eg, balloon angioplasty, radiofrequency ablation), or a combination of these treatments.

Short-term nonsteroidal anti-inflammatory medication is helpful for chest wall pain caused by overuse, trauma, costochondritis, or slipping rib syndrome. In a minority of cases, local injection with anesthetic may be necessary.

Therapeutic trials may be considered in some cases to arrive at a diagnosis. A child with suspected esophagitis may be given an antacid at the time of the pain. If the pain is relieved, further workup and treatment can proceed accordingly. Similarly, a youngster with suspected EIA, particularly if there is a previous history of reactive airways disease, may benefit from a trial of an inhaled bronchodilator at the time of pain.

In the exceedingly common setting of benign chest pain, such as with minor chest wall trauma, mild somatization, or occasional reflux esophagitis, the most important step in management is reassurance of the patient and family that this is not an indication of a serious disorder. It is essential to clarify how one has arrived at this conclusion and why further testing is not appropriate.

A frequent observation in this setting is that most families do not require a definitive diagnosis of the cause of the pain. If a serious disorder is excluded—necessary because 50% of patients believe that chest pain means heart disease—all participants are reassured. Follow-up studies have demonstrated that at least 80% of patients in this category do not seek further medical attention for their chest pain, nor return for follow-up.

Prognosis

The outcome depends on the underlying diagnosis. Most cases of benign chest pain resolve spontaneously, often within a short time of their evaluation. Psychogenic chest pain tends to be recurrent more often than other forms. Even in serious and potentially life-threatening causes of chest pain, early diagnosis and intervention will usually lead to an excellent outcome.

CASE RESOLUTION

The patient and his parents are assured that he has no evidence of a serious medical or psychiatric problem. His heart is strong, his lungs clear, and his circulation good. They are told that chest pain in otherwise healthy children may be mysterious but is common and very rarely a sign of illness. They are told in a gentle but definitive manner that he does not need any further evaluation at this time, but that if the problem does not resolve itself, the child should return for reevaluation.

The boy is delighted to hear that he may return to full sports participation, confirmed in writing to the coach. The parents are very relieved and grateful for the attention and reassurance of the physician. At subsequent office visits for other purposes, he reports no more chest pain.

Selected References

Abdurrahman L, Bockoven JR, Pickoff AS, Ralston MA, Ross JE. Pediatric cardiology update: office-based practice of pediatric cardiology for the primary care provider. *Curr Probl Pediatr Adolesc Health Care*. 2003;33(10):318–347

Angoff GH, Kane DA, Giddins N, et al. Regional implementation of a pediatric cardiology chest pain guideline using SCAMPs methodology. *Pediatrics*. 2013;132(4):e1010–e1017

Cava JR, Sayger PL. Chest pain in children and adolescents. *Pediatr Clin North Am*. 2004;51(6):1553–1568

Eslick GD, Selbst SM, eds. Pediatric chest pain. *Pediatr Clin North Am*. 2010;57 (6, theme issue):1211–1458

Gumbiner CH. Precordial catch syndrome. *South Med J*. 2003;96(1):38–41

Lipsitz JD, Hsu D, Apfel HD, et al. Psychiatric disorders in youth with medically unexplained chest pain versus innocent heart murmur. *J Pediatr*. 2012;160(2):320–324

Massin MM, Bourguignont A, Coremans C, Comté L, Lepage P, Gérard P. Chest pain in pediatric patients presenting to an emergency department or to a cardiac clinic. *Clin Pediatr (Phila)*. 2004;43(3):231–238

Rowe BH, Dulberg CS, Peterson RG, Vlad P, Li MM. Characteristics of children presenting with chest pain to a pediatric emergency department. *CMAJ*. 1990;143(5):388–394

Selbst SM. Chest pain in children. *Pediatrics*. 1985;75(6):1068–1070

Tunaoglu FS, Olguntürk R, Akcabay S, Oguz D, Gücüyener K, Demirsoy S. Chest pain in children referred to a cardiology clinic. *Pediatr Cardiol*. 1995;16(2):69–72

Wiens L, Sabath R, Ewing L, Gowdamarajan R, Portnoy J, Scagliotti D. Chest pain in otherwise healthy children and adolescents is frequently caused by exercise-induced asthma. *Pediatrics*. 1992;90(3):350–353

Zavaras-Angelidou KA, Weinhouse E, Nelson DB. Review of 180 episodes of chest pain in 134 children. *Pediatr Emerg Care*. 1992;8(4):189–193

CHAPTER 94

Hypertension

Gangadarshni Chandramohan, MD, MS, and Sudhir K. Anand, MD

CASE STUDY

A 16-year-old girl is seen in the emergency department with a history of persistent headaches of 2 weeks' duration. She has been having occasional headaches for the past 2 years, which have been treated primarily with acetaminophen. She denies any recent weight loss, hair loss, joint pains, sweating, or palpitations. There is no history of swelling of her eyes or legs or blood noticed in the urine. She was born prematurely at 30 weeks' gestation and stayed in the hospital for 2 weeks. There is no history of urinary tract infection. Her mother (34 years old) and maternal grandma (58 years old) have been on antihypertensives for the past several years. She is an average student at school. There is no known history of drug ingestion. Her diet consists of mostly bread and meat. Also, she regularly eats salty snacks but drinks sodas only occasionally. She never was involved in any physical activity on a regular basis.

The physical examination is remarkable for an obese-looking girl with weight, height, and body mass index above the 95th percentile for age. Pulse is 85 beats/min and blood pressure 158/78 mm Hg in the right arm in supine position. Equal pulses are palpable in all 4 extremities. Blood pressure is 164/92 mm Hg in the right lower extremity. Funduscopic examination reveals evidence of arteriovenous nicking but no papilledema. Chest examination finds normal breath sounds and an active precordium with the apical impulse shifted to the left; no murmurs are heard. The liver is palpable 1 cm below the right costal margin. Neurologic examination is unremarkable; no focal neurologic deficit is present. Urinalysis is normal. Hemoglobin is 11.2 g/dL and hematocrit is 33%. Sodium is 139 mEq/L, potassium 3.8 mEq/L, chloride 102 mEq/L, and bicarbonate 22 mEq/L. Blood urea nitrogen is 15 mg/dL and serum creatinine is 0.9 mg/dL. An electrocardiogram shows left ventricular enlargement. Computed tomography scan of the head is normal.

Questions

1. What is the definition of hypertension in children and adolescents?
2. What are the causes of hypertension in children and adolescents?
3. What is the appropriate evaluation of hypertension in children and adolescents?
4. What are the comorbid conditions and long-term complications associated with essential (primary) hypertension?
5. What is the appropriate emergency treatment of symptomatic hypertension?
6. What is the long-term management of children with essential hypertension?

Hypertension has become a more common problem among children and adolescents over the past few decades because of the increased prevalence of obesity, which is associated with essential (primary) hypertension. Although the increased prevalence of hypertension in children is predominantly due to an increase in essential hypertension, there is a need with childhood hypertension to identify secondary causes. Secondary causes are proportionately more prevalent among young children compared with adolescents and, if identified, may be curable, thereby eliminating the need for lifelong medical treatment. Conversely, essential hypertension typically persists into adulthood and is likely to become a major public health concern in the future. With early intervention, however, the long-term adverse consequences of hypertension are preventable. Children who are expected to be at increased risk for end-organ (heart, central nervous system [CNS], kidneys, and eyes) damage are those with persistently elevated blood pressure (BP) readings, high body mass index (BMI), excessive weight gain, and a family history of hypertension.

Normal Blood Pressure and Definition of Hypertension

Systolic and diastolic BP gradually increase from the newborn period through adolescence; therefore, age-appropriate norms should be used to classify a given BP reading as normal or hypertensive. For example, a BP reading of 118/76 mm Hg would be regarded as normal for a 16-year-old but would signify stage 2 hypertension in a 2-year-old, meaning that this 2-year-old needs urgent medical attention. Blood pressure measurements should be part of routine physical examinations in all children older than 3 years and in all hospitalized children according to American Academy of Pediatrics (AAP) guidelines. The AAP guidelines also recommend that children who are younger than 3 years who have a history of prematurity, congenital heart disease, recurrent urinary tract infections (UTIs), or chronic systemic illnesses should have their BP measured as a routine part of their well-child care. These guidelines have been recently challenged by the US Preventive Services Task Force because they concluded that the current evidence is insufficient to assess the balance of benefits and harms of screening for hypertension in asymptomatic children and adolescents to prevent subsequent cardiovascular disease in childhood or adulthood. In contrast, data from other studies on essential hypertension in childhood show that it is often associated with left ventricular hypertrophy (LVH), increased carotid intimal thickening, and even subtle cognitive changes (Falkner). In view of the conflicting advice, for the present it would be prudent to continue current practice guidelines as recommended by the AAP.

To obtain an accurate BP measurement, an appropriately sized BP cuff should be used; the inner cuff width should be approximately 40% of the arm circumference midway between the olecranon and the acromion, and the length should be greater than 80% around the arm circumference at the same point to avoid inaccurately high readings. There are various other factors that should be taken into consideration while measuring BP to minimize errors, which include patient's posture (sitting versus lying down) and level of the arm in relation to level of the heart (elbow to be at the level of the heart); if it is the first visit, readings from all 4 extremities to rule out coarctation of the aorta should be performed as well. It is also important that the child should remain calm and not be anxious or agitated while the measurement is taken. There are various forms of BP monitors used in pediatric practices, including manual auscultatory aneroid sphygmomanometers and oscillometric automated monitors (which use mean arterial pressure to calculate systolic and diastolic BPs). Oscillometric devices are known to correlate significantly with arterial blood pressure, although there is a tendency for the portable devices to have lower systolic and slightly higher diastolic pressures.

Blood pressure values in children are a continuum, with no clear dividing line between normal and high (tables 94-1 and 94-2). Therefore, the fourth report on high BP in children and adolescents (2004), by using the statistical percentile values, defines hypertension as systolic or diastolic BP of greater than 95th percentile for age, gender, and height on at least 3 occasions (Table 94-3). Furthermore, if the systolic or diastolic BP readings are between the 90th and 95th percentile, it is considered prehypertension. The report further classifies hypertension into 2 categories: stage 1 hypertension, which is when systolic or diastolic BP is persistently between the 95th percentile to 5 mm above the 99th percentiles, and stage 2 hypertension, which is when systolic or diastolic BP is persistently more than 5 mm Hg above the 99th percentile (D_x Box). Because this is a statistical definition, 5% of all children (those with BP readings >95th percentile) would be considered hypertensive.

Epidemiology

The prevalence of persistent hypertension in children based on the current definition is approximately 3% to 5%; however, it can vary depending on the age, ethnicity, geographic distribution, and type of hypertension. The consensus is that the overall prevalence of essential hypertension has been increasing over the past few decades secondary to the increasing prevalence of obesity, cultural factors, and lifestyle changes, which include increases in stress and sedentary lifestyle. Among those who are obese, the prevalence of hypertension has been reported to be up to 30% from some studies, compared with children who are not obese. As in adults, hypertension is more common among African American and Hispanic children compared with white children. Furthermore, adolescents and those from urban cities tend to have higher prevalence compared with younger children and those from rural areas.

Secondary hypertension is more common among infants and young children, whereas essential hypertension is notably more common among adolescents. Children who require hospital admission for their hypertension usually have secondary hypertension, which may have been triggered by an acute event, frequently volume overload. Occasionally, the cause of hypertension is uncertain. In many such children, the acutely increased BP resolves with appropriate medical intervention, and most do not require long-term treatment. Data on prevalence of acute hypertension are sparse because of the transient nature of the condition, and there are no major long-term implications.

Clinical Presentation

Mild or stage 1 hypertension in most children is usually asymptomatic. However, children with moderate to severe hypertension can develop headaches, blurring of vision, and sometimes nosebleeds. Acute presentations of hypertension are divided into 3 categories: hypertensive urgencies, hypertensive emergencies, and hypertensive crisis. Occasionally, the terms *hypertensive emergency* and *hypertensive crisis* are used interchangeably to describe the same situation in which a patient has very elevated BP. *Hypertensive urgency* is defined by the sudden development of elevated BP without evidence of severe end-organ damage but can be symptomatic with headache and vomiting. A *hypertensive emergency*, in comparison, is defined by obvious signs of significant end-organ damage, such as encephalopathy, seizures, papilledema, retinal hemorrhages, or kidney injury, and must be dealt with immediately. Hypertensive crisis is merely a very severe form of hypertension marked by a more than 20% increase in the systolic or diastolic BP above the 95th percentile with clinical evidence of malignant hypertension.

Etiology and Pathophysiology

An increase in BP results from an increase in peripheral resistance or cardiac output or a mixture of the two. The exact cause of hypertension in 90% to 95% of adults is still uncertain; hence, the term essential, primary, or idiopathic hypertension. In the past, hypertension was considered secondary to an underlying disorder in more than 80% of children and fewer than 20% of cases were idiopathic; however, this was true only in children with very severe hypertension. In most obese adolescents with mild increases in BP, no etiology of hypertension is found and they are classified as having essential hypertension.

Table 94-1. Blood Pressure Levels for the 90th and 95th Percentiles of Blood Pressure for Boys Aged 1 Through 17 Years by Percentiles of Height[a]

Age (Year)	BP Percentile ↓	Systolic BP (mmHg) ← Percentile of Height →							Diastolic BP (mmHg) ← Percentile of Height →						
		5th	10th	25th	50th	75th	90th	95th	5th	10th	25th	50th	75th	90th	95th
1	50th	80	81	83	85	87	88	89	34	35	36	37	38	39	39
	90th	94	95	97	99	100	102	103	49	50	51	52	53	53	54
	95th	98	99	101	103	104	106	106	54	54	55	56	57	58	58
	99th	105	106	108	110	112	113	114	61	62	63	64	65	66	66
2	50th	84	85	87	88	90	92	92	39	40	41	42	43	44	44
	90th	97	99	100	102	104	105	106	54	55	56	57	58	58	59
	95th	101	102	104	106	108	109	110	59	59	60	61	62	63	63
	99th	109	110	111	113	115	117	117	66	67	68	69	70	71	71
3	50th	86	87	89	91	93	94	95	44	44	45	46	47	48	48
	90th	100	101	103	105	107	108	109	59	59	60	61	62	63	63
	95th	104	105	107	109	110	112	113	63	63	64	65	66	67	67
	99th	111	112	114	116	118	119	120	71	71	72	73	74	75	75
4	50th	88	89	91	93	95	96	97	47	48	49	50	51	51	52
	90th	102	103	105	107	109	110	111	62	63	64	65	66	66	67
	95th	106	107	109	111	112	114	115	66	67	68	69	70	71	71
	99th	113	114	116	118	120	121	122	74	75	76	77	78	78	79
5	50th	90	91	93	95	96	98	98	50	51	52	53	54	55	55
	90th	104	105	106	108	110	111	112	65	66	67	68	69	69	70
	95th	108	109	110	112	114	115	116	69	70	71	72	73	74	74
	99th	115	116	118	120	121	123	123	77	78	79	80	81	81	82
6	50th	91	92	94	96	98	99	100	53	53	54	55	56	57	57
	90th	105	106	108	110	111	113	113	68	68	69	70	71	72	72
	95th	109	110	112	114	115	117	117	72	72	73	74	75	76	76
	99th	116	117	119	121	123	124	125	80	80	81	82	83	84	84
7	50th	92	94	95	97	99	100	101	55	55	56	57	58	59	59
	90th	106	107	109	111	113	114	115	70	70	71	72	73	74	74
	95th	110	111	113	115	117	118	119	74	74	75	76	77	78	78
	99th	117	118	120	122	124	125	126	82	82	83	84	85	86	86
8	50th	94	95	97	99	100	102	102	56	57	58	59	60	60	61
	90th	107	109	110	112	114	115	116	71	72	72	73	74	75	76
	95th	111	112	114	116	118	119	120	75	76	77	78	79	79	80
	99th	119	120	122	123	125	127	127	83	84	85	86	87	87	88
9	50th	95	96	98	100	102	103	104	57	58	59	60	61	61	62
	90th	109	110	112	114	115	117	118	72	73	74	75	76	76	77
	95th	113	114	116	118	119	121	121	76	77	78	79	80	81	81
	99th	120	121	123	125	127	128	129	84	85	86	87	88	88	89
10	50th	97	98	100	102	103	105	106	58	59	60	61	61	62	63
	90th	111	112	114	115	117	119	119	73	73	74	75	76	77	78
	95th	115	116	117	119	121	122	123	77	78	79	80	81	81	82
	99th	122	123	125	127	128	130	130	85	86	86	88	88	89	90

Table 94-1. Blood Pressure Levels for the 90th and 95th Percentiles of Blood Pressure for Boys Aged 1 Through 17 Years by Percentiles of Height[a], continued

Age (Year)	BP Percentile ↓	Systolic BP (mm Hg) ← Percentile of Height →							Diastolic BP (mm Hg) ← Percentile of Height →						
		5th	10th	25th	50th	75th	90th	95th	5th	10th	25th	50th	75th	90th	95th
11	50th	99	100	102	104	105	107	107	59	59	60	61	62	63	63
	90th	113	114	115	117	119	120	121	74	74	75	76	77	78	78
	95th	117	118	119	121	123	124	125	78	78	79	80	81	82	82
	99th	124	125	127	129	130	132	132	86	86	87	88	89	90	90
12	50th	101	102	104	106	108	109	110	59	60	61	62	63	63	64
	90th	115	116	118	120	121	123	123	74	75	75	76	77	78	79
	95th	119	120	122	123	125	127	127	78	79	80	81	82	82	83
	99th	126	127	129	131	133	134	135	86	87	88	89	90	90	91
13	50th	104	105	106	108	110	111	112	60	60	61	62	63	64	64
	90th	117	118	120	122	124	125	126	75	75	76	77	78	79	79
	95th	121	122	124	126	128	129	130	79	79	80	81	82	83	83
	99th	128	130	131	133	135	136	137	87	87	88	89	90	91	91
14	50th	106	107	109	111	113	114	115	60	61	62	63	64	65	65
	90th	120	121	123	125	126	128	128	75	76	77	78	79	79	80
	95th	124	125	127	128	130	132	132	80	80	81	82	83	84	84
	99th	131	132	134	136	138	139	140	87	88	89	90	91	92	92
15	50th	109	110	112	113	115	117	117	61	62	63	64	65	66	66
	90th	122	124	125	127	129	130	131	76	77	78	79	80	80	81
	95th	126	127	129	131	133	134	135	81	81	82	83	84	85	85
	99th	134	135	136	138	140	142	142	88	89	90	91	92	93	93
16	50th	111	112	114	116	118	119	120	63	63	64	65	66	67	67
	90th	125	126	128	130	131	133	134	78	78	79	80	81	82	82
	95th	129	130	132	134	135	137	137	82	83	83	84	85	86	87
	99th	136	137	139	141	143	144	145	90	90	91	92	93	94	94
17	50th	114	115	116	118	120	121	122	65	66	66	67	68	69	70
	90th	127	128	130	132	134	135	136	80	80	81	82	83	84	84
	95th	131	132	134	136	138	139	140	84	85	86	87	87	88	89
	99th	139	140	141	143	145	146	147	92	93	93	94	95	96	97

Abbreviation: BP, blood pressure.

[a] The 90th percentile is 1.28 SD, 95th percentile is 1.645 SD, and the 99th percentile is 2.326 SD over the mean.

Many factors play a role in the development of essential hypertension. Research reveals variable degrees of alteration in cardiac output, extracellular fluid volume, peripheral resistance, renin-angiotensin system, aldosterone, electrolyte balance, catecholamines, sympathetic nervous system, natriuretic hormones, prostaglandins, kinins, antidiuretic hormone, insulin response, endothelins, nitric oxide (endothelium-derived relaxation factors), and others. Whether these abnormalities are primary or secondary and what their exact role is in the pathogenesis of essential hypertension is still uncertain. Barker's hypothesis of epigenetic transmission, a recently promulgated theory, attributes certain disorders, including childhood hypertension, to altered gene expression from malnutrition or other adverse events during intrauterine life. Epigenetic changes occur as a result of methylation or acetylation of the noncoding gene segment (histones) that can change the chromosomal configuration and result in activation or inhibition of a specific gene transcription (ie, turning the gene on or off). This hypothesis has been further supported by data demonstrating association between fewer nephrons (due to under-expression of genes responsible for branching) in children who were born small for gestational age and later developed hypertension.

Other important factors in the development of hypertension include race, heredity, stress response, sleep apnea, obesity, hyperlipidemia, and increased salt intake. Recently obesity has been strongly implicated in the increase in incidence of hypertension in the United States. Mirroring the increase in obesity, average BPs rose by 1.4 to 3.3 mm Hg between 1990 and 2000. Studies showing that weight reduction in obese patients lowers BP strengthen the

Table 94-2. Blood Pressure Levels for the 90th and 95th Percentiles of Blood Pressure for Girls Aged 1 Through 17 Years by Percentiles of Height[a]

Age (Year)	BP Percentile ↓	Systolic BP (mm Hg) ← Percentile of Height →							Diastolic BP (mm Hg) ← Percentile of Height →						
		5th	10th	25th	50th	75th	90th	95th	5th	10th	25th	50th	75th	90th	95th
I	50th	83	84	85	86	88	89	90	38	39	39	40	41	41	42
	90th	97	97	98	100	101	102	103	52	53	53	54	55	55	56
	95th	100	101	102	104	105	106	107	56	57	57	58	59	59	60
	99th	108	108	109	111	112	113	114	64	64	65	65	66	67	67
2	50th	85	85	87	88	89	91	91	43	44	44	45	46	46	47
	90th	98	99	100	101	103	104	105	57	58	58	59	60	61	61
	95th	102	103	104	105	107	108	109	61	62	62	63	64	65	65
	99th	109	110	111	112	114	115	116	69	69	70	70	71	72	72
3	50th	86	87	88	89	91	92	93	47	48	48	49	50	50	51
	90th	100	100	102	103	104	106	106	61	62	62	63	64	64	65
	95th	104	104	105	107	108	109	110	65	66	66	67	68	68	69
	99th	111	111	113	114	115	116	117	73	73	74	74	75	76	76
4	50th	88	88	90	91	92	94	94	50	50	51	52	52	53	54
	90th	101	102	103	104	106	107	108	64	64	65	66	67	67	68
	95th	105	106	107	108	110	111	112	68	68	69	70	71	71	72
	99th	112	113	114	115	117	118	119	76	76	76	77	78	79	79
5	50th	89	90	91	93	94	95	96	52	53	53	54	55	55	56
	90th	103	103	105	106	107	109	109	66	67	67	68	69	69	70
	95th	107	107	108	110	111	112	113	70	71	71	72	73	73	74
	99th	114	114	116	117	118	120	120	78	78	79	79	80	81	81
6	50th	91	92	93	94	96	97	98	54	54	55	56	56	57	58
	90th	104	105	106	108	109	110	111	68	68	69	70	70	71	72
	95th	108	109	110	111	113	114	115	72	72	73	74	74	75	76
	99th	115	116	117	119	120	121	122	80	80	80	81	82	83	83
7	50th	93	93	95	96	97	99	99	55	56	56	57	58	58	59
	90th	106	107	108	109	111	112	113	69	70	70	71	72	72	73
	95th	110	111	112	113	115	116	116	73	74	74	75	76	76	77
	99th	117	118	119	120	122	123	124	81	81	82	82	83	84	84
8	50th	95	95	96	98	99	100	101	57	57	57	58	59	60	60
	90th	108	109	110	111	113	114	114	71	71	71	72	73	74	74
	95th	112	112	114	115	116	118	118	75	75	75	76	77	78	78
	99th	119	120	121	122	123	125	125	82	82	83	83	84	85	86
9	50th	96	97	98	100	101	102	103	58	58	58	59	60	61	61
	90th	110	110	112	113	114	116	116	72	72	72	73	74	75	75
	95th	114	114	115	117	118	119	120	76	76	76	77	78	79	79
	99th	121	121	123	124	125	127	127	83	83	84	84	85	86	87
10	50th	98	99	100	102	103	104	105	59	59	59	60	61	62	62
	90th	112	112	114	115	116	118	118	73	73	73	74	75	76	76
	95th	116	116	117	119	120	121	122	77	77	77	78	79	80	80
	99th	123	123	125	126	127	129	129	84	84	85	86	86	87	88

Table 94-2. Blood Pressure Levels for the 90th and 95th Percentiles of Blood Pressure for Girls Aged 1 Through 17 Years by Percentiles of Height[a], continued

Age (Year)	BP Percentile ↓	Systolic BP (mm Hg)							Diastolic BP (mm Hg)						
		← Percentile of Height →							← Percentile of Height →						
		5th	10th	25th	50th	75th	90th	95th	5th	10th	25th	50th	75th	90th	95th
11	50th	100	101	102	103	105	106	107	60	60	60	61	62	63	63
	90th	114	114	116	117	118	119	120	74	74	74	75	76	77	77
	95th	118	118	119	121	122	123	124	78	78	78	79	80	81	81
	99th	125	125	126	128	129	130	131	85	85	86	87	87	88	89
12	50th	102	103	104	105	107	108	109	61	61	61	62	63	64	64
	90th	116	116	117	119	120	121	122	75	75	75	76	77	78	78
	95th	119	120	121	123	124	125	126	79	79	79	80	81	82	82
	99th	127	127	128	130	131	132	133	86	86	87	88	88	89	90
13	50th	104	105	106	107	109	110	110	62	62	62	63	64	65	65
	90th	117	118	119	121	122	123	124	76	76	76	77	78	79	79
	95th	121	122	123	124	126	127	128	80	80	80	81	82	83	83
	99th	128	129	130	132	133	134	135	87	87	88	89	89	90	91
14	50th	106	106	107	109	110	111	112	63	63	63	64	65	66	66
	90th	119	120	121	122	124	125	125	77	77	77	78	79	80	80
	95th	123	123	125	126	127	129	129	81	81	81	82	83	84	84
	99th	130	131	132	133	135	136	136	88	88	89	90	90	91	92
15	50th	107	108	109	110	111	113	113	64	64	64	65	66	67	67
	90th	120	121	122	123	125	126	127	78	78	78	79	80	81	81
	95th	124	125	126	127	129	130	131	82	82	82	83	84	85	85
	99th	131	132	133	134	136	137	138	89	89	90	91	91	92	93
16	50th	108	108	110	111	112	114	114	64	64	65	66	66	67	68
	90th	121	122	123	124	126	127	128	78	78	79	80	81	81	82
	95th	125	126	127	128	130	131	132	82	82	83	84	85	85	86
	99th	132	133	134	135	137	138	139	90	90	90	91	92	93	93
17	50th	108	109	110	111	113	114	115	64	65	65	66	67	67	68
	90th	122	122	123	125	126	127	128	78	79	79	80	81	81	82
	95th	125	126	127	129	130	131	132	82	83	83	84	85	85	86
	99th	133	133	134	136	137	138	139	90	90	91	91	92	93	93

Abbreviation: BP, blood pressure.

[a] The 90th percentile is 1.28 SD, 95th percentile is 1.645 SD, and the 99th percentile is 2.326 SD over the mean.

 Dx **Hypertension**

- Blood pressure (BP) elevated above the 95th percentile for age, gender, and height on at least 3 consecutive occasions with the child in a quiet, non-apprehensive state and with BP cuff of appropriate size
- Blood pressure checked in both upper and at least one lower extremity
- Fundus examination: vascular changes, exudates, and papilledema
- Abnormal urinalysis

argument that obesity contributes to hypertension. There also seems to be strong associations between sleep-disordered breathing, sleep apnea, and hypertension.

Recent knowledge from ambulatory BP (ABP) monitoring has contributed significantly to the understanding of hypertension in children by revealing different BP responses under different clinical settings. Ambulatory BP involves using a continuous monitor, such as is done when children have a Holter monitor to detect episodic cardiac arrhythmias. The device particularly assesses changes in BP during sleep and notes whether an individual has dips ("dipper") or no dips ("non-dipper"). The apparatus is somewhat cumbersome, the study is costly, and sleep may be disturbed by the cuff inflation, thereby influencing the results.

Table 94-3. Definitions of Hypertension

Term	Definition
Normal BP	Systolic and diastolic BPs <90th percentile for age, gender, and height
Prehypertension	Average systolic or average diastolic BP between 90th and 95th percentiles for age, gender, and height
	Any BP >120/80 mm Hg regardless of age
Stage 1 hypertension	Average systolic or average diastolic BPs ≥95th percentile to 5 mm above 99th percentile for age, gender, and height with measurements obtained on at least 3 occasions
Stage 2 hypertension	Average systolic or diastolic BP >5 mm above the 99th percentile for age, gender, and height

From National High Blood Pressure Education Program Working Group on High Blood Pressure in Children and Adolescents. The fourth report on the diagnosis, evaluation, and treatment of high blood pressure in children and adolescents. *Pediatrics.* 2004;114(Suppl 2):555–576.

There are 2 different situations in which casual BP measurements in the office setting can significantly differ from ABP or home BP readings: when office BP readings are higher, which is known as white coat hypertension, and when they are lower, which is called masked hypertension. The prevalence and long-term significance of these 2 types of hypertension is still unclear. White coat hypertension is usually considered a benign finding. Some studies, however, show significant association between white coat hypertension and increased left ventricular mass index, but long-term cardiac outcome has not been studied in this population yet. Children with masked hypertension are twice as likely to have a family history of hypertension. If they also have a high pulse rate and BMI, their risk of developing cardiovascular disorders is increased. It is a significant challenge for pediatricians to diagnose these 2 conditions, particularly masked hypertension, in which BP is increased only when away from the usual office or clinic settings. These findings also raise a question about which children need home BP or ABP monitoring to detect these conditions. In the future, we may better understand white coat and masked hypertension and whether there are long-term sequelae of these conditions. Table 94-4 lists diagnostic criteria for normal blood pressure, white coat hypertension, and masked hypertension using an ABP monitor.

Secondary hypertension is more likely to exist in very young children with hypertension, those who meet the criteria for stage 2 hypertension, and those with systemic symptoms of hypertension. The etiology of secondary hypertension varies with the age of the patient and nature of the hypertension (ie, whether the condition is acute or chronic). Renal abnormalities account for 70% to 80% of secondary hypertension in children. The pathogenesis of the hypertension may be related to an increase in extracellular fluid volume (eg, acute glomerulonephritis, chronic renal failure), an increase in renin-angiotensin 2 activity (eg, renal artery stenosis, renin-producing tumor, pheochromocytoma, reflux nephropathy), or a combination of both mechanisms (eg, a patient with chronic renal failure caused by reflux nephropathy). Also, in young children, hypertension may rarely be caused by disorders with a single gene mutation which affects different pathways related to renal sodium handling.

Differential Diagnosis

A reasonable effort should be made to identify the cause of hypertension in all young children who are diagnosed with hypertension because only 30% of them are likely to have essential hypertension. In older children and adolescents with mildly elevated BPs, essential hypertension is the most likely diagnosis but must remain a diagnosis of exclusion (prevalence will vary depending on the type of institution, eg, primary care vs tertiary care vs quaternary care centers). The cause of hypertension is often obvious from a detailed history, complete examination, and simple laboratory tests. However, extensive evaluation is sometimes necessary to determine the etiology of hypertension, especially in cases of genetic disorders or renovascular causes. There are nonsystem-based, miscellaneous causes of hypertension that may be encountered and should be part of the differential diagnosis (boxes 94-1 and 94-2).

Table 94-4. Staging Scheme for Ambulatory Blood Pressure Levels in Children

Staging	Clinic BP[a]	Mean Ambulatory Systolic BP[b]	Systolic BP Load (%)
Normal BP	<95th percentile	<95th percentile	<25
White coat hypertension	>95th percentile	<95th percentile	<25
Masked hypertension	<95th percentile	>95th percentile	>25
High normal BP	>95th percentile	<95th percentile	25–50
Ambulatory hypertension	>95th percentile	>95th percentile	25–50
Severe ambulatory hypertension (at risk for end-organ damage)	>95th percentile	>95th percentile	>50

Abbreviation: BP, blood pressure.

[a] Based on National High Blood Pressure Education Program Working Group on High Blood Pressure in Children and Adolescents. The fourth report on the diagnosis, evaluation, and treatment of high blood pressure in children and adolescents. *Pediatrics.* 2004;114(Suppl 2):555–576.

[b] Based on normative ambulatory blood pressure monitor data adapted from Flynn J, Ingelfinger J, Portman R, eds. *Pediatric Hypertension.* 3rd ed. New York, NY: Humana Press; 2013.

Box 94-1. Causes of Acute or Intermittent Increases in Blood Pressure in Children

Renal Causes
- Acute glomerulonephritis
- Hemolytic uremic syndrome
- Henoch-Schönlein purpura nephritis
- Renal trauma
- Renal artery or vein thrombosis
- After renal biopsy
- Acute obstructive uropathy
- Post-genitourinary surgery
- Blood transfusions in patients with renal failure
- After kidney transplant or with transplant rejection

Drug-Induced Causes
- Corticosteroids
- Amphetamine overdose
- Phencyclidine overdose
- Cocaine overdose
- Anabolic steroids
- Oral contraceptives
- Excessive erythropoietin use in patients with end-stage renal disease
- Cyclosporine A and tacrolimus

Central Nervous System Causes
- Increased intracranial pressure (eg, subdural hematoma, meningitis, tumors)
- Encephalitis
- Poliomyelitis
- Guillain-Barré syndrome
- Porphyria
- Familial dysautonomia

Miscellaneous Causes
- Wrong blood pressure cuff size
- Anxiety, apprehension (white coat hypertension)
- Pain
- Fractures
- Immobilization
- Orthopedic procedures (especially leg lengthening and those requiring traction)
- Abdominal wall defect
- Burns
- Leukemia
- Stevens-Johnson syndrome
- Bacterial endocarditis
- Hypernatremia
- Hypercalcemia
- Heavy metal poisoning

Box 94-2. Causes of Chronic Hypertension in Children

Renal
- Scarred kidney: due to pyelonephritis or vesicoureteral reflux nephropathy
- Chronic glomerulonephritis
- Connective tissue disease: systemic lupus erythematosus, Henoch-Schönlein purpura
- Hydronephrosis
- Congenital dysplastic kidneys, polycystic kidney
- Polycystic kidney disease
- Solitary renal cyst
- Tumors: Wilms, hemangiopericytoma (renin-producing)

Renal Vascular Lesions
- Renal artery stenosis (fibromuscular dysplasia)
- Renal artery thrombosis (especially in the newborn following umbilical artery catheterization)
- Renal vein thrombosis
- Renal artery lesions with neurofibromatosis, tuberous sclerosis

Other Vascular Lesions
- Coarctation of aorta: thoracic, abdominal
- Polyarteritis nodosa and other vasculitides

Endocrine
- Corticosteroid treatment
- Neuroblastoma or other neural crest tumors
- Pheochromocytoma
- Congenital adrenal hyperplasia with 11-β- or 17-α-hydroxylase deficiency
- 11-β-hydroxysteroid dehydrogenase deficiency
- Liddle syndrome
- Primary aldosteronism
- Dexamethasone-suppressible aldosteronism
- Hyperthyroidism
- Hyperparathyroidism
- Cushing syndrome

Central Nervous System
- Intracranial hemorrhage
- Intracranial mass
- Sleep apnea/disordered breathing

Essential (Primary) Hypertension

Evaluation

When a child is identified as having an elevated BP on any occasion, the finding should be verified with at least 2 additional measurements. The physician should also verify that an appropriately sized cuff is being used to take the measurements and that efforts have been made to put the child at ease. Many children develop mild increases of BP (which can extend into the hypertensive range) when they visit a doctor's office because of anxiety or apprehension (white coat hypertension). Sometimes 24-hour ABP readings are necessary to confirm whether hypertension is present. An isolated finding of a mild increase in BP with normal subsequent readings does not indicate hypertension. Once hypertension is confirmed, a detailed history, complete physical examination, and appropriate laboratory evaluation should be performed.

As stated earlier, ABP monitoring may be indicated in the evaluation of hypertension in select children in whom BP readings are consistently increased in the physician's office but the history suggests severe anxiety associated with the visit. Ambulatory BP monitoring may also help in identifying masked hypertension or a prehypertensive state in children by detecting the usual nocturnal dips in BP. Because ABP monitoring is expensive, home BP monitoring twice a day in adults has been shown to be as effective as ABP monitoring and it is currently used by many practitioners. Therefore, home or school BP monitoring should be considered as an alternative by pediatricians who have no access to ABP devices.

History

Information should be obtained about the child's symptoms that may be associated with hypertension, such as headaches and visual difficulties (Questions Box). Inquiry should also be made about the child's history of renal disease, especially previous UTIs, unexplained fevers during infancy and early childhood, edema, hematuria, enuresis or nocturia, duration of gestation, birth weight, and use of umbilical artery catheterization during the newborn period. Information about the child's physical growth; BP recordings during previous physical examinations; eating habits, especially salt intake; use of drugs, especially illicit drugs; and the family's history of hypertension and renal disease should be obtained.

Physical Examination

A thorough examination is essential for determining the etiology of hypertension and the extent of target organ damage caused by hypertension. Poor physical growth or short stature may indicate the presence of an underlying condition, such as Turner syndrome or chronic renal disease with or without renal failure; it may also be the consequence of long-standing severe hypertension alone. Fundus examination is essential to determine if hypertension has been severe and chronic leading to arterial changes, exudate, hemorrhages, or papilledema. Tachycardia may signify heart failure or thyrotoxicosis. The child's pulses should be felt in the upper and lower extremities, and BP should be measured in all 4 extremities to evaluate for coarctation of the aorta and other vascular lesions. A heart murmur may also be present in patients with coarctation of the aorta. Some patients may present in heart failure secondary to chronic severe hypertension or renal disease with fluid retention. The abdomen should be carefully examined for presence of masses caused by cystic kidneys, Wilms tumor, or neuroblastoma and for tenderness, especially in the costovertebral angle. Bruits sometimes may be heard anteriorly, over the lower portions of left or right upper quadrants. in patients with renal artery stenosis. Presence of café au lait or depigmented spots on the skin may signify hypertension secondary to neurofibromatosis or tuberous sclerosis, respectively.

Laboratory Tests

The extent of laboratory evaluation depends on clinical findings, nature of the hypertension (eg, stage 1 or stage 2, acute or chronic), and whether an etiology is apparent or obscure. This can be done in 3 different phases to minimize unnecessary cost and discomfort to patients. Box 94-3 outlines suggested laboratory workups for patients with stage 1 or stage 2 hypertension.

Presence of hematuria, heavy proteinuria, pyuria, or elevated blood urea nitrogen or plasma creatinine would clearly imply a renal disorder as the cause of hypertension and require an appropriate renal evaluation. A kidney biopsy should be performed to diagnose glomerulonephritis, and radiographic investigations, such as ultrasound and nuclear medicine scans, can help identify scarred kidneys, hydronephrosis, cystic kidneys, or tumors.

The presence of electrolyte abnormalities, such as hypokalemia, hypochloremia, or metabolic alkalosis, would indicate the presence of an increased mineralocorticoid hormone on a primary basis (eg, primary aldosteronism, glucocorticoid remediable aldosteronism, adrenogenital syndrome with 11-β- or 17-α-hydroxylase deficiency, Liddle syndrome, 11-β-hydroxysteroid dehydrogenase deficiency, apparent mineralocorticoid excess) (see Box 94-3) or secondary basis to increased renin activity in renovascular hypertension, renin-producing tumor, or reflux nephropathy; these values would also indicate a need to measure plasma renin activity and urinary or plasma aldosterone levels. Endocrine-based causes of hypertension in children are uncommon, and tests like plasma or urinary fractionated metanephrines and catecholamines, plasma cortisol, thyroid-stimulating hormone, and triiodothyronine are measured on an individual basis depending on the clinical evaluation of the patient to rule out neuroendocrine tumors, Cushing syndrome or disease, or hyperthyroidism, respectively.

Imaging Studies

Although electrocardiograms and chest radiographs are often requested to evaluate the effects of hypertension on the heart, in most instances they are normal until the patient enters the late stages of severe hypertension. Echocardiography is now the recommended primary tool for assessing for the presence of target organ damage and, according to the AAP guidelines, is included as part of the initial evaluation of patients with hypertension. In several studies, LVH is present even in children with untreated mild, white coat, or

---

Questions

Hypertension

- Does the child have any symptoms associated with hypertension (eg, headache, dizziness, nosebleed, visual difficulty, shortness of breath)?
- Have blood pressure readings been taken during previous routine physical examinations?
- Has the child had any hematuria, generalized swelling of the body (edema), enuresis (nocturia), burning urination, previous urinary tract infection, or other kidney problems?
- How much salt does the child take? Does he or she love to put extra salt on most foods and frequently like to eat salty foods?
- How has the child been growing?
- Is there a history of use of illicit drugs or oral contraceptives?
- Is there a family history of hypertension or renal disease?

Box 94-3. Laboratory and Radiologic Evaluation of Hypertension

Phase 1: Initial Evaluation (to identify common causes of hypertension and evaluate for cardiac end-organ damage)

1. Urinalysis (urine culture if indicated)
2. Complete blood cell count, serum electrolytes, blood urea nitrogen, and creatinine; lipid profile for obese patients
3. Urine toxicology screening in adolescent children
4. Echocardiography

Phase 2: More Extensive Evaluation (to rule out rare causes of hypertension)

1. Liver profile, calcium, phosphorus, and PTH
2. Plasma renin activity and plasma aldosterone, cortisol, and TSH
3. Plasma fractionated catecholamines and metanephrines
4. Twenty-four–hour urine for creatinine, catecholamines, metanephrines, VMA, HVA, and aldosterone (if plasma aldosterone is high)
5. Renal Doppler ultrasonography
6. Enalapril- or captopril-enhanced iodine-131 mertiatide renal scan
7. Renal arteriography (selective if necessary)

Phase 3: Identify Specific Etiologies (studies done mostly by specialists)

1. Diuretic renal scan, DMSA scan, or voiding nuclear cystogram
2. Renal biopsy
3. Specific imaging studies, including nuclear scan to rule out pheochromocytoma or neuroblastoma
4. Other endocrine, neurology, or cardiology studies

Abbreviations: DMSA, 99mTc dimercaptosuccinic acid; HVA, homovanillic acid; PTH, parathyroid hormone; TSH, thyroid stimulating hormone; VMA, vanillylmandelic acid.

---

masked hypertension, especially when they are overweight. Newer recommendations also include obtaining sleep studies in overweight patients to evaluate for obstructive sleep apnea, which can contribute to the development of hypertension and LVH. Evidence suggests that with appropriate treatment to improve sleep apnea, BP normalizes and end-organ damage is prevented.

If the history, physical examination, and initial investigation do not reveal the etiology of severe hypertension in a young child, renovascular disease should be investigated with a renal Doppler ultrasound, enalapril- or captopril-enhanced iodine-131 mertiatide renal scan, renal vein renin measurements, or selective renal arteriography (sometimes magnetic resonance imaging angiography may be used as a substitute) (see Box 94-3). However, in a patient with suspected renal artery narrowing, interventional renal angiography is the gold standard that can be done not only for diagnostic evaluation but also for therapeutic purposes if these patients require angioplasty or stent placement during the study.

Gene Studies

Gene studies can be done in very rare situations in which a very young child presents with clinical features suggesting a single gene-related condition. Such tests are available only through research laboratories at this time. If the gene study result is positive, it will help rule in a disorder, but if negative, it will not determine other potential genetic defects that involve the same pathway.

Management

As previously stated, an effort should be made to identify a remediable cause in all children diagnosed with hypertension so that an appropriate medical or surgical treatment can be offered.

Patients with stage 1 hypertension can be initially managed with non-pharmacologic measures unless the patient is symptomatic or has significant cardiovascular risk factors, such as diabetes or hyperlipidemia, and a strong family history of hypertension, stroke, or myocardial infarction at a young age. These strategies include supportive care, reduction in sodium intake to about 80 to l00 mEq/day, weight reduction if the child is obese, and biofeedback. The 2004 report also recommends treating obstructive sleep apnea if present. If after a 3- to 6-month observation period BP remains persistently elevated, drug treatment should be initiated and a decision should be made whether the child needs a more thorough laboratory evaluation. Drug therapy may begin with a β-blocker (eg, atenolol), a calcium channel blocker (eg, amlodipine, isradipine), an angiotensin-converting enzyme (ACE) inhibitor (eg, enalapril), an angiotensin 2 blocker (eg, losartan), or a diuretic (eg, hydrochlorothiazide). A child can have more than one risk factor that becomes important when instituting a treatment plan. For example, an obese child with a family history of hypertension may also have chronic kidney disease as well as other risk factors contributing to the development of hypertension or end-organ damage. Therefore, management should be targeted not only toward aggressive control of BP using medications appropriate for a patient with kidney disease but also recommendations for weight reduction, dietary modifications, and increased physical activity. If a patient smokes cigarettes, cessation of smoking is essential as well.

Patients with stage 2 hypertension may require combination therapy or the use of additional drugs, such as α-blockers (eg, prazosin), combined α-β–blockers (eg, labetalol), peripheral vasodilators (eg, hydralazine, minoxidil), or centrally acting drugs (eg, clonidine). The use of one or more of these drugs controls the BP in most patients within a satisfactory range and has a limited number of side effects. Patients with renal artery stenosis can be successfully treated with balloon dilatation of the stenosis or placing a stent. If this procedure is unsuccessful or restenosis occurs, surgical correction of the stenosis is usually successful.

Hypertensive emergencies require immediate and rapid intervention with intravenous (IV) medications such as labetalol, nicardipine, or sodium nitroprusside. Hypertensive urgencies may be treated initially with the mentioned IV medications, oral labetalol, or an ACE inhibitor. In both cases, the aim is to lower the BP by about 20% to 25% of the presenting values in the first 8 hours. Over the following days to weeks, BP can gradually be controlled to come within normal values for age.

Prognosis

The long-term outcome of hypertension in children depends on the underlying etiology. In children with severe hypertension, BP control improves growth and overall well-being. The very long-term

(40–50 years) prognosis for children with persistent, mild essential hypertension is largely unknown; however, adequate BP control should prolong life and reduce cardiovascular, CNS, renal, and retinal morbidity. In untreated or poorly controlled hypertension, the prognosis is poor, especially in combination with obesity and hyperlipidemia, where hypertension is linked with severe cardiovascular morbidity and mortality in adults.

Prevention

While there are no specific predictors for the development of hypertension later in life, it is likely that early childhood health plays a role. Children who are small at birth and undergo rapid catch-up growth seem to have a higher incidence of obesity and hypertension later in life, while breastfed infants have a slower catch-up rate and subsequently have lower rates of hypertension as adults. As a result, it has been postulated that encouraging breastfeeding may have a protective effect. In addition, limiting intake of sodium and caffeine may reduce rates of hypertension in adolescents. Of course, programs aimed at preventing childhood obesity will likely prevent hypertension as well.

CASE RESOLUTION

Because of the elevated blood pressure (BP) and evidence of end-organ dysfunction such as left ventricular hypertrophy (LVH) or focal neurologic deficit, the case presented is a clear-cut stage 2 essential hypertension. However, a possibility of renal artery thrombosis or stenosis secondary to umbilical artery catheter should be taken into consideration. First, dietary modifications (diet low in refined sugar and sodium) and increase in physical activity should be addressed. Because the patient has evidence of LVH and early changes of retinopathy, there is need to initiate appropriate antihypertensive medication to control the BP. A calcium channel blocker or β-blocker can be an initial choice. A renal Doppler ultrasound is an appropriate initial test that can help to determine kidney size, extent of kidney damage, and blood flow to the kidneys.

Selected References

Collins RT, Alpert BS. Pre-hypertension and hypertension in pediatrics: don't let the statistics hide the pathology. *J Pediatr.* 2009;155(2):165–169

Constantine E, Linakis J. The assessment and management of hypertensive emergencies and urgencies in children. *Pediatr Emerg Care.* 2005;21(6):391–397

Dionne JM, Abitbol CL, Flynn JT. Hypertension in infancy: diagnosis, management and outcome. *Pediatr Nephrol.* 2012;27(1):17–32

Falkner B. Hypertension in children and adolescent: epidemiology and natural history. *Pediatr Nephrol.* 2010;25(7):1219–1224

Flynn J. Hypertension in childhood and adolescence. In: Kaplan NM, ed. *Clinical Hypertension.* 9th ed. Philadelphia, PA: Lippincott, Williams & Wilkins; 2006:465–485

Garin EH, Araya CE. Treatment of systemic hypertension in children and adolescents. *Curr Opin Pediatr.* 2009;21(5):600–604

Graettinger WF, Lipson JL, Cheung DG, Weber MA. Validation of portable noninvasive blood pressure monitoring devices: comparisons with intra-arterial and sphygmomanometer measurements. *Am Heart J.* 1988;116(4):1155–1160

Grinsell MM, Norwood VF. At the bottom of the differential diagnosis list: unusual causes of pediatric hypertension. *Pediatr Nephrol.* 2009;24(11):2137–2146

Harshfield GA, Alpert BS, Pulliam DA, Somes GW, Wilson DK. Ambulatory blood pressure recordings in children and adolescents. *Pediatrics.* 1994;94(2 pt 1):180–184

Lande MB, Meagher CC, Fisher SG, Belani P, Wang H, Rashid M. Left ventricular mass index in children with white coat hypertension. *J Pediatr.* 2008;153(1):50–54

Moyer VA; US Preventive Services Task Force. Screening for primary hypertension in children and adolescents: US Preventive Services Task Force recommendation statement. *Pediatrics.* 2013;132(5):907–914

National High Blood Pressure Education Program Working Group on High Blood Pressure in Children and Adolescents. The fourth report on the diagnosis, evaluation, and treatment of high blood pressure in children and adolescents. *Pediatrics.* 2004;114(Suppl 2):555–576

Sorof JM, Lai D, Turner J, Poffenbarger T, Portman RJ. Overweight, ethnicity, and the prevalence of hypertension in school-aged children. *Pediatrics.* 2004;113(3 Pt 1):475–482

SECTION VII

Genitourinary Disorders

CHAPTER 95

Ambiguous Genitalia

Jennifer K. Yee, MD, and Catherine S. Mao, MD

CASE STUDY

A term neonate is being evaluated in the newborn nursery. The mother received prenatal care from the eighth week of gestation, reportedly had no problems during the pregnancy, and took no medications except prenatal vitamins with iron. She specifically denies taking any progesterone-containing drugs. Her previous pregnancy was uneventful, and her 3-year-old son is healthy.

On physical examination, the newborn is active and alert, with normal vital signs. Aside from a minimum amount of breast tissue bilaterally, the physical examination is unremarkable, except for the genitalia. The labioscrotal folds are swollen bilaterally with slight hyperpigmentation and mild rugae. No masses are palpable in the labioscrotal folds. The clitoris/phallus is 1.5 cm in length. Labioscrotal fusion is present, with a very small opening at the anterior aspect. The urethra cannot be visualized.

Questions

1. What conditions should be considered in newborns with ambiguous genitalia?
2. What should families of such newborns be told about the gender of the newborns?
3. What key historical information should be obtained from families of such newborns?
4. What laboratory studies must be obtained to aid in the diagnosis?
5. What psychosocial issues should be addressed with families while neonates are in the newborn nursery?

Ambiguous genitalia result from disorders of sex development (DSD) in newborns and are classified according to chromosomal status and gonads present. This standard classification, using newer nomenclature with previously used nomenclature in parentheses, includes 46,XX DSD (female pseudohermaphroditism) and 46,XY DSD (male pseudohermaphroditism), ovotesticular DSD (true hermaphroditism), and 46,XX testicular DSD or 46,XY gonadal dysgenesis (complete or mixed gonadal dysgenesis). Gonadal dysgenesis in 45,X and 46,XX individuals do not present with ambiguous genitalia but are also classified as DSD.

A multidisciplinary health care team should be involved in the care of newborns with ambiguous genitalia. In addition to the general pediatrician, nurses, social workers, neonatologists, pediatric endocrinologists, geneticists, and surgeons are all significant members of the team. The role of primary care physicians, however, cannot be underestimated because they are always involved in the initial evaluations of the newborns and often have already established relationships with the families.

Epidemiology

The prevalence of ambiguous genitalia in newborns is approximately 1 in 3,000 to 4,000 live births. 46,XX DSD is characterized by female chromosomes (46,XX), normal ovaries and müllerian structures, and virilized external genitalia. The most common DSD, 46,XX DSD is most often caused by congenital adrenal hyperplasia (CAH). Neonatal screening studies suggest that the incidence of CAH is 1 in 5,000 to 15,000.

46,XY DSD occurs in genetic males (46,XY) who have testes but insufficient masculinization of the external genitalia. This disorder most commonly results from androgen insensitivity. Ovotesticular DSD is a rare condition in which ovarian and testicular tissues are present. Seventy percent to 80% of affected individuals have the 46,XX karyotype, and the morphology of the external genitalia varies widely.

46,XY gonadal dysgenesis is characterized by ambiguous genitalia or a female phenotype with a normal XY karyotype. Affected neonates may have a specific gene abnormality that leads to abnormal testicular development and often streak gonads. Reports indicate that this condition is the second most common form of ambiguous genitalia. When affected newborns have chromosomal mosaicism (45,X/46,XY), it is considered to be mixed gonadal dysgenesis.

Clinical Presentation

Variability in the phenotypic as well as clinical presentation of these disorders is considerable (D_x Box). The newborn with ambiguous genitalia may have an enlarged clitoris or small phallus and varying degrees of labioscrotal fusion. Signs of virilization in the female newborn might include hyperpigmented labia and presence of labial rugae. Other findings suggestive of 46,XX DSD are perineal hypospadias or an inguinal hernia. More dramatic presentations, such as severe dehydration and shock in a neonate, are associated with CAH of the salt-wasting form. Females with gonadal dysgenesis often present in adolescence with primary amenorrhea (see Chapter 102). Turner syndrome (45,XO) is a common cause of gonadal dysgenesis and may present with additional clinical features, but 46XX "pure" gonadal dysgenesis is a distinct entity.

Dx **Ambiguous Genitalia**

- Indeterminate or ambiguous genitalia
- Enlarged clitoris or small phallus
- Hyperpigmented, rugated labia majora that may be fused
- Blind-ending or completely absent vaginal pouch
- Phenotypic male neonate with hypospadias or bilateral cryptorchidism
- Phenotypic female neonate with an inguinal hernia or mass

Pathophysiology

To appropriately evaluate and interpret laboratory results of neonates with ambiguous genitalia, it is important to understand the physiology of sexual differentiation and how deviations from this process lead to DSD.

Normal Sexual Differentiation

Normally, before embryos are 6 weeks old, undifferentiated bilateral gonads into which germ cells migrate from the yolk sac have developed. Wolffian and müllerian duct systems are present at this time, making the embryonic gonads of males and females indistinguishable.

If a Y chromosome is present, a testes-determining factor (known as the sex-determining region of the Y chromosome [SRY]) induces differentiation of these gonads into testes by stimulating *SOX9* (SRY-related gene) expression in the gonads, thus blocking female development. This process involves the formation of seminiferous tubules that surround the germ cells. Leydig cells begin to produce testosterone, which in turn acts on the wolffian duct to result in male internal genitalia: vas deferens, epididymis, and seminal vesicles. Concurrently, *SOX9* acts with steroidogenic factor 1, leading to regression of the müllerian ducts secondary to Sertoli cell production of anti-müllerian hormone (AMH; also called müllerian-inhibiting substance). For normal male external genitalia to form, testosterone must be converted to dihydrotestosterone (DHT) via 5-α-reductase. Dihydrotestosterone then combines with a specific androgen receptor, which allows formation of the phallus and scrotum from the previously undifferentiated external genitalia. The process primarily involves growth and fusion. Later in gestation, the testes migrate into the scrotum.

For the undifferentiated gonads to develop into female organs, the Y chromosome must be absent and 2 intact and normal functioning X chromosomes must be present. Because androgens are not produced and there is no AMH, the wolffian duct degenerates and the müllerian duct develops into the internal female structures—fallopian tubes, uterus, and upper vagina. Fusion of undifferentiated external genitalia does not occur in the absence of DHT, so folds and swellings become the labia and the genital tubercle becomes the clitoris. Female differentiation was previously believed to be the default development in the absence of SRY, but recent studies support the existence of female determining factors as well.

Development of Ambiguous Genitalia

Congenital adrenal hyperplasia is the most common cause of virilization of the female and is an autosomal recessively inherited defect. Congenital adrenal hyperplasia is the result of an enzymatic deficiency in the pathway for synthesis of cortisol and aldosterone from cholesterol. The most common of these enzymatic defects is 21-α-hydroxylase deficiency. Other less common defects are 11-β-hydroxylase deficiency and 3-β-hydroxysteroid dehydrogenase deficiency. Lipoid adrenal hyperplasia results from a defect in the steroidogenic acute regulatory protein (StAR) enzyme that transports cholesterol across the mitochondrial membrane for steroid synthesis. A recently identified rare form of CAH is P 450 oxidoreductase deficiency, which can be associated with Antley-Bixler syndrome. Prenatally, circulating levels of androgens are abnormally high from the overproduction of precursors in the steroid synthesis pathways. Hence, the external genitalia of the fetus, which are controlled by androgens, are virilized in the female. Internal female organs, however, are normal because their development is not influenced by androgens. Males may exhibit hyperpigmentation and rugosity but otherwise have normal external genitalia.

The salt-wasting form of 21-α-hydroxylase deficiency is found in approximately two-thirds of patients with classic CAH. As a result of low levels of aldosterone, sodium resorption in the renal tubules is reduced, leading to hyponatremia and hyperkalemia. If this salt-wasting condition goes undiagnosed and untreated, shock and death may result in the first few weeks of life. Newborn screening programs are currently in place in all 50 United States. These programs screen for elevated 17-α-hydroxyprogesterone, targeting identification of patients with 21-α-hydroxylase deficiency, and are less sensitive for detection of neonates with 11-β-hydroxylase deficiency and 3-β-hydroxysteroid dehydrogenase deficiency.

46,XY DSD is secondary to insufficient testosterone production or insensitivity at the cellular level. Androgen insensitivity, the most common cause of this disorder, is the result of an abnormality or a reduction in the number of androgen receptors. Not all affected individuals present with ambiguous genitalia at birth because the spectrum of sensitivity is broad. If the androgen receptor is completely nonfunctional or absent, the external genitalia are those of a normal female (complete testicular feminization). When there is partial function of the androgen receptor, genital ambiguity does occur. This is an X-linked condition so that only 46,XY individuals are affected, but 46,XX females are carriers and pass the mutation to their offspring.

Other causes of 46,XY DSD are inadequate testosterone production secondary to low levels of fetal gonadotropins; defects in testosterone synthesis from enzyme deficiencies or disruption of electron transport; failure to convert testosterone to DHT as a result of 5-α-reductase deficiency; deficient müllerian duct–inhibiting substance, which can be autosomal recessive or X-linked recessive; and intrauterine loss of both testes secondary to torsion or another prenatal event. Causes of testosterone deficiency resulting in 46,XY DSD include CAH due to defects of StAR, P 450 scc, 3-β-hydroxysteroid dehydrogenase, 17-α-hydroxylase, and P 450 oxidoreductase.

While SRY is the considered to be the sex-determining region, defects in SRY explain only approximately 15% of XY gonadal dysgenesis. A loss of function mutation in *SOX9* results in camptomelic dysplasia with XY sex reversal. More recently, an abnormality of a gonad-specific regulatory region of *SOX9* resulted in isolated XY gonadal dysgenesis. Steroidogenic factor 1 mutations have been estimated to account for up to 13% of XY gonadal dysgenesis.

Although most causes of ambiguous genitalia are related to chromosomal abnormalities and inherited enzymatic defects, exogenous sources of hormones can affect the differentiation of sexual organs. In most cases, the effect is minimal and no ambiguity develops. Masculinized female external genitalia can occur, however, depending on the timing and duration of prenatal exposure to androgens or other virilizing drugs. Currently the most commonly used androgens are probably anabolic steroids. A neonate may even be exposed prenatally through transdermal passage to the mother from a family member using androgen creams. An adrenal tumor or poorly controlled CAH in the mother will also lead to virilization of the female fetus. The progestin in birth control pills do not have sufficient androgen action to cause a problem.

Differential Diagnosis

The differential diagnosis of ambiguous genitalia depends on the classification of the DSD (Table 95-1). Some causes of this condition can be life-threatening and therefore must be recognized immediately (eg, salt-wasting CAH).

Table 95-1. Classification and Causes of Ambiguous Genitalia in the Newborn	
Disorder	*Causes*
46,XX DSD	Congenital adrenal hyperplasia
	Maternal androgen ingestion
	Maternal virilizing hormones
	Idiopathic, associated with dysmorphic syndromes
46,XY DSD	Biochemical defects in testosterone biosynthesis (enzyme deficiencies)
	Androgen insensitivity (complete or partial receptor defects)
	5-α-reductase deficiency
	Persistent müllerian duct syndrome
	Gonadotropic failure
	Dysgenetic testes
	Bilateral vanishing testes syndrome
	Idiopathic, associated with dysmorphic syndromes
Ovotesticular DSD	Chimerism
46,XX testicular DSD or 46,XY complete gonadal dysgenesis	Chromosomal mosaicism

Abbreviation: DSD, disorders of sex development.

Evaluation

History

The general obstetric history should be reviewed, although it may not be helpful in all cases. Probably the most important source of information on family history can be derived from family pedigrees (Questions Box). The mother of affected newborns should be interviewed thoroughly for any clinical findings that might suggest the mother as the source of androgens. Undiagnosed chromosomal disorders, consanguinity, and recurrent medical conditions may be established or inferred from the family background.

Physical Examination

A complete physical examination of newborns must be performed in the nursery, in addition to a detailed assessment of genitalia. In particular, the presence of dysmorphic features (eg, microcephaly, low-set ears, micrognathia), which suggests the presence of a chromosomal abnormality, should be appreciated. The areola should be examined for any evidence of hyperpigmentation, and the inguinal area should be palpated for any masses or hernias.

A thorough genital examination should then be performed. The appearance and size of the labioscrotal folds should be noted in terms of pigmentation, presence of rugae, and size. Physicians should keep in mind that normal female labia majora may not completely cover the labia minora and that the labia may be extremely underdeveloped in premature newborns. Practitioners should determine whether any masses are palpable in what appear to be the labia and whether the testes are palpable in what appears to be the scrotum. The size of the phallus/clitoris should be measured; in term neonates, a normal stretched phallus is at least 2.5 cm long, whereas a normal clitoris should not exceed 1 cm. The labioscrotal folds should then be spread apart to look for a vaginal introitus. The presence of posterior labioscrotal fusion, which may preclude this, confirms the

Questions

Ambiguous Genitalia

- Did the mother take any medications containing estrogen, progestational agents, or androgens during the pregnancy? Did she use any other virilizing drugs, such as danazol, during pregnancy?
- Was the mother in contact with anyone using hormonal creams or gels?
- Does the mother have poorly controlled congenital adrenal hyperplasia or an adrenal tumor? Does the mother have any virilizing symptoms that suggest she should undergo an evaluation for these conditions?
- What is the mother's prior obstetric history?
- Did she have any problems with any previous pregnancies?
- Is there a history of any unexplained neonatal deaths, particularly in male offspring?
- Are her other children growing and developing normally?
- Is there a family history of ambiguous genitalia, including microphallus, hypospadias, and cryptorchidism?
- Is there a family history of sterility, female hirsutism, or amenorrhea?
- Are the parents or other family members consanguineous?

suspicion of indeterminate genitalia. The clitoral index (product of clitoral transverse and sagittal dimensions) and the anogenital distance can be determined by an experienced clinician. Limited data on these measurements in normal children are available in the literature. Finally, the location of a urethral meatus should be noted because if hypospadias and cryptorchidism occur together, the chance of DSD is approximately 50%. A rectal examination may help detect the presence of a uterus or prostate but may be difficult.

Laboratory Tests

The most important study to obtain is a karyotype, which can be performed in 24 to 48 hours by many laboratories. Examination of Barr bodies in a buccal smear is not recommended because this test is unreliable. In addition, serum electrolytes should be ordered in the nursery and monitored closely if CAH is suspected. A serum 17-α-hydroxyprogesterone level is mandatory in evaluation for CAH. Other intermediate metabolites, such as 11-deoxycortisol, androstenedione, dehydroepiandrosterone sulfate, and sex steroids (ie, testosterone and DHT) can also be measured to evaluate for androgen excess or deficiency. Measurement of 17-ketosteroids and pregnanetriol in the urine may provide supportive data in newborns with ambiguous genitalia, especially in newborns whose gonads are not palpable.

A human chorionic gonadotropin stimulation test may be performed to measure response in testosterone production if ovotesticular DSD is suspected.

Imaging Studies

Pelvic ultrasonography is effective in determining if müllerian structures are present, but this technique is not as useful for locating the gonads. If the gonads are not palpable, magnetic resonance imaging of the pelvis may be considered. Genitography can aid in visualizing the duct structures under fluoroscopy.

Management

An interdisciplinary team consisting of a pediatrician, pediatric endocrinologist, medical geneticist, urologist, social worker, and psychologist or psychiatrist should be involved in the care of newborns with ambiguous genitalia. All aspects of treatment can then be addressed in an efficient and comprehensive manner. A consensus statement on management of infants with DSD and proposed ethical guidelines for management are available (see Selected References).

Initial Phase: Delivery Room and Newborn Nursery

If the gender of the newborn is uncertain, it should not be assigned in the delivery room. Parents and nursing staff should be notified immediately of the ambiguity, and a unisex name should be assigned, such as "Baby Smith" instead of "Baby Boy Smith" or "Baby Girl Smith." Hospital nameplates should also reflect a gender-neutral status in wording and color. Physicians should congratulate the parents on the birth of their child, then inform them of the genital

ambiguity. Physicians should then reassure parents that they will determine the baby's gender as soon as possible but that additional tests would be necessary to find out. Parents should be encouraged not to speculate on the gender of the newborn in the meantime.

During the initial hours after birth, parents may have difficulty comprehending the condition. An open line of communication must be maintained with the family, even while waiting for test results. Parents should be assured that gender assignment will be made as soon as possible and that more information will follow with test results. Gender assignment can potentially be made within 3 to 5 days or even earlier in some institutions because most preliminary laboratory results are reported in 24 to 48 hours. However, some cases may require more extensive workup, such as a trial of testosterone in partial androgen insensitivity, so gender assignment in these neonates may take more time. The interval of time to gender assignment, therefore, must be individualized. Necessary radiographic studies should be ordered as soon as possible.

Intermediate Phase: Psychologic Issues

Several psychologic issues should be addressed at the time of diagnosis. Alleviation of parental anxiety about the cause of the condition should be the priority; general questions can also be answered. For example, parents may be unclear about what to tell others about the gender of the newborn and find this process very awkward. In addition, parents should be educated about normal sexual differentiation. Pediatricians must emphasize that during the first 6 to 8 weeks of gestation, sexual organs are undifferentiated. Ambiguous genitalia should be explained as overdevelopment or underdevelopment rather than as "freaky" or highly unusual. For parental perspective, genital ambiguity can be compared with another type of birth defect, such as a cardiac septal defect.

Primary care physicians must also assess parents' level of sophistication and their cultural and religious beliefs about gender identity and sexuality. The gender preference for newborns should be addressed. Were the parents hoping for a boy or girl? Do they feel strongly about one gender? The medical team can also help families establish a plan for newborns as to what they want to tell the extended family and in what detail they want to disclose information. After the initial meeting and while awaiting laboratory data, other questions about sexual orientation, puberty, fertility, and self-esteem may arise.

Final Phase: Gender Assignment

After the karyotype is confirmed and the type of DSD has been considered, team members should meet with families to discuss gender assignment before discharge from the hospital. Traditionally, gender assignment was based on size of the phallus, potential response to androgen stimulation, and potential for fertility. More recently, additional factors have been recognized as important in gender assignment, including in utero brain exposure to androgens and likely adult gender identity, quality of sexual function with or without surgery, and psychosocial risk for patient and family in the event of gender dysphoria. Parents must be involved in this decision and must agree with the final outcome. Some investigators strongly believe that gender reassignment and genital surgery should be discussed with the patient at a later date rather than assigned during the neonatal period. Such an approach involves consistent counseling for the patient, open discussion among the family, and a primary care physician willing to work diligently with the patient and family. Support groups should also be offered regardless of the decision about gender reassignment.

Detailed information should be given once again about the origin of the condition. The timing and nature of any future hormonal treatment and surgical procedures should be addressed as well. Parents should be urged to move beyond the issue of ambiguous genitalia once a decision about gender has been made. They must then deal with activities such as birth announcements and inquiries about gender from extended family, siblings, and babysitters. The entire medical team should offer parents encouragement concerning their parenting ability.

Treatment

Hormone replacement therapy is indicated for some newborns with ambiguous genitalia. Cortisol replacement is mandatory in newborns with CAH at daily physiologic doses of 10 to 20 mg/m^2. In newborns with salt-wasting or classic 21-α-hydroxylase deficiency, mineralocorticoid replacement is indicated. Oral fludrocortisone should be administered at doses that suppress plasma renin activity to normal levels without causing hypertension.

Testosterone or estrogen replacement is needed at puberty in disorders in which the gonads failed to develop or were surgically removed. For disorders involving micropenis, injections of testosterone enanthate at regular intervals may be used to increase the length and width of the phallus. Recombinant human growth hormone replacement may also be considered for short stature in mixed gonadal dysgenesis.

Surgical procedures may be necessary in many cases but can be done later in infancy. In partial androgen insensitivity, surgery may be deferred until later in life because of the high rate of gender dysphoria known to occur among these patients. Although laparoscopy or laparotomy may be indicated for a gonadal biopsy, this is generally not needed in the neonatal period for gender assignment. A gonadectomy is indicated prophylactically in all phenotypic females with all or part of a Y chromosome because of the potential for malignant conversion of gonadoblastoma. Clitoral reduction and recession, vaginoplasty, and labioscrotal reduction are usually performed if newborns are to be raised as females. For those to be raised as males, orchiopexy, hypospadias repair, and chordee release are often indicated, but these surgical procedures may be difficult. In some specific cases, however, surgical procedures should be delayed until response to medical treatment is evaluated. For example, in CAH, clitoral size may decrease with glucocorticoid replacement.

Psychologic support for the patient and family will be necessary during the child's growth and development into adulthood. Issues revolving around gender identity, gender role, and sexual orientation require ongoing discussion with the patient and parents. Gender dissatisfaction may occur later in life.

Prognosis

The prognosis for most newborns with ambiguous genitalia is excellent. Problems arise with undiagnosed CAH, which may lead to shock and death in the neonatal period if unrecognized and untreated. Otherwise, children should be able to live long, healthy lives once their families have accepted the diagnosis. Amenorrhea in females and sterility in males or females will need to be addressed during adolescence, at which time psychologic services should be provided.

CASE RESOLUTION

In the case described at the beginning of the chapter, the newborn has ambiguous genitalia. The parents should be informed immediately of this finding, and all references related to gender should be avoided. A karyotype and 17-α-hydroxy-progesterone analyses should be performed immediately. In addition, serial serum electrolytes should be performed starting at 12 to 24 hours of life. The physician should then meet with the family to further discuss disorders of sex development and explain the diagnostic workup. General psychologic services and information about support groups should also be provided.

Selected References

Baxter RM, Vilain E. Translational genetics for diagnosis of human disorders of sex development. *Annu Rev Genomics Hum Genet*. 2013;14:371–392

Creighton S, Chernausek SD, Romao R, Ransley P, Salle JP. Timing and nature of reconstructive surgery for disorders of sex development - introduction. *J Pediatr Urol*. 2012;8(6):602–610

Houk CP, Lee PA. Update on disorders of sex development. *Curr Opin Endocrinol Diabetes Obes*. 2012;19(1):28–32

Hughes IA, Nihoul-Fékété C, Thomas B, Cohen-Kettenis PT. Consequences of the ESPE/LWPES guidelines for diagnosis and treatment of disorders of sex development. *Best Pract Res Clin Endocrinol Metab*. 2007;21(3):351–365

Köhler B, Kleinemeier E, Lux A, et al. Satisfaction with genital surgery and sexual life of adults with XY disorders of sex development: results from the German clinical evaluation study. *J Clin Endocrinol Metab*. 2012; 97(2):577–588

Krone N, Dhir V, Ivison HE, Arlt W. Congenital adrenal hyperplasia and P450 oxidoreductase deficiency. *Clin Endocrinol (Oxf)*. 2007;66(2):162–172

Lee P, Schober J, Nordernström A, et al. Review of recent outcome data of disorders of sex development (DSD): emphasis on surgical and sexual outcomes. *J Pediatr Urol*. 2012;8(6):611–615

Lee PA, Houk CP, Ahmed SF, Hughes IA; International Consensus Conference on Intersex organized by the Lawson Wilkins Pediatric Endocrine Society and the European Society for Paediatric Endocrinology. Consensus statement on management of intersex disorders. International Consensus Conference on Intersex. *Pediatrics*. 2006;118(2):e488–e500

Mieszczak J, Houk CP, Lee PA. Assignment of the sex of rearing in the neonate with a disorder of sex development. *Curr Opin Pediatr*. 2009;21(4):541–547

Ogilvy-Stuart AL, Brain CE. Early assessment of ambiguous genitalia. *Arch Dis Child*. 2004;89(5):401–407

Ottolenghi C, Pelosi E, Tran J, et al. Loss of Wnt4 and Foxl2 leads to female-to-male sex reversal extending to germ cells. *Hum Mol Genet.* 2007;16(23):2795–2804

Sane K, Pescovitz OH. The clitoral index: a determination of clitoral size in normal girls and in girls with abnormal sexual development. *J Pediatr.* 1992; 120(2 Pt 1):264–266

Verkauskas G, Jaubert F, Lortat-Jacob S, Malan V, Thibaud E, Nihoul-Fékété C. The long-term followup of 33 cases of true hermaphroditism: a 40-year experience with conservative gonadal surgery. *J Urol.* 2007;177(2):726–731

Vidal I, Gorduza DB, Haraux E, et al. Surgical options in disorders of sex development (DSD) with ambiguous genitalia. *Best Pract Res Clin Endocrinol Metab.* 2010;24(2):311–324

Wiesemann C, Ude-Koeller S, Sinnecker GH, Thyen U. Ethical principles and recommendations for the medical management of differences of sex development (DSD)/intersex in children and adolescents. *Eur J Pediatr.* 2010;169(6): 671–679

CHAPTER 96

Inguinal Lumps and Bumps

Julie E. Noble, MD

CASE STUDY

A 2-month-old boy presents to your office for evaluation of a lump in his right groin for 1-week duration. The lump has been coming and going, and his mother notices that it is larger when he cries. Today, the lump is prominent, and the infant seems fussy. He has been crying more often and vomited once today. His history is remarkable for having been born at 32 weeks' gestation by spontaneous vaginal delivery. Birth weight was 1,500 g, and he did well in the nursery with no respiratory complications. He was sent home at 4 weeks of age and has had no other medical problems. He breastfeeds well and has normal stools.

Physical examination reveals a well-nourished, irritable infant in no acute distress. His vital signs demonstrate mild tachycardia and temperature to 100°F (37.8°C). His abdomen is soft, and the genitourinary examination is significant for a swelling in the right inguinal area that extends into his scrotum. The mass is mildly tender and cannot be reduced. The rest of the examination is normal.

Questions

1. What are the possible causes of inguinal masses?
2. How does age affect the diagnostic possibilities?
3. How do you differentiate between acute and non-acute conditions?
4. What diagnostic modalities can help with the diagnosis?
5. What are the treatment choices for inguinal masses?
6. Are there long-term consequences?

Inguinal masses occur from disease in normal tissue in the inguinal area or from ectopic tissue, frequently of embryologic origin. A child may present with the chief complaint of an inguinal mass, and the mass may vary in position from anywhere along the inguinal canal to the scrotum or labia (Figure 96-1). Along the inguinal canal, a mass might be an enlarged **lymph node,** a **retractile testis,** an **ovary,** or a **synovial cyst.** At the inguinal ring, a mass might also be a testis or an ovary, or an inguinal hernia. In the scrotum, swelling could be due to a **hernia, hydrocele, varicocele, trauma,** or **testicular pathology.** Labial lesions could be secondary to trauma, an **ectopic ovary, mixed gonadal tissue,** an actual testis as in testicular feminization, or a **Bartholin gland cyst.** The differential diagnosis and subsequent evaluation will vary not only according to the location of the mass and the patient's age but also with the acuity of presentation of the mass.

Epidemiology

Inguinal masses are a fairly frequent complaint in the office setting. The usual cause is an enlarged lymph node, but **hernias and hydroceles** are also common. Surgical repair of hernias and hydroceles are the most common surgical procedures performed in children. The incidence of inguinal hernias has been estimated at 1 to 4 per 100 live births. There is a 60% risk of incarceration in the first 6 months of life. For this reason, surgical correction is recommended early. Hernias are present on the right side in 60% of cases, on the left in 30%, and bilateral in 10%. Of affected children, males outnumber females 4:1. Femoral and direct hernias are more common in girls. Certain conditions are associated with a higher incidence of hernias (Box 96-1). The most significant predisposing factor is prematurity, with hernias reported in 30% of newborns weighing less than 1,000 g at birth.

The other common acute scrotal lesions—**testicular torsion** and **torsion of the appendix testis**—have an incidence of 1:160 in males. Testicular torsion may even occur in utero, but the peak incidence of testicular torsion occurs in the perinatal period and again at puberty. Torsion of the appendix testis is most likely to occur between ages 7

Figure 96-1. The inguinal area.

- Internal inguinal ring
- External inguinal ring
- Testes
- Scrotum

Box 96-1. Conditions Associated With Hernias	
• Abdominal wall defect	• Low birth weight
• Ascites	• Mucopolysaccharidosis
• Connective tissue disease	• Prematurity
• Cystic fibrosis	• Undescended testis
• Family history	• Urologic malformations

and 10 years. **Varicoceles** occur in pubertal and postpubertal males, with a fairly high incidence of up to 15%. **Testicular tumors** are rare in childhood; they occur at an incidence of 0.5 to 2.0 per 100,000 children and account for only 1% of all pediatric solid tumors. But in adolescence, testicular cancer is the most common cause of cancer in young males and may affect as many as 1 in 10,000.

Clinical Presentation

The child with an inguinal mass presents acutely or non-acutely. In the acute presentation, the swelling occurs rapidly and is associated with pain. There may be systemic symptoms of nausea and vomiting. Inguinal pathology should be suspected in any child with abdominal pain. The involved area may be extremely tender. Nonacute masses appear more slowly. Some may be present from birth. They may come and go, especially with crying or straining. Nonacute masses usually are not tender and are not associated with systemic symptoms (D_x Box).

Pathophysiology

Pathophysiological developmental features of an inguinal mass vary depending on the cause of the mass. An enlarged lymph node may result from proliferation of intrinsic lymphocytes or inflammatory infiltrate from infection (lymphadenitis). The etiology of lymphadenopathy is extensive (see Chapter 88). Any of these processes can appear in the inguinal nodes. An enlarged node can also be secondary to metastatic infiltration from another cell line and represent tumor spread.

Dx Inguinal Masses

Acute
- Rapid onset
- Painful
- Tender
- Nausea and vomiting
- Fever
- Overlying skin red
- Cremasteric reflex absent

Non-acute
- Slower onset
- Not painful
- May fluctuate in size
- Cremasteric reflex present

A hydrocele develops secondary to failure of obliteration of the patent processus vaginalis during embryologic development. During the 27th to 28th weeks of gestation, the testicle, gubernaculum, and processus vaginalis descend from the peritoneum through the inguinal canal into the scrotum. The processus vaginalis begins closing prior to birth and attaches to the testis, forming the tunica vaginalis testis. The closure is complete by 1 to 2 years of age. Failure of closure results in a hydrocele (a peritoneal connection with fluid) or a hernia, with intra-abdominal contents. Either may bulge into the inguinal canal and scrotum. If the hernia cannot be reduced and abdominal contents are at risk for vascular compromise, the hernia is termed *incarcerated*. This condition is a surgical emergency.

Sometimes a parent may misinterpret a normal testicle in the process of descent as an abnormal mass. A delay in the normal descent process of the testis occurs occasionally, and the testicle may not be in the scrotum at the time of birth. Torsion of the testis after it has reached the scrotum can occur in the newborn if the testis twists on the spermatic cord. Similarly, the testicle can also twist in the pubertal period on its own vasculature within the tunica vaginalis. This is frequently secondary to a high attachment of the tunica vaginalis to the spermatic cord, allowing the testis to hang freely, like a bell clapper. Both types of torsion cause vasculature compromise and an ischemic testis.

Likewise, a vestigial remnant called the appendix testis can twist, resulting in vascular compromise of that localized part of the testis.

Pathologically, a traumatic scrotal mass is usually a hematoma, although testicular rupture may occur if the tunica albuginea is torn as a result of trauma. Testicular neoplasms in prepubertal children tend to be germ cell tumors. Yolk sac tumors, teratomas, and mixed germ cell tumors with infiltration of their respective cell lines are the usual diseases found.

A varicocele, another scrotal mass, is caused by increased pressure within the venous drainage of the testicle with subsequent dilatation of the veins, producing a mass. Because of the anatomy of the venous drainage, 90% of varicoceles occur on the left side.

Infections of the epididymis or testis can cause an inflammatory infiltrate and swelling. In the female, infection of Bartholin gland in the labia creates an abscess and leads to an acute, painful mass.

Differential Diagnosis

Location, acuity, and patient age aid in establishing the differential diagnosis.

Non-acute masses, which have a slow onset and are not painful, include lymphadenopathy, a retractile testis, hydrocele, hernia, varicocele, tumor, and ectopic ovary.

Acute masses that have a sudden onset and are associated with pain include epididymitis, orchitis, testicular torsion, traumatic hematoma, torsion of the appendix testis, lymphadenitis, and incarcerated hernia (Box 96-2).

Skin changes can mimic an acute scrotal mass. Henoch-Schönlein purpura, a vasculitis of unclear etiology, can develop in the scrotal area. Scrotal edema can also occur acutely.

Box 96-2. Differential Diagnosis of Inguinal Masses

Non-acute	*Acute*
• Ectopic ovary	• Bartholin abscess
• Hernia	• Epididymitis
• Hydrocele	• Henoch-Schönlein purpura
• Lymphadenopathy	• Idiopathic scrotal swelling
• Retractile testis	• Incarcerated hernia
• Synovial cyst	• Lymphadenitis
• Testicular tumor	• Orchitis
• Varicocele	• Testicular torsion
• Venous aneurysm	• Torsion of appendix testis
	• Trauma

Testicular torsion occurs most commonly in the newborn period and again at puberty. Incarcerated hernias are seen most often in the first 6 months of life. Varicoceles are noted almost always at adolescence and are located in the upper left area of the scrotum. Testicular tumors are also much more common in adolescence.

The gender of the patient will influence the differential diagnosis of the lesion as well as the workup.

Evaluation

History

A thorough, focused history will help define the differential diagnosis (Questions Box). Inquiring about systemic symptoms should always be included and, if positive, may suggest a more generalized process such as a tumor or systemic infection. Symptoms of dysuria would point to epididymitis or orchitis. A history of trauma or possible sexual abuse should always be sought. Hernias and testicular torsion may have a family history positive for the same condition.

Physical Examination

A complete physical examination should always be performed in assessing any pediatric complaint. Evidence of diffuse adenopathy may be present. With an inguinal mass, a concentrated, thorough

Questions

Inguinal Masses

- How long has the mass been present?
- Is it painful?
- Does it come and go?
- Was there a history of trauma?
- Does the child have dysuria?
- Is there fever or vomiting?
- Are there any other masses?
- Has the child had any lower extremity infections?
- Is there a history of renal disease?
- Is there a history of preterm delivery?
- Is there a positive family history?

examination of the inguinal area and lower extremity is needed. A lower extremity lesion may indicate a reactive adenopathy. If the mass is not apparent on inspection and it comes and goes, ask the parent to point to its location. Observe the skin for evidence of erythema, swelling, or bruising. Gently palpate the inguinal canal to see if you can feel a mass, then assess the scrotal or labial area. If the mass is of acute onset, observe the scrotum and try to localize the tenderness. An incarcerated hernia, testicular torsion, torsion of the appendix testis, epididymitis, and orchitis are extremely tender. If there is torsion of the appendix testis, there may be a classic blue dot at the upper pole of the testis. Try to elicit a cremasteric reflex. If present, it virtually eliminates testicular torsion. If the testis has a horizontal lie, it may indicate a bell clapper type of abnormal fixation. The pain of epididymitis and orchitis is relieved partially when the testis is elevated (Prehn sign). Transilluminating the mass may be helpful. A fluid-filled mass, such as a hydrocele, will definitely transilluminate; incarcerated bowel may also transilluminate.

Any mass should be accurately measured. Evaluating the borders of an inguinal mass is important. A hydrocele does not extend into the inguinal canal; therefore, the top border can be felt below the pubis. A hernia will extend into the inguinal canal, so an upper border will not be apparent. Reduction of any hernia with gentle pressure should be attempted. To detect a hernia that is not readily apparent, causing the infant to cry increases intra-abdominal pressure and may demonstrate the hernia. An older child should be asked to stand and cough while the inguinal canal is palpated. A varicocele, which feels like a bag of worms, is a non-tender mass over the spermatic cord and is readily palpated if the teen is in a standing position.

Laboratory Tests

Laboratory tests should be directed toward the most likely diagnosis as determined by the history and physical examination.

If an infection is suspected, a complete blood cell count (CBC) should be obtained. If the infection is thought to be epididymitis or orchitis, a urinalysis and urine culture, along with tests for gonorrhea and chlamydia, should also be obtained. If lymphadenopathy is suspected, a CBC, mononucleosis test, cat-scratch disease test, and possible biopsy may be necessary. An inguinal mass in a female may be a normal testes, and chromosomal evaluation may be indicated to diagnose a disorder of sexual differentiation (see Chapter 95). If a tumor is suspected, the α-fetoprotein level, which is elevated in 90% of yolk sac tumors, and β-human chorionic gonadotropin should be assayed.

Imaging Studies

Ultrasound can be helpful in defining inguinal masses and is the best test to define scrotal contents. It can be useful in differentiating between a hydrocele or hernia and enlarged lymph nodes where a characteristic central echolucent area can be seen. It gives accurate information in evaluating tumors. Ultrasound is the imaging test of choice and can provide information in identifying a mass as ovarian or testicular because the ovary is smaller and more echogenic and may have follicular cysts. Color Doppler ultrasonography is the most accurate test in evaluating the scrotum when symptoms are acute to identify a testicular fracture and also assess blood flow in testicular torsion but has a longer time frame and may not be practical in the acute setting. Nuclear imaging may be possible but also has a long time frame. If incarceration of a hernia is suspected, a flat plate radiograph of the abdomen is helpful to detect signs of intestinal obstruction. Computed tomography and magnetic resonance imaging are only moderately effective in evaluations and generally not recommended.

Management

Many inguinal masses require surgical treatment. Acute symptoms involving the scrotum present a surgical emergency. There may not be time to perform diagnostic studies. If there is a high probability of a testicular torsion, the scrotum should be surgically explored immediately. Surgery within 4 to 8 hours of symptom onset has an excellent rate of a viable testis. If surgery is beyond 8 hours, the possibility of a viable testis is progressively worse. After 48 hours it is unlikely that the testis will be salvaged. If the testis is nonviable, it is removed. Torsion of the appendix testis does not need to be explored if the diagnosis is certain.

Surgical intervention may also be indicated with scrotal trauma, which can cause torsion or testicular rupture. A urologic referral is indicated for assessment.

All hernias require surgical repair at some time. Immediate surgery is indicated for an incarcerated hernia that cannot be reduced. If it is reduced, elective surgical repair can be scheduled. There is controversy regarding the indications for surgery on the contralateral side. An infant younger than 1 year has a 20% chance of developing a hernia on the other side, and most surgeons repair both sides at the same time. Other accepted indications for exploration of the unaffected side include preterm infant, twin gestation, left-sided hernia, increased abdominal pressure, and female gender. Currently, some surgeons use laparoscopy at the time of the hernia repair to define a patent processus vaginalis on the opposite side and repair it if patency is found. Hydroceles do not have to be repaired surgically unless they persist beyond 1 year of age. This persistence implies a peritoneal connection and an impending hernia, so repair is indicated. A fracture of the testicle also dictates the need for surgical repair. Varicoceles are removed if there is significant pain, the testicle shows growth retardation, there is bilateral disease, or the teen has a solitary testis. Subinguinal microsurgical varicocelectomy can now be performed preserving lymphatic drainage. All testicular tumors are removed. Additional antitumor therapy is dependent on the stage and cell line of the tumor.

Infectious inguinal masses are treated according to the specific bacteriologic diagnosis.

Prognosis

After surgical treatment for an inguinal hernia or testicular torsion, the child generally does well. The most significant long-term complication of hernia surgery is subsequent impaired testicular function, and decreased testicular size is noted in up to 27% of cases. Damage to the vas deferens and testicular vessels may impair spermatogenesis and result in a higher incidence of impaired fertility. Surgery for testicular torsion may also be associated with subsequent infertility, particularly if an affected testis is left in place. Two-thirds of affected testicles demonstrate atrophy. If there is loss of a testis, the physician should offer a prosthesis in the future because there can be significant psychologic implications.

There is a low risk of recurrence of a hernia following repair. Increased abdominal pressure and history of incarcerated hernia predispose to recurrence with the rate being as high as 12% in children with ventriculoperitoneal shunts. A hydrocele may develop following varicocele repair.

CASE RESOLUTION

In the case presented at the beginning of the chapter, the infant's history of prematurity associated with a mass that comes and goes most likely indicates an inguinal hernia. With the additional symptoms of pain, fever, and vomiting and the findings of an inflamed, non-reducible mass on examination, there is a high likelihood that the hernia is incarcerated. The infant is taken to the operating room, where this diagnosis is confirmed. The hernia is reduced and repaired, and the intestine is noted to be viable. The contralateral side is explored and found to be normal. The infant makes an uneventful recovery.

Selected References

Adelman WP, Joffe A. Consultation with the specialist: testicular masses/cancer. *Pediatr Rev.* 2005;26(9):341–344

Cavanaugh RM Jr. Screening for genitourinary abnormalities in adolescent males. *Pediatr Rev.* 2009;30(11):431–437

Delaney LR, Karmazyn B. Ultrasound of the pediatric scrotum. *Semin Ultrasound CT MR.* 2013;34(3):248–256

Gatti JM, Murphy JP. Acute testicular disorders. *Pediatr Rev.* 2008;29(7):235–241

Haynes JH. Inguinal and scrotal disorders. *Surg Clin North Am.* 2006;86(2):371–381

Lambert SM. Pediatric urological emergencies. *Pediatr Clin North Am.* 2012;59(4):965–976

Maisonet L. Inguinal hernia. *Pediatr Rev.* 2003;24(1):34–35

Merriman LS, Herrel L, Kirsh AJ. Inguinal and genital anomalies. *Pediatr Clin North Am.* 2012;59(4):769–781

Mesrobian HG, Balcom AH, Durkee CT. Urologic problems of the neonate. *Pediatr Clin North Am.* 2004;51(4):1051–1062

Palmer LS. Pediatric urologic imaging. *Urol Clin North Am.* 2006;33(3):409–423

CHAPTER 97

Hematuria

Elaine S. Kamil, MD

CASE STUDY

A 6-year-old boy is brought to the office for a school entry examination. He was the full-term product of an uncomplicated pregnancy, labor, and delivery. Although he has had 4 or 5 episodes of otitis media, he has generally been in good health. He has never been hospitalized or experienced any significant trauma. He has no known allergies, has been fully immunized, and is developmentally normal. However, his mom reports that he has complained of occasional mild abdominal pain.

In addition, the physical examination is completely normal. The boy's height and weight are at the 75th percentile, and his blood pressure is 100/64 mm Hg. Screening tests for hearing and vision are completely normal.

The boy's hematocrit is 42. His urinalysis comes back with a specific gravity of 1.025, pH 6, 2+ blood, and trace protein. Microscopic examination shows 18 to 20 red blood cells per high-power field; 0 to 1 white blood cells per high-power field; and a rare, fine, granular cast.

Questions

1. What disease entities cause hematuria?
2. How should hematuria be evaluated?
3. How does the approach to hematuria differ in children who complain of dark or red urine?
4. What is the appropriate follow-up of children with asymptomatic microscopic hematuria?

Hematuria is a common problem in pediatrics, and primary care physicians should have a clear understanding of its pathophysiology, etiology, evaluation, and therapy. Hematuria can be caused by a serious medical problem, or it may only be an incidental finding with no potential for impairment of patients' health. In general, hematuria is categorized as gross or microscopic. The etiology and approach to hematuria vary with its severity and symptomatology. Gross hematuria is defined as red or brown urine caused by the presence of red blood cells (RBCs). Microscopic hematuria is defined as 3 or more consecutive urine samples with a positive dipstick and 6 or more RBCs per high-power field in a fresh, spun urine sample.

Epidemiology

The incidence of **gross hematuria** is about 1.3 in 1,000 patient visits (Table 97-1). In one series, the causes in about half of the patients were readily apparent from the intake history or physical examination. The incidence of gross hematuria may increase in the community during an epidemic of a disease, such as acute glomerulonephritis, a condition often associated with gross hematuria. In another series, approximately 30% of children with gross hematuria had glomerular diseases, most commonly immunoglobulin (Ig) A nephropathy. The incidence of kidney stones, another cause of hematuria, is increasing in the pediatric population.

Microscopic hematuria is a more common pediatric problem. Prevalence rates for persistent microscopic hematuria range from 0.5% to 2.0%, but 4% to 5% of school-aged children may have microscopic hematuria on a single voided specimen. The incidence is artificially increased in the summer because at that time children tend

Table 97-1. Etiology of Gross Hematuria in an Unselected Pediatric Population	
Causes	**Patients (%)**
Readily Apparent	
Documented UTI	26
Perineal irritation	11
Meatal stenosis with ulcer	7
Trauma	7
Coagulopathy	3
Stones	2
Total	56
Other	
Suspected UTI	23
Recurrent gross hematuria	5
Acute nephritis	4
Ureteropelvic junction obstruction	1
Cystic cystitis	<1
Epididymitis	<1
Tumor	<1
Unknown	9
Total	44

Abbreviation: UTI, urinary tract infection.

Modified with permission from Ingelfinger JR, Davis AE, Grupe WE. Frequency and etiology of gross hematuria in a general pediatric setting. *Pediatrics.* 1977;59(4):557–561.

to visit pediatricians for camp physicals and preparticipation sports physicals that typically include a screening urinalysis.

Clinical Presentation

Children with gross hematuria present with the sudden appearance of red or brown urine, which may be associated with flank or urethral pain or with a history of trauma.

Children with microscopic hematuria may have urinary complaints (eg, dysuria). In children who appear well, microscopic hematuria is usually detected on screening dipstick examination or on urinalysis obtained for other indications.

Pathophysiology

Gross Hematuria

Gross hematuria occurs because of the presence of large numbers of RBCs in the urine. Blood may enter the urine because of rupture of blood vessels following trauma or inflammation in the glomeruli or interstitial regions of the kidney. It may also occur as a result of severe inflammation of the bladder wall.

Causes of gross hematuria are listed in Box 97-1. The presence of casts in the urine suggests the diagnosis of glomerulonephritis. The most common causes of glomerulonephritis in children include acute postinfectious glomerulonephritis, anaphylactoid purpura, IgA nephropathy, membranoproliferative glomerulonephritis (MPGN), dense deposit disease, and systemic lupus erythematosus (SLE).

Common causes of gross hematuria in the absence of RBC casts include urinary tract infection **(UTI) from bacteria or some viruses, renal trauma, bleeding diathesis** (eg, hemophilia, idiopathic thrombocytopenic purpura), **renal tumors, obstruction of the urinary tract, renal stones, hypercalciuria,** or **hemolytic uremic syndrome (HUS).** A hemangioma in the urinary tract is an extremely rare cause of gross hematuria. In endemic areas, gross hematuria may be caused by schistosomiasis. Another rare cause of gross hematuria is nutcracker phenomenon caused by left-sided renal vein congestion from compression of the renal vein by the superior mesenteric artery. The symptoms of nutcracker phenomenon are distinctive: intermittent gross hematuria associated with left-sided flank pain that is relieved by lying down. Another cause is urethrorrhagia, with which children, typically prepubertal boys, pass bloody urine, usually at the end of their voiding and frequently accompanied by spots of blood in the underwear.

Microscopic Hematuria

Microscopic hematuria occurs when small numbers of RBCs enter the urine via tiny ruptures in the glomerular capillary walls or in the capillaries of the tubulointerstitium or bladder lining. One study showed that otherwise healthy children with microscopic hematuria had increased erythrocyte deformability, making it easier for RBCs to slip through the glomerular capillaries. For purposes of discussion, the following causes of microscopic hematuria are considered: infectious, structural, traumatic, glomerular, and interstitial.

Box 97-1. Common Causes of Gross Hematuria in Pediatric Patients

Glomerular Causes
- IgA nephropathy
- Acute post-infectious GN
- Lupus nephritis
- Membranoproliferative GN
- Dense deposit disease
- Anaphylactoid purpura GN
- Alport syndrome
- Thin basement membrane disease
- Rapidly progressive GN
- Vasculitis, ANCA positive
- Anti-glomerular basement membrane disease
- Hemolytic uremic syndrome

Hematologic Causes
- Sickle cell disease or trait or hemoglobin C
- Hemophilia
- Thrombocytopenia
- Thrombosis (renal arterial or venous)

Other
- Hypercalciuria
- Munchausen by proxy
- Urethrorrhagia

Structural Causes
- Renal trauma
- Tumor
- Obstruction
- Renal stones
- Polycystic kidney disease
- Foreign bodies

Vascular Abnormalities
- Hemangiomas
- Nutcracker phenomenon
- Arteriovenous malformations

Infectious Causes
- Bacterial urinary tract infection
- Viral cystitis
- Schistosomiasis
- Tuberculosis

Interstitial Diseases
- Acute interstitial nephritis
- Tubulointerstitial nephritis with uveitis

Abbreviations: ANCA, antineutrophil cytoplasmic autoantibody; GN, glomerulonephritis; IgA, immunoglobulin A.

Separate consideration of the causes of microscopic and gross hematuria is often helpful, although significant overlap exists. The presence of gross hematuria typically calls for a more rapid, and usually more extensive, evaluation.

Urinary tract infection is one of the most common **infectious causes** of hematuria. Bacterial infections of the bladder or kidney occur much more frequently than viral cystitis. Adenovirus is the most common viral cause of hemorrhagic cystitis and is usually associated with dysuria. Other viral causes include cytomegalovirus, parvovirus 19, and BK polyomavirus nephropathy. Vaginitis in girls and prostatitis in teenaged boys may also result in hematuria.

Any type of congenital obstructive uropathy may lead to massive dilatation of the urinary tract, which makes the urinary tract more susceptible to bleeding, even with trivial trauma. **Chronic urinary tract obstruction** in children (eg, posterior urethral valves, congenital ureteropelvic junction obstruction) is often asymptomatic. In the past, these conditions were typically diagnosed when children presented with UTIs or gross hematuria after relatively trivial trauma. Now they are commonly diagnosed after a prenatal ultrasound reveals hydronephrosis. Nevertheless, urinary tract obstruction may be detected during an evaluation for asymptomatic microscopic hematuria.

Any **tumor** of the genitourinary tract may be associated with gross and microscopic hematuria. Pelvic tumors rarely cause urinary obstruction in children, although such tumors frequently cause obstruction in adults. Children with Wilms tumor, the most common childhood renal tumor, usually present with an abdominal mass but may experience hematuria.

Congenital renal malformations are quite common. Any of these may be associated with hematuria and include polycystic kidney disease, renal dysplasia, medullary sponge kidney, and simple cysts. Patients with polycystic kidney disease may even have severe, painful hematuria.

Vascular problems may lead to hematuria. Hemangiomas of the kidney, bladder, or ureter are very rare but may bleed. Arteriovenous malformations also occur infrequently. Hematuria may be a sign of a renal artery or vein thrombosis, particularly in sick neonates.

Young children are more susceptible to **renal injury,** which may result in hematuria, than older children or adults because their kidneys are relatively less protected by the rib cage. In addition, children may insert foreign objects into the urethra and bladder that cause pain and hematuria. Microscopic hematuria has also been described after extremely vigorous exercise, such as marathon running. Child abuse or Munchausen syndrome by proxy should be considered if any suspicions are raised on the basis of the history or physical examination.

Hypercalciuria is another cause of microscopic hematuria. Children with hypercalciuria often have a family history of urinary calculi. Calcium oxalate crystals may be present on microscopic examination of the urine. A urinary calcium-creatinine ratio is best obtained on a first morning, fasting urine sample with reminders to the family that the child should empty his bladder before going to bed. Urinary calcium excretion varies with age. Normal values are listed in Table 97-2.

There are 2 types of hypercalciuria: absorptive and renal leak. Children with absorptive hypercalciuria over-absorb calcium from the gastrointestinal tract, probably because of an exquisite sensitivity to vitamin D, and can be treated with a reduced calcium diet to the recommended daily allowance for age. Children with renal leak hypercalciuria have an inherently higher rate of urinary calcium excretion and may require thiazide diuretics to reduce urinary calcium excretion. **Interstitial nephritis,** usually from drug exposure, may also cause hematuria. Generally, patients with interstitial nephritis may exhibit other signs of tubular disease, such as glycosuria, polyuria, or proteinuria.

Glomerular disease may cause gross or microscopic hematuria. Etiologies include acute or chronic glomerulonephritis, such as acute postinfectious glomerulonephritis, MPGN, dense deposit disease, antineutrophil cytoplasmic antibody–associated vasculitis, IgA nephropathy, SLE, thin basement membrane disease, and Alport syndrome. The RBCs originating from glomeruli are dysmorphic, and these patients often have RBC casts when the urine is carefully examined.

Sickle cell disease, sickle cell trait, and hemoglobin C trait have been associated with gross or microscopic hematuria.

Differential Diagnosis

When children complain of gross hematuria or red urine, practitioners must first determine if they have hematuria or pigmenturia by using a urine dipstick. If the dipstick result is negative for blood, the dark urine is due to dyes, drugs, or pigments (Table 97-3). If the dipstick is positive for blood, the red color is caused by intact RBCs, hemolyzed RBCs, hemoglobin, or myoglobin; the clarification is based on microscopic examination of fresh, spun urine.

Children whose dipstick results are positive for blood but show no RBCs may have hemoglobinuria or myoglobinuria, or the urine may have been improperly handled on the way to the laboratory. Hemoglobinuria may be seen with acute autoimmune hemolytic anemia, drug-induced hemolysis, paroxysmal nocturnal hemoglobinuria, a mismatched blood transfusion, cardiopulmonary bypass, freshwater drowning, and, in some cases, HUS. Myoglobinuria is seen in individuals with rhabdomyolysis. Acute rhabdomyolysis can

Table 97-2. Normal Values for Urinary Calcium-Creatinine Ratios[a]		
Age	**Urine Calcium-Creatinine**	**24-Hour Urine Calcium**
Preterm	≤0.82	≤8.9 mg/kg/d[b]
<7 mo	≤0.86	
7–18 mo	≤0.60	
19 mo–6 y	≤0.42	
6 y–adult	≤0.22	<4 mg/kg/d

[a]Samples for calcium-creatinine ratio should be obtained on a fasting, first-voided morning specimen. The calcium and creatinine concentrations must be in the same units (eg, milligrams per deciliter) before the ratio is calculated.
[b]For healthy preterm newborns taking no medications. Calcium excretion varies with diet and phosphorus intake and it is higher if patients are treated with furosemide, xanthines, or glucocorticoids.

Table 97-3. Distinguishing Hematuria From Pigmenturia			
Problem	**Urine Color**	**Dipstick**	**Microscopic Appearance**
Hematuria	Red, brown, or red-brown	Positive	Red blood cells
Hemoglobinuria	Red, brown, or red-brown	Positive	Negative
Myoglobinuria	Red, brown, or red-brown	Positive	Negative
Porphyrins	Red	Negative	Negative
Exogenous pigments[a]	Red or orange	Negative	Negative

[a]Some common exogenous pigments include phenytoin, beets, rifampin, nitrofurantoin, sulfas, amitriptyline, methyldopa, phenothiazine, and chloroquine.

occur after a crush injury or a very prolonged seizure and in certain susceptible individuals with an inborn error of muscle metabolism. Myoglobinuria may also be seen with the myositis associated with influenza infections. Free hemoglobin and myoglobin are toxic to the renal epithelial cells, mandating a generous fluid intake and close monitoring. Serum appears clear in myoglobinuria and pink in hemoglobinuria.

Evaluation

Gross Hematuria

History

The history is crucial to an accurate, efficient, and cost-effective evaluation of patients with hematuria (Questions Box). The family should be questioned carefully about trauma (to trunk, abdomen, or perineum), recent skin infection or pharyngitis, dysuria, and abdominal or flank pain. The presence of gross hematuria at the onset or at the end of urination is associated with bleeding from the urethra or bladder trigone. Parents should be asked whether their children appear "puffy." A family history of hematuria, kidney disease, hearing loss, SLE, bleeding diathesis, hemolytic anemia, or inborn error of muscle metabolism may be important.

Physical Examination

A complete physical examination is also essential. Blood pressure should be measured accurately. The skin should be examined thoroughly for rashes or petechiae; the abdomen should be checked carefully for renal masses or tenderness; the genitalia should be examined thoroughly for signs of trauma, masses, or rashes (see Chapter 132); and the joints should be checked carefully for signs of arthritis. Fundi should be examined for any hypertensive changes. Children should be assessed for the presence of edema. Short stature could be a sign of previously undiagnosed chronic renal insufficiency.

A careful cardiac and chest examination is necessary to detect signs of congestive heart failure (CHF), a finding sometimes seen in acute glomerulonephritis.

Laboratory Tests

Studies have shown that careful microscopic examination of a urine sample can help determine whether bleeding originates from the upper or lower urinary tract. Red blood cells originating in the glomerulus have a dysmorphic appearance. The first morning urine sample is the most reliable but is not appropriate in some settings, such as after a motor vehicle crash. Sometimes gross hematuria is so substantial that spinning the urine results in a large pellet of debris that is difficult to examine. In such instances, it is prudent to examine an unspun sample. The presence of RBC casts indicates glomerulonephritis, but the absence of such casts does not rule out this condition.

If the urine shows RBC casts or if there are other features suspicious for glomerulonephritis, the evaluation should include an antistreptolysin-O (ASO) titer, antinuclear antibody (ANA), C3, complete blood cell count (CBC) and differential with platelet count, blood urea nitrogen (BUN) and creatinine, serum albumin, and a random urine for a urinary total protein-creatinine ratio. However, RBC casts may not always be seen in glomerulonephritis.

If the urine shows only large numbers of RBCs, no RBC casts, and no bacteriuria, a CBC with differential and platelet count, urine culture, and prothrombin time (PT) and partial thromboplastin time (PTT) should be obtained. A sickle cell test should be considered as well. Hypercalciuria can be evaluated by collecting a first morning sample for calcium-creatinine ratio; a more extensive evaluation to assess risk factors for kidney stones should include a 24-hour urine for a stone risk profile that includes urinary calcium, citrate, uric acid, and oxalate.

Imaging Studies

If the urine has large numbers of RBCs, a renal ultrasound should be obtained. With gross hematuria and a history of serious trauma, an abdominal computed tomography scan should be performed. Computed tomography scan without contrast is also an excellent modality to detect kidney stones. Children with RBC casts should have a chest radiograph to evaluate for evidence of CHF. Special renal Doppler ultrasound studies are indicated if nutcracker phenomenon is being considered in the differential.

Microscopic Hematuria

The evaluation of microscopic hematuria is similar to that of gross hematuria. Figure 97-1 outlines an approach to the evaluation of microscopic hematuria.

History and Physical Examination

Because many conditions may cause gross or microscopic hematuria, the same historical questions apply to both conditions, and the same careful physical examination is indicated.

Laboratory Tests

Generally, initial evaluation includes a urine culture and a careful microscopic examination of the urine on a fresh sample. If the culture is negative, hematuria is minimal with no associated proteinuria, and children are otherwise healthy, the urinalysis should be repeated once or twice over the following 2 weeks. Red blood cell casts always signify a glomerular origin for the RBCs. Casts are best preserved in acidic, concentrated urine. Thus, the first morning urine is the best sample to examine for casts. Red blood cell morphology

---

Questions

Hematuria

- Has the child suffered any recent trauma?
- Has the child had fever or dysuria?
- Does the child have any flank or abdominal pain?
- Does the child have any rashes, joint pains, or edema?
- Does the child have a family history of hematuria, kidney disease, kidney stones, or gross hematuria?
- Is there a family history of bleeding disorders or inborn errors of muscle metabolism?

Figure 97-1. **Evaluation of asymptomatic, microscopic hematuria.** Abbreviations: ASO, antistreptolysin-O; BUN, blood urea nitrogen; CBC, complete blood cell count; PT, prothrombin time; PTT, partial thromboplastin time; RBCs, red blood cells.

should be assessed. Red blood cells originating in the glomerulus are **dysmorphic** and of smaller caliber, whereas those that come from lower downstream appear like normal **biconcave** disks. Although RBC morphology is best appreciated with the use of a polarizing microscope, with experience, dysmorphic RBCs can be recognized using an ordinary microscope. Red blood cells of glomerular origin have a mean cell volume of 50 μL or less. In contrast, RBCs of non-glomerular origin have a mean cell volume of 80 to 90 μL. The presence of a special form of dysmorphic erythrocyte, the G1 cell, is even more specific for glomerular bleeding. These cells are doughnut shaped and contain one or more blebs on their surfaces. However, the majority of urinary microscopic examinations are now being performed by machine, and urine microscopy is becoming a lost art. Many medical schools and residency programs no longer teach students how to perform urine microscopy.

Clotting ability should be determined with a platelet count, PT, and PTT. A sickle cell test should be performed. Renal function should be screened with a BUN and creatinine, and a urine calcium-creatinine ratio should be determined. A C3, ANA, and ASO titer should also be checked. If a urine dipstick shows more than a trace of protein, a urinary protein-creatinine ratio should also be determined, preferably on a first morning sample. If there is a family history of renal disease, a hearing screen should be ordered. All immediate family members should have their urine checked for blood.

If a bloody urine sample is analyzed with a Coulter counter, characteristic distribution curves are seen for glomerular and non-glomerular hematuria. This test is not readily available, however.

Imaging Studies

A renal ultrasound should be performed to rule out structural abnormalities and tumors. Chest radiographs should be obtained if acute glomerulonephritis is suspected.

Renal Biopsy

The definitive diagnosis of the etiology of hematuria may require a kidney biopsy. Generally, pediatric nephrologists perform kidney biopsies only in selected instances after ruling out non-glomerular causes for the hematuria. Indications for renal biopsy in a child with hematuria would include an associated abnormal urinary protein excretion, decreased renal function, recurrent macroscopic hematuria, persistently depressed serum complement levels, serologic evidence for SLE, positive ANCA testing, hypertension, or a family history suggestive of Alport syndrome or renal insufficiency of unknown etiology.

Glomerular Diseases Associated With Hematuria

Glomerulonephritis

Acute and chronic glomerulonephritis are associated with hematuria. The diagnosis of acute postinfectious glomerulonephritis requires a nephritic urine sediment (RBCs, RBC casts), a low serum complement, and an elevated streptococcal titer (ASO titer, antideoxyribonuclease B, or positive streptozyme). It is important to document that the serum complement returns to normal within 3 months because MPGN or dense deposit disease may present in a similar way. The serum complement is chronically depressed in MPGN and dense deposit disease.

The most common form of glomerulonephritis in children is **acute poststreptococcal glomerulonephritis.** Many cases are asymptomatic, however, and do not come to the attention of physicians. The resulting hematuria, which may be gross or microscopic, is rarely seen before the age of 2 years. The condition is most commonly diagnosed in preschool-aged and school-aged children, who typically present with gross hematuria, often with some edema and hypertension. The hypertension may be severe, and occasionally children even have hypertensive seizures. The edema results from transient, acute renal failure with salt and fluid retention.

Most children with acute poststreptococcal glomerulonephritis recover completely and have an excellent long-term prognosis. Proteinuria is rarely severe enough to cause nephrotic syndrome, and renal failure is rarely serious enough to require dialysis. If hypertension occurs, the chest radiograph often shows some degree of pulmonary edema, even in the absence of overt clinical signs of CHF. Any hypertension requires treatment. Other infections cause postinfectious glomerulonephritis, but they are less common and overall less well characterized.

The most common form of chronic glomerulonephritis that affects children is **IgA nephropathy.** On kidney biopsy, patients have mesangial proliferation with mesangial deposits of IgA as the dominant Ig. In later stages, glomerulosclerosis and interstitial fibrosis are apparent. More than one-third of adults with IgA nephropathy develop end-stage renal disease; the percentage of children who progress to this point is less well known. Gross hematuria in IgA nephropathy is occasionally so severe that patients may pass clots and have flank pain. The presence of persistent proteinuria is considered a poor prognostic sign.

Other forms of primary chronic glomerulonephritis include **MPGN, dense deposit disease, mesangial proliferative glomerulonephritis,** and **membranous nephropathy,** which is technically not a form of glomerulonephritis because it usually lacks a significant proliferative component. Children with these diseases present with hematuria almost always associated with heavy proteinuria.

Secondary forms of glomerulonephritis include the nephritis of SLE, anaphylactoid purpura, and nephritis associated with various vasculitides such as Wegener granulomatosis and pauci-immune crescentic glomerulonephritis (ANCA-positive glomerulonephritis). An ANCA panel is indicated in children with glomerulonephritis and decreased renal function. Children with lupus tend to present with multisystem disease but may have only renal manifestations of the disease. Antinuclear antibody is a good screening test for lupus. If the ANA is positive, C3, C4, anti–double-stranded DNA, and an antiglobulin (Coombs) test should be checked.

Anaphylactoid Purpura

Anaphylactoid purpura, also called Henoch-Schönlein purpura, is almost always accompanied by the classic cutaneous vasculitis rash, which is prominent over the lower arms and lower extremities. Abdominal pain may be severe, and affected patients are at risk for the development of intussusception. Children with anaphylactoid purpura have microscopic hematuria, which usually clears over time but is occasionally associated with heavy proteinuria and nephrotic syndrome. Children with associated proteinuria are at risk for developing progressive renal disease. All children with anaphylactoid purpura should have their urine monitored for cessation of hematuria or development of proteinuria. Children with heavy proteinuria and suspected anaphylactoid purpura should have a diagnostic renal biopsy.

Hemolytic Uremic Syndrome

Hemolytic uremic syndrome is a disease characterized by thrombotic thrombocytopenic purpura, thrombocytopenia, and acute renal failure. It typically follows a prodrome of bloody diarrhea from acute colitis caused by a verotoxin-producing strain of *Escherichia coli* (O157:H7), among others, or other enteropathogenic bacteria. The verotoxin is toxic to human endothelial cells. The damaged endothelial cells incite the deposition of fibrin within the glomerular capillaries. These fibrin thrombi lead to the shearing of RBCs and consumption of platelets. Several other organisms, such as pneumococcus and *Shigella,* may precipitate HUS. In atypical cases of HUS, the precipitating event may be an upper respiratory infection. Some cases of atypical HUS are familial. Children present with pallor and severe abdominal pain. Urine output may be diminished as a result of renal failure, and in many cases dialysis is required. Hypertension may be severe.

Other Glomerular Diseases

Alport syndrome, thin basement membrane disease (benign familial hematuria), focal segmental glomerulosclerosis (FSGS), and minimal change disease (MCD) are also associated with hematuria. Alport syndrome is a disease in which thinning and duplication of the glomerular basement membranes occur. The renal involvement eventually leads to end-stage renal disease in males (less commonly in females). Patients or their family members often have nerve deafness or keratoconus. The inheritance of Alport syndrome varies by kindred; it may be autosomal-dominant, autosomal-recessive, or X-linked. The X-linked inheritance is by far the most common mode of inheritance, with female carriers being much less severely affected than affected males. Thin basement membrane disease also is characterized by thinning of the glomerular basement membrane, but the glomeruli are otherwise normal, and the clinical course is usually benign. Patients with MCD and FSGS typically present with nephrotic syndrome but may also have microscopic hematuria.

Management

Gross Hematuria

The management of gross hematuria depends on the underlying cause. Children with a history of trauma should be placed on bed rest pending surgical consultation (see Chapter 65). If the evaluation indicates acute glomerulonephritis and if children are not hypertensive, they can be followed carefully as outpatients with monitoring of blood pressure and renal function with consultation with a pediatric nephrologist. Children with coagulopathies require specific treatment of their bleeding disorders (eg, intravenous gamma globulin for idiopathic thrombocytopenic purpura). If kidney stones are found, after the acute episode has passed, children should have an evaluation for stone risk factors.

If some degree of renal insufficiency is present, children should promptly be referred to a pediatric nephrologist to rule out more unusual causes of glomerulonephritis, for consideration of renal biopsy, and for treatment.

Microscopic Hematuria

Laboratory test results other than urinalysis may be negative in otherwise healthy children with microscopic hematuria. Some of these children may be recovering from subclinical cases of postinfectious glomerulonephritis, which can cause microscopic hematuria for up to 1 year. Others may have early IgA nephropathy and not yet have significant proteinuria, and some may have thin basement membrane disease or Alport syndrome. As long as children have normal renal function, normal urinary calcium excretion, normal blood pressure, a negative renal ultrasound, no significant proteinuria, and all other tests are normal, it is safe to monitor them every 3 to 6 months until the problem resolves. Healthy children with an otherwise negative workup who show no change in their clinical state for a period of 1 year may subsequently be monitored annually. If hypercalciuria is detected, a low-calcium diet or treatment with thiazide diuretics may be tried. Increased urinary microalbuminuria has been shown to be predictive of glomerular lesions in children with isolated microscopic hematuria.

Prognosis

The prognosis for children with hematuria depends on the underlying cause. Gross hematuria is more often associated with serious renal disease, such as acute glomerulonephritis, HUS, or renal trauma. Even so, most children with gross hematuria have a good prognosis, provided the diagnosis is rapidly discovered and appropriate specific therapy is given. Children with persistent microscopic hematuria who have no family history of the condition, have a negative evaluation, and do not develop hypertension or proteinuria have an excellent long-term prognosis, though a recent study has shown a small but significantly increased incidence of end-stage kidney disease over 22 years in 16- to 25-year-olds with persistent asymptomatic isolated microscopic hematuria.

CASE RESOLUTION

The boy in the opening scenario shows no worrisome clinical signs, such as hypertension or significant proteinuria. His urine should be rechecked twice more, and if the hematuria persists, his evaluation should follow the algorithm in Figure 97-1.

Selected References

Adams ND, Rowe JC. Nephrocalcinosis. In: Bailie MD, ed. *Clinics in Perinatology.* Philadelphia, PA: WB Saunders; 1992:179–195

Assadi FK. Value of urinary excretion of microalbumin in predicting glomerular lesions in children with isolated microscopic hematuria. *Pediatr Nephrol.* 2005;20(8):1131–1135

Bergstein J, Leiser J, Andreoli S. The clinical significance of asymptomatic gross and microscopic hematuria in children. *Arch Pediatr Adolesc Med.* 2005;159(4):353–355

Greenfield SP, Williot P, Kaplan D. Gross hematuria in children: a ten-year review. *Urology.* 2007;69(1):166–169

Hoppe B, Kemper MJ. Diagnostic examination of the child with urolithiasis and nephrocalcinosis. *Pediatr Nephrol.* 2010;25(3):403–413

Ingelfinger JR, Davis AE, Grupe WE. Frequency and etiology of gross hematuria in a general pediatric setting. *Pediatrics.* 1977;59(4):557–561

Kashtan CE. Alport syndrome and thin glomerular basement membrane disease. *J Am Soc Nephrol.* 1998;9(9):1736–1750

Lettgen B, Wohlmuth A. Validity of G1-cells in the differentiation between glomerular and non-glomerular haematuria in children. *Pediatr Nephrol.* 1995;9(4):435–437

Meglic A, Kuzman D, Jazbec J, Japelj-Pavesić B, Kendra RB. Erythrocyte deformability and microhematuria in children and adolescents. *Pediatr Nephrol.* 2003;18(2):127–132

Pan CG. Evaluation of gross hematuria. *Pediatr Clin North Am.* 2006;53(3):401–412

Patel HP, Bissler JJ. Hematuria in children. *Pediatr Clin North Am.* 2001;48(6):1519–1537

Piqueras AI, White RH, Raafat F, Moghal N, Milford DV. Renal biopsy diagnosis in children presenting with haematuria. *Pediatr Nephrol.* 1998;12(5):386–391

Sargent JD, Stukel TA, Kresel J, Klein RZ. Normal values for random urinary calcium to creatinine ratios in infancy. *J Pediatr.* 1993;123(3):393–397

Savige J, Rana K, Tonna S, Buzza M, Dagher H, Wang YY. Thin basement membrane nephropathy. *Kidney Int.* 2003;64(4):1169–1178

Tsukahara H, Yoshimoto M, Morikawa K, Okada T, Kuroda M, Sudo M. Urinary erythrocyte volume analysis: a simple method for localizing the site of hematuria in pediatric patients. *J Pediatr.* 1989;115(3):433–436

Vivante A, Afek A, Frenkel-Nir Y, et al. Persistent asymptomatic isolated microscopic hematuria in Israeli adolescents and young adults and risk for end-stage renal disease. *JAMA.* 2011;306(7):729–736

Walker BR, Ellison ED, Snow BW, Cartwright PC. The natural history of idiopathic urethrorrhagia in boys. *J Urol.* 2001;166(1):231–232

Youn T, Trachtman H, Gauthier B. Clinical spectrum of gross hematuria in pediatric patients. *Clin Pediatr (Phila).* 2006;45(2):135–141

CHAPTER 98

Proteinuria

Elaine S. Kamil, MD

CASE STUDY

A 14-year-old boy is brought to the office for a preparticipation sports physical examination. He has been previously healthy but had one hospital admission at the age of 2 years for treatment of a fractured humerus. He has no acute complaints. The family history is positive for diabetes mellitus in the paternal grandfather and lung cancer in the maternal grandfather. It is negative for renal disease or hypertension. The boy's height and weight are at the 75th percentile for age, and his blood pressure is 110/70 mm Hg.

On physical examination he is a well-developed, well-nourished, athletic teenager. No abnormal findings are present. The complete blood cell count reveals a hemoglobin of 14.8 g/dL, a hematocrit of 48.3%, and a white blood cell (WBC) count of 8,400/mm³ with a normal differential. The urine has a pH of 5, a specific gravity of 1.025, and 3+ protein on dipstick. The rest of the dipstick is negative. Microscopic examination shows 0 to 1 WBC count per high-power field and 0 to 2 hyaline casts per low-power field.

Questions

1. What conditions cause proteinuria?
2. When should children with proteinuria undergo further evaluation?
3. What type of evaluation should be carried out to assess proteinuria?
4. When should children with proteinuria be referred to a pediatric nephrologist?

A small amount of **protein** is normally present in the urine. In children, normal urine protein excretion is less than 100 mg/m²/24 hours or 4 mg/m²/hour. Urine protein levels increase somewhat under certain conditions, such as vigorous exercise, febrile illnesses, accidental trauma, and congestive heart failure (CHF). Urinary protein excretion in children is also affected by age, gender, and body habitus. Most of the protein in the **glomerular filtrate** is reabsorbed by the tubular cells. Pathologic amounts of protein are present in the urine when the **glomerular leak** of protein is increased, when the **tubules fail to reabsorb** the protein filtered by the glomerulus, or if **inflammation in the renal interstitium** leads to the addition of tubular proteins to the urine.

Urinary protein is initially detected by **urine dipstick,** but this method may produce false-positive results in alkaline or in highly concentrated urine. A dipstick positive for protein of 1+ in concentrated urine may not correlate with an abnormal 24-hour urinary protein excretion, whereas a dipstick of 1+ in very dilute urine may be associated with an abnormal 24-hour urinary protein excretion. Proteinuria is more accurately determined by performing a timed urine collection or a random sample for chemical determination of the ratio of urinary total protein concentration divided by the urinary creatinine concentration (urine TP/Cr).

Epidemiology

The prevalence of **proteinuria** depends on how the condition is defined. In a Texas study, 10 mg/dL of proteinuria was found consistently in the urine of 2% to 3% of children in 3 consecutive urine samples. When 50 mg/dL was used as the cutoff for proteinuria, however, only 0.4% to 0.7% of boys and 0.4% to 2.5% of girls had proteinuria in 2 of 3 consecutive samples. The prevalence of proteinuria increased with age. In Finland, about 11% of school-aged children had at least one episode of proteinuria of 25 mg/dL by dipstick when the urine was tested 4 times. Approximately 2.5% of the children had proteinuria on 2 of 4 occasions.

Clinical Presentation

Proteinuria is a laboratory finding that may present incidentally on a screening urinalysis or be detected during the evaluation of a complaint, such as edema, that may be caused by kidney disease. When proteinuria is detected as an incidental finding in otherwise normal children, the laboratory evaluation of the proteinuria should be delayed until its persistence is confirmed on repeat dipstick, preferably on a first morning urine sample (D$_x$ Box). **Edematous children** with proteinuria most likely have renal lesions or, more rarely, CHF. Additional findings on examination could include the presence of

Dx Proteinuria

- Presence of dipstick proteinuria (>1+ confirmed on 3 occasions)
- Random urine total protein-creatinine ratio greater than 0.2 or 24-hour urine protein greater than 4 mg/m²/hour
- Orthostatic proteinuria (assessed through separate measurement of afternoon and first morning urine for total protein-creatinine ratios)

hypertension, ascites, pleural effusions, or the rash of systemic lupus erythematosus or anaphylactoid purpura.

Edema in the absence of significant proteinuria can be seen in conditions causing hypoproteinemia, such as liver or inflammatory bowel disease, or during allergic reactions.

Pathophysiology

The glomerular capillaries are adapted to permit the filtration of minimal amounts of plasma proteins, particularly those with a small molecular radius. Approximately 320 mg of albumin and 360 mg of lower molecular weight proteins are filtered by the glomerular capillaries each day. Ninety-five percent of this is reabsorbed by the proximal tubular cells. Normally, children may excrete up to 100 mg/m^2/day of protein. Urinary protein excretion is increased in newborns to about 240 mg/m^2/day and in adolescents to about 300 mg/m^2/day. Adults may normally excrete up to 150 mg of protein per day. Only 10% to 15% of this is albumin; the rest of the proteins are other plasma proteins and urinary glycoproteins.

When increased proteinuria results from glomerular disease, higher levels of urinary proteins are primarily caused by the enhanced filtration of albumin. Abnormal urinary protein excretion is a marker of chronic kidney disease, and attempts to improve proteinuria with angiotensin-converting enzyme inhibition in this setting has been shown to slow the progression of glomerular diseases. Protein excretion may be increased transiently by any condition that raises intra-glomerular capillary pressure, such as CHF, strenuous exercise, epinephrine use, fever, or surgery. Children and adults with very early diabetic nephropathy or early end-organ damage from hypertension will show elevated urinary microalbumin-creatinine ratios. Children with diabetes or hypertension should have regular determination of urinary microalbumin-creatinine ratios to detect early, reversible glomerular damage.

Orthostatic proteinuria, which affects some children, is a poorly understood, benign condition. Individuals excrete pathologic amounts of protein in their urine while they are upright, but their urinary protein excretion returns to normal when they are recumbent. This condition seems to be more common in athletic individuals. Normal children exhibit a diurnal variation in urinary protein excretion, but that variation is exaggerated in children with orthostatic proteinuria. In a recent careful study of 91 healthy Hispanic and non-Hispanic white children, aged 6 to 19 years, in an American Southwestern city, 19.8% of children had orthostatic proteinuria. It was more common in boys older than 10 years, and in those with a body mass index above the 85th percentile for age. Orthostatic proteinuria may be caused by increased pressure in the renal vasculature while patients are upright. Several investigators have shown partial obstruction of the left renal vein by entrapment between the aorta and superior mesenteric artery in patients with orthostatic proteinuria while they are standing.

Differential Diagnosis

The proteinuria may be **physiological** (secondary to fever, CHF), **transient, orthostatic, tubular** (as seen in allergic interstitial nephritis), or **glomerular.** Aminoaciduria as a form of tubular proteinuria may occur, as is seen in certain inborn errors of metabolism.

Evaluation

History

It is important to elicit a complete history (Questions Box) in children with proteinuria. When asking about a history of swelling, the practitioner should note that subtle periorbital edema may be present only in the early morning hours. If the proteinuria is detected at a routine screening examination, the conditions under which the urine was obtained should be determined. Children may have been sick with a high fever or have just participated in an athletic event such as a track meet.

Physical Examination

The physical examination should include a determination of blood pressure and measurement of height and weight. A careful assessment for edema should be made. The skin should be examined for signs of rashes such as that seen in Henoch-Schönlein purpura or healing impetigo. The joints should be inspected for any signs of swelling or joint inflammation. The abdominal examination should include a careful search for ascites or organomegaly.

Laboratory Tests

The extent of the laboratory evaluation depends on the child's general health (eg, the child is ill with another problem), the amount of proteinuria on dipstick, and whether the child has edema. The suggested evaluation is outlined in Figure 98-1. In non-edematous, otherwise healthy children, it is prudent to examine the urine sediment and, if negative, recheck the dipstick in a few days. If proteinuria of 1+ is consistently present and no hematuria is evident, a first-stage

---

Questions

Proteinuria

- Was the mother's pregnancy remarkable in any way? What was the child's birth like?
- Did the child have any neonatal problems that may indicate possible renal damage? Was the child preterm? Did the child have intrauterine growth restriction?
- Is any swelling apparent in areas such as the ankles, abdomen, or periorbital region?
- Has the child had any recent illnesses, particularly pharyngitis or impetigo?
- Does the child have a history of joint pains and skin rashes, especially the adolescent patient who may be at greater risk of having a collagen vascular disease?
- Has the child had any previous urinary tract infections, urinary abnormalities, or dark urine?
- Does the child have a history of hypertension or weight loss or gain?
- Is there a family history of renal disease?
- Does the child have diabetes mellitus?

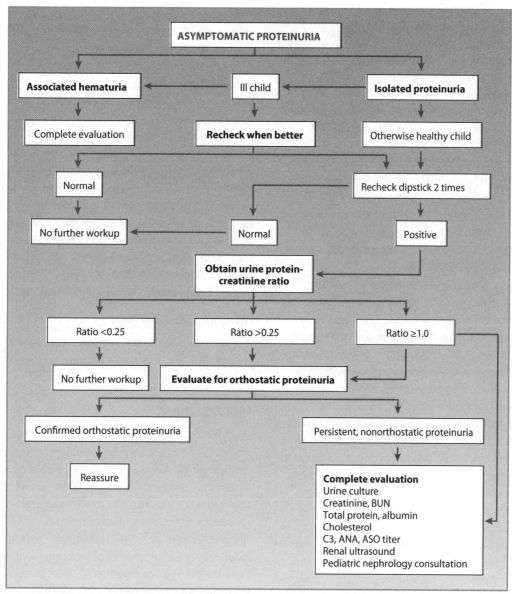

Figure 98-1. Suggested evaluation of children with asymptomatic proteinuria. Abbreviations: ANA, antinuclear antibody; ASO, antistreptolysin-O; BUN, blood urea nitrogen.

evaluation is indicated. If children are ill with a fever or are hospitalized with a serious illness, it is often appropriate to delay evaluation of the proteinuria until the acute illness is under control, providing no associated hematuria, hypoproteinemia, hypertension, or azotemia is present.

In healthy ambulatory patients with persistent, isolated dipstick proteinuria on 3 occasions, it is important to quantitate the proteinuria (Box 98-1). This may be done simply by ordering a urine TP/Cr. If the ratio is abnormal (>0.2), children need to be evaluated first for orthostatic proteinuria, which can be ruled out in several ways. The simplest evaluation involves checking a urine dipstick on a first-voided morning sample and again on an afternoon specimen. This procedure should be repeated on 2 different days. It is critical to be sure that children empty their bladders before going to bed because urine produced during the evening when they are nonrecumbent may contain protein and give an inaccurate result. If the

dipstick for protein from the morning urine is negative on a concentrated acid urine and if the afternoon sample is positive for protein on a concentrated acid urine, the child most likely has orthostatic proteinuria.

A more accurate way of checking for orthostatic proteinuria involves the determination of urine TP/Cr ratios on the first morning and afternoon urine samples. A diagnosis of orthostatic proteinuria can be made if the ratio is normal on the recumbent sample and elevated on the daytime sample. The most accurate way of diagnosing orthostatic proteinuria entails collecting 2 timed urine samples, one during the hours that children are up during the day and the other while they are in bed at night. In most instances of orthostatic proteinuria in children, the total urinary protein excretion is less than 1 g. The urine collected in the recumbent period should contain less than 50 mg/m^2 of protein. If these 2 timed samples meet the criteria for orthostatic proteinuria, they do not need to be

Box 98-1. Methods for Assessment of Urinary Protein

Detection of proteinuria by dipstick is only semiquantitative. This examination is affected by urinary pH and concentration; therefore, more definitive tests are warranted if a patient's urine consistently shows dipstick proteinuria. The sulfosalicylic acid (SSA) turbidity test is also semiquantitative. When SSA is added to an aliquot of urine, it precipitates urinary proteins. The amount of turbidity is graded on a scale of 0 to 4+.

Urinary protein is most accurately quantitated by a chemical determination on a timed urine collection (usually 24 hours). The concentration (measured in milligrams per deciliter) is multiplied by the total urine volume to determine the milligrams of protein excreted in 24 hours. Twenty-four–hour urine samples are difficult to collect in young children. However, several studies have shown that a random urine sample for a protein-creatinine ratio correlates well with the 24-hour urinary protein excretion. The ratio is determined by dividing the urine protein concentration (milligrams per deciliter) by the urine creatinine concentration (milligrams per deciliter). The units must be the same for each component. The urinary protein-creatinine ratio is normally less than 0.2. A ratio of 3.5 or greater in an adult or greater than 1.0 in children indicates nephrotic range proteinuria. A recent study has found that proteinuria in combination with leukocyturia (by dipstick) is likely to indicate more significant noninfectious renal inflammation.

Occasionally, it is important to determine whether proteinuria has a tubular or glomerular basis. In these instances, a urinary β_2-microglobulin is helpful. β_2-microglobulin, a very small protein that is freely filtered at the glomerular level, is nearly completely reabsorbed by the proximal tubules. In instances of tubular injury, such as interstitial nephritis, acute kidney injury, or nephrotoxic renal injury, urinary β_2-microglobulin is increased. With glomerular proteinuria, urine protein electrophoresis shows a heavy preponderance of albumin. The urine microalbumin-creatinine ratio is an excellent indicator of glomerular proteinuria. It is readily available in most laboratories and will detect minimal but pathologic amounts of glomerular proteinuria such as that seen in early diabetic nephropathy and with early hypertensive glomerular damage.

repeated. It is important to remember, however, that even in renal disease, proteinuria improves somewhat when patients are recumbent.

If children do not have orthostatic proteinuria, a 24-hour urine protein excretion may be determined. If the collection of a 24-hour urine sample is impractical, the urine TP/Cr ratio is a reliable alternative. Blood chemistries (eg, blood urea nitrogen [BUN], creatinine) should be obtained to determine renal function. Electrolyte status should be assessed with total carbon dioxide as well as serum total protein, albumin, and cholesterol. Serologies should be obtained for antinuclear antibodies, C3, antistreptolysin-O titer, and hepatitis B surface antigen if children come from a population at risk for hepatitis B.

Twenty-four–hour urine protein excretion should be less than 4 mg/m^2/hour. Neonates may excrete as much as 150 mg/m^2/12 hours, however. Table 98-1 gives a summary of normal urinary protein excretion. If children have nephrotic range proteinuria or

symptoms consistent with nephrotic syndrome (heavy proteinuria accompanied by hypoalbuminemia and hypercholesterolemia), they require further evaluation for nephrotic syndrome (see Chapter 150). If they do not have nephrotic-range proteinuria, abnormal tubular proteinuria should be ruled out. A normal urinary β_2-microglobulin rules out tubular proteinuria. In general, consultation with a pediatric nephrologist is recommended if children have an abnormal 24-hour urinary protein excretion (see Table 98-1). If the proteinuria exceeds 1 g/day or if any other minor signs of renal dysfunction or hematuria are present, a biopsy is warranted. A recent study from Japan showed that in children with constant isolated proteinuria, a urine TP/Cr ratio of >0.5 was predictive of more than minimal glomerular abnormalities on kidney biopsy. Sometimes, otherwise healthy children with small amounts of isolated proteinuria of less than 750 to 1,000 mg/day are followed by the pediatric nephrologist without a kidney biopsy. However, if this degree of proteinuria persists for 1 year or more, a renal biopsy is warranted.

Imaging Studies

A renal ultrasound should be obtained to rule out any structural abnormalities but may not be indicated in the child with simple orthostatic proteinuria.

Management

Most children with normal renal function and normal blood pressure whose evaluation reveals physiological or orthostatic proteinuria should have repeat urinalysis on an annual basis. If the proteinuria worsens or if hematuria develops, a repeat evaluation of renal function is indicated. Children whose initial evaluation reveals persistent, significant proteinuria require careful follow-up to detect and monitor signs of serious renal disease. This follow-up should include repeat blood pressure measurement and urinalysis every 3 months and repeat chemistries (BUN, creatinine, serum albumin) and urine Tp/Cr ratios every 6 months. These children should be managed in consultation with a pediatric nephrologist, whose experience is helpful in reassessing the need for kidney biopsy.

Children with physiological or orthostatic proteinuria who have minimal, persistent proteinuria should be able to follow a full school schedule and be allowed to participate in sports, provided there are no other contraindications. The usual immunization schedule should

Table 98-1. Urinary Protein Excretion by Age

Age	24-Hour Urine Protein (mg)	Urine Protein-Creatinine Ratio
Premature newborn	14–60	—
Full-term newborn	15–68	—
2–23 mo	17–85	≤0.50
2–4 y	20–121	≤0.2
4–10 y	26–194	≤0.2
10–16 y	29–238	≤0.2

not be interrupted, and children should follow a regular diet. No increase in dietary protein is necessary to compensate for the minimal amounts of protein lost in the urine. Results of recent studies in nephrotic patients have found that a high-protein diet may actually increase urinary protein losses.

Prognosis

The outlook for children with proteinuria depends entirely on the underlying cause of the proteinuria. Children whose proteinuria is associated with edema or hematuria are more likely to have significant renal disease, such as glomerulonephritis, and the prognosis may be less favorable. If the proteinuria is due to a form of chronic glomerulonephritis, children may ultimately develop end-stage renal disease. In individuals with glomerular diseases, persistent proteinuria is a strong risk factor for progressive loss of renal function. If the proteinuria is physiological or orthostatic, however, the long-term prognosis is excellent. The likelihood that these children will develop renal functional impairment is no greater than for the rest of the general population.

CASE RESOLUTION

In the case presented at the beginning of the chapter, odds are that the evaluation of the healthy teenaged boy with isolated proteinuria will reveal that he has orthostatic proteinuria, and his long-term prognosis is good.

Selected References

Abitbol C, Zilleruelo G, Freundlich M, Strauss J. Quantitation of proteinuria with urinary protein/creatinine ratios and random testing with dipsticks in nephrotic children. *J Pediatr.* 1990;116(2):243–247

Brandt JR, Jacobs A, Raissy HH, et al. Orthostatic proteinuria and the spectrum of diurnal variability of urinary protein excretion in healthy children. *Pediatr Nephrol.* 2010;25(6):1131–1137

Ginsberg JM, Chang BS, Matarese RA, Garella S. Use of single voided urine samples to estimate quantitative proteinuria. *N Engl J Med.* 1983;309(25): 1543–1546

Hama T, Nakanishi K, Shima Y, et al. Renal biopsy criteria in children with asymptomatic constant isolated proteinuria. *Nephrol Dial Transplant.* 2012; 27(8):3186–3190

Hogg RJ, Portman RJ, Milliner D, Lemley KV, Eddy A, Ingelfinger J. Evaluation and management of proteinuria and nephrotic syndrome in children: recommendations from a pediatric nephrology panel established at the National Kidney Foundation conference on proteinuria, albuminuria, risk, assessment, detection, and elimination (PARADE). *Pediatrics.* 2000;105(6):1242–1249

Houser MT, Jahn MF, Kobayashi A, Walburn J. Assessment of urinary protein excretion in the adolescent: effect of body position and exercise. *J Pediatr.* 1986;109(3):556–561

Koss S, Perl A, Wieder A, Frank R, Vento S, Trachtman H. Proteinuria and renal disease: prognostic value of urine dipstick testing for leukocytes. *Pediatr Nephrol.* 2006;21(4):584–587

Pradhan M, Kaplan BS. Proteinuria. In: Kaplan BS, Meyers KEC, eds. *Pediatric Nephrology and Urology: The Requisites in Pediatrics.* Philadelphia, PA: Elsevier; 2005:103–109

Ragazzi M, Milani G, Edefonti A, Burdick L, Bianchetti MG, Fossali EF. Left renal vein entrapment: a frequent feature in children with postural proteinuria. *Pediatr Nephrol.* 2008; 23(10):1837–1839

Reuben DB, Wachtel TJ, Brown PC, Driscoll JL. Transient proteinuria in emergency medical admissions. *N Engl J Med.* 1982;306(17):1031–1033

Trachtman H, Bergwerk A, Gauthier B. Isolated proteinuria in children. Natural history and indications for renal biopsy. *Clin Pediatr (Phila).* 1994;33(8): 468–472

Vehaskari VM. Mechanism of orthostatic proteinuria. *Pediatr Nephrol.* 1990;4(4): 328–330

Yoshikawa N, Kitagawa K, Ohta K, Tanaka R, Nakamura H. Asymptomatic constant isolated proteinuria in children. *J Pediatr.* 1991;119(3):375–379

CHAPTER 99

Urinary Tract Infections

Gangadarshni Chandramohan, MD, MS, and Sudhir K. Anand, MD

CASE STUDY

A 2-year-old girl is brought to the office with a 1-day history of fever (temperature 103°F [39.4°C]), vomiting, and mild diarrhea. There was no history of any change in her urinary habits and she still wears diapers. The child has been somewhat irritable but fully alert.

Physical examination reveals an ill-appearing toddler. Her temperature is 102.6°F (39.2°C), heart rate is 122 bpm, respiratory rate is 30 breaths per minute, and blood pressure is 90/60 mm Hg. The neck is supple. Head, eye, ear, nose, throat, chest, heart, abdominal, and genital examinations are normal. Urinalysis shows specific gravity 1.025, pH 6.0, leukocyte esterase and nitrite both strongly positive, protein trace, and blood trace; the sediment has 15 to 20 white blood cells and 2 to 4 red blood cells per high-power field. The Gram stain shows more than 100,000 gram-negative rods, and the urine culture result is pending.

Questions

1. What are the possible diagnoses of children with positive leukocyte esterase or nitrite on urinalysis?
2. What are the indications for hospital admission of children with urinary tract infections (UTIs)?
3. What antibiotics are used in the treatment of UTIs?
4. What is the appropriate diagnostic workup for children with suspected UTIs? When are renal ultrasound, technetium Tc 99m succimer renal scan, and voiding cystourethrogram included in the evaluation?
5. If workup reveals vesicoureteral reflux, how should children be managed over the long term?

Urinary tract infection (UTI) is now the most common serious bacterial infection that affects infants and children. A UTI may be asymptomatic, associated with urinary symptoms, or occasionally complicated by sepsis. In most children, UTIs resolve completely with appropriate antibiotic therapy. However, in children with underlying anatomic abnormalities (eg, vesicoureteral reflux) or delayed or inadequate antibiotic treatment, UTIs may result in renal scarring that can sometimes lead to hypertension or, rarely, end-stage renal disease.

Urinary tract infection is a nonspecific, generic term implying significant bacteriuria, irrespective of the site of bacterial growth in the urinary tract. In many young children with bacteriuria, clinical findings overlap and precise classification cannot be easily made. Some commonly used terms are clarified as follows.

Asymptomatic, covert, and **screening bacteriuria** are synonymous terms usually used when bacteriuria is detected during surveys of healthy children. However, some affected children may actually have urinary symptoms on close questioning.

Cystitis implies infection of the bladder only. Its major feature is voiding symptoms (ie, dysuria, frequency, urgency, enuresis, and foul-smelling urine). Fever, if present, is usually low-grade, and lower abdominal pain also may be seen

Acute pyelonephritis is infection of renal parenchyma characterized by systemic symptoms such as high fever, chills, flank pain, and vomiting in addition to dysuria.

Recurrent UTI generally refers to reinfection with a new organism (can be the same or a different species). This condition is a common problem, especially in the first year after initial UTI. Reinfection with the same organism is infrequent and may indicate underlying structural problems of the urinary tract, the presence of stones, or inappropriate antibiotic therapy.

Chronic pyelonephritis is a term that has been used in various ways. Ideally, it should be employed only after renal biopsy specimens reveal renal scarring on histology due to repeated infections. Practically, the term often refers to scarred kidneys as demonstrated by nuclear medicine studies or reduced kidney function.

Urethritis implies infection of the urethra and is usually seen in the setting of sexually transmitted infections. The usual symptoms are dysuria and urethral discharge.

Epidemiology

Bacteriuria is detected in approximately 1% of girls and 2% of boys during routine screening of healthy newborns and young infants. Approximately 1% of girls continue to have asymptomatic bacteriuria throughout childhood. Bacteriuria in boys older than 1 year is very uncommon. In most affected infants and children, bacteriuria resolves spontaneously with time and does not lead to renal damage.

Symptomatic UTI occurs in approximately 2.5% of children annually and accounts for more than 1 million office visits per year. Up to about 7% girls and 2% boys have culture-proven symptomatic UTI by age 6 years. Before the age of 1 year, UTI recurs in 75% of infants. After 1 year of age, 40% of girls and 30% of boys develop recurrent UTIs following the first episode. In early infancy, UTI is about twice as common in boys than girls and about 10 times more common in uncircumcised boys than circumcised boys. After the first 6 months of life, the incidence of symptomatic UTI becomes considerably higher in females than males, and the difference between circumcised and uncircumcised males disappears. Among vaccinated febrile infants, UTI is the source of fever in approximately 4% to 8% of patients, even in those who have upper respiratory infection symptoms.

Clinical Presentation

Signs and symptoms of UTI in neonates and young infants are usually nonspecific and include fever, irritability, poor weight gain (or weight loss), diarrhea, vomiting, and jaundice. Occasionally, bacteremia or sepsis with temperature instability, cyanosis, and disseminated intravascular coagulation may occur. Older children often have similar signs and symptoms, and they are often able to describe abdominal or flank pain, dysuria, frequency, urgency, enuresis, foul-smelling or cloudy urine, and occasionally gross hematuria (D$_x$ Box).

Pathophysiology

The pathogenesis of UTI involves interaction between various bacterial factors and protective host factors (Ragnarsdóttir and Svanborg).

Bacterial Factors

Escherichia coli accounts for 80% to 90% of first infections. The remainder are caused by other gram-negative enteric bacilli (eg, *Proteus, Klebsiella, Enterobacter*) and gram-positive cocci (eg, enterococci, *Staphylococcus saprophyticus*). Rarely, *Morganella morganii, Proteus mirabilis, Providencia stuartii,* and *Serratia* spp can cause infection in young children as well. Most organisms that cause UTI originate from the fecal flora. *S saprophyticus* (a coagulase-negative staphylococcus) infections are primarily seen in adolescents with UTI. Nosocomial infection can be caused by *Citrobacter, Enterobacter, Enterococcus,* and *Pseudomonas.*

Microorganisms that cause UTI usually enter the urinary tract by an ascending route. To initiate colonization and infect the urinary tract, these organisms must first adhere to uroepithelium so they are not swept away during voiding. Bacterial adhesion in *E coli* is mediated by fimbriae, which are fine, hairlike proteins emanating from the bacterial cell wall. One important type of fimbriae, called P-fimbriae, adheres to receptors (Gal-Gal) on the uroepithelium, and some studies have shown that women and children with recurrent UTI have increased numbers of these receptors. In most young children with normal anatomy, acute pyelonephritis is caused by *E coli* with P-fimbriae. In most patients with VUR and scarred kidneys, however, the infection is caused by *E coli* lacking P-fimbriae. Hence, the role of P-fimbriae in the pathogenesis of renal scarring is uncertain. Additionally, many of these bacteria, which are typically extracellular organisms, are able to survive and flourish intracellularly by taking advantage of the host cell's nutrients and evading immune defenses. Other bacterial virulence factors include K and H antigens, colicin, and hemolysin, but their role in the pathogenesis of UTI is not clearly defined.

Host Factors

There are many unalterable host factors that contribute to the pathogenesis of UTI, including age, sex, genetics, anatomy, and immune response to infection. Females seem to be at increased risk because the female urethra is shorter than the male urethra and closer to the anus. As previously stated, the uroepithelium of older girls and adult women who develop recurrent UTI binds *E coli* more avidly than uroepithelium from non-susceptible patients. In addition, individuals with certain P and Lewis blood groups develop more UTIs than others. Urinary obstruction or other anomalies may contribute to the development of UTIs in about 2% of girls and 5% of boys, especially infants.

Vesicoureteral reflux signifies retrograde passage of urine from the bladder to the ureter. After passage through the bladder wall, the normal ureter tunnels under the bladder mucosa for approximately 2 cm before it opens into the bladder lumen. Under normal circumstances, the submucosal segment is compressed when the bladder is filled and during voiding, preventing reflux of urine into the ureter. Most VUR is primary and caused by a congenital abnormality of the ureterovesical junction, with the ureter having a short submucosal segment and more laterally placed openings. Reflux may also occur in the presence of normal ureteral anatomy when bladder pressures exceed 40 cm of water, as seen in patients with posterior urethral valves or neurogenic bladders. Vesicoureteral reflux is graded on a scale of 1 through 5, with stage 5 being the most severe (Figure 99-1).

The incidence of VUR in normal infants is generally stated to be less than 2%; however, recent studies suggest that the incidence of low-grade VUR in normal children is much higher and in fact may be similar to that in children with UTI. In infants with UTI, the incidence of VUR is about 25% to 50%; in school-aged children, about 25% to 30%; and in adolescents, about 10% to 15%. These figures suggest that, with increasing age and maturation of the bladder wall, VUR often spontaneously resolves. Vesicoureteral reflux may also be a familial disorder and has been reported in 10% to 30%

Dx **Urinary Tract Infection**

- Abdominal pain
- Burning or pain on urination
- Urgency
- Frequency
- Fever
- Leukocyturia
- Positive urine culture

Figure 99-1. Grading of vesicoureteral reflux by vesicoureterogram based on international classification. 1, Ureter only. 2, Ureter, pelvis, and calyces, but without dilatation. 3, Mild or moderate dilatation of ureter and mild or moderate dilatation of renal pelvis, but no or slight blunting of fornices. 4, Moderate dilatation or tortuosity of the ureter with moderate dilatation of renal pelvis and calyces and complete obliteration of the sharp angles of fornices, but maintenance of papillary impressions in most calyces. 5, Gross dilatation and tortuosity of ureters, renal pelvis, and calyces; papillary impressions are no longer visible in most calyces.

of siblings of index cases. The incidence of UTI is increased in the presence of VUR probably because of incomplete emptying of the bladder; the urine refluxed into the ureters or kidneys returns to the bladder via the abnormally tunneled ureters at the end of voiding. This also provides infected urine direct access to the kidneys, which can lead to pyelonephritis and potential renal scarring.

Intuitively, it would seem that the greater the severity of VUR in children with UTI, the greater the likelihood of renal scarring. Recently, however, it has been clearly recognized that many neonates (especially boys) with antenatal VUR, even in the absence of UTI, have congenital dysplastic renal parenchymal defects, which had been misidentified as infective scars. Therefore, it is now presumed that the progression of renal scarring in this group occurs as a result of the natural course of the congenital defect with or without a superimposed UTI.

While there are many predisposing host factors that cannot be changed, there are several behavioral issues that are often associated with UTI in older children. School-aged children with frequent complaints of dysuria or recurrent UTIs who do not have a history of UTI as infants should be questioned for symptoms of *dysfunctional voiding,* a term often applied in the setting of children (especially girls) who have no neurologic or anatomic abnormalities but who exhibit abnormal voiding behavior. These girls will often hold their urine for so long that they need to rush to the bathroom only to incompletely empty their bladder, leading to urinary stasis and the potential for infection. Additionally, constipation and abnormal stooling patterns are frequently associated with dysfunctional voiding and can also lead to the development of UTI.

Differential Diagnosis

In infants and young children, symptoms of UTI are often nonspecific. Thus, a high degree of suspicion for UTI must be maintained. An acute abdomen may rarely be confused with UTI. Some children

with dysuria may have chemical irritation from exposure to materials such as bubble baths. Overweight girls may retain urine in their labial folds, which can cause maceration, urethral irritation, or vulvitis. Similarly, some young girls do not sit with their legs spread wide enough on the toilet, which can lead to reflux into the vagina and cause post-void dribbling with subsequent urethral irritation or vulvitis. In these cases, urinalysis and urine culture findings usually help differentiate UTI from vulvitis or urethral irritation.

Evaluation

History

In all infants and young children with fever without an apparent source, urinalysis, urine Gram stain, and urine culture should be obtained to evaluate for UTI prior to initiating antibiotics. If febrile children younger than 2 years do not appear to be ill, workup should be based on risk assessment. For girls, the risk factors associated with UTI are white race, younger than 12 months, temperature at or above 102.2°F (39°C), fever for more than 2 days, and no source of infection; for boys, risk factors associated with UTI are race other than African American, temperature at or above 102.2°F (39°C), fever for more than 24 hours, or no other evident source of infection. If there is a high likelihood of having UTI based on risk assessment of an individual child, antibiotics can be initiated after obtaining a urine culture; otherwise, it is acceptable to watch until the culture results are available. In older children, a history of fever, dysuria, frequency, abdominal pain, and nausea and vomiting is suggestive of UTI (Questions Box). History of previous UTIs, abnormal voiding, and constipation should also be sought.

Physical Examination

The abdomen should be examined for masses and tenderness, the genitalia for local lesions, and the lumbosacral area for anomalies such as deep sacral dimples. Blood pressure should be measured to evaluate for hypertension.

Laboratory Tests

The diagnosis of UTI is established by documenting significant bacteria in a urine specimen sent for culture. In young infants, the specimen should always be obtained by bladder puncture or catheterization. In infants and children, because of the risk of contamination, a bag urine sample is not reliable. In older children with

Questions

Urinary Tract Infection

- Does it hurt when the child urinates? Does the child scream when urinating?
- Does the child void more frequently?
- Does the urine have an unusual odor?
- Has the child had previous urinary infections?
- Does the child have a good urinary stream, or does the child dribble?

bladder control, a midstream urine collection is satisfactory. The diagnosis of UTI should never be based on the presence or absence of white blood cells alone. Although most older children with symptomatic UTI have pyuria, many neonates and young infants with UTI (25%–50%) may not manifest this finding. Furthermore, leukocyturia may occur in other renal disorders in the absence of UTI. A positive urinary nitrite test is suggestive of UTI, but the false-negative rate is nearly 50%.

Most patients with UTI (>85%) have urine bacterial counts greater than 100,000/mL on a voided specimen (ie, significant bacteriuria), although some adult women and teenage girls with symptomatic recurrent UTI have catheterized or "clean catch" urine colony counts less than 1,000/mL. In general, this has not been observed in young children. Colony counts between 10,000 and 100,000/mL obtained via clean catch are generally unlikely to be significant unless children have symptoms of UTI, associated leukocyturia, or cultures that are pure growths of a single organism. Any growth of an organism from a suprapubic tap is considered significant. A colony count of at least 10,000/mL in samples obtained by catheterization is usually necessary to diagnose a UTI. However, in most children with UTIs, urine collected by either of these techniques grows more than 50,000 organisms/mL.

C-reactive protein is usually increased in infants and children with high fever and clinical findings suggestive of acute pyelonephritis. Several other laboratory studies, including erythrocyte sedimentation rate, urinary lactic acid dehydrogenase isoenzymes, urinary concentrating ability, and antibody-coated bacteria, have been used with varying success to differentiate upper (renal) from lower (bladder) UTI in older children and adults. Overall, the reliability of these studies in pediatric patients, especially infants and young children, is not adequate to recommend their routine use. More recently, there has been some focus on serum procalcitonin, and preliminary studies suggest that it might have some predictive value in terms of pyelonephritis and VUR.

Imaging Studies

Although there is controversy concerning the recommendations, the most recent position statement from the American Academy of Pediatrics (AAP) (2011) states that children younger than 2 years should have renal and bladder ultrasonography done after the first UTI; however, routine voiding cystoureterogram (VCUG) should not be performed unless there is evidence of hydronephrosis, scarring, or other anomalies suggestive of obstructive uropathy or high-grade reflux as well as other atypical complex situations, or if there are recurrent UTIs. The 2 ultrasound studies detect structural renal and bladder anomalies and VUR in most patients. In girls, nuclear VCUG instead of contrast VCUG is an acceptable alternative. Renal ultrasound can be performed as soon as feasible after diagnosis. If indicated, VCUG may be done once there is clinical evidence that the UTI is resolving, or it may be delayed 4 to 6 weeks depending on clinical circumstances. Antibiotic prophylaxis, according to the AAP guidelines, must be administered until completion of the

studies. An excretory urogram (intravenous pyelogram) is no longer recommended.

In the past, some authorities recommended a routine technetium Tc 99m succimer renal scan to differentiate upper from lower tract infection. Although the test result is positive in 60% to 90% of children with a clinical diagnosis of acute pyelonephritis, the cost of the nuclear scan, the high dose of radiation, and the fact that therapy is usually not altered preclude the routine use of this study. The scan is most helpful in a child in whom the diagnosis of acute pyelonephritis is in doubt or when used in follow-up to detect development of renal scars, especially in patients with VUR and recurrent UTI.

Management

All newborns and infants younger than 2 months with UTIs should be treated with parenteral **antibiotics,** starting with broad-spectrum antibiotic coverage such as ceftriaxone, cefotaxime, or ampicillin and gentamicin, pending results of sensitivity studies. Infants and children older than 2 months who appear well and are able to tolerate liquids may receive oral antibiotics on an outpatient basis. Most physicians recommend cephalexin for the first infection until the results of bacterial sensitivity tests are available and treatment is continued for 10 days. In older children with clear-cut lower tract infection, shorter courses of trimethoprim-sulfamethoxazole are also effective. One should be aware of the local E coli resistance patterns, however, because some communities have a high incidence of E coli resistant to trimethoprim-sulfamethoxazole. Children who appear toxic or are vomiting should be admitted to the hospital and started on parenteral antibiotics until they show clinical improvement, at which time they can be sent home on oral therapy.

Although recent studies have suggested that antibiotics do not necessarily prevent infections or renal scarring and may cause increased risk of resistant infections, most children with VUR are still placed on low-dose antibiotics (trimethoprim-sulfamethoxazole, cephalexin, or nitrofurantoin) that are continued for 12 to 18 months following treatment for an acute infection. At the end of this period, a radionuclide VCUG is repeated to determine whether reflux has resolved. Development of new renal scars can be best detected by technetium Tc 99m succimer renal scanning.

Surgery is not necessary in most infants with VUR, including many with severe disease (grades 4 and 5) because most grade 1 through 3 and some grade 4 and 5 reflux in infants disappears with increasing age. In children older than 5 years with grade 4 or 5 reflux, the rate of disappearance with medical treatment is much lower (about 20%–25%). The results of the Randomized Intervention in Children With Vesicoureteral Reflux Study show no difference in the rate of renal scarring between prophylactic medical treatment and surgery. Therefore, surgical reimplantation of the ureter is usually recommended only for those patients who have poor adherence with prophylaxis or breakthrough infections, especially if the upper tract is involved. This latter group seems to have benefited the most from surgery.

An alternate to surgical reimplantation, Deflux is a gel composed of dextranomers and hyaluronic acid that can be injected endoscopically into the ureters. It was approved by the US Food and Drug Administration in September 2001 after having been used extensively throughout Europe with great success. Most pediatric urologists agree that Deflux should be used for persistent grades 2 through 4 reflux, while grade 1 can be managed expectantly. Severe grade 5 reflux usually requires surgical intervention.

Prognosis

In most children, UTI is a minor illness with very few long-term or serious consequences. However, UTI commonly reoccurs, especially during the first year following the initial UTI. Repeat urine cultures should be obtained during follow-up assessments in all children with grade 4 or 5 (high-grade) VUR, first at 1- to 2-month intervals and later at 3- to 4-month intervals for at least 1 year or until disappearance of reflux.

Risk factors for the development of renal scars and eventual hypertension or, rarely, renal failure include young age (<1 year), recurrent episodes of acute pyelonephritis, delay in starting effective antibiotic therapy, high-grade reflux, and anatomic or neurogenic obstruction. If repeat infection is prevented in these children, however, development of fresh scars is uncommon, and renal function and growth remain normal. As a group, infants and children younger than 2 years with UTI and high-grade VUR are more likely to develop calyceal clubbing and renal scarring, whereas progressive renal scarring as a result of UTI or reflux after 5 years of age is relatively less common., As prevention of renal scars following UTI remains the most important objective, it is important that until the results of more appropriately designed studies become available, VUR and UTI be considered as risk factors for renal scarring and each child be treated with prudence. Until the new guidelines from the Randomized Intervention in Children with Vesicoureteral Reflux study become available, each case of UTI should be assessed on an individualized basis to determine the necessity for prophylaxis antibiotic.

CASE RESOLUTION

In the case history, the young girl is hospitalized because of the vomiting. She is started on intravenous ceftriaxone and improves in 48 hours. Her inpatient renal ultrasound is normal, and she is discharged home with oral antibiotics. Because this is her first episode of UTI with no evidence of abnormal findings on ultrasound, a voiding cystoureterogram is not indicated, At this point, prophylactic antibiotics are not considered because of her history and her normal renal ultrasound.

Selected References

American Academy of Pediatrics Subcommittee on Urinary Tract Infection, Steering Committee on Quality Improvement and Management. Urinary tract infection: clinical practice guideline for the diagnosis and management of the initial UTI in febrile infants and children 2 to 24 months. *Pediatrics*. 2011; 128(3):595–610

Conway PH, Cnaan A, Zaoutis T, Henry BV, Grundmeier RW, Keren R. Recurrent urinary tract infections in children: risk factors and association with prophylactic antimicrobials. *JAMA*. 2007;298(2):179–186

Doré-Bergeron MJ, Gauthier M, Chevalier I, McManus B, Tapiero B, Lebrun S. Urinary tract infections in 1 to 3-month-old infants: ambulatory treatment with intravenous antibiotics. *Pediatrics*. 2009;124(1):16–22

Feld LG, Mattoo TK. Urinary tract infections and vesicoureteral reflux in infants and children. *Pediatr Rev*. 2010;31(11):451–463

Hannula A, Venhola M, Renko M, Pokka T, Huttunen NP, Uhari M. Vesicoureteral reflux in children with suspected and proven urinary tract infection. *Pediatr Nephrol*. 2010;25(8):1463–1469

Hoberman A, Charron M, Hickey RW, Baskin M, Kearney DH, Wald ER. Imaging studies after a first febrile urinary tract infection in young children. *N Engl J Med*. 2003;348(3):195–202

Ragnarsdóttir B, Svanborg C. Susceptibility to acute pyelonephritis or asymptomatic bacteriuria: host-pathogen interaction in urinary tract infections. *Pediatr Nephrol*. 2012;27(11):2017–2029

CHAPTER 100

Vaginitis

Monica Sifuentes, MD

CASE STUDY

An 11-year-old girl is brought to your office with vaginal itching for 1 week and a yellow discharge on her underwear for the past 4 days. The girl reports no associated abdominal pain, vomiting, or diarrhea. She has no urinary problems and also denies any history of sexual abuse. Although she occasionally bathes with bubble bath, she most often takes showers. Except for the vaginal complaint, she is healthy, and she takes no medications.

The physical examination is notable for a soft, nontender abdomen with no organomegaly. Bowel sounds are audible in all quadrants. The genitalia are sexual maturity rating (Tanner stage) 2. The labia majora and minora and the clitoris all appear normal, and the hymen is annular in shape with a smooth rim. A scant amount of yellow discharge, along with minimal perihymenal injection, is noted at the vaginal introitus. The anal examination is normal, with an intact anal wink.

Questions

1. What are the most common causes for vaginal discharge in prepubescent and pubescent girls? How do they differ?
2. What basic historical information must be obtained from all females whose chief complaint is vaginal discharge?
3. What specific methods are used to perform a gynecologic examination in prepubescent and pubescent girls?
4. What is the appropriate laboratory evaluation for prepubescent and pubescent girls who complain of vaginal discharge? How does this evaluation differ for pubescent girls who are sexually active?
5. What are the various treatment options for girls with vaginitis?

Vaginal discharge is not an uncommon occurrence in prepubescent and pubescent girls. Practitioners are largely responsible for differentiating between a physiologic discharge, or leukorrhea, and a pathologic discharge, which occurs, for example, with a bacterial or yeast infection. In cases of an abnormal discharge, the possibility of sexual abuse needs to be considered and investigated appropriately (see Chapter 132). Primary care physicians should become familiar with the various causes of vaginal discharge in prepubescent and pubescent girls. More importantly, they should be comfortable performing gynecologic examinations in these patients so that the appropriate treatment can be initiated.

Vulvovaginitis, which is often used interchangeably with vaginitis or vulvitis, signifies inflammation of the perineal area, often accompanied by vaginal discharge. The discharge may be bloody, malodorous, or purulent, depending on the etiology (Table 100-1).

Epidemiology

Vulvovaginitis is a common gynecologic complaint in prepubescent girls. Most cases of vulvovaginitis in this age group result from **nonspecific inflammation;** vaginal cultures show normal flora in 33% to 85% of such cases. The incidence of more specific **bacterial causes,** such as group A beta-hemolytic streptococcus (GABHS), has been reported in approximately 10% to 20% of patients. However, its occurrence seems to be seasonal, and confirming the diagnosis depends on the use of proper culturing techniques using the

Table 100-1. Characteristics and Specific Causes of Vaginal Discharge

Color	Consistency	Amount	Cause
Clear/white	Thin	Variable	Physiologic leukorrhea; bacterial vaginosis
White	Cottage cheese–like	Moderate	*Candida*
White/yellow	Variable	Variable	Chemical irritation, pinworms, *Chlamydia trachomatis,* bacterial vaginosis
Yellow/green	Thick	Moderate–profuse	*Neisseria gonorrhoeae,* foreign body, *Trichomonas vaginalis,* group A beta-hemolytic streptococci
Bloody	Variable	Variable	*Shigella,* group A beta-hemolytic streptococci, foreign body

appropriate media. Other bacterial causes include **respiratory pathogens,** such as *Haemophilus influenzae, Neisseria meningitidis,* and *Streptococcus pneumoniae,* and **enteric organisms,** such as *Shigella* and *Yersinia enterocolitica.* A positive culture for **sexually transmitted pathogens** such as *Chlamydia trachomatis* or *Neisseria gonorrhoeae* can be found in approximately 5% of children who are evaluated for child sexual abuse. Higher figures have been reported from selected centers and when data from adolescent victims are included. These organisms are not considered part of the normal flora in prepubescent girls. Vaginal and rectal infections with *C trachomatis* can be acquired perinatally but usually are not considered perinatally acquired after 2 to 3 years of age.

Parasitic infections may also lead to vaginal symptoms. Twenty percent of females with a rectal infestation of *Enterobius vermicularis,* the organism known as pinworm, have vulvovaginitis. Affected patients often complain of anal pruritus in addition to the vaginal discharge. **Mycotic infections** with organisms such as *Candida albicans* also can cause symptoms in prepubescent girls, although many of these girls have a previous history of recent oral antibiotic use, diabetes mellitus, immunosuppression, or other risk factors.

Clinical Presentation

Prepubescent and pubescent girls with vulvovaginitis most commonly present with a vaginal discharge, which may be white, purulent (ie, yellow or green), or serosanguineous. Its consistency can range from smooth and thin to thick and cottage cheese–like. The discharge may also be malodorous. In addition, girls may complain of associated pruritus, erythema, urinary problems such as dysuria and increased frequency, and abdominal pain (D_x Box). Sexually active pubescent girls with vaginitis from a sexually transmitted infection (STI) (eg, gonorrhea) generally have a more profuse, purulent discharge.

Pathophysiology

Prepubescent girls are at risk for developing vulvovaginitis for anatomic and physiologic reasons. Unlike pubertal girls and young women, prepubescent girls have no pubic hair and a smaller labial fat pad to protect the vaginal introitus. The labia minora are small and tend to open when girls are in a squatting position, thereby exposing the vaginal introitus. The relative proximity of the anus to the vagina in young girls also contributes to vaginal contamination with enteric organisms. More importantly, poor hygienic practices (ie, wiping back to front after urination or defecation) can further compound the problem.

In addition, the normal physiology of the vaginal epithelium in prepubescent girls predisposes to vaginitis and vulvar inflammation. The unestrogenized vaginal epithelium is relatively thin, immature, and easily traumatized. Also, the pH of the vagina is neutral to alkaline, compared with the acidic environment of the vagina in adult females. Local antibody production also may be lacking in the vagina of prepubescent girls. Vulvar skin is also easily irritated by soaps,

medications, chemicals such as bubble baths, and close-fitting clothing. Girls who are overweight may be particularly susceptible to perineal irritation and subsequent inflammation of the area.

Differential Diagnosis

A vaginal discharge is normal at 2 distinct times in prepubescent girls: shortly after birth, secondary to the effects of maternal estrogen, and approximately 6 months to 1 year before the onset of menarche (physiologic leukorrhea), which occurs, in most girls, by sexual maturity rating (SMR) (Tanner stage) 4. Other causes of vaginal discharges in prepubescent and pubescent girls are presented in Box 100-1.

Evaluation

Prepubescent Girls

History

A complete history should be obtained in all girls with a vaginal discharge (Questions Box). Practitioners should inquire about the

---

Dx — Vaginitis

- Non-physiologic vaginal discharge
- Profuse, malodorous, or purulent vaginal discharge
- Perineal erythema
- Vaginal pruritus or irritation
- Dysuria

Box 100-1. Causes of Vaginal Discharge in Prepubescent and Pubescent Girls

Prepubescent Girls
- Estrogen withdrawal (neonates)
- Nonspecific vulvovaginitis
- Chemical irritation secondary to soaps and detergents
- Mechanical irritation from nylon panties or tight-fitting clothes
- Foreign body in vagina
- Poor hygiene
- Pinworms
- Yeast infection (eg, *Candida*)
- Bacterial infection (eg, group A beta-hemolytic streptococcus, nonencapsulated *Haemophilus influenzae, Shigella* sp, *Salmonella* sp, *Yersinia*)
- Sexually transmitted infection (eg, gonococcal infection, chlamydial infection, trichomoniasis, human herpesvirus, human papillomavirus)
- Congenital abnormality (eg, ectopic ureter [local inflammation])
- Acquired abnormality (eg, labial fusion [pooling of urine in vagina])
- Urethral prolapse
- Systemic illness (eg, scarlet fever, measles, varicella, Kawasaki disease, Crohn disease)
- Vulvar skin disease: lichen sclerosis, contact dermatitis, psoriasis, zinc deficiency

Pubescent Girls
- Physiologic leukorrhea
- Foreign body in vagina (eg, retained tampon or condom)
- Yeast infection (eg, *Candida)*
- Bacterial infection (eg, group A beta-hemolytic streptococcus, *Staphylococcus aureus*)
- Sexually transmitted infection (eg, gonococcal infection, chlamydial infection, trichomoniasis, bacterial vaginosis)
- Chemical irritation (eg, douches, spermicides, latex [condoms])
- Local trauma (eg, penile studs)

Vaginitis

Questions

Prepubescent Girls

- What is the color of the discharge?
- What is the consistency of the discharge?
- How profuse is the discharge?
- Is the discharge malodorous?
- How long has the discharge been present?
- How often does the discharge occur (ie, is it found on the panties daily)?
- Are there any associated problems (eg, dysuria, abdominal pain, enuresis, anal pruritus)?
- What types of laundry soaps or detergents are used?
- Does the child take bubble baths?
- Has the child had any recent illnesses or treatment with oral antibiotics?
- Does the child clean herself after using the toilet, or does she require help?
- In what direction does she tend to wipe after a bowel movement?
- Is there a concern for, or history of, child sexual abuse?
- Has there been any recent behavioral changes (eg, nightmares, tears, recurrent abdominal pain)?
- What has the family done to treat the discharge?

Pubescent Girls (all of the above questions plus the following)

- What is the reproductive history (menstrual and sexual)?
- Does the adolescent douche or use scented panty liners?
- Does the adolescent use or share sex toys?
- Is there a history of sexual assault or abuse?
- If appropriate, is the adolescent using any form of barrier or hormonal contraception? When was the last episode of unprotected intercourse?
- How many sexual partners has the patient had?
- Does the patient or partner have any history of a previous sexually transmitted infection, including hepatitis B or C?

appearance of the discharge, its duration, and the relative amount. A profuse, purulent discharge is probably more consistent with one specific etiology (eg, N gonorrhoeae) than is a scant, thin discharge that suggests a nonspecific etiology. The existence of urinary problems also should be determined. Pooling of urine in the vagina secondary to labial fusion can lead to vulvovaginitis in addition to a urinary tract infection. Changes in bowel or bladder habits and sudden changes in behavior, such as nightmares or inappropriate stranger anxiety, also should be noted. Such changes in behavior warrant a further inquiry into the possibility of sexual abuse, regardless of the practitioner's index of suspicion. Depending on the information disclosed and the age of the patient, a decision might be made to interview the child and parents independently. Other points to discuss include the type of detergents or soaps used for laundry as well as for bathing because these may be irritating. Any recent illnesses also should be documented as a possible source of autoinoculation or, if oral antibiotics were prescribed, as a reason for the alteration of the normal vaginal flora. In addition, patients' hygienic practices should be reviewed. Adolescent patients should always be interviewed alone (see Chapter 6). In particular, a reproductive history must be obtained, keeping in mind that puberty and sexual activity alter normal vaginal flora.

Physical Examination

Although the genital examination is the priority, a complete physical examination should be performed. This not only allows clinicians to identify other abnormal physical findings, but it also alleviates some of the anxiety often associated with a genital examination. Because most vaginal discharges in prepubescent girls result from nonspecific vulvovaginitis, visualization of the cervix with a speculum is not indicated. Regardless of the gender of the examiner, a chaperone is recommended during the genital examination, particularly in postpubertal patients.

The overall demeanor of the young patient at the onset of the genital examination should be noted. Overly compliant, apathetic behavior in children may be a cause for concern for sexual abuse, especially in the context of a chronic or recurrent purulent vaginal discharge.

On physical examination, the patient's SMR must be noted and recorded. In addition, the external genitalia should be examined closely for the presence of any lesions or evidence of erythema. Chronic changes in labial skin, such as those associated with constant scratching, also should be documented.

Girls should be placed in the modified lithotomy or batrachian (frog leg) position, and the labia majora should be gently spread apart to visualize the hymen. The knee-chest position also can be used, depending on the comfort level of the practitioner as well as the patient. If the labia cannot be spread apart, the girl may have labial fusion or adhesions. Perihymenal and periurethral erythema and injection should be noted, in addition to any evidence of edema, trauma, or abnormal masses such as urethral prolapse. Hymenal size and appearance should be carefully evaluated for any evidence of suspected sexual abuse (see Chapter 132). The appearance, consistency, and amount of the vaginal discharge, including the presence or absence of an odor, also should be documented. These findings may vary depending on the characteristics and cause of the discharge. Finally, the anus should be inspected for tone and any evidence of trauma or abnormal lesions such as genital warts. An anal wink is normally elicited. Although not usually indicated, a rectal examination should be performed in an attempt to palpate a foreign body or mass in those patients with a chronic or bloody vaginal discharge. If the examiner cannot adequately visualize the perineum, vulva, and vaginal introitus using the batrachian (supine) or knee-chest position and the patient has persistent or significant symptoms, an examination under anesthesia may be warranted.

Laboratory Tests

Laboratory studies are often unnecessary in prepubescent girls with a nonspecific, non-bloody vaginal discharge, diffuse vulvar erythema, and no suspicion or history of sexual abuse. A vaginal culture for isolation of GABHS is indicated in girls with an abrupt onset of a serosanguineous discharge and a history of a systemic illness. The cellophane tape test may be helpful in diagnosing a pinworm infection in girls with associated vulvar or anal pruritus. A potassium hydroxide (KOH) wet mount reveals pseudohypha if a monilial infection is present, although this diagnosis is often made clinically.

If the discharge is purulent, persistent, or malodorous or if sexual abuse is suspected, vaginal cultures must be obtained for *N gonorrhoeae* and *C trachomatis*. For suspected cases of sexual abuse or assault, culture remains the gold standard because of the risk of a false-positive result with non-amplified probe tests (direct immunofluorescent smears, enzyme immunoassays) and nucleic acid amplification tests (NAATs). With genital and anal specimens, false-positive results can occur because of cross-reaction with fecal flora. In certain cases, a normal saline wet mount to check for mobile trichomonads may be indicated.

Pubescent Girls

History

In adolescent or pubescent girls with vaginal discharge, physicians should inquire about a history of sexual activity or assault in addition to other information that relates to their condition (see Questions Box). Questions concerning the possible acquisition of an STI also must be asked in a nonjudgmental, confidential manner.

Physical Examination

Pubescent girls with an uncomplicated history who have never been sexually active should be examined in a similar fashion as the prepubescent female. The external genitalia should be examined to evaluate the SMR of the patient and the presence of any lesions or anatomic abnormalities. Perihymenal or periurethral erythema and hymenal size and appearance should be noted. In the absence of a mucopurulent or bloody discharge, a speculum examination is generally not warranted.

In addition to an overall physical examination, a complete external genital and speculum examination is indicated in symptomatic, sexually active girls (ie, history of lower abdominal pain, severe dysmenorrhea, or vaginal discharge). The purpose of the speculum examination is to visualize the cervix, properly obtain vaginal and cervical specimens, and examine the vagina for lesions (eg, condylomata acuminata). A bimanual examination also should be performed to check for cervical motion tenderness as well as adnexal masses or uterine tenderness, which are associated with pelvic inflammatory disease (PID).

Laboratory Tests

Pubescent girls who are not sexually active should have a laboratory evaluation similar to that described for prepubescent girls. Sexually active adolescents, however, warrant a more thorough evaluation to establish the etiology of their symptoms and investigate for cervicitis. In general, if a speculum examination is being performed in these adolescents, a single-swab endocervical sample should be obtained and sent for gonorrhea and chlamydia via NAATs (eg, ligase chain reaction, polymerase chain reaction). Urine or a vaginal swab also should be sent for *N gonorrhoeae* and *C trachomatis* in those adolescents who refuse a pelvic examination or for screening purposes in the asymptomatic sexually active patient. Recommendations have changed for teenagers regarding the age at which cervical cancer screening (Pap smear) is indicated (see Chapter 42 for details). A culture or direct fluorescent antibody test for herpes simplex is indicated only if the history of exposure is positive and ulcerative or vesicular lesions are present.

Other causes of vaginal symptoms can be determined by the pH and microscopic analysis of a fresh sample of the vaginal discharge. A normal saline wet mount should be made using a sterile, saline-moistened swab, especially if a nonspecific discharge is present or bacterial vaginosis (BV) is a concern. In addition, motile or static trichomonads may be seen on a wet mount as well as white blood cells. A 10% KOH mount is appropriate in cases of suspected candidiasis. Mixing 10% KOH with the discharge may also produce a "fishy" odor (positive "whiff test"), which is consistent with BV and sometimes a trichomonad infection. In addition, a vaginal pH greater than 4.5 is commonly seen with BV or trichomoniasis, although it is not specific. Commercial kits to evaluate for BV, trichomoniasis, and candida via nucleic acid probes are available for the office setting where pH paper, KOH, and microscopic analysis of vaginal fluids is not possible. A Gram stain of any purulent material may lead to an early diagnosis of gonococcal cervicitis. Serologies for syphilis should also be obtained in adolescents with suspected (symptomatic) or proven STIs. In addition, these patients should be offered annual testing for HIV.

Management

Management of a **nonspecific vaginal discharge** is aimed at relieving the uncomfortable symptoms associated with this type of inflammation. Prepubescent girls should be instructed to **discontinue use of all chemical irritants,** including bubble baths and harsh soaps, in the genital area. Warm water **sitz baths** should be recommended once or twice daily for approximately 1 week or until the patient feels better. A small amount of A + D ointment or similar emollient can be used to protect the vulvar skin and promote healing. In addition, girls should be instructed in **proper hygiene** (eg, wiping front to back after a bowel movement, appropriate hand washing). The use of cotton or cotton-crotch underwear and loose-fitting skirts or pants should be encouraged. Occasionally, a persistent, nonspecific vaginal discharge lasting longer than 2 to 3 weeks' duration may benefit from a 10-day course of oral antibiotics such as amoxicillin, amoxicillin-clavulanate, or clindamycin. Girls who are obese with poor hygiene are especially prone to recurrences of vulvovaginitis.

Antifungal medications such as **clotrimazole** (Lotrimin) or **miconazole** (Monistat) cream may be prescribed if a monilial infection is present. Empiric treatment may be warranted in children or adolescents with a previous history of oral antibiotic usage, diabetes mellitus, or other chronic conditions that may alter the normal vaginal flora.

Pinworms are treated with a single oral dose of **albendazole, 400 mg,** or **pyrantel pamoate** (Antiminth), 11 mg/kg/dose (to a maximum of 1 g). Most authorities recommend repeat treatment after 2 weeks to kill worms that may have hatched after the first dose. Bedding and clothing should be laundered and dried in a dryer.

If a retained foreign body is suspected in a prepubescent girl, an examination under general anesthesia may be necessary. Alternatively, practitioners can attempt vaginal irrigation in a cooperative child by placing a small feeding tube at the hymenal opening and injecting warm saline. Toilet paper is the most commonly retrieved material in prepubescent girls.

Pubescent girls who are not sexually active should be treated in a similar fashion as prepubertal girls. If the discharge is consistent with a diagnosis of physiologic leukorrhea, practitioners should reassure patients and educate them about other issues related to puberty (eg, menarche, body odor). Sexually active adolescents with positive vaginal cultures, NAATs, or highly suspicious vaginal discharges should receive treatment depending on the suspected or causal organism (see Chapter 101 for details concerning treatment). Table 100-2 briefly outlines current recommendations.

Any disclosure of molestation by prepubescent or pubescent girls must be reported to the appropriate authorities. In addition, abnormal physical findings and positive cultures for STIs in prepubescent and pubescent girls who have never been sexually active must be reported to law enforcement and investigated.

Prognosis

In most prepubescent girls, vaginitis resolves spontaneously or after appropriate treatment with no permanent sequelae. In contrast, pubescent girls treated for vulvovaginitis or uncomplicated cervicitis from an STI continue to be at future risk for the development of PID, HIV, and pregnancy given their high-risk behavior, inconsistent use of barrier contraception (eg, condoms), and recurrent exposure to STIs.

CASE RESOLUTION

In the case presented at the beginning of the chapter, the girl and her parents should be assured that the discharge is consistent with a nonspecific process. She should be instructed to take sitz baths for 1 week, discontinue bubble baths and the use of soap in the genital area, and wear loose-fitting clothes with cotton underwear. The girl should be reexamined in 1 to 2 weeks for resolution of her symptoms. No laboratory studies are warranted at this time.

Table 100-2. Treatment Recommendations for Adolescents With Infectious Vaginal Discharge

Organism	Treatment[a]
Neisseria gonorrhoeae	Ceftriaxone, 250 mg intramuscularly, once, PLUS treatment for Chlamydia trachomatis
Chlamydia trachomatis[b]	Azithromycin, 1 g orally, once, or doxycycline, orally, 100 mg twice a day for 1 week
Trichomonas vaginalis	Metronidazole, 2 g orally, once, or tinidazole, 2 g orally, once
Bacterial vaginosis	Metronidazole, 500 mg, orally twice a day for 7 days; or clindamycin cream 2%, one applicator-ful intravaginally at bedtime for 7 days; or metronidazole gel 0.75%, one applicatorful intravaginally once a day for 5 days
Candida albicans	1% clotrimazole cream 5 g intravaginally for 7–14 days; 2% clotrimazole cream 5 g intravaginally for 3 days; 2% miconazole cream 5 g intravaginally for 7 days; 4% miconazole cream 5 g intravaginally for 3 days; 0.4% terconazole cream 5 g intravaginally for 7 days; 0.8% terconazole cream 5 g intravaginally for 3 days; fluconazole, 150 mg orally once

[a]For a complete list of treatment options, refer to Workowski KA, Berman S; Centers for Disease Control and Prevention. Sexually transmitted diseases treatment guidelines, 2010. *MMWR Recomm Rep.* 2010;59(RR-12):1–110.

[b]May be associated with vaginal discharge because it causes cervicitis.

Selected References

Braverman PK, Breech L; American Academy of Pediatrics Committee on Adolescence. Gynecologic examination for adolescents in the pediatric office setting. *Pediatrics.* 2010;126(3):583–590

Burstein GR, Murray PJ. Diagnosis and management of sexually transmitted diseases among adolescents. *Pediatr Rev.* 2003;24(4):119–127

Emans SJ. Vulvovaginal problems in the pre-pubertal child. In: *Emans, Laufer, Goldstein's Pediatric and Adolescent Gynecology.* 6th ed. Philadelphia, PA: Lippincott Williams & Wilkins; 2012:42–59

Farhi D, Wendling J, Molinari E, et al. Non-sexually related acute genital ulcers in 13 pubertal girls: a clinical and microbiological study. *Arch Dermatol.* 2009; 145(1):38–45

Fortin K, Jenny C. Sexual abuse. *Pediatr Rev.* 2012;33(1):19–32

Jacobs AM, Alderman EM. Gynecologic examination of the prepubertal girl. *Pediatr Rev.* 2014;35(3):97–105

Kokotos F. Vulvovaginitis. *Pediatr Rev.* 2006;27(3):116–117

Stricker T, Navratil F, Sennhauser FH. Vulvovaginitis in prepubertal girls. *Arch Dis Child.* 2003;88(4):324–326

Sugar NF, Graham EA. Common gynecologic problems in prepubertal girls. *Pediatr Rev.* 2006;27(6):213–223

Syed TS, Braverman PK. Vaginitis in adolescents. *Adolesc Med Clin.* 2004;15(2): 235–251

Workowski KA, Berman S; Centers for Disease Control and Prevention. Sexually transmitted diseases treatment guidelines, 2010. *MMWR Recomm Rep.* 2010; 59(RR-12):1–110

CHAPTER 101

Sexually Transmitted Infections

Monica Sifuentes, MD

CASE STUDY

A 17-year-old male presents with a small red lesion on the tip of his penis. He noticed an area of erythema a few weeks before, but it resolved spontaneously. He reports no fever, myalgia, headache, dysuria, or urethral discharge. He is sexually active and occasionally uses condoms. He did not use a condom during his last sexual encounter 2 weeks ago, however, because his partner uses oral contraception. The adolescent has never been treated for any sexually transmitted infections (STIs) and is otherwise healthy. His partners are exclusively female.

On examination, he is a sexual maturity rating (Tanner stage) 4 circumcised male with a 2- to 3-mm vesicle on the glans penis. Minimal erythema is present at the base of the lesion, and there is no urethral discharge. The testicles are descended bilaterally, and no masses are palpable. Bilateral shotty, non-tender, inguinal adenopathy is evident.

Questions

1. What conditions are associated with vesicles in the genital area?
2. What risk factors are associated with the acquisition of STIs during adolescence?
3. What screening tests should be performed in patients with suspected STIs?
4. What recommendations regarding partners of patients with STIs should be given?
5. What issues of confidentiality are important to address with adolescents who desire treatment for STIs?

Most teenagers in the United States have their first sexual experience before they graduate from high school. In the 2011 national Youth Risk Behavior Survey conducted by the Centers for Disease Control and Prevention (CDC), nearly half of all students in high school reported having had sexual intercourse during their lifetime, with 6% of students nationwide reporting sexual intercourse for the first time before age 13 years. More importantly, nearly 18% of boys and 13% of girls in grades 9 to 12 reported having had 4 or more sexual partners during their life. The consequences of sexual activity in adolescents include increased rates of bacterial and viral sexually transmitted infections (STIs), unintended pregnancy, and the possible acquisition of long-term infections such as HIV in the 15- to 24-year age group. Without adequate antiretroviral therapy, the average time from acquisition of HIV infection to the development of AIDS is approximately 10 years, but some people may progress through this latency phase faster. Given the complex nature of these consequences, the clinician must be skilled and comfortable in obtaining a complete sexual history in teenaged patients and in diagnosing and treating common STIs.

Increasing levels of sexual activity directly affect STI trends in adolescents. Other influential factors include multiple (sequential or concurrent) sexual partners; inconsistent and incorrect use of condoms and other barrier methods; experimentation with drugs, including alcohol, which results in poor judgment concerning sexual activity; poor compliance with antibiotic regimens; and biological factors, such as an earlier age of menarche and the presence of cervical ectopia in adolescent females. The feeling of invulnerability and the associated risk-taking behavior that occurs during adolescence make most sexual encounters spontaneous rather than premeditated. As a result, preventive measures are forgotten, ignored, or overlooked by this age group, allowing adolescents to disregard the possible consequences of their actions. Other factors influencing STI trends are related to societal norms. Traditionally, educational materials and STI services have not been readily available to adolescents in some areas of the United States, unlike other industrialized countries. Many teens also have difficulty accessing comprehensive health care in their communities and are concerned about confidentiality when obtaining medical services for sensitive issues. In addition, the depiction of casual sexual relationships in television sitcoms, music videos, and motion pictures may play a major role in glamorizing sex. Advances in technology via unlimited Internet access also gives teenagers the opportunity to communicate with peers that were previously unreachable and access health information that is unfiltered and may be misleading.

Epidemiology

The overall prevalence of STIs in adolescents is difficult to estimate because not all STIs are reportable, many infections are asymptomatic, and collected data may not include specific subsets of the population such as teens younger than 15 years. It has been estimated, however, that nearly 50% of all new STIs diagnosed annually in the United States occur among teenagers and young adults aged 15 to 24 years. *Chlamydia* remains the most common cause of cervicitis and urethritis in adolescents, with age-specific rates highest among girls and young women 15 to 24 years of age and young men 20 to

24 years of age. Additionally, studies have shown that certain adolescent subpopulations are at greater risk for chlamydial infection, such as homeless and incarcerated youth, socioeconomically disadvantaged youth, teenagers attending family planning clinics, and pregnant adolescents. Complications of untreated chlamydial cervicitis occur in 10% to 30% of cases and include pelvic inflammatory disease (PID), ectopic pregnancy, chronic pelvic pain, and infertility. Epididymitis, a result of urethral infection, occurs in 1% to 3% of infected males. Other conditions that are uncommon but may occur in males as a result of an infection with chlamydia include proctitis, prostatitis, and reactive arthritis (formerly called Reiter syndrome).

Teenagers have the highest incidence of **gonorrhea** of any age group, although prevalence rates have decreased since 2001. The highest rates of gonorrhea reportedly occur in adolescent females, young men in their early 20s, young adult inner-city minorities, incarcerated youth, men who have sex with men, and prostitutes. A large number of sexual partners, injection drug use, exposure to prostitutes, and casual sexual contacts also contribute to the risk of infection. In 2011, the CDC reported gonorrhea rates to be highest among adolescents and young adults compared with the rest of the population, particularly among teenaged girls and young women. The incidence of gonorrhea in 15- to 19-year-old women was 556.5 per 100,000. Men aged 15 to 19 years had the second highest rates of gonorrhea (248.6 per 100,000) compared with men aged 20 to 24 years, who had even higher rates of gonorrhea (450.6 per 100,000). Of the more than 1 million cases of PID reported annually in the United States, 20% to 30% are in sexually active adolescents. The risk of developing PID is increased severalfold in this age group compared with adult women for several reasons: failure to use condoms consistently, multiple new partners within the previous 12 months, and a history of other STIs. Additionally, according to the National Survey of Family Growth, girls who initiated vaginal intercourse at younger than 15 years had the highest prevalence of PID. Complications of PID, such as tubo-ovarian abscess (TOA) formation, are more likely to occur in adolescents as a result of late presentation, delayed diagnosis, difficulty accessing health care, and non-adherence with prescribed treatment regimens.

Although the rate of primary and secondary **syphilis** declined from 1990 to 2000, the number of cases is now increasing, primarily among young men. During 2005, the incidence of syphilis was highest among women in the 20- to 24-year-old age group and among men in their mid-30s. In 2012, however, young men aged 20 to 24 years had the highest rates of syphilis. Studies have shown that people with syphilis, as well as other STIs causing genital ulcers, also are at increased risk for HIV acquisition.

Human papillomavirus (HPV) is the most common STI in the United States, with the highest infection rates among adolescents and young adults. Recent studies report the prevalence in sexually active adolescents to range from 30% to 60% and to decline with age. The prevalence of HPV in adolescents varies widely for 2 reasons: infection with HPV is often latent and generally regresses spontaneously, and HPV is not a reportable condition. Behavioral and biological risk factors for HPV infection have been identified and include early age of sexual initiation, unprotected intercourse with multiple sexual partners, partner's number of sexual partners, a lack of consistent condom use, and a history of another STI such as genital herpes, which may facilitate HPV acquisition by compromising mucosal integrity. Cigarette use also increases the risk of infection and HPV-related disease, as does an altered immune system.

Infection with **human herpesvirus 2** is underestimated and is the most common cause of genital ulcerative disease in the United States. Reportedly, human herpesvirus 2 occurs in approximately 4% of whites and 17% of African Americans by the end of their teenage years.

As of 2011, there are more than 35,000 adolescents and young adults in the United States living with a diagnosis of **HIV**. Because the time from acute HIV infection to immunosuppression is, on average, 10 years for untreated adolescents, estimates of asymptomatic or early HIV infection are often based on reported cases of **AIDS** in young adults in their 20s. AIDS in adolescents occurs primarily in males and ethnic minorities. Most of these individuals are infected through sexual contact or injection drug use. Teen subpopulations who are at particularly high risk for acquiring HIV are youth who have male-to-male sexual contact; are bisexual, transgendered, or homeless or a runaway; are injection drug users; are incarcerated; are mentally ill; are in the foster care system; or have been sexually or physically abused.

Clinical Presentation

Adolescents with an STI may go to their physicians with specific complaints related to the genitourinary system, such as painful urination or vaginal discharge. They also may report more generalized complaints, like fever and malaise, especially in cases of primary human herpesvirus infection or during the viremic phase of HIV acquisition (D_x Box: Sexually Transmitted Infections). In addition,

Sexually Transmitted Infections

Males
- Dysuria
- Urethral discharge or pain
- Testicular pain
- Presence of any lesions in the genital area such as ulcers, vesicles, or warts
- Sexual partner who has a sexually transmitted infection (STI)

Females
- Dysuria
- Abnormal vaginal discharge
- Intermenstrual or irregular vaginal bleeding
- Dysmenorrhea
- Dyspareunia
- Postcoital bleeding
- Lower abdominal pain
- Systemic symptoms such as fever, nausea, vomiting, malaise
- Presence of any lesions in the genital area such as ulcers, vesicles, or warts
- Sexual partner who has an STI

some teenagers will use a vague complaint as an opportunity to visit their primary care practitioner with the hope that the physician inquires about sexual behaviors. It may be only then that the adolescent will disclose his or her true concern about an infection if the physician appears genuinely interested and nonjudgmental.

Pathophysiology

A number of biological factors contribute to the increased prevalence rates of STIs in adolescents, particularly in females. At the onset of puberty, the columnar epithelial cells in the vagina transform to squamous epithelium, while columnar cells at the cervix persist (Figure 101-1). With increasing age, the squamocolumnar junction recedes into the endocervix. In adolescent females, however, this junction, referred to as ectopia, is often located at the vaginal portion of the cervix and is relatively exposed, which places these females at particular risk for gonococcal and chlamydial infections. The infectious organisms preferentially attach to cervical columnar cells and infect them. Of note is that the use of oral contraceptives also prolongs this immature histologic state.

The cytologic changes seen in cervical cells of adolescents with HPV infection are also believed to be age-related. The immature cervical metaplastic or columnar cells seem to be more highly vulnerable to infection and neoplastic changes. In addition, exposure to other cofactors (eg, tobacco use, multiple episodes of new HPV infections) is likely to promote the development of squamous intraepithelial neoplasia (SIN) and cervical carcinoma. Not all young women exposed to HPV develop lesions or progress to SIN, however, and most will not remain positive for HPV throughout their lifetime.

The presence of genital ulcers has been shown to facilitate the transmission and acquisition of HIV. Such ulcers provide a point of entry past denuded epithelium. In addition, it is hypothesized that many activated lymphocytes and macrophages are located at the base of the ulcer and are therefore susceptible to infection by HIV.

Pelvic inflammatory disease usually develops from an ascending mixed polymicrobial infection, often related to an untreated STI of the cervix and vagina. The infection spreads contiguously upward to the upper genital tract, resulting in inflammation, scarring, and crypt formation in the fallopian tubes. The most common causal organisms, which account for more than half of the cases of PID in most series, are *Chlamydia trachomatis* and *Neisseria gonorrhoeae*. Other agents include *Escherichia coli*, other enteric flora, and microbes implicated in bacterial vaginosis, such as *Mycoplasma hominis*, *Mycoplasma genitalium*, *Ureaplasma urealyticum*, *Bacteroides* species, and anaerobic cocci. Viruses such as HIV and human herpesvirus can facilitate the process of this ascending infection by disrupting normal immunologic barriers to infection, such as altering the vaginal pH and flora and the cervical mucus barrier.

Differential Diagnosis

Most patients with STIs present with 1 of 5 clinical syndromes: urethritis/cervicitis, epididymitis, PID, genital ulcer disease, or genital warts, all of which can be easily diagnosed (Box 101-1). Other conditions that mimic STIs, however, must be considered,

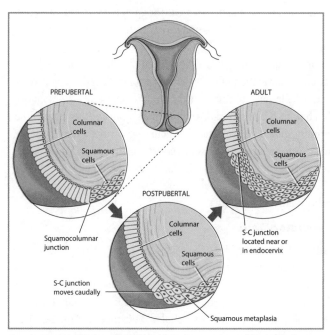

Figure 101-1. Development of the cervical squamocolumnar (S-C) junction, from puberty to adulthood.

Box 101-1. Differential Diagnosis of Sexually Transmitted Infection by Clinical Syndrome

Urethritis
- *Neisseria gonorrhoeae*
- Nongonococcal disease
  - —*Chlamydia trachomatis*
  - —*Ureaplasma urealyticum*
  - —*Trichomonas vaginalis*
  - —Human herpesvirus
  - —Yeasts

Cervicitis
- *C trachomatis*
- *N gonorrhoeae*
- *T vaginalis*
- Human herpesvirus (especially primary type 2)

Pelvic Inflammatory Disease
- *N gonorrhoeae*
- *C trachomatis*
- Anaerobes
- Gram-negative rods
- Streptococci
- *Mycoplasma hominis*
- *U urealyticum*

Vaginitis
- *T vaginalis*
- *Candida albicans* and other yeast
- *Gardnerella vaginalis*

Genital Ulcers
- *Treponema pallidum* (syphilis)
- Human herpesvirus 1 and 2
- *Haemophilus ducreyi* (chancroid)
- *C trachomatis* (lymphogranuloma venereum)

Genital Warts
- *T pallidum* (condyloma latum)
- Human papillomavirus (condyloma acuminatum)

Proctitis
- *N gonorrhoeae*
- *C trachomatis*
- *T pallidum*
- Human herpesvirus
- Particular to homosexual youth (in addition to the above)
  - —Hepatitis A and B virus
  - —*Shigella*
  - —*Campylobacter*
  - —*Giardia lamblia*
  - —*Entamoeba histolytica*

Pharyngitis
- *N gonorrhoeae*
- Human herpesvirus 1 and 2

particularly in certain cases in which the adolescent denies sexual activity or where the disorder does not respond to routine medical management. These disorders include **mucocutaneous ulcers** associated with systemic lupus erythematosus and Behçet syndrome. Often, systemic disorders such as these can be ruled out historically, although a minimal workup might be necessary. **Benign oral lesions,** such as aphthous ulcers, also can be confused with herpetic ulcers. When evaluating an adolescent female with acute lower abdominal pain, surgical conditions such as **appendicitis, ovarian torsion,** and **ectopic pregnancy** must be ruled out. In the sexually active male with testicular pain, **testicular torsion** must be cautiously considered and thoroughly evaluated before a diagnosis of acute epididymitis is made.

Evaluation

In all sexually active adolescents, a complete history, including a sexual history, should be obtained (Questions Box). Because sexual identity and sexual behavior may differ, risk assessment for an STI, particularly HIV, should be based on a review of actual sexual behavior (eg, anal intercourse) rather than on an adolescent's stated sexual orientation at the time of the visit. A detailed gynecologic history also should be reviewed with females, including any recent changes in menstrual bleeding and dyspareunia. The rest of the history should then focus on the particular complaint and any associated symptoms. Sexually active adolescents should have a complete physical examination, including a thorough genital examination. Although diagnostic tests should be determined by the adolescent's risk for a specific STI based on historical and physical findings, one must keep in mind that many adolescent patients are asymptomatic, and

screening for common STIs such as chlamydia and gonorrhea should be performed at least annually on all sexually active teenagers through noninvasive urine or vaginal nucleic acid amplification testing (NAAT). Adolescents at higher risk (eg, a history of STI, multiple partners, men who have sex with men) should be screened every 6 months.

Urethritis and Epididymitis

History

Because infectious urethritis is more common in young men, all sexually active adolescent males should be asked about the presence of dysuria, urethral discharge, and urethral erythema or pruritus. In females, symptoms such as dysuria and increased urination may appear more gradually and are reported more frequently than other symptoms like meatal edema, erythema, or urethral discharge, which are rarely noticed in girls. General urinary symptoms such as acute urinary frequency or urgency are uncommon with urethritis, especially in males, but all patients should be asked about these symptoms. More often, urethritis is asymptomatic, and the diagnosis is made by routine annual screening in sexually active adolescents or through known contact with a partner with an STI (eg, *C trachomatis, N gonorrhoeae*).

To diagnose acute epididymitis, sexually active males should be asked about testicular pain and swelling. Symptoms associated with urethritis may be present or may have preceded the scrotal symptoms.

Physical Examination

In males, the urethra should be the focus of the genital examination. The presence of a urethral discharge and its consistency (ie, mucopurulent or purulent) should be noted. Any other urethral or genital lesions also should be assessed. The epididymis, spermatic cord, and testes should be palpated carefully for tenderness and swelling.

In females, a full pelvic examination should be performed after careful examination of the external genitalia for any ulcerative or wart-like lesions. Urethritis is most often caused by *C trachomatis*, but human herpesvirus and trichomoniasis can be other causes. The urethra should be inspected for edema, erythema, or any evidence of a discharge prior to speculum insertion. The presence or absence of a vaginal or endocervical discharge also should be noted during the pelvic examination, but its absence does not rule out the possibility of an STI.

Laboratory Tests

Although less desirable to the adolescent male, a Gram stain of the urethral discharge may confirm the diagnosis of urethritis in males. The specimen should be obtained using a Dacron or cotton swab because calcium alginate inhibits the growth of *Chlamydia*. The presence of gram-negative, intracellular diplococci with the typical "kidney bean" morphology is indicative of an infection with *N gonorrhoeae* (gonococcal urethritis). Five or more polymorphonuclear (PMN) leukocytes per oil immersion field but no organisms

---

Questions

Sexually Transmitted Infections

- Are you currently in a relationship?
- Are you sexually active?
- At what age did you begin to have sex?
- Do you have sex with men, women, or both?
- How many partners have you had? When was your last contact?
- Have you ever been forced to have sex, had sex while under the influence of alcohol or drugs, or exchanged sex for food, shelter, money, or drugs?
- Do you or your partner(s) use contraception? What type?
- Do you or your partner(s) use drugs or alcohol?
- Have you or any of your sexual contacts ever been diagnosed with a sexually transmitted infection? Did you and they receive treatment?
- Do you have abdominal pain, dysuria, increased urinary frequency, or hesitancy?
- Have you noticed any ulcers, blisters, warts, or other bumps in the genital area? Are the lesions painful?
- For females: Do you have a vaginal discharge or itching? Is sex uncomfortable or painful? Do you have bleeding between periods or after intercourse?
- For males: Do you have a discharge from your penis? Any testicular pain or swelling? Any associated burning or itching?

indicates the more common type of infection, nongonococcal urethritis, usually found in males. In 15% to 40% of cases, nongonococcal urethritis is caused by *C trachomatis.* If no PMN leukocytes are seen on Gram stain or if the patient is asymptomatic, assessment for leukocyte esterase with a urine dipstick should be made using the first 10 to 15 mL of a first-voided urine specimen. The sediment also should be examined under the microscope to determine if more than 10 white blood cells per high-power field are present. A routine urine culture is generally not recommended in males and may be of little help in females unless the physician is suspicious of a urinary tract infection.

Screening tests using urine or vaginal samples are considered standard of care for detecting gonorrhea and *C trachomatis,* especially in asymptomatic sexually active adolescents. These non-culture tests rely on amplification of DNA (ie, polymerase chain reaction [PCR] and ligase chain reaction) and are highly sensitive and convenient for screening teenagers because the test can be performed on a routine patient-obtained urine or a physician/patient-obtained vaginal specimen. A disadvantage is that these tests are costly and may have a greater potential for false-positive results, making a definitive diagnosis questionable in a judicial setting. In the adolescent population, however, NAATs are definitely more acceptable than tests requiring a direct urethral swab specimen and can be used to confirm chlamydial or gonococcal urethritis for screening or diagnostic purposes.

Color duplex Doppler ultrasound may be necessary to make an accurate diagnosis of epididymitis, especially if there is any consideration for testicular torsion in the adolescent male. Whether the diagnosis is questionable or confirmed, a urologic consultation should be obtained immediately.

Cervicitis

History

Cervicitis in females is parallel to urethritis in males. Because cervicitis is a local infection, systemic symptoms may not occur, which makes asymptomatic infections, especially with *C trachomatis,* very common. However, a variety of important historical points and associated complaints should be addressed in all female sexually active teenagers. Is a vaginal discharge present? If so, does it have an odor or color? Is the patient experiencing any urinary frequency, urgency, or dysuria? Has she had any non-menstrual vaginal bleeding or spotting, including postcoital bleeding or dyspareunia from endocervicitis? A known exposure to other STIs also must be ascertained. Is the current partner symptomatic or receiving antibiotic treatment? Does the patient or her current or past partners have a history of an STI?

More generalized symptoms, such as moderate lower abdominal pain (acute or chronic) associated with nausea, vomiting, and fever, may indicate a complication of untreated or undetected cervicitis, such as PID. Additional symptoms associated with disseminated gonococcal infection such as fever, arthritis, and rash should be investigated as well as the involvement of other areas of the body (eg sore throat).

Physical Examination

After completing the full physical examination with particular attention to the patient's skin, pharynx, hands, fingers, and joints, the physician should then focus on the genitourinary examination. The sexual maturity rating should first be noted, and the external genitalia should be examined for the presence of any lesions or inflammation of the perineum. Any urethral erythema or discharge also should be noted. The presence of a vaginal discharge can be assessed more completely when performing the speculum examination, which should be performed in all sexually active adolescent females with vaginal or persistent lower urinary tract complaints.

During the speculum examination, the vaginal mucosa should be inspected, the presence of a vaginal discharge identified, and the appearance of the cervical os documented. The physician should determine whether a purulent or mucopurulent exudate is visible in the endocervical canal and look for any evidence of cervical friability or sustained endocervical bleeding as a swab is gently passed through the cervical os to perform the NAAT. A swab of the vaginal discharge should be collected for a wet mount examination, if necessary. Cervical inflammation must be differentiated from normal adolescent ectopia. A presumptive diagnosis of mucopurulent cervicitis is made when there is a copious discharge from the cervical os, cervical erosion, or friability. A bimanual examination also must be performed to evaluate for cervical motion tenderness (CMT), adnexal masses or fullness, and uterine tenderness.

Laboratory Tests

According to the CDC, NAATs for *N gonorrhoeae* and *C trachomatis* are preferred for the diagnostic evaluation of cervicitis and can be performed on vaginal, urine, or endocervical specimens. If a pelvic examination is being performed, an endocervical or vaginal swab specimen for NAATs can be collected by direct visualization. A Gram stain of the discharge also can be performed to detect the presence of gram-negative diplococci or PMN leukocytes. The presence of 30 or more PMN leukocytes per oil immersion field is presumptively positive for cervicitis. A wet mount to diagnose associated STIs, such as trichomoniasis, is recommended, especially if the discharge is foul smelling or frothy. Adolescents who are diagnosed with a new STI or engaged in other high-risk behaviors, such as unprotected sex, multiple sexual partners, inconsistent or incorrect condom use, or young men who have sex with men, also should receive testing for other STIs such as HIV, syphilis, and viral hepatitis.

Pelvic Inflammatory Disease

History

When considering a diagnosis of PID, the history should include a discussion of known risk factors, such as unprotected sexual activity, including the number of sexual partners, especially new partners in the previous 2 months; a previous history of an STI or recent exposure to an STI; the type and consistency of contraceptive use; and the timing of the last menstrual cycle because most women present with PID during the first half of their menstrual cycle. The physician also should ask patients about the presence of symptoms that are often associated with PID: the onset, duration, quality, and location of abdominal pain; urinary symptoms that may indicate concomitant urethritis; intermenstrual bleeding; dysmenorrhea or dyspareunia; abnormal vaginal discharge; right upper quadrant pain; and systemic symptoms such as nausea, vomiting, fever, and malaise. The classic symptoms of PID, which include pelvic or lower abdominal pain, vaginal discharge, fever, and irregular vaginal bleeding, may not be present. More often, symptoms are nonspecific or vague, and the clinician must maintain a high index of suspicion in any sexually active female with acute or subacute pelvic or lower abdominal pain.

Physical Examination

Classic signs of acute PID include fever with lower abdomen pain and tenderness of the cervix, uterus, or adnexa. However, the clinical presentation can vary from vague discomfort to severe disease. A thorough physical examination should be completed before performing the pelvic examination to exclude other common causes of lower abdominal pain. This should include a review of the vital signs, looking for fever or tachycardia. The blood pressure also must be reviewed carefully because hypotension can be seen with a ruptured ectopic pregnancy, which may present with similar symptoms including abdominal pain and vaginal bleeding. The abdomen should be assessed for tenderness and guarding. The location of the pain is particularly relevant because certain acute surgical conditions, such as appendicitis, ovarian torsion, and ectopic pregnancy, are important considerations in the differential diagnosis of PID. In addition, right upper quadrant pain is consistent with perihepatitis, or Fitz-Hugh–Curtis syndrome, which can be seen with a gonorrheal or chlamydial infection. The speculum examination should then be performed, looking for a mucopurulent endocervical exudate or any evidence of cervicitis (cervical friability or erosion). The bimanual examination is also an important part of the physical examination. The cervix should be carefully palpated for any evidence of CMT and the uterus for tenderness or adnexal masses.

Laboratory Tests

The diagnosis of PID is based on clinical findings and a high index of suspicion, after other causes for pelvic or lower abdominal pain have been excluded. Previous CDC criteria for the diagnosis of PID included 3 major components: lower abdominal pain, CMT, and adnexal tenderness. Current recommendations now outline one or more minimum clinical criteria and 5 additional criteria to support the diagnosis (D_x Box: Pelvic Inflammatory Disease). Particularly when evaluating an adolescent for PID, early conservative treatment and maximum sensitivity for subtle clinical findings are paramount to avoid a delayed or missed diagnosis. A NAAT for *N gonorrhoeae* and *C trachomatis* should be sent on the endocervical or vaginal swab specimen obtained during the pelvic examination. If readily available, a Gram stain of any cervical discharge should be performed. The specimen should be examined microscopically for PMN

Dx Pelvic Inflammatory Disease

Pelvic or lower abdominal pain and one or more of the following minimum criteria on pelvic examination:

- Cervical motion tenderness
- Uterine tenderness
- Adnexal tenderness

Additional Findings

- Oral temperature >38.3°C (101°F)
- Abnormal vaginal or cervical mucopurulent discharge
- Presence of abundant numbers of white blood cells on saline microscopy of vaginal secretions
- Elevated erythrocyte sedimentation rate or C-reactive protein
- Laboratory documentation of cervical infection with *Neisseria gonorrhoeae* or *Chlamydia trachomatis*

Specific Criteria for the Diagnosis

- Inflammatory tubal mass or tubo-ovarian complex seen on magnetic resonance imaging or transvaginal ultrasound, or evidence of pelvic infection (tubal hyperemia) via Doppler
- Histologic evidence of endometritis on endometrial biopsy
- Laparoscopic abnormalities consistent with pelvic inflammatory disease

From Workowski KA, Berman S; Centers for Disease Control and Prevention. Sexually transmitted diseases treatment guidelines, 2010. *MMWR Recomm Rep.* 2010;59(RR-12):1–110

leukocytes as well as gram-negative, intracellular diplococci. The presence of numerous PMN leukocytes per oil immersion field is one of the clinical criteria for making a diagnosis of PID. (See Laboratory Tests under Urethritis and Epididymitis.)

Other laboratory studies to obtain include a complete blood cell count with differential and a sedimentation rate or C-reactive protein, although in some cases the laboratory tests are normal. A urine pregnancy test should be performed to exclude the possibility of a concomitant intrauterine or ectopic pregnancy. Additionally, a urinalysis and urine culture should be obtained, as well as a serologic test for syphilis. HIV testing also should be offered to the adolescent female. Testing for viral hepatitis is recommended in the patient who has not been immunized against hepatitis B or who has exposure to injection drug use (hepatitis C).

Laparoscopy may be performed to make a definitive diagnosis of PID or to obtain cultures directly from the fallopian tubes in cases in which the diagnosis is equivocal or the patient is not improving on standard antimicrobial therapy. A gynecologist should be consulted immediately for these challenging cases.

Imaging Studies

A transvaginal ultrasound may help exclude diagnoses such as ectopic pregnancy or ovarian torsion and also can aid in the detection of complications associated with PID, such as TOA. Fluid in the cul-de-sac may be seen on ultrasound; however, it is not specific for the diagnosis of PID.

Genital Ulcers

History

Probably the most important information to obtain from the adolescent with genital ulcers is whether they are painful. A painless chancre on the penis, around the mouth, in the oropharynx, or on the external genitalia in females is consistent with syphilis. If the lesions are painful or are associated with a grouped vesicular eruption, human herpesvirus is the likely cause. The presence of systemic symptoms such as fever, chills, headache, or malaise also is important to discern because these symptoms can be seen with a primary infection with human herpesvirus or secondary syphilis. Generalized complaints, however, are associated with secondary syphilis only 50% of the time. A history of adenopathy, localized or generalized, also must be noted, along with dysuria, which may be present in females with human herpesvirus. In addition, a history of a viral-like illness accompanied by a rash should be explored further. A diffuse maculopapular rash, especially on the palms and soles, is a classic sign of secondary syphilis. Because a nonspecific rash also can be seen with primary HIV infection, all possible exposures to other STIs should be reviewed with the teenager.

Physical Examination

All adolescents who present with chancres, or ulcers, should receive a complete physical examination. The skin, including the palms and soles, should be examined closely for any dull red to reddish-brown macular or papular lesions. The oropharynx should be carefully checked for chancres or blisters. All lymph nodes should be palpated for pain, enlargement, or induration. Suppurative or fluctuant nodes are often associated with chancroid caused by *Haemophilus ducreyi*. The genital examination should focus on the appearance of the lesions. The following questions should be asked of the patient: Are the lesions ulcerative, clustered, and painful (human herpesvirus or chancroid)? Are they associated with grouped vesicles on an erythematous base (human herpesvirus)? Is tender inguinal adenopathy present (human herpesvirus or chancroid)? Or is there a single, painless, indurated chancre with a clean base and a sharply defined, slightly elevated border (syphilis)? The lymph nodes associated with this syphilitic type chancre are often non-tender but enlarged. Other less common STIs produce genital ulcers that are often painful and deep and may be accompanied by some purulence. Adenopathy can be quite impressive with chancroid and lymphogranuloma venereum (*C trachomatis*).

Laboratory Tests

The necessary diagnostic tests depend on the patient's clinical picture. However, all adolescents who present with an ulcerative lesion should have dark-field microscopy performed for syphilis or direct fluorescent antibody testing of the lesions, which is also available and very specific. Nontreponemal serologic tests for syphilis, such as the Venereal Disease Research Laboratory (VDRL) or rapid plasma reagin (RPR) tests, should be done if direct examination is not available or the clinical appearance of the ulcer is nonspecific. In cases of early primary syphilis in which the VDRL or RPR may not be reactive initially, the test should be repeated in 1 week. Treponemal tests, such as the fluorescent treponemal antibody absorption test, should be used only as confirmatory tests and not for screening purposes.

Viral cell culture and PCR are the preferred human herpesvirus tests for persons who seek treatment for genital ulcers or other mucocutaneous lesions. Samples should be obtained from the base of a fresh unroofed vesicle. Human herpesvirus monoclonal antibody can be performed in older lesions that may be culture-negative and can differentiate between types 1 and 2. Human herpesvirus serology is generally not helpful. Given the well-described correlation between genital ulcers and HIV, it is recommended that all patients with a diagnosis of syphilis be tested for HIV as well. Conversely, annual syphilis screening may not be indicated for all teens but is currently recommended for an adolescent with multiple sexual partners; a history of injection drug use; a history of sex with men, women, or both; or a previously diagnosed STI.

Genital Warts

History

Risk factors for HPV infection should be assessed in all sexually active adolescents regardless of their immunization status. These include a history of multiple sexual partners, younger than 25 years, a previous history of STIs, lack of consistent condom use, pregnancy, altered immune response, and tobacco use. Symptoms may include pruritus, pain, or dyspareunia, but often the condition is asymptomatic. Adolescents may palpate a lesion on the external genitalia, complain of local irritation, or note bleeding from larger, traumatized lesions, depending on their location.

Physical Examination

A complete pelvic examination should be performed on all sexually active female adolescents who complain of lower abdominal pain, vaginal discharge, or intra-menstrual or postcoital vaginal bleeding, or who express concern with "something they felt" in the genital area. Before the speculum is inserted, the external genitalia should be carefully inspected for lesions. Genital warts, or condylomata acuminata, most commonly appear on squamous epithelium as irregular polypoid masses with an irregular, cauliflower-like surface that may coalesce into larger lesions. They are usually located at the posterior introitus, labia minora, and the vestibule in females, and may be found on the cervix and vagina as well. In males, warts are found more commonly on the circumcised penile shaft, glans, or corona, as well as under the foreskin of the uncircumcised penis. They also may appear as flat, flesh-colored papules on the scrotum and anus. Because this is a common location for lesions, the anus should be inspected carefully in males and females. Intra-anal warts are seen in persons who have receptive anal intercourse, but they can also occur in men and women who do not have a history of anal sexual contact. Condylomata plana are subclinical lesions that are not grossly visible but are apparent on colposcopy and histology. Condylomata lata are flat, flesh-colored warts that occur in moist areas (anus, scrotum, vulva) and may be associated with other signs of secondary syphilis.

Laboratory Tests

The diagnosis of genital warts is often made by visual inspection and generally does not require confirmation by biopsy. A biopsy may be required in specific instances, such as an uncertain diagnosis, the lesions are not improving or worsen with standard therapy, the lesion is atypical, the patient is immunocompromised, or the warts appear pigmented, indurated, bleeding, or ulcerated. A definitive diagnosis of HPV infection is based on detection of viral nucleic acid or capsid protein. Tests that detect specific types of HPV DNA are available but are not routinely recommended because this information would not alter the clinical management of the condition, except in extraordinary circumstances.

Subclinical HPV infection can be detected using 3% to 5% acetic acid, Schiller iodine, and colposcopy. In the past, suspicious areas of white epithelium or a specific vascular pattern consistent with HPV infection were biopsied. However, this procedure is no longer recommended because prospective studies have shown that many cervical and anogenital lesions, if left untreated in adolescents, resolve spontaneously. For this reason, in 2009, the American College of Obstetricians and Gynecologists modified its recommendations for screening for cervical cancer in young women to begin at 21 years of age. Of note, the American Cancer Society continues to recommend that young women start cervical screening with Papanicolaou tests 3 years after the onset of vaginal intercourse and no later than age 21 years (see Chapter 42 for details).

Nucleic acid amplification tests for the detection of gonorrhea or chlamydia can be performed on urine, endocervical, or vaginal specimens. Additionally, a nontreponemal antibody test for syphilis (RPR or VDRL) is indicated. An HIV antibody test should be offered to all adolescents who are deemed at risk.

A urinalysis for asymptomatic hematuria is indicated in males with visible condylomata. Its presence would indicate a urethral or meatal lesion.

Management

Although many states differ with regard to the details of health care delivery for adolescents, all 50 states including the District of Columbia allow health care professionals to evaluate and treat adolescents for an STI without parental consent, except for unusual circumstances. Routine laboratory screening for common STIs is recommended at least annually in all sexually active adolescents and as indicated for those who are symptomatic or require more frequent testing. Positive laboratory results for gonorrhea, chlamydia, syphilis, chancroid, and HIV/AIDS are reportable diseases in every state. Notification of all partners within 60 days of the onset of symptoms or diagnosis of infection or, if greater than 60 days, the last sexual partner is usually anonymous and carried out by local public health officials. Contacts are informed that a partner has been diagnosed with an STI and are instructed to be evaluated and receive appropriate treatment.

The complete treatment of the sexual partners of patients diagnosed with an STI is extremely important to prevent reinfection. However, because partners are often asymptomatic and do not seek treatment, and persistent and recurrent infection rates are reported to be particularly high among adolescents, expedited partner therapy (EPT) is now advocated in many states. Expedited partner therapy is the practice of treating the sex partners of persons with STIs without an intervening formal medical evaluation or professional prevention counseling. An extension of EPT, patient-delivered partner therapy, is another practical means for providing patients with medications or prescriptions for their partners. Care must be taken when treating the female partners of men with gonorrhea or chlamydia without an examination because of the potential for undiagnosed PID in the female partner. Therefore, as per CDC guidelines, EPT for female partners should include a review of the symptoms of PID and advice on when to seek medical attention in addition to accepting prescribed medications. Antibiotic recommendations and dosing schedules for the inpatient treatment of PID are noted in Box 101-2, as well as in chapters 100 (Table 100-2) and 132 (Table 132-1) for other infections. The outpatient management of PID in adolescents with mild to moderate disease has been supported by the 2010 CDC treatment guidelines; however, individual physician judgment of the teen's ability to adhere to an outpatient regimen is crucial to prevent short- and long-term sequelae. For further details about specific conditions and therapies, consult Selected References at the end of this chapter, specifically the 2010 CDC treatment guidelines.

Box 101-2. Parenteral Regimens for the Inpatient Treatment of Pelvic Inflammatory Disease

Parenteral Regimen A

Cefotetan, 2 g IV every 12 h

or

Cefoxitin, 2 g IV every 6 h

plus

Doxycycline,[a] 100 mg PO or IV every 12 h

Parenteral Regimen B

Clindamycin 900 mg IV every 8 h

plus

Gentamicin loading dose IV or IM (2 mg/kg body weight), followed by a maintenance dose of 1.5 mg/kg every 8 h (Single daily dosing 3–5 mg/kg may be substituted.)

The above regimens are continued for 24–48 hours after the patient improves clinically. On discharge from the hospital, doxycycline is continued orally for a total of 14 days. Clindamycin, 450 mg PO 4 times a day, can be used as an alternative to complete 14 days of treatment.

When tubo-ovarian abscess is present, clindamycin or metronidazole with doxycycline is recommended rather than doxycycline alone.

Abbreviations: IM, intramuscularly; IV, intravenously; PO, orally.

[a]Doxycycline should be administered orally when possible because of the pain associated with IV infusion.

In addition to antimicrobial therapy, management of an adolescent with an STI should include preventive services and counseling on risk reduction in a nonjudgmental and developmentally appropriate manner. In addition, the patient's primary language, culture, sexual orientation, sexual practices, and age should be taken into account. Adolescents with a first-time STI as well as those with recurrent STIs should be educated about disease transmission, consequences of delayed treatment, and methods for the prevention of acquiring new and recurrent infections (eg, abstinence, condom use, limiting the number of sexual partners, modifying sexual behaviors, pre-exposure immunization [Gardasil and Cervarix]). The risk for acquiring other specific STIs, such as HIV, also should be addressed. The physician should spend time with adolescents with recurrent STIs and explore the reasons why preventive methods have failed in the past. Several factors are extremely important to consider, including an untreated or undisclosed partner, poor sexual judgment secondary to substance use or abuse, and non-adherence to previously prescribed treatment regimens.

Except in pregnant women, test of cure (repeat testing 3 to 4 weeks after completion of therapy) is not strictly indicated in most routine cases of gonorrhea and chlamydia infection in which the physician is certain the patient has been treated with an appropriate antibiotic regimen and the partners have been prescribed therapy or will be evaluated appropriately. Most posttreatment infections are the result of reinfection rather than treatment failure and occur because the sex partner did not receive treatment or from the initiation of sexual activity with a new infected partner. Because repeat infections can increase the risk of long-term complications associated with PID and the rate of reinfection in adolescents is so high, the CDC recommends that patients with gonorrhea and chlamydia be retested as early as 3 weeks to 3 months after treatment. Further, if combination therapy of ceftriaxone and either doxycycline or azithromycin is not available for the treatment of uncomplicated genital, rectal, and pharyngeal gonococcal infection, a test of cure is recommended 1 week after treatment if alternative regimens with oral cefixime or azithromycin alone are used (2012 CDC updated guidelines).

Prognosis

If diagnosed and treated in a timely manner, the prognosis for most STIs is good, especially with the advent of observed single-dose oral therapies for the most common uncomplicated STIs in adolescents. Short-term sequelae of PID, however, regardless of treatment, include TOA and Fitz-Hugh–Curtis syndrome (perihepatitis), exposure to radiologic procedures, and prolonged hospitalization. Long-term consequences of PID are chronic abdominal or pelvic pain, ectopic pregnancy, and tubal infertility, for which prevention of recurrent infection is crucial. Currently, there is no pharmacologic agent to eradicate human herpesvirus, HIV, or HPV, although acyclovir, famciclovir, and valacyclovir are useful in treating the signs of primary herpes and reducing the incidence of recurrences. Long-term safety

of valacyclovir or famciclovir for longer than 1 year currently is unknown. The prognosis for HIV is variable, depending on the individual's disease progression at the time of diagnosis and his or her adherence to antiretroviral therapy. Recurrence of HPV lesions is not uncommon because the virus cannot be eradicated completely despite appropriate treatment.

CASE RESOLUTION

In the case presented at the beginning of the chapter, a diagnosis of human herpesvirus infection can be made clinically. The adolescent should be counseled with regard to the mode of transmission, the natural history of primary versus recurrent infection, and the role of antiviral agents. A first-void urine sample should be checked for leukocyte esterase or polymorphonuclear leukocytes and sent for nucleic acid amplification testing for the detection of gonorrhea and chlamydia. A serum rapid plasma reagin or Venereal Disease Research Laboratory test should be performed as well as a thorough assessment for HIV risk. HIV testing should be offered, allowing the patient time to ask questions or decline testing. The adolescent should be given a return appointment in 1 to 2 weeks to review laboratory results, discuss possible treatment options for recurrent human herpesvirus infection, and explore risk-reduction behavior.

Selected References

American Academy of Pediatrics Committee on Pediatric AIDS. Adolescents and HIV infection: the pediatrician's role in promoting routine testing. *Pediatrics.* 2011;128(5):1023–1029

Berlan ED, Holland-Hall C. Sexually transmitted infections in adolescents: advances in epidemiology, screening, and diagnosis. *Adoles Med State Art Rev.* 2010;21(2):332–346

Centers for Disease Control and Prevention. *Expedited Partner Treatment in the Management of Sexually Transmitted Diseases.* Atlanta, GA: US Department of Health and Human Services; 2006

Centers for Disease Control and Prevention. *Sexually Transmitted Disease Surveillance 2011.* Atlanta, GA: US Department of Health and Human Services; 2012

Comkornruecha M. Gonococcal infections. *Pediatr Rev.* 2013;34(5):228–234

English A. Sexual and reproductive health care for adolescents: legal rights and policy challenges. *Adolesc Med State Art Rev.* 2007;18(3):571–581

Goyal M, Hersh A, Luan X, et al. Are emergency departments appropriately treating adolescent pelvic inflammatory disease? *JAMA Pediatr.* 2013;167(7):672–673

Haamid F, Holland-Hall C. Overview of sexually transmitted infections in adolescents. *Adolesc Med State Art Rev.* 2012;23(1):73–94

Hogben M, Burstein GR. Expedited partner therapy for adolescents diagnosed with gonorrhea or chlamydia: a review and commentary. *Adolesc Med Clin.* 2006;17(3):687–695

Lehmann C, D'Angelo LJ. Human immunodeficiency virus infection in adolescents. *Adolesc Med State Art Rev.* 2010;21(2):364–387

Niccolai LM, Hochberg AL, Ethier KA, Lewis JB, Ickovics JR. Burden of recurrent Chlamydia trachomatis infections in young women: further uncovering the "hidden epidemic." *Arch Pediatr Adolesc Med.* 2007;161(3):246–251

Siqueira LM. Chlamydia infections in children and adolescents. *Pediatr Rev.* 2014;35(4):145–154

Trager JD. Sexually transmitted diseases causing genital lesions in adolescents. *Adolesc Med Clin.* 2004;15(2):323–352

Trent M. Pelvic inflammatory disease. *Pediatr Rev.* 2013;34(4):163–172

Trent M. Status of adolescent pelvic inflammatory disease management in the United States. *Curr Opin Obstet Gynecol.* 2103;25(5):350–356

Wellington MA, Bonnez W. Consultation with the specialist: genital warts. *Pediatr Rev.* 2005;26(12):467–471

Workowski KA, Berman S; Centers for Disease Control and Prevention. Sexually transmitted diseases treatment guidelines, 2010. *MMWR Recomm Rep.* 2010;59(RR-12):1–110

CHAPTER 102

Menstrual Disorders

Monica Sifuentes, MD

CASE STUDY

A 16-year-old girl presents with a 9-day history of vaginal bleeding. She has no history of abdominal pain, nausea, vomiting, fever, dysuria, or anorexia, and she reports no dizziness or syncope. Her menses usually last 4 to 5 days and, in general, occur monthly. Her last menstrual period was 3 weeks ago and was normal in duration and flow. Menarche occurred at 14 years of age. She is sexually active, has had 2 partners, and reportedly uses condoms "most of the time." Neither she nor her current partner has ever been diagnosed with or treated for a sexually transmitted infection (STI). She has no family history of blood dyscrasia or cancer and no history of chronic illness and takes no medications.

On physical examination, she is in no acute distress. Her temperature is 98.4°F (36.9°C). Her heart rate is 100 beats/min, and her blood pressure is 110/60 mm Hg. Her body mass index is at the 50th percentile. The physical examination, including a pelvic examination, is unremarkable except for minimal blood noted at the vaginal introitus.

Questions

1. What menstrual disorders commonly affect adolescent girls?
2. What factors contribute to the development of menstrual disorders, particularly during adolescence?
3. What relevant history should be obtained in adolescents with menstrual or pelvic complaints?
4. What treatment options are currently available for primary dysmenorrhea?
5. What conditions must be considered in adolescents with abnormal vaginal bleeding?
6. How is abnormal uterine bleeding managed in adolescent patients?

Gynecologic concerns and complaints are common reasons for adolescent girls to visit their primary care physicians. The challenge for pediatricians is to differentiate between an organic etiology, a functional condition, and psychogenic complaints. When this cannot be readily done or if the physical examination is equivocal, multiple diagnostic procedures may be performed, often with variable results. In addition, many pediatricians are uncomfortable evaluating gynecologic problems in adolescents and performing pelvic examinations, which contributes to this diagnostic dilemma. The purpose of this chapter is to review some of the more common gynecologic conditions affecting the adolescent girl and to highlight the significant historical and physical findings associated with each problem. For a discussion of the infectious conditions that cause pelvic pain, see Chapter 101.

Epidemiology

The overall prevalence of menstrual disorders during adolescence is estimated to be 50%, with the most common gynecologic complaint being dysmenorrhea, or painful menstruation. At least 70% to 90% of women have some pain associated with menses regardless of the degree of discomfort. Although most menstruating women report mild to moderate discomfort, severe dysmenorrhea occurs in 10% to 15% of women and has been reported to be responsible for significantly limiting daily activity in these females. Uterine anomalies or pelvic abnormalities such as endometriosis can be found in approximately 10% of adolescents and young women with severe dysmenorrhea.

Prevalence estimates concerning premenstrual syndrome (PMS) are difficult to assess because most studies in adolescents are retrospective and self-reports can be unreliable and misleading. In these studies, between 30% and 75% of older adolescents report significant PMS-type complaints. An estimated 20% to 40% of adult women experience PMS symptoms bothersome enough to impair daily functions, and 5% to 10% have debilitating symptoms. Other menstrual problems in adolescents include abnormal uterine bleeding, vaginal discharge, and amenorrhea.

Several factors contribute to the occurrence of gynecologic problems during adolescence. The average age of menarche in the United States remains at 12.5 years (range: 9–16 years), although the age of onset of puberty has decreased in some racial groups and in children with obesity. Bleeding may be irregular or prolonged initially in young adolescents because a majority of early menstrual cycles may be anovulatory and irregular, especially during the first few years after menarche. Once ovulatory cycles are established, however, bleeding problems may resolve, but menstrual symptoms such as pain, headache, bloating, and vomiting may predominate. Early sexual activity among adolescents and associated sexually transmitted infections (STIs) also may contribute to the presence of certain gynecologic conditions in this age group, particularly vaginitis, abnormal vaginal bleeding, and pelvic pain.

Clinical Presentation

Adolescents with menstrual disorders may present in a variety of ways. They may have specific symptoms, such as heavy vaginal bleeding, irregular periods, or painful menses, or more general complaints, such as fatigue, dizziness, and syncope (D_x Box). In addition, adolescents or their parents may have questions or concerns about delayed pubertal development and primary or secondary amenorrhea.

Pathophysiology

Puberty and the Normal Menstrual Cycle

Figure 102-1 depicts the menstrual cycle, which typically lasts for 21 to 35 days, with a mean length of approximately 28 days. Normal duration of menses is 4 to 7 days. Blood loss is usually 30 to 40 mL per cycle, and most women do not lose more than 60 mL per cycle. Regular ovulatory cycles usually do not occur until 2 to 3 years after menarche, although 10% to 20% of cycles can remain anovulatory as long as 5 years after menarche. Of note, it has been reported that girls with earlier menarche establish regular ovulatory menstrual cycles more rapidly than girls with later menarche.

One-quarter of females begin menstruating when they reach sexual maturity rating (SMR) (Tanner stage) 3 of sexual maturation, but approximately two-thirds do not menstruate until they reach SMR 4 breast and genital development. It is important to note that several other processes occur before the onset of menstruation. Thelarche, or the beginning of breast development, takes place approximately 2 to 3 years before menarche, and growth acceleration usually begins about 1 year before thelarche.

Menstrual Disorders

Primary Dysmenorrhea
- Painful menstruation.
- Lower abdominal pain associated with menstruation, usually worse on the first few days of bleeding.
- Associated back pain.
- Pain sometimes accompanied by nausea, vomiting, fatigue, headache, bloating, and diarrhea.
- Symptoms began 6 to 12 months after menarche.

Abnormal Uterine Bleeding
- Prolonged bleeding (>8 days) *or*
- Excessive bleeding (>6 tampons/pads per day) *or*
- Frequent uterine bleeding (≤21 days)
- No demonstrable organic etiology
- Normal laboratory studies, except may have anemia

Primary Amenorrhea
- No spontaneous menstruation in a girl of reproductive age
- Absence of menarche by age 16 years in a girl with normal pubertal development *or*
- Absence of menarche by age 14 years in a girl with no secondary sexual development *or*
- Absence of menarche within 1 to 2 years of reaching full sexual maturation (sexual maturity rating 5)

Dysmenorrhea

Dysmenorrhea is often accompanied by other symptoms such as nausea, vomiting, diarrhea, bloating, low back pain, and headaches. It can be classified as primary or secondary. Primary dysmenorrhea occurs in the absence of any pelvic pathology and is most commonly seen in older adolescents once ovulatory cycles are established. Secondary dysmenorrhea refers to painful menses associated with some underlying pelvic pathology, such as pelvic inflammatory disease (PID), endometriosis, ovarian cysts or tumors, or cervical stenosis. A complete list of causes of secondary amenorrhea can be found in Box 102-1. In adolescents, endometriosis is the most common cause of secondary dysmenorrhea.

Numerous studies have shown that cell membrane phospholipids, endometrial prostaglandins, and leukotrienes play a role in the pathogenesis of primary dysmenorrhea. After ovulation, fatty acids build up in the phospholipids of the cell membrane in response to the production of progesterone. Arachidonic acid as well as other omega-7 fatty acids are then released after the onset of progesterone withdrawal before menstruation. A cascade of prostaglandins and leukotrienes is initiated in the uterus during menses, which leads to an inflammatory response. Prostaglandin $F_2\alpha$, produced locally by the endometrium from arachidonic acid, is a potent vasoconstrictor and myometrial stimulant that causes uterine contractions, leading to tissue ischemia and pain. Another prostaglandin, $E_{2\alpha}$, causes hypersensitivity of the pain nerve terminals in the uterine myometrium. The cumulative effect of these prostaglandins may cause the pain of primary dysmenorrhea. Hormonal and endocrine factors also may play a role in the etiology of primary dysmenorrhea because ovulatory cycles with estrogen and progesterone are necessary for development of the condition.

Most cases of primary dysmenorrhea begin 1 to 2 years after menarche, and symptoms gradually increase until patients reach their early-20s. Parity and advancing age are associated with a decrease in symptomatology.

Abnormal Uterine Bleeding

Abnormal uterine bleeding (formerly called dysfunctional uterine bleeding) is defined as abnormal or excessive endometrial bleeding in the absence of any pelvic pathology. Menstruation is considered excessive if the cycles are short (<21 days) and the bleeding is prolonged (≥8 days). Although abnormal uterine bleeding is the most common cause of abnormal or excessive vaginal bleeding in adolescents, it should be considered a diagnosis of exclusion. Other causes of abnormal bleeding should first be investigated by obtaining a thorough history, performing a complete physical examination, and obtaining laboratory studies as indicated.

Abnormal uterine bleeding is usually the result of anovulatory, immature menstrual cycles. In adolescents, 50% of menstrual cycles are anovulatory within the first 2 years of menarche. If menarche occurs later in adolescence (ie, at SMR 5), this period of anovulation reportedly lasts even longer. Most cases of abnormal uterine bleeding in adolescence are thought to result from the delayed maturation of the hypothalamic-pituitary-ovarian axis. Normally, a positive

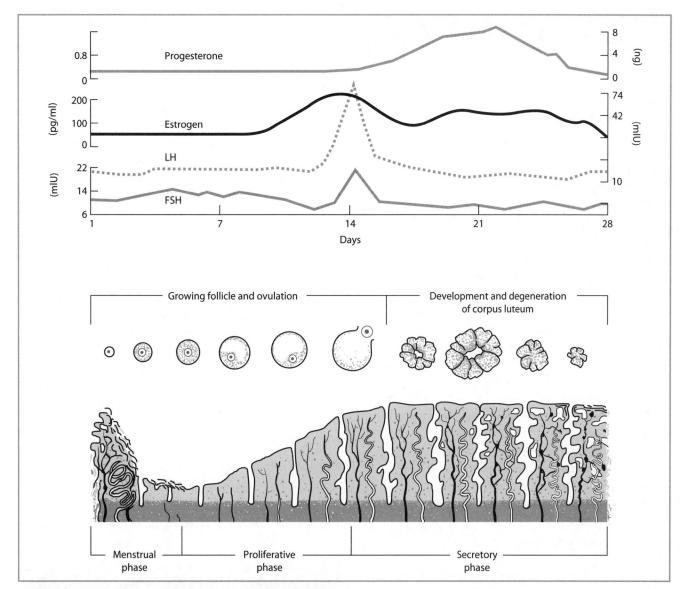

Figure 102-1. The normal ovulatory menstrual cycle. Abbreviations: FSH, follicle-stimulating hormone; LH, luteinizing hormone.

feedback mechanism develops with rising estrogen levels, resulting in a surge in luteinizing hormone (LH) and follicle-stimulating hormone, which triggers ovulation. The progesterone-producing corpus luteum then stimulates development of the secretory endometrium, with subsequent shedding after approximately 14 days if no fertilization occurs (menses). With anovulation, there is no progesterone-producing corpus luteum and, therefore, no development of a secretory endometrium. Thus, estrogen remains unopposed, and proliferative endometrium continues to accumulate. Finally, when the tissue can no longer maintain its integrity, it sloughs. In addition, without progesterone, the normal vasospasm that helps limit endometrial bleeding does not occur. Hence, bleeding is prolonged, frequent, and heavy.

Premenstrual Syndrome

Premenstrual syndrome refers to a group of physical, cognitive, affective, and behavioral symptoms that occur 1 to 2 weeks prior to menses (during the luteal phase of the menstrual cycle) and resolve within

a few days following the onset of menstruation. A variety of mechanisms have been proposed, including an increased sensitivity to the normal cyclic fluctuations in steroid hormones and releasing factors and alterations in neurotransmitters such as endorphins, γ-aminobutyric acid, and serotonin. The exact etiology remains unknown, however, despite multiple studies aimed at pinpointing the cause of this complex condition. In addition to hormonal factors, the role of vitamin deficiencies remains undocumented in the medical literature.

Amenorrhea

Amenorrhea is defined as the lack of spontaneous menstruation in women of reproductive age. Like dysmenorrhea, it can be considered primary or secondary. Traditionally, **primary amenorrhea** was defined by the following criteria: (1) an absence of menarche by age 16 years in girls with otherwise normal pubertal development, (2) an absence of menarche by the age of 14 years in girls with no secondary sexual development, and (3) an absence of menarche

---

Box 102-1. Differential Diagnosis of Common Menstrual Disorders

Dysmenorrhea (Primary and Secondary)

- Endometriosis
- PID
- Uterine myomas, polyps, or adhesions
- Adenomyosis
- Ovarian cysts or tumors
- Presence of an intrauterine device
- Cervical stenosis or strictures
- Congenital malformations (ie, septate uterus, imperforate hymen)

Abnormal Vaginal Bleeding

- Abnormal uterine bleeding: anovulation
- Complications of pregnancy: spontaneous/threatened/incomplete abortion, ectopic pregnancy, hydatidiform mole
- Infections of the lower and upper genital tract: PID, cervicitis/vaginitis
- Blood dyscrasia and thrombocytopenia: vWD, ITP, leukemia, platelet defects, leukemia, aplastic anemia
- Endocrine disorders: hypothyroidism and hyperthyroidism, hyperprolactinemia, late-onset 21-hydroxylase deficiency, Cushing or Addison disease, PCOS
- Vaginal anomalies: carcinoma
- Cervical/uterine abnormalities: endometriosis, polyp, hemangioma, sarcoma
- Ovarian abnormalities: ovarian failure, tumors, cysts
- Systemic illness: IBD, malignancy, SLE, diabetes mellitus
- Foreign body: retained condom or tampon, IUD
- Medications: aspirin, anticoagulants, hormonal contraception, androgens
- Trauma or sexual assault

Amenorrhea (Primary and Secondary)

- Pregnancy
- Systemic abnormalities: endocrinopathies (hypothyroidism, Cushing syndrome), chronic diseases (IBD, sickle cell disease), poor nutrition (anorexia nervosa), obesity, intense exercise, stress, drugs (opiates, valproate)
- Hypothalamic lesions: tumors, infiltrative lesions (TB, CNS leukemia)
- Pituitary lesions: prolactinoma, drugs causing elevated prolactin (marijuana, cocaine), cranial irradiation
- Ovarian failure: gonadal dysgenesis (Turner syndrome), autoimmune failure (associated with diabetes mellitus, adrenal insufficiency, thyroid and celiac disease), radiation- or chemotherapy-induced oophoritis, galactosemia
- Congenital abnormalities of the reproductive tract: imperforate hymen, transverse vaginal septum, absence or abnormality of the uterus, complete androgen insensitivity syndrome (46,XY-testicular feminization), Mayer-Rokitansky-Küster-Hauser syndrome
- Androgen excess: PCOS, benign ovarian androgen excess

Abbreviations: CNS, central nervous system; IBD, inflammatory bowel disease; ITP, idiopathic thrombocytopenic purpura; IUD, intrauterine device; PCOS, polycystic ovary syndrome; PID, pelvic inflammatory disease; SLE, systemic lupus erythematosus; TB, tuberculosis; vWD, von Willebrand disease.

---

within 1 to 2 years of reaching SMR 5 pubic hair. Causes of primary amenorrhea range from congenital anatomic anomalies to genetic and endocrine conditions. However, because many of these disorders can be diagnosed and treated earlier than 16 years of age, guidelines have been modified addressing when menstrual conditions should be evaluated. Current guidelines encourage a more proactive medical evaluation for girls who lack menses by the age of 15 or more than 3 years after the onset of secondary sexual development. In addition, absence of secondary sexual characteristics by age 13 is considered abnormal (Box 102-2). A detailed discussion of each of the etiologies that cause primary amenorrhea is beyond the scope of this chapter; see Selected References for more information.

Secondary amenorrhea occurs in girls who have already established menstruation but have had 3 or more consecutive months of amenorrhea. The most common cause of secondary amenorrhea is pregnancy, which must be ruled out in all adolescents presenting with this complaint, regardless of their acknowledgment of sexual activity. Other causes include systemic illnesses, significant changes in weight, stress, intense physical exertion, eating disorders (eg, anorexia nervosa), and certain medications such as phenothiazines, glucocorticoids, and heroin. Although polycystic ovary syndrome (PCOS) is another common cause of secondary amenorrhea in young adult women, it is often characterized by a wide range of menstrual irregularities, including abnormal uterine bleeding, oligomenorrhea, and amenorrhea of perimenarcheal onset.

Vaginal Discharge

Vaginal discharge can be normal (physiologic), nonspecific, or related to a particular bacterial or viral pathogen. A thin, white discharge, known as leukorrhea, occurs approximately 6 months to 1 year prior

---

Box 102-2. Menstrual Conditions That May Require Evaluation

Menses that

- Have not started within 3 years of thelarche
- Have not started by 13 years of age with no signs of pubertal development
- Have not started by 14 years of age with
  — Signs of hirsutism *or*
  — A history or physical examination suggestive of excessive exercise or eating disorder *or*
  — Concerns about an outflow tract obstruction or anomaly
- Have not started by 15 years of age
- Are regular, occurring monthly, then become markedly irregular
- Occur more frequently than every 21 days or less frequently than every 45 days
- Occur 90 days apart even for one cycle
- Last longer than 7 days
- Require frequent pad/tampon changes (soaking more than 1 every 1–2 hours)

Modified from American Academy of Pediatrics Committee on Adolescence, American College of Obstetricians and Gynecologists Committee on Adolescent Health Care. Menstruation in girls and adolescents: using the menstrual cycle as a vital sign. *Pediatrics.* 2006;118(5):2245–2250.

to the onset of menarche. A purulent, malodorous, or bloody discharge is considered abnormal, however. Etiologies are varied and may be infectious, inflammatory, or traumatic (see chapters 100 and 101).

Differential Diagnosis

The differential diagnosis of common menstrual disorders is extensive and can be found in Box 102-1. Other etiologies of pelvic pain include mid-cycle menstrual disorders (eg, mittelschmerz), urinary tract infections, complications of untreated or inadequately treated PID, and abdominal conditions such as inflammatory bowel disease and irritable bowel syndrome. Psychogenic pain also should be considered as a cause of recurrent pelvic pain and may be secondary to depression, anxiety, previous sexual abuse, or another psychologic condition.

Evaluation

History

A thorough history should be obtained in adolescent girls with suspected menstrual disorders because many non-gynecologic conditions can affect menses as well. A complete psychosocial assessment also should be performed. The acronym **HEADDSSS** (*h*ome environment, *e*mployment and education, *a*ctivities, *d*iet, *d*rugs, *s*afety, *s*exual activity/sexuality, *s*uicide/depression) serves as a useful tool when interviewing adolescents (see Chapter 6).

Most of the interview should then focus on the gynecologic history (Box 102-3), including pattern of menstrual bleeding, and any associated problems (Questions Box). With primary dysmenorrhea, pain that radiates to the anterior thighs or the lower back is not uncommon, although other emergent etiologies must be explored if the patient presents acutely. The color of the blood may be helpful when assessing abnormal vaginal bleeding. Brown or dark blood may be associated with a cervical obstruction or endometriosis,

---

Box 102-3. Gynecologic History

- Age at menarche
- Date of last menstrual period
- Regularity of menses
- Duration and pattern of bleeding
- Amount of flow (number of pads/tampons used per day and amount of saturation)
- Associated menstrual symptoms such as bloating, headache, lower abdominal pain, and cramping
- Maternal and sibling gynecologic history
- Treatment of menstrual symptoms
- Sexual activity (consensual and nonconsensual)
- Age at debut
- Number of partners and ages
- Date of last sexual encounter
- Protected versus unprotected vaginal or anal intercourse
- Current method of contraception

Questions

Menstrual Disorders

Dysmenorrhea

- What is the pain like?
- Does it always occur with menses?
- When did the pain first begin in relation to menarche?
- How frequently does the pain occur?
- How long does the pain last?
- Are any symptoms associated with the pain (eg, nausea, vomiting, diarrhea, headache)?
- Does the adolescent miss a lot of school or work as a result of painful menses?
- Do the painful menses interfere with other activities?
- What does the adolescent do for the pain? Has she tried any medications or complementary or alternative remedies?
- Is there a maternal or sibling history of painful menses?
- Is there a family history of endometriosis?

Abnormal Vaginal Bleeding

- What was the age at menarche?
- Does the adolescent have any symptoms of anemia?
- Is she fatigued, easily tired, dizzy, or short of breath?
- Has she experienced any syncopal episodes?
- Does the adolescent have any history of blood loss in the urine or stool?
- Is there any evidence or a family history of a bleeding disorder (eg, easy bruising, bleeding from the gums or nares)?
- Does the adolescent have any symptoms of pregnancy (eg, breast tenderness, nausea, fatigue)?
- Is there any known exposure to sexually transmitted infections?
- Is there a marked change in the adolescent's weight? Has the adolescent been on any diets recently?
- Is the adolescent using any medications such as aspirin, oral contraceptives, long-acting progestational agents, psychotropic medications, or anticoagulants?
- Does the adolescent have a history of a systemic illness such as systemic lupus erythematosus, diabetes mellitus, or renal disease? Does the adolescent have a history of trauma?
- Is the bleeding cyclic in nature?
- Is there breakthrough bleeding throughout the cycle?
- Is there a family history of bleeding disorders, type 2 diabetes mellitus, polycystic ovary syndrome, or thyroid disease?

Amenorrhea

- Has the adolescent ever had a period?
- Has she noticed any other changes associated with puberty (eg, breast development, pubic hair, growth spurt)?
- Does she have any other symptoms such as galactorrhea, weight loss, or hirsutism?
- Has the adolescent experienced significant changes or stressors in her life (eg, parental divorce, new school)?
- How often does the adolescent exercise?
- What is the adolescent's typical diet or are there any dietary restrictions (eg, vegetarian)?
- Is the adolescent taking any medications, including contraception?
- Does the adolescent have a history of headaches or visual changes?
- Does the review of systems reveal anything suggestive of a chronic illness such as Crohn disease?

whereas red or pink blood is found with most other conditions. More importantly, the timing of the bleeding is extremely significant. Cyclic bleeding beginning at menarche is more consistent with the presence of a blood dyscrasia. In contrast, breakthrough bleeding throughout the cycle may indicate an infection, endometriosis, or perhaps a polyp. The passing of blood clots on rising in the morning is not uncommon secondary to the vaginal pooling of blood while the patient is supine. Clots throughout the day, however, are not normal and require further investigation.

Physical Examination

A complete physical examination, including an evaluation for stigmata of a systemic illness, must be performed in adolescent girls with suspected menstrual disorders. Patients' height and weight should be plotted on the growth chart and compared with previous measurements. Depending on the SMR, physicians can then determine if they have experienced their expected growth spurt. Body mass index ($[weight, kg]/[height, m]^2$) also should be calculated and compared with previous values, especially in girls with amenorrhea. Vital signs, including orthostatic measurements, are a screen for significant blood loss with resultant anemia and are especially important to review in patients with excessive vaginal bleeding or amenorrhea as the result of restrictive eating (eg, hypothermia, severe bradycardia, orthostatic hypotension). The skin should be inspected for any evidence of androgen excess (eg, hirsutism, acne), insulin resistance (acanthosis nigricans), bruising, or petechiae. The thyroid gland should be palpated for masses or any evidence of hypertrophy, and the abdomen and suprapubic area also should be palpated for masses.

In addition, the SMR of the breasts should be noted and compared with pubic hair development, particularly in adolescents with primary amenorrhea. Other signs compatible with gonadal dysgenesis include webbed neck, broad shield-like chest, short fourth metacarpal, and an increased carrying angle of the arms. The presence or absence of galactorrhea also should be noted. The external genitalia should then be carefully inspected for clitoral size (normal clitoral glans width 2–4 mm) and patency of the hymen. Passing a cotton swab gently through the vaginal introitus can help determine vaginal length as well as the presence of a transverse or longitudinal vaginal septum. A bimanual or rectoabdominal examination may be performed in adolescents who are not sexually active to ensure the presence of a normal vagina, uterus, and adnexa. A speculum examination is generally not necessary for the non–sexually active adolescent with suspected abnormal uterine bleeding or simple primary dysmenorrhea. If the sexually active teen is asymptomatic, screening for STIs, particularly chlamydia and gonorrhea, can be performed noninvasively using a voided urine sample or vaginal swab, and the pelvic examination can be deferred. However, in adolescents who are sexually active and have an abnormal vaginal discharge, inter-cycle menstrual bleeding, history of dyspareunia, or lower abdominal pain, a complete pelvic and bimanual examination is mandatory.

Laboratory Tests

The performance of laboratory studies depends on the particular menstrual complaint. No laboratory studies initially are necessary for primary dysmenorrhea because the diagnosis is usually based on the clinical history and physical examination. The same is true for PMS. The laboratory evaluation for primary amenorrhea depends on the presence or absence of associated secondary sexual characteristics. For a full discussion of the diagnostic evaluation of primary and secondary amenorrhea, refer to Selected References.

In the case of abnormal vaginal bleeding, baseline studies must include a hemoglobin or hematocrit. Other initial laboratory studies should include a complete blood cell count to evaluate the red cell indices and platelets, a reticulocyte count, and a urine pregnancy test. Further diagnostic studies depend on the severity of the anemia and findings on history and physical examination. These may include coagulation studies (prothrombin time/partial thromboplastin time), erythrocyte sedimentation rate, and thyroid function tests. Other tests for the evaluation of a blood dyscrasia, such as a von Willebrand factor (measured with ristocetin cofactor activity and antigen), factor VIII, and fibrinogen, should be performed in the patient presenting with severe anemia, especially at menarche or shortly thereafter. The studies should be performed in consultation with a pediatric hematologist and obtained prior to the administration of any estrogen-containing medications, which may affect the results of certain assays. If the patient is sexually active and a pelvic examination is performed, an endocervical specimen can be obtained for nucleic acid amplification tests (NAATs) for *Chlamydia trachomatis* and *Neisseria gonorrhoeae*. Nucleic acid amplification tests of the urine or a vaginal swab to screen for gonorrhea and chlamydia are also available (eg, ligase chain reaction, polymerase chain reaction). Follicle-stimulating hormone, LH, prolactin, thyroid-stimulating hormone, testosterone, free testosterone, and dehydroepiandrosterone sulfate studies should be performed in patients with a history of chronic anovulation or in whom androgen excess is suspected (ie, PCOS).

Imaging Studies

A transabdominal or transvaginal pelvic ultrasound can be helpful in patients with abnormal vaginal bleeding or amenorrhea if a mass is suspected or palpated on physical examination. Complex congenital obstructive anomalies, such as a longitudinal vaginal septum with hemi-obstruction, cervical agenesis or stenosis, or a partially obstructing uterine septum, may require magnetic resonance imaging (MRI) if pelvic ultrasonography is inconclusive. Plain radiographs are not indicated. An MRI of the head may be indicated in the adolescent with amenorrhea if the patient presents with central nervous system (CNS) symptoms or the serum prolactin is elevated.

Management

With each of these adolescent gynecologic conditions, effective treatment is multifaceted and includes patient and parent education, reassurance about the ease with which the condition can be treated, and appropriate medications for those conditions requiring therapy. In general, a **menstrual calendar** or diary initially can be very helpful with most gynecologic conditions to confirm the severity of the bleeding and to assess the pattern of each menstrual cycle.

Dysmenorrhea

General modalities in the treatment of primary dysmenorrhea include education about menstruation, proper nutrition, application of heat (heating pad), simple exercise, and psychologic support. In addition, transcutaneous electrical nerve stimulation has been shown to have some efficacy as a non-pharmacologic therapy for primary dysmenorrhea. It has been reported to work by blocking efferent pain stimuli.

For mild to moderate symptoms of dysmenorrhea, over-the-counter **nonsteroidal anti-inflammatory drugs (NSAIDs),** such as ibuprofen and naproxen sodium, are appropriate for pain management and can also reduce blood loss. Physicians most often suggest that patients use ibuprofen initially because it is safe as well as efficacious when taken in appropriate doses and frequency. The dose is 400 to 600 mg every 6 to 8 hours. Ibuprofen should be taken at the onset of the menstrual cycle and continued for 24 to 72 hours or for the usual duration of symptoms. Girls who are unable to take the medications at the onset of menses secondary to vomiting can be instructed to start the NSAID 1 to 2 days before menses actually occurs.

For moderate to severe dysmenorrhea in patients who are not sexually active and do not desire birth control, a faster acting NSAID, such as naproxen, may be an alternative choice (Table 102-1). The major mechanism of action of NSAIDs is the inhibition of prostaglandin synthesis. Side effects of these drugs, which most commonly relate to the gastrointestinal tract, are nausea, vomiting, and dyspepsia. These reactions can be minimized by taking the medication with food or an antacid. Other adverse reactions include renal effects; skin reactions, such as erythema multiforme and urticaria; and CNS effects, including headache and dizziness. Contraindications to NSAID use include peptic ulcer disease, clotting disorders, and renal disease. All NSAIDs should be administered with food and taken for 3 to 4 menstrual cycles before their efficacy is evaluated.

Table 102-1. Nonsteroidal Anti-inflammatory Drugs in the Treatment of Primary Dysmenorrhea

Generic	Trade Name(s)	Dosage
Ibuprofen	Motrin, Advil	400–600 mg every 6–8 h for 24–72 h
Naproxen	Aleve, Naprosyn	440 mg at onset, then 220 mg every 8–12 h 500 mg at onset, then 250 mg every 6–8 h
Naproxen sodium	Anaprox	550 mg at onset, then 275 mg every 6–8 h
Mefenamic acid	Ponstel	500 mg at onset, then 250 mg every 6 h

Low-dose combination oral contraceptives are indicated in adolescents with moderate or severe dysmenorrhea who are sexually active or in patients whose symptoms are not sufficiently relieved by NSAIDs alone and whose own medical or family history does not preclude their use. Oral contraceptives decrease the production of prostaglandins by inhibiting ovulation as well as endometrial growth. Because the symptoms of dysmenorrhea are prevented only after several cycles of oral contraceptive pill (OCP) usage, patients should be told not to expect complete resolution of symptoms during the first month of treatment. Most adolescents who fit the classic clinical presentation of primary dysmenorrhea do not warrant a pelvic examination prior to initiating oral contraceptives. If an adolescent is sexually active, routine STI screening can be performed using a vaginal swab or urine-based NAATs. Reevaluation after 2 to 3 cycles is indicated to document adherence and resolution or improvement of symptoms.

Thirty or 35 µg of ethinyl estradiol–containing monophasic oral contraceptives should be used for a minimum of 3 to 4 months. If symptoms do not improve, an NSAID can be added to the treatment regimen. Oral contraceptives are more than 90% effective in cases of severe dysmenorrhea, and physicians should emphasize this hormonal benefit to patients and their parents. Although 20 µg of ethinyl estradiol–containing OCP formulations are now available, the literature remains inconclusive concerning their first-line use for primary dysmenorrhea.

If the patient continues to have dysmenorrhea despite the judicious use of NSAIDs and oral contraceptives, a search for other pelvic pathology, such as endometriosis, is warranted and the patient should be referred to a gynecologist for further evaluation and possible laparoscopy.

Abnormal Uterine Bleeding

The management of abnormal uterine bleeding depends on the severity and frequency of the bleeding and the degree of anemia (Table 102-2). The goal of treatment is 4-fold: to control the bleeding, to correct the anemia, to replenish iron stores, and to prevent further episodes of bleeding. Patients with mild or moderate anemia can be treated as outpatients with weekly to monthly follow-up depending on how quickly the bleeding is controlled. Although monophasic **combination oral contraceptives** are appropriate in the treatment of abnormal uterine bleeding if the condition is moderate or if birth control is desired, **other hormone regimens,** such as estrogen (alone) or synthetic progestin (alone), also can be used. This is especially important in adolescents who have a medical contraindication or disinterest in combined OCP therapy. **Supplemental oral iron therapy** is also required in all teens that are anemic.

Most adolescent girls with severe bleeding and anemia require a more extensive evaluation, and such patients usually are hospitalized for appropriate parenteral therapy and possible blood transfusion. Occasionally, intravenous conjugated estrogens may be required every 4 to 6 hours for the first 24 hours to stop severe acute hemorrhage. Otherwise, in cases of moderate to severe

Table 102-2. General Guidelines for the Management of Abnormal Uterine Bleeding in Adolescents			
	Mild Anemia (BP, HR stable)	*Moderate Anemia* *(BP, HR stable, moderate flow)*	*Severe Anemia* *(BP stable, increased HR, heavy flow)*
Hemoglobin (g/dL)	>11	8–10	≤7
Management	Reassurance, menstrual calendar, supplemental iron twice daily, COCP 1 pill daily (if sexually active) Consider NSAID to help reduce blood loss.	Initially, 3-4 monophasic COCPs (30–35 μg ethinyl estradiol and potent progestational agent[a]) every 6-8 h for 2–3 d or until bleeding stops; take with antiemetic; taper to every 12 h for 2–3 d, then every day once bleeding has stopped; skip placebos in first pill pack; then cycle for minimum of 3-6 mo; oral iron supplementation Consider NSAID to help reduce blood loss.	Hospitalization if signs of hypovolemia or severe anemia; consider IV estrogen until bleeding stops; begin 3–4 monophasic COCPs (50 μg or 30–35 μg ethinyl estradiol and potent progestational agent[a]) every day with antiemetic and taper as with moderate anemia over next 21 d; skip placebo pills for at least 1 mo or until hemoglobin has normalized; then cycle with monophasic COCPs (30–35 μg ethinyl estradiol) for 6–12 mo; oral iron supplementation
Follow-up	2 mo	2–3 wk, then every 2–3 mo	1–2 wk, then every mo

Abbreviations: BP, blood pressure; HR, heart rate; COCP, combination oral contraceptive pill; IV, intravenous; NSAID, nonsteroidal anti-inflammatory drug.

[a]Potent progestin: norgestrel or levonorgestrel.

anemia, a combination OCP containing 30 or 35 μg of ethinyl estradiol is initiated 3 to 4 times a day; the progesterone component is necessary to stabilize the endometrium. In addition, an antiemetic is often required 1 hour prior to the OCP during the first few days of therapy. Once bleeding is controlled, the frequency of OCP administration can be tapered, and adolescents can continue a monophasic combined oral contraceptive daily, skipping the placebo pills for at least the first cycle, and then switch to a lower-dose combination oral contraceptive for at least 6 cycles total. Studies have demonstrated that 20% to 25% of adolescents who require hospitalization for severe anemia within the first year following menarche have an underlying coagulopathy and therefore warrant a thorough investigation. In cases of abnormal uterine bleeding in which oral contraceptives are used but patients do not desire birth control, oral contraceptives should not be stopped until at least 3 months after the anemia has resolved to ensure restoration of iron stores.

Surgical treatment, such as dilatation and curettage, is rarely indicated in the adolescent patient and is reserved for patients refractory to aggressive medical treatment.

Premenstrual Syndrome

Although various sources have advocated many different treatment regimens for the management of PMS, no definitive studies have been reported, and no single effective treatment has been found. Therapies for mild to moderate symptoms include diet modification for patients who complain predominantly of bloating, promotion of regular aerobic exercise, education about menstrual physiology and the relationship of changing hormones to symptoms, stress management, and cognitive-behavior therapy or group therapy. Calcium supplementation (1,200 mg daily) and vitamin D have been reported to improve symptoms. Other vitamin and mineral supplements as well as certain herbal preparations require

more definitive research before definitively recommending their usage. Of note, some therapies that had been used extensively in the past also have been associated with undesirable outcomes, such as the development of peripheral neuropathy with pyridoxine (B_6) at high doses. Combined OCPs, NSAIDs, and spironolactone may be helpful if physical symptoms predominate. Other medications that may be used when mood symptoms predominate and are significantly impairing function are selective serotonin reuptake inhibitors such as fluoxetine. While shown to be effective in scientific double-blind studies of women with symptoms of PMS, anxiolytics, specifically alprazolam, are not generally used in adolescents due to the possible development of drug dependency.

Vaginitis

See chapters 100 and 101 for a discussion of the management of vaginal discharge in adolescents.

Prognosis

Most adolescents with common menstrual complaints who receive aggressive, appropriate care are usually symptom-free after 3 to 4 months of continuous therapy. Complications associated with oral contraceptive use and NSAIDs are rare in this otherwise healthy patient population. Symptoms associated with an immature hypothalamic-pituitary-ovarian axis, such as anovulatory bleeding and abnormal uterine bleeding, may also resolve spontaneously but generally respond favorably to hormonal management. The prognosis for adolescents with amenorrhea depends in part on the underlying etiology.

Resource

Center for Young Women's Health: www.youngwomenshealth.org

CASE RESOLUTION

In the case presented at the beginning of the chapter, more information should be obtained to exclude the numerous other causes of abnormal vaginal bleeding in the adolescent before a diagnosis of abnormal uterine bleeding can be made. Questions about breast tenderness, galactorrhea, weight loss, fatigue, visual changes, prolonged bleeding, and easy bruising can be particularly important. If the adolescent has no other complaints, a hemoglobin or hematocrit as well as a complete blood cell count and a pregnancy test should be performed. An endocervical, vaginal, or urine specimen should be sent for nucleic acid amplification tests for gonorrhea and chlamydia. Depending on the degree of anemia and the desire for contraception, the adolescent should be placed on twice-daily iron supplementation and oral combined hormonal therapy for at least 3 months.

Selected References

Adams Hillard PJ, Deitch HR. Menstrual disorders in the college age female. *Pediatr Clin North Am.* 2005;52(1):179–197

American Academy of Pediatrics Committee on Adolescence, American College of Obstetricians and Gynecologists Committee on Adolescent Health Care. Menstruation in girls and adolescents: using the menstrual cycle as a vital sign. *Pediatrics.* 2006;118(5):2245–2250

American Academy of Pediatrics Committee on Sports Medicine and Fitness. Medical concerns in the female athlete. *Pediatrics.* 2000;106(3):610–613

Bloomfield D. Secondary amenorrhea. *Pediatr Rev.* 2006;27(3):113–114

Bordini B, Rosenfield RL. Normal pubertal development: part II: clinical aspects of puberty. *Pediatr Rev.* 2011;32(7):281–292

Braverman PK. Premenstrual syndrome and premenstrual dysphoric disorder. *J Pediatr Adolesc Gynecol.* 2007;20(1):3–12

Chumlea WC, Schubert CM, Roche AF, et al. Age at menarche and racial comparisons in US girls. *Pediatrics.* 2003;111(1):110–113

Ellis MH, Beyth Y. Abnormal vaginal bleeding in adolescence as the presenting symptom of a bleeding diathesis. *J Pediatr Adolesc Gynecol.* 1999;12(3):127–131

Gray SH. Menstrual disorders. *Pediatr Rev.* 2013;34(1):6–18

Gray SH, Emans SJ. Abnormal vaginal bleeding in adolescents. *Pediatr Rev.* 2007;28(5):175–182

Harel Z. Dysmenorrhea in adolescents and young adults: etiology and management. *J Pediatr Adolesc Gynecol.* 2006;19(6):363–371

Hillard PJ. Consultation with the specialist: dysmenorrhea. *Pediatr Rev.* 2006;27(2):64–71

James AH, Kouides PA, Abdul-Kadir R, et al. Von Willebrand disease and other bleeding disorders in women: consensus on diagnosis and management from an international expert panel. *Am J Obstet Gynecol.* 2009;201(1):12.e1–12.e8

Laufer M. Gynecologic pain: dysmenorrhea, acute and chronic pelvic pain, endometriosis, and premenstrual syndrome. In: Emans SJ, Laufer MR, eds. *Emans, Laufer, Goldstein's Pediatric and Adolescent Gynecology.* 6th ed. Philadelphia, PA: Lippincott Williams & Wilkins; 2012:238–271

Peacock A, Alvi NS, Mushtaq T. Period problems: disorders of menstruation in adolescents. *Arch Dis Child.* 2012; 97(6):554–560

Slap GB. Menstrual disorders in adolescence. *Best Pract Res Clin Obstet Gynaecol.* 2003;17(1):75–92

CHAPTER 103

Disorders of the Breast

Monica Sifuentes, MD

CASE STUDY

A 2-year-old girl is brought to the office for bilateral breast swelling first noticed 3 weeks ago by her mother. The swelling is non-tender and does not appear to be increasing in size. There is no history of galactorrhea. The child is otherwise healthy, takes no medications, and is not using any estrogen-containing creams or other products.

On physical examination, vital signs are normal, and the child is at the 50th percentile for height and weight. A 1.5-cm, firm, non-tender mass is palpated below her left nipple. Below the right nipple, a 1-cm, non-tender mass of similar consistency is present. There is no discharge from either nipple and no areolar widening. The abdomen is soft with no masses palpated. The genitalia are those of a normal prepubescent female with no pubic hair and vaginal mucosa that appears red and not estrogenized.

Questions

1. What is premature thelarche, and how can it be differentiated from true precocious puberty?
2. What are the most common causes of breast hypertrophy in the infant?
3. When does pubertal breast development normally occur in females?
4. What are the most common causes of breast masses in adolescent females and how should they be managed?
5. How can physiologic pubertal gynecomastia be differentiated from pathologic causes of gynecomastia in adolescent males?

Breast disorders can occur in all pediatric age groups. The neonate may present to the pediatrician with bilateral breast hypertrophy and galactorrhea or mastitis. A bewildered parent might bring in a young prepubertal daughter because of early breast development. An anxious adolescent female may notice for the first time that her breasts are asymmetric, or she may feel a lump beneath the skin. An adolescent male can present with unilateral or bilateral gynecomastia that causes him severe psychologic distress. Whatever the underlying cause, breast problems can be disconcerting at any age. Primary care physicians should be equipped to differentiate between normal variants of growth and pathologic conditions in newborns, infants, children, and adolescents. Although rare, significant disorders can then be diagnosed and treated appropriately.

Epidemiology

Breast problems range from congenital anomalies and benign disorders related to hormonal stimulation to breast masses and tumors. Serious disorders such as breast cancer are practically unheard of in children and adolescents, although inappropriate breast enlargement or gynecomastia as a sign of another neoplastic process is not uncommon.

Benign breast hypertrophy can occur in 60% to 90% of neonates and is seen in male and female term neonates. It may occur unilaterally or bilaterally. Occasionally there is a nipple discharge, particularly in the case of well-intentioned family members who try to "extract the milk," inadvertently promoting the central secretion of prolactin and oxytocin via breast stimulation.

Congenital anomalies of the breast include polythelia, athelia, polymastia, and amastia. Polythelia, or extra accessory nipples, can be found anywhere along the embryonic mammary ridge ("milk line") from the axilla to the groin and is seen in 2% of the general population (Figure 103-1). Reportedly, abnormalities of the urologic and cardiovascular systems have been associated with polythelia. Polymastia refers to supernumerary breasts along the milk line and is seen less frequently than polythelia. The usual locations for supernumerary breasts are below the breast on the chest or the upper abdomen. Polythelia and polymastia may be familial and can occur bilaterally as well as unilaterally. Problems associated with breast development such as a tuberous breast deformity also can be thought of as a congenital anomaly, although it is not manifested until later in puberty when breast growth is noted to be underdeveloped or abnormal in appearance. The breasts have the appearance of a tuberous plant root, with an elevated submammary fold, narrow breast base, and "herniation" of glandular tissue through the areolae, which are unusually large.

Amastia (congenital absence of glandular breast tissue) and athelia (absence of a nipple) are rare occurrences, but their presence often is associated with other anomalies of the chest wall, such as pectus excavatum. Amastia (Figure 103-2) also is seen in Poland syndrome, which includes absence of the ipsilateral pectoral muscles, various rib

Figure 103-1. Polythelia. Supernumerary nipples along the embryonic mammary ridge (milk line).

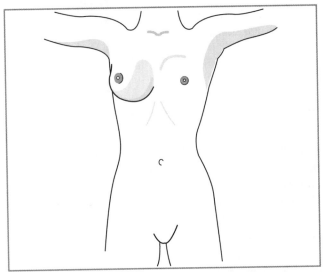

Figure 103-2. Amastia. Unilateral (left) complete absence of breast tissue.

deformities and upper limb defects such as syndactyly (webbed fingers), and radial nerve aplasia.

Premature thelarche is isolated unilateral or bilateral breast development in girls between 1 and 4 years of age without other signs of sexual maturation (eg, pubic hair, estrogenized vaginal mucosa, acceleration of linear growth). It has been estimated that 60% of cases occur between 6 months and 2 years of age and that a diagnosis after 4 years of age is uncommon. In contrast, precocious puberty is the appearance of any sign of secondary sexual maturation before age 8 in white girls with a normal body mass index or age 9 in boys. In young females, this involves breast or pubic hair development, and in males, pubic hair or testicular enlargement. Despite well-documented ethnic variation among children, 7 years is considered the lower acceptable age limit for the onset of puberty in non-Hispanic African American and Mexican American girls.

Gynecomastia commonly occurs in males progressing through puberty and is often called transient or physiologic pubertal gynecomastia. An estimated 70% of adolescent males are said to be affected, with a peak incidence between ages 13 and 14. This generally corresponds to sexual maturity rating (SMR) (Tanner stage) 3 to 4 genital and pubic hair development in the young male. Like breast development in the pubertal female, transient pubertal gynecomastia may be asymmetric, although concurrent or sequential involvement of both breasts can occur. It is uncommon for pubertal gynecomastia to occur beyond 17 or 18 years of age.

In the adolescent female, breast masses are not uncommon; however, clinically significant lesions are rare. Breast cancer per se has an estimated annual incidence of 0.1 in 100,000 adolescents. In most patient series through age 20 years, the most common benign breast tumor is a fibroadenoma, which has been reported in 60% to 95% of biopsied lesions. Two-thirds of these lesions are located in the lateral quadrants of the breast, with most in the upper outer quadrant. Their peak incidence is in late adolescence (17–21 years of age), and they tend to occur more commonly in African American females. Reportedly, 10% to 15% of cases are bilateral. In addition, 25% of cases involve multiple fibroadenomas.

Fibrocystic changes are the second most common histologic diagnosis after fibroadenomas. Other breast masses include solitary cysts, abscesses, lipomas, and phyllodes tumors (also known as cystosarcoma phyllodes), an extremely rare, rapidly growing, painless breast tumor that is nearly always benign and clinically can be confused with fibroadenoma, except for its aggressive growth. If malignant, however, cystosarcoma phyllodes can metastasize hematogenously to the lungs.

Malignancy is reported in less than 1% of excised lesions. There are fewer than 50 cases of primary breast cancer in children and adolescents reported in the literature to date. Rhabdomyosarcoma and fibrosarcomas are among the other rarely reported primary tumors of the breast in adolescents. Metastatic cancer of the breast is more common than primary breast cancer and has been reported in children with primary hepatocellular carcinoma, leukemia, Hodgkin and non-Hodgkin lymphoma, neuroblastoma, and rhabdomyosarcoma. Of note is the increased lifetime risk for radiation-induced breast cancer in girls and adolescents who receive chest wall radiation during peak breast development (10–16 years of age) typically administered during treatment for Hodgkin lymphoma. According to the literature, it takes an average of 20 years for breast cancer to develop in about 40% of treated girls.

Normal Breast Development

In the adolescent female, the first sign of puberty is breast development or thelarche. This begins with the appearance of a breast bud beneath the areola. Under the influence of estrogen, there is an increase in the adipose tissue along with the beginning of ductal and stromal growth. Progesterone initiates alveolar budding and lobular growth and contributes to the development of secretory lobules and alveoli. The alveoli are later lined by milk-secreting cells under the influence of prolactin when full maturation occurs during the first pregnancy.

The normal progression of breast growth is divided into 5 stages or SMRs. These descriptions are used to follow normal breast development, which occurs parallel with and generally precedes pubic hair development. It usually takes 2 to 4 years for the completion of breast development, although, as in all aspects of puberty, variations do occur. The practitioner should keep in mind that many females will remain in SMR 3 or 4 breast development until pregnancy. Additionally, especially between SMR 2 and 4, significant breast asymmetry can be quite common in the adolescent without indicating a pathologic process. Once both breasts are fully mature and reach SMR 5, adequate catch-up growth usually has occurred.

Clinical Presentation

Neonates with breast disorders usually present in the first few weeks of life with bilateral breast enlargement that may be asymmetric (D_x Box). There may be an associated clear or cloudy nipple discharge. If an infection is present, the overlying skin may be warm and erythematous. Fever or other nonspecific symptoms such as poor feeding and irritability also may be present because mastitis involves the entire breast bud and, although rare, septicemia can occur.

In prepubertal females, benign premature thelarche will present as unilateral or bilateral non-tender subareolar swelling without the appearance of other secondary sexual characteristics. In contrast, girls with precocious puberty may have axillary hair, nipple and areola enlargement and thinning, and pubic hair in addition to early breast development. Adolescent females with a breast problem often will complain of a unilateral breast lump noted incidentally by the teenager. It may be tender, fluctuant, firm, rubbery, or nodular. The adolescent also may complain of painful breasts (mastalgia) that can be cyclic in nature. For most breast masses, the overlying skin is normal, but occasionally skin changes do occur. Rarely, an associated nipple discharge may be present.

Because most breast masses occur in females, gynecomastia is particularly anxiety provoking in young adolescent males. It usually appears as a unilateral or bilateral 2- to 3-cm firm mass beneath the areola, which may or may not be tender. There may be irritation of the skin of the nipple from prolonged clothing friction. Galactorrhea rarely accompanies pubertal gynecomastia and may indicate self-

Dx Breast Disorder

Neonates, Infants, Prepubescent Children, and Adolescent Males
- Unilateral or bilateral subareolar mass
- Possible associated nipple discharge
- Skin changes, such as erythema in neonates and infants

Adolescent Females
- Firm, rubbery, freely movable mass
- Possible tenderness
- Breast asymmetry
- Skin changes such as shininess, venous distention, or dimpling (rare)
- Possible associated nipple discharge

stimulation; illicit drug use including cannabis, opiates, benzodiazepines, and amphetamines; or exposure to other medications.

Pathophysiology

Neonatal breast hypertrophy seems to be a response to maternal estrogen exposure in utero. Constant stimulation can lead to persistent swelling, galactorrhea, and overt infection (mastitis). Of note, if galactorrhea is present, it should not persist beyond the first few weeks of life. In general, preterm neonates are less responsive to maternal hormones and, therefore, breast hypertrophy occurs less often in this age group. It also may be delayed for weeks.

Benign premature thelarche is a variation of normal pubertal development with transient elevations in estrogen levels from functional ovarian cysts or fluctuations in pituitary gonadotropin secretion. Often, the breast enlargement occurs without other estrogen effects, such as an increase in uterine size or changes in the appearance of the external genitalia. In general, no linear growth or bone age advancement is associated with this condition. Current research is examining the potential role of leptin and its influence on sex steroids in the development of premature thelarche as well as pubertal gynecomastia.

Central precocious puberty is due to early activation of the hypothalamic-pituitary-gonadal axis and the secretion of gonadotropin-releasing hormone (GnRH)–dependent pituitary gonadotropins in a pulsatile pattern. Although a search for an underlying central nervous system (CNS) or gonadal abnormality may be undertaken, most cases in females are idiopathic. In contrast, fewer than 10% of males with precocious puberty do not have an identifiable cause, and it has been reported that approximately half of boys with precocious puberty have an identifiable intracranial process. Central nervous system tumors cause precocious puberty by impinging on the neuronal pathways that inhibit the GnRH pulse generator in childhood. Cranial irradiation, received as a part of tumor therapy, also can lead to central sexual precocity. Pseudo-precocious puberty is GnRH-independent and is caused by the extrapituitary secretion of gonadotropins or the secretion of gonadal steroids independent of pulsatile GnRH stimulation. (See Muir in Selected References for a general review of precocious puberty.)

The cause of fibroadenomas in adolescent females is postulated to be an abnormal sensitivity to estrogen. Observations supporting this hypothesis include the presence of estrogen receptors in the tumor and an increased incidence of this type of tumor during late adolescence. Thus prolonged exposure to estrogen may play a role in its development. Enlargement can occur during pregnancy or toward the end of the menstrual cycle.

The definition of gynecomastia is an increase in the glandular and stromal tissue of the male breast. Physiologic gynecomastia is thought to occur from a transient imbalance between estrogen and androgens during puberty. Alterations in the ratio of these hormones leads to an increase in estrogen relative to testosterone. Certain medications can cause elevations in serum prolactin and lead to gynecomastia or galactorrhea (Box 103-1). Some illicit drugs, such as marijuana, contain phytoestrogens that can mimic

Box 103-1. Causes of Galactorrhea

- Mechanical stimulation of the nipple
- Medications
  — Opiates
  — Estrogens
  — Digitalis
  — Butyrophenones (haloperidol)
  — Phenothiazines
  — Risperidone
  — Metoclopramide
  — Isoniazid
  — Reserpine
  — Cimetidine
  — Benzodiazepines
  — Tricyclic antidepressants
- Illicit drugs
  — Marijuana
  — Heroin
- Hypothalamic-pituitary disorders

Box 103-2. Differential Diagnosis of Precocious Puberty

- Central (true)—gonadotropin-releasing hormone (GnRH)–dependent
- Idiopathic
- Central nervous system
  — Tumor
    - Optic and hypothalamic gliomas (often associated with neurofibromatosis), hypothalamic hamartoma, astrocytoma, ependymoma, craniopharyngioma
  — Lesion
    - Congenital defects, hydrocephalus, cyst in the third ventricle
  — Insult
    - Postinfectious encephalitis or meningitis, static encephalopathy
  — Infection
    - Abscess, tuberculous granulomas of the hypothalamus
  — Head trauma
  — Sequela of cranial radiation
  — Sarcoid granuloma
- Endocrine
  — Hypothyroidism
  — Secondary to GnRH-independent precocious puberty (21-hydroxylase deficiency, Albright syndrome)
  — Peripheral (pseudo-)—GnRH-independent
  — Adrenal
    - Tumor
    - 21- or 11-hydroxylase deficiency
- Gonadal
  — Tumor
    - Albright syndrome
    - Familial testotoxicosis
  — Ectopic human chorionic gonadotropin–secreting tumor
  — Exogenous steroids

estrogen or stimulate estrogen receptor sites. Specific medications such as spironolactone and cimetidine interfere with androgen receptors or induce inhibition of enzymes needed in steroid synthesis.

Differential Diagnosis

The differential diagnosis of breast disorders in children and adolescents depends on gender and age at onset. In addition, the presence or absence of other secondary sexual characteristics is helpful to differentiate between a variation of normal pubertal development and a pathologic process.

Infants and Children Younger Than 9 Years

In prepubertal children, the differential diagnosis of isolated early breast development includes exposure to exogenous sources of estrogen such as skin creams that may contain tea tree or lavender oil, makeup, and medications (oral contraceptives).

For patients with suspected precocious puberty, other etiologies must be considered in addition to exogenous hormones (Box 103-2). Central nervous system tumors, lesions, and insults are among the most common causes. Congenital tumors such as hypothalamic hamartomas are especially important to rule out because they often present before age 3 years. Other CNS tumors to consider are neurofibromas, optic gliomas, astrocytomas, and ependymomas. Specific CNS lesions include cysts in the area of the third ventricle and congenital brain defects. Hydrocephalus, postinfectious encephalitis or meningitis, head trauma, and static cerebral encephalopathy also can lead to sexual precocity. Endocrine disorders include primary hypothyroidism, estrogen-producing tumors of the ovary or adrenal gland, and ovarian cysts.

Adolescents

The differential diagnosis of breast masses in adolescent females is extensive (Box 103-3). Conditions can be distinguished from one another based on the location of the lesion; its texture, mobility, and size; and how rapidly it is enlarging.

According to some authors, gynecomastia can be classified as type 1, 2, and 3, which is determined by findings on physical examination. Type 1 is consistent with benign pubertal hypertrophy. The differential diagnosis for types 2 and 3 includes physiologic gynecomastia (no evidence of an underlying disease process); organic disorders such as hyperthyroidism, liver disease, and testicular neoplasms; and side effects of medications or drugs of abuse (Box 103-4).

Persistent galactorrhea can be caused by several conditions in addition to excessive stimulation of the nipple from sexual activity or constant friction from jogging without a support bra. Other etiologies include neurologic, hypothalamic, pituitary, and endocrine disorders. Common causes in the adolescent female are prolactin-secreting tumors and hypothyroidism. Drugs that induce

Box 103-3. Causes of Breast Masses in the Adolescent Female

- **Fibroadenoma**
- **Breast abscess**
- **Breast cyst**
- Juvenile (giant) fibroadenoma
- Cystosarcoma phyllodes (benign)
- Fat necrosis (secondary to trauma)
- Lipoma
- Hematoma
- Intraductal papilloma
- Adenocarcinoma
- Rhabdomyosarcoma
- Angiosarcoma
- Lymphoma
- Cystosarcoma phyllodes (malignant)

Box 103-4. Causes of Type 2 Gynecomastia in the Adolescent Male

- Idiopathic
- Tumors
  — Seminomas (40% of germ-cell tumors), Leydig cell tumor, teratoma, feminizing adrenal tumor, hepatoma, bronchogenic sarcoma (ectopic human chorionic gonadotropin production)
- Thyroid dysfunction (hyperthyroidism and hypothyroidism)
- Renal failure and dialysis
- Chronic liver disease/cirrhosis of the liver
- Klinefelter syndrome (XXY)
- Testicular feminization syndrome (partial androgen insensitivity syndrome)
- Drugs (medications and substances of abuse)
  — Marijuana, amphetamines, heroin, methadone
  — Alcohol
  — Anabolic steroids/androgens
  — Estrogens, testosterone
  — Growth hormone
  — Cimetidine, ranitidine
  — Omeprazole
  — Digitalis
  — Spironolactone
  — Phenytoin
  — Tricyclic antidepressants
  — Anxiolytics: diazepam, buspirone
  — Risperidone
  — Selective serotonin reuptake inhibitors
  — Cancer chemotherapeutic agents: alkylating agents, methotrexate
  — Isoniazid
  — Ketoconazole
  — Highly active antiretroviral treatment
- Pseudogynecomastia (adipose tissue in obese male)

galactorrhea in females are the same ones that can cause gynecomastia in males (see boxes 103-1 and 103-4).

Evaluation

History

In the infant or child, the history should focus on endogenous as well as exogenous sources of estrogen (Questions Box). In addition, it is important to ascertain from the parents whether a growth spurt has occurred as well as if other physical features of puberty have appeared. With teenagers, it is important to inquire about medications, complementary and alternative therapies including herbal remedies, supplements, and illicit drug use as well as systemic illness. All adolescent patients should be interviewed alone, especially when being asked about illicit substance use (see Chapter 136). The adolescent male may feel particularly embarrassed given the nature of his visit; thus, the clinician should be especially patient and supportive during the interview.

Physical Examination

The physical examination includes an assessment of the patient's linear growth, especially in cases of suspected precocious puberty. The height and weight should be plotted on the growth curve and compared with previous measurements. Accelerations in height occur in sexual precocity. Excessive weight gain also should be noted; obesity can simulate breast enlargement in young females and gynecomastia in males, and adipose tissue can be mistaken for breast development if the tissue is not palpated correctly.

The extent of the breast examination depends on the age of the patient. In infants and young children, the breast tissue should be measured and the size recorded so that growth can be monitored over time. Consistency of the tissue and mobility also should be evaluated. Breast growth as a result of neonatal breast hypertrophy and benign premature thelarche is non-tender, firm, and freely mobile.

The nipple should be examined for a clear or cloudy discharge by gently compressing each one separately.

In the adolescent female, the breast examination should include visual inspection of the breasts as well as palpation of any lesions and axillary nodes. Ideally, this would be performed in the sitting and supine positions, as is done in adult women. Most adolescent females, however, may be uncomfortable with so extensive an examination. The physician must take the time to explain the reasons for the examination to help the patient feel less self-conscious. Male physicians always should have a female staff member present to chaperone during the breast examination. In contrast, it is often left to the discretion of the individual female physician as to whether or not to have a chaperone present.

Visual inspection should assess for SMR, appearance of the skin, breast symmetry, and evidence of trauma. Shiny skin or superficial venous distention on one breast would indicate the possible presence of an underlying large mass. A peau d'orange (orange peel)

Breast Disorder

Prepubertal Children

- At what age was the breast mass first noted?
- Does it seem to be increasing in size?
- Is it tender or erythematous?
- Is there associated discharge from the nipple?
- Has the child been exposed to any estrogen-containing skin creams, medications, or other products?
- Is the child or adolescent using any herbal supplements, such as ginseng or fennel, or products that contain tea tree or lavender oil?
- In the male patient, is he taking any medications known to cause gynecomastia, such as digoxin, omeprazole, or isoniazid?
- Is the child experiencing any neurologic symptoms such as headaches, ataxia, or visual disturbances?
- Is there a history of head trauma, central nervous system infection, or insult?
- Has the parent noted any other signs of early pubertal development (eg, pubic hair, acne, sudden increase in height)?

Adolescent

- When was the breast mass first noticed, and where is it located?
- Does it seem to be increasing in size?
- Is the lesion tender?
- Is there a history of trauma to the breast?
- Is there any discharge from either nipple?
- In the female, when was the last menstrual period?
- Is there a history of headache or visual disturbances?
- Are there any signs or symptoms of systemic illness, such as weight loss?
- Is there a family history of breast cancer in a first-degree relative, particularly the mother? What was her age at diagnosis?
- Is there a history of chest wall radiation or treatment with chemotherapeutic agents?
- In the male, is he taking any medications that can cause gynecomastia, such as cimetidine?
- Is the adolescent male using anabolic steroids?
- Is the adolescent using any other illicit substances such as marijuana or heroin?
- Is there a family history of gynecomastia or abnormal sexual development?

appearance of the skin or erythema and warmth should be noted as a sign of an infiltrative lesion or infection, respectively.

Palpation of the breast mass can be accomplished with the patient in the supine position using 1 of 3 methods. Using the second, third, and fourth fingers of one hand, the examiner should gently palpate each breast in a pattern of concentric circles, spokes of a wheel, or vertical and horizontal lines. The location of the mass should be noted; a mass beneath the areola might indicate an intraductal lesion, whereas the upper outer quadrant is the classic location for a fibroadenoma. The consistency of the lesion is important. Is it firm, rubbery, and fluctuant, or irregular and lumpy? Is it freely movable or attached to the chest wall? Fibroadenomas tend to be non-tender, firm, discrete, freely movable, and rubbery. A tender, poorly defined mass is consistent with a contusion; a hematoma is more sharply defined with associated skin ecchymoses. Fat necrosis can develop

after trauma and is painless, firm, well circumscribed, and mobile. The size of the mass should be measured and recorded. One must keep in mind that tumor size does not generally correlate with malignant potential. Tender, diffuse, cord-like thickening, which may feel like a beanbag, may be indicative of fibrocystic breast changes. The mean age of presentation of fibrocystic breast changes is mid-adolescence. This condition may involve one or both breasts, is more apparent around the time of menses, and may be exacerbated by the consumption of caffeinated beverages. Limiting caffeine consumption may provide symptomatic relief. Finally, each nipple should be gently squeezed to check for a discharge. If present, note whether it is clear, milky, or bloody. A serosanguineous or sanguineous discharge would indicate the presence of an intraductal mass. In addition, a retracted nipple indicates involvement of the areolar area.

In the adolescent male, the breast tissue should be gently palpated in the supine position to distinguish between fat deposition without glandular proliferation in the overweight patient (pseudogynecomastia or adipomastia) and true gynecomastia. Type 1 gynecomastia presents as a unilateral or bilateral freely mobile subareolar nodule, which is generally up to 3 cm in size. Enlargement beyond the areolar perimeter is consistent with type 2; type 3 resembles SMR 3 breast development in girls. The breast tissue associated with types 1 and 2 also is firm and rubbery and may be tender to palpation, whereas type 3 has a consistency similar to female breast tissue.

The examiner should palpate for axillary lymphadenopathy. Although most clinicians think of its association with breast cancer, it also may be found with infection or necrosis of a benign tumor. In the adolescent male, in addition to palpation of the breast tissue, it is important to evaluate liver size and texture as well as determine the SMR of the genitalia to determine whether pubertal development is consistent with the gynecomastia. The testicles should be palpated carefully for size and consistency and the presence of masses, nodules, or asymmetry. Any evidence of atrophy (decrease in testicular size) should be noted. In addition, findings suggestive of hypothyroidism or hyperthyroidism, liver disease, or other stigmata suggestive of a syndrome must be investigated.

A detailed neurologic examination including examination of the fundi should be performed, especially in children with sexual precocity to confirm or detect a CNS disorder.

Laboratory Tests

The laboratory workup for breast disorders is dictated by the findings on history and physical examination. Isolated neonatal breast hyperplasia and premature thelarche require no laboratory studies. Although serum gonadotropin concentrations (luteinizing hormone and follicle-stimulating hormone) and estradiol levels can be obtained in girls with precocious puberty, definitive demonstration of an activated hypothalamic-pituitary axis generally requires the administration of a GnRH stimulation test by the subspecialist. In addition, a morning testosterone level should be ordered in boys. Based on these results, further studies may be indicated, such as a serum human chorionic gonadotropin (hCG) level.

For most breast lesions in adolescent females, no laboratory studies are needed. A fine-needle aspiration (FNA) of the lesion may be performed for those cases that seem to be cystic or if the diagnosis is uncertain. The aspirated fluid should be sent for cytologic analysis if the mass does not completely disappear with this procedure. Sometimes it is necessary to perform another procedure, such as a core needle biopsy, to relieve patient and parental anxiety or to better identify the etiology of the mass. An excision biopsy of the mass allows for more accurate histologic information but is rarely indicated for most lesions.

In the healthy adolescent male with no evidence of systemic illness, no history of medication use or illicit substance abuse, and a normal physical examination including the testicular examination, no further laboratory studies are necessary. If pubertal gynecomastia and other systemic illnesses are ruled out, an endocrine workup is appropriate to elucidate the cause of non-pubertal gynecomastia. This should begin with morning serum levels of hCG, LH, FSH, and serum testosterone and estradiol because circadian variation may affect their interpretation. Dehydroepiandrosterone sulfate, thyroid function tests, renal function studies, and liver enzymes also may be useful. If these laboratory studies are normal, the diagnosis is idiopathic gynecomastia. If they are abnormal, consultation with a pediatric endocrinologist or adolescent medicine specialist should occur.

A pregnancy test and serum prolactin level should be ordered in the adolescent female with galactorrhea, regardless of the menstrual history.

Imaging Studies

Hand and wrist radiographs to determine the child's bone age should be obtained in children with a diagnosis of precocious puberty. In addition, boys should have magnetic resonance imaging (MRI) of the brain to evaluate for a CNS lesion or structural abnormality in the hypothalamus or pituitary gland. Depending on the history, an MRI may be indicated in some girls. Pelvic ultrasound, although rarely necessary, can be performed to rule out the presence of an ovarian tumor or cyst in girls with precocious puberty.

Mammograms are not helpful in the pediatric age group, especially in adolescents, and are not recommended as part of the evaluation of a breast mass. They can be very difficult to interpret because of the dense fibro-glandular breast tissue of female adolescents. In addition, the risk of breast malignancy in an otherwise healthy adolescent girl is negligible. A breast ultrasound is the primary imaging modality for the evaluation of a breast mass for several reasons: it accurately confirms the presence of the mass and helps distinguish between a cystic lesion and a solid mass. Ultrasound is noninvasive and causes no pain for the anxious teenager. It can also provide more accurate measurement of the size of the lesion and its location prior to the FNA or core needle biopsy. Finally, specific characteristics of the lesion such as the shape, margins, and presence of microcalcification can help to differentiate benign and malignant lesions.

A testicular ultrasound to search for a tumor is indicated in the adolescent male if the level of serum hCG or estradiol is elevated or if a testicular mass is noted on physical examination. Other imaging studies for the evaluation of gynecomastia generally are not useful.

Management

In neonates, mastitis most often is caused by *Staphylococcus aureus* and group B streptococcus. Gram-negative bacilli also have been reported. Parenteral antibiotics should be initiated when the diagnosis is made. Incision and drainage of a breast abscess is rarely indicated and should only be undertaken by an experienced surgeon familiar with the anatomy of the breast to minimize the likelihood of injury to the affected breast bud.

Congenital anomalies such as polythelia and polymastia do not require any treatment. If, however, the patient or parent wants the tissue removed for aesthetic or psychologic reasons, it is recommended to do so before puberty. Reconstructive surgery for amastia, as in Poland syndrome, is typically delayed until late adolescence to allow full development of the unaffected breast.

Although no treatment is required for benign premature thelarche, parents need to be reassured that the condition is self-limited. The patient should be reexamined periodically to check for any further progression of puberty, such as persistent breast growth, the appearance of pubic hair, or a growth spurt.

The treatment for central precocious puberty is directed at controlling the secondary sexual development with GnRH agonists. When GnRH is administered continuously, gonadotropin secretion decreases. Currently, leuprolide acetate is the only GnRH agonist available for use in the United States. Children should be followed every 1 to 3 months in conjunction with a pediatric endocrinologist to monitor their progression and response to therapy.

Unless otherwise indicated by the type of tumor, children with a CNS lesion as a cause of precocious puberty usually do not require neurosurgical intervention. Therapy should focus on minimizing the degree of growth acceleration and the development of secondary sexual characteristics.

Most breast masses in adolescent females are small, well demarcated, firm or rubbery, and non-tender and can be managed with the "wait and watch" approach. The patient can be followed every 3 to 4 months, preferably allowing a few menstrual cycles to pass between each visit. If there is no change in the lesion or just a small increase in its size, no studies or procedures are indicated because it is most likely a fibroadenoma. As previously noted, an FNA or core needle biopsy may be requested to relieve the anxiety for the parents and the teenager that accompanies the presence of a breast lesion and to confirm the diagnosis. Total excision of the tumor mass and a careful histologic evaluation may be warranted in some cases, especially if the mass is painful or rapidly enlarging and exceeds 3 cm, but excision is generally unnecessary in most instances. According to the literature, if findings on physical examination, imaging, and biopsy are consistent with a benign lesion, the diagnosis of a benign mass can be made with 99% accuracy. If this is the case, no further procedures are indicated and follow-up with the patient can occur every 6 months to 1 year. Surgical removal of progressively enlarging tumors over several months, such as a giant fibroadenoma, is important. This type of fibroadenoma is greater than 5 cm in size at onset or appears soon after menarche and accounts for 4% to 10% of fibroadenomas of the breast. When the lesion becomes very large, an acceptable cosmetic result is more difficult. Accordingly, giant fibroadenomas should be removed shortly after the time of diagnosis rather than waiting and watching. Of note, any adolescent patient with a palpable breast mass and a past history of malignant disease or family history of breast cancer should be evaluated aggressively and referred to a pediatric surgeon or breast surgeon directly for a diagnostic excisional biopsy.

The primary treatment for physiologic pubertal gynecomastia, or type 1, is reassurance for the adolescent male and his family that the condition is self-limited and should regress spontaneously within 1 to 2 years, although some sources report up to 3 years. The teenager should be told explicitly that he is not "becoming a girl." In most cases, he should be reexamined periodically (every 6 months) until resolution occurs. Type 2 gynecomastia may need surgical reduction of the mammary gland, although some studies have shown success with medical therapy. The off-label use of 10 to 20 mg of tamoxifen orally twice a daily for 3 months has been shown in some cases to decrease breast tenderness and pain, followed by a decrease in breast tissue. Plastic surgery intervention may be warranted for cases of persistent breast growth or moderate to severe gynecomastia (SMR 3–4 breasts) in the older adolescent with psychologic difficulties related to the condition. Surgical intervention currently involves a combination of ultrasonic liposuction and direct excision of the breast tissue beneath the nipple and areola. The young man may benefit from concurrent psychologic counseling as well.

Other underlying causes for gynecomastia should be treated accordingly, and any drugs or medications contributing to the condition or associated galactorrhea should be discontinued, if possible.

Prognosis

The prognosis of a breast disorder in the child or adolescent depends on the particular lesion. In general, most lesions, such as neonatal breast hyperplasia and premature thelarche, are self-limited and resolve on their own. Breast development persists for 3 to 5 years in 50% of cases of premature thelarche, but in one retrospective study, most cases regressed within 6 months to 6 years after the diagnosis. Aside from the short stature that may accompany idiopathic central precocious puberty, these females also tend to have a good prognosis. Fibroadenomas in the adolescent female can recur but typically are benign and have no proven link to the development of breast cancer. Most cases of pubertal gynecomastia in the adolescent male resolve within 1 to 2 years.

CASE RESOLUTION

The child in the case study has a diagnosis of premature thelarche. She has no known exposure to exogenous sources of estrogen or alternative therapies that are associated with breast growth and has isolated breast tissue development with no other secondary signs of pubertal maturation. Her parents should be informed of this diagnosis and reassured that the condition is self-limited and does not indicate that the child is starting puberty. The child should be scheduled for a follow-up visit in 3 to 4 months to remeasure the breast buds and reexamine the genitalia for the appearance of pubic hair as well as to monitor the patient's linear growth.

Selected References

Bock K, Duda VF, Hadji P, et al. Pathologic breast conditions in childhood and adolescence: evaluation by sonographic diagnosis. *J Ultrasound Med*. 2005; 24(10):1347–1357

De Silva NK. Breast disorders in the female adolescent. *Adolesc Med State Art Rev*. 2012;23(1):34–52

De Silva NK, Brandt ML. Disorders of the breast in children and adolescents, part 1: disorders of growth and infections of the breast. *J Pediatr Adolesc Gynecol*. 2006;19(5):345–349

De Silva NK, Brandt ML. Disorders of the breast in children and adolescents, part 2: breast masses. *J Pediatr Adolesc Gynecol*. 2006;19(6):415–418

Diamantopoulos S, Bao Y. Gynecomastia and premature thelarche: a guide for practitioners. *Pediatr Rev*. 2007;28(9):e57–e68

Ezer SS, Oguzkurt P, Ince E, Temiz A, Bolat FA, Hicsonmez A. Surgical treatment of the solid breast masses in female adolescents. *J Pediatr Adolesc Gynecol*. 2013; 26(1):31–35

Frazier AL, Rosenberg SM. Preadolescent and adolescent risk factors for benign breast disease. *J Adolesc Health*. 2013;52(5 Suppl):S36–S40

Granada C, Omar H, Loveless MB. Update on adolescent gynecology. *Adolesc Med State Art Rev*. 2013;24(1):133–154

Greydanus DE, Matytsina L, Gains M. Breast disorders in children and adolescents. *Prim Care*. 2006;33(2):455–502

Joffe A. Gynecomastia. In: Neinstein LS, ed. *Adolescent Health Care: A Practical Guide*. 5th ed. Baltimore, MD: Lippincott Williams & Wilkins; 2008:180–184

Kennedy RD, Boughey JC. Management of pediatric and adolescent breast masses. *Semin Plast Surg*. 2013;27:19–22

Ma NS, Geffner ME. Gynecomastia in prepubertal and pubertal men. *Curr Opin Pediatr*. 2008;20(4):465–470

Muir A. Precocious puberty. *Pediatr Rev*. 2006;27(10):373–381

Nordt CA, DiVasta AD. Gynecomastia in adolescents. *Curr Opin Pediatr*. 2008; 20(4):375–382

Rosenfield RL, Lipton RB, Drum ML. Thelarche, pubarche, and menarche attainment in children with normal and elevated body mass index. *Pediatrics*. 2009; 123(1):84–88

Orthopedic Disorders

CHAPTER 104

Developmental Dysplasia of the Hip

David P. Zamorano, MD; Andrew K. Battenberg, MD; and Steven Donohoe, BS

CASE STUDY

A 4-month-old girl is seen for her routine health mainte-nance visit. She is doing well and has no complaints. The results of the entire examination are within normal limits except for limited external rotation and abduction of the left hip, which is approximately 45 degrees, in compari-son to that of the right hip, which is almost 90 degrees.

Questions

1. What factors are responsible for normal growth and development of the hip joint?

2. What specific physical maneuvers help in the evaluation of infants with decreased range of motion of the hip?

3. What are the clinical findings of hip dislocation during and after the neonatal period?

4. What are some of the conditions often seen in conjunction with hip dysplasia that may be noted on physical examination?

5. What is the appropriate diagnostic workup of infants with suspected hip dysplasia?

Developmental dysplasia of the hip (DDH) is a common pediatric orthopedic concern that requires a thorough understanding of nor-mal development, anatomic pathology, natural history, and treat-ment. While previously referred to as congenital dislocation of the hip, the term was changed because DDH defines a spectrum of hip pathology, ranging from congenital dysplasia of the hip to partial dislocation of the femoral head (hip subluxation), acetabular dys-plasia, and complete dislocation of the femoral head from the true acetabulum. Developmental dysplasia of the hip may exist at birth or develop during infancy. In a newborn with DDH, the femoral head dislocates into and out of the acetabulum. In an older child, the fem-oral head remains dislocated, leading to secondary changes in the head, acetabulum, and lateral pelvic wall where the displaced fem-oral head articulates. When DDH is recognized and treated appro-priately, children potentially develop completely normally. If the diagnosis is missed or delayed, however, children may suffer signif-icant morbidity, including severe degenerative hip disease.

Epidemiology

Historically, the incidence of DDH is 1 in 1,000 live births. The liter-ature has observed that pediatricians diagnose DDH in 8.6 in 1,000 live births and orthopedic surgeons in 1.5 in 1,000 live births, while the use of ultrasound has resulted in the diagnosis of 25 in 1,000 live births. Hip instability in the neonate is estimated to range from 11.5 to 17 per 1,000 live births. Approximately 60% of these cases resolve by 1 week of age, and 90% resolve by 2 months of age. Approximately 60% of infants affected by DDH are firstborn.

Girls are affected 5 times more frequently than boys. Ethnic vari-ations exist, with incidence highest among the Native American Navajo, followed by whites and African Americans. Approximately 20% of all DDH occurs in infants born in the breech position. A pos-itive family history of DDH increases the risk by 10%. A female born in the breech position has a 1 in 35 chance of having DDH.

The left hip is involved in 60% of children with DDH, the right hip in 20% of cases, and 20% of cases are bilateral. Developmental dysplasia of the hip has an increased association with lesions of mechanical molding, such as congenital torticollis (approximately 8% of affected children may have DDH), metatarsus adductus (approximately 2%–10% of these children may have DDH), and tali-pes calcaneovalgus.

Clinical Presentation

The clinical presentation and signs of DDH in children vary with age. In neonates, diagnosis is made primarily by the physical examina-tion (eg, Ortolani and Barlow maneuvers). In older infants, asym-metric skinfolds, limitation of hip abduction, and a positive Galeazzi sign are classic signs of DDH. Physical signs, which become more obvious once children are walking, include waddling gait, limping, and toe-walking (D_x Box).

Pathophysiology

Developmental dysplasia of the hip encompasses a wide variety of conditions ranging from hip instability to dislocation. For normal growth and development of the hip joint to occur, there must be a

Dx   Developmental Hip Dysplasia

- Breech presentation
- Oligohydramnios
- Female gender
- Positive family history or ethnic background
- Persistent hip asymmetry (asymmetric skinfolds, abduction of one hip and adduction of the other)
- Lower-limb deformity (limp, toe-walking)
- Torticollis

genetically determined balance of growth of the acetabular and triradiate cartilages and a well-located and centered femoral head. In a normal hip at birth, there is a tight articulation between the femoral head and acetabulum; however, in DDH or dislocation, this tight articulation is lost. Dysplasia refers to (1) a hip that is dislocated but can be relocated or (2) a hip with a positive Ortolani sign, meaning it can be provoked to dislocate. The term *dislocation* refers to any hip with a negative Ortolani sign, meaning that the hip is not reducible and is associated with secondary adaptive changes such as shortening, decreased abduction, and asymmetric skinfolds.

Dysplasia of the acetabulum is also associated with hip instability. The dysplastic acetabular cavity is shallower with a more vertical inclination angle (Figure 104-1). Although most dislocations occur at or near the time of delivery, this abnormal development of the acetabular cavity helps explain why dislocations can also occur later in infancy. Late hip dislocations are reported in 3% to 8% of affected infants.

The etiology of DDH is poorly defined but is thought to be multifactorial, involving genetic and intrauterine environmental factors. The primary **intrauterine environmental factors** are tight maternal abdominal and uterine musculature, breech presentation (causes abnormal hip flexion leading to dislocation of the femoral head), and positioning of the fetal hip against the mother's sacrum (causing increased femoral adduction leading to dislocation of the

Figure 104-1. In developmental dysplasia of the hip, inclination angle is increased. Because the acetabulum is more vertical-orientated, the hip articulation is less stable.

femoral head). In utero mechanical factors relate to molding and restriction of fetal movement. It is believed that the tight, unstretched maternal abdomen and uterine musculature of primigravidae may restrict fetal movement, thus predisposing firstborns to DDH. The increased occurrence of other conditions thought to be secondary to molding (eg, congenital muscular torticollis) with DDH supports this theory of space restriction. **Physiological factors** relate to ligamentous laxity and inherent instability of the hip at birth. In utero, there is a growth rate discrepancy between the femoral head and acetabulum. The femoral head grows more rapidly so that neonates are born with only 50% of their femoral heads covered by the acetabulum. Additionally, there is diffuse ligamentous laxity in the final 4 weeks of gestation in preparation for birth, including laxity of the hip capsule. Female neonates may be even more sensitive to maternal hormones such as estrogen and relaxin, which are thought to be responsible for this generalized physiological laxity. **Environmental factors** that may predispose newborns and infants to DDH include swaddling with the legs in extension and adduction, which is still practiced in some societies (eg, Navajos in North America who use cradle boards). This was also practiced in Japan until 1975, and after teaching proper swaddling methods they recorded a 5-fold decrease in the incidence of DDH. Other factors include muscle contractures due to neuromuscular disease, such as cerebral palsy.

Differential Diagnosis

The differential diagnosis of DDH depends on the age of the child and the presenting complaint. Newborns and infants may have a "click" on abduction of the hip that represents the snapping of a ligament rather than the reduction of the dislocated hip into the joint. Infants who have limited abduction may have a neuromuscular disorder such as spastic diplegia, a form of cerebral palsy affecting the lower extremities. Older children who present with gait disturbances such as limp, waddling gait, or toe-walking may have neuromuscular conditions, fractures, or infection (eg, osteomyelitis, septic arthritis).

Evaluation

History

Family history of DDH should be reviewed, and a careful neonatal history should be taken, including presentation (eg, breech vs vertex), type of delivery, history of prenatal problems (eg, oligohydramnios), and presence of congenital torticollis or metatarsus adductus (Questions Box).

Physical Examination

It is important to evaluate the hip joint for instability or dislocation throughout the first year of life or until the child begins to walk. It is also important to assess for other causes of hip instability, as this could potentially change treatment approach and prognosis. This includes a neurologic examination to assess for spasticity associated with cerebral palsy, a neck examination to assess for torticollis, a

Developmental Hip Dysplasia

Questions

- Was the neonate a breech presentation?
- Does the child have any muscular problems, such as torticollis?
- When did the gait disturbance begin?
- Does anything make the child's gait better or worse?
- Is the child in any pain?
- Did any member of the family have hip dysplasia?

cutaneous examination to assess for changes associated with spinal disorders like spina bifida, and a foot examination for conditions like metatarsus adductus. The **Ortolani and Barlow maneuvers** may be used in the neonatal period to evaluate for DDH (Figure 104-2). Both tests are performed with newborns in a supine position and the hips and knees flexed to 90 degrees. Neonates should be quiet and relaxed because both tests require a cooperative child for adequate results.

The Ortolani maneuver, also referred to as the *click of entry,* is a diagnostic test used to detect reduction of a dislocated femoral head. To perform, the examiner gently abducts the hip and lifts the femoral head anteriorly. A positive sign is a palpable "clunk," felt when a dislocated femoral head is reduced. This "clunk" differs from the audible hip click, which is due to non-pathologic processes, such as ligamentous snapping. Each leg should be examined separately, not simultaneously.

The Barlow maneuver, also referred to as the *click of exit,* is another diagnostic test; it identifies a dislocatable femoral head in an unstable or dysplastic acetabulum. To perform the maneuver, the hips are adducted and a posterior force is placed along the longitudinal axis of the femur. Subluxations or dislocations are readily palpable. The Ortolani and Barlow maneuvers are rarely used after 6 to 8 weeks of age because the surrounding soft tissues and muscles adapt to the dislocated hip, making it more difficult to reduce.

If the diagnosis of DDH or dislocation is not made shortly after birth, there is a different set of physical findings, including asymmetry of hip abduction that is secondary to adductor muscle shortening and contracture on the affected side. Limited hip abduction is the most reliable late diagnostic sign.

As the femoral head dislocates posteriorly, the thigh is shortened on the affected side, producing relative limb shortening and asymmetry of the gluteal, thigh, and labial folds. Asymmetric gluteal folds result from bunching of skin and subcutaneous tissue on the affected side; however, asymmetric skinfolds have not been shown to be reliable signs and assessment for DDH requires further evaluation. **Galeazzi sign** is noted when the femoral head displaces laterally and proximally, causing apparent shortening of the femur on the affected side. On examination, a positive Galeazzi sign may be observed with discrepancy in knee heights noted when infants are supine, the sacrum flat on the examination table, and hips and knees bent (Figure 104-3).

In children of walking age, the physician may notice a limp because of the relative leg length discrepancy. Children may try to disguise the limp by toe-walking. A Trendelenburg test may be positive. Normally, when a child stands on one leg, the hip abductors straighten the pelvis and keep the center of gravity over the femoral head. If the abductors are weak, the weight shifts to the opposite side, causing it to droop. The gait abnormality classically associated with unilateral hip dislocation in a child of walking age is called the Trendelenburg gait. A child with bilateral involvement may display hyperlordosis and a waddling gait.

Figure 104-2. Ortolani and Barlow maneuvers. A, Ortolani (reduction) maneuver. B, Barlow (dislocation) maneuver.

Figure 104-3. Late signs in the diagnosis of developmental dysplasia of the hip. A, Asymmetry of thigh folds. B, Asymmetry of hip abduction. C, Discrepancy of knee heights.

Imaging Studies

Radiologic and ultrasound evaluations may aid in the diagnosis. Hip ultrasonography helps to confirm the diagnosis and to identify more subtle forms of the disorder. In some European countries, ultrasound is used as a primary screening modality, but in the United States it is only recommended to be used in the setting of high-risk newborns (ie, female born breech) or in a newborn with a click that has not resolved after 2 weeks of observation. Ultrasonography is the only diagnostic test that allows real-time evaluation and a 3-dimensional view of the neonate's hip. Reliable radiograph changes begin to

become evident by 4 to 6 months of age, when the ossific nucleus of the femoral head appears in most infants (Figure 104-4). A flat, shallow acetabulum and delayed ossification of the femoral head are the simplest and most easily recognizable findings.

Classification

One of the most commonly used classification systems for severity of persistent DDH into adulthood was developed by John F. Crowe in the late 1970s. The Crowe classification (Table 104-1) assumes that the ratio of femoral head diameter to pelvic height is 1:5. Using this assumption, any proximal migration of the femoral head can be noted based on its relationship to 3 major landmarks identified on an anteroposterior radiograph of the pelvis: (1) inferior margin of the acetabulum (teardrop); (2) pelvic height (distance from iliac crest

Figure 104-4. Radiographic findings associated with developmental dysplasia of the hip. The left hip is dislocated. The femur is lateral and proximal, the acetabulum is shallow and flat, and there is delayed ossification of the femoral head, as evidenced by the absence of the ossific nucleus on the left.

Table 104-1. Crowe Classification for Developmental Dysplasia of the Hip in Adults	
Crowe Classification Group	**Description**
1	Proximal displacement <0.1% of pelvic height OR Subluxation <50%
2	Displacement of 0.10%–0.15% OR Subluxation 50%–75%
3	Displacement of 0.15%–0.20% OR Subluxation 75%–100%
4	Displacement >20% OR Subluxation >100%

Adapted with permission from Crowe JF, Mani VJ, Ranawat CS. Total hip replacement in congenital dislocation and dysplasia of the hip. *J Bone Joint Surg Am.* 1979;61(1):15–23.

to ischial tuberosity); and (3) medial head-neck junction (distance from head-neck junction to the teardrop). The amount of migration of the femoral head is directly related to the severity of the hip dysplasia, and this will guide prognosis and treatment.

Management

The need for repeat examinations of the hips during the first year of life cannot be overemphasized. Children suspected of any hip instability or any child with less than 60 degrees of hip abduction should be evaluated with appropriate imaging studies and referred to an orthopedic surgeon for further evaluation. An orthopedic surgeon can aid the primary care physician in the diagnosis and management of DDH.

The goal of treatment is to return the femoral head to its normal position within the acetabulum and restore normal hip functioning. The common practice of triple diapering should be discouraged because it is unreliable, often delays definitive therapy, and may produce complications, such as avascular necrosis of the femoral head.

The management of DDH is divided into 5 different treatment groups.

1. Newborn to 6 months
2. Infant (6–18 months)
3. Toddler (18–36 months)
4. Child and juvenile (3–8 years)
5. Adolescent to young adult (beyond 8 years)

The **Pavlik harness** is the primary method of treating DDH during infancy. This device has evolved as the clear method of choice for treatment of newborns and infants with DDH and has become accepted as the standard of treatment worldwide. The Pavlik harness consists of a chest strap, shoulder straps, and anterior and posterior stirrup straps that maintain the hips in flexion and abduction while restricting extension and adduction (Figure 104-5). When properly used, the harness holds the hips in a flexed and abducted

Shoulder Strap

Chest Strap

Abduction Strap

Abduction Strap

Leg Strap

Figure 104-5. **Pavlik harness.**

position while allowing newborns and infants to move their legs within safe limits of abduction and adduction until stability is achieved. In the newborn with DDH, the harness should be worn for 23 hours daily until the clinical and radiographic examinations are normal. The harness must be worn for a minimum of 3 months by infants 3 months and younger, whereas infants and children 4 months or older usually wear the harness for a period of double their age. A newborn with a diagnosis of true dislocation must wear the harness full time until the dislocatable hip has stabilized in the acetabulum.

The harness should be applied and monitored by an orthopedic surgeon because inappropriate application may lead to adverse outcomes, such as inferior dislocation and, the most serious, avascular necrosis of the femoral head. Parents play a key role in the successful use of the harness and must be educated on the disease process and the proper use of the harness. Overall, the Pavlik harness has an 85% to 95% success rate; however, it loses efficacy as the child ages because of soft tissue contractures that develop in previously untreated individuals.

If this treatment method is ineffective or if the diagnosis is not made until after 6 months of age, **traction** followed by open or closed **reduction and spica cast immobilization** may be used. Good results are more difficult to obtain with increasing age, especially after children are walking, because chronic dislocation leads to more permanent pathologic changes to femoral, acetabular, and soft tissue anatomy. Operative treatment is required in children older than 18 months to safely reduce the dislocated hip and to surgically re-create normal anatomy. These procedures include **femoral shortening, acetabuloplasty** to correct acetabular dysplasia, and **capsulorrhaphy** (suturing the joint capsule).

Prognosis

The prognosis of DDH depends on age at the time of diagnosis and severity of the deformity. The long-term prognosis for satisfactory hip function is good for children when DDH is recognized early and treated appropriately. Generally children with DDH that is diagnosed after the first year of life have a poorer prognosis for satisfactory hip function than those with DDH that is diagnosed during infancy. Left untreated, the prognosis differs based on the type of DDH. In general, a patient with unilateral dislocation will have a worse prognosis than a patient with bilateral dislocation because of the associated limb-length discrepancy, asymmetric motion and strength, gait abnormalities, and subsequent degeneration of the ipsilateral knee. Although controversial, it is generally accepted that patients with chronic subluxation have the worst prognosis due to femoral point loading in the partially dislocated hip; this point loading leads to early arthritis. Regardless of where a patient is on the spectrum of DDH, if left untreated, it will result in disability ranging from limp to pain and stiffness in the hip, and early onset degenerative joint disease in adult life.

> ## *CASE RESOLUTION*
>
> The infant presented in the case study has less than 60 degrees of abduction of the left hip, a sign of developmental dysplasia of the hip. An anteroposterior view of the pelvis may be ordered to confirm the diagnosis. Regardless of the radiographic findings, the infant should be referred to an orthopedic surgeon for further evaluation and management. If hip dislocation is confirmed, the initial treatment will involve bracing with the Pavlik harness.

Selected References

American Academy of Pediatrics Committee on Quality Improvement, Subcommittee on Developmental Dysplasia of the Hip. Clinical practice guideline: early detection of developmental dysplasia of the hip. *Pediatrics.* 2000;105(4):896–905

Aronsson DD, Goldberg MJ, Kling TF Jr, Roy DR. Developmental dysplasia of the hip. *Pediatrics.* 1994;94(2 Pt 1):201–208

Ballock RT, Richards BS. Hip dysplasia: early diagnosis makes a difference. *Contemp Pediatr.* 1997;14:108–117

Bialik V, Bialik GM, Blazer S, Sujov P, Wiener F, Berant M. Developmental dysplasia of the hip: a new approach to incidence. *Pediatrics.* 1999;103(1):93–99

Bond CD, Hennrikus WL, DellaMaggiore ED. Prospective evaluation of newborn soft-tissue hip "clicks" with ultrasound. *J Pediatr Orthop.* 1997;17(2):199–201

Bracken J, Tran T, Ditchfield M. Developmental dysplasia of the hip: controversies and current concepts. *J Paediatr Child Health.* 2012;48(11):963–973

Guille JT, Pizzutillo PD, MacEwen GD. Developmental dysplasia of the hip from birth to six months. *J Am Acad Orthop Surg.* 2000;8(4):232–242

Hensinger RN. Congenital dislocation of the hip. Treatment in infancy to walking age. *Orthop Clin North Am.* 1987;18(4):597–616

Mooney JF, Emans JB. Developmental dislocation of the hip: a clinical overview. *Pediatr Rev.* 1995;16(8):299–304

Novacheck TF. Developmental dysplasia of the hip. *Pediatr Clin North Am.* 1996;43(4):829–848

Rális Z, McKibbin B. Changes in shape of the human hip joint during its development and their relation to its stability. *J Bone Joint Surg Br.* 1973;55(4):780–785

Shipman SA, Helfand M, Moyer VA, Yawn BP. Screening for developmental dysplasia of the hip: a systematic literature review for the US Preventive Services Task Force. *Pediatrics.* 2006;117(3):e557–e576

Theophilopoulos EP, Barrett DJ. Get a grip on the pediatric hip. *Contemp Pediatr.* 1998;15:43–65

Vitale MG, Skaggs DL. Developmental dysplasia of the hip from six months to four years of age. *J Am Acad Orthop Surg.* 2001;9(6):401–411

Wientroub S, Grill F. Ultrasonography in developmental dysplasia of the hip. *J Bone Joint Surg Am.* 2000;82-A(7):1004–1018

Yiannakopoulos CK, Chougle A, Eskelinen A, Hodgkinson JP, Hartofilakidis G. Inter- and intra-observer variability of the Crowe and Hartofilakidis classification systems for congenital hip disease in adults. *J Bone Joint Surg Br.* 2008;90(5):579–583

CHAPTER 105

Intoeing and Out-toeing: Rotational Problems of the Lower Extremity

David P. Zamorano, MD; Andrew K. Battenberg, MD; and Steven Donohoe, BS

CASE STUDY

A 3-year-old girl is brought to the office. Her mother is concerned because beginning a few months ago, her daughter's feet appeared to "turn in" when she walked. The girl has never walked like this before, and she has no history of trauma, fever, pain, or swelling in the joints. The physical examination is within normal limits except for the intoeing gait.

Questions

1. How can observation of children's gait help determine the etiology of their intoeing and out-toeing (rotational problems)?
2. What are the common causes of intoeing and out-toeing?
3. Does evaluation of intoeing and out-toeing require any laboratory or radiologic studies?
4. What is the natural history of most rotational problems?

Benign rotational variations of the lower extremities such as intoeing (pigeon toe) and out-toeing are seen in many healthy children. Although rotational problems that produce intoeing and out-toeing may initially be physically alarming, spontaneous resolution occurs in most cases. They are a common cause of parental concern during infancy and childhood; however, they rarely lead to physical limitation. Most of these children can be managed adequately by primary care physicians and do not need orthopedic referral. A thorough understanding of the normal rotational variations that occur in children younger than 10 years is essential to proper treatment and patient and parent education. More importantly, a general understanding is imperative to identify more serious underlying structural problems.

Specific terminology used to describe limb positioning is as follows. **Version** is normal variation in limb rotation, whereas **torsion** refers to abnormal conditions (ie, >2 standard deviations above or below the mean). **Adduction** is movement toward the midline, in contrast to **abduction,** which is movement away from the midline. **Varus angulation** is deviation toward the midline, whereas **valgus angulation** is deviation away from the midline. An **inverted** foot is one turned toward the midline on its long axis. An **everted** foot is one turned away from the midline on its long axis.

Epidemiology

In neonates or young infants, intoeing is most likely the result of clubfoot (talipes equinovarus), isolated metatarsus adductus, or metatarsus varus. The incidence of clubfoot is 1 in 1,000 live births, with a male to female ratio of 2:1. The condition is bilateral in approximately 50% of cases. The incidence of metatarsus adductus, a much more common problem, is about 1 in 500 live births. It is often bilateral. Internal tibial torsion is the primary cause of intoeing in the second year of life, and femoral torsion accounts for most cases of this condition during early childhood.

Physiological out-toeing is classically evident in infants who have not yet begun to walk and is the most common cause of bilateral out-toeing. In older infants and children, however, lateral tibial torsion is believed to be the most common cause of out-toeing.

Clinical Presentation

Children with congenital clubfoot, metatarsus adductus, and metatarsus varus present with intoeing during infancy. Congenital clubfoot is usually evident at birth. A severe medial, midline, plantar crease is present, and the foot appears C-shaped, with the heel and forefront turned inward (Figure 105-1). The affected foot is small,

Figure 105-1. Congenital clubfoot (talipes equinovarus).

wide, and stiff, and the lower leg appears small due to hypoplasia of the calf muscles. In contrast to clubfoot, only the forefoot turns inward in metatarsus adductus and varus.

Tibial torsion is apparent during the second year of life. In affected children, the feet turn inward during ambulation, but the knees are straight because the deformity is distal to the knee. Medial femoral torsion is evident at 3 to 4 years of age and usually affects girls. Affected children can sit in the "W" position with both legs behind them. As the child walks, the knees and the feet appear to turn inward because the deformity is proximal to the knee.

Physiological out-toeing is seen in infancy. Classically, parents note that when they hold their child in a standing position, both feet turn outward. Approximately 5 degrees of out-toeing is normal after age 3 years. Further degrees of out-toeing may be due to lateral tibial torsion.

Pathophysiology

Several factors are involved in the etiology of rotational conditions. Most of these deformations are caused by intrauterine positioning. Genetics are also believed to play a role in the development of rotational problems, as parents may often have the same rotational deformity as their children. Other contributing factors include **bony and neuromuscular abnormalities** in clubfoot and certain sleeping and sitting positions in metatarsus adductus and medial tibial torsion. For example, sleeping in the prone position with the legs internally rotated may worsen internal tibial torsion or metatarsus adductus.

During the early intrauterine period, internal rotation of the lower extremity brings the big toe to the midline. However, during the later intrauterine period, infancy, and childhood, external rotation predominates. Alterations in this normal lateral process are

caused by genetic and environmental factors, including intrauterine molding and sleep positions. Conditions influenced by intrauterine position, such as metatarsus adductus and developmental dysplasia of the hip, are sometimes found in the same children.

Congenital clubfoot is most commonly an isolated birth defect and is considered idiopathic. Two major etiologies have been proposed: (1) a germline defect in the talus results in abnormal bony development leading to plantar flexion, inversion, soft tissue contractures, and hypoplasia of the calf muscles and the bones of the foot, and (2) clubfoot represents the final common pathway of disruption anywhere along the neuromuscular unit, including the central nervous system, peripheral nerves, and muscles. Additionally, genetics are believed to play a major role given that 25% of all cases are familial and there is 33% concordance of identical twins. Environmental factors, including intrauterine position and molding, are also thought to contribute.

Intoeing is usually caused by benign conditions such as metatarsus adductus, excessive internal tibial torsion, and excessive femoral torsion. Less frequently, patients have pathologic conditions such as clubfoot, skewfoot, hip disorders, and neuromuscular diseases. Out-toeing is typically caused by external rotation contracture of the hip, external tibial torsion, or external femoral torsion. We will now review the conditions associated with rotational variations in children.

Intoeing

Metatarsus Adductus and Metatarsus Primus Varus

Metatarsus adductus, with or without internal tibial torsion, is the most common cause of intoeing from birth to 1 year of age. It is a functional deformity in which the forefoot is adducted with respect to the hindfoot with a neutral or slightly valgus heel. It is the most common pediatric foot problem referred to orthopedic surgeons and occurs in 1 in 500 live births and in 1 in 20 siblings of patients with metatarsus adductus. The rate is higher in males, twin births, and preterm babies. Numerous theories exist as to the cause of metatarsus adductus, including in utero positioning, sleeping position of the baby, muscle imbalance, and medial cuneiform abnormality.

Presenting complaints include cosmesis, intoeing gait, or excessive shoe wear. On physical examination, the foot appears C-shaped with a concave medial border and convex lateral border. The forefoot can be brought into the neutral position by stroking the lateral border of the foot or by gently straightening it. Metatarsus adductus can be classified into flexible or inflexible based on physical examination. Most cases of flexible metatarsus adductus resolve spontaneously and do not require splinting, bracing, or special shoes. However, patients with rigid metatarsus adductus should undergo early casting; uncommonly, resistant cases may require surgery.

Congenital **metatarsus primus varus** is a bony abnormality characterized by an isolated adducted first metatarsal. Unlike flexible metatarsus adductus, metatarsus varus is a fixed deformity. The foot cannot be brought into the neutral position, and there is a deep vertical skin crease along the medial border of the tarsometatarsal joints. Because it is a more rigid deformity, early casting is recommended and persistent deformity requires surgery.

Skewfoot or Congenital Metatarsus Varus

Skewfoot, also known as *serpentine metatarsus adductus,* is characterized by adducted metatarsals combined with a valgus deformity of the heel and plantar flexion of the talus. It is theorized that improper casting of metatarsus adductus or clubfoot may result in a skewfoot; however, most cases are idiopathic. Patients present with pain or callus formation under the head of the talus and base of the fifth metatarsal. Some feet undergo spontaneous correction, while surgery is indicated for a persistently symptomatic foot.

Dynamic Abductor Hallucis/Searching Toe

Dynamic abductor hallucis/searching toe, also known as *wandering* or *atavistic* toe, can cause intoeing. Children with a so-called searching toe have a big toe that points medially when they walk. Unlike the other causes of intoeing, which are structural and present at rest, this condition is a dynamic deformity. Searching toe results from the contraction of the abductors of the big toe during the stance phase of gait, which pulls the toe toward the midline. It usually resolves with age and subsequent development of fine motor coordination.

Clubfoot

Congenital **clubfoot,** a pathologic deformity of the foot, may be identified at birth (see Figure 105-1). Clubfoot may be an isolated deformity or seen in association with other neuromuscular anomalies such as arthrogryposis, myelomeningocele, amniotic band syndrome, cerebral palsy, or poliomyelitis.

The diagnosis of congenital clubfoot is made at birth on the basis of 3 conditions: forefoot varus, heel varus, and ankle equinus. Clubfoot can range in severity from a rigid deformity, in which the forefoot cannot be passively abducted into a neutral position, to nonrigid deformities, in which the forefoot can be gently brought toward the midline. Normal dorsiflexion of the ankle helps distinguish severe forms of metatarsus varus from clubfoot.

Internal Tibial Torsion

Internal tibial torsion is the most common cause of intoeing from ages 1 to 3 years, thought to be caused by intrauterine positioning, and usually first noticed by parents when their child begins to walk. Parents often complain that the child is clumsy and trips frequently. The condition is bilateral in two-thirds of affected children; when unilateral, it more commonly affects the left leg. Observation of gait reveals that the knees point forward but the feet turn inward. Because the knees are straight, the site of the rotational deformity is below this joint. If the feet are normal and no metatarsus adductus or varus is present, the rotational deformity can be isolated to the lower leg. It is important to measure the thigh-foot and trans-malleolar axes in the physical examination. Expectant observation is recommended because the natural history of internal tibial torsion strongly favors spontaneous resolution by 4 years of age.

Internal Femoral Torsion

Internal femoral torsion is the most common cause of intoeing in children presenting at 3 to 6 years of age, tends to occur in females, and is usually bilateral. Children generally present when parents notice worsening intoeing in a child who has no previous history of intoeing. Although excessive medial femoral torsion may be present at birth, it is often masked by the external rotatory forces present during infancy. Children with excessive internal femoral torsion characteristically sit with their legs in the "W" position and run with an eggbeater-type motion. While no association between internal femoral torsion and degenerative joint disease has been shown, some studies suggest there is an increased association with knee pain. This is seen most often in "miserable malalignment syndrome," a combination of internal femoral torsion and external tibial torsion. No treatment is necessary for most cases of femoral torsion, which usually resolves by 8 years of age.

Out-toeing

Physiological Out-toeing

Out-toeing of infancy, which is most commonly seen in children who are just learning to walk, is caused by intrauterine positioning that leads to external rotatory contractures of the soft tissues surrounding the hip. This condition may be perpetuated in children who sleep in the prone, frog-leg position, which holds the hips in external rotation and prevents normal stretching of the external rotators. Although both feet turn outward when infants stand, the lateral rotation of both hips is normal on examination (Figure 105-2). More serious conditions, such as slipped capital femoral epiphysis, hip dysplasia, or coxa vara, are less common but should be considered.

Figure 105-2. Physiological out-toeing of infancy.

External Tibial Torsion

This condition may be suspected in children who are 3 to 5 years of age, but detection can often be delayed until late childhood or adolescence. This condition tends to be unilateral, most often affects the right side, and generally worsens over time. Increased external tibial torsion is often associated with neuromuscular conditions, such as myelodysplasia and poliomyelitis. As the condition progresses, patients can develop disability and pain in the form of patellofemoral pain and instability. Some studies have even shown an association between external tibial torsion and degenerative joint disease of the knee.

Adolescent Hallux Valgus

This condition is well-described in the adult population but is beginning to be seen more often in the adolescent population. It is far more common in females, and studies have shown that up to 75% of affected patients have an affected mother. It is thought to be caused by a triad of deformities: (1) abnormal bone growth, or exostosis, over the medial side of the first metatarsal head; (2) valgus deformity of the hallux; and (3) associated metatarsus primus varus. The etiologic factors for development of this deformity are similar to adults. The main contributing intrinsic factor is increased ligamentous laxity of the foot. The most common extrinsic factor is improper shoe wear. It has long been accepted that shoes with a narrow toe box, especially shoes with high heels, are highly associated with hallux valgus. Other extrinsic factors commonly associated with hallux valgus are neuromuscular disorders, like cerebral palsy.

The most common presenting complaint is pain over the medial aspect of the great toe metatarsal head. This is usually the result of pressure and chronic friction over the area. This can lead to gait abnormalities and limit the patient's ability to participate in regular activity.

Differential Diagnosis

Intoeing and out-toeing may be classified according to anatomic level and usual age at presentation (Table 105-1). These conditions may be localized to 1 of 4 areas: toe, foot, tibia, and femur. If intoeing

problems are placed in chronologic order by age of presentation, the affected area follows a toe-to-femur sequence.

Evaluation

History

The clinical history must delineate the onset, duration, and progression of any structural problems. The typical natural history of benign rotational conditions shows improvement over time, whereas a more serious condition would have a more progressive deformity. Relevant family and birth history, including gestational age, length of labor, complications, Apgar scores, birth weight, and length of hospital stay, should be noted. These details may heighten suspicion for cerebral palsy or the presence of hereditary disorders, such as vitamin D–resistant rickets, mucopolysaccharidoses, achondroplasia, epiphyseal dysplasia, or metaphyseal dysplasia, that may affect rotational profiles. A thorough developmental history is important because developmental delays may be a sign of underlying neuromuscular or neurologic disorders (Questions Box). It is also important to determine whether the rotational problems cause marked functional impairment in the patient; this includes problems with tripping, pain, or shoe wear difficulties.

Physical Examination

Normal variability in the lower extremities of young children must be differentiated from more serious structural problems. A detailed physical examination, including assessment of gait and neurologic and musculoskeletal function, is essential for making the correct diagnosis. This evaluation should include examination of the hips for signs of developmental dysplasia, which may be associated with metatarsus adductus (see Chapter 104). Observation of the child's stature and body-to-limb ratio is also useful because short stature or disproportionate body-to-limb ratio may suggest a skeletal dysplasia.

Evaluation of postural conditions requires static and dynamic physical examination. Static examination includes an overall evaluation of the patient and a rotational profile. The child's rotational profile, as described by Staheli, consists of 5 components (Figure 105-3). The 5 components of this profile are internal and external hip rotation, thigh-foot axis, trans-malleolar axis, heel-bisector line, and foot progression angle during gait (Figure 105-4).

Table 105-1. Site and Age of Onset of Rotational Problems of the Lower Extremity in Children

Problem	Site of Problem	Age of Onset
Intoeing		
Searching toe	Toe	Infancy
Clubfoot	Foot	Birth
Metatarsus adductus/varus	Foot	Birth/infancy
Medial tibial torsion	Tibia	Toddler stage (12–24 mo)
Medial femoral torsion	Femur	Early childhood (3–5 y)
Out-toeing		
Physiological out-toeing	Hips	Infancy
Lateral tibial torsion	Tibia	Childhood

Questions

Intoeing and Out-toeing

- Is there any family history of intoeing or out-toeing?
- What is the birth history? Was the child a breech presentation?
- At what age did the child begin walking?
- When did the rotational deformity appear? Is it getting better or worse?
- Does the rotational problem produce any disability (eg, tripping or falling a great deal when walking or running)?
- Has any previous treatment been tried?
- In what position does the child sleep? In what position does the child sit?

Figure 105-3. **Rotational profile. (Reproduced with permission from Wenger DR, Rang M.** *The Art and Practice of Children's Orthopedics.* **New York, NY: Raven Press; 1993.)**

Figure 105-4. **Evaluation of foot progression angle.**

Hip rotation in infants averages 40 degrees of internal rotation and 70 degrees of external rotation. By 10 years of age, internal hip rotation averages 50 degrees and external rotation 45 degrees. Internal rotation measuring between 70 and 90 degrees is evidence of femoral torsion.

The **thigh-foot axis** consists of the rotation of the tibia and hindfoot in relation to the longitudinal axis of the thigh and indicates the amount of tibial torsion. In infants, the thigh-foot angle averages 5 degrees internal (range: −30 to +20 degrees). Excessive internal tibial torsion spontaneously resolves by 3 to 4 years of age, and by 8 years of age the thigh-foot axis averages 10 degrees external.

The **trans-malleolar axis** also aids in determining the amount of tibial torsion. It is formed by the angle at the intersection of an imaginary line from the lateral to medial malleolus and a second line from the lateral to medial femoral condyles. At gestational age 5 months, the fetus has an average of 20 degrees of internal tibial torsion. During development, the tibia externally rotates to an average final adult position of 23 degrees of external rotation.

The **heel-bisector line** examines the foot and is a line drawn through the midline axis of the hindfoot and forefoot. In a neutral foot, the heel-bisector line passes through the second web space.

Finally, the **foot progression angle during gait** is the angle of the foot relative to an imaginary straight line in the patient's path (see Figure 105-4). Patients who intoe are assigned a negative value and patients who out-toe are assigned a positive value. This value represents the sum total effect of the child's structural alignment and dynamic torsion forces resulting from muscle forces.

The examination of infants with clubfoot should include a careful examination of the back for signs of possible spinal dysraphism (eg, skin dimples, hairy patches) and a thorough neurologic examination.

Internal tibial torsion may be diagnosed by having children sit at the end of the examination table with both knees flexed to 90 degrees and palpating the medial and lateral malleoli with the thumb and index finger. Normally, the medial malleolus lies anterior to the lateral malleolus (approximately one fingerbreadth). If the lateral malleolus is on the same plane or anterior to the medial malleolus, internal tibial torsion is indicated.

The diagnosis of tibial torsion can also be made by measuring the thigh-foot angle (Figure 105-5). Measurement of the thigh-foot angle involves having children lie prone on the examination table and observing the relationship of the long axis of the foot compared with the axis of the thigh as viewed from above. The shape of the foot itself can also be assessed with children in this position. Slight internal rotation is normal as children first learn to walk.

Diagnosis of medial femoral torsion can be made by observing children's gaits and measuring hip rotation. For example, when a child with medial femoral torsion ambulates, the knees and feet appear to turn inward. Internal and external hip rotation are evaluated with the child in a prone position, the pelvis flat, and the knees flexed 90 degrees (Figure 105-6). The degrees of normal rotation vary with age (see Figure 105-3). During childhood, internal hip rotation greater than 70 degrees implies medial femoral torsion.

Imaging Studies

Routine imaging studies are not necessary for rotational deformities. Imaging studies may be considered by the orthopedic surgeon in severe deformities when operative correction is being considered.

Figure 105-5. Evaluation of the thigh-foot axis. A, Observation with the child in the prone position is best. B, Determination of the thigh-foot axis. C, Assessment of the shape of the foot.

Figure 105-6. Evaluation of hip rotation. A, The child is prone and knees are flexed to 90 degrees. B, Medial rotation is measured. C, Lateral rotation is measured.

In patients with clubfoot, radiographs are used to assess the relationship and development of the bones and to monitor cast correction.

Management

Intoeing

Metatarsus adductus generally resolves spontaneously, but stretching exercises for the foot may be advisable, particularly if parents are anxious to "do something." Parents are instructed to manipulate the foot with each diaper change. Because most cases resolve within the first 3 months of life, referral to an orthopedic surgeon should be made if the deformity is still present at 3 to 4 months of age. Cast correction may be required for rigid deformities or deformities that persist beyond 3 to 4 months. Shoe modifications (eg, putting shoes on the wrong foot) should be avoided because they have not been shown to have any long-term benefits.

Because metatarsus varus may progress when children begin walking, referral to an orthopedic surgeon should be made as soon as the condition is detected. Serial casting followed by corrective shoes or inserts is the first line of treatment, and surgery is rarely required. Treatment for medial tibial torsion is rarely required because this problem generally corrects with time when children learn to walk. Night splinting, although still occasionally instituted, has not been shown to affect the natural history of this condition. If the deformity is severe, persists without improvement beyond the age of 18 months, or persists after the child has been walking for 1 year, referral to an orthopedic surgeon should be made. Surgical correction (eg, tibial rotational osteotomy) may be required if the deformity is severe or persists beyond 8 to 10 years of age.

Like other conditions that produce intoeing, medial femoral torsion generally does not require treatment. Even if it persists into adulthood, it usually produces no disability, nor does it increase the risk for degenerative arthritis in the involved joint. Nonoperative treatment is ineffective. Surgical correction may be required if there is a history of repeated falls, severe gait problems, marked cosmetic deformity, anterior anteversion greater than 50 degrees, or internal hip rotation greater than 80 degrees. A derotational femoral osteotomy is the only effective method of treatment. It should not be performed until children are at least 8 to 10 years of age.

Clubfoot, unlike other problems, is a pathologic deformity that requires treatment. Treatment, which should begin during the first week of life, consists of serial manipulations of the foot and casting. Several months of casting may be required to attain full correction. Surgery is often required for resistant or recurrent cases. As many as 50% to 75% of patients with clubfoot may eventually require surgery. Surgery is usually delayed until infants are 6 to 12 months of age.

Out-toeing

Physiological out-toeing of infancy is a rotational problem that spontaneously resolves when children learn to walk. Most cases resolve by 18 months of age. Severe lateral tibial torsion may require surgical correction with a tibial derotational osteotomy.

In hallux valgus, the main concern is often cosmesis. Encouraging proper shoe wear or use of orthotics will lead to improvement in the deformity, but it can be difficult for adolescents to adhere to these recommendations. If the patient fails nonsurgical treatment or is noncompliant, the patient should be referred to an orthopedic surgeon to discuss operative correction.

Prognosis

Because the lower extremity rotates laterally with growth, the natural history of internal rotational problems, such as internal tibial torsion and medial femoral torsion, is resolution over time. In contrast, lateral tibial torsion may become worse with time.

The prognosis for most rotational problems is excellent. Parental reassurance and education on the natural history of these deformities may decrease anxiety and prevent unnecessary visits to specialists. Functional disability or degenerative arthritis is not commonly associated with persistence of these conditions.

Left untreated, clubfoot often leads to considerable pain and disability. The affected foot can be difficult to fit with shoes. Additionally, clubfoot can be unsightly and cause children significant emotional distress.

CASE RESOLUTION

The girl described in the case study seems to have medial femoral torsion because she has no history of rotational problems. Her entire leg turns in when she walks. Internal hip rotation greater than 70 degrees confirms the diagnosis. The mother can be reassured that this is a normal, age-related phenomenon that will most likely resolve over time. The child can be reevaluated in 4 to 6 months. Orthopedic referral is not required at this time.

Selected References

Craig CL, Goldberg MJ. Foot and leg problems. *Pediatr Rev.* 1993;14(10): 395–400

Delahay J. Adolescent hallux valgus. In: McCarthy JJ, Drennan JC, eds. *Drennan's The Child's Foot and Ankle.* 2nd ed. Philadelphia, PA: Lippincott Williams & Wilkins; 2010:270–279

Dobbs MB, Gurnett CA. Update on clubfoot: etiology and treatment. *Clin Orthop Relat Res.* 2009;467(5):1146–1153

Fuchs R, Staheli LT. Sprinting and intoeing. *J Pediatr Orthop.* 1996;16(4): 489–491

Hoekelman RA. Foot and leg problems. In: Hoekelman RA, ed. *Primary Pediatric Care.* 4th ed. St Louis, MO: Mosby; 1997:1097–1105

Hoffinger SA. Evaluation and management of pediatric foot deformities. *Pediatr Clin North Am.* 1996;43(5):1091–1111

Lincoln TL, Suen PW. Common rotational variations in children. *J Am Acad Orthop Surg.* 2003;11(5):312–320

Staheli LT. Lower positional deformity in infants and children: a review. *J Pediatr Orthop.* 1990;10(4):559–563

Wenger DR, Rang M. *The Art and Practice of Children's Orthopedics.* New York, NY: Raven Press; 1993

CHAPTER 106

Angular Deformities of the Lower Extremity: Bowlegs and Knock-knees

Carol D. Berkowitz, MD; Andrew K. Battenberg, MD; and Nima Eftekhary, MD

CASE STUDY

During the routine health maintenance examination of a 2-year-old, you observe moderate to severe bilateral bowing of both legs. The child's mother reports that her son began walking at 10 months. She has not noticed problems with his gait and says he does not trip or fall excessively. On examination, the boy's weight is greater than the 95th percentile for age, but otherwise he appears to be a healthy African American child.

Questions

1. What types of angular deformities affect children's lower extremities?
2. How does children's age help determine whether they have physiological or pathologic angular deformities?
3. What clinical measurements can help distinguish physiological from pathologic angular deformities?
4. To what extent are radiographs used in the routine assessment of angular deformities?

With normal growth and development, the angular alignment of children's legs progresses through a series of developmental stages—from relative bowlegs to knock-knees and eventually straight legs. Rotational problems such as intoeing and out-toeing are deformities in the transverse plane that occur when a bone rotates internally or externally along its long axis (Figure 106-1). Angular deformities such as bowlegs and knock-knees are deformities in the frontal plane. In bowleg deformity, the legs distal to the knees are angled or tilted toward the midline (tibial varus), whereas they are tilted away from the midline of the body in knock-knee deformity (tibial valgus) (Figure 106-2). Variations in the knee angle that fall outside the normal range (eg, more than ±2 standard deviations of the mean) are referred to as *genu varum* for bowlegs and *genu valgum* for knock-knees. Appreciation of the normal developmental sequence in conjunction with a careful history and physical examination can help pediatricians identify pathologic cases of bowlegs and knock-knees and initiate prompt treatment (D$_x$ Box).

Epidemiology

Bowlegs and knock-knees are common in infants and children. While babies are all born bowlegged, parents usually don't appreciate this finding until infants begin to walk. Knock-knees occur less

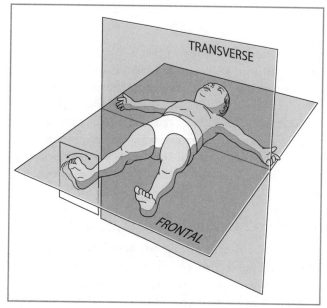

Figure 106-1. Select body reference and rotational planes. Rotational problems are deformities in the transverse plane. Angular deformities are in the frontal plane.

Figure 106-2. Varus and valgus deformities of the lower extremities. A, Bowleg deformity. B, Knock-knee deformity.

 Pathologic Bowlegs and Knock-Knees

- Asymmetric deformity
- Inconsistency with the normal sequence of angular development
- Stature less than the fifth percentile for age
- Severe deformity (>10 cm intermalleolar or intercondylar distance)
- History of rapid progression
- Presence of other musculoskeletal abnormalities

frequently than bowlegs, are seen more often in females, and are commonly associated with generalized ligamentous laxity. Though the frequency of these conditions is generally unknown, one study of more than 3,000 children aged 7 to 11 years found a prevalence of 7.9% for bowlegs and 2% for knock-knees. Males were 3 times more likely than females to have bowlegs, while females were twice as likely to have knock-knees. Pathologic cases of bowlegs and knock-knees are uncommon and are defined by the degree of the angulation.

Clinical Presentation

Children with **bowlegs** have a characteristic wide-based stance with increased distance between the knees. They may walk with a waddling gait. Intoeing may be noted as a result of associated internal tibial torsion. Evaluation is required for pathologic bowlegs when the intercondylar distance (distance between the knees) is more than 10 cm with the child lying supine with the medial malleoli touching.

Severe **knock-knees** may produce an awkward gait with the knees rubbing. Children may walk with both feet apart in an effort to avoid knee-to-knee contact. They may need to place one knee behind the other to stand with both feet together. Evaluation for pathologic knock-knees is warranted when the intermalleolar distance (distance between the ankles) is more than 10 cm with the child lying supine with the knees touching.

Pathophysiology

The normal variation in the angular alignment of the lower extremities changes with age. During the first 2 years of life, relative bowing of the legs is common. Although physiological bowing of the lower leg may be appreciated at birth, it is most prominent during the second year of life, when it most commonly involves the tibia and the femur. When associated with internal tibial torsion, the deformity may appear more striking. Physiological knock-knees develop between 3 and 4 years of age. The knock-knee stage resolves somewhere between 5 and 7 years of age, when normal adult alignment develops. A slight knock-knee appearance remains in normal adults. Bowlegs or knock-knees that develop outside of this sequence require further evaluation for pathologic causes.

The **tibiofemoral angle,** the angle between the long axis of the femur and the long axis of the tibia, is used to assess the angular alignment of the leg. At birth the tibiofemoral angle is approximately 15 degrees varus, and it decreases to 0 degrees between the ages of 18 and 24 months. By 3 to 4 years, the angle peaks at about 10 degrees of valgus angulation. Then between 5 and 7 years it decreases to the normal range of about 7 to 9 degrees in girls and 4 to 6 degrees in boys (Figure 106-3).

Differential Diagnosis

The most common causes of genu varum and genu valgum are presented in Box 106-1. Physiological bowlegs and knock-knees are usually bilateral, and they occur in a sequence that follows the normal developmental pattern. Lateral bowing of the tibia is commonly noted during the first year of life. Bowlegs (involving the femur and the tibia) are pronounced during the second year, and knock-knees become prominent between 3 and 4 years of age. This is the normal sequence of angular development. Most cases of bowlegs are the result of normal physiological processes, tibia vara (Blount disease), and rickets. Common causes of pathologic knock-knees are severe renal rickets and previous fractures of the proximal tibia.

Tibia vara (Blount disease), a growth disturbance involving the posterior-medial aspect of the proximal tibia (physis, epiphysis, and metaphysis), is the most common cause of pathologic bowlegs and is due to idiopathic undergrowth of the medial side of the tibia. There are 2 forms of the disease: early-onset (or infantile) and late-onset, which are defined by disease development before or after 4 years of age. The late-onset form is further subdivided into juvenile (4–10 years of age) and adolescent (>10 years of age). At all ages, tibia vara is more common in African Americans.

The infantile form, initially classified by Langenskiöld, is bilateral 80% of the time and is associated with internal tibial torsion. The etiology is believed to involve mechanical stress on the growth plate, thus converting physiological bowlegs to pathologic varus. Affected children are often obese, in the upper growth percentiles,

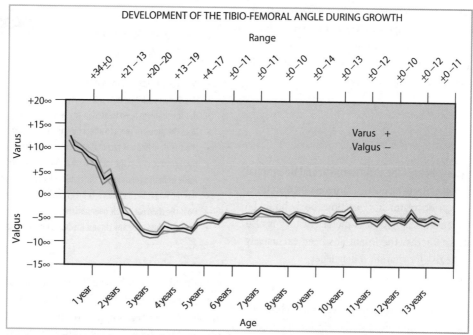

Figure 106-3. Development of the tibiofemoral angle. (Reproduced with permission from Salenius P, Vankka E. The development of the tibiofemoral angle in children. *J Bone Joint Surg Am.* **1975;57[2]:259–261.)**

Box 106-1. Common Causes of Genu Varum and Genu Valgum

Genu Varum

- Physiological bowlegs
- Rickets (vitamin D deficiency [nutritional] or vitamin D resistance [hereditary])
- Tibia vara (Blount disease)
- Achondroplasia
- Metaphyseal dysplasia
- Trauma, infection, or tumor of the proximal tibia (resulting in malunion or partial physeal arrest)
- Excessive prenatal fluoride ingestion

Genu Valgum

- Physiological knock-knees
- Rickets (renal osteodystrophy)
- Trauma, infection, or tumor of the distal femur or proximal tibia (resulting in malunion or partial physeal arrest)
- Paralytic conditions (eg, myelodysplasia, polio, cerebral palsy) leading to contracture of the iliotibial band
- Osteogenesis imperfecta
- Rheumatoid arthritis of the knee

and early walkers, which puts early stress on the growth plate. Blount disease produces a sharp angulation at the proximal tibia, whereas physiological bowlegs lead to a gradual curvature of the legs involving the femur and tibia. Six stages of radiograph progression based on the degree of epiphyseal depression and metaphyseal fragmentation at the proximal tibia have been identified (Langenskiöld staging). It may be difficult to distinguish between early stages of tibia

vara and physiological bowlegs, though criteria have been established to help predict infantile tibia vara in children presenting with idiopathic bowed legs: (1) a body mass index greater than or equal to 22 and (2) a tibial metaphyseal-diaphyseal angle greater than or equal to 10 degrees. These criteria have been shown to have a sensitivity of 95%, specificity of 100%, positive predictive value of 100%, and negative predictive value of 98%.

The late-onset form of tibia vara is less common than the juvenile form and is usually unilateral. Knee pain, rather than deformity, is the most common presenting sign. It is more common in males than females, and affected children are generally obese but have a normal height. Although the etiology is unclear, it is believed that in predisposed obese adolescents, repetitive trauma due to excess weight leads to decreased growth of the medial tibial physis.

Rickets, a disease of the growing skeleton, is a disorder caused by abnormal calcium and phosphorus metabolism that produces inadequate bone mineralization. Rickets takes several forms, including vitamin D–deficient (nutritional) rickets, vitamin D–resistant (hereditary) rickets (the most common form), and severe renal osteodystrophy. Signs of rickets include short stature, poor muscle tone, joint pain, and angular deformities of the lower extremities. Nutritional rickets may occur in infants who are exclusively breastfed and not supplemented with vitamin D. The alignment at the time of onset of disease determines the direction of angulation. For example, vitamin D–deficient or vitamin D–resistant rickets generally has an early onset and is more often associated with bowlegs. Children with rickets and bowlegs, unlike those with tibia vara, are late walkers and often have evidence of growth impairment. Renal osteodystrophy, which usually has a later onset, results in genu valgum (knock-knees).

Pathologic processes, including trauma (fractures), infections, and tumors, involving the proximal tibia are additional potential causes of bowlegs and knock-knees. Overgrowth or malunion following fractures of the proximal tibial metaphysis most commonly results in genu valgum rather than genu varum.

Evaluation

History

A family history, an assessment of the child's growth and nutritional history, and a description of the deformity, its progression over time, effect on function, and prior treatment (Questions Box) should be obtained from the parents or caregivers. A dietary history is also important, particularly whether the infant has been exclusively breastfed because of the risk for vitamin D deficiency.

Physical Examination

Physical examination begins with a general screening of children's nutritional growth and developmental status. Children's growth parameters (height, weight, head circumference) should be measured and plotted on standard growth curves. Limb length should be measured bilaterally, using the distance from the anterior superior iliac spine of the pelvis to the medial malleolus of the ankle as a direct measurement of "true" leg length. The rotational status of the lower limb should be assessed because internal tibial torsion is often associated with genu varum (see Chapter 105). Children should be observed standing and ambulating to determine the alignment of the legs in the coronal and sagittal planes. The intercondylar and intermalleolar distances can be measured with the child supine to determine the presence of excessive bowlegs or knock-knees (see Clinical Presentation on page 694). The intercondylar and intermalleolar distances should be followed every 6 months to monitor the progression of the deformity.

Laboratory Tests

Most children with physiological angulation do not require any laboratory studies. A general metabolic screening, including hemoglobin, calcium, phosphorus, vitamin D level, creatinine, and alkaline phosphatase, may be ordered if a systemic or metabolic abnormality is suspected.

Imaging Studies

Radiographs are usually performed in the evaluation of bowlegs or knock-knees if pathology is suspected. True pathology is more likely if the deformity is unilateral, painful, very asymmetric, or progressing at an accelerated rate. If obtained, radiographs should include the entire lower extremity so that the alignment of the femur and tibia may be assessed. Children should be standing, and a single radiograph of both legs should be taken that includes the hip and the ankle. Radiographs centered on the knee or ankle are also helpful in determining if the physeal plate is open. Pathologic conditions such as rickets (osteoporosis, metaphyseal fraying, cortical thinning, widening of the growth plates), tibia vera (Blount disease) (beaking

---

Questions

Pathologic Bowlegs and Knock-knees

- When was the deformity first noticed?
- Has it changed? If so, how fast?
- Has the problem been treated in any way?
- Does the problem seem to affect how the child walks?
- Has the child had any recent illness or trauma in the affected leg?
- Does anyone else in the family have a similar problem?
- Aside from this condition, is the child growing and developing normally?
- Has the infant been exclusively breastfed?
- Does the child eat a well-balanced diet?
- Does the child have any chronic medical problems such as kidney disease?

---

of the medial metaphysis of the proximal tibia), various bone dysplasia, and forms of dwarfism can usually be ruled out by radiographs. An increased uptake of the proximal medial aspect of the tibia on bone scan may help differentiate early infantile tibia vera from extreme physiological bowlegs. If pathology within the joint or premature arrest of physes is suspected, a computed tomography scan or magnetic resonance imaging can detect minor defects that may not be apparent on conventional radiography.

Management

Angular deformities within normal developmental limits should be managed with continual observation and reassessment. The severity of the deformity should be documented, and children should be followed at 3- to 6-month intervals until the condition resolves. Physicians should **reassure parents** that bowlegs and knock-knees are normal developmental variations that resolve spontaneously with time. Special diets, braces or shoe wedges, arch supports, and bars are generally best avoided; they have not been shown to affect the normal developmental sequence.

Children with physiological varus may be followed clinically until 18 months to 2 years of age. Pathology should be suspected if correction has not begun by this time or if the angulation is progressive. Children with more than 10 degrees of valgus or with an intermalleolar distance greater than 10 cm after 8 to 9 years of age may require further evaluation. Children with suspected cases of pathologic bowlegs and knock-knees require **referral to an orthopedist** for evaluation.

Although treatment of tibia vera in children younger than 3 to 4 years may consist of **bracing** if the deformity is mild and identified early, **surgery** is often necessary. Surgery involves an osteotomy to realign the tibia. Failure to do so may result in damage to the medial aspect of the knee over time. Medical management, such as administration of vitamin D for nutritional rickets, is of primary importance in the treatment of the various forms of rickets. Surgical correction, such as osteotomies to correct varus or valgus deformities, should be reserved until medical management has been maximized because even severe deformities may resolve with conservative management.

Additionally, guided growth by the less invasive means of epiphyseal stapling (hemi-epiphysiodesis) can be used to restrict growth on one half of the physis, with unrestricted growth on the other half of the physis. This leads to a correction in the angular deformity over time. The ideal patient for this intervention is one with a severe, pathologic angular deformity with open physes.

Prognosis

Physiological bowlegs and knock-knees spontaneously resolve without further sequelae. Although knock-knees are primarily a cosmetic problem, degenerative arthritis may rarely be a late complication. Though there is no evidence of a causal relationship between malalignment of the knee and development of osteoarthritis, biomechanical and gait studies suggest that malalignment can contribute to the development of osteoarthritis. Genu varum increases load in the medial compartment of the knee during gait, and genu valgum increases load in the lateral compartment of the knee. Surgical correction may be required for adolescents with severe deformity to prevent such late complications.

CASE RESOLUTION

The boy described in the case history should be evaluated for pathologic causes of genu varum, especially tibia vera (Blount disease), for the following reasons:
- His age is at the upper limit of normal for bowlegs and his deformity is severe.
- He is African American.
- He has a history of early walking.
- He is obese.

A standing radiograph of the lower extremities should be obtained, and the boy should be referred to an orthopedist for further evaluation and management.

Selected References

Bruce RW Jr. Torsional and angular deformities. *Pediatr Clin North Am.* 1996; 43(4):867–881

Eggert P, Viemann M. Physiologic bowlegs or infantile Blount's disease. Some new aspects on an old problem. *Pediatr Radiol.* 1996;26(5):349–352

Henderson RC. Tibia vara: a complication of adolescent obesity. *J Pediatr.* 1992; 121(3):482–486

Karimi-Mobarake M, Kashefipour A, Yousfnejad Z. The prevalence of genu varum and genu valgum in primary school children in Iran 2003-2004. *J Med Sci.* 2005; 5:52–54

Kling TF Jr. Angular deformities of the lower limbs in children. *Orthop Clin North Am.* 1987;18(4):513–527

Mankin KP, Zimbler S. Gait and leg alignment: what's normal and what's not. *Contemp Pediatr.* 1997;14:41–70

Sabharwal S. Blount disease. *J Bone Joint Surg Am.* 2009;91(7):1758–1776

Saran N, Rathjen KE. Guided growth for the correction of pediatric lower limb angular deformity. *J Am Acad Orthop Surg.* 2010;18(9):528–536

Scherl SA. Common lower extremity problems in children. *Pediatr Rev.* 2004; 25(2):52–62

Scoles PV. Lower extremity development. In: *Pediatric Orthopedics in Clinical Practice.* 2nd ed. Chicago, IL: Year Book Medical Publishers; 1988:82–121

Scott AC, Kelly CH, Sullivan E. Body mass index as a prognostic factor in development of infantile Blount disease. *J Pediatr Orthop.* 2007;27(8):921–925

Wilkins KE. Bowlegs. *Pediatr Clin North Am.* 1986;33(6):1429–1438

CHAPTER 107

Orthopedic Injuries and Growing Pains

Sara T. Stewart, MD

CASE STUDY

A 6-year-old boy has a 1-week history of leg pains. He wakes up at night and cries because his legs hurt, yet during the day he is fine, with no pain or movement limitations. He has no history of trauma, fever, or joint swelling. The family history is negative for rheumatic or collagen-vascular disease. The boy's height and weight are at the 50th percentile for age, he is afebrile, and the physical examination is unremarkable.

Questions

1. What is the differential diagnosis of leg pains in school-aged children?
2. What laboratory or radiographic studies are appropriate for children with leg pains?
3. How do musculoskeletal injuries in children differ from those in adults (eg, type of injury sustained, location of injury)?
4. How does one decide the extent of the diagnostic workup in a child with extremity pain?
5. What physiological factors cause musculoskeletal injury patterns to change with age?

Children by nature are active and explorative. They experience cuts, scrapes, minor injuries, and pain routinely. Because primary care physicians are often the first to examine children with injuries, they play an important role in making the preliminary diagnosis and assessing the need for further evaluation and treatment. The more common complaints and injuries seen in pediatricians' offices are discussed in this chapter: growing pains, pulled elbow (also called nursemaid's elbow), and fractures, including growth plate injuries. The evaluation of children with limp is discussed in Chapter 109.

Epidemiology

The term **growing pains** is somewhat misleading because there is no evidence that these pains are associated with growth. The period of middle childhood, when growing pains are diagnosed, is not the period of most rapid growth in the child. *Leg aches* or *idiopathic leg pain* may be better terms, but growing pains is the most widely used term.

The prevalence of growing pains is not well defined but seems to be between 15% and 30% of all children. They are seen most commonly in children between the ages of 4 and 14 years, and girls are affected more frequently than boys.

Pulled elbow, nursemaid's elbow, or radial head subluxation is the most common joint injury in childhood. It occurs most commonly in children 1 to 4 years of age, with a peak incidence between 2 and 3 years of age. Other ligament and tendon injuries are relatively uncommon in prepubertal children due to the relative strength of these structures in comparison to the growth plate of the adjacent developing bone. Most commonly, fractures involving the growth plate occur before ligamentous injury. When joint dislocations and ligamentous injury occur in children (with the exception of pulled elbow), they are usually caused by significant trauma.

Trauma and injury are significant causes of morbidity and mortality in childhood. Injuries are the most common reason for hospitalization in children and adolescents younger than 18 years and are the leading cause of death beyond the first year of life. Musculoskeletal problems account for 15% of all injuries and most commonly occur in the upper extremity. Fractures are perhaps the most common significant form of musculoskeletal injury in children who present to physicians for evaluation and treatment.

Clinical Presentation (D$_x$ Box)

Children with growing pains typically present with a history of intermittent, poorly localized pain in the bilateral lower extremities that occurs at night over a long period. The pain most commonly involves the calves and anterior thighs, never the joints. Symptoms usually resolve over several minutes, and in the morning the child has normal activity.

Pulled elbow is characterized by a sudden onset of elbow pain associated with the traumatic event and subsequent decreased use of the arm. At the time of presentation for medical care, a child with pulled elbow typically appears well, aside from a refusal to use the affected arm. The child typically holds the arm close to the body with

Dx Growing Pains and Orthopedic Injuries

Growing Pains
- Age between 4 and 14 years
- Normal growth and development
- Intermittent pain or aches in the legs
- Occurrence of symptoms at night
- Pain poorly localized to the anterior thighs, calves, and behind the knees; absence of joint involvement
- Absence of limp, disability, or inflammation
- Response to supportive measures such as heat and massage

Pulled (Nursemaid's) Elbow
- Age between 1 and 4 years
- Elbow pain of acute onset
- History of sudden longitudinal traction on an extended and pronated arm
- Forearm held in a position of flexion and pronation
- Lack of spontaneous movement of the elbow

Fractures
- Obvious deformity
- Swelling or tenderness over the fracture site
- Limited range of movement or absence of movement of the affected extremity

Figure 107-1. Pulled (nursemaid's) elbow. The sudden traction on the outstretched arm pulls the radius distally, causing a tear in the annular ligament at its attachment to the radius. A portion of the ligament becomes trapped within the joint as the traction is released and the arm recoils. A, Mechanism of injury. B, Pathology. C, Method of reduction (hyperpronation).

the elbow in slight flexion and the forearm pronated. There is usually no gross deformity, swelling, or overlying skin trauma, and the child typically refuses to supinate the forearm during examination. There may also be point tenderness laterally over the radial head.

An underlying **fracture** is strongly indicated by obvious deformity or lack of spontaneous movement in the extremity in question. Localized swelling, tenderness, and limited range of movement may all be signs of a fracture.

Pathophysiology

Growing pains are recurrent aches or pains localized most commonly to the muscles of the legs and occasionally to the muscles of the arms of children. The pain is located deep within the extremity and not in the joints. Etiology remains unclear. Emotional and psychologic stress, a low pain threshold, bone fatigue, and myalgia secondary to exercise or physical activity have all been implicated as possible contributory factors.

Pulled elbow is a subluxation of the radial head caused by a rapid and forceful extension and pronation of the forearm. This mechanism most commonly occurs when a caregiver pulls a child toward himself or herself and the child resists, wanting to go in the other direction. As illustrated in Figure 107-1, the subluxation occurs due to tearing of the annular ligament, with trapping of the ligament between the radius and the capitulum humeri. This injury is seen primarily in young children because the attachment of the ligament to the bone becomes thicker with age and growth.

Because of anatomic and physiological differences (eg, presence of cartilaginous growth plate as well as thicker periosteum and greater

plasticity of the skeleton), fracture patterns seen in children often differ from those in adults. Additionally, fractures may influence long-term growth and development of the affected limb in a growing child.

Fractures are classified based on anatomic location, type of fracture, and degree of angulation or displacement. Fracture location may be described as diaphyseal, metaphyseal, or epiphyseal/growth plate depending on the portion of the bone involved (figures 107-2 and 107-3). Fractures may be open or closed. In closed fractures, the skin over the fracture site is intact, whereas in open fractures, the skin is broken. When 2 bone fragments are displaced relative to each other, the direction and degree of displacement are based on the distal fragment.

The Salter-Harris classification is used most commonly to classify growth plate injury (Table 107-1, Figure 107-4). Approximately 15% of all fractures in children involve the growth plate. Type 1 and 2 fractures are the most common fractures involving the growth plate. Type 3 and 4 fractures involve the epiphysis and are considered to be intra-articular. Type 5 fractures are uncommon and are caused by a crush injury to the growth plate. Initial radiographs in type 1 and 5 fractures may appear normal because bone fragments are not displaced. Because of involvement of the growth plate, there is a risk of growth arrest with any physis injury. The risk is variable, however, depending on the type of injury.

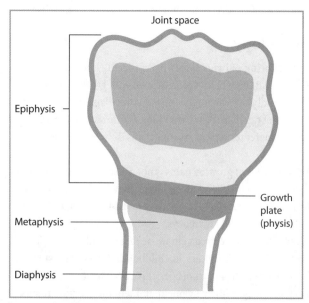

Figure 107-2. Anatomy of a long bone.

Joint space

Epiphysis

Metaphysis

Diaphysis

Growth plate (physis)

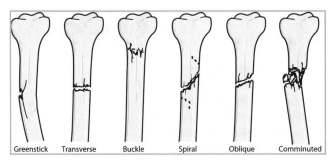

Figure 107-3. Non-epiphyseal plate fractures.

Figure 107-4. Salter-Harris classification of epiphyseal plate fractures.

Differential Diagnosis

The diagnosis of **growing pains** is one of exclusion. Leg pain in children has many causes (Box 107-1). If they are limited to vague pains in the legs at night with no associated limp or signs of inflammation, the differential diagnosis may be limited to growing pains, general systemic diseases such as leukemia, benign bone tumors such as osteoid osteoma, and perhaps fibromyalgia. Leukemic infiltration of the bones may cause leg pain before systemic signs such as fever, weight loss, and adenopathy are present. Osteoid osteoma, a benign bone tumor that most commonly occurs in adolescent boys, characteristically causes pain that is worse at night and is usually relieved by anti-inflammatory medications. The pain may be localized in one

place, however, unlike with growing pains. Fibromyalgia, which is probably underdiagnosed in the pediatric population, is a well-recognized cause in adults of chronic, generalized limb pain without a clear, organic source. It is seen more commonly in adolescents than in younger children. This benign, intermittent musculoskeletal pain syndrome is associated with multiple tender "trigger points," stiffness, fatigue, and a non-restorative sleep pattern.

When evaluating for **pulled elbow,** an elbow fracture should be ruled out. Certain fractures and specific features of fractures deserve mention (see Figure 107-3). Fractures that often occur during childhood include clavicular fractures (the most common childhood fracture and most commonly fractured bone from birth trauma) and spiral fractures of the distal tibia—the "toddler's fracture." This fracture typically occurs in children who have not been walking long, eg, those between 9 months and 3 years of age. It is thought to be

Table 107-1. Long Bone Fracture Patterns Seen in Children

Type	Description
Non-epiphyseal Plate Fractures	
Complete	Both sides of the bone fractured; type depends on direction of fracture line.
Transverse	Perpendicular to long axis of the bone
Oblique	At an angle to long axis of the bone
Spiral	Zigzag course around the bone
Comminuted	Fractures with 3 or more fragments (rare in children)
Buckle or torus	Bone compression causes it to bend or buckle rather than break; occurs at junction of metaphysis and diaphysis.
Greenstick	Cortex broken on tension side but intact on compression side
Bowing	Deformation of bone caused by bending without fracturing
Classic metaphyseal lesion	Fracture of distal, poorly mineralized metaphysis, perpendicular to long axis of bone; previously termed bucket-handle or chip fracture
Epiphyseal Plate Fractures (Salter-Harris Classification)	
Type 1	Horizontal fracture through the physis
Type 2	Fracture through the physis, extending into the metaphysis
Type 3	Fracture through the epiphysis, extending into the physis
Type 4	Fracture through the epiphysis, physis, and metaphysis
Type 5	Crush injury of the physis

Box 107-1. Common Causes of Leg Pain in Children

Growing Pains (Leg Aches, Idiopathic Leg Pains)	***Collagen Disease***
Trauma	• Juvenile rheumatoid arthritis
• Fracture	• Dermatomyositis
• Compartment syndromes	• Fibromyalgia
• Soft tissue injury	• Rheumatic fever
• Muscle strain/sprain	***Other Musculoskeletal Causes***
Infection	• Legg-Calvé-Perthes disease
• Cellulitis	• Slipped capital femoral epiphysis
• Soft tissue abscess	• Osgood-Schlatter disease
• Myositis	• Transient synovitis of the hip
• Osteomyelitis	• Osteochondritis dissecans
• Septic arthritis	• Patellofemoral stress/ chondromalacia patellae
Neoplasia	• Generalized ligamentous laxity and joint hypermobility
• Malignant bone tumors (eg, osteosarcoma, Ewing sarcoma)	***Miscellaneous Causes***
• Leukemia	• Sickle cell disease pain crisis
• Metastatic disease (eg, lymphoma, neuroblastoma)	• Psychosomatic conditions
Benign Bone Lesions	
• Osteoid osteoma	
• Bone cysts	
• Langerhans cell histiocytosis	

caused by a rotational force on the lower leg, which could occur as an ambulatory child falls in a twisting motion. Often, when the child presents for medical care, the parents are unaware of a history of trauma and the chief complaint is that the child refuses to bear weight on the affected leg. Elbow fractures, including supracondylar humerus, as well as lateral and medial condyle fractures, occur commonly due to a fall directly on the elbow or on an outstretched hand. These fractures require careful attention to neurovascular status because of the risk of associated injury to the median or radial nerve or brachial artery, leading to Volkmann ischemic contracture. A Monteggia fracture is a dislocation of the radial head in association with an ulnar shaft fracture. Long bone fractures in preambulatory children, rib fractures, classic metaphyseal lesions, and the presence of multiple fractures in one child are all concerning for non-accidental trauma and should prompt a more thorough evaluation of possible physical abuse (see Chapter 131).

Because of the relative weakness of the physis compared with the surrounding ligaments, trauma sustained near joints may be more likely to cause a type 1 Salter-Harris growth plate fracture rather than ligamentous injury (eg, sprain, strain). Therefore, it is important to include this type of fracture in the differential diagnosis of children with point tenderness near the end of a long bone because this injury does require cast immobilization.

Evaluation

Accurate diagnosis of pediatric orthopedic injuries is often challenging because children may be not only poor "historians" but also uncooperative with examinations, especially if they are experiencing pain.

History

A thorough history is essential for the accurate diagnosis of growing pains and orthopedic injuries (Questions Box: Growing Pains and Questions Box: Orthopedic Injuries). A complete history of the events related to the injury, including what happened after the injury was sustained, should be obtained.

Physical Examination

The physical examination of children with suspected **growing pains** should include evaluation for signs of systemic disease such as fever, lymphadenopathy, hepatosplenomegaly, abnormal growth, and generalized weakness or fatigue. Leg length and circumference should be measured. The legs should be palpated and range of motion assessed in the hip, knee, and ankle.

Children with suspected **pulled elbow** should be observed for how they hold the affected arm compared with the unaffected arm. They should be evaluated for limited active motion at the elbow and resistance to attempts at passive movement, especially supination. No swelling should be present, but there may be tenderness over the radial head. The shoulder and wrist should also be well examined.

It is important to undress children with suspected **fractures** and perform a complete physical examination. Simply examining the involved extremity is insufficient. The presence of a deformity, point

---

Growing Pains — Questions

- When (ie, what time of day) does the pain typically occur?
- How long has the pain been occurring?
- Does the pain resolve and then recur in any predictable manner?
- Where is the pain? Does it change location?
- Does anything make the pain better or worse?
- Is the child sick in any other way?
- Does the pain interfere with the child's activities?
- Does the parent notice any changes such as swelling or redness in the child's legs?

Orthopedic Injuries — Questions

- How did the injury occur?
- How long ago was the injury sustained? When did the symptoms begin?
- Was the incident witnessed by an adult?
- How strong was the injuring force? What direction did it come from?
- What was the position of the affected extremity at the time of the injury?
- Did the child experience any head trauma or loss of consciousness?
- What, if any, first aid was administered at the scene?
- Has the child been able to move the affected extremity since the injury occurred?

---

tenderness, or limitation of motion supports the diagnosis of a fracture. All long bones should be palpated, and the presence of bruises and scars should be noted because these may indicate child abuse. Examination of the involved extremity includes inspection of the overlying skin for swelling, lacerations, or punctures. The degree of active and passive motion and strength compared with the uninvolved side should be noted. In cases of suspected leg injuries, the child's gait should be observed, if possible. Assessment of neurovascular function distal to the injury includes evaluation of capillary refill, peripheral pulses, and motor and sensory function.

Laboratory Tests

A complete blood cell count and erythrocyte sedimentation rate (ESR) may be considered for children with leg pains that do not resolve or for children with symptoms that are atypical for growing pains. Rheumatologic screening tests can be ordered based on abnormalities in these tests (eg, elevated ESR or white blood cell count). Laboratory tests, if obtained, should be normal if a child is diagnosed with growing pains. Routine laboratory studies are not necessary in the evaluation of pulled elbow or fractures. However, because fractures of the femur are often associated with significant blood loss, it is important to monitor the hematocrit in these patients.

Imaging Studies

If leg pains persist and interfere with routine activity, radiographs or a bone scan of the legs may be considered. Radiographic evaluation is not required for children with pulled elbow if presentation is typical and reduction is successful. Radiographs, if taken in such children, are usually completely negative because the dislocation is often corrected during positioning for radiographs. However, radiographs should be obtained in children with suspected fractures. Fractures involving the growth plate, especially Salter-Harris type 1 and 5 fractures, may be particularly difficult to diagnose radiographically because the growth plate is primarily cartilaginous and, hence, radiolucent. A bone scan or follow-up radiograph may be used to diagnose suspected fractures when initial radiographs are negative.

Management

Parental education and reassurance about the benign nature of **growing pains** are important. The pains themselves usually respond to **supportive measures** such as heat, massage, and analgesia. Stretching exercises for the legs have also been recommended. Referral to an orthopedist should be considered if the pain is severe and persistent and physical examination and laboratory workup fail to reveal a specific diagnosis.

Pulled elbow is one of the few medical conditions that has a dramatic, immediate cure. To treat the elbow, the annular ligament must be reduced back to its anatomic position, and there are 2 common methods of reduction. In both methods, the elbow is stabilized with application of pressure laterally over the radial head with the thumb of the medical practitioner. In the first method, there is rapid, firm hyperpronation of the forearm. In the second, the forearm is firmly supinated, then the elbow is flexed. While both methods of reduction have high success rates, several studies suggest superiority of the hyperpronation method. A click may be heard or felt as the radial head is reduced, and relief of pain is usually immediate for those children treated shortly after the injury. Return of function may require up to 30 minutes, however. If treatment is delayed, such rapid relief of symptoms may not be seen. Following reduction, the parents should be advised that the child may need mild pain medication. Some physicians recommend short-term immobilization in a sling or splint to facilitate soft tissue healing. If reduction is unsuccessful, consider the possibility of obtaining radiographs and referring the patient for orthopedic consultation.

Most **fractures** should be referred to an orthopedic surgeon for evaluation and treatment unless the primary care physician is experienced in reducing and casting fractures. Several techniques are used in fracture management. **Closed reduction** is the nonoperative reduction or realignment of fracture fragments. **Open reduction** implies that an incision has been made to expose the fracture and proceed with manipulating the bone fragments into place. Fixation, or stabilization of the fracture with any type of device, may be required following the reduction. This is termed **internal fixation** if the device is under the skin and **external fixation** if the device begins outside of the skin but passes through the skin to bone. Indications for open reduction include failure of closed reduction, need for precise anatomic reduction, and complex multisystem trauma.

Certain fractures are common in pediatrics. Most clavicular fractures do not require reduction and can be treated with immobilization in a sling for 4 to 8 weeks. Elbow fractures (eg, lateral condyle and supracondylar humeral fractures) are at particular risk for neurovascular compromise and often necessitate open reduction to achieve anatomic reduction. Distal forearm fractures are usually managed with closed reduction and casting, but forearm fractures in the middle and proximal thirds of the bone may be harder to reduce in the office setting. Stable metacarpal and phalangeal fractures can be splinted in an aluminum splint or taped to an adjacent finger ("buddy taping"). The metacarpophalangeal joints should be maintained in 50 to 90 degrees of flexion, and the interphalangeal joints should be in about 20 degrees of flexion to minimize stiffness. Unstable finger fractures may require open reduction and pin fixation.

Femoral shaft fractures in infants and children can be managed with closed reduction and spica cast placement. As children become older, a fixation device may be required in addition to the closed reduction. Open reduction is necessary on rare occasions. Closed reduction and cast immobilization are usually used in the management of tibial shaft fractures. Short cast immobilization may be required for metatarsal fractures, and buddy taping is used for stable toe fractures.

Because of the potential for infection, open fractures are orthopedic emergencies that require immediate attention and orthopedic consultation. Careful debridement of the wound is required. Antibiotics should be administered, and tetanus immunization may be given based on a review of the immunization history.

Prognosis

Growing pains resolve over time without sequelae. Recurrence of pulled elbow is common, occurring again in up to one-third of patients. Therefore, parents should be cautioned about pulling children's arms or lifting them by one hand. Fractures in children generally heal faster and remodel (the spontaneous correction of deformity) better than equivalent fractures in adults. Vascular and nerve injuries and growth disturbances are potential complications of fractures and their management. Compartment syndrome, a potentially serious vascular injury, may also develop.

Growth plate injuries require special attention because of the potential for subsequent growth abnormalities of the affected bone. Prognosis of growth plate fractures depends on the type of injury sustained. Salter-Harris type 1 and 2 fractures generally have a good prognosis for long-term healing and growth. The severity of the injury and accuracy of reduction determine the prognosis of type 3 and 4 fractures. Growth arrest is common following type 5 fractures because the physis itself is injured.

CASE RESOLUTION

The child presented in the case study has the benign condition commonly referred to as growing pains. Management involves parental education and reassurance. Local heat, massage, and analgesia (using ibuprofen) may be recommended.

Selected References

Boutis K. Common pediatric fractures treated with minimal intervention. *Pediatr Emerg Care.* 2010;26(2):152–162

Browner EA. Nursemaid's elbow (annular ligament displacement). *Pediatr Rev.* 2013;34(8):366–367

Kerssemakers SP, Fotiadou AN, de Jonge MC, Karantanas AH, Maas M. Sport injuries in the paediatric and adolescent patient: a growing problem. *Pediatr Radiol.* 2009;39(5):471–484

Krul M, van der Wouden JC, van Suijlekom-Smit LW, Koes BW. Manipulative interventions for reducing pulled elbow in young children. *Cochrane Database Syst Rev.* 2012;1:CD007759

Laine JC, Kaiser SP, Diab M. High-risk pediatric orthopedic pitfalls. *Emerg Med Clin North Am.* 2010;28(1):85–102

Weiser P. Approach to the patient with noninflammatory musculoskeletal pain. *Pediatr Clin North Am.* 2012;59(2):471–492

CHAPTER 108

Sports-Related Acute Injuries

Monica Sifuentes, MD; Andrew K. Battenberg, MD; and Steven Donohoe, BS

CASE STUDY

A 15-year-old female basketball player complains of 6 months of intermittent pain in her left knee. Occasionally the knee gives out while she is playing ball. The teen denies any associated swelling or erythema over the joint. She is able to walk with no problem and reports no history of direct trauma to the area. She is otherwise healthy.

On physical examination, she is a well-developed, well-nourished teenaged girl in no acute distress. The examination is normal except for mild pain to direct palpation of the left patella. No swelling, erythema, or effusion of the knee joint is evident, and the left hip, knee, and ankle have full range of motion. The back is straight.

Questions

1. What are some of the most common orthopedic complaints in adolescent patients, and why do they occur in this age group?
2. What is the pathophysiology of overuse syndromes?
3. What is the purpose of the preparticipation physical evaluation?
4. What conditions disqualify adolescents from participation in competitive sports?
5. What are the current recommendations for the treatment and rehabilitation of acute soft tissue injuries?

Many adolescents with varying degrees of athletic ability participate in sports during their junior high and high school years. Some choose to continue this participation at the college level. Regardless of the ultimate goal, team sports are an important means by which children and adolescents can experience winning and losing. Individuals learn the importance of group participation and develop interactive skills with other team members. They are exposed to the concept of physical fitness, which can improve body image as well as self-esteem.

Participation in athletics carries significant risks, however. Injuries, inappropriate coaching, and aggressive training sessions are not uncommon occurrences that may have long-term sequelae for young athletes. Primary care practitioners are responsible not only for the evaluation of children prior to their participation in sports but also for the diagnosis, treatment, and prevention of athletic injuries.

Epidemiology

Recent estimates indicate that approximately 38 million young athletes participate in organized sports in the United States each year. Of these, 4 million athletes younger than 14 years and 2 million high school–aged athletes are treated for a sports injury annually. These numbers have increased dramatically over the last 20 years. This increase is thought to be multifactorial, including an increase in the number of female athletes following the passage of Title IX, a new emphasis on year-round competition, single-sport focus, and increased training intensity. Several studies have attempted to quantify the overall injury rate associated with athletic participation. In general, the rate of injury for 13- to 19-year-olds is 7% to 11%. Approximately 20% of those injured sustain a significant injury. For boys, the sport with the highest injury rate in all age groups is football, followed by basketball and soccer. In girls, roller-skating and gymnastics account for the most injuries. Gender differences between boys and girls have been found in some studies depending on the sport. Overall, boys tend to have more shoulder-related injuries, whereas girls tend to have more knee and ankle injuries and more problems with overuse syndromes. Reports indicate that the severity of sports-related injuries increases with age. Along with the increased incidence of injuries, there has been an emergence of sports-related injuries previously thought to be very rare in the pediatric population. For example, anterior cruciate ligament (ACL) injuries are being seen with increased frequency in this demographic, especially among high school–aged girls. Treatment of such injuries are complicated in skeletally immature individuals because of the need to preserve growth potential.

Preparticipation Physical Evaluation

The goal of the preparticipation physical evaluation (PPE) is the identification of any physical conditions or abnormalities that may predispose young athletes to injury. Examples include a history of concussion with head trauma or an incompletely healed sprain.

The PPE consists of 2 parts: (1) a review of the patient's current health and medical history, including sports injuries and family history relating to participation in strenuous exercise, and (2) a complete physical examination with a focus on the musculoskeletal system. Known as a "2-minute orthopedic examination," the musculoskeletal examination is a detailed assessment of all muscle groups, assessing their strength, tone, and function. Congenital or acquired deformities should also be noted. The American Academy of Pediatrics (AAP) has developed a form specifically for the PPE visit (see Chapter 35).

Disqualification from participation in specific sports is appropriate in certain situations. Competitive sports are classified according to their degree of contact or impact and how strenuous they are. Recommendations differ depending on the adolescent's medical condition and the type of sport the athlete desires to play. For details of these recommendations, see Selected References on page 709. Fortunately, many young athletes are healthy and rarely need to be restricted from participation.

Clinical Presentation

Older children and adolescents with sports-related injuries usually present to the practitioner with specific complaints of pain or swelling in a particular joint (D$_x$ Box). In addition, they may complain of nonspecific musculoskeletal pain occurring in certain areas, such as the lower back or shoulder. Other complaints may include a limp, decreased range of motion of an extremity, or an inability to participate in a desired activity without pain.

Pathophysiology

Adolescents, unlike adults, are particularly susceptible to injury because their bones and joints are not fully mature. Most injuries during adolescence involve the epiphysis, which is the weakest point of the musculoskeletal system. In addition, the presence of congenital anomalies, such as leg-length discrepancies or hip rotation abnormalities, puts the young athlete at further risk for injury. Biomechanical and neuromuscular factors, hormonal influences, and anatomic differences have also been proposed reasons for higher rates of some injuries in young female athletes compared to young male athletes. For example, patellofemoral pain syndrome, which presents as knee pain exacerbated by activity, is a very common problem in adolescent females, affecting nearly 1 in 10 of those who are active. Contributing biomechanical factors include tight iliotibial bands, weak gluteal strength, and a relative genu valgum due to wider female hips. This combination leads to valgus stresses at the knee, internal rotation of the femur, and abnormal patellar tracking, which puts the athlete at greater risk for patellofemoral syndrome.

Most orthopedic injuries are the result of macro-trauma or microtrauma. Sprains are an example of macro-trauma, whereas overuse syndromes can be considered microtrauma. **Macro-trauma** occurs from complete or partial tearing of muscle, ligaments, or tendons and is often associated with acute injuries. In contrast, **microtrauma** is usually produced by chronic repetitive trauma to a particular area, leading to inflammation and ultimately to pain. This most commonly occurs in soft tissues such as the muscles and tendons but can occur in bone as well.

Definitions

A **sprain** is a stretching injury of a ligament or the connective tissue that attaches bone to bone. A **strain** is a stretching injury of a muscle or its tendon, which is the connective tissue that attaches muscle to bone. **Tendinitis** is an inflammation of the tendon. **Apophysitis** is an inflammation of the apophysis, which is the site of ligament or tendon attachment to growth cartilage (eg, Osgood-Schlatter disease [apophysitis of the tibial tubercle], Sever disease [calcaneal apophysitis]). A **stress fracture** is an incomplete fracture often occurring in the bones of the legs and feet from repetitive trauma to the area. It is believed that the pain associated with shin splints may be caused in part by atypical stress fractures of the distal tibia.

Overuse syndromes occur from repetitive microtrauma to the musculoskeletal system secondary to excessive or biomechanically incorrect activity. They are usually the result of training errors in which athletes are "trying to do too much too fast." Common syndromes in adolescents include Osgood-Schlatter disease, shin splints (medial tibial stress syndrome), and patellofemoral syndrome (chondromalacia patellae).

Grading of Sports Injuries

Sprains can be classified according to the degree of injury and most commonly occur in the knee or ankle. Assigning a grade that describes the injury is useful when considering the prognosis of a particular injury. Consultants also find these grades helpful. Grade 1 through 3 is the usual classification used for sprains: grade 1 generally refers to stretching of the ligament, grade 2 a partial tearing of the ligament, and grade 3 a complete tearing of the ligament. Stability of the joint, range of motion, and degree of pain and swelling determine the grade of the sprain. The grading system for **strains,** on the other hand, is based on an assessment of strength. Because strains do not usually cause joint instability, criteria for grading strains are different than for sprains and may be more subjective. A description of these 2 grading systems appears in Table 108-1.

Dx Orthopedic Injury

- Joint pain or swelling
- Tenderness to palpation of the affected joint
- Decreased range of motion of the affected joint or extremity
- May or may not have associated bruising of the skin overlying the injury

---

Table 108-1. General Classification of Sprains and Strains

	Joint	Range of Motion	Weight Bearing	Pain	Swelling
Sprains					
Grade 1	Stable	Normal	Normal	+	+
Grade 2	Stable	↓	↓	++	++
Grade 3	Unstable	↓↓	↓↓	+++	+++
	Strength	Palpable Defect	Pain		
Strains					
Grade 1	>4/5	−	+		
Grade 2	3/5–4/5	+/−	++		
Grade 3	<3/5	+/−	+++		

Box 108-1. Differential Diagnosis Based on the Site of Injury

Back Injuries

- Muscle strain
- Spondylolysis
- Epiphyseal injury
- Herniated disks

Injuries to the Upper Extremity

- Acromioclavicular sprains
- Sternoclavicular sprains
- Glenohumeral dislocation
- Glenohumeral subluxation
- Impingement syndrome
- Acute elbow injuries
- Olecranon bursitis
- Lateral epicondylitis
- Flexor-pronator tendinitis
- Wrist sprains
- Scaphoid fractures
- Hamate fractures
- Finger injuries

Injuries to the Lower Extremity

- Iliac crest contusion
- Iliac apophysitis
- Quadriceps contusion
- Femoral stress fracture
- Medial/lateral ligament sprains
- Anterior cruciate ligament sprain
- Posterior cruciate ligament sprain
- Patellar dislocation/subluxation
- Prepatellar bursitis
- Patellofemoral stress syndrome
- Patellar tendinitis
- Osgood-Schlatter disease
- Shin splints
- Ankle sprains
- Achilles tendinitis
- Calcaneal apophysitis
- Plantar fasciitis

Questions

Sports-Related Injuries

- What is the acuity of the injury?
- What activity or sport was the patient engaged in at the time of the injury?
- How often has the patient engaged in this sport or particular activity in the past?
- Were there any new additions to the routine this time?
- Did the pain begin after a single injury or after repetitive activity?
- If the injury is related to a repetitive activity, does the pain occur at a specific time during this activity?
- What was the mechanism of injury?
- Is the pain incapacitating?
- Has a similar injury ever occurred in the past?
- How was the injury treated?
- Was there any pain following the previous injury?
- Does the patient feel as if he or she has completely recovered?
- How was this current injury managed acutely?
- Has the patient altered daily activity in any way to compensate for this problem?

Differential Diagnosis

The differential diagnosis of orthopedic conditions depends on the anatomic site of the injury or complaint and the mechanism of injury. Box 108-1 lists some of the more common orthopedic conditions by location. Anomalies of skeletal development, such as congenital angular deformities of long bones and soft tissue abnormalities like Ehlers-Danlos syndrome, should be considered as possible etiologies for overuse syndromes. Other non-orthopedic conditions, such as collagen-vascular diseases, infections, and tumors, may present with joint or bone symptomatology.

Evaluation

History

The history should focus on the musculoskeletal system and how the injury occurred (Questions Box).

Physical Examination

The physical examination should focus on the musculoskeletal system. If, however, teenagers have not had a physical examination within the past year, a complete physical examination should first be performed to exclude any systemic condition that might manifest itself initially as musculoskeletal pain. This is especially important in adolescents with chronic or systemic complaints, such as intermittent extremity pain, swelling of an affected joint, and fever.

In general, any pain or swelling of an affected joint or muscle should be noted. If there is history of acute trauma, an area of ecchymosis or joint effusion may be seen. The affected joint should be tested for range of motion and joint laxity to determine the degree of sprain. Special testing for ligament laxity should be performed (Figure 108-1). For the knee, the most common method is the drawer test for anterior and posterior movement of the knee joint. However, the Lachman test has gained considerable popularity as it has been shown to be a more sensitive and specific test for ACL injuries. The patient is examined in a supine position on an examining table and the knee, ligaments, and tibia are assessed. It is important to note that in the setting of a recent injury, soft tissue swelling and guarding due to pain can limit the efficacy of these tests. Additionally, a large knee effusion is evidence of significant intra-articular pathology, such as a fracture or ligament rupture.

Muscle spasms and diminished range of motion in an adjacent joint should be noted because these may be signs of a strain injury. Strength of the strained muscle(s) should be assessed, and any pain with palpation or range of motion should be noted. A palpable defect of the muscle suggests complete rupture of the muscle, whereas muscular contusions are associated with localized pain, soft tissue swelling, or hematoma. Pinpoint tenderness over a particular bone may indicate a fracture or, if at the site of a tendon insertion, inflammation. Reviewing the mechanism of injury and the timing of the symptoms is often helpful in differentiating between a fracture and tendinitis.

Laboratory Tests

A complete blood cell count and erythrocyte sedimentation rate may be helpful in adolescents with a history of chronic joint pain or swelling. If the results are abnormal, further workup is indicated to distinguish between a collagen-vascular disease such as systemic lupus erythematosus, an infection such as osteomyelitis, or, rarely, an arthritic disorder such as juvenile idiopathic arthritis.

Figure 108-1. Maneuvers used to determine stability of the knee joint. A, Anterior drawer test: Anterior force is applied. B, Posterior drawer test: Posterior force is applied. C, Medial ligament stability: Lateral force is applied.

Imaging Studies

A plain radiograph of the involved joint or bone is often the only necessary diagnostic study to perform. Because ankle sprain is such a common occurrence, it is important to understand when a radiograph is needed to rule out fracture: The Ottawa ankle rules are guidelines for obtaining radiographs in acute ankle injury, are approximately 100% sensitive, and have been validated for use in children older than 6 years (Box 108-2). Plain radiographs of joints above and below the symptomatic area are also sometimes indicated.

Box 108-2. Ottawa Ankle Rules

- Obtain ankle radiograph if ANY of the following:
  —Bone tenderness at posterior edge or tip of lateral malleolus
  —Bone tenderness at posterior edge or tip of medial malleolus
  —Bone tenderness along distal 6 cm of tibia or fibula
  —Inability to bear weight immediately after injury AND in emergency department for 4 steps
- Obtain foot radiograph if ANY of the following:
  —Bone tenderness at base of the fifth metatarsal
  —Bone tenderness at navicular bone
  —Inability to bear weight immediately after injury AND in emergency department for 4 steps

---

One example is the Maisonneuve fracture, a fracture of the proximal fibula near the knee that can occur with serious ankle injury; this fracture can be missed if a knee radiograph is not obtained in addition to ankle views. In general, advanced diagnostic tests such as computerized tomography scanning have limited value in the evaluation of an acute soft tissue injury. Magnetic resonance imaging may be indicated for injuries that do not improve despite adequate treatment and rehabilitation. See Chapter 109 for a discussion of imaging studies used to evaluate a child presenting with limp.

Management

With soft tissue injuries, the aim of acute management is to limit the extent of bleeding and inflammation that occur in the first 48 to 72 hours following the injury. The mnemonic **RICE** (rest, ice, compression, elevation) is helpful. Rest should be explained as "relative rest" because athletes should be allowed to do whatever they want as long as they are pain-free during or within 24 hours of the activity. Ice should be placed in a plastic bag and applied directly to the skin for a continuous 20 minutes. Longer periods of icing are discouraged because this can result in peripheral nerve palsy from cryoinjury. Patients should ice the injury 3 to 4 times a day for the first 48 hours and then at least once daily until the swelling or pain is gone. Compression is especially important and should be started as quickly as possible. When applying compression bandages, wrapping should begin distal to the injury and should proceed proximally; this prevents trapping of edema and swelling distal to the compression wrap, allowing proper drainage of injured tissue. Elevation of the injured extremity should occur as often as possible. The use of this plan for soft tissue injuries facilitates early healing and allows rehabilitation to proceed more quickly.

Anti-inflammatory or analgesic medications, such as ibuprofen, aspirin, and naproxen, are useful in controlling the symptoms of pain and swelling. For adolescent patients, dosages are similar to those used in adults: aspirin, 650 to 1,000 mg every 6 hours; ibuprofen, 400 to 800 mg every 6 to 8 hours; naproxen, 500 mg twice daily. To minimize gastrointestinal side effects, the medication should be administered with a snack or milk. Ideally, these drugs should be used for 7 to 10 days. Corticosteroids, oral or parenteral, are not indicated in the management of overuse injuries or acute trauma to the extremities.

After the acute phase, therapy is aimed at rehabilitation and resolution of any edema or hematoma (Box 108-3). Athletes should slowly begin range-of-motion exercises as tolerated. Full tissue

---

Box 108-3. Principles of Rehabilitation

- Resolution of hematoma
- Resolution of edema
- Regain full range of motion or flexibility
- Regain full muscle strength and endurance
- Regain agility and coordination
- Regain cardiovascular endurance

healing may take 6 to 8 weeks, but most young athletes do not have to wait that long to return to athletic activity.

Modified activity, depending on the degree of tissue damage, should initially be recommended in athletes who have suffered from overuse syndromes. Complete rest is rarely indicated. Participation in another sport such as swimming or cycling is often preferable to complete immobilization. In addition to the use of anti-inflammatory agents, physical therapy is another important therapeutic modality. Cryotherapy, whirlpool, or alternating heat and ice treatments can be helpful. Reconditioning should be continued after 3 to 12 weeks of modified activity, depending on the degree of recovery. This entails gradual strengthening and flexibility training as well as reevaluation of previous modes of training to minimize the risk of reinjury (Box 108-4). Additional aspects to consider are strength imbalances and biomechanics such as those that occur in patellofemoral syndrome. By identifying specific musculoskeletal imbalances, the clinician can suggest stretches and strengthening exercises specific to the patient's deficits.

Prevention

Injury prevention is an important aspect of sports medicine with which the primary practitioner should be familiar. Part of injury prevention includes the recognition of risk factors associated with sports injuries. In general, risk factors can be divided into 2 subgroups: modifiable and non-modifiable. Non-modifiable risk factors include gender, individual physical features, and the type of sport. Modifiable risk factors include flexibility, alignment, strength, endurance, and proprioception. Because many injuries are the result of "trying to do too much too soon," proper physical **training and conditioning** are essential, no matter how fit the athlete appears. Stretching, warm-up and cooldown exercises, and the type of equipment used for the sport should be reviewed with the athlete during the sports physical visit. The type of sport to be played should also be reviewed and, if participating in a contact sport, the adolescent should be **matched with other athletes** based on weight and pubertal development rather than age. Some studies suggest that such matching will greatly reduce the risk of injury to the smaller, less mature athlete. Because an old or incompletely healed injury is a significant risk factor for reinjury, all **previous injuries should receive proper treatment and rehabilitation** before the athlete returns to play. **Protective equipment,** especially for collision and contact sports, as well as for those involving a ball or racquet, also should be emphasized to athletes and their parents. In addition, the AAP recommendation of **avoiding strength and weight training** until the athlete reaches sexual maturity rating (Tanner stage) 5 of pubertal development should be endorsed to prevent the risk of serious injury. **Education on the hazards of anabolic steroid use and creatine** also may be indicated.

Prognosis

Orthopedic injuries in young athletes and active adolescents have a great capacity for healing if given the opportunity. Early medical intervention to prevent irreversible tissue damage ensures complete recovery in most cases. Long-term sequelae are associated with repeated trauma, incompletely treated cases, and chronic inflammatory changes. Some conditions, however, such as Osgood-Schlatter disease, will resolve even without treatment and do not lead to any permanent damage to the joint.

CASE RESOLUTION

In the case presented, the teenager has symptoms and physical findings consistent with patellofemoral pain syndrome (traditionally referred to as chondromalacia patellae). Because plain radiographs are usually not helpful in confirming the diagnosis, none are necessary at this time. Management should include strength training for the quadriceps muscles, activity modification, nonsteroidal anti-inflammatory medication, and ice compresses after activity.

Selected References

American Academy of Pediatrics, American Academy of Orthopaedic Surgeons. *Care of the Young Athlete.* Anderson SJ, Harris SS, eds. 2nd ed. Elk Grove Village, IL: American Academy of Pediatrics; 2010

American Academy of Pediatrics Council on Sports Medicine and Fitness. Strength training by children and adolescents. *Pediatrics.* 2008;121(4):835–840

Batra AS, Hohn AR. Consultation with the specialist: palpitations, syncope, and sudden cardiac death in children: who's at risk? *Pediatr Rev.* 2003;24(8):269–275

Brenner JS; American Academy of Pediatrics Council on Sports Medicine and Fitness. Overuse injuries, overtraining, and burnout in child and adolescent athletes. *Pediatrics.* 2007;119(6):1242–1245

Carry PM, Kanai S, Miller NH, Polousky JD. Adolescent patellofemoral pain: a review of evidence for the role of lower extremity biomechanics and core instability. *Orthopedics.* 2010;33(7):498–507

Dowling S, Spooner CH, Liang Y, et al. Accuracy of Ottawa ankle rules to exclude fractures of the ankle and midfoot in children: a meta-analysis. *Acad Emerg Med.* 2009;16(4):277–287

Emery CA. Risk factors for injury in child and adolescent sport: a systematic review of the literature. *Clin J Sport Med.* 2003;13(4):256–268

Frank JS, Gambacorta PL. Anterior Cruciate Ligament Injuries in the Skeletally Immature Athlete: Diagnosis and Management. *J Am Acad Orthop Surg.* 2013; 21: 78–87

Koutures CG, Gregory AJM; American Academy of Pediatrics Council on Sports Medicine and Fitness. Injuries in youth soccer. *Pediatrics.* 2010;125(2):410–414

Box 108-4. Rehabilitation of Musculoskeletal Injuries[a]

Four Phases of Rehabilitation

- Limit additional injury and control pain and swelling (RICE mnemonic).
- Improve strength and flexibility (range of motion) of the injured structures.
- Progressively improve strength, flexibility, proprioception, and endurance training until near-normal function is attained.
- Return to exercise and sports symptom-free.

[a]Modified from Hergenroeder AC. Prevention of sports injuries. *Pediatrics.* 1998;101(6):1057–1063.

Labella C, Carl R. Preventing knee ligament injuries in young athletes. *Pediatr Ann.* 2010;39(11):714–720

LaBella CR. Common acute sport-related lower extremity injuries in children and adolescents. *Clin Pediatr Emerg Med.* 2007;8:31–42

Metzl JD. Managing sports injuries in the pediatric office. *Pediatr Rev.* 2008; 29(3):75–85

Metzl JD. Preparticipation examination of the adolescent athlete: part 1. *Pediatr Rev.* 2001;22(6):199–204

Metzl JD. Preparticipation examination of the adolescent athlete: part 2. *Pediatr Rev.* 2001;22(7):227–239

Rodenberg RE, Cayce K, Hall S. Your guide to a dreaded injury: the ACL tear. *Contemp Pediatr.* 2006;23:26–39

Stiell IG, Greenberg GH, McKnight RD, Nair RC, McDowell I, Worthington JR. A study to develop clinical decision rules for the use of radiography in acute ankle injuries. *Ann Emerg Med.* 1992;21(4):384–390

Stricker PR. *Sport Success Rx! Your Child's Prescription for the Best Experience: How to Maximize Potential AND Minimize Pressure.* Elk Grove Village, IL: American Academy of Pediatrics; 2006

CHAPTER 109

Evaluation of Limp

Andrea Fang, MD, and Marianne Gausche-Hill, MD

CASE STUDY

A 6-year-old boy who has a 2-day history of right knee pain and limp is brought to the office. No history of knee trauma, swelling, redness, or associated fever is present. The medical history is unremarkable. The boy is afebrile, and his height and weight are at the 10th percentile for age. Examination of the right leg reveals decreased abduction and internal rotation of the hip; the knee is normal. The boy limps when he walks and favors his right leg.

Questions

1. What is the differential diagnosis of painful and painless limp in children?
2. What is the differential diagnosis of knee pain in children?
3. What laboratory and radiographic tests are indicated in the evaluation of children with limp?
4. What is the appropriate management of children with suspected infectious causes of limp?

A limp is a gait disturbance that occurs when an effort is made to minimize weight bearing on an affected leg so that pain and instability are reduced. The disturbance may be secondary to muscle weakness, deformity, pain, or a combination thereof. Muscle weakness may be caused by primary muscle disease, neurologic conditions, or disuse atrophy. Structural causes of limp include leg-length discrepancy and joint stiffness, while painful causes of limp include trauma, synovitis, infection (ie, bone, joint, or soft tissue), or neoplasm. A limp can be a sign of significant underlying disease, and accurate diagnosis and appropriate management are essential to prevent potentially serious morbidity.

Epidemiology

A limp may be due to pain originating in a leg or to pain referred from the abdomen or spine. Age often defines the diagnostic possibilities because certain disorders are seen more frequently in particular age groups. Infectious causes of limp occur more frequently in infants and young children, and noninfectious causes are more common in school-aged children and adolescents (Box 109-1).

Clinical Presentation

A painful limp usually has an acute onset and may be associated with systemic signs such as fever, especially when the etiology is infectious. Toddlers may simply refuse to walk or walk with a slow, cautious gait when they are in pain rather than limp. Non-painful limp often has an insidious onset and is commonly caused by weakness (eg, muscular dystrophy) or deformity (eg, leg-length discrepancy).

Pathophysiology

Normal gait has 2 phases: stance and swing. During the stance phase, both feet are on the ground as one foot heel strikes while the

Box 109-1. Differential Diagnosis of Limp in Children		
1–3 y	**4–10 y**	**≥11 y**
Painful Limp	*Painful Limp*	*Painful Limp*
Septic arthritis/ osteomyelitis	Septic arthritis/ osteomyelitis	Trauma
Transient synovitis	Transient synovitis	Septic arthritis/ osteomyelitis
Intervertebral diskitis	Trauma	Slipped capital femoral epiphysis (SCFE)
Juvenile idiopathic arthritis (JIA)	Legg-Calvé-Perthes disease (LCPD) (acute phase)	Osgood-Schlatter disease
Neoplasia (leukemia, metastatic disease)	Intervertebral diskitis	JIA
Trauma (toddler's fractures)	JIA	Sickle cell pain crisis
Child abuse	Sickle cell pain crisis	Neoplasia (leukemia, primary bone tumor, metastatic disease)
Painless Limp	Neoplasia (leukemia, primary bone tumor, metastatic disease)	*Painless Limp*
Developmental hip dysplasia	*Painless Limp*	SCFE
Neuromuscular disease (cerebral palsy)	LCPD (chronic phase)	Leg-length discrepancy
Leg-length discrepancy	Developmental hip dysplasia	Neuromuscular disease (cerebral palsy, muscular dystrophy)
	Neuromuscular disease (cerebral palsy, muscular dystrophy)	Scoliosis
	Leg-length discrepancy	

opposite foot moves to pre-swing; during the swing phase, one foot is not touching the ground as the limb is moved forward. Stance phase is shortened in limp to decrease the amount of time spent in bearing weight on the affected side or to minimize instability.

Normal adult gait is smooth and efficient, requiring the coordinated actions of the muscles of the legs and pelvis. Normal gait in children varies according to age and developmental maturity. Toddlers typically walk with a broad-based, tiptoe, "bouncing" gait with arms abducted for balance. They may initiate the stance phase with either toe or heel strike. By 2 years of age, children should initiate the stance phase consistently with heel strike. Children who are 3 to 4 years of age should exhibit normal adult gait with reciprocating arm swing most of the time.

Several types of abnormal gaits are recognized. An **antalgic gait** has a characteristic shortened stance phase due to pain. A **Trendelenburg gait** is caused by weakness of the hip abductors (gluteus medius) with which the pelvis dips down during stance phase, producing a swaying type of gait. A tiptoe or **toe-to-heel** gait is normal in children for several months after they learn to walk. Persistence of such a gait beyond 2 years of age is abnormal and may result from idiopathic heel-cord contracture or contracture secondary to cerebral palsy.

Differential Diagnosis

Trauma is a frequent cause of limp in children and adolescents. In toddlers, a fall may not be witnessed; therefore, they can present with limp or refusal to walk and have an occult fracture, such as a **toddler's fracture** (Figure 109-1). This is an oblique or spiral fracture of the middle or distal tibia, which occurs after a fall or jump involving a twisting motion. Toddlers are at risk for such injuries because of their unsteady gait. Standard anteroposterior (AP) and lateral radiograph views are usually obtained to determine if a fracture is present. They can initially be normal, and oblique views may be helpful. Follow-up radiographs or a bone scan may be necessary to make the diagnosis. Older children will usually be able to recall a specific injury and localize pain to a specific area. Individuals who have tenderness over open growth plates should be splinted and warrant close follow-up even with normal radiographs, as there is a

possibility of a Salter-Harris type 1 fracture, which occurs through the growth plate and may not be radiographically apparent.

Painless limp in toddlers may be due to **developmental hip dysplasia, cerebral palsy,** or **leg-length discrepancy** (anisomelia). As a result of developmental hip dysplasia, children may have a Trendelenburg gait secondary to leg-length discrepancy or to weakness of the hip abductors. Children with spastic cerebral palsy often walk on their toes because of increased tone or heel-cord contractures. Functional or apparent leg-length discrepancies may result from pelvic obliquity or spinal deformity. Children with true leg-length inequality compensate by walking on tiptoe on the shorter side or bending the knee on the longer side. Limb discrepancies may be managed with orthotics (eg, heel lifts) for mild cases, and surgical lengthening or shortening procedures may be necessary for more severe cases.

Transient synovitis of the hip is a benign, self-limited inflammatory process involving the synovial lining and one of the most common causes of limp in the young child. The exact cause of the inflammation is not known. There has been an association with certain upper respiratory infections, but no infectious agent has been identified. A higher incidence has also been noted in children who were subsequently diagnosed with Legg-Calvé-Perthes disease (LCPD) than the general population. This may be related to misdiagnosis or the use of traction for transient synovitis, a practice no longer in use. Age varies, but it typically affects children 4 to 10 years old, although it can present outside this age range. Males are affected approximately twice as often as females. Individuals usually present with acute onset of unilateral hip pain associated with a limp. There can be referred pain to the anterior thigh or knee. Associated systemic symptoms, such as fever, are rare or absent and should prompt an investigation for another cause. The leg may be held in a position of abduction, flexion, and external rotation to reduce intracapsular pressure and associated pain. Symptoms are usually unilateral, but in fewer than 10% of cases, there is bilateral involvement, often with one side being more symptomatic than the other.

Transient synovitis is a diagnosis of exclusion and must be differentiated from more concerning diagnoses such as septic arthritis. Consequently, laboratory evaluation typically consists of complete blood cell count (CBC), erythrocyte sedimentation rate (ESR), and C-reactive protein (CRP). The results are usually within normal limits or slightly elevated. Radiographs are often obtained, which are usually normal or show signs suggestive of an effusion. An ultrasound is often performed to look for the presence of an effusion within the joint, which can be noted in this condition. If an arthrocentesis is performed, the fluid in transient synovitis usually has a white blood cell (WBC) count of less than 50,000/mm³ and a negative Gram stain. Individuals with normal laboratory values or with a fluid aspirate not suggestive of septic arthritis (when arthrocentesis has been performed) are typically managed with supportive care and close follow-up within 24 to 48 hours. Rest and nonsteroidal anti-inflammatory agents are the mainstays of therapy. Virtually all children recover within 3 to 10 days with no significant sequelae.

Figure 109-1. Toddler's fracture. (Courtesy of Michael Diament, MD.)

Recurrence rates can be as high as 69% within the first year of an episode synovitis.

Septic arthritis occurs when there is an infection within the joint space. In children, this usually occurs in the face of bacteremia, with hematogenous spread to the highly vascular synovial membrane. It can also occur from contiguous spread of an adjacent infection (eg, osteomyelitis) or by direct inoculation (eg, surgery, penetrating trauma). *Staphylococcus aureus* remains the most common pathogen identified across all age groups, with increasing incidences of community-acquired methicillin-resistant strains. Infants younger than 2 months can also be infected by neonatal pathogens, such as *Streptococcus agalactiae* (eg, group B streptococcus [GBS]) and gram-negative enteric organisms (eg, *Escherichia coli*). Septic joints in children between 2 months and 5 years are usually caused by *S aureus*, *Streptococcus pyogenes*, *Streptococcus pneumoniae,* and *Kingella kingae*. Children older than 5 years will usually have infections caused by *S aureus* or *S pyogenes*. *Neisseria gonorrhoeae* infections can be seen in sexually active adolescents.

Infants and children will often present with fever, decreased use of the affected extremity, limp, or refusal to walk. The most commonly affected joint is the hip, which is classically held in a position of abduction, flexion, and external rotation to reduce intracapsular pressure and associated pain. Passive range of motion typically elicits significant discomfort and resistance. Parents of infants may notice increased crying with manipulation of the legs with activities such as diaper changing.

Subtle or early cases can often present a diagnostic challenge because there can be significant clinical and laboratory overlap with transient synovitis. Unfortunately, there is no highly sensitive or specific laboratory test that can readily distinguish these 2 entities. Temperature higher than 101.3°F (38.5°C) was shown to be the single best predictor of septic arthritis in one study, with no children diagnosed with transient synovitis having a temperature above 101.3°F (38.5°C). Other predictors include refusal to bear weight, ESR greater than 40 mm/hour, a CRP greater than 2.0 mg/dL, and serum WBC count greater than 12,000/mm³. The presence of 1 of these 5 factors was associated with a probability of having septic arthritis of around 37%, while the presence of all 5 factors was associated with a probability of 98%. Imaging often consists of plain radiographs and ultrasound. Radiographs usually are non-diagnostic but may demonstrate joint-space widening suggestive of an effusion. Ultrasound will usually demonstrate the presence of an effusion.

Analysis of synovial fluid remains the gold standard for the diagnosis of septic arthritis, and arthrocentesis of any effusion under sedation or anesthesia is indicated if there is a clinical suspicion of septic arthritis. A WBC count greater than 50,000/mm³ within the fluid aspirate is generally considered diagnostic of septic arthritis; however, elevated counts can be seen in certain rheumatologic conditions. The presence of bacteria on Gram stain of joint aspirate regardless of WBC count suggests infection. Routine cultures of joint aspirate as well as peripheral blood cultures should be sent. In addition, with the increasing recognition of *K kingae* as a causative agent in septic arthritis, joint aspirations should be directly inoculated into blood culture bottles to enhance isolation because this organism is difficult to recover with standard culture techniques. In most studies, only around 50% of joint aspirate cultures grew out an identifiable pathogen. In one study, close to 50% of the aspirates that were sterile on standard culture media grew out *K kingae* from blood cultures. Other studies suggest sending a polymerase chain reaction (PCR) assay or a nasopharyngeal and throat culture, given this is often an area of colonization for patients with *K kingae* infections.

Complications occur in 10% to 25% of all cases of septic arthritis of the hip, increasing when delays of 5 days or more have passed before initiation of therapy. These complications include abnormal bone growth, permanent limp, unstable articulation of the affected joint, and decreased range of motion.

Osteomyelitis is an infection of the bone that is typically caused by a bacterial organism. Close to 50% of pediatric cases of osteomyelitis occur in children younger than 5 years. Most cases of osteomyelitis in children occur from hematogenous deposition of bacteria into the bone marrow during a transient episode of bacteremia. Other cases may be caused from contiguous spread of an adjacent infection or direct inoculation. Osteomyelitis most commonly begins in the highly vascularized metaphysis of long bones of young children. The femur, tibia, and pelvis account for most cases. As with septic arthritis, *S aureus* remains the most common organism identified across all age groups, with an increasing incidence of methicillin-resistant *S aureus* (MRSA). Other organisms include *S pyogenes, S pneumoniae,* and *K kingae*. Young infants can also be infected by neonatal pathogens such as GBS and enteric gram-negative organisms. Individuals with sickle cell disease (SCD) are at increased risk to be infected with *Salmonella*. *Haemophilus influenzae* type b should also be considered in unvaccinated children.

Children often present with pain or localized symptoms at the affected site. More than half will have a fever. Younger children may present with limp, reduced range of motion, or refusal to bear weight. If there is subperiosteal spread, there may be erythema, warmth, and swelling at the affected site.

Laboratory tests can be supportive of a diagnosis of osteomyelitis but are usually not specific. Typically, a CBC, ESR, and CRP are obtained along with blood cultures. Leukocytosis may be present, but in more than half the cases, the WBC count can be normal. Inflammatory markers are elevated in up to 90% of cases. A CRP greater than 10 mg/L (1.0 mg/dL) may also increase the suspicion for osteomyelitis complicated by septic arthritis. Blood cultures are positive in 40% to 55% of cases. Given the importance of discerning the causative organism, consider ordering PCR assays for *K kingae* given its increasing incidence and difficulty to isolate. Radiographs are often normal or show only soft-tissue changes early in the course of the disease. Periosteal reactions and lytic lesions are usually not present until day 10 to 21 into the disease. Bone scans can be helpful in the preverbal child or in individuals who cannot localize their pain. Magnetic resonance imaging (MRI) has become the study of choice, with a reported sensitivity of 97%. It is very useful for distinguishing between bone and soft-tissue infections.

Diskitis refers to an inflammatory process involving the intervertebral disks. This disease typically occurs in children younger than 5 years. It occurs almost exclusively in the lumbar region, causing progressive limp, back pain, and refusal to walk. Most children are afebrile. It is thought to occur in younger children because of the presence of vascular channels in the cartilaginous region of the disk space as well as abundant intraosseous arterial anastomoses. These vascular channels disappear with age. Laboratory studies are often nonspecific, with slight elevations in the peripheral WBC count and ESR. Radiographs are abnormal in most cases (75%), with decreased vertebral disk space and erosion of adjacent vertebral end plates being the most common abnormalities seen. Bone scans will demonstrate nonspecific increased marker uptake in the affected area. Computed tomography scans rarely provide a specific diagnosis and are not generally used. Magnetic resonance imaging will demonstrate characteristic inflammatory changes and allow for differentiation from other conditions, such as vertebral osteomyelitis.

The exact etiology of diskitis is not known, and the treatment is somewhat controversial. Several authors propose that it is the result of an infectious process and warrants antibiotic therapy. Others propose that it is simply a benign self-limited inflammatory disease because most cultures are sterile and patients can recover without any antimicrobial therapy. In most cases, broad spectrum antibiotics and strategies to prevent kyphosis are initiated.

Legg-Calvé-Perthes disease is an idiopathic avascular necrosis of the femoral head. The exact etiology is unclear but involves some disruption in the vascular supply of the capital femoral epiphysis. This is most commonly seen in children 3 to 12 years old (median age 7 years). Boys are affected 4 to 5 times more than girls. It is usually unilateral but can be bilateral in up to 15% of cases. Children typically present with a chronic intermittent limp that can be painful or painless. It is not uncommon for the child to be symptomatic for months before a diagnosis is made. Pain is usually worsened with internal rotation and abduction.

Laboratory tests are usually normal. Radiographs early in the course of the disease may be negative or show widening of the joint space. In later stages, radiographic findings include an increased density and decreased size of the femoral head (necrosis), patchy areas of radiolucency near the epiphysis (fragmentation), and flattening of the femoral head (reconstitution) (Figure 109-2)

Slipped capital femoral epiphysis (SCFE) is a displacement or slipping of the femoral epiphysis from the neck of the femur through the open physis (growth plate). This is the most common hip disorder affecting adolescents. It is more common in boys than girls and occurs more frequently among African Americans and Hispanics than whites. Typical age of onset is 9 to 16 years. Individuals are often noted to be overweight and frequently present with a chief complaint of knee pain. They will often have an antalgic gait. The foot is noted to be externally rotated in severe slips but may be neutral or pigeon-toed in mild slips. Examination of the knee will be normal without discomfort, despite the complaint of knee pain. Passive flexion of the hip will often result in obligate external rotation. There will usually be pain with internal rotation. A SCFE is stable when the individual can walk with or without crutches; an unstable SCFE occurs when the child cannot walk. Laboratory testing is not indicated. Radiographs of the hip in the AP and batrachian (frog-leg) positions reveal the diagnosis in approximately 80% of cases. Early radiographic findings include widening of the physis and later reveal slippage (Figure 109-3). Both hips should be viewed because up to 20% of SCFEs are bilateral. Ultrasound in experienced hands has been shown to be an effective diagnostic tool (sensitivity of 95%). Computed tomography scan and MRI can reveal the presence of a slip. Magnetic resonance imaging is much more sensitive and can detect physeal widening in the pre-slip condition.

Osgood-Schlatter disease (OSD), or traction apophysitis of the tibial tubercle, is an overuse injury of the knee seen most commonly in adolescent athletes. Repetitive microtrauma causes partial avulsion of the patellar tendon at its insertion on the tibia. Individuals will typically present with a localized bony prominence, swelling, and tenderness over the tibial tubercle at the insertion of the patellar tendon. Radiographs are commonly performed to rule out other pathology and will typically demonstrate soft tissue swelling or edema of the skin and tissues, as well as ossific fragments within the tendon (Figure 109-4).

A limp can also result from certain systemic disease processes, such as **juvenile idiopathic arthritis, SCD,** and **neoplastic disease.** Juvenile idiopathic arthritis may involve multiple joints, and there is usually evidence of inflammation (eg, warmth, swelling or effusion, redness). The pain is usually worse in the morning and improves

Figure 109-2. Legg-Calvé-Perthes disease. (Courtesy of Michael Diament, MD.)

Figure 109-3. Slipped capital femoral epiphysis. (Courtesy of Michael Diament, MD.)

Figure 109-4. Osgood-Schlatter disease. (Courtesy of Michael Diament, MD.)

throughout the day. **Sickle cell disease** is now detected on newborn screen, and most patients know of their diagnosis. Acute pain crises with SCD can affect multiple areas, resulting in significant discomfort, limp, and refusal to walk. Careful consideration for infectious etiologies (ie, osteomyelitis) is necessary in the highly febrile or ill child with SCD who presents with a limp or bone pain. In addition, SCD patients are at risk of avascular necrosis of the hip secondary to vasoocclusive episodes. Neoplastic disease processes such as leukemia or primary bone tumors (eg, Ewing sarcoma, osteosarcoma) can present with bone pain and limp. The presence of pallor, petechiae, disseminated lymphadenopathy, or hepatosplenomegaly may suggest the presence of leukemia. The peripheral CBC will usually show the presence of blasts and varying degrees of involvement of the various cell lines (ie, anemia, thrombocytopenia). Primary bone tumors may present with bony deformities or overlying soft-tissue swelling. Radiographs will often reveal characteristic bony lesions, which may require an MRI to ascertain involvement. Computed tomography scans may be necessary to look for metastases. Individuals may require referral to an orthopedist for biopsy to ascertain a definitive diagnosis and possible amputation. Referral to an oncologist will be necessary to initiate appropriate therapy, including chemotherapy or radiation.

Evaluation

History

The history should focus on the time of onset of the limp, its chronicity, and the degree of disability it produces. Often, a history of trauma is provided, even when a non-traumatic cause is present.

Young toddlers are often falling as they learn how to walk, and parents will frequently relay some trivial or unrelated injury. Delayed motor development may be a sign of neuromuscular disease such as cerebral palsy, whereas a history of loss of motor milestones may indicate muscular dystrophy or spinal cord tumor. It is important to remember that pelvic pathology may be referred to the hip, and hip pathology is often referred to the knee or thigh.

Physical Examination

Physical examination begins with observation for any overt deformities (eg, leg-length discrepancy, joint swelling). All joints should be palpated, and the presence of swelling, tenderness, erythema, or warmth should be noted. A thorough evaluation of the hips is essential in children with knee pain. The type of gait abnormality may be determined by observing children walk or run.

Children should be examined supine and standing, if possible. Standing children can be assessed for pelvic obliquity and spinal deformities. Range of motion of the hips, knees, ankles, and feet can be checked in supine children, comparing the affected side with the non-affected side. Deep tendon reflexes and muscle strength should be assessed, and leg-length measurements should also be made as indicated. Children should be supine for a true measurement of leg length, taken as the distance from the anterosuperior iliac spine to the medial malleolus. A discrepancy of more than 2 cm is considered significant in adults. The significance of discrepancies can be confirmed by imaging studies.

Laboratory Tests

Laboratory procedures are usually necessary in children with an acute onset of limp, especially in those with refusal to bear weight. Complete blood cell count, CRP, and ESR are useful markers of systemic disease or significant inflammation. There can be significant overlap between the differing etiologies, and no single screening test reliably distinguishes between the various inflammatory and infectious causes of limp. Blood and local cultures (eg, joint fluid, bone) may be useful in the evaluation of suspected infectious entities. Additional testing for rheumatologic causes may be clinically indicated, such as antinuclear antibody or rheumatoid factor (see Chapter 148).

Imaging Studies

Radiographs are the most commonly used imaging study. A minimum of 2 views should be obtained. Examination of the hip involves imaging in the AP view as well as the batrachian (frog-leg) position. Both hips should be radiographed for comparison and to assess for the presence of bilateral disease. Ultrasound is helpful if there is concern about an effusion within the joint space and can also be used to guide diagnostic and therapeutic interventions (eg, arthrocentesis). Computed tomography scan can sometimes provide useful information, but MRI is being used with increasing frequency because of its superior resolution and lack of radiation. Bone scans may be helpful in the early stages of disease when radiographs are typically normal or when there is difficulty establishing a localized area of involvement.

Management

Management depends on the etiology. Management of septic arthritis consists of surgical drainage and intravenous (IV) antibiotics. Empiric therapy typically consists of a antistaphylococcal penicillin (eg, nafcillin, oxacillin). If there are high rates of community-acquired MRSA in the region, clindamycin or vancomycin may be necessary until sensitivities can be performed. The addition of a third-generation cephalosporin is indicated in the newborn period pending Gram stain and culture results or when *N gonorrhoeae* is suspected in adolescents. Length of therapy is typically 2 to 4 weeks of IV antibiotics. Prognosis is generally good with prompt diagnosis and management within 4 days of symptom onset.

Initial management of osteomyelitis also consists of IV antibiotics. Occasionally, surgery may be indicated, particularly if there is a subperiosteal or soft-tissue abscess or sequestrums present. In communities where methicillin-susceptible *S aureus* is more prevalent, empiric antibiotic therapy consists of a antistaphylococcal penicillin (eg, nafcillin, oxacillin) or a first-generation cephalosporin (eg, cefazolin). In areas where community-acquired MRSA is of concern, clindamycin or vancomycin may be necessary. Neonates and individuals with SCD require the addition of a third-generation cephalosporin pending culture results. In individuals with a presumed pseudomonal infection, an extended spectrum β-lactam (eg, ceftazidime, cefepime, piperacillin/tazobactam) plus an aminoglycoside are indicated. Four to 6 weeks of antibiotic therapy is currently recommended. There is increasing data that supports switching to oral antibiotics after receiving as little as 2 to 4 days of parenteral therapy if compliance is likely, an organism has been identified, clinical improvement is noted, the patient is afebrile, and the inflammatory markers have begun to normalize. Oral dosages 2 to 3 times those normally recommended for non-bony infections are often used for β-lactam antibiotics. Other oral antibiotics (eg, clindamycin, trimethoprim-sulfamethoxazole, fluoroquinolone) have excellent bioavailability, and the usual oral dosages may be used. Amoxicillin should be considered in children younger than 4 years who have not been vaccinated to cover *H influenzae*. Consultation with an infectious disease specialist is often indicated.

Supportive measures with nonsteroidal anti-inflammatory agents are generally indicated for the management of diskitis. Broad-spectrum antibiotics are generally given and addition of anti-staphylococcal antibiotics should also be considered and have been shown to speed symptom improvement. A brace may be helpful for support and pain relief. Most patients recover without any complications.

Prompt referral to an orthopedist is indicated in cases of LCPD. The goal of treatment of LCPD is to maintain full joint mobility and prevent deformity of the femoral head. Bed rest and immobilization decrease the pain and help restore range of motion. Traction and abduction casts or braces are used to contain the femoral head within the acetabulum in an effort to maintain its spherical shape. Surgical correction of gross deformities of the femoral head may be necessary in severe cases. Benefits of surgery are more likely to be seen with patients younger than 6 years.

Treatment for SCFE consists of surgical reduction and stabilization with placement of screws through the epiphysis. The screws are typically left in place and do not need to be removed. Non–weight bearing is maintained until early callus is seen on the posterior-inferior metaphysis and the pain has resolved. Gradual and progressive weight bearing is allowed, and progression to full weight bearing usually occurs 3 to 4 months after fixation. No running or jumping is allowed until the physis closes.

Treatment of OSD consists of rest, ice, nonsteroidal anti-inflammatory agents, and strengthening exercises of the quadriceps and hamstring muscles. Surgical treatment is rarely indicated and is reserved for those patients who do not respond to conservative therapy.

Prognosis

The prognosis depends on the etiology of the limp, rapid diagnosis, and appropriate therapy.

The prognosis is good in most cases of septic arthritis and osteomyelitis if the infection is diagnosed early and treated appropriately. Prognosis of osteomyelitis is usually good, with less than 0.1% mortality and less than 2% of patients who receive at least 3 weeks of antibiotic therapy developing chronic osteomyelitis. Treatment of chronic disease can be difficult, often necessitating prolonged courses of antibiotics (up to 6–12 months) and multiple surgeries for debridement. Rare complications include disturbances in bone growth, limb-length discrepancies, arthritis, abnormal gait, and pathologic fractures. Prognosis is also worse if treatment is delayed, the patient is younger, or the infection involves the hip, ankle, or knee. The main complication is degenerative arthritis of the hip. Patients require regular follow-up with orthopedics the first year after diagnosis.

Prognosis of LCPD is related to the degree of femoral head involvement and age at onset of the disease. Children younger than 6 years have the best prognosis. The risk of development of degenerative arthritis in adulthood increases in children whose disease is more extensive and whose condition is diagnosed later (ie, after 8 years of age).

If patients with SCFE are untreated, the potential for further slipping of the femoral head remains until the growth plate closes. Potential treatment-related complications of SCFE include chondrolysis of the femoral head and acetabulum, avascular necrosis, and fracture at the site of pin placement. In general the prognosis is good and is based on the degree of slippage. The main complication is the development of avascular necrosis of the femoral head, which typically leads to degenerative hip disease later in life. This occurs in up to 15% of slips and is more common in an unstable SCFE. Only 7% of patients in the moderate-slip category have a poor outcome compared with 24% of patients in the severe-slip category.

In about 5% to 10% of cases, OSD may become chronic, with persistent swelling and tenderness. In such cases, a radiograph may show the formation of an ossicle over the tibial tubercle; this ossicle may require surgical resection.

CASE RESOLUTION

In the case described at the beginning of the chapter, the child's history and physical examination seem to be consistent with Legg-Calvé-Perthes disease. The child's knee pain is actually secondary to hip pathology. The diagnosis may have been missed if the physician had not examined the hips and noted the abnormality in range of motion. Anteroposterior and batrachian (frog-leg) radiographs of the hips were taken, which showed widening of the joint space. Orthopedic consultation was obtained, and hospitalization for bed rest and ensured immobilization were recommended.

Selected References

Caird MS, Flynn JM, Leung YL, Millman JE, D'Italia JG, Dormans JP. Factors distinguishing septic arthritis from transient synovitis of the hip in children. A prospective study. *J Bone Joint Surg Am.* 2006;88(6):1251–1257

Copley LA. Pediatric musculoskeletal infection: trends and antibiotic recommendations. *J Am Acad Orthop Surg.* 2009;17(10):618–626

Dahl MT. Limb length discrepancy. *Pediatr Clin North Am.* 1996;43(4):849–865

Dartnell J, Ramachandran M, Katchburian M. Haematogenous acute and subacute paediatric osteomyelitis: a systematic review of the literature. *J Bone Joint Surg Br.* 2012;94(5):584–595

Do TT. Transient synovitis as a cause of painful limps in children. *Curr Opin Pediatr.* 2000;12(1):48–51

Dodwell ER. Osteomyelitis and septic arthritis in children: current concepts. *Curr Opin Pediatr.* 2013;25(1):58–63

Dormans JP, Moroz L. Infection and tumors of the spine in children. *J Bone Joint Surg Am.* 2007;89(Suppl 1):79–97

Faust SN, Clark J, Pallett A, Clarke NM. Managing bone and joint infection in children. *Arch Dis Child.* 2012;97(6):545–553

Fernandez M, Carrol CL, Baker CJ. Discitis and vertebral osteomyelitis in children: an 18-year review. *Pediatrics.* 2000;105(6):1299–1304

Frank G, Mahoney HM, Eppes SC. Musculoskeletal infections in children. *Pediatr Clin North Am.* 2005;52(4):1083–1106

Gholve PA, Cameron DB, Millis MB. Slipped capital femoral epiphysis update. *Curr Opin Pediatr.* 2009;21(1):39–45

Gholve PA, Scher DM, Khakharia S, Widmann RF, Green DW. Osgood Schlatter syndrome. *Curr Opin Pediatr.* 2007;19(1):44–50

Gutierrez K. Bone and joint infections in children. *Pediatr Clin North Am.* 2005;52(3):779–794

Henrickson M, Passo MH. Recognizing patterns in chronic limb pain. *Contemp Pediatr.* 1994;11:33–62

Hurley JM, Betz RR, Loder RT, Davidson RS, Alburger PD, Steel HH. Slipped capital femoral epiphysis. The prevalence of late contralateral slip. *J Bone Joint Surg Am.* 1996;78(2):226–230

Kocher MS, Mandiga R, Zurakowski D, Barnewolt C, Kasser JR. Validation of a clinical prediction rule for the differentiation between septic arthritis and transient synovitis of the hip in children. *J Bone Joint Surg Am.* 2004;86-A(8):1629–1635

Koop S, Quanbeck D. Three common causes of childhood hip pain. *Pediatr Clin North Am.* 1996;43(5):1053–1066

Laine JC, Kaiser SP, Diab M. High-risk pediatric orthopedic pitfalls. *Emerg Med Clin North Am.* 2010;28(1):85–102

Lehmann CL, Arons RR, Loder RT, Vitale MG. The epidemiology of slipped capital femoral epiphysis: an update. *J Pediatr Orthop.* 2006;26(3):286–290

Loder RT. Controversies in slipped capital femoral epiphysis. *Orthop Clin North Am.* 2006;37(2):211–221

Luhmann SJ, Jones A, Schootman M, Gordon JE, Schoenecker PL, Luhmann JD. Differentiation between septic arthritis and transient synovitis of the hip in children with clinical prediction algorithms. *J Bone Joint Surg Am.* 2004;86-A(5):956–962

MacEwen GD, Dehne R. The limping child. *Pediatr Rev.* 1991;12(9):268–274

Nguyen NA, Klein G, Dogbey G, McCourt JB, Mehlman CT. Operative versus nonoperative treatments for Legg-Calvé-Perthes disease: a meta-analysis. *J Pediatr Orthop.* 2012;32(7):697–705

Nouri A, Walmsley D, Pruszczynski B, Synder M. Transient synovitis of the hip: a comprehensive review. *J Pediatr Orthop B.* 2014;23(1):32–36

Peltola H, Pääkkönen M. Acute osteomyelitis in children. *N Engl J Med.* 2014;370(4):352–360

Ranson M. Imaging of pediatric musculoskeletal infection. *Semin Musculoskelet Radiol.* 2009;13(3):277–299

Renshaw TS. The child who has a limp. *Pediatr Rev.* 1995;16(12):458–465

Reynolds RA. Diagnosis and treatment of slipped capital femoral epiphysis. *Curr Opin Pediatr.* 1999;11(1):80–83

Schmit P, Glorion C. Osteomyelitis in infants and children. *Eur Radiol.* 2004;14(Suppl 4):L44–L54

Shah SS. Abnormal gait in a child with fever: diagnosing septic arthritis of the hip. *Pediatr Emerg Care.* 2005;21(5):336–341

Vazquez M. Osteomyelitis in children. *Curr Opin Pediatr.* 2002;14(1):112–115

Yagupsky P. *Kingella kingae:* from medical rarity to an emerging pediatric pathogen. *Lancet Infect Dis.* 2004;4(6):358–367

CHAPTER 110

Musculoskeletal Disorders of the Neck and Back

Carol D. Berkowitz, MD; Andrew K. Battenberg, MD; and Nima Eftekhary, BS

CASE STUDY

A 4-week-old boy is brought to the office by his mother, who complains that her son always holds his head tilted to the right. She reports that he has held it in this position for about 1 week and prefers to look mainly to the left. The infant is the 8-lb, 8-oz product of a term gestation born via forceps extraction, and he had no complications in the neonatal period. He is feeding well on breast milk and has no history of fever, upper respiratory symptoms, vomiting, or diarrhea.

On examination, the head is tilted toward the right side with limited lateral rotation to the right and decreased lateral side bending to the left. Except for the presence of a small mass palpable on the right side of the neck, the examination is within normal limits.

Questions

1. What laboratory or radiologic studies are indicated in infants with torticollis?
2. What is the differential diagnosis of torticollis in infants?
3. What are some of the common musculoskeletal abnormalities that may be seen in association with torticollis?
4. What are other common musculoskeletal problems in children and adolescents?
5. What is the current recommended management of children and adolescents with idiopathic scoliosis?

Children with disorders of the spine can present with deformity, back pain, or occasionally both. Nontraumatic congenital and developmental deformities of the spine are frequently encountered in pediatric practice. Torticollis and scoliosis are 2 of the most common disorders in children that present as spinal deformity. **Torticollis,** or wry neck, is a positional abnormality of the neck resulting in abnormal tilting and rotation of the head. **Scoliosis** refers to any lateral curvature of the spine that measures more than 10 degrees as determined by an anteroposterior (AP) radiograph of the spine. Scoliosis can be divided into 3 categories: infantile (birth–3 years), juvenile (3–10 years), and adolescent. **Back pain** is a far less common complaint in children than in adults. When such pain occurs in children, it usually signals the presence of organic disease. However, in adolescents, musculoskeletal strain is a common etiology.

Epidemiology

Some degree of spinal asymmetry is seen in about 2% to 5% of the population.

The most common type of **torticollis** seen in children is congenital muscular torticollis. The incidence is estimated to be between 1% and 2% and is increased in breech presentations (1.8% vs 0.3% in vertex presentation). It is associated with developmental dysplasia of the hip (DDH) in as many as 10% to 20% of affected infants. Family history may be positive in up to 10% of cases.

Acquired torticollis is much more common in older children and is usually secondary to trauma or infection, including cervical lymphadenitis, retropharyngeal abscess, myositis, and even upper respiratory tract infections. Episodes of benign paroxysmal torticollis, which often begin in the first year of life and generally resolve by 5 years of age, may have a familial basis. An association with benign paroxysmal vertigo and migraines has been noted.

Infantile scoliosis is rare in the United States and usually spontaneously resolves. The prevalence of juvenile **scoliosis** among school-aged children is 3% to 5%. A right thoracic single curve is the most common curve seen by physicians. Seventy-five percent to 80% of cases of structural scoliosis are idiopathic, 10% are due to neuromuscular causes, 5% are congenital, and the remaining 5% to 10% are due to trauma or miscellaneous causes. Scoliosis that begins in childhood affects boys and girls equally, and affected boys actually outnumber girls during the first 3 years of life. However, idiopathic scoliosis that develops after the age of 10 years is more common in girls than boys, with a ratio estimated between 5:1 and 7:1. In children with cerebral palsy, the incidence of scoliosis is increased, and it is found in about 20% of all cases.

Back pain is quite uncommon in preadolescent children. Unlike in adults, where it is often difficult to identify the cause of back pain, most cases of back pain in children have an identifiable etiology.

Clinical Presentation

Although **torticollis** may be noted at birth, it usually manifests at 2 to 4 weeks of age. Newborns and infants with congenital muscular torticollis present with a characteristic head tilt toward the affected side with the chin pointing toward the opposite side; this positioning is secondary to unilateral fibrosis and contracture of the sternocleidomastoid muscle (Figure 110-1). Unrecognized or untreated cases of torticollis may present as plagiocephaly (see Chapter 73) or facial asymmetry during infancy. Benign paroxysmal torticollis of infancy may present as recurrent episodes of head tilt that may be associated with vomiting, ataxia, agitation, or malaise (D$_x$ Box).

No obvious deformity may be noted in mild **scoliosis.** Asymmetry of shoulder heights, scapular prominence or position, and waistline or pelvic levelness may all be signs of scoliosis (see D$_x$ Box) (Figure 110-2A). Back pain is reported in 25% of adolescents with

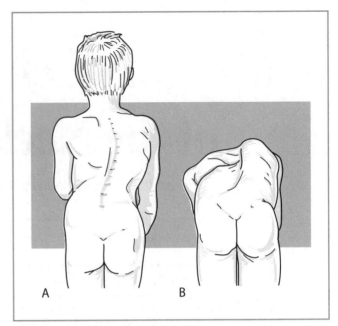

Figure 110-2. Scoliosis. A, Child with scoliosis (rear view). B, Child with scoliosis performing bend test.

idiopathic scoliosis. Scoliosis may be detected during school-based screening programs or preparticipation sports physical evaluations.

When pain is present, further examination for some other cause (eg, bone tumors, spondylolysis, spondylolisthesis) is warranted.

Preverbal children with **back pain** may present with limp or refusal to bear weight or walk.

Pathophysiology

Torticollis may be congenital or acquired. The etiology of congenital muscular torticollis is unknown. It is believed to be caused by intrauterine positioning or trauma to the soft tissues of the neck during delivery, which results in venous occlusion and ischemia of the sternocleidomastoid muscle. This leads to edema and degeneration of the muscle fibers with eventual fibrosis of the muscle body. However, one prospective study of 821 patients with congenital muscular torticollis found that 55% of patients had a sternocleidomastoid tumor, 34% of patients had thickening and tightness of the sternocleidomastoid muscle, and 11% had head tilt without tumor or thickening of the sternocleidomastoid muscle. Deformities of the face and skull may result if the condition is left untreated. Plagiocephaly (cranial asymmetry), with flattening of the face on the affected side and flattening of the occiput on the contralateral side, is seen most commonly.

Unlike kyphosis and lordosis, which are curves in the AP plane, **scoliosis** is a lateral curvature of the spine occurring in the frontal plane. Scoliosis can be functional (nonstructural) or structural. In functional scoliosis, there is no fixed deformity of the spine and the apparent curvature disappears with lying down or with forward flexion. Individuals with leg-length discrepancies appear to have scoliosis but have no spinal abnormality. Structural scoliosis may be

Figure 110-1. Torticollis. Infant with congenital muscular torticollis showing head tilt.

  Torticollis and Scoliosis

Torticollis
- Head tilt
- Limited range of motion of the neck
- Contracture of the sternocleidomastoid muscle
- Plagiocephaly (congenital torticollis)
- Firm, non-tender, mobile mass within the body of the sternocleidomastoid muscle (congenital torticollis)

Scoliosis
- Lateral curvature of the spine
- Some pain
- Back or truncal asymmetry

idiopathic or caused by various underlying disorders. The cause of idiopathic scoliosis is unknown, and there appears to be a higher incidence of scoliosis in other family members. In addition, there are reports of lower levels of melatonin in patients with scoliosis, compared with age-matched controls. This finding has not been confirmed and its relationship to the scoliosis is unclear. Abnormalities of fibrillin have also been seen in some patients with scoliosis, a finding also reported in patients with Marfan syndrome. In structural scoliosis, as the spine curves laterally it forces the vertebrae to rotate, resulting in deformity of attached structures. For example, a "rib hump" may be produced due to scoliosis in the thoracic spine (Figure 110-2B). Pelvic obliquity or flank prominence may be produced when the curvature is in the lumbar spine.

Differential Diagnosis

The differential diagnosis of congenital and acquired **torticollis** is presented in Box 110-1. Congenital muscular torticollis is the most common cause of congenital torticollis. Acquired torticollis is seen primarily in older infants and children and may appear in association with nystagmus and head nodding, a clinical triad referred to as spasmus nutans. Cervical lymphadenitis is a common cause of acquired torticollis in children 1 to 5 years of age, whereas trauma to the soft tissues or muscles of the neck is seen more frequently in school-aged children. Acute episodes (eg, benign paroxysmal

torticollis of infancy) must be differentiated from chronic conditions (eg, Sandifer syndrome, rheumatoid arthritis).

Functional or nonstructural **scoliosis** may be secondary to poor posture, leg-length discrepancies, or muscle spasm. Structural scoliosis can be classified into idiopathic, congenital, neuromuscular, and miscellaneous forms (Box 110-2). Idiopathic scoliosis, which is by far the most common type of structural scoliosis, may be divided into 3 categories based on age: infantile (0–3 years), juvenile (3–10 years), and adolescent (>10 years). The adolescent form occurs most frequently, accounting for up to 85% of cases.

Congenital scoliosis results from anomalies of the spine such as hemivertebrae or failure of vertebral segmentation. The incidence of cardiac and renal anomalies is increased. Although neuromuscular scoliosis is most often seen in children with spastic cerebral palsy, it may also be apparent in other conditions, such as poliomyelitis, meningomyelocele, muscular dystrophy, Friedreich ataxia, and spinal muscular atrophy. The miscellaneous causes of scoliosis are uncommon and include trauma, metabolic disorders, and neurocutaneous diseases.

The most common causes of **back pain** in children may be classified into 5 categories (Box 110-3). When pain is significant enough that a child presents to the emergency department, common causes include trauma (25%), muscle strain (24%), sickle cell crisis (13%), idiopathic cause (13%), urinary tract infection (5%), and viral syndrome (4%). Other infectious causes, such as diskitis, occur much more frequently in children than adults. Because the spine of children is smaller and has greater flexibility and ligamentous strength, children have a lower risk of traumatic injury than adults. Common causes of back pain in adults, such as musculoskeletal back pain (ie, muscle strain) and herniated disks, are uncommon in children. Predisposed individuals often experience their first episode of musculoskeletal back pain during adolescence or young adulthood, and children, as a whole, account for only 1% to 4% of all herniated disks.

Box 110-1. Common Causes of Torticollis

Congenital
- Congenital muscular torticollis
- Pterygium coli (skin web)
- Occipitocervical spine anomalies (eg, Klippel-Feil syndrome)

Acquired
- Infectious
- Cervical lymphadenitis
- Retropharyngeal abscess
- Osteomyelitis of cervical vertebrae
- Traumatic
- Atlantooccipital, atlas-axis (C1-C2), or C2-C3 subluxation
- Cervical musculature injury (spastic torticollis)
- Cervical spine fractures
- Neurologic
- Tumors (posterior fossa or cervical cord)
- Dystonic drug reactions
- Syringomyelia
- Ocular disturbances (strabismus, nystagmus)
- Other
- Spasmus nutans
- Sandifer syndrome (hiatal hernia with gastroesophageal reflux)
- Benign paroxysmal torticollis of infancy
- Rheumatoid arthritis
- Hysteria
- Soft tissue tumors of the neck

Box 110-2. Common Causes of Scoliosis

Functional Scoliosis
- Poor posture
- Leg-length discrepancies
- Muscle spasm
- Herniated disk
- Back injury

Structural Scoliosis
- Idiopathic
- Congenital
- Neuromuscular
- Miscellaneous
- Trauma (eg, fractures or dislocations of the vertebrae)
- Intraspinal tumors
- Metabolic disorders (eg, juvenile osteoporosis, osteogenesis imperfecta, mucopolysaccharidosis)
- Neurocutaneous syndromes (eg, neurofibromatosis)
- Marfan syndrome

Box 110-3. Common Causes of Back Pain in Children

Infectious
- Myalgia (eg, influenza)
- Diskitis (more common in children <5 years of age)
- Vertebral osteomyelitis (pyogenic, tuberculosis [Pott disease])
- Referred pain (pyelonephritis, pneumonia)

Inflammatory
- Rheumatologic diseases (juvenile rheumatoid arthritis, ankylosing spondylitis)
- Crohn disease/ulcerative colitis/psoriatic arthritis
- Disk space calcification

Neoplastic
- Primary vertebral and spinal tumors (eg, Ewing sarcoma, osteosarcoma, neuroblastoma)
- Metastatic disease (eg, neuroblastoma)
- Benign tumors (eg, eosinophilic granuloma, osteoid osteoma)

Developmental
- Spondylolysis, spondylolisthesis (adolescents)
- Scheuermann kyphosis (adolescents)

Traumatic
- Herniated nucleus pulposus (disk herniation)
- Ligamentous or muscle strain (eg, overuse syndromes)
- Compression fracture of vertebrae

Other
- Sickle cell crisis
- Osteoporosis (eg, rickets, osteogenesis imperfecta)
- Child abuse
- Psychogenic

Evaluation

History

A careful history may provide clues to diagnosis and etiology (Questions Box). Back pain is reported in about 25% of adolescents with scoliosis.

Physical Examination

In children with suspected **torticollis,** a thorough examination with specific attention to the head and neck region should be performed. Limited head rotation toward the affected side with decreased lateral side bending to the opposite side may occur. During the first 4 to 6 weeks of life, a firm, non-tender mobile mass (or pseudotumor) may be palpated within the body of the sternocleidomastoid muscle; the mass gradually regresses by 6 months of age. Because torticollis is associated with DDH, the hips should be examined for stability. A neurologic examination should also be performed to look for any neurologic deficits that may be signs of an underlying tumor. Fever or signs of inflammation point to infectious causes. Because torticollis may be secondary to visual disturbances such as strabismus, a careful eye examination is warranted. The presence of nystagmus or head nodding suggests spasmus nutans.

Screening for **scoliosis** should be part of the routine health maintenance examination of school-aged children and adolescents.

Questions

Torticollis, Scoliosis, and Back Pain

Torticollis
- Is there any family history of torticollis?
- What type of delivery did the mother have (ie, cesarean or vaginal)? Were forceps required?
- When was the head tilt first noticed?
- Does the infant move his or her neck in all directions, or does he or she always prefer to look in one direction?
- Does the infant have any recent history of trauma to the head or neck area?
- Is the head tilt persistent or does it come and go?
- Has the infant been sick or febrile?
- Does the child have nystagmus or head bobbing?

Scoliosis
- Is there a family history of scoliosis?
- Have the parents noticed the curvature of the spine? If so, how old was the child when the condition was first noted?
- Has the curvature increased since it was first noticed?
- Does the child have any back pain?
- Has the child had any previous treatment for the condition?
- (If appropriate) Has the child begun menstruating?
- Is the child complaining of neurologic symptoms?
- Does the child have concerns about cosmesis?

Back Pain
- How long has the child had the pain?
- Where is the pain localized?
- Is the pain persistent or does it come and go?
- Does the pain radiate anywhere (eg, down the legs)?
- Is the child limping or having difficulty walking?
- Has the child lost any motor milestones (eg, skills such as walking or standing that he or she could previously perform)?
- What makes the pain better? What makes it worse?
- Has there been any recent history of trauma or has the child begun participating in a new sport or physical activity?
- Has the child had a fever?
- Has the child had any problems with bowel or bladder function?
- Is the child taking any medication?

Children should be examined with the back fully exposed. The posture should be observed from the front, back, and both sides. The presence of any skin lesions such as café au lait spots should be noted. Any midline skin defects such as dimples or hair patches should also be noted because they are often associated with underlying spinal lesions. The spine should be palpated for any signs of tenderness, and a complete neurologic examination should be performed.

The back should be observed for asymmetry of the shoulders, scapulae, or pelvis. Physicians should have children bend forward at the waist to an angle of 90 degrees with the knees straight and the palms held together. This maneuver accentuates the curvature of structural scoliosis and emphasizes the rotational deformity of the spine. For example, in thoracic scoliosis, a characteristic rib hump is apparent on the convex side of the curve. An inclinometer can be used to determine the degree of scoliosis. More than 7 degrees of angulation correlates with a Cobb angle of 20 degrees and warrants referral to an orthopedist.

Scoliosis is described in terms of the primary or major curve, which is predominantly thoracic. The major curve may be accompanied by a secondary or minor curve, which is predominantly lumbar and often compensates the primary curve. The location is defined by the apical vertebra (eg, T2-T11 = thoracic, T12-L1 = thoracolumbar), the direction of the curvature by the side of convexity, and the severity indicated by the degree of curvature as measured on the spinal radiograph. Curves greater than 15 degrees are abnormal. Mild scoliosis is defined as curvature of less than 20 degrees, moderate as 20 to 40 degrees, and severe as greater than 40 to 45 degrees.

The evaluation of **back pain** begins with observation of children's posture and gait. Any midline skin lesions should be noted. A thorough general physical examination is important because referred pain (eg, pancreatitis, pyelonephritis, nephrolithiasis) may be causing the symptoms in the back. The spine should be palpated for any signs of tenderness. A complete neurologic examination should be performed, and any motor or sensory deficits should be noted. The motor examination should emphasize evaluation of the hips and the lower extremities, including range of motion and strength.

Laboratory Tests

In cases of **congenital torticollis,** laboratory studies are rarely necessary. In acquired torticollis, if any infection is suspected, a complete blood cell count (CBC) and blood and local cultures may aid in the diagnosis.

No specific laboratory tests are required in the evaluation of idiopathic **scoliosis.** Specific laboratory studies may be performed in the evaluation of other forms of scoliosis as indicated by the history and physical examination (eg, a urine metabolic screen for suspected metabolic disturbances).

Laboratory assessment for **back pain** depends on the history and physical examination. A CBC, blood culture, and erythrocyte sedimentation rate may be useful in the evaluation of suspected infectious etiologies. Rheumatologic studies such as a rheumatoid factor or human leukocyte antigen typing may help in the diagnosis of rheumatologic conditions. If the back pain is of acute onset, studies such as a urinalysis or serum amylase would help determine if the pain is referred, for example, in pyelonephritis or pancreatitis.

Imaging Studies

Radiographs are generally not useful in children with suspected **torticollis** unless bony anomalies are suspected. Anteroposterior and lateral views of the cervical spine can identify subluxation of C1-C2; however, yield is less than 1%. Ultrasound evaluation may reveal the location of a sternocleidomastoid mass. Magnetic resonance imaging (MRI) of the sternocleidomastoid muscle mass may be considered if an underlying condition (eg, branchial cleft cyst) is suspected. Computed tomography scan or MRI of the head or cervical spinal cord would be indicated if a neurologic tumor is suspected.

Routine radiographs are not required in the evaluation of all children with mild scoliosis (ie, minor degrees of curvature noted on physical examination). It may be best to obtain radiographs after orthopedic

evaluation is complete. Standing posteroanterior (PA) and lateral spine radiographs are used to determine the location and direction of the curvature, measure the degree of asymmetry (Cobb angle), and evaluate the vertebrae. Shoe lifts should be used prior to radiography to compensate for leg-length discrepancies. Repeat radiographs of the spine are used to follow the progression of the curvature over time. Because the risk of curve progression before skeletal maturity is a primary concern, hand and wrist radiographs should be taken to assess bone age in prepubertal children with scoliosis. Magnetic resonance imaging is recommended in individuals with rapid progression of their curve at more than 1 degree per month. Magnetic resonance imaging should include cervical, thoracic, and lumbar spine to identify deformities such as an Arnold-Chiari malformation or a tethered cord.

As with scoliosis, routine radiographs are not indicated in all cases of **back pain.** Various radiologic studies may be ordered depending on the suspected diagnosis. Radiographs may be useful in the evaluation of suspected vertebral abnormalities such as spondylolysis and spondylolisthesis. However, these conditions may represent incidental findings and not be the source of the back pain. If diskitis is suspected, a bone scan may be more appropriate than radiographs. Similarly, a bone scan or MRI is useful in the evaluation of suspected vertebral tumors.

Management

Treatment of congenital muscular **torticollis** consists of **passive stretching exercises** of the neck. With the neck in a neutral position (ie, not hyperextended), the head is bent to one side so that the ear on the side opposite to the contracted muscle is brought to the shoulder, or the chin is lowered to touch the shoulder on the affected side. These exercises are done 3 times per week, with each session consisting of 3 repetitions of 14 manual stretches of the affected sternocleidomastoid muscle. In addition, **changing the placement of the crib** in relation to the nursery door and **repositioning toys and mobiles** in the crib stimulate children to look toward the side opposite the preferred gaze. Children should also be fed with their chin turned toward the shoulder of the affected sternocleidomastoid muscle. Torticollis resolves spontaneously in most infants. When the deformity persists beyond the age of 1 to 2 years, **surgical release** of the contracted muscle may be indicated.

Management of acquired torticollis depends on etiology. The evaluation and treatment of many of these conditions can be complex and often require consultation with specialists in head and neck surgery, neurology, and orthopedic surgery.

Management of **scoliosis falls into 3 groups: observation, bracing, and surgery. Observation** involves **close follow-up** with careful repeat examinations and radiographic studies. Children who have not undergone their rapid growth phase are at greatest risk of marked progression of their curve. The Risser sign is used to assess the degree to which skeletal maturation has progressed. The sign is based on the degree of ossification of the iliac apophysis, with a Risser 0 signifying no ossification and a Risser 5 representing full ossification. An initial consultation with an orthopedic surgeon is generally advisable, even in minor degrees of curvature. The goal of follow-up is early detection of curvature with implementation of treatment to prevent or reduce curve progression. Children with curves less than 20 to 25 degrees should be monitored for progression with assessment every 4 to 6 months at a specialist clinic to monitor for curve progression. Only PA radiographs are taken at each subsequent visit to minimize radiation exposure. Curves between 25 and 45 degrees do not require bracing in skeletally mature individuals (Risser 4 or 5) but should be braced (eg, with Milwaukee brace) in growing children (Risser 0 or 1). The goal of **bracing** is not to correct any existing curvature but to prevent further curve progression. The efficacy of bracing is determined by adherence to the regimen; however, poor compliance is common. **Surgery** (eg, the Harrington rod, posterior spinal fusion) may be indicated for children with curves greater than 45 to 50 degrees. These curves have a high likelihood of progression regardless of the patient's age and skeletal maturity. The goals of surgery include arrest of curve progression, improved cosmesis, and improvement of the deformity. The development of pedicle screws has advanced the process of spinal fusion.

Although the management of **back pain** is diagnosis dependent, **rest** and **immobilization** are principles of treatment that apply in many instances. In the management of diskitis, antistaphylococcal antibiotics may be necessary in addition to immobilization. If spondylolisthesis and spondylolysis do not respond to rest and immobilization, operative stabilization may be required. In adolescents with low back pain related to muscular injury, conservative treatment, including bed rest, heat, and anti-inflammatory medications, may be tried for 1 to 2 weeks followed by a gradual return to normal activity. It is not advisable to institute such treatment in younger children without pursuing a more extensive evaluation or consultation with an orthopedic surgeon because the risk of serious disease is significant in this age group.

Prognosis

Congenital muscular **torticollis** responds to conservative management in about 90% of infants. The asymmetry of the face and skull also corrects over time once the contracture of the sternocleidomastoid muscle resolves. Spasmus nutans, a condition that develops between 4 and 12 months of age, usually resolves spontaneously by 3 years of age.

The direction and location of the curvature in **scoliosis** do not change with age, but the degree of curvature may remain stable or progress. Factors associated with a high risk of curve progression include female gender, positive family history for scoliosis, younger age at diagnosis (especially before the adolescent growth spurt), and a larger curve at the time of diagnosis. In addition, a double curve is more likely to progress than a single curve, and a thoracic curve is more likely to progress than a lumbar curve. Left untreated, severe scoliosis can produce cardiopulmonary impairment or cosmetic deformity, which may lead to low self-esteem and poor body image. Decreased exercise tolerance has been reported in individuals with curves as small as 20 degrees. Individuals with infantile and juvenile scoliosis experience increased mortality from pulmonary and cardiac conditions during their 40s and 50s.

Most cases (80%–90%) of low **back pain** in adolescents and young adults resolve spontaneously in 2 to 8 weeks. It is important for patients to learn how to prevent recurrence by improving posture, learning how to lift heavy objects appropriately, and instituting a program of exercises to help strengthen the abdominal and back muscles.

CASE RESOLUTION

The history of the infant presented in the opening case study is consistent with congenital muscular torticollis. Physical examination helps confirm the diagnosis. The hips should be evaluated thoroughly because of the association of congenital muscular torticollis with developmental dysplasia of the hip. A program consisting of neck stretching exercises and repositioning of interesting toys and objects in the infant's crib to the side opposite the preferred gaze should be instituted. The infant can be reevaluated in 2 to 3 weeks to monitor progress.

Selected References

Altaf F, Gibson A, Dannawi Z, Noordeen H. Adolescent idiopathic scoliosis. *BMJ.* 2013;346:f2508

Ballock RT, Song KM. The prevalence of nonmuscular causes of torticollis in children. *J Pediatr Orthop.* 1996;16(4):500–504

Boachie-Adjei O, Lonner B. Spinal deformity. *Pediatr Clin North Am.* 1996;43(4):883–897

Cheng JC, Au AW. Infantile torticollis: a review of 624 cases. *J Pediatr Orthop.* 1994;14(6):802–808

Davids JR, Wenger DR, Mubarak SJ. Congenital muscular torticollis: sequela of intrauterine or perinatal compartment syndrome. *J Pediatr Orthop.* 1993;13(2):141–147

Davis PJ, Williams HJ. The investigation and management of back pain in children. *Arch Dis Child Educ Pract Ed.* 2008;93(3):73–83

Epps HR, Salter RB. Orthopedic conditions of the cervical spine and shoulder. *Pediatr Clin North Am.* 1996;43(4):919–931

Epstein JA, Epstein NE, Marc J, Rosenthal AD, Lavine LS. Lumbar intervertebral disk herniation in teenage children: recognition and management of associated anomalies. *Spine (Phila Pa 1976).* 1984;9(4):427–432

Glancy GL. Advances in idiopathic scoliosis in children and adolescents. *Adv Pediatr.* 2007;54:55–66

Kautz SM, Skaggs DL. Getting an angle on spinal deformities. *Contemp Pediatr.* 1998;15:111–128

Lenke LG, Betz RR, Harms J, et al. Adolescent idiopathic scoliosis: a new classification to determine extent of spinal arthrodesis. *J Bone Joint Surg Am.* 2001;83-A(8):1169–1181

Lowe TG, Edgar M, Margulies JY, et al. Etiology of idiopathic scoliosis: current trends in research. *J Bone Joint Surg Am.* 2000;82-A(8):1157–1168

Payne WK 3rd, Ogilvie JW. Back pain in children and adolescents. *Pediatr Clin North Am.* 1996;43(4):899–917

Ramirez N, Johnston CE, Browne RH. The prevalence of back pain in children who have idiopathic scoliosis. *J Bone Joint Surg Am.* 1997;79(3):364–368

Selbst SM, Lavelle JM, Soyupak SK, Markowitz RI. Back pain in children who present to the emergency department. *Clin Pediatr (Phila).* 1999;38(7):401–406

Stewart DG Jr, Skaggs DL. Consultation with the specialist: adolescent idiopathic scoliosis. *Pediatr Rev.* 2006;27(8):299–306

Tomczak KK, Rosman NP. Torticollis. *J Child Neurol.* 2013;28(3):365–378

Weinstein SL, Dolan LA, Wright JG, Dobbs MB. Effects of bracing in adolescents with idiopathic scoliosis. *N Engl J Med.* 2013;369(16):1512–1521

Gastrointestinal Disorders

CHAPTER 111

Vomiting

George Gershman, MD

CASE STUDY

A 6-week-old boy who has been vomiting after each meal for 3 days is brought to the office. He is breastfed, afebrile, and otherwise well. The history of the pregnancy and birth are normal. His birth weight was 3,500 g, and his current weight is 4,500 g. The physical examination is unremarkable. The mother nurses the infant in the office. Although he feeds hungrily and well, he vomits about 5 minutes after the feeding. The vomiting is projectile, and the vomitus shoots across the room. The vomitus contains curdled milk. On reexamination of the abdomen, a small mass is felt in the right upper quadrant.

Questions

1. What is the mechanism of vomiting, and how does it differ from regurgitation and rumination?
2. What are the common causes of vomiting in infants?
3. What are the common causes of vomiting in older children?
4. What is the significance of bilious vomiting?
5. What are the unique features of vomiting related to increased intracranial pressure?
6. What are some strategies for the management of vomiting in older children?

Vomiting is a common complaint of infants and children and led Thomas Phaire to write, "Many tymes the stomake of ye child is so feble that it cannot retayne eyther meate or drynke…" (*The Boke of Chyldren*, 1544). Vomiting is defined as the forceful ejection of the stomach contents through the mouth. The mechanism involves a series of complex, neurologically coordinated events under the control of the central nervous system (CNS). In contrast, regurgitation is the effortless bringing up of 1 or 2 mouthfuls of food without distress or discomfort. This is a frequent symptom of gastroesophageal reflux in infants (see Chapter 112). Rumination, a form of autostimulation, is the voluntary induction of regurgitation. It is most often noted in infants between the ages of 3 and 6 months. Rumination occurs in infants with developmental delays or with a disturbed mother-infant relationship. It is said that affected infants always smell like vomitus, which may be on the clothing, but that vomiting is rarely seen because the presence of another person provides distraction.

Rumination should be considered in infants from deprived environments (eg, neglectful homes). Cases of rumination have been described in premature newborns who were maintained in a neonatal intensive care unit after they no longer needed vigilant care from the nursing staff. Incubators, which were cut off from the outside environment, contributed to the isolation and subsequent rumination. The condition resolved once the newborns were held and nurtured.

Epidemiology

Fifty percent of infants have spitting up or vomiting as an isolated complaint and fewer than 5% of these infants have significant underlying disease. Vomiting occurs less frequently in older children, who often experience acute, self-limited illnesses, such as gastroenteritis.

Clinical Presentation

Infants and children may present with vomiting as an isolated complaint or in association with other symptoms, including faintness, diaphoresis, sweating, pallor, tachycardia, fever, anorexia, abdominal pain, or diarrhea (D_x Box). When vomiting has persisted over a period, weight loss or failure to thrive (FTT) may occur. Neurologic symptoms, including headache and gait disturbances, may be noted in children with CNS problems. Other neurologic symptoms of altered muscle tone, lethargy, seizures, or coma in young infants suggest inborn errors of metabolism.

Pathophysiology

Vomiting is a reflex reaction that occurs in response to numerous stimuli, such as enteric infections, toxins, drugs, chemotherapy, and

Vomiting

- Vomiting
- Nausea
- Abdominal pain
- Anorexia
- Diarrhea
- Headache
- Fever
- Lethargy

radiation. The final common pathway involves expulsion of food from the relaxed stomach into the mouth due to coordinated contraction of the abdominal wall, respiratory muscles, increased intra-abdominal and thoracic pressure, and relaxation of the lower and upper esophageal sphincters.

Anything that delays gastric emptying may be associated with vomiting. Gastric emptying may be delayed by a high-fat meal, swallowed mucus (eg, maternal mucus after birth, nasal mucus with an upper respiratory infection), fever, infection, and malnutrition. Delayed gastric emptying may develop with long-standing diabetes mellitus.

Vomiting can be divided into 3 phases: nausea, retching, and emesis. However, nausea may occur without retching and vomiting, and retching may occur without vomiting.

Nausea is a significant and difficult-to-define discomfort related to the sensation of a need to vomit. It can be produced by various stimuli (eg, bacterial toxins, drugs, intestinal distention, visceral pain, unpleasant memories, labyrinthine stimulation, noxious odors, visual stimulations, unpleasant taste, increased cerebral pressure). Peripheral receptors in the stomach and the small and large intestines detect emetic stimuli; distention and contractions are recognized by mechanoreceptors, and toxins are sensed by chemoreceptors. Emetic stimuli may also originate from the obstructed or inflamed bile ducts, peritoneal inflammation, mesenteric vascular occlusion, pharynx, and heart. Vagal pathways mediate emetic responses to a variety of peripheral stimuli. Most afferent vagal fibers project to the nucleus tractus solitarius and some to the area of postrema or dorsal vagal motor nucleus. The serotonergic pathway plays the central role in nausea induced by peripheral stimuli.

The area postrema on the dorsal surface of the medulla close to the fourth ventricle is considered the chemoreceptor trigger zone to a variety of neurochemical stimuli. Bacterial toxins, drugs, toxic products of metabolic disorders, and radiation therapy may induce nausea by stimulation of numerous central receptors: dopamine D_2, muscarinic M_1, histaminergic H_1, serotonergic 5-HT3, and vasopressinergic subtypes located in the area postrema. However, afferent excitation of multiple brain sites, including the nucleus tractus solitarius, dorsal vagal and phrenic nuclei, medullary nuclei controlling respiration, hypothalamus, and amygdala, is responsible for coordinated activities of various organs and muscles and the induction of retching and emesis.

Retching is the second phase of vomiting. It is produced by concurrent contractions of inspiratory thoracic, diaphragmatic, and abdominal muscles against the closed glottis. The generated high positive intra-abdominal pressure forces gastric contents into the esophagus and herniates the gastric cardia into the thorax. At this phase, the high negative thoracic pressure prevents emesis of gastric fluids.

Emesis is the final stage of vomiting. Synchronous contractions of the inspiratory and expiratory muscles generate high positive intrathoracic pressure sufficient to produce expulsion of gastric contents into the mouth. Oral propulsion of the vomitus is facilitated by the elevation of the hyoid bone and larynx. Airways are protected from aspiration by glottis closure. Elevation of the soft palate prevents passage of the vomitus into the nasal cavities. Hyperventilation may occur before emesis. During vomiting, breathing is suppressed.

With emesis, retrograde giant contractions originate from the middle of the small intestine. Intestinal contents move into the stomach, causing duodenogastric reflux. Within the stomach, the fundus remains flaccid, but the antrum and pylorus contract. Relaxation of the lower esophageal sphincter also occurs.

In children with pyloric stenosis, duodenogastric reflux is prevented by hypertrophy of the pylorus. Projectile vomiting is facilitated by giant, often-visible contractions of the antrum and relaxation of the proximal stomach and low esophageal sphincter. Nausea is not associated with vomiting related to pyloric stenosis, and affected infants are frequently eager to eat immediately after vomiting.

Vomiting induced by increased intracranial pressure (ICP) is also not associated with nausea. In addition, such vomiting frequently occurs first thing in the morning on awaking and on an empty stomach. Regurgitation is a return of undigested food back up the esophagus to the mouth without the force and displeasure associated with vomiting. It could be manifested by visible spitting up after feeding or be silent. Clinical evidence of regurgitation is not always associated with gastroesophageal reflux disease.

Differential Diagnosis

Vomiting can be a manifestation of gastrointestinal (GI), renal, metabolic, allergic, and CNS disorders. Some conditions respond to medical management, and others mandate surgical intervention (Box 111-1). The green color of the vomitus, referred to as bilious vomiting, is a serious sign, usually indicative of intestinal obstruction distal to the major duodenal papilla and of the need for surgical intervention. Bilious vomiting can also occur in children with pseudo-obstruction syndrome or acute pancreatitis and other conditions leading to paralytic ileus.

The presence of blood in the vomitus is another ominous sign and is discussed in Chapter 113.

Box 111-1. Differential Diagnosis of Vomiting in Infancy	
Medical Conditions	• Inborn errors of metabolism
• Gastroenteritis	• Congenital adrenal hyperplasia
• Ingestion of maternal blood or mucus	• Infections (eg, otitis media, urinary tract)
• Overfeeding	
• Food allergies	
• Gastroesophageal reflux	
Surgical Conditions	
• Atresia/stenosis of gastrointestinal tract	• Congenital megacolon (Hirschsprung disease)
• Pyloric stenosis	• Intussusception
• Volvulus	• Appendicitis

The most common cause of vomiting is acute viral or bacterial gastroenteritis. Acute gastroenteritis is discussed in greater detail in Chapter 114. In cases that are not related to acute gastroenteritis, considering the age of the patient is the best approach to the differential diagnosis of vomiting.

Newborns and Infants

Vomiting in neonates may be associated with the ingestion of irritants such as maternal blood or mucus. Either of these substances delays gastric emptying. Structural anomalies of the GI tract may also cause vomiting in neonates. The onset of symptoms is directly related to the level of obstruction—the higher the structural obstruction, the earlier the onset of vomiting. Lesions of the esophagus, such as esophageal atresia, may be evident in the delivery room, with an unsuccessful attempt to pass a nasogastric tube. Lower GI lesions, such as ileal atresia, may not present for several days. These lesions require surgical intervention. Infants with atretic lesions may also have a history of polyhydramnios or a single umbilical artery.

Overfeeding is the most common reason for spitting up in young infants. Frequently, infants who present with vomiting are actually experiencing spitting up or regurgitation. Overfeeding is less likely to occur in breastfed infants because they have better control of their satiety. The physician should approach breastfed infants who are vomiting with care and concern.

Mothers of bottle-fed infants may feel that the volume of formula consumed by their infants is insufficient. Some non-nursing mothers feel the need to reinsert a nipple in the infant's mouth, and infants who are still interested in sucking (nonnutritive sucking) continue to feed, often exceeding the capacity of the stomach.

Food allergies are another common cause of vomiting during infancy. Infants with cow's milk formula intolerance may experience vomiting. At least 30% of these infants are also allergic to soy protein. Associated symptoms such as diarrhea, rhinorrhea, eczema, and growth failure frequently occur.

Gastroesophageal reflux is a common cause of regurgitation. It is described in detail in Chapter 112.

Achalasia is a rare cause of vomiting during infancy. It is defined as an absence of effective esophageal peristalsis and coordinated relaxation of the low esophageal sphincter. Ingested food that is unable to pass into the stomach may be regurgitated. Children with achalasia usually do not present until later in childhood, although they may have a prenatal history of polyhydramnios, a sign suggesting an abnormal swallowing pattern, even in utero.

Metabolic disorders, including inborn errors of metabolism and endocrine problems, may also be associated with vomiting. For example, children with galactosemia may present with vomiting as well as with jaundice, dehydration, cataracts, and hepatomegaly. Other inborn errors of metabolism include methylmalonic acidemia, disorders of the urea cycle, phenylketonuria, maple syrup urine disease, renal tubular acidosis, hypercalcemia, and diabetes insipidus. Some of these disorders induce symptoms suggestive of sepsis, such as lethargy and seizures.

Male newborns with congenital adrenal hyperplasia (CAH) may present with vomiting and electrolyte disturbance, symptoms indicative of adrenal insufficiency. Affected male newborns usually present at about 10 to 14 days of age with vomiting and hyperkalemia (which should not be attributed to hemolysis of the specimen); hyponatremia develops later. In females, CAH is usually detected in the newborn nursery because of ambiguous genitalia. Diagnosis of this potentially lethal condition is critical to ensure the institution of replacement therapy and survival of affected newborns and infants.

Vomiting may be induced by infection in parts of the body other than the GI tract. Most notably, urinary tract infections (UTIs) in infants may cause projectile vomiting, a symptom highly suggestive of pyloric stenosis. These infants are usually febrile and the diagnosis is considered when the urinalysis or culture is positive. Otitis media may also be associated with vomiting.

Vomiting, especially if unrelated to meals, may occur with increased ICP. In young infants, this suggests the possibility of an intracranial hemorrhage, such as occurs with abusive head trauma.

Pyloric stenosis, a condition caused by hypertrophy of the muscle surrounding the pyloric channel, is the most common surgical condition associated with vomiting in infancy. The condition affects males significantly more frequently than females and usually appears in newborns and infants between the ages of 2 weeks and 2 months. Factors that are known to increase the risk of pyloric stenosis include being firstborn, male, and a greater birth weight and early exposure to erythromycin. The emesis is projectile and non-bilious and frequently contains curdled milk, which reflects delayed gastric emptying, a problem caused by failure of the hypertrophied pylorus to relax. Affected newborns and infants have an intact appetite and are eager to eat. In some newborns and infants, starvation leads to few bowel movements and constipation; in others, there may be small, frequent, mucus-laden stools (starvation diarrhea) that represent intestinal juice. If pyloric stenosis is not diagnosed promptly, newborns and infants may fail to gain weight or may exhibit FTT. Symptoms suggestive of pyloric stenosis may result from an antral membrane or duplication of the GI tract.

Children

Vomiting in children is frequently associated with gastroenteritis. Infections elsewhere in the body, particularly UTIs, streptococcal pharyngitis, and otitis media, are also associated with vomiting. Labyrinthitis presents with vomiting associated with dizziness. Older children with new-onset diabetes mellitus may present with vomiting. Vomiting may also appear in children who are already known to be diabetic; this is particularly true when ketosis is present. Slow gastric emptying (gastroparesis) is a complication of long-standing diabetes mellitus. Vomiting is also a component of peptic ulcer disease, which is described in more detail in Chapter 116.

Vomiting may be a major symptom of CNS-related problems, such as tumors, infections, hydrocephalus, malformations, and other causes of increased ICP. As previously noted, vomiting in CNS-related conditions is often unrelated to meals and may not be associated with nausea. Autonomic epilepsy and migraine headaches are also associated with vomiting. Cyclic vomiting is an condition characterized by recurrent episodes of vomiting with intervals of complete wellness between attacks. There is a frequent association of cyclic vomiting syndrome with a family history of migraine headaches. Emotional upset and other factors, such as infection and physical exhaustion, can precipitate events. As a rule, cyclic vomiting syndrome lasts an average of 2½ to 5½ years, resolving in late childhood or early adolescence. A few patients continue to be symptomatic through adulthood

Vomiting is one of the hallmarks of Reye syndrome, a disorder that involves an encephalopathy in association with fatty infiltration of the liver. The etiology of the condition is unclear, but the root of the disorder seems to be related to mitochondrial dysfunction. Affected children usually have a history of viral illness, most commonly influenza or chickenpox. Following a period of recovery, they experience altered consciousness with vomiting. Hepatic enzymes and serum ammonia are elevated. Aspirin, which uncouples oxidative phosphorylation, is apparently linked to Reye syndrome, epidemiologically as well as theoretically. There has been a marked reduction in the incidence of Reye syndrome related to the decrease in the use of aspirin as well as for children vaccinated against varicella and influenza.

Certain medications, including theophylline, erythromycin, and digitalis, may also be associated with vomiting. Some of these medications cause transient relaxation of the lower esophageal sphincter; others affect the chemoreceptor trigger zone.

Familial dysautonomia (also called Riley-Day syndrome), a rare condition that affects Jewish individuals, results in vomiting. The disorder is inherited in an autosomal-recessive manner and consists of an imbalance in the autonomic nervous system. Children experience intractable vomiting in addition to excess perspiration, inability to produce tears, difficulty swallowing and chewing, and cold hands and feet. They also have hyperpyrexia and hypertension. These children require fluid replacement and management with antiemetics.

Surgical conditions such as appendicitis, gall bladder disease, and twisted ovarian cysts are discussed in Chapter 116.

Adolescents

Vomiting during the adolescent years may be caused by any of the previously mentioned conditions. In addition, adolescents may develop vomiting in association with intentional ingestion of illicit drugs or alcohol. Many adolescents have incorrect notions of the sexual activity needed to initiate pregnancy. Teenaged girls, who have been vomiting, especially for a time, should be evaluated for pregnancy, regardless of their disclosed sexual activity status.

Adolescents with eating disorders, particularly bulimia, vomit but may not disclose their vomiting. They may ingest emetics, such as ipecac, to help control their weight (see Chapter 137).

Evaluation

History

A complete history is essential for correct diagnosis (Questions Box). A positive family history of vomiting may suggest a diagnosis of food

---

Questions

Vomiting

- What is the nature of the vomiting (eg, projectile, bilious, non-bilious)?
- How long has the child been vomiting?
- Are any symptoms, such as fever, diarrhea, dizziness, or lethargy, associated with the vomiting?
- What is the relationship of the vomiting to meals?
- Does the vomiting occur at night, indicating possible hiatal hernia and gastroesophageal reflux?
- Is there a family history of migraine headache?
- Is the child taking any medications?
- Have any measures been taken to relieve the vomiting?

---

intolerance or allergy, gastroesophageal reflux or peptic ulcer disease, migraine, or familial dysautonomia.

Physical Examination

The examination can show the effect of vomiting on children's growth. The weight may provide evidence of the chronicity of the process; weight loss suggests a protracted course. Evidence of other infections, such as otitis media or pneumonia, may also be apparent. An abnormal neurologic examination would suggest a CNS process or an inborn error of metabolism. The fundi of the eyes should be assessed for the presence of papilledema or retinal hemorrhages. Nystagmus may be noted in children with labyrinthitis or CNS disturbances. The examination of the abdomen may show abdominal distention due to surgical or nonsurgical conditions such as congenital megacolon (Hirschsprung disease); malrotation; adhesions after previous surgery; pancreatitis; celiac disease; chronic idiopathic constipation; and abdominal, pelvic, or retroperitoneal masses.

Laboratory Tests

Laboratory assessment is determined by the differential diagnosis. If gastroenteritis or enterocolitis is suspected, an examination of the stools for leukocytes and occult blood is appropriate. Specimens for bacterial or viral cultures or viral antigen detection can be submitted. A complete blood cell count may support the diagnosis of infection or reveal signs of anemia. In breastfed neonates and infants, vomited blood should be evaluated using the Apt test to determine whether it came from the mother or infant.

Electrolytes should be obtained in infants or children with a history of significant vomiting and may confirm dehydration, acid-base imbalance, or electrolyte disturbance. Infants with pyloric stenosis who vomit stomach contents develop a hypochloremic-hypokalemic alkalosis. A urinalysis also may show evidence of dehydration as well as signs of a UTI. Tests for inborn errors of metabolism, such as urine for acid analysis, are appropriate if this is suspected.

Imaging Studies

Radiographic procedures, such as an esophagogram or upper GI series, are the procedure of choice for the diagnosis of esophageal and duodenal atresia and intestinal malrotation. An abdominal ultrasound is most effective in the diagnosis of pyloric stenosis or intussusception. A flat plate of the abdomen may show stomach distention, a "double bubble" (air in the stomach and duodenum), or a paucity of intestinal air in cases of high-level obstruction. Consultation with a pediatric gastroenterologist may lead to additional diagnostic tests, such as 24- to 48-hour esophageal pH, or combine esophageal pH and impedance monitoring and upper GI endoscopy.

Management

The initial step in the management of vomiting infants or children is to ensure adequate hydration and integrity of the cardiovascular bed. This may require the administration of intravenous fluids. Oral rehydration is the mainstay of therapy in infants and children whose vomiting is related to gastroenteritis. Small, frequent feedings with clear fluids are better tolerated than large, infrequent feedings, although the latter may be necessary in infants with diarrhea because each feeding may result in a bowel movement. Antiemetics such as phenothiazines are discouraged in children because of the high incidence of side effects, including dystonic posturing. Drugs commonly used in pediatric practice include antihistamines, dopamine D_2, and serotonin 5-HT3 receptor antagonists. Oral ondansetron is frequently used as a single dose to manage the vomiting seen in acute viral gastroenteritis in the pediatric emergency department or as repeated doses for hospitalized children with other conditions associated with vomiting.

Further management depends on the diagnosis. Bacterial infections should be treated with the appropriate antibiotics. Surgical conditions, such as pyloric stenosis or intussusception, should be managed urgently. Inborn errors of metabolism require consultation with a geneticist and dietary manipulation. Congenital adrenal hyperplasia should be managed in consultation with an endocrinologist. This condition necessitates replacement hormonal therapy.

Prognosis

Most cases of acute vomiting resolve spontaneously or are readily managed once the underlying condition is diagnosed. The overall prognosis is therefore quite good.

Protracted vomiting may result in starvation and FTT, however. Severe vomiting may cause tears in the esophagus and lead to hematemesis (Mallory-Weiss syndrome). Obstructive causes of vomiting in infants respond to surgical intervention.

CASE RESOLUTION

The infant in the case study exhibits signs and symptoms consistent with pyloric stenosis. The boy is a healthy, vigorous breastfed infant, and his weight gain of 1,000 g in 6 weeks (average: 25 g/d) is normal. The vomitus is curdled, indicating that it has been in the stomach for more than 3 hours. Gastric emptying is delayed. The presence of a mass in the right upper quadrant is also consistent with the diagnosis. An ultrasound would confirm the finding. It would be equally appropriate to feed the infant nothing by mouth, start intravenous fluids, and obtain surgical consultation.

Selected References

Boles RG. High degree of efficacy in the treatment of cyclic vomiting syndrome with combined co-enzyme Q10, L-carnitine and amitriptyline, a case series. *BMC Neurol.* 2011;11:102

Chandran L, Chitkara M. Vomiting in children: reassurance, red flag, or referral? *Pediatr Rev.* 2008;29(6):183–192

Chong SK. Gastrointestinal problems in the handicapped child. *Curr Opin Pediatr.* 2001;13(5):441–446

Fedorowicz Z, Jagannath VA, Carter B. Antiemetics for reducing vomiting related to acute gastroenteritis in children and adolescents. *Cochrane Database Syst Rev.* 2011;(9):CD005506

Freedman SB, Adler M, Seshadri R, Powell EC. Oral ondansetron for gastroenteritis in a pediatric emergency department. *N Engl J Med.* 2006;354(16):1698–1705

Gershman G. Approach to the child with gastroesophageal reflux. In: Osborn LM, DeWitt TS, First LR, Zenel JA, eds. *Pediatrics.* Philadelphia, PA: Mosby; 2005:658–665

Li BU, Lefevre F, Chelimsky GG, et al. North American Society for Pediatric Gastroenterology, Hepatology, and Nutrition consensus statement on the diagnosis and management of cyclic vomiting syndrome. *J Pediatr Gastroenterol Nutr.* 2008;47(3):379–393

Li BUK. Nausea, vomiting and pyloric stenosis. In: Walker WA, Kleinman RE, Sanderson IR, Goulet OJ, et al, eds. *Pediatric Gastrointestinal Disease, Pathophysiology, Diagnosis, Management.* 5th ed. Vol 1. Philadelphia, PA: BC Decker; 2008:127–138

Lee LY, Abbott L, Mahlangu B, Moodie SJ, Anderson S. The management of cyclic vomiting syndrome: a systematic review. *Eur J Gastroenterol Hepatol.* 2012;24(9):1001–1006

CHAPTER 112

Gastroesophageal Reflux

George Gershman, MD

CASE STUDY

A 15-month-old boy presents with a history of vomiting small amounts of food 3 to 4 times per week. The emesis occurs most often after meals. There does not seem to be any pain or discomfort with the vomiting. He has been otherwise healthy, with an uneventful course as an infant, good weight gain, and no hospitalizations. There is no history of pneumonia or abdominal pain. Physical examination is normal, with no anemia or urinary tract disease noted on laboratory assessment.

Questions

1. What are the characteristics of gastroesophageal reflux?
2. What is the difference between gastroesophageal reflux and gastroesophageal reflux disease (GERD)?
3. What groups of children are at risk for GERD?
4. What is the appropriate workup for an infant with suspected GERD?
5. What is the appropriate management of infants and children with gastroesophageal reflux and GERD?
6. What is the natural history of gastroesophageal reflux in children?

Gastroesophageal reflux (GER) is the retrograde movement of gastric contents from the stomach into the esophagus which could reach the pharynx or mouth, with or without emesis. It is not a disease per se; rather, it is a sign of various conditions ranging from a normal physiological process occurring a few times per day in healthy infants to the manifestation of several diseases, including gastroesophageal reflux disease (GERD), food allergy, increased intracranial pressure, seizure disorders, or infections. Most episodes of reflux in healthy individuals are brief (last less than 3 minutes), often follow meals, and cause few or no symptoms. Gastroesophageal reflux may be expressed clinically with esophageal and extra-esophageal symptoms: regurgitation (reflux of gastric content to the pharynx or mouth) and vomiting (a forceful expulsion of the regurgitant from the mouth) or cough, wheezing, or aspiration pneumonias, respectively. Gastroesophageal reflux is common in infants: at least half of healthy infants experience some degree of GER. The incidence of GER reaches a peak between 4 to 6 months of age. By 18 months of age, most infants become asymptomatic.

Although this process is common in the first year of life, it typically does not pose a problem unless it fails to resolve between 18 to 24 months of age. In contrast, children with GERD suffer from recurrent GER associated with esophageal or extra-intestinal pathology: esophagitis, Barrett syndrome, aspiration pneumonia, or asthma and corresponding clinical conditions such as poor weight gain, chronic cough, wheezing, and sleep apnea. While GER may require only anticipatory guidance and monitoring, GERD necessitates further evaluation and medical therapy. Thus, although GER could be a sign of GERD, it is important to distinguish these 2 entities for proper patient care.

Epidemiology

Most infants with GER or GERD brought in for medical care became symptomatic before 6 months of age. Regurgitation occurs at least once daily in half of infants younger than 3 months and in nearly two-thirds of infants by 4 months. By 12 months, only 5% of infants will remain symptomatic. Little is known about prevalence of GERD in children and adolescents. A recent cross-sectional observational study in more than 10,000 children and adolescents in France revealed the prevalence of GERD as 6%. One retrospective study in the United States showed that 5% to 8% of children and adolescents suffered from weekly symptoms of GERD.

High-Risk Groups

Patients with neurologic injury have a higher prevalence of GERD. Management of these individuals requires a more aggressive approach. They are more likely to have esophagitis or aspiration. Infants who have undergone repair of esophageal atresia also have more severe disease, with at least half requiring antireflux surgery. Chronic respiratory disease such as cystic fibrosis is associated with GERD. Gastroesophageal reflux disease is described in two-thirds of patients with asthma, but this association is controversial. It is not clear whether the altered physiology of these diseases causes reflux or if reflux exacerbates the pulmonary dysfunction. Similar triggers for asthma and GERD are described, so it may be that they are coexisting and unrelated. Recent studies with intraluminal impedance monitoring (see Evaluation on page 735) show that nonacid reflux occurs frequently in patients with asthma. This would help to explain the lack of success of therapy aimed at acid suppression in this group of patients.

Clinical Presentation

The most frequent presentation for infants with GER is recurrent non-forceful and small volume emeses (D$_x$ Box). Vomiting typically occurs after feeding and does not seem to disturb the patient. Some parents report a link between fussiness and crying with feeding, but this is not reproducible in trials comparing symptoms with pH studies. Further symptoms such as poor weight gain, anemia, or swallowing difficulties could be linked to GERD. Sandifer syndrome is a rare presentation of GERD in infants, with characteristic paroxysmal movements involving spasmodic torticollis and dystonia. Nodding and rotation of the head, neck extension, gurgling, writhing movements of the limbs, and severe hypotonia can also be witnessed. Infants and children can develop extra-esophageal manifestations of GERD such as nighttime cough, sleep apnea, wheezing, and recurrent pneumonia. Children older than 8 years and adolescents may have symptoms of adult-type GERD: frequent heartburn, chest and abdominal pain, and dysphagia.

Pathophysiology

There are many factors involved in the pathophysiology of reflux disease. Many of them change as the child grows. This helps explain the improvement in infant GER over time. Motility and pressure differentials between the esophagus and stomach control the flow of gas and liquid across the lower esophageal sphincter (LES). Regurgitant is allowed into the distal esophagus multiple times daily in all ages by *transient LES relaxations.* Increased frequency or duration of these relaxations, rather than low LES pressure, is felt to be a major cause of GERD. Transient LES relaxations are mediated by a brain stem reflex involving the vagal nerve and release of nitric oxide.

Position of the gastroesophageal junction and its relationship to the diaphragmatic crura play an important role. The opposed crura have a "pinchcock" action that works with the esophagogastric angle, or "angle of His", to prevent reflux. As this angle becomes more open or obtuse, reflux may increase. Disruption of this anatomic association, as seen with hiatal hernia, predisposes individuals to reflux.

Inappropriate relaxations of the LES that are too frequent or prolonged expose the esophageal mucosa to noxious material. Swallowed saliva and coordinated esophageal peristalsis neutralizes the regurgitant and sweeps it into the stomach. Inflammation of the esophagus may disrupt this process by decreasing peristaltic activity. Lack of mucus secretion by the esophageal mucosa and poor esophageal clearance increase the risk of esophagitis by precipitating exposure of esophageal mucosa to hydrochloric acid, pepsin, bile acids, and pancreatic enzymes.

Before food or secretions can move out of the esophagus, the stomach must be ready to accept it. The fundus normally relaxes without an increase in pressure. Dysfunction of this fundic accommodation or delay in gastric emptying can increase pressure in the stomach and exacerbate reflux. The volume of ingested feedings is noted to be a factor in infants. Based on the size of their stomachs, infants typically take twice the volume of older children. This leaves more material in the stomach at any given time, potentially increasing intragastric pressure.

Differential Diagnosis

A diverse group of symptoms, each with its own list of potential diagnoses, are associated with reflux disease. Regurgitation and vomiting are the most commonly reported symptoms. Many of the causes of vomiting in the newborn can be separated from reflux with a history and physical examination (Box 112-1). Forceful, bilious, or

---

Box 112-1. Common Non-reflux Causes of Vomiting

Infections
- Sepsis
- Meningitis
- Urinary tract infection
- Otitis media

Obstruction
- Pyloric stenosis
- Malrotation
- Intussusception

Gastrointestinal
- Eosinophilic esophagitis
- Peptic ulcer disease
- Achalasia
- Gastroparesis
- Gastroenteritis
- Gall bladder disease
- Pancreatitis
- Celiac disease
- Pill esophagitis
- Crohn disease

Metabolic/Endocrine
- Galactosemia
- Fructose intolerance
- Urea cycle defects
- Diabetic ketoacidosis

Toxic
- Lead poisoning

Neurologic
- Hydrocephalus and shunt malfunctions
- Subdural hematoma
- Intracranial hemorrhage
- Tumors
- Migraine

Allergic
- Dietary protein intolerance

Respiratory
- Post-tussive emesis
- Pneumonia

Renal
- Obstructive uropathy
- Renal insufficiency

Cardiac
- Congestive heart failure

Other, Seen in Adolescents
- Recreational drugs
- Alcohol
- Pregnancy

Other
- Overfeeding
- Self-induced vomiting

Dx **Presenting Signs and Symptoms of Gastroesophageal Reflux Disease**

- Regurgitation
- Vomiting
- Fussiness or sleep disturbance
- Poor weight gain
- Hematemesis or anemia
- Odynophagia or dysphagia
- Asthma/apnea/aspiration

bloody emesis is not typical of reflux. Fussiness and crying are non-specific symptoms with etiologies ranging from infantile colic to meningitis. Eosinophilic esophagitis (E_oE) should be considered in toddlers and children with recurrent emesis and atopic dermatitis, food allergy, or asthma and older children and adolescents with dysphagia. Children with E_oE may also suffer from recurrent food impaction in the esophagus. The primary therapy of E_oE focuses on dietary manipulation and the elimination of identified foods to which the child is allergic.

Evaluation

Infants who fit into the definition of "happy spitter" (normal-appearing, thriving child with recurrent emesis) do not required any diagnostic workup. It is important to reassure parents and encourage proper feeding technique. However, the presence of red flag symptoms such as bilious vomiting, poor weight gain, food avoidance, chronic cough, unexplained anemia, or significant chest or abdominal pain should prompt thorough diagnostic evaluation.

History

Targeted questions about the timing and volume of feedings and their relationship to regurgitation can help build the case for reflux. Specific attention should be paid to respiratory symptoms such as nighttime cough or previous episodes of pneumonia. Difficulties with feeding and swallowing should be outlined carefully. Gagging or dysphagia with different consistencies of food should be noted. Family history of reflux, especially as an infant, may be helpful. Clinical questionnaires, including the Infant Gastroesophageal Reflux Questionnaire, have been validated but do not predict prognosis or severity. They are more useful in the research setting.

Physical Examination

One should perform a full physical examination, including an observance of feeding. Neurologic deficits or delay should be noted. The abdomen should be carefully palpated for masses or distension. Growth parameters should be reviewed longitudinally and the child's body habitus, particularly the amount of subcutaneous tissue, should be noted.

Laboratory Tests

Most patients with reflux will need no laboratory testing. Urinalysis and culture is reasonable in an infant with sudden onset of emesis. Children with large-volume emesis or weight loss should be assessed for acidosis or other electrolyte abnormalities. Markers of kidney and liver function are reasonable to obtain. Anemia workup should be initiated in a child who is pale, irritable, and undernourished.

Intra-esophageal pH Monitoring

Currently, measurement of the intra-esophageal pH for periods of 24 to 48 hours is considered the gold standard for the diagnosis of GERD. This is performed by placing a catheter trans-nasally into the distal esophagus to measure the intraluminal pH as the patient records the symptoms, such as cough and pain. Meals are also recorded. Monitoring of pH can be performed safely in all age groups, and certain parameters of this procedure do correlate with esophagitis. It does not detect nonacid reflux, making its utility in linking respiratory disease to GERD questionable. It may be combined with multichannel sleep studies to investigate apnea or nighttime symptoms. A wireless device that attaches to the esophageal mucosa has been used in children. The device can be placed with or without endoscopy, but the size of the capsule may prohibit its use in smaller children.

Combined Multiple Intraluminal Impedance and pH Monitoring

Impedance monitoring is being used more often to diagnose GER in children. This technology involves the placement of a catheter transnasally into the esophagus for measurement of ionic conductivity, which is low when the esophagus is empty and increases when it contains liquid. The catheter has multiple sensors that can detect the direction of liquid flow. Decrease of intra-esophageal impedance by liquids moving from the distal sensors upward determines reflux. The addition of a pH sensor to the distal end of the catheter allows the defining of reflux as acid or nonacid. It is superior to pH monitoring alone for evaluation of the temporal relation between symptoms and GER. This study is especially attractive in breastfed or bottle-fed infants to eliminate the buffering effect of human milk or formula on gastric acid to detect nonacid reflux.

Upper Gastrointestinal Series

This test is not useful for the diagnosis of GERD because of low sensitivity and specificity. It should be used only to confirm or rule out anatomic abnormalities such as malrotation, esophageal or intestinal webs, or hiatal hernia that may cause symptoms similar to those of GERD.

Nuclear Scintigraphy

The test is based on administration of an age-appropriate feeding of technetium-labeled food. It is designed to assess gastric emptying and detect the reflux of a tracer in the esophagus. The standards for interpretation of this test are poorly established. According to limited published literature, scintigraphy may have a role in the diagnosis of pulmonary aspiration in patients with chronic and refractory respiratory symptoms. A negative test result does not rule out possible pulmonary aspiration of refluxed material. Gastric emptying studies by themselves do not confirm the diagnosis of GERD and are recommended only in individuals with symptoms of gastric retention. Nuclear scintigraphy is not recommended for the routine evaluation of pediatric patients with suspected GERD.

Endoscopy With Biopsy

Endoscopy of the upper GI tract allows direct visualization of the esophagus and obtaining mucosal biopsies. The presence and severity of esophagitis can be documented. Other disease processes, including infection, E_oE, and Crohn, can be detected. Biopsies should always be taken, even in the absence of macroscopic findings.

Management

Infants who are thriving with no symptoms other than regurgitation or vomiting will benefit primarily from alleviation of parental anxiety. Discussion involving the normal course and benign nature of GER may be all that is required. The infant should be followed up by a pediatrician until the resolution of symptoms. Referral to a pediatric gastroenterologist should be considered when GERD is suspected.

Lifestyle Changes

Life in recumbence has its disadvantages for infants, namely allowing the esophagus and stomach to reside at the same level. This concept has led to the use of positioning in infants. There are multiple positions used, including prone, prone at a 30-degree angle, or supine at a 30-degree angle. The only proven position seems to be prone. Unfortunately, this position has been associated with a higher rate of sudden infant death syndrome (SIDS) in infants. The practitioner must balance the risk of GERD with that of SIDS in the individual patient. The 30-degree supine position does not seem to be more effective in decreasing reflux than the flat supine position, but there is conflicting evidence on this point.

Infants with reflux are often put through "formula roulette." Cow's milk or soy-based formulas are employed and some progress to partially digested or elemental formulas. There is a select group of infants with regurgitation that have cow's milk protein intolerance who may respond to a 2-week trial of hypoallergenic formula. This is more likely in the patient with a family history of atopy. Nearly half of infants intolerant of milk protein will also exhibit symptoms with soy; thus, protein hydrolysate formulations may be of more use. There is no indication for lactose-free cow's milk formulas in this patient population. Rice cereal may be used as a thickening agent. This does not change findings on esophageal pH monitoring, but it may decrease the frequency of regurgitation. Patients with poor weight gain will benefit from the increased caloric density of the thickened formula. One tablespoon of rice cereal per 2 oz of formula will increase the content from 20 to 27 cal/oz. Increasing amounts of rice cereal will increase the viscosity and caloric density, but this also increases osmolarity. Excessively concentrated formulas may worsen vomiting. Nipples used with thickened formula will need to be tailored by crosscutting, but this may lead to increases in coughing or gagging. Formulas containing commercial "anti-regurgitant" agents are now available. Although no more effective than rice cereal for regurgitation, they do not increase the caloric density and may require less energy to pull from the nipple. This must be balanced with the unknown long-term risks of these newer ingredients as well as the increased cost.

Environmental and dietary factors have been studied in the older child and teenager. Currently only caffeine, chocolate, and spicy foods that provoke symptoms should be avoided. Obesity and exposure to tobacco smoke have also been implicated.

Medications

The pharmacologic agents used in reflux disease are felt to be safe and, therefore, sometimes used empirically without diagnostic confirmation (Table 112-1). Although this approach may be useful in adolescents for up to 4 weeks, it should be used with caution in infants or young children. There is emerging evidence of harm from acid suppression, especially proton pump inhibitors (PPIs), although acid suppression is the mainstay of treatment. The goal is to reduce exposure of the esophagus to acid. There are 3 main types of drugs that can be used: antacids, H_2-receptor antagonists (H_2RAs), and PPIs. The only clinically effective antacids are those that contain aluminum, which has been associated with bone and nervous system toxicity, especially in infants. H_2-receptor antagonists inhibit acid production in the gastric parietal cell. They are effective in the healing of esophagitis; however, tachyphylaxis has been seen as early as 1 week after initiation. Further complicating this class of medications are side effects such as fussiness that may be mistaken for reflux symptoms. Cimetidine and famotidine have the most evidence for effective and safe use in pediatrics.

Proton pump inhibitors bond and deactivate hydrogen, irreversibly inhibiting hydrogen potassium adenosinetriphosphatase, the final pathway of gastric acid. Proton pump inhibitors should be taken 30 minutes prior to a meal so that the drug is in the bloodstream in the largest concentration at mealtime. Omeprazole, lansoprazole, and esomeprazole have been studied in children. No PPI has been approved for use in infants younger than 1 year. Proton pump inhibitors may be used as the initial drug or following failure of H_2RAs.

There are emerging studies in children and adults showing adverse effects from long-term acid suppression. Up to 14% of

Table 112-1. Pharmacologic Agents Used for Reflux Disease		
Drug	**Pediatric Dose**	**Adverse Effects**
Cimetidine	20–40 mg/kg/d, divided 3–4 times per d	Hypotension, gynecomastia, reduced hepatic metabolism of other drugs, neutropenia, agranulocytosis, thrombocytopenia
Famotidine	0.5–1 mg/kg/d divided every day to twice per d	Headache, dizziness, constipation, diarrhea
Omeprazole	0.7–3.3 mg/kg/d divided every d to twice per d	Headache, diarrhea, abdominal pain, nausea, rash, vitamin B_{12} deficiency, constipation
Lansoprazole	15 mg (weight <30 kg) 30 mg (weight >30 kg)	Headache, nausea, constipation, diarrhea, abdominal pain, proteinuria, hypotension, elevated transaminases
Metoclopramide	0.1 mg/kg/dose 4 times per d before meals	Drowsiness, restlessness, dystonia, gynecomastia, galactorrhea
Erythromycin	3–5 mg/kg/dose 3–4 times per d before meals	Diarrhea, vomiting, cramps, antibiotic effect, pyloric stenosis

patients can have side effects of headache, diarrhea, constipation, or nausea. Increased rates of community-acquired pneumonia, gastroenteritis, and necrotizing enterocolitis have been described. Adult studies have shown increased hip fractures and vitamin B_{12} deficiency, suggesting malabsorption secondary to hypochlorhydria, but these have not been reproduced in children. Further studies are needed to understand the significance of these adverse effects. Currently, the efficacy of empiric therapy with PPI in children is not established and empiric therapy should be used with caution, especially in young children. Administration of long-term acid suppression without a diagnosis is inadvisable. When acid suppression is required, the smallest effective dose should be used.

Prokinetic agents are indicated in the patient with evidence of delayed gastric emptying. Cisapride, a mixed serotonergic agent, was the model drug for this class. It has been shown to improve reflux symptoms and pH parameters in infants. However, it has been associated with QT prolongation and arrhythmia with some deaths. The use of cisapride has been severely restricted since 2000. Other drugs in the group are less likely to improve reflux but are still widely used. Metoclopramide also has mixed serotonergic effects, in addition to anti-dopaminergic and cholinomimetic actions. Adverse effects, including central nervous system complications, limit the use of this drug; it now carries a black box warning from the US Food and Drug Administration. Erythromycin is a motilin receptor agonist that is also used less commonly in GERD. There is evidence that its use in pregnancy or young infants may increase the risk of pyloric stenosis. Many interactions have been seen with this macrolide antibiotic, which also limits its use. Thus, potential adverse effects of currently available prokinetic agents outweigh the potential benefits of these medications for treatment of GERD.

Buffering agents, alginate, and sucralfate are useful on demand for occasional heartburn. Chronic use of buffering agents or sodium alginate is not recommended for GERD because some have absorbable components that may have adverse effects with long-term use. Special caution is required in infants.

Antireflux Procedures

Patients who continue to have reflux on maximum medical therapy or those who have serious extra-esophageal manifestations, such as recurrent aspiration, should be considered for surgery. Patients requiring long-term drug therapy may also be selected for surgery. The most popular procedure is the Nissen fundoplication. The laparoscopic approach to fundoplication is used widely and entails a full wrap of the fundus of the stomach around the esophagus to increase LES tone and create a more acute angle of His. More than 90% of patients remain symptom-free up to 11 years postoperatively. Complications, including gas bloat, dumping syndrome, and dysphagia, are reported at variable frequencies. Failure rates are higher in neurologically impaired children and those with esophageal atresia repair. There are several other fundoplication procedures that have variable degrees of wrapping.

Significant delay in gastric emptying may require an additional surgical procedure at the gastric outlet. Pyloroplasty enhances the exit from the stomach. There is some concern that fundoplication itself results in accelerated gastric emptying and additive effects of pyloroplasty might result in dumping of gastric contents into the duodenum too rapidly, but this has not been shown to be a significant problem, and this procedure should be given strong consideration in infants or children with documented moderate or severe delayed gastric emptying.

Endoscopic antireflux procedures have mixed results in adults. The most studied and effective is trans-oral incisionless fundoplication (TIF), which involves placing sutures through the gastroesophageal junction, pleating the mucosa and reinforcing LES. Pediatric experience with TIF is limited to a few dozen cases. The preliminary results showed that the procedure is safe and efficacious in a highly selected group of older children and adolescents.

Prognosis

Complications arising from untreated GERD include esophagitis, Barrett syndrome, strictures, and esophageal adenocarcinoma and aspiration. However, most infants with GER have a more favorable outcome. Regurgitation resolves in most children by 18 months and is absent by 24 months in 98%. There is some evidence that a portion of patients who become asymptomatic will continue to have abnormal histology in the esophagus at follow-up endoscopy. Therefore, it is unclear if the disease process continues into later childhood. Future studies that follow infants with reflux longitudinally into adulthood will be of great benefit. There is much to be learned in the area of nonacid reflux and its role in respiratory disease as intraluminal impedance becomes more widely used.

Children with persistent reflux symptoms into later childhood have a worse prognosis. Patients with a history of esophageal atresia repair or severe neurologic injury may have a poor prognosis, often requiring high-dose medication or antireflux surgery. They are more likely to suffer from complications of GERD.

CASE RESOLUTION

This child has infrequent emesis that does not impose any threat to his health. This is a classic example of the so-called "happy spitter" who does not need a workup unless the symptoms persist beyond the second year of life.

Selected References

Michail S. Gastroesophageal reflux. *Pediatr Rev.* 2007;28(3):101–110

Rosen R. Gastroesophageal reflux in infants: more than just a pHenomenon. *JAMA Pediatr.* 2014;168(1):83–89

Rudolph CD, Hassall E. Gastroesophageal reflux. In: Walker WA, Goulet O, Kleinman RE, Sherman PM, Shneider BL, Sanderson IR, eds. *Pediatric Gastrointestinal Disease: Pathophysiology, Diagnosis, Management.* 5th ed. Hamilton, Ontario, Canada: BC Decker Inc; 2008:59–72

Vandenplas Y. Gastroesophageal reflux. In: Wyllie R, Hyams JS, Kay M, eds. *Pediatric Gastrointestinal and Liver Disease.* 4th ed. Philadelphia, PA: Elsevier; 2012:232–247

Vandenplas Y, Rudolph CD, Di Lorenzo C, et al. Pediatric gastroesophageal reflux clinical practice guidelines: joint recommendations of the North American Society for Pediatric Gastroenterology, Hepatology, and Nutrition (NASPGHAN) and the European Society for Pediatric Gastroenterology, Hepatology, and Nutrition (ESPGHAN). *J Pediatr Gastroenterol Nutr.* 2009;49(4):498–547

van der Pol RJ, Smits MJ, van Wijk MP, Omari TI, Tabbers MM, Benninga MA. Efficacy of proton-pump inhibitors in children with gastroesophageal reflux disease: a systematic review. *Pediatrics.* 2011;127(5):925–935

CHAPTER 113

Gastrointestinal Bleeding

George Gershman, MD

CASE STUDY

A 4-year-old boy is evaluated for intermittent passing of bright red blood from the rectum for 2 weeks. Blood coats the stool or appears as a spot after a bowel movement. The mother reports no vomiting, diarrhea, loss of appetite, weight loss, fever, or abdominal pain. The boy has no history of constipation, straining, or pain with defecation and is taking no medications. The family has no pets and has not traveled recently.

On physical examination, the boy is a well-appearing, energetic, interactive youngster. Weight and height are at the 75th percentile for age. The abdomen is soft, flat, and non-tender, and bowel sounds are normally active. No organomegaly or masses are evident. No rashes, bruising, or hemangiomas are present. No tags, fissures, or fistulas are seen on close visual inspection of the perianal area. Digital rectal examination reveals normal sphincter tone, and a small, mobile, pealike mass is palpable in the rectal vault. A film of bright red blood is present on the glove after the examination. A complete blood cell count with platelet count and a prothrombin and partial thromboplastin time determination yield normal results.

Questions

1. What is a proper way to assess the children with gastrointestinal (GI) bleeding?
2. What are the specific characteristics of upper and lower GI tract bleeding?
3. What age-related conditions account for upper and lower GI tract bleeding in children?
4. What is the appropriate approach to the child with GI bleeding?
5. How does the physician decide what type of management is appropriate for a given patient?

Bleeding from the gastrointestinal (GI) tract in infants and children is always stressful and frightening for patients and their parents. It can also be challenging for a physician, especially if bleeding is severe, though fortunately, life-threatening GI bleeding is rare in pediatric practice. However, a pediatrician or emergency department physician should be prepared to initiate effective resuscitation and a diagnostic workup focusing on common age-specific causes of GI bleeding. The primary goal of this approach is a reduction of morbidity associated with significant hemorrhage.

Epidemiology

The incidence of bleeding from the upper GI tract (upper GI bleeding) among infants and children is unknown. Clinical experience suggests that the incidence in children is significantly less than in adults. This assertion is supported indirectly by epidemiologic data from the United Kingdom and United States, which indicate that the incidence of upper GI bleeding in adults younger than 29 years is approximately 18 to 23 per 100,000 adults per year, which is almost 4 to 5 times lower than among older age groups. However, the risk of upper GI bleeding is higher (between 6.2% and 10.2%) in infants and children admitted to pediatric intensive care units.

Despite the fact that rectal bleeding is quite common in pediatric practice, the epidemiology of this problem is not well established. In one study, rectal bleeding was a chief complain of 0.3% of all visits to a tertiary emergency department during a 10-month period.

Clinical Presentation

Bleeding into the GI tract can be manifest as hematemesis, melena, occult bleeding, or hematochezia.

Hematemesis is vomiting of bright-red "fresh" blood or "coffee ground" (dark-brown) "old" blood exposed to hydrochloric acid. Usually, hematemesis reflects acute bleeding from the esophagus, stomach, or proximal duodenum. Swallowed maternal blood in neonates and epistaxis in older children should be ruled out to avoid unnecessary invasive procedures.

Melena is characterized as liquid, coal-black, shiny, sticky, tarry, foul-smelling stool. It suggests bleeding from the upper GI tract. Occasionally, bleeding from the ileum can be associated with melena. However, in this case, the stool is black but not tarry. Melena suggests a minimum loss of 50 to 100 mL in adults or 2% of the blood volume in children. Stool may remain black or tarry for a few days after massive hemorrhage even though active bleeding has ceased.

Occult bleeding is the presence of an invisible quantity of blood in stool. It is usually chronic, recurrent losses of small amounts of blood, which often lead to severe microcytic anemia. The most commonly used technique for detection of blood in stool is the Hemoccult stool test. This test is based on the chemical reaction of a dye (guaiac) with peroxidase-containing substances and hydrogen peroxide. It is not specific for the presence of blood (hemoglobin) in stool. False-positive results could be secondary to peroxidase activity in food products such as cantaloupes, radishes, bean sprouts, cauliflower, broccoli, grapes, and red meat or iron preparations. False-negative results of the Hemoccult test are associated with prolonged colonic transient time and bacterial degradation of hemoglobin to porphyrin, which does not have peroxidase activity.

Currently, fecal immunochemical test is available for detection of blood in stool based on labeling of human hemoglobin by specific antibodies. The test does not require a special diet. It is more specific for the detection of bleeding from the colon due to enzymatic digestion of the hemoglobin from the upper GI tract.

Hematochezia is the passage of bright-red or maroon-colored blood from the rectum. This may be pure blood, bloody diarrhea, or blood mixed with stool. As a rule, it is a sign of lower GI bleeding from the distal colon or, less frequently, from the right colon or distal ileum. Rarely, hematochezia may occur in children with massive bleeding from the duodenum.

Pathophysiology

Compensatory responses to acute bleeding facilitate a restoration of depleted intravascular volume, maintenance of a normal cardiac output (CO) and adequate oxygenation of vital organs (ie, brain, heart, lungs, and adrenal gland), and mobilization of internal energy stores.

Two parameters determine the degree of compensation: volume of blood loss and velocity of bleeding.

Mild Blood Loss (<15% of Circulatory Volume) or Class 1 Bleeding

Relatively slow blood loss of less than 15% of the blood volume triggers redistribution of depot blood from the venous system to the systemic circulation and a shift of extracellular fluids into the vascular space. Adequate CO without changes in heart rate and blood pressure is maintained and there are no hemodynamic abnormalities. However, a rapid blood loss (even <10% of blood volume) may compromise CO and trigger tachycardia and other compensatory mechanisms to restore normal blood circulation.

Moderate Blood Loss (Between 15% and 30% of Circulating Volume) or Class 2 Bleeding

Blood loss of more than 15% of the blood volume leads to tachycardia, an increased systemic vascular resistance caused by activation of the sympathetic nervous system and hypothalamic-pituitary-adrenomedullary axis. In children, CO depends on heart rate rather than stroke volume due to a smaller ventricular mass. With hemorrhage, tachycardia is the principal mechanism for maintenance of an adequate CO in pediatric patients; however, prolonged tachycardia increases myocardial oxygen demand and decreases diastolic-dependent coronary perfusion. This eventually leads to cardiovascular decompensation if fluid resuscitation is delayed or insufficient.

Normal blood pressure and adequate perfusion of vital organs in children with moderate bleeding is maintained by increased systemic vascular resistance and redistribution of blood from skin, muscle, splanchnic organs, and kidney to the brain, heart, lungs, and adrenal gland due to local production of adenosine, nitric oxide, and prostaglandins. Therefore, blood pressure is a poor indicator of cardiovascular homeostasis in children with moderate GI bleeding. In contrast, persistent tachycardia is the red flag of pending cardiovascular collapse.

Severe Blood Loss (>30% of Circulating Volume) or Class 3 Bleeding

Failure of compensatory mechanisms and decreased CO leads to hypotension and tissue hypoxia. Compensatory tachypnea contributes to respiratory alkalosis in the initial phase of severe bleeding. Tissue hypoxia compromises mitochondria functional capacity to generate energy as adenosine triphosphate. This leads to metabolic acidosis due to excessive production of lactic acid and cellular death.

Hypoperfusion of the kidney causes acute spasm of the preglomerular arterioles and acute tubular necrosis and renal failure. Hypoxia and excessive cytokine production can induce liver failure—sudden onset of jaundice due to hepatocellular necrosis, elevation of transaminases, coagulopathy, hypoglycemia, and encephalopathy. Myocardial ischemia is a common consequence of severe bleeding. Sepsis, thrombotic microangiopathy, and a systemic inflammatory response syndrome may occur in the late stages of uncontrolled or inadequately treated severe hemorrhage.

Evaluation

The initial assessment of the child with suspected GI bleeding should be focused on signs of hemodynamic instability and clues for the etiology of bleeding. Four major questions must be answered promptly.

1. Is the patient stable?
2. Is the bleeding real?
3. What is the source of bleeding?
4. What is the best treatment option?

The first and the most important step in the initial assessment of the child with suspected GI bleeding is recognition of hemodynamic instability (Box 113-1).

A prompt assessment of estimated blood loss and the degree of hemodynamic instability should be done using objective criteria, such as mental status, skin color, capillary refill, pulse, blood pressure, and orthostatic maneuvers (Table 113-1). Special attention should be focused on tachycardia and narrowed pulse pressure, which are the earliest signs of impending shock. Hypotension usually occurs in the late phase of shock in children and is an ominous finding. The value of the initial hematocrit may not accurately reflect the severity of blood loss. First, the hematocrit does not fall immediately with hemorrhage due to proportionate reductions of plasma and red cell volumes. Second, the hematocrit begins to fall due to compensatory restoration of the intravascular volume by the shift of extra vascular fluids into the vascular bed. This process begins shortly after the onset of bleeding; however, it is not complete for 24 to 72 hours. At this point, plasma volume is larger than normal and the hematocrit reaches its true nadir, assuming that bleeding has stopped.

Box 113-1. Procedural Management of Gastrointestinal Bleeding

Endoscopic Hemostasis of Non-varicose Bleeding
Indications
- Active bleeding from a gastric or duodenal ulcer
- Stigmata of recent bleeding: a non-bleeding visible vessel in the ulcer base and a densely adherent clot
- Bleeding arteriovenous malformation
- Bleeding after polypectomy

Methods
- Injection of vasoconstrictive agent
- Thermal coagulation
  — Bipolar coagulation
  — Heater probes
  — Argon plasma coagulation device
- Metal clips

Endoscopic Hemostasis of Varicose Bleeding
Indications
- Active bleeding from esophageal or gastric varices
- History of bleeding secondary to portal hypertension
- Failure of shunting procedure

Techniques
- Sclerotherapy
- Endoscopic varicose ligation

Polypectomy
Indication
- Juvenile polyps <3 cm
- Multiple polyps <2 cm

Table 113-1. Clinical Manifestations of Gastrointestinal Bleeding According to Blood Loss Volume

Symptoms and Signs	Blood Loss		
	<15%	15%–30%	>30%
Normal appearance	+	–	–
Anxiety	–	+	+
Disorientation	–	–	+
Lethargy	–	–	+
Tachycardia	–	+ +	+
Pallor	–	+	+ +
Livedo reticularis	–	+	+ +
Cold extremities	–	+	+
Capillary refill >2 sec	–	+	+
Hypotension	–	–	+
Narrowed pulse pressure	–	+	+
Elevated diastolic pressure	–	+	–
Low diastolic pressure	–	–	+

Differential Diagnosis

There are 3 essential components of the diagnosis of GI bleeding.
- Confirmation that bleeding is real
- Allocation of the bleeding area to the upper versus lower GI tract
- Detection of the specific cause of bleeding

Red staining of emesis or stool can be induced by cranberries, cranberry juice, cherries, strawberries, beets, tomatoes, candies, amoxicillin, phenytoin, and rifampin. Bismuth preparations, activated charcoal, iron, spinach, blueberries, and licorice can simulate bleeding by staining emesis and coloring stool black. An appropriate history, a normal physical examination, and guaiac-negative stool are sufficient to rule out a true bleeding episode.

It is important to remember that hematemesis or melena can be secondary to epistaxis. History of recent tonsillectomy and adenoidectomy, nasal allergies, dry environment, or nose-picking habits increases the probability of epistaxis. Thorough examination of the nose and oropharynx can help to establish the right diagnosis.

Detailed history and physical examination help narrow the diagnostic workup. For example, treatment with nonsteroidal anti-inflammatory drugs (NSAIDs) is a risk factor for acute gastric ulcers and bleeding from the stomach. Jaundice, hepatomegaly, spider hemangiomas, prominent vessels of the abdominal wall, or ascites are the signs of chronic liver disease and suggestive of portal hypertension. However, GI bleeding in a febrile child with hemodynamic instability and jaundice could be secondary to sepsis-related coagulopathy or acute liver failure.

Careful assessment of the perineum can reveal anal fissures, fistulas, or perianal inflammation.

If the source of bleeding is not obvious, the placement of a nasogastric tube is very useful. A tube with the largest bore tolerable should be placed for adequate gastric lavage. A 10F to 12F sump tube is a reasonable choice for small children; a 14F to 16F tube is reasonable for older patients. Room-temperature saline is the optimal fluid for irrigation. Iced saline lavage is no longer recommended because it compromises platelet function at the bleeding site and may induce hypothermia (especially in infants) with subsequent clinically significant arrhythmia. A bloody or coffee ground aspirate indicates upper GI bleeding, if epistaxis was ruled out. The absence of blood in the stomach does not exclude upper GI bleeding because the source of hemorrhage can be in the duodenum. The presence of coffee ground fluid in gastric aspirate, which promptly clears by gastric lavage, suggests that bleeding has stopped. Failure to obtain clear return on gastric lavage indicates ongoing bleeding.

Results of blood tests give some clues to the nature of bleeding. Low hemoglobin and hematocrit with normal mean corpuscular volume (MCV) are typical for acute blood loss. Elevated blood urea nitrogen suggests volume depletion and absorption of the blood proteins in the small intestine, which supports the diagnosis of upper GI bleeding. Very low hemoglobin, hematocrit, and MCV in a hemodynamically stable patient are consistent with chronic GI blood loss.

Knowledge of common causes of GI bleeding in an age-specific group of children helps with diagnostic strategy (Table 113-2).

Table 113-2. Common Causes of Gastrointestinal Bleeding in Children

Age	Upper GI Bleeding	Lower GI Bleeding
Neonates (0–30 d)	• Swallowed maternal blood • Stress ulcers/sepsis • Hemorrhagic gastritis • Hemorrhagic disease of the newborn	• Necrotizing enterocolitis • Midgut volvulus • Congenital megacolon (Hirschsprung disease) • Vascular malformation
Infants (30 d–6 mo)	• Cow's milk or soy protein allergy • Esophagitis • Prolapse gastropathy	• Anal fissure • Allergic proctitis or enterocolitis • Intestinal lymphoid hyperplasia • Intussusception
Infants and children (6 mo–6 y)	• Epistaxis • Esophagitis • Prolapse gastropathy • Portal hypertension • Drug-induced ulcers • Gastritis • Mallory-Weiss tear	• Anal fissures • Intussusception • Meckel diverticulum • Intestinal lymphoid hyperplasia • Polyps • Infectious colitis • Hemolytic uremic syndrome • Henoch-Schönlein purpura
Children and teenagers (7–18 y)	• Epistaxis • Drug-induced gastropathy and acute ulcers • Peptic ulcer • Esophagitis • Gastritis • Portal hypertension	• Infectious colitis • Ulcerative colitis • Crohn disease • Anal fissure • Polyps

Abbreviation: GI, gastrointestinal.

In general, endoscopy is the method of choice for the diagnosis of the specific causes of acute and chronic GI bleeding related to mucosal and submucosal lesions of the GI tract. The choice of the particular type of endoscopic procedure is related to suspected pathology. Upper and lower GI endoscopy and enteroscopy are routine methods for diagnosis of diseases such as acute or peptic ulcers, esophagitis, gastritis, esophageal varices, vascular malformations, ulcerative colitis, Crohn disease, polyps, and other causes of GI bleeding. Capsule endoscopy is the minimally invasive method of endoscopic investigation of the entire small intestine. It is used for diagnosis of GI bleeding of obscure origin, usually after negative results of conventional endoscopic procedures.

Radiographs and abdominal ultrasound are useful for diagnosis of structural abnormalities such as intussusception, necrotizing enterocolitis, and malrotation.

Technetium 99m pertechnetate scan is the diagnostic procedure of choice in children with suspected Meckel diverticulum. It is 85% sensitive and 95% specific.

A tagged red blood cell scan and angiography are alternative methods used in children with active GI bleeding of obscure origin, especially when vascular anomalies or hemobilia are suspected.

Age-Associated Causes of GI Bleeding

Neonates

In healthy breastfed neonates and infants, hematemesis could be caused by swallowed maternal blood. In such cases, careful examination of maternal breast and areola can lead to correct diagnosis. In addition, the Apt test can be useful, especially in the first 3 to 4 weeks of postnatal life while concentration of fetal hemoglobin is still high. The test is based on the chemical reaction of adult hemoglobin with sodium hydroxide, which leads to a color change from bright red to yellow or crusty brown. Fetal hemoglobin is resistant to hydroxylation, and blood from the infant remains bright red.

Acute gastric or duodenal ulcers should be suspected in sick premature or full-term asphyxiated or septic newborns or patients with intracerebral bleeding, increased intracranial pressure, congenital heart disease, respiratory failure, or hypoglycemia. The typical scenario includes sudden onset of hematemesis or melena and signs of hemodynamic instability. Occasionally, severe upper GI bleeding can occur in healthy full-term neonates within the first few days of life.

Gastrointestinal bleeding is a common manifestation of necrotizing enterocolitis. The warning signs of necrotizing enterocolitis are abdominal distention, feeding intolerance with increased gastric residuals, mild diarrhea, hematochezia, or stool positive for occult blood.

Plain radiographs can be diagnostic if they show pneumatosis intestinalis or gas in the portal vein.

Rare causes of GI bleeding in the first month of life include congenital megacolon (Hirschsprung disease), midgut volvulus, duplication cyst, vascular malformation, and hemorrhagic disease of the newborn, particularly in breastfed neonates who did not receive vitamin K.

Infants Up to First 6 Months of Age

One of the leading causes of GI bleeding in infants younger than 6 months is cow's milk or soy protein allergy. The spectrum of symptoms includes recurrent vomiting, hematemesis, failure to thrive, and diarrhea with guaiac-positive stools or hematochezia.

Exclusively breastfeeding infants may develop similar symptoms on rare occasions. Elimination of cow's milk, eggs, peanuts, fish, and tree nuts from maternal diet may lead to resolution of allergic symptoms in the breastfeeding infant. For infants with persistent symptoms or whose mothers are unable to restrict their diet according to current recommendations and for formula-fed infants with cow's milk protein allergy, hypoallergenic (extensively hydrolyzed and free amino acid–based) formulas can be used to relieve the symptoms. Most infants with GI manifestations of cow's milk protein allergy will improve within the first 2 weeks of treatment.

An anal fissure is another common cause of bleeding in infants. The diagnosis is made by careful examination of the anus.

Intermittent rectal bleeding with streaks of frank blood mixed with normal-appearing stool can be secondary to intestinal lymphoid hyperplasia of the colon or terminal ileum. During endoscopy, multiple hemispheric smooth nodules of less than 4 mm can be found in clusters or diffusely throughout the GI tract. It is considered an excessive reaction of the GI tract lymphatic tissue (lymphoid follicles and Peyer patches) to food-related or other antigens. Spontaneous regression of lymphoid follicles is quite common. In addition to parental reassurance, an elimination diet for breastfeeding mothers is a reasonable initial treatment. Feeding with extensively hydrolyzed protein formula is the next therapeutic step. Corticosteroid therapy is restricted to infants with a severe form of this disease—recurrent abdominal pain, significant anemia, persistent rectal bleeding, diarrhea, and failure to thrive. In such cases, immunodeficiency has to be excluded.

Esophagitis should be suspected as a cause of bleeding in infants with a history of recurrent emesis and interrupted feeding patterns associated with crying, irritability, or arching. Patients with repaired esophageal atresia with or without tracheoesophageal fistula are at higher risk of severe reflux disease and esophagitis. Bleeding induced by esophagitis is usually recurrent and not intensive. The patients may have hematemesis with streaks of blood or guaiac-positive stool.

Infants or older children can develop minor bleeding due to prolapse of gastric mucosa into the esophagus through the gastroesophageal junction (prolapse gastropathy). This condition is manifested by recurrent emesis with food and appearance of flecks of denatured blood at the end of vomiting. The presence of large amounts of frank blood or clots at the end of recurrent emesis suggests a more serious problem, such as Mallory-Weiss tear.

Infants and Children Younger Than 7 Years

Several diseases have a higher incidence in this age group compared with other children.

The signs and symptoms of **portal hypertension** are a large-volume hematemesis, history of omphalitis secondary to catheterization of the umbilical vein, presence of splenomegaly or hepatosplenomegaly, and other stigmata of chronic liver disease, such as jaundice, spider angiomas, caput medusa, and ascites. Esophageal varices are the most common site of bleeding in children with intrahepatic-sinusoidal and extrahepatic-presinusoidal forms of portal hypertension. Two-thirds of children with portal hypertension will bleed before 5 years of age. The diagnosis is based on the presence of esophageal or gastric varices or hypertensive gastropathy during an upper GI endoscopy.

Intussusception, which is more common in the first 2 years of life, is strongly considered in infants and children with sudden onset of severe, cramping abdominal pain intercepted by pain-free episodes and currant jelly stools. A lead point is often present in children older than 2 years. Diagnosis is confirmed by ultrasonography (positive: concentric circles or the target-shaped sign) or barium enema. Hydrostatic reduction of intussusceptions is successful in more than 90% of children.

Meckel diverticulum is the most common congenital anomaly in children. It is estimated that approximately 2% of infants have a remnant of the omphalomesenteric duct. However, fewer than 5% of children will develop complications, including GI bleeding. The predominant location of Meckel diverticulum is the distal ileum (40–60 cm above the ileocecal valve). Ectopic tissue is present in up to 80% of symptomatic patients. Gastric mucosa is the most common type of ectopia. The cause of bleeding is peptic ulceration at the junction of the ectopic gastric mucosa and normal ileum, the so-called marginal ulcer. Bleeding can be massive, but it may cease spontaneously secondary to contraction of the splanchnic vessels in response to hypovolemia. This phenomenon explains the intermittent nature of bleeding from Meckel diverticulum. Bleeding is usually painless but sometimes coincides with recurrent abdominal pain.

The diagnostic procedure of choice is a technetium 99m pertechnetate scan.

Juvenile polyps may occur in as many as 1% of children, with peak incidence from 2 to 5 years of age. The common clinical presentation is recurrent, painless bleeding with a small amount of blood on formed stool. Diarrhea and tenesmus can occur when the polyp is large and located in the left colon.

Typical juvenile polyps are smooth, rounded, and red. Polyps of less than 1 cm are usually sessile; polyps larger than 1 cm have short or long stalks. Juvenile polyps are composed of normal but cystically dilated crypts embedded in an abundant lamina propria. Colonic mucosa adjacent to the large polyp has distinguished, so-called "chicken skin" appearance. Colonoscopy is indicated due to the high incidence (almost 50%) of coexisting of the rectal polyps with polyps in the more proximal portions of the colon.

Endoscopic polypectomy is the treatment of choice. There is a general consensus that a single juvenile polyp is not a premalignant condition. Therefore, removal of a solid juvenile polyp is curative. Surveillance colonoscopy is not indicated unless the child develops a new episode of rectal bleeding.

Hemolytic uremic syndrome (HUS) should always be suspected in infants and toddlers with bloody diarrhea, which is present in three-quarters of children with epidemic HUS. In two-thirds of these children, *Escherichia coli* O157:H7 can be isolated. Bloody diarrhea in HUS results from hemorrhagic colitis caused by the presence of endothelial damage produced by verotoxin and Shiga toxin and submucosal hemorrhages. Tenesmus is common. Diffuse, severe abdominal pain with peritoneal signs can occur.

The presence of the so-called thumbprinting sign on a contrast enema or a computed tomography scan reflects a submucosal hemorrhage of the colon. Colitis-related symptoms last no longer than a week, followed by signs of hemolytic anemia and oliguria. Known GI complications of HUS are intussusception, pancreatitis, and intestinal obstruction. Small or large bowel perforation may occur during peritoneal dialysis, which may be performed to manage the acute renal failure that can accompany HUS.

Henoch-Schönlein purpura is most common in children younger than 7 years; the median age is 4 years. It should be suspected in children with sudden onset of severe diffuse abdominal pain, vomiting, and hematochezia following a viral illness during the winter and early spring and about a week after the appearance of purpuric-type skin lesions on the buttocks or lower extremities.

On rare occasions, GI manifestations may precede the skin rash. Severe anemia is uncommon. The small and large bowels have different degrees of hemorrhagic lesions. These may be apparent on a small bowel radiograph series or contrast enema with coarsening of folds and thumbprinting. Abdominal pain and hematochezia are self-limited. Treatment with corticosteroids is controversial, although it may shorten the course of GI symptoms of abdominal pain by 1 or 2 days.

Children 7 Years and Older

The common causes of GI bleeding in this age group are listed in Table 113-2.

Drug-induced gastritis or acute ulcer should be strongly suspected in children treated with NSAIDs or oral steroids. The degree of bleeding ranges from mild to moderate. Typical clinical presentation is the sudden onset of abdominal discomfort followed by hematemesis or melena. Two types of lesions can occur: gastropathy or acute gastric ulcers due to alteration of the mucosal microcirculation, and mucosal cytoprotection related to suppression of local synthesis of prostaglandins. The incidence of NSAID-related GI bleeding is much higher in patients with *Helicobacter pylori* gastritis. Therefore, eradication of *H pylori* infection is recommended before long-term therapy with NSAIDs.

Although **peptic ulcer disease** is relatively rare in pediatric patients, it accounts for at least one-third of the cases of upper GI bleeding in school-aged children. Most bleeding ulcers are located in the duodenal bulb. At least 80% of bleeding episodes from duodenal ulcers cease spontaneously. However, if the bleeding is arterial, it may become life-threatening. Urgent endoscopy is necessary as soon as the patient becomes more stable after fluid resuscitation.

Risk factors for recurrent bleeding are large ulcer (>2 cm), location of the ulcer on the posteroinferior wall of the duodenal bulb, blood spurting from the base of the ulcer, a visible vessel, or an adherent clot. In these circumstances, the risk of recurrent bleeding is relatively high even after initially successful endoscopic hemostasis and acid suppression with intravenous (IV) infusion of proton pump inhibitors. The most critical time for re-bleeding is the first 3 days following the initial hemostasis.

The risk of recurrent bleeding is minimal in children with a clear base ulcer or a pigmented spot sign, a small flat thrombus in the center of an ulcer. Endoscopic hemostasis is not indicated in these cases. Hemodynamically stable children without the endoscopically identified risk factors can be managed safely on an outpatient basis.

Colitis is the most common cause of rectal bleeding in older children and teenagers. Infectious colitis is by far more common than inflammatory bowel disease. In general, bacterial colitis is an acute, self-limited disorder manifested by sudden onset of fever, tenesmus, and bloody diarrhea lasting from 5 to 7 days.

Chronic diarrhea (lasting ≥2 weeks) is usually associated with chronic inflammatory bowel disease. Rare causes of chronic infectious colitis are *Yersinia enterocolitica,* tuberculosis, *Entamoeba*

histolytica, Strongyloides stercoralis, and opportunistic infections in immunocompromised patients.

Clostridium difficile colitis should be ruled out, especially in children treated with antibiotics or hospitalized patients.

Ulcerative colitis usually presents with insidious onset of diarrhea, nocturnal diarrhea, and subsequent hematochezia. Clinical manifestations of moderate to severe forms of ulcerative colitis include bloody diarrhea, abdominal cramps, urgency to defecate, malaise, anorexia with weight loss, intermittent low-grade fever, and some degree of anemia and hypoalbuminemia.

Crohn disease has a more indolent onset associated with abdominal pain, diarrhea, poor appetite, and weight loss. Diarrhea is not grossly bloody unless there is bleeding from an anal fistula or colitis that is diffuse or left-sided.

Differentiation between bacterial colitis and the early stage of chronic inflammatory bowel disease is always a challenge. A high index of suspicion and negative bacterial stool culture results, including *Yersinia* species and other rare pathogens, are essential parts of early diagnosis. The definitive diagnosis of chronic inflammatory bowel disease is based on the results of upper and lower GI endoscopy including multiple biopsies.

Management

It is imperative to initiate **resuscitation** of the hemodynamically unstable patient almost immediately before any diagnostic procedure is considered. Two large-bore peripheral IV lines or a central line should be placed and secured. Blood has to be typed and cross-matched and sent for baseline laboratory assessment of hemoglobin, hematocrit, MCV, platelet count, electrolytes, creatinine, blood urea nitrogen, liver enzymes, and clotting factors. Oxygen supplementation and large boluses of saline target restoration of circulation and tissue oxygenation. The volume of isotonic solution should be sufficient to improve tachycardia and reverse narrow pulse pressure. Blood transfusion is indicated for patients with

- Persisted tachycardia, abnormal pulse pressure, or orthostatic hypotension after replacement of 15% to 20% of blood volume with isotonic solution
- Estimated blood loss of 30% or more
- Hemoglobin of 6 g/dL or less
- Uncontrolled bleeding
- Hemorrhagic shock
- Hemoglobin of 7 to 9 g/dL in children with chronic heart and lung diseases and signs of hypoxia

Packed red cells are the product of choice for replacement of blood loss. Matched whole blood is preferred for patients with massive bleeding. Fresh-frozen plasma is indicated for children with suspected or documented clotting factor deficiency, including those with acute or chronic liver disease. Platelet transfusion is indicated in rare cases of severe bleeding with estimated blood loss of more than 50% of the patient's blood volume or children with active hemorrhage and platelet count less than 50,000/mm³. Early blood transfusion is reasonable for children with active bleeding and known chronic heart or lung diseases. Monitoring of vital signs is a more accurate way to assess the effect of blood transfusion than monitoring of hematocrit soon after transfusion. It is reasonable to wait 6 hours before checking a posttransfusion hematocrit.

Octreotide (a synthetic somatostatin analogue) is effective adjuvant medical therapy of severe bleeding from esophageal or gastric varices. It should be given to the child with active hemorrhage and any evidence of chronic liver disease or previously diagnosed portal hypertension. The initial IV bolus of 1 μg/kg is followed by continuous infusion of octreotide with the initial rate of infusion as 1 μg/kg/h. The dose can be increased every 6 hours up to 5 μg/kg/h.

Endoscopic hemostasis is a gold standard therapy for moderate to severe upper GI bleeding related to peptic ulcer disease, esophageal or gastric varices, and vascular malformation.

Surgery should be reserved for children with severe uncontrolled bleeding from a known source or specific disorders, such as Meckel diverticulum.

Prognosis

The prognosis for infants and children with GI bleeding depends on the condition causing the bleeding. Early, aggressive treatment of the consequences of blood loss is essential to decreasing morbidity and mortality. Generally, prognosis is good, and overall mortality is less than 5%.

CASE RESOLUTION

The young child in the case study with episodic, painless rectal bleeding has a juvenile polyp. The polyp was palpable on digital rectal examination. A colonoscopy was negative for additional polyps. Polypectomy was performed without complications. Histologic examination of the removed neoplasm confirmed the diagnosis of juvenile polyp.

Selected References

Abd El-Hamid N, Taylor RM, Marinello D, et al. Aetiology and management of extrahepatic portal vein obstruction in children: King's College Hospital experience. *J Pediatr Gastroenterol Nutr.* 2008;47(5):630–634

Boyle JT. Gastrointestinal bleeding in infants and children. *Pediatr Rev.* 2008; 29(2):39–52

Durno CA. Colonic polyps in children and adolescents. *Can J Gastroenterol.* 2007;21(4):233–239

du Toit G, Meyer R, Shah N, et al. Identifying and managing cow's milk protein allergy. *Arch Dis Child Educ Pract Ed.* 2010;95(5):134–144

Goyal A, Treem WR, Hyams JS. Severe upper gastrointestinal bleeding in healthy full-term neonates. *Am J Gastroenterol.* 1994; 89(4):613–616

Gugig R, Rosenthal P. Management of portal hypertension in children. *World J Gastroenterol.* 2012;18(11):1176–1184

Kalach N, Bontems P, Koletzko S, et al. Frequency and risk factors of gastric and duodenal ulcers or erosions in children: a prospective 1-month European multicenter study. *Eur J Gastroenterol Hepatol.* 2010;22(10):1174–1181

Reveiz L, Guerrero-Lozano R, Camacho A, Yara L, Mosquera PA. Stress ulcer, gastritis, and gastrointestinal bleeding prophylaxis in critically ill pediatric patients: a systematic review. *Pediatr Crit Care Med.* 2010;11(1):124–132

Sagar J, Kumar V, Shah DK. Meckel's diverticulum: a systemic review. *J R Soc Med.* 2006;99(10):501–505

CHAPTER 114

Diarrhea

George Gershman, MD

CASE STUDY

A 10-year-old boy is evaluated for a 10-lb weight loss, fatigue, poor appetite, abdominal and joint pain, and bloody diarrhea for the last 5 months. He reports 5 to 7 bowel movements per day and frequent awaking at night due to the urge to defecate. He describes the stool as liquid and mushy with streaks of blood and mucus. Bowel movements are associated with tenesmus and the feeling of incomplete defecation. There are no ill contacts or history of recent travel. Vital signs are normal. The patient appears pale and malnourished. The mucous membranes are moist without ulcers. The abdomen is soft with mild tenderness in the left hypogastric area. Bowel sounds are active. The rectal examination is unremarkable except for the presence of gross blood.

Questions

1. What are the major categories of diarrhea?
2. What are the common infectious agents that cause diarrhea in infants and children?
3. What are the manifestations of acute and chronic diarrhea?
4. What conditions lead to prolonged diarrhea in infants and children?
5. How is diarrhea managed in infants and children?

The word *diarrhea* is derived from Greek "to flow through," and is associated with increased volume of loose stool and frequency of bowel movements. However, the number of bowel movements and consistency of stool varies significantly from person to person and type of diet. For example, some healthy breastfed infants have a bowel movement once per week, whereas others may pass stool 7 to 10 times a day. The stool of breastfed infants is usually more loose than that of bottle-fed babies.

Diarrhea is a manifestation of various disorders such as acute and chronic infection, chronic inflammatory bowel disease, food allergy or sensitivity, enzyme deficiency, hormonal imbalance, drug side effects, mucosa atrophy, and short bowel syndrome that affect absorption of nutrients and water from the small and large intestines or abnormal secretion of fluids into the intestinal lumen.

Epidemiology

Diarrhea is very common throughout the world. In the United States, acute gastroenteritis is second in frequency only to upper respiratory infections. According to the World Health Organization, 2.5 million children in Latin America, Asia, and Africa die annually from dehydration secondary to diarrhea. In contrast, approximately 400 children die from this condition in the United States each year. These children often come from lower socioeconomic classes.

In the United States, each child experiences an average of 0.9 episodes of diarrhea per year unless enrolled in a child care facility. In that case, the number increases to up to 3.2 episodes per year, a figure similar to that of children in developing nations. The leading cause of diarrhea in children in developing nations is infection with viruses, bacteria, or parasites. The severity of the infection is influenced by the underlying state of nutrition. An episode of acute gastroenteritis can precipitate severe malnutrition in marginally intact children. The fecal-oral route is the major path for the spread of infectious diarrhea. In developing nations, poor sanitation and contaminated drinking water perpetuate the problem. In the United States, contaminated food supply, such as the contamination of eggs and poultry with *Salmonella*, is associated with the spread of bacterial gastroenteritis. Puppies have been found to be a reservoir of *Campylobacter*.

Definitions

Diarrhea is defined as stool mass more than 10 g/kg/day in infants and more than 200 g/day in older children.

Acute diarrhea is characterized by the sudden onset with resolution of diarrhea within 2 weeks.

Persistent diarrhea implies an acute onset of diarrhea that lasts at least 14 days. The definition is based on acute onset diarrhea that continues beyond the expected duration of an infectious etiology.

Chronic diarrhea is defined as diarrhea lasting at least 14 days and associated with specific causes (eg, celiac disease, inflammatory bowel diseases).

Clinical Presentation

Presenting symptoms include frequent, watery stools, which may contain blood or mucus. Affected children may experience fever, vomiting, bloating, and abdominal pain. Signs and symptoms of dehydration, such as decreased skin turgor, dry mucous membranes, depressed fontanel, diminished tearing, and tachycardia, may be present. Persistent diarrhea may be associated with weight loss and failure to gain weight at an appropriate rate (D$_x$ Box).

Pathophysiology

The consistency of stool depends on the stool's water content. The movement of water through the wall of the intestine is always related to the movement of electrolytes because no active transport of water occurs. The absorption of water is associated with the active transport of sodium, and the secretion of water is associated with the electrogenic transport of chloride. Regulatory mechanisms of water and electrolyte transport across the intestine require integration of the enteric nervous system, cells in the lamina propria, and epithelial cells. This complex system works through the generation of hormone peptides, active amines, arachidonic acid metabolites, and nitric oxide. The bulk of absorbed water crosses the intestinal epithelium between the cells (tight junctions) following the osmotic gradient generated by the transport of nutrients and electrolytes. Thus, diarrhea is the reversal from the normal status of absorption to exaggerated secretion. This can be induced by 2 processes: excessive osmotic load generated by ingestion of nonabsorbable sugars, such as lactulose, or malabsorption of lactose or other nutrients, which generates an abnormal osmotic pressure inside the lumen of the intestine and water leak into the gut; and active secretion of enterocytes secondary to direct action of viral or bacterial products or toxins and different substances on the cells, particularly in the crypt areas.

Osmotic diarrhea occurs whenever digestion or absorption is impaired. In general, it is relatively small-volume diarrhea, which is dependent on oral intake and abolished with fasting. The most common causes of osmotic diarrhea are malabsorption of carbohydrate due to excessive consumption (eg, concentrated formulas, carbonated beverages) or decreased production of brush-border enzymes or the presence of nonabsorbable substances such as lactulose, sorbitol, or magnesium salts in the intestinal lumen; decreased absorptive capacity of the intestine due to acute or chronic inflammation of the small bowel mucosa (eg, acute viral gastroenteritis, cow's milk protein allergy, bacterial overgrowth, giardiasis, celiac disease); lack of pancreatic enzymes or bile acid; and decreased absorptive capacity of the small intestine secondary to congenital or acquired short bowel syndrome. Recent data suggest that disruption of the differentiation of intestinal enteroendocrine cells has profound effects on the nutrient absorption by the small intestine.

In general, non-absorbed nutrients create an osmotic load that stimulates water leak into the intestinal lumen across the tight junction. In addition, unabsorbed nutrients, such as carbohydrates, are the substrate for fermentation by colonic bacteria with liberation of short-chain organic acids, which create a secondary osmotic load in the large intestine and exacerbation of osmotic diarrhea.

Secretory diarrhea can be induced by any process, which creates a state of active intestinal secretion. In general, secretory diarrhea is associated with intestinal loss of large volumes of fluids, which continues despite cessation of eating. Secretory diarrhea can be induced by bacterial, viral (eg, rotavirus, HIV), or protozoon (*Cryptosporidium parvum* in immunocompromised children) infection or excessive secretion of several hormones and neuropeptides such as serotonin, histamine, and cholecystokinin. Secretory diarrhea is also seen with certain tumors, such as ganglioneuroblastoma, and congenital disorders of fluid and electrolyte metabolism, such as congenital chloride diarrhea. The classic example of secretary diarrhea is infection with enterotoxigenic *Escherichia coli* and *Vibrio cholerae*. Both bacteria produce toxins that bind to specific enterocyte membrane receptors and activate adenylate cyclase, and production of cyclic adenosine monophosphate (by cholera toxin and heat-labile toxin from enterotoxigenic *E coli*) or cyclic guanosine monophosphate (by heat-stable toxin produced by *E coli*). The ultimate pathway involves the opening of chloride channels and massive water loss. Secretory diarrhea is particularly common in developing nations, where it is related to infection with organisms such as enterotoxin *E coli* and *V cholerae*. In the United States, the most common cause of secretory diarrhea is rotavirus infection. Vasoactive intestinal peptide-secreting tumors such as ganglioneuroma and neuroblastoma must be considered in the diagnosis in children with persistent secretory diarrhea.

In reality, osmotic and secretory components are present in many cases of diarrhea.

Motility disorders such as pseudo-obstruction syndrome or colonic inertia can be associated with persistent nonspecific diarrhea.

Inflammatory diarrhea occurs acutely with certain infections or chronic inflammatory bowel disease. **Steatorrhea** refers to the presence of an excessive amount of fat in stools. Approximately 95% of the fat content of food should be absorbed. In infants younger than 12 months, 10% of ingested fat may appear in the stool. Fat malabsorption occurs with problems of the small intestine, including giardiasis, chronic liver and pancreatic disorders such as biliary atresia, and cystic fibrosis.

Differential Diagnosis

Acute Diarrhea

The major cause of diarrhea in infants and children is **acute gastroenteritis,** most commonly with a **viral infection.** The most

---

Dx **Diarrhea**

- Liquid stools
- Frequent stools
- Blood in stool
- Mucus in stool
- Fever
- Poor weight gain or weight loss
- Dehydration
- Vomiting
- Abdominal pain

common virus is rotavirus, which usually occurs during the winter months, hence the term winter vomiting syndrome. Infants present with a history of antecedent mild upper respiratory symptoms, followed by fever and vomiting. Watery diarrhea, which is usually free of blood or mucus, then occurs. About 10% of infected infants have signs of otitis media. Dehydration may also occur secondary to rotavirus infection. It is typically mildly hypernatremic, with serum sodium values of about 150 mEq/L. Enteric adenovirus is the second most common viral pathogen causing diarrhea. In the summer months, enteroviral infections may produce similar pathology.

The most common **bacterial agents** associated with gastroenteritis in the United States are *Shigella, Salmonella,* and *Campylobacter. Aeromonas,* a common pathogen in developing countries, is recovered in less than 1% of cases of diarrhea in the United States.

Campylobacter produce signs of colitis, with blood and mucus in the stools. Patients are usually febrile and experience abdominal cramps. As a rule, children infected with *Shigella* are sicker, with higher levels of fever and more marked leukocytosis. In addition, infants and toddlers are particularly prone to seizures. Infection with *Salmonella* may also be associated with high fever. Stools may be mucus-laden, and inflammation of the small intestine may be evident. Parasitic infections, particularly with *Giardia lamblia, Entamoeba histolytica,* and *C parvum,* may be associated with diarrhea and may follow a more protracted course. Infestation with these organisms does not usually result in fever.

Infectious conditions that do not affect the gastrointestinal (GI) tract (otitis media and urinary tract infection) may also be associated with diarrhea. Sixty percent of children with hepatitis A develop diarrhea in the first week of illness. Other conditions may also result in diarrhea. In newborns, infection with *E coli* may produce epidemic outbreaks of large, explosive, watery, green stools without blood. These outbreaks may result in closure of newborn nurseries. Changes in stool consistency in conjunction with feeding intolerance and abdominal distention could be related to necrotizing enterocolitis. It mostly affects preterm newborns. Although the exact etiology of necrotizing enterocolitis remains unknown, ischemia or reperfusion injury, exacerbated by activation of proinflammatory intracellular cascades, gut immaturity, and specifics of intestinal flora in premature newborns are the main factors. Feeding intolerance, bloody stools, pneumatosis intestinalis, and air in the portal vein are the hallmarks of the disorder. Enterocolitis may also occur in infants with Hirschsprung disease (congenital megacolon). Adrenal insufficiency, as well as certain inborn errors of metabolism such as galactosemia, may lead to diarrhea. In general, other symptoms such as vomiting occur. Infants may present in shock because of hypovolemia related to dehydration.

Food intolerance may result in diarrhea in infants as well as in older children. Overfeeding or the ingestion of large quantities of fruit juices, dried fruits, or sorbitol-containing products can produce osmotic diarrhea. Food allergies may also be associated with malabsorption. Infants with cow's milk protein allergy can suffer from diarrhea, growth retardation, anemia, hypoproteinemia, edema, respiratory symptoms, and eczema. Eosinophilia and elevated levels of immunoglobulin E are uncommon in infants with cow's milk protein allergy. Because 25% to 50% of cow's milk protein–allergic children are also soy protein–allergic, symptoms of diarrhea may not abate when soy formula is offered. However, soy formula does help infants with lactase deficiency. Congenital lactose intolerance is an extremely rare disorder. Acquired lactase deficiency is fairly common, especially in certain racial groups; it is reported in 10% of whites, 70% to 80% of African Americans, and 90% of Asians. The disorder is associated with diarrhea, cramping, bloating, and abdominal pain after consumption of lactose. The stool has an acid pH, floats because it contains air, and is positive for reducing substances. Lactase deficiency may occur following an episode of acute gastroenteritis, when the brush border of the small intestine has been disrupted.

Persistent Diarrhea

Infants and children may have a protracted course of loose stools following an episode of acute gastroenteritis. Risk factors for persistent diarrhea are

- Caloric and protein malnutrition
- Vitamin A and zinc deficiency
- Prior infection such as measles
- Male gender and young age (between 6 and 24 months)
- Young maternal age

In most cases, no cause for persistent diarrhea can be detected, but infestation with *Shigella* or enterotoxigenic *E coli* may be a contributing factor. The possibility of infection with HIV should be considered in infants and children with protracted diarrhea, especially in geographic areas where disease prevalence is high. Certain children with acute diarrhea have such a modified diet (eg, clear fluids) that they develop starvation stools. These slimy, dark green or golden stools represent the secretion of the small intestine. Starvation stools do not have a fecal odor. Insufficient fat in the diet may contribute to starvation diarrhea.

Chronic Diarrhea

Inflammatory bowel disease, which occurs more commonly in older children and adolescents, is associated with chronic diarrhea. Ulcerative colitis presents with infiltration of the lamina propria with inflammatory cells, distortion of the glands, and crypt abscesses. Fever, weight loss, and anorexia are often present. Diarrhea is the hallmark of the disease, and patients experience tenesmus as well as mucus-laden and bloody stools. Inflammation always affects the rectum. It can be localized in the left colon (left-side colitis) or spread out through the entire large intestine (pancolitis).

Crohn disease may also lead to chronic diarrhea, although lower abdominal pain aggravated by defecation may be a more prominent part of the medical history. Affected individuals frequently experience extraintestinal manifestations of the disease, such as fever, anorexia, weight loss or growth retardation, recurrent stomatitis, uveitis, arthralgia and arthritis, and clubbing. Perianal disease, such as fistulas, may be noted in 30% of patients.

Irritable bowel syndrome may lead to chronic diarrhea in infants and children. Affected children do not suffer from diarrhea at night, which is a sign of infectious or secretory diarrhea. Partially formed first stool in the morning and increased frequency during the day is the classic history. Bowel movement tends to occur after each meal, suggesting a prominent gastrocolic reflex. Children may have 3 to 10 stools per day, which may be mucus-laden and contain undigested vegetable fiber. Alternating periods of constipation may occur. Affected children appear well throughout this illness, without weight loss, growth impairment, fever, leukocytosis, steatorrhea, or protein malabsorption. Their appetite remains good. Treatment of this type of chronic diarrhea involves the use of a high-residue diet to add bulk to the stool and thereby prevent small, frequent stools. Different probiotics have been used lately for treatment of irritable bowel syndrome in children with various success rates.

Other frequent causes of chronic diarrhea are a consumption of large amount of fruit juice or carbonated beverages and side effects of medications such as antibiotics or nonsteroidal anti-inflammatory drugs.

There are many rare conditions that can lead to chronic diarrhea, such as autoimmune enteropathy, microvillus inclusion disease, and intestinal polyposis. Chronic diarrhea may also be associated with **maldigestion,** as with cystic fibrosis, or **malabsorption,** as with celiac disease or gluten enteropathy.

Newborns with **cystic fibrosis** may present with meconium ileus or, rarely, with acute appendicitis. Failure to thrive is common among patients with cystic fibrosis despite the fact that many of them have voracious appetites. Stools are large, bulky, and foul-smelling secondary to the steatorrhea. Isolated GI complaints are reported in 15% to 20% of patients with cystic fibrosis. Rectal prolapse is not uncommon. Most affected children also suffer from recurrent pneumonia and chronic pulmonary disease.

Celiac disease is related to an allergy to the gliadin portion of the wheat protein, gluten. This protein is also found in barley, rye, and oat. Characteristically, villous flattening is apparent on small intestinal biopsy. This flattening restricts the absorptive capacity of the intestine and leads to malabsorption. Children with the classic form of celiac disease have short stature, pale skin, sparse hair, protuberant abdomen, and wasted buttocks. In recent reports, subtle signs of celiac disease have been recognized and usually reflect growth failure, anemia, iron and folate deficiency, short stature, abnormal liver enzymes, dental enamel defects, osteoporosis, delayed puberty, and neurologic abnormalities. Symptoms appear a few months after grains are introduced into the diet, usually between the ages of 9 and 12 months. Stools are mushy, bulky, and foul-smelling. Fat content in the stool may be 2 to 3 times the normal level.

Evaluation

History

A careful history should be obtained (Questions Box).

Questions

Diarrhea

- How long has the diarrhea been present?
- How frequent are the bowel movements?
- What is the consistency of the stools?
- Is diarrhea related to eating, which is a sign of osmotic diarrhea, or does it occur even if the child does not eat, which is a sign of secretory diarrhea?
- Do the stools contain any blood or mucus, which suggests a bacterial or parasitic infection?
- Is the child febrile?
- Does the child have any symptoms associated with the diarrhea?
- Does the child have a history of recent travel or exposure to animals?
- Is anyone at home ill?
- Has the child experienced any change in the frequency of urination, which is an important measure of the state of hydration?
- What is the child's diet now? What has it been?

Physical Examination

Children should be assessed for the presence of dehydration: altered vital signs, delayed capillary refill, decreased skin turgor, a sunken fontanel, dry mucous membranes, and reduced tearing. Persistent severe skin changes in the perianal area should trigger a further workup to rule out acrodermatitis enteropathica. Perianal fissures may be present in Crohn disease. Evidence of growth retardation should be determined by assessing growth parameters. Failure to gain weight over a period of months should trigger the workup of GI disorders such as chronic inflammatory bowel disease, celiac disease, or cystic fibrosis.

Laboratory Tests

Stool assessment, a major component of the evaluation, involves 4 steps. First, the stool is evaluated for its quantity as well as its gross appearance. Undigested pieces of fruits and vegetables in the stool of toddlers are often a sign of poor chewing. Small, threadlike bodies that resemble worms are concretions of bile and are common in the stool of infants. The change in stool volume with fasting can also be checked. Reduced volume while fasting is consistent with osmotic diarrhea.

Second, the stool is subjected to chemical and microscopic analyses to detect the presence of unabsorbed nutrients such as carbohydrates and fats. The presence of carbohydrates may be detected using a small amount of stool liquefied in about 1 mL of water. A Clinitest tablet is added to the sample, and a change in color from blue to green or orange is indicative of the presence of undigested carbohydrate. If the main source of dietary sugar is sucrose, as determined by the history, the specimen must be hydrolyzed by heating with hydrochloric acid. If the specimen sits around for too long, the presence of bacteria in the stool may break down the carbohydrate and lead to a false-negative result. The presence of fat can be determined qualitatively and quantitatively. The stool may be examined under a microscope with just water or using a Sudan or carmine red stain. If there are 10 or more globules of fat per high-power field, a quantitative fat analysis over a 3-day period should be undertaken. Ten percent of children with abnormal stool fat on microscopic assessment have a normal 3-day quantitative stool fat value. A fecal elastase test is a valid alternative to 3 days of fecal stool collection.

Third, the stool is examined for the presence of blood and leukocytes. Blood may be present in the stool but originate from excoriations in the diaper area rather than from the GI tract. To assess for leukocytes in the stool, the mucous component of the stool should be smeared on a glass slide and stained with methylene blue. More than 2 to 4 leukocytes per high-power field is abnormal and suggests a bacterial infection. The sensitivity of the fecal leukocyte test is 85%, but the specificity is only 50% to 60%. Absence of leukocytes or erythrocytes in the stool signifies a very low probability of an invasive bacterial infection (predictive value of a negative test is 95%). A stool specimen should be submitted for culture and may be evaluated for ova and parasites. Stool analysis using Rotazyme will detect rotavirus. Fecal calprotectin and lactoferrin are sensitive and specific tests to assess the activity of chronic intestinal inflammation.

Fourth, stool is assessed for levels of sodium and potassium and stool osmolality to calculate the so-called ion gap (ion gap = stool osmolarity – [(Na + K) × 2). An ion gap exceeding 100 mOsm/kg and low sodium concentration in the stool (<40 mEq/L) is typical for osmotic diarrhea. On the contrary, an ion gap equal to or lower than 100 mOsm/kg and a sodium concentration in stool higher than 70 mEq/L is consistent with secretory diarrhea.

Additional studies, especially in the face of dehydration or fever, include serum electrolytes, complete blood cell count, urinalysis, and urine culture. Upper GI endoscopy with a small bowel biopsy is indicated for diagnosis of diseases such as celiac disease or other causes of persistent or chronic malabsorptive diarrhea. Colonoscopy should be considered after consultation with a gastroenterologist if inflammatory bowel disease or familial polyposis is suspected.

Management

Initial management of children with gastroenteritis involves **adequate oral hydration and correction of electrolyte deficits** (see Chapter 56). Intravenous fluid therapy may be necessary in children who cannot tolerate an adequate oral fluid volume. Children with significant dehydration may require admission to the hospital. Less severely affected children may be managed as outpatients using oral rehydrating solutions such as Pedialyte or Infalyte. Alternatively, parents can be advised to make oral rehydrating solutions by using water (1 L), sugar (4–8 teaspoons), and salt (½ teaspoon).

Dietary manipulation in the treatment of diarrhea is somewhat controversial. Traditionally, affected children have been placed on clear fluids for 1 or 2 days, with a gradual return to a more regular diet with time. A **BRAT diet** (*b*ananas, *r*ice or *r*ice cereal, *a*pplesauce, *t*ea or *t*oast) was often recommended because of the intrinsic binding properties of these particular foods. Recent studies recommend a full resumption of a normal diet, including dairy products, as the way to ensure adequate nutrition during the acute illness. A high-fat, low-carbohydrate diet accelerates improvement. A lactose-free diet is beneficial for infants and children with persistent diarrhea.

Antimicrobial therapy is indicated for infection with certain pathogens such as *Campylobacter*, *E histolytica*, *G lamblia*, and *Shigella*. Antimicrobial agents are used to treat *Salmonella* infection in certain populations such as neonates, immunodeficient children, and children with sickle cell anemia.

Antidiarrheal agents are not usually recommended for the management of diarrhea in children. Diarrhea is believed to be the body's way of eliminating a toxic substance that has been ingested. In addition, the diarrhea often progresses in spite of the medication, which has its most binding effect after the illness has subsided, leading to constipation.

Children with chronic diarrhea secondary to a specific condition should be managed as dictated by the particular disorder.

Prognosis

Most cases of diarrhea in infants and children in the United States are self-limited and resolve without problems. More chronic cases may lead to malnutrition. Enteral feedings or hyperalimentation may be used to ensure a good outcome. Some children require consultation with a pediatric gastroenterologist.

CASE RESOLUTION

In the case study, chronic bloody diarrhea, abdominal pain, weight loss, and other constitutional symptoms point toward the diagnosis of chronic inflammatory bowel disease. The patient should be referred to a pediatric gastroenterologist for further workup and adequate treatment.

Selected References

Chiou E, Nurko S. Functional abdominal pain and irritable bowel syndrome in children and adolescents. *Therapy*. 2011;8(3):315–331

Grimwood K, Forbes DA. Acute and persistent diarrhea. *Pediatr Clin North Am*. 2009;56(6):1343–1361

Guandalini S, Kahn SA. Acute diarrhea. In: Walker WA, Goulet OJ, Kleinman RE, et al, eds. *Pediatric Gastrointestinal Disease, Pathophysiology, Diagnosis, Management*. 5th ed. Philadelphia, PA: BC Decker; 2008:253–264

Guarino A, De Marco G. Persistent diarrhea. In: Walker WA, Goulet OJ, Kleinman RE, et al, eds. *Pediatric Gastrointestinal Disease, Pathophysiology, Diagnosis, Management*. 5th ed. Philadelphia, PA: BC Decker; 2008:265–274

Koletzko S, Osterrieder S. Acute infectious diarrhea in children. *Dtsch Arztebl Int*. 2009;106(33):539–548

Lee KS, Kang DS, Yu J, Chang YP, Park WS. How to do in persistent diarrhea of children?: concepts and treatments of chronic diarrhea. *Pediatr Gastroenterol Hepatol Nutr*. 2012;15(4):229–236

Limbos MA. Approach to the child with diarrhea. In: Osborn LM, DeWitt TG, First LR, Zenel JA, eds. *Pediatrics*. Philadelphia, PA: Mosby; 2005:627–633

Reilly NR, Fasano A, Green PH. Presentation of celiac disease. *Gastrointest Endosc Clin N Am*. 2012;22(4):613–621

Walker-Smith JA. Chronic diarrhea. In: Lifschitz CH, ed. *Pediatric Gastroenterology and Nutrition in Clinical Practice*. New York, NY: Dekker; 2002:685–700

Zella GC, Israel EJ. Chronic diarrhea in children. *Pediatr Rev*. 2012;33(5):207–218

CHAPTER 115

Constipation

Doron D. Kahana, MD, and Khalid M. Khan, MD

CASE STUDY

A 9-year-old girl is brought to the office by her mother complaining of bloody stool. The mother reports that the blood is bright red and seen on the toilet paper and dripping into the bowl—there is no blood mixed into the stool. The child complains of perianal pain that is burning during defecation and says that the bleeding is noted toward the end of the bowel movement. On further history, the child has been complaining of intermittent, colicky abdominal pain, mostly in the afternoon and evening, which are relieved with bowel movements, which are reported to be infrequent, with multiple skipped days in between. The mom recalls that the toilet has been plugged a few times after the patient used it. There has been no weight loss and the child eats an age-appropriate diet that is high in pasta, cheese, processed meat, breads, and candy. The child at times is gassy and looks bloated, but otherwise she is healthy, growing and developing normally. On examination, vital signs are normal; patient is at the 65th percentile in height and 80th percentile in weight. Abdomen is soft and non-tender but mildly full in the left lower quadrant. Perianal examination reveals a deep anal fissure, and rectal examination reveals a firm fecal mass. The rest of the examination is normal.

Questions

1. What is the definition of constipation?
2. How is the stooling pattern related to diet?
3. What conditions are associated with constipation?
4. How do familial factors influence stooling patterns?
5. What is the management of chronic constipation?

Constipation is a common and significant complaint that accounts for approximately 3% of visits to pediatric clinics and up to 25% of pediatric gastroenterology visits. Constipation is often associated with fecal incontinence and abdominal pain, can cause significant distress to the child and family, and has a significant effect on health care costs. Stools that are dry, hard, and difficult to pass define constipation. While reduced *frequency* of stooling is a common characteristic of constipation, it is not a universal characteristic. The guidelines of the North American Society for Pediatric Gastroenterology, Hepatology and Nutrition define constipation as "a delay or difficulty in defecation, present for two or more weeks and sufficient to cause significant distress to the patient." This definition is less stringent that the Rome III criteria, which divide the entity into 2 groups, based on age of the patient, with children younger than 4 years needing to meet 2 criteria for at least 1 month and those older than 4 years for at least 2 months. The 6 Rome III criteria are defecation frequency 2 times or fewer per week, fecal incontinence, retentive posturing, pain during defecation, large-diameter stools, and palpable rectal fecal mass. Average stooling frequency is 3 to 4 per day during the first weeks of life and decreases to 1 to 2 per day with introduction of table foods by 1 year of age. After age 4 and into adulthood, normal stool frequency can range from 3 per day to 3 per week.

Many factors influence the frequency of stooling in normal newborns, infants, and young children, including diet, familial pattern of intestinal motility, personal sensitivity, hygiene habits, hydration status, variable stressors, and intake of medications. Exclusively breastfed newborns and infants may have long intervals (sometimes several days) between normal bowel movements, usually starting in the third month of life, although the stool will remain loose and seedy. Introduction of solids starting at 6 months of age is often associated with additional slowdown in bowel frequency, and functional constipation may initiate as early as this time.

Functional constipation is defined as constipation in the absence of organic disease; however, it is important to note that chronic constipation is also a condition that begets disease and, thus, must be treated appropriately. Constipation is one of a number of unique medical conditions that create a positive feedback loop—stool withholding results in worsening constipation as stretch receptors accommodate a distended rectum and contractile forces fail to result in a complete evacuation.

In infancy, peristaltic motility may be weak or poorly coordinated, and the lack of physical mobility or ambulation requires the infant to exert a physiological effort (ie, Valsalva maneuver) to allow passage of stool. Parents may interpret "straining" as a sign of constipation despite the passage of soft, normal stools. Therapy in such cases, if necessary, is usually nonmedical and involves manual stimulation of the anal sphincters and bringing of the knees toward the chest in a "bicycle kick." Older infants and toddlers may have constipation secondary to food intolerance, such as cow's milk protein allergy, and removal of the inciting agent may result in complete resolution. Toilet training can prove to be a challenge, especially in constipated toddlers, and stressful parent-child interactions may result in resistance to toilet train on the part of the child.

Commonly, chronic constipation in childhood is triggered by a painful evacuation that results in an unpleasant experience. School-aged children may elect to withhold stool because of fear of toileting outside the home or because of social stressors (eg, parental divorce, bullying). Assessment of the etiology of constipation requires a careful medical history to determine the age of onset, characteristic of the stool, and presence of contributing or confounding factors. Comorbidities, such as anal fissures or overflow encopresis, may develop over time and usually signify a more chronic course.

Epidemiology

Functional constipation is a common problem in childhood, with an estimated prevalence of 3% worldwide. Prevalence of constipation in infants is lower, but it increases between the ages of 2 and 4 years. The onset often coincides with toilet training and dietary changes and is partially a product of increased colonic transit time. Prevalence of constipation in infants and toddlers is equal among males and females, but it becomes 3 times more frequent in boys than girls by age 5 years. Fecal soiling is a significant comorbidity and is reported in up to one-third of females and half of all males with severe, chronic constipation (see Chapter 55).

Clinical Presentation

Infants often present with infrequent stooling, with some parents reporting facial grimacing and grunting during defecation as well as apparent discomfort or fussiness with bowel movements, defined by Rome III as *infant dyschezia*. History of delayed passage of meconium or onset of symptoms before 1 month of age, recurrent vomiting, poor weight gain, or family history of congenital megacolon (Hirschsprung disease) or cystic fibrosis indicate the need for further evaluation. Toddlers usually present complaining of abdominal pain and reporting the passage of hard or large stools. School-aged children may present with fecal soiling, which usually represents overflow incontinence (only 10%–15% of all cases of encopresis are non-fecal retentive). Parents describe a stool-withholding posture in which the legs are clamped together and the gluteal muscles are contracted in an effort to suppress defecation (Figure 115-1). Poor appetite and episodic vomiting in severe cases are secondary to a persistent sense of fullness from a dilated and impacted colon. In infants, toxic megacolon from Hirschsprung disease can present with lethargy and signs of sepsis, peritoneal signs, and bloody diarrhea. Hydronephrosis, urinary tract infections, and enuresis are also historically associated with chronic constipation and an impacted colon.

Physical examination should include growth parameters, abdominal examination, perianal inspection, digital rectal examination, inspection of the lumbosacral region, and neurologic evaluation for tone and deep tendon reflexes. The abdomen may be distended and contain a fecal mass on palpation; anal position must be confirmed, and the presence of stool present around the anus or on the undergarments, erythema, rash, skin tags, or fissures should be noted. Lumbosacral dimple, hair tuft, gluteal cleft deviation, or sacral agenesis must be excluded.

Figure 115-1. Child exhibiting retentive posture.

Pathophysiology

What Is the Colon?

The colon is a muscular organ that processes dietary residue through bacterial fermentation, salvaging nutrients and reabsorbing more than 90% of the water that enters, and prepares stool for transient storage and eventual excretion (Figure 115-2). Fermented food residue produces gas (eg, hydrogen, methane) and short-chain fatty acids; the latter provide colonocytes with readily available fuel (via butyric acid) that enters the portal circulation for calorie salvage in the liver (eg, propionic and acetic acids). The fermentation process may release other micronutrients and vitamins (eg, vitamins K_2 and B_{12}, folic acid, biotin) and is thus an important component of colonic function.

Normal Physiology

Digested food normally takes about 2 to 6 hours to reach the cecum from the duodenum (following gastric emptying, which has a normal half-time of 60–90 minutes). The propagation of food in the small intestine occurs via peristaltic waves called the migrating motor complex. Once chyme is in the cecum, peristalsis slows down, and it may take several hours or days for it to be expelled as stool. The longer the transit time, the more extensive the water resorption and the more likely it is for the stool to be dry and hard. The rectosigmoid is the

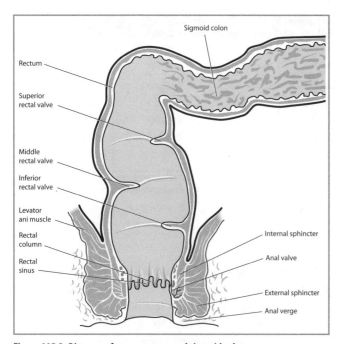

Figure 115-2. Diagram of anus, rectum, and sigmoid colon.

sensing organ that initiates the process of defecation and can store stool until it is socially acceptable to expel it. Contraction and emptying of the rectosigmoid is stimulated by eating, a process called the *gastrocolic reflex*. In the rectum, the pelvic floor muscles (levator ani, puborectalis) regulate fecal retention and defecation. The puborectalis suspends the rectosigmoid and imposes constraints that facilitate voluntary stool retention (continence). Continence is also promoted by contraction of the internal and external anal sphincters.

Defecation

The urge to defecate is signaled by the propulsion of feces from the sigmoid colon to the rectum. Distention of the rectum causes relaxation of the internal anal sphincter; the external anal sphincter and puborectalis must voluntarily relax under parasympathetic conditions. The pelvic floor muscles descend, permitting straightening of the anus and rectum (see Figure 115-2). Thus, defecation is facilitated by squatting or sitting and by increasing intra-abdominal pressure. The urge to defecate can be consciously repressed by voluntary contraction of the external anal sphincter and likely subconscious sympathetic reflex inhibition and contraction of the puborectalis muscle. The process of defecation is learned early in childhood and remains spontaneous throughout life. The spontaneity of this process may be lost for a variety of reasons, including secondary to trauma, pelvic floor dysfunction, pseudo-obstruction, or surgical resection.

The Vicious Cycle of Constipation

If the urge to defecate is suppressed, the rectosigmoid and eventually the entire colon will become dilated and impacted, and defecation may become difficult. The increased caliber of the colonic lumen makes contractions weaker and less effective in propagating stool. Moreover, the constipated child may become desensitized to rectal distention. Eventually, delayed defecation leads to formation of hard, bulky stool, which makes defecation difficult and painful. The child learns to tighten the external anal sphincter and gluteal muscles, pushing feces higher into the rectal vault and suppressing the urge to defecate—this is the vicious cycle of constipation (Figure 115-3). In children, the initiating event may be a painful evacuation, possibly after an acute illness (eg, cold, respiratory infection) or a course of antibiotics. Intentional and prolonged suppression of defecation is an important factor in the pathogenesis of chronic constipation.

Familial Factors

Some families are predisposed to constipation. Concordance for constipation is 4 times more common in monozygotic twins than dizygotic twins. It may be related to increased absorption of water or an unusually long or poorly motile colon. Poor sensitivity to a critical rectal volume or the need for a particularly large rectal volume may delay the initiation of defecation in genetically predisposed individuals.

Differential Diagnosis

The differential diagnosis of constipation can be divided into congenital versus acquired and then into the following etiologic categories: anatomic; neurologic; hormonal; infectious/toxic; drug-induced/metabolic; functional; and other, such as genetic or allergic (Box 115-1). Functional constipation is often supported by a history that includes poor dietary and hydration habits, stool-withholding behavior, and a normal physical examination. Dietary history may reveal high consumption of cow's milk (>24 oz/day), cheese, or sugary fruit juice, as well as poor intake of fruits, vegetables, and whole grains. Stool withholding is most commonly seen in young, school-aged children and often is a product of a stressful environment such as a new sibling, a move, parental struggles, or a new school environment.

Chronic constipation that is resistant to medical therapy should not be ignored. Conditions such as congenital megacolon (Hirschsprung

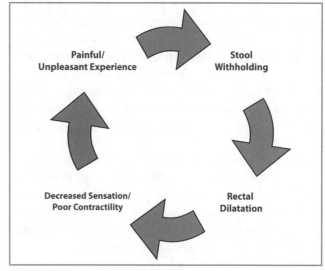

Figure 115-3. The vicious cycle of constipation.

					Drug-Induced/	
Anatomic	*Neurologic*	*Hormonal*	*Other*	*Infectious/Toxic*	*Metabolic*	*Functional*
• Anal stenosis • Imperforate anus • Ectopic anus • Postsurgical stricture	• Congenital megacolon (Hirschsprung disease) • Cerebral palsy • Hypotonia • Spina bifida (occulta) • Meningomyelocele • Sacral agenesis • Intestinal pseudo-obstruction syndrome	• Hypothyroidism • Panhypopituitarism • Multiple endocrine neoplasia • Pheochromocytoma	• Cystic fibrosis • Celiac disease • Cow's milk protein allergy or sensitivity	• Postinfectious ileus • Botulism	• Analgesics (opioids) • Antacids • Anticholinergics • Bismuth • Iron • Cholestyramine • Hypocalcemia • Hyperkalemia	• Dehydration • Stool withholding • Stress • Anxiety • Fear of painful evacuation

Box 115-1. Differential Diagnosis of Constipation

disease) and congenital intestinal malrotation can present past the neonatal period and may lead to intestinal devastation (eg, volvulus, ischemia). Several conditions are particularly important to consider when evaluating constipation in infants, including congenital megacolon, hypothyroidism, anal stenosis or atresia, meningomyelocele (occulta), and cerebral palsy. Failure to pass meconium or a delay in the passage of meconium beyond 24 hours should raise suspicion for a congenital or genetic aberration (eg, congenital megacolon, cystic fibrosis).

Congenital megacolon (Hirschsprung disease) is an intestinal motility disorder resulting from aganglionosis of the myenteric plexus that affects the rectosigmoid. In rare cases, the entire colon is involved, although in the majority of cases, the distribution is distal to proximal. The severity of the disease and complexity of surgical treatment is directly proportional to the length of the affected colon. When ganglion cells are missing in the very distal portion of the rectum, the disorder may resemble chronic idiopathic constipation, often recalcitrant to medical therapy. The prevalence of congenital megacolon is about 1 in 5,000 live births and may account for up to 3% of all cases of constipation referred to a gastroenterologist. Physical examination of a patient with congenital megacolon may reveal some degree of abdominal distention and an empty rectal vault. In infants, a rectal examination frequently induces a gush of air and an explosive stool due to digital bypass of the diseased lumen. Early recognition of this condition is important to prevent the development of toxic megacolon and enterocolitis, a condition that carries high morbidity and significant mortality. Congenital megacolon may be seen in conjunction with syndromes such as Down (trisomy 21), Smith-Lemli-Opitz, and Waardenburg, and several genetic mutations in the receptor tyrosine kinase gene *RET* have been described as responsible for the pathogenic mechanism.

Infants with hypothyroidism secondary to hypopituitarism may also present with constipation and are not diagnosed through the newborn screening process because of normal (ie, low) levels of thyroid-stimulating hormone. These children may appear clinically normal or display some of the features of hypothyroidism (eg, large fontanel, umbilical hernia, coarse facies, macroglossia).

Anal stenosis, imperforate anus with a perineal fistula, or an anteriorly displaced anus may not be recognized immediately in the newborn period because the condition may be very subtle. Anorectal malformations occur in about 1 in 7,000 live births, which reinforces the need for a perianal and rectal examination with every constipated child.

Severe constipation that begins prior to toilet training is more suggestive of an organic etiology, such as congenital megacolon, malrotation, or pseudo-obstruction. Pseudo-obstruction may present in older children with a history of intermittent constipation, abdominal distention, pain, nausea, and vomiting. Onset of constipation around the time of toilet training, when stooling had been normal in the past, suggests functional constipation.

Constipation may develop in some children in association with the use of medications such as iron or bismuth (eg, Pepto-Bismol), codeine or other narcotics, chemotherapeutic agents (eg, vincristine), and agents with anticholinergic properties (eg, pseudoephedrine, imipramine).

Evaluation

History

Commonly associated historical signs and symptoms of constipation include abdominal pain (especially during and after meals), abdominal distention, excessive flatulence, hard stools, dyschezia (painful evacuations), bright-red blood per rectum, toilet plugging, and urinary symptoms (eg, enuresis, recurrent infections) (Questions Box). Overflow incontinence may mislead the clinician to a differential diagnosis for chronic diarrhea. Fecal soiling due to stool retention and overflow is noted in many children with severe, chronic constipation, although a complete physical examination in such a setting should reveal a stool mass in the lower left abdominal quadrant and an impacted colon or rectum on digital manipulation. As with all conditions that present with abdominal pain, it is important to screen for the presence of recurrent mouth sores, skin rashes, joint pain, weight loss, bloody or mucous stools, incomplete evacuations, and tenesmus (rectal spasm accompanied by a strong urge to defecate, often with the passing of blood or mucus). Family history of

Constipation — **Questions**

- What is the child's stooling pattern? How often does the child have a bowel movement? What is the appearance and consistency of the stool?
- What was the child's age when the problem began?
- What makes up the child's diet?
- Does the child take any medications?
- Does the child have any symptoms associated with constipation, such as recurrent abdominal pain? If so, how long have these been occurring?
- Has the child been sick recently with any illnesses that might cause constipation?
- Has the child recently experienced any changes in routine that could cause constipation?
- Is there a family history of constipation?
- How old was the child when he or she was toilet trained?
- Is there any bleeding with stooling?
- Is there pain with stooling?
- Have any remedies such as laxatives, enemas, or suppositories been used to relieve the symptoms?

inflammatory bowel disease, celiac disease, irritable bowel syndrome, constipation, and atopy (eg, food allergy) should also be noted with every child presenting with abdominal pain.

Physical Examination

The physical examination in cases of functional constipation is usually normal. If the child is complaining of abdominal pain, ask the child to indicate the area of greatest pain with one finger. In functional disease, the child most often will point directly to the umbilicus. Palpation may reveal a firm stool mass in the left lower quadrant that is classically non-tender. Consistency and color of the stool in the rectum will vary, but a hard and dry stool is strongly suggestive of stool impaction. An empty rectum should raise suspicion for an organic etiology. Digital manipulation followed by an "explosive" passage of stool is suggestive of congenital megacolon (Hirschsprung disease). The back of the child should be inspected for a sacral dimple or a hair tuft, especially in infants, as this may be a sign of occult spinal cord anomaly.

Signs of pallor, mouth sores, hepatosplenomegaly, arthritis, or skin rashes may suggest another underlying disease process.

Laboratory Tests

Malnourishment is possible if the child consumes a restricted diet (eg, >24 oz of cow's milk or soda per day) or has a suggestive physical examination (eg, pallor, dry skin). Iron deficiency anemia and mineral deficiencies (eg, calcium, zinc) are signs of poor nutritional intake. A lipid panel may reveal high triglycerides (from excessive sugar intake) and low high-density lipoprotein (from poor-quality fat intake). Thyroid function may require evaluation in certain cases. Routine laboratory testing for hypothyroidism, celiac disease, and hypercalcemia is not recommended in children without alarm symptoms.

Imaging Studies

A flat plate of the abdomen is usually not indicated but may help on a clinical level by showing the child and parents the significant amount of stool present. Anatomic studies, such as a barium enema to evaluate for malrotation, a congenital stricture, imperforate anus, or congenital megacolon, may be indicated if history or physical examination is concerning. It is recommended for barium enema to be performed without a prior clean-out to sensitize the study for the presence of a transitional zone. Evidence does not support the routine use of magnetic resonance imaging of the spine in patients with constipation without other neurologic abnormalities.

Further Tests

Anorectal manometry and a suction rectal biopsy may be carried out by a gastroenterologist to help diagnose congenital megacolon (Hirschsprung disease); however, only a full-thickness rectal biopsy will confirm the presence or absence of aganglionosis and must be performed by a surgeon. Colonic manometry can also measure colonic peristaltic waves and help diagnose pseudo-obstruction and other dysmotility disorders. Evidence is conflicting for the role of allergy testing to diagnose cow's milk protein allergy or other food sensitivities.

Management

In the Primary Care Setting

Most cases of constipation can be evaluated and managed by primary care physicians. In functional constipation, the mainstay of management involves a 3-pronged approach of dietary therapy, behavioral modification, and medications (Figure 115-4).

Diets that predispose to constipation are rich in simple carbohydrates (eg, sugar), refined and processed carbohydrates (eg, pasta), saturated fat (eg, fried food), processed meat (eg, hot dogs), and dairy (especially milk and cheese). Dietary therapy should begin by decreasing the intake of these food items and increasing the intake of fruit,

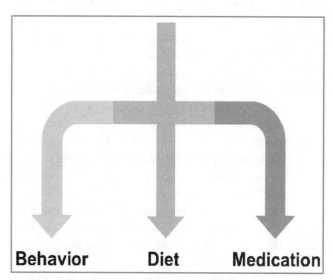

Figure 115-4. Three-pronged management of constipation.

Box 115-2. Dietary Therapy in Chronic Constipation						
Avoid/Decrease			**Introduce/Increase**			
Simple/Processed Carbohydrates	**Fat**	**Meat/Dairy**	**Fruit/Nectar**	**Dried Fruit**	**Vegetables/Roots**	**Legumes/Tree Nuts/Seeds**
• Sugar • Corn syrup • Soda • White bread • White rice • Pastries/biscuits • Pasta/macaroni • Potato/corn chips	• Fried food • Saturated fat • Trans fat • Animal fat • Gravy • Vegetable oil	• Processed meat • Red meat • Ground beef • Cold cuts • Cow's milk • Cheese • Cream	• Pears • Plums • Papaya • Peaches • Pineapple • Apples • Berries • Cantaloupe	• Prunes • Raisins • Apricots • Cranberries • Cherries • Dates	• Asparagus • Broccoli • Cauliflower • Carrots • Spinach • Yams • Parsnip • Celery • Beets	• Red beans • Garbanzo beans • Peas • Cashews • Almonds • Walnuts • Pistachios • Sunflower seeds • Flaxseed

vegetables, whole grains, legumes, and tree nuts. Prune juice and fruit nectars (eg, pear, peach, apricot) may be supplemented, are well tolerated and effective, and may be mixed with the child's favorite drink. Most fruit, such as pears, papaya, and cantaloupe, as well as vegetables, roots, and tree nuts are high in beneficial fiber. Dried fruit (eg, raisins, cranberries) are rich in sorbitol and thereby cathartic. It is important to continuously introduce new food items to the diet, especially fruit and vegetables. Introduction of certain foods, such as whole-grain breads and brown rice, may need to be gradual and require some adjustment but will render lifelong benefits (Box 115-2).

Behavior modification can be challenging, but it is absolutely essential to breaking the vicious cycle. Teaching of proper toilet hygiene to the child should be done in a firm and consistent manner; engaging the child with a sticker or star chart may help. In short, it is recommended that the child sit on the toilet once or twice daily for 8 to 10 minutes at a time, preferably after a meal (taking advantage of the gastrocolic reflex). Longer toilet sitting should be discouraged because it may lead to perianal disease such as a fissure or hemorrhoids. Even if the child fails to have a bowel movement with each toilet sitting, good toilet hygiene will make the experience routine and hopefully help prevent further reluctance to use the toilet. Biofeedback is useful when available, especially in children with encopresis or paradoxical contraction of the external anal sphincter.

Medications are generally safe and largely over the counter (Box 115-3). The 2 most commonly used medications are polyethylene glycol (PEG 3350), a nonabsorbable high–molecular weight synthetic polymer (non-fermentable), and lactulose, a nonabsorbable high–molecular weight sugar (fermentable). Both work by helping the colon retain water and thus prevent the complete dehydration of stool. Lactulose is a prebiotic that is fermented into short-chain fatty acid and can beneficially lower stool pH; however, the process may cause gassiness and bloating in some patients, and therefore dosing may need to be increased gradually. Suppositories or enemas are often avoided nowadays, as is manual disimpaction, because high-dose polyethylene glycol administration showed equal efficacy with less invasiveness. Mineral oil is useful in lubricating hard stool and decreasing the pain associated with fissures; however, it should not be given to infants or neurologically impaired

patients because of risk of aspiration and chemical pneumonitis. Dietary fiber supplements (ie, prebiotics), such as psyllium husk, guar gum, inulin, and fructosan, are helpful for maintenance therapy. Probiotics, notably the strains *Lactobacillus reuteri, L plantarum, Bifidobacterium longum, B breve,* and *B animalis* subsp *Lactis,* have also shown usefulness in the therapy of constipation.

The most important element in the management of functional constipation is persistence and long-term therapy. Several months of medication and follow-up (eg, 6–12) are often needed, as the colon needs to heal from a chronic injury to regain regularity. Dietary changes and toilet hygiene should be incorporated into a healthy lifestyle and practiced into adulthood.

When to Refer to a Gastroenterologist

Constipation that is refractory to medical therapy should not be ignored. Although uncommon, anatomic aberrations (eg, malrotation), congenital megacolon (Hirschsprung disease), and intestinal pseudo-obstruction may present after infancy and lead to toxic megacolon or intestinal or colonic volvulus, resulting in intestinal ischemia and devastation. These conditions may require surgical

Box 115-3. Pharmaceutical and Supplement Therapy in Constipation		
Osmotic Laxatives	**Psyllium Husk**	**Prebiotics/Probiotics**
• Polyethylene glycol • Lactulose • Magnesium hydroxide • Phosphate	• Bulking agents • Guar gum • Bran • Calcium polycarbophil • Methylcellulose	• Inulin • Fructo-oligosaccharide • *Lactobacillus reuteri, L plantarum* • *Bifidobacterium longum, B animalis, B breve*
Lubricant/Detergent	**Stimulants**	**Enemas/Suppositories**
• Mineral oil • Docusate sodium	• Senna • Bisacodyl	• Phosphate • Saline • Mineral oil • Glycerin

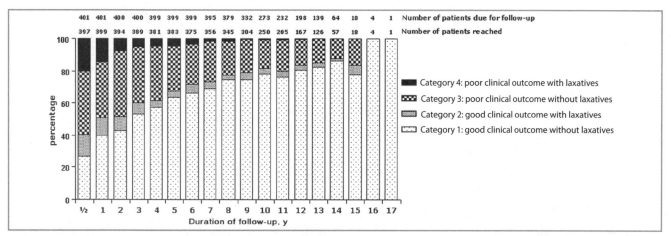

Figure 115-5. Clinical outcomes of patients according to follow-up year, divided into the 4 defined outcome categories. Numbers in the upper row above the bars show the numbers of patients due for follow-up evaluation each year. Numbers in the second row show the numbers of patients reached for follow-up evaluation each year. (Reproduced from Bongers ME, van Wijk MP, Reitsma JB, Benninga MA. Long-term prognosis for childhood constipation: clinical outcomes in adulthood. *Pediatrics.* 2010;126[1]:e156–e162.)

intervention and long-term follow-up and thus should be referred to a specialist. Special attention should be paid to infants with persistent constipation because of the high risk of serious conditions such as congenital megacolon or malrotation.

Prognosis

Prognosis varies with etiology. Functional constipation is usually amenable to routine management, but treatment failures are reported in 20% of children with functional fecal retention, and some long-term studies suggest persistence of symptoms for 25% to 50% of children. A long delay in presentation increases the risk of poor clinical outcome. Age at presentation and stooling frequency are also strong predictors of clinical outcome. Relapse rate at 1 year, after a successful initial intervention, is less than 5% but increases to 10% to 40% after 5 to 7 years, with significantly higher rates for women. Long duration of symptoms, poor self-esteem, and prior sexual abuse are among risk factors for a poor prognosis. Nonetheless, long-term studies largely show 2 important conclusions: prolonged laxative use is important, and dietary and behavioral modifications are ultimately successful in weaning laxative use (Figure 115-5).

CASE RESOLUTION

The child in the case study has functional constipation with a fissure. The bleeding is very distal and bright red blood is noted on the toilet paper and in the bowl, not mixed into the stool. The belly pain is visceral, related to gas distention and stool retention, and relieved with defecation. Gassiness implies stool retention and fermentation in the colon. Normal appetite and growth parameters are reassuring. The rectal examination establishes the diagnosis of an anal fissure and no further testing is necessary for this child at this point.

Selected References

Bae SH. Long-term safety of PEG 4000 in children with chronic functional constipation: a biochemical perspective. *Korean J Pediatr.* 2010;53(7):741–744

Bardisa-Ezcurra L, Ullman R, Gordon J; Guideline Development Group. Diagnosis and management of idiopathic childhood constipation: summary of NICE guidance. *BMJ.* 2010;340:c2585

Biggs WS, Dery WH. Evaluation and treatment of constipation in infants and children. *Am Fam Physician.* 2006;73(3):469–477

Bongers ME, van Wijk MP, Reitsma JB, Benninga MA. Long-term prognosis for childhood constipation: clinical outcomes in adulthood. *Pediatrics.* 2010;126(1): e156–e162

Coccorullo P, Strisciuglio C, Martinelli M, Miele E, Greco L, Staiano A. Lactobacillus reuteri (DSM 17938) in infants with functional chronic constipation: a double-blind, randomized, placebo-controlled study. *J Pediatr.* 2010;157(4): 598–602

Del Piano M, Carmagnola S, Anderloni A, et al. The use of probiotics in healthy volunteers with evacuation disorders and hard stools: a double-blind, randomized, placebo-controlled study. *J Clin Gastroenterol.* 2010;44(Suppl 1):S30–S34

El-Hodhod MA, Younis NT, Zaitoun YA, Daoud SD. Cow's milk allergy related pediatric constipation: appropriate time of milk tolerance. *Pediatr Allergy Immunol.* 2010;21(2 Pt 2):e407–e412

Liem O, Harman J, Benninga M, Kelleher K, Mousa H, Di Lorenzo C. Health utilization and cost impact of childhood constipation in the United States. *J Pediatr.* 2009;154(2):258–262

Loening-Baucke V. Prevalence, symptoms and outcome of constipation in infants and toddlers. *J Pediatr.* 2005;146(3):359–363

Maffei HV, Vicentini AP. Prospective evaluation of dietary treatment in childhood constipation: high dietary fiber and wheat bran intake are associated with constipation amelioration. *J Pediatr Gastroenterol Nutr.* 2011;52(1):55–59

North American Society for Pediatric Gastroenterology, Hepatology and Nutrition. Evaluation and treatment of constipation in children: summary of updated recommendations of the North American Society for Pediatric Gastroenterology, Hepatology and Nutrition. *J Pediatr Gastroenterol Nutr.* 2006;43(3): 405–407

Plunkett A, Phillips CP, Beattie RM. Management of chronic functional constipation in childhood. *Pediatr Drugs.* 2007;9(1):33–46

Raghunath N, Glassman MS, Halata MS, Berezin SH, Stewart JM, Medow MS. Anorectal motility abnormalities in children with encopresis and chronic constipation. *J Pediatr.* 2011;158(2):293–296

CHAPTER 116

Abdominal Pain

George Gershman, MD

CASE STUDY

A 16-month-old previously healthy boy was brought to the emergency department by his parents, who reported sudden onset of recurrent loud crying episodes lasting 10 to 15 minutes and a single episode of non-bloody, non-bilious vomiting over the last 12 hours. During each episode, the child was inconsolable, then fell asleep, only to awake crying again and moving his legs toward the abdomen as though he had abdominal pain. He refused to eat and looked exhausted. He also passed 2 bloody, mucus-like bowel movements. Three days prior to the current illness, the child had acute viral gastroenteritis. In the emergency department, the temperature and vital signs were normal except for mild tachycardia. Weight and height were at the 50th percentile. The physical examination revealed a slightly distended and tender abdomen. Bowel sounds were normal. There was no evidence of hepatosplenomegaly or ascites. The rectal examination showed an empty rectal vault and a small amount of gross blood.

Questions

1. What types of abdominal pain occur in children?
2. What characteristics distinguish functional from organic abdominal pain?
3. What are the common organic causes of recurrent abdominal pain in children?
4. What functional gastrointestinal disorders manifest with recurrent abdominal pain in children?

Abdominal pain is one of the most common symptoms of childhood and may be acute or chronic. Acute abdominal pain resolves within 4 weeks since onset of symptoms. Most children with acute abdominal pain have self-limiting conditions such as viral or bacterial gastroenteritis. However, a sudden onset of abdominal pain can be caused by serious, life-threatening conditions (eg, acute appendicitis, intussusception, hemolytic uremic syndrome). *Chronic abdominal pain* is defined as pain that persists for at least 2 months. The majority of children with chronic abdominal pain have so-called functional abdominal pain (FAP). The criteria for childhood FAP must include all of the following criteria: presence of abdominal pain at least once per week for 2 or more months prior to diagnosis; episodic or continuous nature of abdominal pain; insufficient criteria for other functional gastrointestinal (GI) disorders and absence of anatomic abnormalities; and inflammatory, metabolic, and neoplastic process related to the patient's symptoms. Children with FAP experience intermittent or continued non-localized abdominal pain equally. The onset of pain is usually not associated with defecation. Children with FAP and loss of daily function fall into the category of FAP syndrome. The term FAP should not suggest that affected children are malingerers or their symptoms are fictitious. An organic etiology is found in fewer than 10% of school-aged children with chronic or recurrent abdominal pain (RAP). However, failure to recognize these conditions or delayed therapy can have devastating effects.

Epidemiology

According to community and school-based studies, up to 38% of children and adolescents experience abdominal pain weekly, with up to 24% of children reporting symptoms persisting longer than 8 weeks. Abdominal pain is the essential part of several functional GI disorders, such as irritable bowel syndrome (IBS), functional dyspepsia, and abdominal migraine, as well as organic disorders, which occur with variable frequency in different age groups.

Pathophysiology

There are 3 main reasons for acute or chronic organic abdominal pain: inflammation, distention of the viscera, and ischemia.

Abdominal pain can originate from abdominal viscera (visceral pain), parietal peritoneum, abdominal wall, retroperitoneal skeletal muscles (somatic pain), and extra-abdominal sites (so-called referred pain). Impulses of visceral pain are carried out primarily by small, unmyelinated, slow-conducting afferent C fibers incorporated into the autonomic sensory pathways. Each visceral organ receives dual sympathetic and parasympathetic innervations. Sensory fibers associated with the sympathetic nervous system traverse prevertebral (celiac, superior and inferior mesenteric ganglion) and paravertebral ganglion and terminate in the spinal cord. Sensory fibers contained in the vagus and pelvic nerves (parasympathetic branch of the autonomic nervous system) terminate in the brain stem and lumbosacral spinal cord, respectively. Sensory fibers from visceral organs that connect with the spinal column terminate within spinal segments 4 to 5. This explains why visceral pain is poorly localized and often perceived along the midline as a dull or aching sensation. For example, the onset of acute appendicitis is usually manifested by pain in the periumbilical or epigastric areas before the pain migrates to the right lower quadrant. It is frequently accompanied by symptoms of autonomic disturbance (eg, nausea, pallor).

Somatic pain is induced by irritation of the parietal peritoneum and supportive tissue. Signals from the pain receptors (nociceptors) are transmitted for the most part by rapid conducting myelinated A delta fibers responsible for tactile, thermal, and chemical stimulation and discrimination of location and intensity of stimuli. As a result, somatic pain is well localized, intense, and sharp. The important characteristic of somatic pain is aggravation by movement. Therefore, the child with somatic abdominal pain is likely to lie still, in contrast with the restless patient with visceral pain.

The classic example of referred pain is abdominal pain induced by inflammation of parietal pleura at the onset of pneumonia as the result of shared central projections of the parietal pleura and abdominal wall.

The location of abdominal pain is determined by the level of spinal cord connection with the corresponding visceral organs through the afferent sensory fibers. The structures of foregut origin, such as distal esophagus, stomach, duodenum, liver, and pancreas, are innervated by the nerves that enter the spinal cord at the T5 to T9 segments. Pain from these organs is perceived between the xiphoid and umbilicus. The structures related to the primitive midgut (small intestine, appendix, and right colon) project the afferent fibers to the T8 to T9 segments of the spinal cord. As a result, the associated pain affects the periumbilical area. The structures related to the embryonic hindgut, including the left colon and rectum, share the innervations, which involve spinal segments T10 to L1 and allocate the pain to between the umbilicus and symphysis pubis.

Radiation of the pain may be helpful in diagnosis (eg, pain related to acute cholecystitis or biliary colic often refers to the area just under the inferior angle of the right scapula or above the right clavicle). Another example of referred pain is pain between the scapulae and middle back region in patients with pancreatitis.

The pathophysiology of FAP is different from acute or chronic organic abdominal pain. The genesis of FAP is related to abnormalities in the enteric nervous system and dysregulation of the brain-gut interaction. It is now believed that children with FAP may have abnormal responses to normal physiologic functions related to meals as well as intestinal distention during peristalsis, associated hormonal changes, and psychologic conditions like anxiety and parental separation.

Research data suggest that visceral hyperalgesia is the key element in the pathophysiology of FAP. This theory implies sensitization of the various receptors associated with afferent innervation of the GI tract by an infectious or allergic process or abnormal processing of afferent signals by the central nervous system.

Clinical Presentation

Children who experience abdominal pain may present with pain that may be characterized as persistent or intermittent, waxing and waning or steady and unrelenting, sharp or dull, and worsened or unaffected by movement. They may have associated complaints, including

vomiting, diarrhea, constipation, fever, weight loss, headache, and anorexia (D$_x$ Box).

Pain from distention of smooth muscle also waxes and wanes, is poorly localized, and is unaffected by motion. Distention of any hollow viscus, including the stomach, intestines, biliary tree, fallopian tubes, or ureters, can result in such symptomatology. A classic example of such pain is renal colic, in which the patient is writhing because of the discomfort.

Differential Diagnosis

In assessing the possible disease entities that may account for abdominal pain, patient age and duration of symptoms are the key differential components. Location of the pain may provide a clue to the etiology. Disease affecting the stomach is usually appreciated in the epigastrium. Duodenal problems are noted between the xiphoid and umbilicus, small intestinal pathology is appreciated in the periumbilical area, and cecal inflammation may be felt from the epigastrium to McBurney point. Disease in the colon is less specifically noted but is usually felt in the hypogastrium. Pain related to the urinary bladder and rectum may project to suprapubic or sacral areas. Pain may also be referred to the back. Renal colic is noted in the back but more in a lateral or costovertebral angle site.

Acute and Chronic Abdominal Pain

Young Infants: Medical Conditions

A unique disorder of infants, **colic** has been referred to as paroxysmal fussiness of infancy. The onset of symptoms is usually between 2 and 4 weeks of age, with resolution by 3 to 4 months. Although RAP seems to be present, abdominal pain has never been established as the cause of colic. Colic is characterized by fussiness and crying. Symptoms usually appear after feeding, particularly late in the day around dinnertime. Infants cry, clench their fists, and flex their legs. A gas-cry–air-swallowing cycle seems to occur. The symptoms may respond to a number of measures, including rhythmic motion and anti-gas medications. Infants with colic usually appear well otherwise and often have accelerated weight gain secondary to repeated feeding made in efforts to quiet them.

Abdominal pain may also occur with **food allergy,** particularly cow's milk protein allergy. Generally, symptoms such as vomiting,

 Abdominal Pain

- Abdominal pain
- Abdominal wall rigidity
- Abdominal tenderness
- Vomiting
- Alterations in bowel sounds
- Diarrhea or constipation
- Anorexia
- Fever

diarrhea, Hemoccult-positive stools, failure to thrive, rhinitis, eczema, pallor, irritability, and a positive family history of allergies are associated with food allergies. Disaccharidase deficiency may result in abdominal pain, but diarrhea is also usually present.

Young Infants: Surgical Conditions

Intussusception occurs in infants 3 months and older. The infant may have been previously well or experienced a recent bout of diarrhea. Vomiting is reported in about 50% of patients, and pallor is frequently present. Lethargy is not an uncommon associated symptom. An etiology is noted in fewer than 2.5% of affected infants, although a lead point (lymphoma or Meckel diverticulum) may be found in 5% to 10% of older children. The intussusception most often involves the area around the ileocecal valve. Compression of the vessels within the bowel wall may lead to necrosis and gangrene. The presence of blood and mucus in the stools gives a "currant jelly" appearance, although the initial stool is often normal, having been the stool that was present in the rectum prior to the intussusception.

Abdominal examination of affected children may be benign except for pain over the area of the intussusception or may reveal the presence of a mass. Bowel sounds may be increased secondary to the obstruction. Rectal examination may reveal blood and presence of a mass. Fever and leukocytosis may also be noted. A radiograph of the abdomen is usually nonspecific. Intussusception is diagnosed by abdominal ultrasound or barium enema. Hydrostatic reduction is the treatment of choice of intussusception; it is successful in approximately 90% to 95% of children. Failure of hydrostatic reduction or associated complications is related to delayed diagnosis and severe edema and necrosis of the affected bowel.

School-aged Children: Medical Conditions

Functional abdominal pain. As noted previously, most children with RAP suffer from functional GI disorders. According to the clinical presentation, functional GI disorders can be subdivided into 5 categories: FAP, FAP syndrome, functional dyspepsia, IBS, and abdominal migraine. Children with FAP usually do not have association of pain with eating, defecation, menses, or exercise. It is occasionally triggered by a new environment, difficulties at school, or domestic problems. The pain is usually periumbilical and can be quite severe. It can be recurrent or continuous and may affect daily activity.

Irritable bowel syndrome in children is characterized by abdominal discomfort or pain associated with 2 or more symptoms: improvement after defecation, and onset of pain associated with a change in frequency or in form of stool. Symptoms that cumulatively support the diagnosis of IBS are 4 or more stools per day or 2 or fewer stools per week, lumpy or hard or loose or watery stool, straining, urgency or feeling of incomplete evacuation, passage of mucus, or bloating or feeling of abdominal distention. Children with IBS are often anxious and express multiple somatic complaints. Although many children seem to outgrow FAP and IBS, long-term follow-up studies suggests that a significant number remain symptomatic into adulthood.

Children with functional dyspepsia experience persistent abdominal pain or RAP or discomfort centered in the upper abdomen (above the umbilicus). Pain is not relieved by defecation or associated with the onset of change in stool frequency or consistency. Dyspeptic symptoms may follow a viral illness. Pain is often relieved by medical inhibition of gastric secretion. Children with functional dyspepsia may suffer from nausea, early satiety, postprandial fullness, vomiting, and a sense of bloating.

Abdominal migraine is characterized by paroxysmal episodes of intense, acute periumbilical pain that last for one to several hours. Pain is often incapacitating. Children return to their usual state of health for weeks to months between the paroxysms of pain. The pain interferes with normal activities and is often accompanied by pallor, anorexia, photophobia, headache, nausea, and vomiting. There is an increased incidence of maternal migraine in children with abdominal migraine.

As mentioned previously, an organic etiology is found in fewer than 10% of school-aged children with RAP. Alarming symptoms and signs of organic diseases are persistent right upper and right lower quadrant pain, pain that wakes the child from sleep, dysphagia, persistent vomiting, arthritis, perirectal disease, GI blood loss, nocturnal diarrhea, involuntary weight loss, deceleration of linear growth, delayed puberty, unexplained fever, and family history of inflammatory bowel disease, celiac disease, or peptic ulcer disease.

Peptic ulcers may develop in children in 3 situations. Acute infantile ulcers may occur in newborns secondary to stress and hypoxia. Stress ulcers may occur in children who are the victims of trauma, including burns and hypoxia (eg, after submersion). The routine use of histamine H_2-receptor antagonists or proton pump inhibitors has reduced the incidence of ulcers in hospitalized critically ill children.

The most common type of ulcer in children is acute, drug-induced ulcerations of the stomach and the duodenum due to nonsteroidal anti-inflammatory drugs or corticosteroids. Chronic or peptic ulcers may develop in prepubertal children and teenagers with no apparent precipitating factors. A positive family history of peptic ulcer disease is reported in 25% to 50% of children. Unlike the classic ulcer symptoms of adults, in which pain occurs on an empty stomach and is relieved by eating, children may find that ulcer-related pain is not associated with the specific clinical pattern. Positive family history, microcytic anemia, and Hemoccult-positive stools should raise a clinical suspicion and prompt referral of the child to the pediatric gastroenterologist. There is clear evidence linking ulcer disease and infection with *Helicobacter pylori* in adults. The relationship between *H pylori* and peptic ulcer disease in children is not so strong, though two-thirds of pediatric patients with endoscopic evidence of peptic ulcer disease have infection with *H pylori*.

Mesenteric adenitis may produce symptoms indistinguishable from appendicitis, although affected children may not appear as ill. Nausea and vomiting and a history of an antecedent upper respiratory infection are often present.

Parenteral infections such as tonsillitis or pneumonia may present with fever and abdominal pain. In addition, hepatitis may result in pain and tenderness localized to the right upper quadrant in association with anorexia. Hepatitis in children is usually due to hepatitis A, and many infected young children are anicteric.

Pancreatitis produces abdominal pain that is often referred to the back. In the past, mumps was the most common cause of pancreatitis. Other infections such as hepatitis B, Epstein-Barr virus and coxsackievirus B, and *Mycoplasma pneumoniae* are the common infectious etiologies of acute pancreatitis.

Acute pancreatitis can be induced by some medications (eg, steroids, chemotherapeutic agents). Familial and recurrent forms of pancreatitis are also reported. Trauma, particularly from injuries sustained as a result of an impact against handlebars of bicycles, is a common cause. In children with pancreatitis and no apparent etiology, trauma related to child abuse should be considered.

Parasitic infestations, particularly with *Giardia lamblia,* may produce abdominal pain, often with bloating and diarrhea.

Genitourinary problems may result in abdominal pain. An abnormal urinalysis provides clues to the etiology. Renal stones occur infrequently in children, and boys are more often affected than girls. In two-thirds of affected children, stones are detected incidentally or in association with a urinary tract infection (UTI). Stones may be composed of calcium phosphate or oxalate, magnesium, uric acid, cystine, or xanthine. In addition to flank or abdominal pain, patients may also experience hematuria, fever, recurrent UTI, and persistent pyuria.

Hematologic and vascular disorders such as sickle cell disease, rheumatic fever, and Henoch-Schönlein purpura may also present with abdominal pain. Sickle cell anemia should be considered in African American children with abdominal pain. Pain may be related to vaso-occlusive events including bowel ischemia and splenic infarction or cholecystitis. Henoch-Schönlein purpura, which is also referred to as anaphylactoid purpura, is characterized by a hemorrhagic skin rash, joint pain, and renal abnormalities in addition to abdominal pain. This pain may result from a number of processes, including vasculitis and ischemia of the bowel wall, edema of the bowel wall, and intussusception of the small intestine.

Diabetes mellitus may lead to abdominal pain secondary to cramping of accessory muscles of respiration during a bout of ketoacidosis.

Acute intermittent porphyria is an uncommon cause of abdominal pain in children. The pain is often colicky and may be associated with constipation, nausea, and vomiting. Neurologic symptoms such as pain or paresthesia in the extremities may be present. Often, symptoms are precipitated by the ingestion of medications (eg, barbiturates, sulfa drugs). Some antispasmodic medications, such as Donnatal elixir, contain phenobarbital and can precipitate an attack. The diagnosis is made by evaluating urine for the presence of protoporphyrins.

Primary peritonitis is secondary to infection with *Streptococcus pneumoniae* and is seen in children with nephrotic syndrome, cirrhosis, and sickle cell disease, and in young girls with fever, abdominal pain, and vaginal discharge.

School-aged Children: Surgical Conditions

Appendicitis is the most common surgical condition that produces abdominal pain in school-aged children. Appendicitis may even occur in newborns, in whom it is seen in association with conditions such as cystic fibrosis and congenital megacolon (Hirschsprung disease) that lead to diminished passage of stool. The condition is frequently difficult to diagnose in children younger than 3 or 4 years for 2 reasons: examination of such young children for pain is difficult and symptoms are similar to those of acute gastroenteritis (ie, fever, abdominal pain, anorexia). Classically, patients complain of periumbilical pain that localizes to the right lower quadrant in 1 to 5 hours. They often have a low-grade fever, with a temperature of 100.4°F (38°C). Vomiting and increased urinary frequency may occur. Stooling is variable.

Physical examination may reveal guarding and localized pain as well as rebound tenderness. A positive psoas or obturator sign may be present, indicating inflammation of these muscles. Tenderness may also be noted on rectal examination. Leukocytosis more than 10,000/μL is also usually present. A radiograph of the abdomen may reveal 1 of 4 signs: a fecalith in the appendix (appendicolith), air in the cecum (sentinel loop), blurring of the shadow of the psoas muscle, or edema of the abdominal wall on the right side. A chest radiograph is also useful to rule out the presence of pneumonia, which may produce symptoms that mimic appendicitis.

Meckel diverticulum may be responsible for abdominal pain in a number of ways. It may serve as the lead point for an intussusception, cause symptoms of ulcer disease (pain or hemorrhage) secondary to the presence of ectopic gastric mucosa, or become acutely inflamed as in appendicitis. Meckel diverticulum follows the rule of 2s: it affects 2% of the population, is 2 feet from the ileocecal valve, is 2 inches in length, and is 2 times more common in males than in females.

Adolescents

In female adolescents, **gynecologic problems** such as torsion of the ovary, mittelschmerz, dysmenorrhea, and pelvic inflammatory disease must be considered as causes of abdominal pain. In addition, pain may result from gall bladder disease secondary to cholelithiasis or cholecystitis. Cholelithiasis is also a consideration in previously pregnant adolescent patients with abdominal pain and fatty food intolerance.

Evaluation

History

A thorough history should be obtained (Questions Box). A detailed description of pain may suggest a specific etiology. For example, pain worsened by eating can occur in children with gastroesophageal reflux disease, gastritis, cholecystitis, or pancreatitis. Nocturnal pain or pain relieved by a meal is more common in children with peptic ulcer disease. Pain relieved by defecation is suggestive of IBS. Pain aggravated by defecation raises suspicion of chronic inflammatory bowel disease. Localization of abdominal pain is an

Abdominal Pain

Questions

- What is the nature of the pain? Is it sharp or dull, well or poorly localized, intermittent or relentless, or worsened or unaffected by movement?
- How often does the pain occur?
- How long has the pain been present?
- Do any maneuvers, such as eating or lying down, reduce the symptomatology?
- Is the pain related to meals in any way? Is it worse after eating?
- Are there any symptoms such as fever, weight loss, anorexia, vomiting, diarrhea, constipation, dysuria, or headache associated with the pain?
- Does anyone else in the family have similar symptoms?
- Does the pain occur at night and on weekends?
- Is there a history of travel?

important additional diagnostic clue; FAP is usually localized along the midline or periumbilical area. Associated symptoms such as fever, weight loss, anorexia, vomiting, diarrhea, leukocytosis, and an elevated sedimentation rate also suggest an organic etiology.

Physical Examination

The physical examination should include an assessment of the severity of the pain. Children should be observed when they do not suspect that they are being watched. For example, a child who stands up and hops around when the physician leaves the room may have pain with a psychosomatic basis. Detection of abdominal tenderness may be ascertained during auscultation of the abdomen by pressing down with the stethoscope.

A rectal examination is also an integral part of the evaluation. In prepubescent girls with genitourinary symptoms or adolescent females, a genital assessment should be included.

Growth parameters should be evaluated for evidence of impairments, especially in children with RAP. Abnormal findings such as abdominal masses or perianal skin tags are clues to an organic etiology. Children who appear vigilant and keep their eyes open during the examination often have organic problems.

Laboratory Tests

The laboratory assessment is determined by the differential diagnosis. In general, laboratory tests include a complete blood cell count, a urinalysis, and an erythrocyte sedimentation rate (in recurrent cases). In children with suspected lactose intolerance, a hydrogen breath test is recommended by some physicians, although a trial of dietary manipulation or use of exogenous lactase (eg, Lactaid) may be more cost-effective. Other laboratory tests, such as serum amylase or liver function studies, are appropriate if pancreatitis or hepatitis is suspected. Detection of H pylori antigen in the stool supports the diagnosis of H pylori. Stool evaluation for occult blood and parasites is also helpful. Consultation with a gastroenterologist should be considered in patients suspected of having ulcer disease or inflammatory bowel disease. Specialists may order diagnostic procedures such as endoscopy to arrive at the diagnosis.

Imaging Studies

In general, a flat plate of the abdomen should be obtained, especially if an acute surgical condition is suspected. An abdominal computed tomography scan can be useful in some children with right low quadrant pain to confirm the diagnosis of acute appendicitis. Abdominal ultrasound and a barium enema are indicated to diagnose intussusception. Technetium scans help detect Meckel diverticulum if ectopic gastric mucosa is present. Ultrasonography is useful in suspected cases of cholelithiasis and cholecystitis. It may also detect pancreatic edema or pseudocyst, hydronephrosis, or abdominal masses.

Management

Management depends on the suspected cause of the abdominal pain. Medical conditions warrant treatment with **pharmacologic agents.** Peptic ulcer disease requires H_2 blockers such as cimetidine, proton pump inhibitors such as omeprazole, or cytoprotective agents like sucralfate. Infection with H pylori is managed with a combination of different antibiotics with proton pump inhibitors and bismuth preparations. Urinary tract infections should be treated with antibiotics. Conditions such as appendicitis mandate **surgical intervention.**

The management of children with RAP is challenging. A 3-tiered empiric trial has been suggested for children in whom no distinct cause is identified. First, a high-fiber diet should be implemented. This helps alleviate the abdominal pain symptoms of children with IBS. Second, antacids, H_2 blockers, or proton pump inhibitors are used empirically to see if symptoms respond to decreased acid levels. Third, a trial of Lactaid or a lactose-free period may also be implemented. A low dose of tricyclic antidepressant (eg, amitriptyline 0.1–0.2 mg/kg) has been used successfully in children with FAP.

Prognosis

In general, the prognosis for children with acute abdominal pain is good, although it varies depending on the condition. In 30% to 50% of children with RAP, symptoms resolve within 2 to 6 weeks of diagnosis. Thirty percent to 50% of affected children experience abdominal pain as adults, although the pain does not limit their activities. As adults, these individuals may experience IBS or other chronic nonspecific complaints, such as headache, backache, and chronic pelvic pain.

CASE RESOLUTION

In the case study, the boy has the classic symptoms of intussusception. It is not uncommon for the onset of ileocolic intussusception to follow acute gastroenteritis. Symptoms are related to the bowel ischemia. The child should receive intravenous hydration and a prompt diagnostic procedure (ie, a contrast enema or abdominal ultrasound followed by hydrostatic reduction of intussusception). The patient may be a candidate for surgical reduction of intussusception if attempts of nonsurgical treatment fail.

Selected References

American Academy of Pediatrics Subcommittee on Chronic Abdominal Pain. Chronic abdominal pain in children. *Pediatrics*. 2005;115(3):812–815

Chiou E, Nurko S. Management of functional abdominal pain and irritable bowel syndrome in children and adolescents. *Expert Rev Gastroenterol Hepatol*. 2010;4(3):293–304

Hyman PE, Milla PJ, Benninga MA, Davidson GP, Fleisher DF, Taminiau J. Childhood functional gastrointestinal disorders: neonate/toddler. *Gastroenterology*. 2006;130(5):1519–1526

Paul SP, Candy DS. Clinical update: recurrent abdominal pain in children. *Community Pract*. 2013;86:48–51

Rasquin A, Di Lorenzo C, Forbes D, et al. Childhood functional gastrointestinal disorders: child/adolescent. *Gastroenterology*. 2006;130(5):1527–1537

Saps M, Seshadri R, Sztainberg M, Schaffer G, Marshall BM, Di Lorenzo C. A prospective school-based study of abdominal pain and other common somatic complaints in children. *J Pediatr*. 2009;154(3):322–326

Vlieger AM, Benninga MA. Chronic abdominal pain including functional abdominal pain, irritable bowel syndrome and abdominal migraine. In: Walker's *Pediatric Gastrointestinal Disease: Pathophysiology—Diagnosis—Management*. 5th ed. Philadelphia, PA: BC Decker; 2008:715–728

Yang WC, Chen CY, Wu HP. Etiology of non-traumatic acute abdomen in pediatric emergency departments. *World J Clin Cases*. 2013;1(9):276–284

CHAPTER 117

Jaundice

Doron D. Kahana, MD, and Khalid M. Khan, MD

CASE STUDY

A 4-week-old boy is brought to the office for a routine weight check because he is breastfeeding. He was the product of a full-term, normal, spontaneous vaginal delivery, with a birth weight of 3,600 g. He has been feeding well, exclusively at the breast, with loose stools following each feeding. On physical examination, the infant weighs 4,900 g. The examination is normal except that the boy appears jaundiced. On further questioning, the mother states that her son was jaundiced shortly after birth, but she was told that the bilirubin level was all right. She thinks the jaundice may be more noticeable now. His stool is yellow and pasty, though sometimes it seems lighter in color.

Questions

1. What are the common causes of unconjugated hyperbilirubinemia in young infants?
2. What are the common causes of conjugated hyperbilirubinemia in young infants?
3. What are the usual causes of jaundice in older children and adolescents?
4. What is the appropriate management of hyperbilirubinemia in breastfed infants?
5. What are the diagnostic studies that are done to determine the etiology of jaundice?

Jaundice is a condition that occurs when bilirubin reaches a level in the blood that makes it visibly apparent. In newborns, this level is 5 mg/dL. In older children and adolescents, jaundice becomes apparent at serum bilirubin levels of 2 mg/dL. The term **physiologic jaundice** is used to denote the jaundice that normally occurs following birth. In full-term neonates, bilirubin reaches its peak of about 6 mg/dL between the second and fourth days of life. Levels above 10 mg/dL are probably not physiological. Bilirubin generally returns to a normal level (<1 mg/dL) by 12 days of age. Premature newborns experience their peak level of bilirubin, which may be up to 10 to 12 mg/dL, between the fifth and seventh days of life. Levels above 14 mg/dL are probably not physiological. Levels may be elevated in premature neonates for up to 2 months.

Although physiologic jaundice, a benign finding, affects all newborns, other, more serious disorders may present with jaundice in the newborn period. The physician must be able to differentiate between physiologic and pathologic causes of jaundice to ensure appropriate intervention and management. New-onset jaundice in older children and adolescents is never physiological and the natural history will be determined by the underlying disorder.

Epidemiology

Physiologic jaundice is nearly universal in neonates because of the rapid turnover of red blood cells and the relative immaturity of the liver giving rise to unconjugated hyperbilirubinemia. The most notable disorder associated with higher levels of unconjugated bilirubin in the newborn period is hemolysis from maternal antibodies to the baby's blood group (eg, ABO incompatibility). **Breastfeeding jaundice** results from inadequate milk intake, mild dehydration, and mild elevation in the level of conjugated bilirubin. The condition should be distinguished from pathologic cholestasis. **Breast milk jaundice** is different from breastfeeding jaundice and affects about 1% of breastfed newborns and infants. Factors in the maternal milk as well as the immature neonatal microflora that promote recirculation of bilirubin from the gut (enterohepatic circulation) give rise to unconjugated hyperbilirubinemia. Various illnesses, particularly bacterial infections, also may precipitate jaundice in newborns. Cholestasis, defined physiologically as a reduction in canalicular bile flow, is manifested as conjugated hyperbilirubinemia. Neonatal cholestasis, seen in a small number of cases of neonatal jaundice, may be caused by neonatal hepatitis (often without a discernible cause), extrahepatic biliary atresia (BA), or genetic and metabolic diseases. Jaundice occurs much less frequently in the postneonatal period and is most often secondary to viral hepatitis (see Chapter 118).

Clinical Presentation

Children with jaundice have yellow skin, conjunctiva, and mucous membranes. In newborns, the coloration may not be appreciated by parents because of its gradual onset and the parents' inexperience. The finding may be apparent in otherwise asymptomatic newborns and infants during routine health maintenance visits but may go unappreciated by the examining clinician. In addition to the yellow color, children with jaundice may also present with symptoms related to the cause of the jaundice, including vomiting, anorexia, failure to thrive, acholic (pale, poorly pigmented) stools, dark urine, fatigue, and abdominal pain or fullness and rickets (D_x Box).

Dx Jaundice

- Yellow skin, mucous membranes, and conjunctiva
- Tenderness in the right upper quadrant of the abdomen
- Hepatomegaly
- Anorexia
- Acholic stools
- Vomiting
- Pruritus

Pathophysiology

Bilirubin, a red pigment found primarily in bile, forms from the breakdown of heme-containing compounds, mainly hemoglobin, but also muscle myoglobin, cytochromes, catalases, and tryptophan 2,3-dioxygenase. Disruption along any point in the synthesis and transport of bilirubin or anatomic obstruction in the processing and excretion of bile may result in increased levels of bilirubin and the appearance of jaundice (Figure 117-1). After the breakdown of hemoglobin, unconjugated bilirubin is taken up by the hepatocyte plasma membrane carrier, bilitranslocase, and bound to intracellular

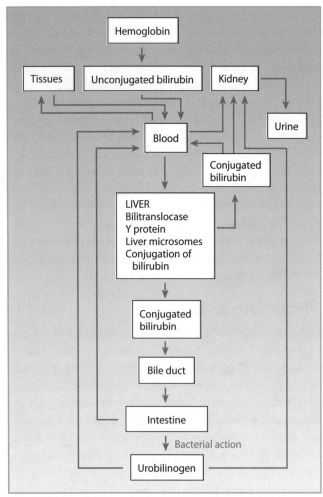

Figure 117-1. The bilirubin pathway.

proteins (Y proteins or glutathione S-transferase). Uptake depends on hepatic blood flow and the presence of the necessary binding proteins. Once in the liver, unconjugated bilirubin is conjugated by the enzyme glucuronosyltransferase. Conjugated bilirubin, which is water soluble, can be eliminated through the kidneys, while unconjugated bilirubin is not water soluble and can be taken up in tissues and stored. Following conjugation, bilirubin passes into the bile through the bile canaliculi. It then moves to the gastrointestinal tract, where some of it may be reabsorbed (enterohepatic circulation) or acted on by bacteria to form urobilinogen and stercobilinogen, which may appear in the urine or stool, respectively.

In neonates, a number of factors contribute to physiologic jaundice. First, increased destruction of red blood cells occurs because red blood cell survival in neonates is only 70 to 90 days, as opposed to 120 days in older children. Second, hepatic uptake is lower, likely a result of decreased levels of hepatic proteins as well as decreased hepatic blood flow. Levels of glucuronosyltransferase do not reach adult values until the second week of life; as a result, conjugation of bilirubin occurs at a slower rate. Gilbert syndrome is an autosomal-recessive disorder characterized by low physiologic levels of glucuronosyltransferase; these individuals remain prone to jaundice at times of illness, stress, and starvation. Prolonged jaundice may occur in some breastfed newborns and infants and is likely related to poor caloric or fluid intake, weight loss and catabolism, slow passage of meconium, or immature intestinal microflora. Breast milk jaundice is different, an unconjugated hyperbilirubinemia, and thought to result from milk components such as pregnanetriol, which blocks glucuronosyltransferase (see Chapter 26 for more information about breastfeeding). In older children, similar mechanisms may act to cause an increase in the bilirubin level. Hemolytic anemias (eg, glucose-6-phosphate dehydrogenase [G6PD] deficiency, pyruvate kinase deficiency [PKD]) may lead to increased red blood cell destruction. Inflammatory or infectious processes involving the liver, such as hepatitis, may impair the ability of the liver to excrete bilirubin. Pharmaceutical and toxicologic agents may also interfere with the ability of the liver to metabolize bilirubin.

Differential Diagnosis

The differential diagnosis of jaundice in children involves 3 criteria: age, the type of hyperbilirubinemia (conjugated or unconjugated), and, if the hyperbilirubinemia is conjugated, the nature of the obstruction (intrahepatic or extrahepatic). The latter 2 factors are particularly important in determining the etiology of jaundice in neonates and young infants. A diagrammatic representation of the differential diagnosis of jaundice in children is shown in figures 117-2, 117-3, and 117-4.

Neonates and Infants Younger Than 8 Weeks

Unconjugated Hyperbilirubinemia

Jaundice occurs universally in all newborns, but marked elevation of bilirubin levels (>15 mg/dL) and presence of jaundice in the first 24 hours of life or beyond 2 weeks of age warrant assessment. When

Figure 117-2. Differential diagnosis of jaundice (unconjugated hyperbilirubinemia) in neonates and infants (during the first 8 weeks of life). Abbreviations: G6PD, glucose-6-phosphate dehydrogenase; Hgb, hemoglobin; IDM, infant of diabetic mother; SGA, small for gestational age.

stenosis, duodenal atresia, annular pancreas, and jejunal atresia, may lead to jaundice, perhaps because of starvation and decreased levels of glucuronosyltransferase. Genetic and hematologic disorders should also be considered in the differential diagnosis.

Crigler-Najjar syndrome type 1 is an autosomal-recessive disorder characterized by an absence of glucuronosyltransferase and thus severe unconjugated hyperbilirubinemia with bilirubin levels approaching 50 mg/dL soon after birth. **Crigler-Najjar syndrome type 2 is also autosomal recessive but characterized by a reduced function of glucuronosyltransferase;** bilirubin levels average 20 mg/dL and persist beyond 2 weeks in the absence of hemolysis. Because of very high bilirubin levels, type 1 disease may lead to kernicterus unless managed with exchange transfusion. Phototherapy, cholestyramine resin, and eventual liver transplantation are additional therapies. **Hematologic problems** may also produce jaundice in the neonatal period. Such problems are most often associated with blood group (usually Rh or ABO) incompatibility between mothers and newborns, but some minor blood group determinants can also precipitate similar problems. Jaundice occurs in affected newborns and infants because of the rapid destruction of red blood cells, which release hemoglobin that converts to bilirubin. Hemolytic anemias, such as spherocytosis, will result in jaundice, as will conditions that result in polycythemia (increased red blood cells in the circulation), such as maternal-neonate or twin-twin transfusions, neonates who are small for gestational age, delayed clamping of the umbilical cord, neonates of diabetic mothers, and neonates with hyperviscosity syndrome.

Conjugated Hyperbilirubinemia

When more than 15% of the total bilirubin is direct, jaundice is categorized as conjugated (or direct) hyperbilirubinemia. This is always pathologic and warrants further investigation. Total parenteral nutrition is the most common cause of conjugated hyperbilirubinemia in the neonatal intensive care unit, is most likely related to the lipid component of the total parenteral nutrition, but does not usually present a diagnostic dilemma. The institution of oral feedings helps reverse the process. In other cases, determination of whether the

less than 15% of the total bilirubin is conjugated (direct hyperbilirubinemia), unconjugated hyperbilirubinemia is present. This is determined by measuring the levels of total and direct (ie, conjugated) bilirubin in the blood (bilirubin fractionation). **Physiologic jaundice** is associated with unconjugated hyperbilirubinemia and typically does not require an investigation. The hematologic workup of affected newborns and infants is normal. Jaundice related to inadequate human milk intake is called *breastfeeding jaundice,* which may resemble physiologic jaundice and occurs during the first week of life, whereas with *breast milk jaundice,* bilirubin levels rise during the second week of life when physiologic jaundice is improving. Breast milk jaundice usually peaks by the age of 4 weeks and can last up to 12 weeks. Levels may reach as high as 25 to 30 mg/dL, possibly posing a threat to the developing brain. In those cases, there may be a need to stop breastfeeding and introduce formula or phototherapy.

Conditions associated with slow intestinal transit time and increased enterohepatic circulation, such as hypothyroidism, also may result in jaundice. High intestinal obstructions, such as pyloric

Figure 117-3. Differential diagnosis of jaundice (conjugated hyperbilirubinemia) in neonates (during the first 8 weeks of life). Abbreviation: UTI, urinary tract infection.

infectious causes include enteroviruses, reovirus 3, parvovirus B19, human herpesvirus 6, adenovirus 2, *Listeria monocytogenes,* and tuberculosis. Differentiating among these conditions is usually done on the basis of culture, polymerase chain reaction, or serology testing. Certain physical and epidemiologic findings may help to distinguish these entities. Syphilis is more common in developing nations; jaundice may appear within the first 24 hours of life or later on. Infection with *L monocytogenes* may be associated with the presence of focal granulomas on the posterior pharynx; similar granulomas may be evident in the liver.

Metabolic diseases and **inborn errors of metabolism** may also lead to hepatitis. Most of these conditions are inherited in an autosomal-recessive manner and are relatively rare. In addition to jaundice, newborns and infants may present with vomiting, irritability, lethargy, anorexia, hepatomegaly, hypoglycemia, failure to thrive, bleeding, or cataracts. Galactosemia may be detected through neonatal screening or may present as *E coli* sepsis. Newborns and infants with hereditary

problem is intrahepatic or extrahepatic is the major consideration. Intrahepatic involvement represents a spectrum of conditions from inflammation (hepatitis), to inadequate formation of the bile ducts (biliary hypoplasia), to the destruction of the bile ducts (BA).

Hepatitis is inflammation of the liver usually caused by an infection in the liver, although infection elsewhere in the body (eg, sepsis, urinary tract infection [UTI] in neonates and young infants) may also cause jaundice. Urinary tract infections are usually caused by *Escherichia coli.* The hepatic involvement resolves with appropriate antibiotic therapy of the primary infection.

Primary liver infection in the neonatal period may be caused by a number of pathogens, collectively abbreviated as **TORCHS** (*t*oxoplasmosis, *o*ther agents, *r*ubella, *c*ytomegalovirus [CMV], *h*uman herpesvirus, *H*IV, *s*yphilis); the most common culprits are CMV and human herpesvirus. Neonates infected prenatally often have low birth weights, hepatosplenomegaly, petechial rashes, and ocular findings such as cataracts and chorioretinitis. Maternal transmission of hepatitis B is a possible etiology of neonatal cholestasis, but hepatitis C is usually asymptomatic in the neonate. Hepatitis A may cause an acute infection but rarely manifests as jaundice in neonates. **Other**

fructose intolerance present after exposure to fructose, sucrose, or sorbitol usually past the neonatal period. α_1-Antitrypsin deficiency may account for 20% to 30% of cases of idiopathic neonatal liver disease and up to 10% of neonatal cholestatic disease depending on the population. Inborn errors of metabolism (eg, glycogen storage disease, tyrosinemia, phenylketonuria) generally present with conjugated (direct) hyperbilirubinemia, while inborn errors of erythrocyte metabolism (PKD or G6PD deficiency) present with unconjugated (indirect) hyperbilirubinemia.

Other genetic conditions that lead to jaundice in newborns include lysosomal storage disease (eg, infantile Gaucher disease, Niemann-Pick disease, Wolman disease) and cystic fibrosis. The latter can cause cholestatic jaundice because of the presence of inspissated bile in the bile canaliculi. About half of the newborns and infants with cystic fibrosis have meconium ileus, meconium peritonitis, or intestinal atresia. "Plugged" bile ducts, when bilirubin production overwhelms the drainage system, may be seen with severe hemolytic anemia as well. Drugs may also induce intrahepatic cholestasis. A number of syndromes are associated with persistent intrahepatic cholestasis. Alagille syndrome (arteriohepatic dysplasia) is characterized

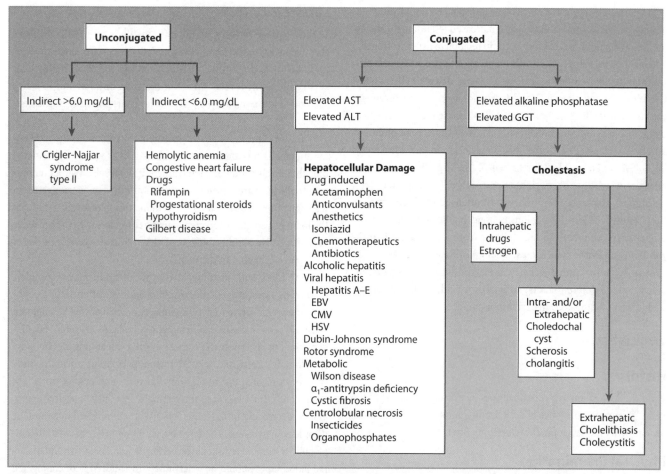

Figure 117-4. Differential diagnosis of jaundice in older infants, children, and adolescents. Abbreviations: ALT, alanine aminotransferase; AST, aspartate aminotransferase; CMV, cytomegalovirus; EBV, Epstein-Barr virus; GGT, γ-glutamyltransferase; HSV, herpes simplex virus.

by dysmorphic facies, skeletal and cardiovascular anomalies, and a paucity of intralobular bile ducts; the incidence is 1 in 100,000 live births. Progressive familial intrahepatic cholestasis (which are mostly a result of autosomal-recessive defects in bile acid transporters) and bile acid synthetic defect, together with Alagille syndrome (which is autosomal dominant), account for a total of about 10% of cases of neonatal cholestasis. Not surprisingly, as the etiologies for more of these cases are identified through genetic and metabolic testing, fewer cases are labeled *idiopathic neonatal hepatitis.*

Extrahepatic BA accounts for about 25% of cases of cholestasis in newborns and is characterized by ascending obliteration of the biliary tree. Newborns and infants are often well until 3 to 6 weeks of age, when they develop conjugated (direct) hyperbilirubinemia. The incidence is 1 in 14,000 live births and diagnosis must be prompt for surgical correction to be successful long term. Surgery after 2 months of age is unfortunately associated with liver failure and the future need for transplantation. It has been postulated that some primary insults, such as α_1-antitrypsin deficiency, metabolic disorders, or viral infections such as CMV and human herpesvirus, may be the inciting event leading to BA. Choledochal cysts appear as dilatations of the biliary tree and obstruct the passage of bile. They usually present outside of the infancy period with bilious emesis.

Older Infants, Children, and Adolescents

The approach to the differential diagnosis of jaundice in older infants and children is similar to the process in neonates and young infants. After determining the fractionation of the bilirubin, the differential diagnosis is suggested by the bilirubin level. Unconjugated hyperbilirubinemia is usually caused by hemolysis, and the level of indirect bilirubin helps clarify the differential diagnosis. Patients with levels below 6 mg/dL may have hemolytic anemia; a haptoglobin and peripheral blood smear should help solidify the diagnosis. Patients whose indirect bilirubin is greater than 6 mg/dL may have **Crigler-Najjar syndrome type 2** and respond favorably to phenobarbital. **Congestive heart failure** and **hypothyroidism** may also produce unconjugated hyperbilirubinemia to varying degrees. **Gilbert disease,** the most common inherited cause of unconjugated hyperbilirubinemia with a prevalence of 5%, is caused by reduced activity of the enzyme glucuronosyltransferase, which conjugates bilirubin. Bilirubin levels may rise to about 5 mg/dL in response to stress and starvation. Many different drugs, including rifampin and birth control pills, may also be associated with hyperbilirubinemia (usually indirect).

Conjugated (direct) hyperbilirubinemia may result from cholestasis and hepatocellular inflammation or injury. Cholestasis is characterized by high levels of alkaline phosphatase, mildly to moderately elevated transaminases, and increased γ-glutamyltransferase. Intrahepatic cholestasis can occur in relation to drugs (estrogens) and alcohol, as well as genetic disorders, such as **progressive familial intrahepatic cholestasis (PFIC or Byler disease).** This condition is divided into types 1, 2, and 3, depending on gene involvement. In this disorder, liver cells are less able to secrete bile. Extrahepatic cholestasis is seen with cholelithiasis or other obstructions of the biliary tree, such as a cyst. Cholelithiasis may occur in individuals with hemolytic anemia (black or brown pigment gallstones) and in adolescents who are overweight or postpartum (usually cholesterol gallstones). Hepatocellular injury most often results from hepatitis (see Chapter 118), including infectious, alcoholic, nonalcoholic steatohepatitis, and drug-induced. Rarer disorders include **Dubin-Johnson** and **Rotor syndromes.** Metabolic diseases such as Wilson disease, α_1-antitrypsin deficiency, and cystic fibrosis should be considered in the differential diagnosis of every older child presenting with direct (conjugated) hyperbilirubinemia.

Evaluation

History

A careful history must be obtained, documenting the timing of the onset of jaundice, presence of fever, feeding intolerance, pale stools, and growth and development (Questions Box).

Physical Examination

Patients should be evaluated for evidence of dysmorphism, organomegaly (liver or spleen), ocular anomalies, developmental delay, abnormal heart sounds (eg, murmur), rash, hearing deficits, or lymphadenopathy. Unique facial features (eg micrognathia, ocular anomalies) or a cardiac defect may suggest a genetic disorder such as PFIC or Alagille syndrome. Spleen enlargement is noted in hemolytic disorders and some inborn errors of metabolism, while isolated liver enlargement suggests hepatitis. Rashes and lymphadenopathy are associated with certain infectious conditions, including congenital infections (TORCHS) in newborns and infectious mononucleosis in adolescents.

Questions

Jaundice

- What associated symptoms are present?
- How long have the symptoms been present?
- Does the child have a fever, which may suggest the presence of an infection?
- What is the color of the stools (acholic stools suggest obstruction)?
- Does the child have a family history of jaundice, hepatitis, or consanguinity?
- What is the child's diet? If a newborn or an infant, is he or she breastfed or formula-fed?
- When did the parents first notice the jaundice?
- Has the child been jaundiced previously?
- Has the child been vaccinated against hepatitis A and B?
- Is there a history of foreign travel or shellfish ingestion?

Laboratory Tests

In the newborn nursery, noninvasive methods are used to measure the level of jaundice. The Jaundice Meter uses reflectance spectrophotometry to determine the skin color and correlates highly with serum bilirubin levels. An icterometer is another noninvasive method that uses an acrylic plastic color chart placed against a neonate's nose.

The aim of the laboratory assessment is to discover where bilirubin metabolism is abnormal. Total bilirubin as well as fractionated bilirubin levels should be determined. If the levels of direct (conjugated) bilirubin are elevated, consultation with a pediatric gastroenterologist should be considered. Demonstration of a yellow color to the foam of a shaken specimen of urine correlates with the presence of conjugated hyperbilirubinemia. Urine test strips also readily detect conjugated bilirubin in the urine.

In children with unconjugated hyperbilirubinemia, a complete blood cell count with reticulocyte count and evaluation of the peripheral smear confirm hemolytic anemia. A normal or low hemoglobin is usually seen in the face of hemolytic anemia. An elevated reticulocyte count or an abnormal peripheral blood smear indicates hemolysis. Hemolytic anemias with abnormal peripheral smears include spherocytosis, elliptocytosis, stomatocytosis, and pyknocytosis (see Chapter 86). The levels of serum haptoglobin, which binds free hemoglobin, decreasing its oxidative activity, are diminished in hemolytic disorders. In neonates, a hemoglobin level should be obtained, an antiglobulin (Coombs) test should be performed, and newborn and maternal blood types should be determined. In children with conjugated hyperbilirubinemia, tests should be performed to determine if infections such as bacteremia, UTI, congenital infection (TORCHS), or hepatitis are present. Evaluation for metabolic diseases should also be obtained by assessing urine for the presence of reducing substances, organic acids, and bile acid metabolites. A sweat chloride test and α_1-antitrypsin level should be considered. The status of liver function can be determined by evaluating aspartate aminotransferase, alanine aminotransferase, γ-glutamyltransferase, and alkaline phosphatase. To assess synthetic liver function, one should test prothrombin time, total protein, albumin, glucose, cholesterol, and ammonia.

Imaging Studies

The anatomy of the biliary tree can be evaluated using ultrasound, which is usually sensitive enough to visualize a choledochal cyst. A "triangular cord sign" is a specific but not very sensitive sign seen on ultrasound for the diagnosis of BA. A triangular-shaped echogenicity demonstrates the atretic ductal remnant in the area cephalad to the portal vein bifurcation. Other imaging tests, including excretion studies (biliary scintigraphy by radioisotope, ie, hepatobiliary iminodiacetic acid scan) and cholangiogram, can be used to help differentiate hepatitis from BA. Consultation with a pediatric gastroenterologist or pediatric surgeon may be appropriate.

Liver Biopsy

A histologic evaluation may be necessary if laboratory results have not defined an etiology. A detailed review by an experienced pathologist may be diagnostic and save the neonate from exploratory surgery.

Management

The management of jaundice depends on the cause of the condition. Physiologic jaundice and jaundice secondary to breastfeeding usually require no intervention. Breastfeeding jaundice is potentially preventable. Advise the mother to initiate breastfeeding within 1 hour of life with continuous rooming-in, breastfeed every 2 to 3 hours, and promptly respond to hunger cues, and discourage supplementation with water or sugar water. Monitor urine output. If bilirubin levels are greater than 20 mg/dL, interrupting breastfeeding for 24 to 48 hours will successfully lower bilirubin levels, but support and counseling are mandatory to ensure that breastfeeding resumes. Studies suggest that the use of a casein hydrolysate formula (eg, Nutramigen) may lead to a greater degree of reduction in the level of bilirubin than the use of a whey-predominant formula (eg, Enfamil). Some practitioners use **bilirubin-reducing lights,** but available data do not support imminent neurologic damage even when bilirubin levels climb as high as 25 to 30 mg/dL. Newer phototherapy techniques involve the use of woven fiber-optic pads that can be used in the home. Increasing the exposure of the neonate to phototherapy by using standard phototherapy above and a fiber-optic pad below is more effective than either modality alone. Clinical trials are demonstrating the efficacy of a single intramuscular dose of Sn-mesoporphyrin in treating and preventing neonatal hyperbilirubinemia. Sn-mesoporphyrin, a **metalloporphyrin,** blocks heme oxygenase, the first step in the production of bilirubin. Sn-mesoporphyrin may be especially helpful in situations in which blood transfusions are prohibited by parents for religious reasons or known hemolytic disease will put the neonate at risk for kernicterus.

Neonates who are preterm or ill or have hemolysis may be at greater risk from elevated bilirubin levels. **Exchange transfusion** may be indicated in addition to phototherapy and hydration. Preterm neonates should receive exchange transfusions when the bilirubin reaches the newborn's weight (eg, 11 mg/dL in a 1,100-g newborn). Intravenous immunoglobulin may prevent the need for exchange transfusion in babies with hemolysis due to blood group or Rh incompatibility by reducing hemolysis.

Diet and nutrition can be an integral part to supporting a neonate with conjugated hyperbilirubinemia. Formulas that fortify with medium-chain triglycerides (eg, Neocate, Pregestimil, Alimentum) will allow for fat absorption independent of bile acids. Supplementation with fat-soluble vitamins A, D, E, and K is essential. Vitamin D (25) hydroxide levels are easy to check and can act as a surrogate marker for the others. If galactosemia is suspected, switch to soy formula, pending results of the newborn screen.

Medications play a limited role in the management of jaundice. **Phenobarbital** may speed up hepatic excretion of bilirubin, even in cases of hemolytic anemia. This drug is also useful in the management of jaundice caused by certain genetic conditions, such as Crigler-Najjar syndrome. Appropriate **antibiotics** should be used to combat infections associated with jaundice (eg, cholangitis). For relief of pruritus, ursodeoxycholic acid (15–30 mg/kg/day), hydroxyzine, or rifampin may be offered.

Infants with BA may require **surgery** to link the surface of the liver to the intestinal tract, allowing for passage of bilirubin directly into the lumen of the small intestine (ie, portoenterostomy). Adolescents with gallbladder disease may also require surgical intervention (ie, cholecystectomy).

Prognosis

Most newborns and infants with elevated bilirubin levels have physiologic, breastfeeding, or breast milk jaundice. Prognosis is excellent in these conditions and usually does not require significant intervention. In recent years, concern has arisen about a recrudescence of kernicterus, including cases in breastfed, healthy term neonates and infants. Early discharge from the nursery and late follow-up may have contributed to this debilitating complication. Physicians should pursue an appropriate assessment of hyperbilirubinemia in jaundiced newborns and infants and not simply ascribe the symptoms to breastfeeding. Other conditions may require further medical or surgical intervention. Children with metabolic abnormalities usually require lifelong nutritional intervention. Those with hepatic disease may succumb to their hepatic dysfunction or need a liver transplantation. Newborns and infants who undergo surgical correction of BA prior to 6 weeks of age have a better prognosis than those who undergo surgery after age 6 weeks. These children should be monitored for recurrent episodes of cholangitis, which will promote cirrhosis and the eventual need for liver transplantation.

Older infants, children, and adolescents who develop jaundice often have self-limited conditions that spontaneously resolve, most commonly viral syndromes that affect the liver (eg, Epstein-Barr virus, hepatitis A).

CASE RESOLUTION

In the case study, fractionation of the bilirubin revealed 7 mg/dL of conjugated and 3 mg/dL of unconjugated bilirubin; hemoglobin, peripheral blood smear, and haptoglobin were all normal, as was a neonatal genetic screen. An ultrasound was positive for the triangular cord sign and could not detect a gallbladder. Nuclear scintigraphy scan showed decreased activity in the intestine, and liver biopsy showed bile duct hyperplasia and an inflammatory infiltrate. Biliary atresia was strongly suspected and an open cholangiogram confirmed the condition; portoenterostomy was performed. The infant was started on fat-soluble vitamins (A, D, E, K) and antibiotics for cholangitis prophylaxis.

Selected References

Balistreri WF, Bezerra JA. Whatever happened to "neonatal hepatitis"? *Clin Liver Dis.* 2006;10(1):27–53

Bhutani VK, Wong RJ. Bilirubin neurotoxicity in preterm infants: risk and prevention. *J Clin Neonatol.* 2013;2(2):61–69

Brumbaugh D, Mack C. Conjugated hyperbilirubinemia in children. *Pediatr Rev.* 2012;33(7):291–302

Farrant P, Meire HB, Mieli-Vergani G. Ultrasound features of the gall bladder in infants presenting with conjugated hyperbilirubinemia. *Br J Radiol.* 2000;73(875): 1154–1158

Harb R, Thomas DW. Conjugated hyperbilirubinemia: screening and treatment in older infants and children. *Pediatr Rev.* 2007;28(3):83–91

Hartley JL, Davenport M, Kelly DA. Biliary atresia. *Lancet.* 2009;374(9702): 1704–1713

Hartley JL, Gissen P, Kelly DA. Alagille syndrome and other hereditary causes of cholestasis. *Clin Liver Dis.* 2013;17(2):279–300

Maisels MJ. Neonatal jaundice. *Pediatr Rev.* 2006;27(12):443–454

Palermo JJ, Joerger S, Turmelle Y, Putnam P, Garbutt J. Neonatal cholestasis: opportunities to increase early detection. *Acad Pediatr.* 2012;12(4):283–287

Schulz S, Wong RJ, Vreman HJ, Stevenson DK. Metalloporphyrins – an update. *Front Pharmacol.* 2012;3:68

St-Jules DE, Watters CA, Iwamoto LM. Use of fish oil-based lipid emulsions in infants with intestinal failure-associated liver disease: a case series. *Infant Child Adolesc Nutr.* 2014;6(1):6–13

Suchy FJ, Sokol RJ, Balistreri WF. *Liver Disease in Children.* 3rd ed. Cambridge, UK: Cambridge University Press; 2007

Sun S, Chen G, Zheng S, et al. Analysis of clinical parameters that contribute to the misdiagnosis of biliary atresia. *J Pediatr Surg.* 2013;48(7):1490–1494

Watchko JF. Identification of neonates at risk for hazardous hyperbilirubinemia: emerging clinical insights. *Pediatr Clin North Am.* 2009;56(3):671–687

CHAPTER 118

Viral Hepatitis

ChrisAnna M. Mink, MD

CASE STUDY

A 15-year-old boy is brought to the office with a 1-week history of intermittent fever, vomiting, diarrhea, and diffuse abdominal pain. His mother reports the appearance of "yellow eyes and skin" on the day before the visit. Her son was previously in good health, and he has not seen a physician in several years. He is taking no medications and has no known ill contacts. He has no history of recent travel outside the United States and denies any unusual food ingestions. Mom reports that he frequently eats at a local fast-food restaurant with his soccer team, but his family does not eat there. He has one ear piercing and denies sexual activity, drug use, or tattoos.

The physical examination is significant for a temperature of 101.4°F (38.6°C), pulse of 100 beats/min, and blood pressure of 110/63 mm Hg. The teen is a well-developed, well-nourished male with yellow skin and sclera. The abdomen is soft, with mild diffuse tenderness, most notably over the right upper quadrant, and normal bowel sounds. The liver edge is palpated 5 cm below the right costal margin, and no splenomegaly is present. The rectal examination is normal, with guaiac-negative stool.

Questions

1. What are the most common causes of viral hepatitis in children and adolescents?
2. What is the appropriate evaluation for children and adolescents with suspected hepatitis?
3. What complications are associated with viral hepatitis?
4. What treatments are currently available for viral hepatitis, and how does treatment differ depending on the specific etiology?

Hepatitis is an inflammation of the liver that can occur as the result of an exposure to a toxin, such as a chemical or drug, or an infectious agent. Viruses are the most common cause of hepatitis in children and adolescents, and previously most cases in the United States were the result of hepatitis A virus (HAV), hepatitis B virus (HBV), or hepatitis C virus (HCV). With the advent of routine immunization for pediatric and adolescent age groups for HAV and HBV, the incidence of both infections has dramatically declined. Routine immunizations have reduced the occurrence of infection, as well as complications and long-term consequences, especially for hepatitis B. All 3 of these unrelated viruses can produce an acute illness characterized by nausea, malaise, abdominal pain, and jaundice. Hepatitis B virus and HCV also can produce a chronic infection that is associated with an increased risk for chronic liver disease and hepatocellular carcinoma.

Other common viruses that can cause hepatitis in children in the United States are Epstein-Barr virus (EBV), cytomegalovirus (CMV), varicella-zoster virus (VZV), adenovirus, enteroviruses, and human herpesvirus; however, their contribution to the overall morbidity and mortality associated with infectious hepatitis is minimal. Hepatitis D (as coinfection with hepatitis B) and hepatitis E are more commonly seen in other parts of the world.

Epidemiology

In 2011, nearly 6,000 cases of viral hepatitis were passively reported in the United States to the Centers for Disease Control and Prevention (CDC). Most cases were caused by HAV or HBV, with approximately 1,200 cases attributed to HCV. This reflects a more than 80% decline in HAV and HBV from the peak incidence in 1995. The number of cases of HCV is increased, which is primarily attributed to a rise in infections among adolescents and young adults in Eastern and Midwestern states, many of whom have a history of intravenous (IV) drug use. In addition, concerted efforts to investigate cases more actively to increase ascertainment of hepatitis cases by states and local public health officials were funded by the CDC. The total number of acute and chronic hepatitis cases is probably underestimated as a result of under-recognition and underreporting but likely exceeds 25,000.

Although the incidence of HAV and HBV infections are declining, children younger than 15 years continue to have one of the highest incidence rates of infectious hepatitis. Both genders are equally affected. Certain situations are associated with increased risk for infection with HAV, including crowded living conditions, chronic care facilities, military institutions, prisons, child care centers, travelers to endemic areas, and high-risk sexual practices (eg, commercial sex workers, men who have sex with men). Poor personal hygiene and inadequate sanitation are also risk factors. In approximately 50% of hepatitis A cases, however, the source of infection is unknown. Hepatitis A is found worldwide, but specific locations are associated with an increased incidence of the disease, including Central and South America, Africa, the Mediterranean region, and Asia.

Groups at high risk for HBV infection include illicit parenteral drug users, commercial sex workers, men who have sex with men, heterosexuals with multiple sexual partners, health care workers, neonates born to infected mothers, recipients of hemodialysis, household contacts of carriers of HBV, and immigrants from HBV-endemic areas. Individuals who live in crowded environments with poor hygienic standards, such as institutions for the developmentally disabled or correctional facilities, are also at risk for HBV infection. No risk factors are identified in 40% of cases. Worldwide, approximately 5% of the population (ie, 350 million people) is chronically infected with HBV. Individuals with chronic hepatitis B are the primary reservoirs for infection. Areas with the highest incidence of hepatitis B include Southeast Asia, most of Africa, the Pacific Islands, China, and parts of the Middle East.

Approximately 10% to 15% of primary infections with HBV result in a chronic carrier state. The younger children are when they are infected with HBV, the more likely they are to become chronic carriers. Between 70% and 90% of neonates born to infected mothers become carriers, and at least 50% of children infected before the age of 5 years become carriers. Boys have a greater risk of becoming carriers than girls, though the reason for this disparity is not known.

Hepatitis C virus accounts for 20% to 40% of all viral hepatitis in all age groups. High-risk individuals are recipients of transfusions of blood or blood products, recipients of organ or tissue transplants, IV drug users, health care workers with blood exposure, hemodialysis patients, and, infrequently, sexual or household contacts of infected persons. No identifiable source can be found in at least 35% of cases. In the pediatric population, recipients of blood and blood products before 1992, clotting factor concentrates before 1987 (eg, people with hemophilia), dialysis patients, institutionalized children, and high-risk newborns (eg, maternal history of IV drug abuse, sexually transmitted infections [STIs], or HIV coinfection) are most likely to be at risk for HCV infection.

Because hepatitis D only occurs as a coinfection with HBV, high-risk groups are the same, with the exclusion of health care workers and homosexual males. High prevalence rates occur in Eastern Europe, Central Africa, southern Italy, and the Middle East.

Hepatitis E virus (HEV) infection is endemic in developing countries such as Mexico, Central and Southeast Asia, North Africa, China, and India. No cases of HEV infection acquired in the United States have been reported. In endemic regions, HEV is the most common cause of symptomatic hepatitis in children. Young and middle-aged adults are most commonly affected, and HEV infection is especially severe for pregnant women.

Clinical Presentation

Children with acute hepatitis generally present with complaints suggestive of a flu-like illness, including fever, malaise, decreased appetite, nausea, and vomiting. They may also report diffuse abdominal pain. Unlike adults, in whom jaundice is a common finding, pediatric patients, particularly infants and young children, are frequently anicteric. Hepatomegaly is often found on physical examination, though not universally, and there may be varying degrees of right upper quadrant discomfort (D_x Box). A nonspecific macular rash,

Hepatitis

- Diffuse abdominal pain
- Nonspecific symptoms (eg, fever, malaise, anorexia, nausea, vomiting)
- Jaundice (not necessarily in all cases)
- Dark urine and light-colored stool
- Pain or tenderness over the liver area
- Hepatomegaly

papulovesicular acrodermatitis (Gianotti-Crosti syndrome), and arthralgia can also occur in the course of HBV infection.

Pathophysiology

Hepatitis A

Hepatitis A virus is a picornavirus composed of single-stranded RNA with only one serotype. The most common modes of transmission are through close personal contact and contaminated food and water. This generally occurs by fecal contamination and oral ingestion. Shellfish, such as raw oysters, clams, and mussels, are a frequent source of infection. Infected food handlers may also transmit the disease.

The average incubation period for hepatitis A is 28 to 30 days (range: 15–50 days). Peak viral secretion occurs before the onset of jaundice. The virus is shed in the stool 2 to 3 weeks before the onset of jaundice and up to 1 week after its appearance. However, most young children are anicteric, so infections often go unnoticed during this highly contagious period (Figure 118-1). The duration of illness is usually 2 to 4 weeks. A prolonged course or relapse occurs in 10% to 20% of adult cases. A chronic carrier state for HAV does not exist, though

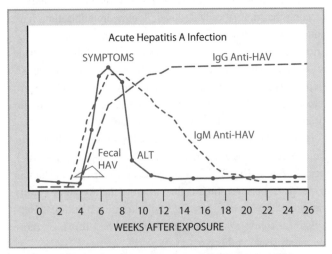

Figure 118-1. Course of acute hepatitis A infection. Abbreviations: HAV, hepatitis A virus; Ig, immunoglobulin. (Reproduced with permission from Tabor E. Etiology, diagnosis and treatment of viral hepatitis in children. In: Aronoff SC, Hughes WT, Kohl S, Speck WT, Wald ER, eds. *Advances in Pediatric Infectious Diseases*. Chicago, IL: Year Book Medical Publishers; 1988.)

fulminant infections can occur. Lifelong immunity is conferred after a single infection. Mortality is rare, especially in children.

Hepatitis B

Hepatitis B virus is a double-stranded DNA virus in the *Hepadnaviridae* family. The disease is usually spread by contact with infected blood or blood products, but it can also occur through close interpersonal contact. Although hepatitis B surface antigen (HBsAg) is found in numerous body secretions (eg, blood and blood products, feces, urine, tears, saliva, semen, human milk, vaginal secretions, cerebrospinal and synovial fluid), only serum, semen, vaginal secretions, and saliva have been proven contagious. No fecal-oral transmission occurs. Transmission is facilitated through percutaneous inoculation (eg, tattooing, IV drug use) and exposure of cuts in the skin and mucous membranes to contaminated fluids on objects such as razors and utensils. Sexual transmission occurs via semen, vaginal secretions, and saliva. Perinatal vertical transmission occurs in neonates whose mothers are acutely infected or chronic carriers. Although the exact mode of transmission is unclear for household contacts, postnatal infection from household exposure has been reported.

The average incubation period for HBV infection is 3 to 4 months (range: 1–6 months). Figure 118-2 depicts the typical course of acute hepatitis B, along with the course of the chronic carrier state.

Hepatitis C

Hepatitis C virus is a single-stranded RNA virus in the *Flavivirus* family; it is able to mutate rapidly, thus escaping detection by the host's immune system. Like HBV, HCV can be spread through contact with contaminated blood and blood products. Conditions associated with HCV infection in children and adolescents include hemophilia and hemoglobinopathies such as thalassemia and sickle cell disease (possibly due to increased exposure to blood products), a history of malignancy, administration of hemodialysis or solid organ transplantation, and IV drug use. Vertical transmission can occur but seems to be infrequent (1%–5% of neonates born to HCV-infected mothers). Contaminated immune globulin (Ig) administered between April 1, 1993, and February 23, 1994, has been implicated as a source of HCV infection. Transmission of infection via household and sexual contact has been demonstrated as well.

The incubation period is variable, ranging from 2 weeks to 6 months, and averages 6 to 7 weeks. Most affected children are anicteric as well as asymptomatic. If symptomatic infection is present, it is usually mild, insidious, and indistinguishable from infections caused by HAV or HBV. Jaundice occurs in only 25% of patients. Fulminant hepatitis is extremely uncommon.

Hepatitis D

Acute hepatitis D, or delta hepatitis, is caused by a distinct single-stranded RNA virus that requires HBsAg for replication. The virus and a delta antigen are enclosed in an envelope of HBsAg. Transmission is similar to HBV, but vertical transmission is uncommon. Hepatitis D occurs as a coinfection with HBV or a superinfection in a chronic carrier of HBV. Acute disease is usually more severe and

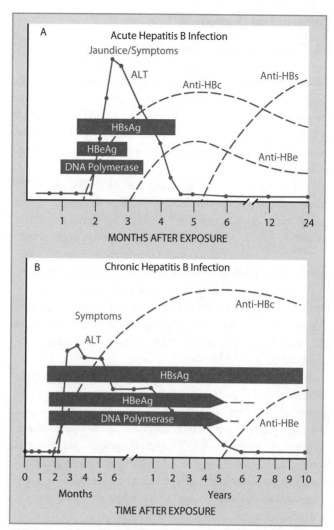

Figure 118-2. Course of hepatitis B infection. A, Acute hepatitis B infection. B, Chronic hepatitis B infection. Abbreviations: ALT, alanine aminotransferase; HBc, hepatitis B core; HBe, hepatitis B e; HBeAg, hepatitis B e antigen; HBs, hepatitis B surface; HBsAg, hepatitis B surface antigen. (Reproduced with permission from Tabor E. Etiology, diagnosis and treatment of viral hepatitis in children. In: Aronoff SC, Hughes WT, Kohl S, Speck WT, Wald ER, eds. *Advances in Pediatric Infectious Diseases.* Chicago, IL: Year Book Medical Publishers; 1988.)

carries a higher risk of fulminant hepatitis than hepatitis B infection alone.

Hepatitis E

Hepatitis E virus is caused by an enterically transmitted RNA virus. Transmission is primarily through contaminated drinking water and fecal-oral spread, especially during rainy or monsoon seasons in endemic areas.

The incubation period ranges from 2 to 9 weeks, with most cases of acute infection being self-limited. Mortality is low in endemic populations, except in pregnant women. Nearly all cases of HEV infection in the United States have been reported in travelers to endemic areas.

Differential Diagnosis

The differential diagnosis of hepatitis depends on the patient's age, possible exposures, and immunization history. Possible infectious causes in neonates include overwhelming bacterial sepsis, VZV, and congenital infections (TORCHES [*t*oxoplasmosis, *r*ubella, *C*MV, *h*uman herpesvirus, *H*IV, *e*nteroviruses, and *s*yphilis]), in addition to HBV infection. Perinatal transmission of HAV is rare. Genetic disorders and anatomic abnormalities causing biliary obstruction (eg, biliary atresia) should also be considered (see Chapter 117).

In older infants and children, in addition to HAV, HBV, and HCV, other viral etiologies include EBV, CMV, enteroviruses (including coxsackieviruses), adenovirus, VZV, human herpesvirus, and, less commonly, rubella, rubeola, and HIV. Acute or chronic anemias such as sickle cell disease can also cause hepatomegaly and jaundice. Noninfectious conditions to consider include drug-induced hepatitis (eg, treatment with prescribed medications such as isoniazid or phenytoin), toxin ingestion (eg, acetaminophen, herbal remedies), and conditions such as cystic fibrosis, α_1-antitrypsin deficiency, Wilson disease, and other congenital disorders such as Caroli disease (intrahepatic dilation of the bile ducts).

In adolescents, viral etiologies to consider are similar to those listed for children. Other infectious processes to consider in the adolescent age group include biliary tract infections, bacterial sepsis, Fitz-Hugh–Curtis syndrome (liver inflammation associated with pelvic infections, especially with *Chlamydia trachomatis*, *Neisseria gonorrhea*, or *Mycoplasma hominis*.) The list of prescribed and illicit drugs that may cause liver toxicity is extensive and includes oral contraceptives, seizure medications, alcohol, inhalants, acetaminophen, and tetracycline.

Evaluation

History

A comprehensive history should be obtained in children of all ages (Questions Box). A dietary and travel history is essential, especially when considering HAV and HEV.

For neonates and young infants, a complete maternal and obstetric history should be obtained and include the following questions: Does the mother have any history of IV drug use? Does the mother come from an area where hepatitis is highly endemic, such as Southeast Asia? Did the mother receive prenatal care? Was hepatitis B screening performed prenatally or at delivery? Did the mother have any known STIs or sexual contacts with hepatitis B–infected individuals, or did she have multiple sexual partners?

The physician should ask adolescents about sexual activity, STIs, and the number of sexual partners. In addition, it is important to inquire about parenteral drug use and tattoos.

Physical Examination

Most children with viral hepatitis are asymptomatic and generally do not present for medical evaluation. For symptomatic children, there are no clues on examination to aid in differentiating the causes.

Questions

Hepatitis

- Does the child have any history of fever, malaise, anorexia, or weight loss?
- Has the child experienced any vomiting or diarrhea?
- Is any abdominal pain or discomfort present? If so, in what location?
- Are yellow eyes or any changes in skin color apparent? If so, for how long?
- Is the color of the urine dark and the stool light?
- What is the child's recent travel history?
- Has the child ingested any shellfish in the previous 1 to 2 months?
- Has the child been in contact with any individuals with hepatitis or jaundice (including sexual contacts)?
- Is the child taking any medications (eg, isoniazid)?
- Does the child have a history of transfusion with blood or blood products?
- Is the adolescent sexually active, or has the adolescent had any known exposure to sexually transmitted infections (STIs)?
- Does the adolescent have a history of intravenous (IV) drug use?
- Does the mother have a history of hepatitis, IV drug use, STIs, or multiple sexual partners?

However, a complete physical examination should be performed to help rule out other etiologies. All vital signs should be recorded. The temperature is important, especially if children have a recent history of fever. In children who are vomiting, signs of dehydration (eg, tachycardia, evidence of orthostatic hypotension, dry mucous membranes, tenting of the skin, sunken eyes, lethargy) should be noted. Growth parameters, particularly weight, should be obtained and compared with previous measurements, if available.

The skin should be examined for jaundice; evidence of pruritus (eg, excoriations), which may be associated with elevated bilirubin; or a nonspecific rash. Icterus of the sclera, tympanic membranes, and palate should also be noted. The abdomen should be palpated for tenderness and organomegaly, particularly hepatomegaly. The liver span should also be determined by percussion because it will help monitor the patient's progress. Splenomegaly, which is not typically found in hepatitis, indicates a different diagnosis, such as leukemia, or another infectious cause, such as EBV or CMV. A rectal examination should be performed to look for masses or blood in the stool, which may suggest a neoplastic etiology.

A neurologic examination is important to document any signs of encephalopathy from hyperammonemia, which occurs more commonly in chronic liver disease or fulminant hepatic failure.

Laboratory Tests

The initial laboratory tests needed are directed by the severity of illness in the child at presentation. At a minimum, these include liver function tests (LFTs) (alanine aminotransferase, aspartate aminotransferase, γ-glutamyltransferase, and total and direct bilirubin) and coagulation studies (prothrombin time /partial thromboplastin time). Monitoring PT is particularly useful because of its rapid turnaround time and predictive utility; if the value is greater than 3 seconds above the upper limit of normal (international normalized ratio

>1.5), prognosis is poor. Serologic testing for hepatitis A (HAV-IgM and HAV-IgG) and hepatitis B panel (HBsAg, anti-HBs, hepatitis B e antigen [HBeAg], anti-HBe, and hepatitis B core antibody) should also be performed. Nucleic acid amplification testing, such as polymerase chain reaction (PCR) to detect hepatitis B DNA, is also available. Diagnostic antibody patterns for HAV and HBV are shown in figures 118-1 and 118-2.

Serum antibody to HCV (anti-HCV) should be sent, especially for individuals with risk factors for infection. A confirmatory test such as a recombinant immunoblot assay, which measures antibody to various regions of the HCV genome, is generally performed if a screening enzyme immunoassay is positive, as false-positive enzyme immunoassays may occur. Hepatitis C virus serologic assays detect IgG anti-HCV antibody; IgM tests are not available. Hepatitis C virus RNA PCR has generally replaced the immunoblot for confirmatory testing, and PCR can also be used in other situations (eg, testing an immunocompromised individual who may not make antibodies).

Serologic markers for hepatitis D (IgM and IgG anti–hepatitis D virus) can be sent when concurrent HBV infection is evident. Isolation of the hepatitis D antigen in the liver, however, is the gold standard test for diagnosis of hepatitis D. Other serologic testing may be performed as indicated by history (eg, testing for syphilis with rapid plasma reagin for sexually active teens or victims of sexual abuse). A complete blood cell count and comprehensive metabolic panel may be needed in ill-appearing children, especially with signs of dehydration. A urinalysis for bilirubin should be done. In severe or complicated cases of viral hepatitis, additional testing, such as liver biopsy or ultrasound, may be indicated. For these cases, consultation with specialists in infectious diseases and hepatology is needed.

Management

For most cases of acute HAV, HBV, or HCV infection, therapy consists of **supportive care.** These illnesses are usually self-limited, and no specific therapy is indicated. Adequate nutrition and hydration are of primary importance. Therefore, the **intake of sufficient food and fluids** should be ensured. A low-protein diet during the acute phase of the illness may be considered. The use of **antipyretics** such as acetaminophen or ibuprofen for fever usually does not pose a problem in patients with mild disease and acutely elevated LFTs. However, because it is metabolized by the liver, it is preferable to limit the use of acetaminophen. Physical activity should be limited until patients feel better and LFTs return to normal. Children and adolescents can return to school when they are no longer jaundiced; they may also resume a normal diet at that time.

In children with more severe symptoms, IV hydration and an antiemetic may be indicated. Hospitalization is required for children who are moderately to severely dehydrated, are unable to tolerate fluids, or have evidence of fulminant liver failure. Treatment is aimed at correcting any metabolic abnormalities or electrolyte disturbances, including hypoglycemia. Coagulopathies should be corrected with vitamin K, fresh frozen plasma, and cryoprecipitate. Total parenteral nutrition may be required to maintain caloric needs.

Consultation with a pediatric gastroenterologist is important for management of children with acute fulminant liver failure or chronic, active hepatitis. Although no specific treatments are available for fulminant acute viral hepatitis, a few treatment options are now approved for treating children with chronic infection with HBV and HCV. Treatment options for both infections include immunomodulators such as interferon-α (IFN-α), available as IFN-α-2b and pegylated recombinant IFN-α-2a. For hepatitis B, 5 antiviral agents are available, including entecavir, lamivudine, telbivudine (nucleoside analogues), and tenofovir and adefovir (nucleotide analogues), and ribavirin is available for treatment of HCV. Generally, treatments are given as combination regimens under direction of a specialist. Choosing to treat and with what regimen depend on the child's age, underlying health status, and degree of viral activity. All treatment regimens are associated with adverse effects. Most pediatric patients with chronic HCV infection are asymptomatic and do not usually warrant treatment.

Children and adolescents with HBV and HCV chronic infection and their parents should be counseled to avoid hepatotoxic medications and alcohol. Their parents should be informed of the possibility of transmission to others, and patients should refrain from donating blood, organs, tissue, or semen. In addition, sexually active adolescents should be informed of the possible risk to sexual partners. Toothbrushes and razors should not be shared among household contacts. Most children with chronic HBV and HCV infection should not be excluded from child care centers because of their infection. Possible reasons for exclusion of HBV-infected children include biting behaviors, bleeding disorders, and generalized dermatitis. Because children with chronic HBV and HCV infection are at risk for the development of serious liver disease, they should be followed regularly by their physician in conjunction with a pediatric gastroenterologist experienced in caring for these children.

Prevention

All children should routinely receive immunizations for HBV (starting as early as birth) and for HAV (starting at 12 months of age). For older children and adolescents, review of their immunization records should be performed at all medical encounters, and catch-up doses of hepatitis A and B vaccine should be provided. In the United States, some states require proof of hepatitis B vaccination for school enrollment.

Hepatitis A

Routine **immunization** for children starting at the age of 12 months has been recommended by the Advisory Committee on Immunization Practices and American Academy of Pediatrics since late 2006. In 1995, target groups were given hepatitis A vaccine, which led to a more than 85% decline in disease incidence. **Hand washing** by food handlers, medical personnel, and child care workers is one of the primary methods for prevention of the spread of HAV. **Contact precautions** should be used for hospitalized patients for at least 1 week after onset of symptoms. Active immunization with hepatitis A vaccine or passive immunization with Ig is recommended as postexposure prophylaxis for all people who have had intimate exposure to infected individuals. The hepatitis A vaccine and Ig may be administered at the same time in different sites. Postexposure Ig is generally not indicated for contacts at school or work, but Ig is indicated for HAV-exposed infants younger than 12 months, as they are not candidates for HAV vaccine. The dose of Ig is 0.02 mL/kg within 48 hours of exposure, given no later than 2 weeks after exposure. Immune globulin is 80% to 90% effective in prevention of clinical HAV disease. Pre-exposure prophylaxis with vaccine or Ig is recommended for travelers to endemic areas. If the stay is less than 3 months, the dose of Ig is 0.02 mL/kg; for longer stays, the dose is 0.06 mL/kg every 5 months. Two inactivated hepatitis A vaccines have been licensed in the United States for use in children 12 months and older, as well as for adults. The vaccine efficacy is greater than 94% for preventing clinical HAV disease. The 2 licensed vaccines seem to be interchangeable. Two doses of the vaccine are recommended and should be given initially and 6 to 12 months later. Combination vaccine against HAV and HBV is licensed for individuals older than 18 years.

In addition to routine childhood immunization, specific other groups for whom hepatitis A vaccine is recommended include travelers to endemic areas who are older than 12 months, individuals with chronic liver disease, men who have sex with men, users of injection and illicit drugs, and those at occupational risk of exposure. Other potential recipients include child care center staff and attendees, hospital personnel, food handlers, and individuals with hemophilia.

Hepatitis B

Preventive strategies for hepatitis B include universal immunization of all neonates beginning shortly after birth and pre-exposure and postexposure prophylaxis. In addition, vaccination of selected individuals at increased risk and catch-up vaccination for unimmunized adolescents, especially those at high risk, is recommended.

Passive immunization with **hepatitis B immunoglobulin (HBIG)** is recommended for infants born to known HBsAg-positive mothers or mothers whose status is unknown. Passive immunization is also recommended for susceptible individuals who are sexual partners of persons with acute hepatitis B infections, household contacts (including children <1 year who have received <2 doses of vaccine), and those who experience mucosal or percutaneous exposure to HBsAg-positive blood. Unimmunized victims of sexual assault or abuse should receive HBIG if the offender is known to be HBsAg-positive. Simultaneous active immunization with the hepatitis B vaccine is recommended in these cases.

Immunization with the hepatitis B vaccine (active immunization) is currently recommended for all newborns, infants, children, and adolescents not previously immunized, IV drug users, men who have sex with men, individuals receiving blood or blood products regularly (eg, people with hemophilia), children in chronic care facilities, household contacts of chronic carriers, and health care professionals. The standard schedule consists of 3 doses. Newborns should receive the first dose before discharge from the nursery or shortly

thereafter, the second dose 1 to 2 months later, and the third dose at 6 to 18 months of age. Infants should not receive the third dose before 6 months of age. Dosing intervals for other individuals are similar, and for adolescents (11–15 years of age), a 2-dose regimen using Recombivax is US Food and Drug Administration approved.

Perinatal vertical transmission of HBV can be prevented by giving newborns HBIG (0.5 mL intramuscularly) within 12 hours after birth and hepatitis B vaccine concurrently (at a different site) prior to discharge. This practice prevents approximately 90% of chronic infections in neonates born to mothers with HBsAg and HBeAg. Post-immunization serologic screening is recommended, however, for these infants at 1 year of age because approximately 5% become carriers despite appropriate preventive vaccination. Special schedules for active and passive immunizations against HBV should be consulted for premature neonates who weigh less than 2,000 g.

Hepatitis C

No vaccine exists for the prevention of HCV infection. Because Ig is manufactured from plasma that is HCV-antibody negative, it is not recommended for prophylaxis.

Current recommendations include screening individuals with risk factors for HCV infection (see Pathophysiology), neonates born to HCV-infected women, recipients of Ig between April 1993 and February 1994, and children with clinical hepatitis found not to have hepatitis A or B.

Hepatitis D

Prevention of HBV infection through universal vaccination is the most important means of controlling hepatitis D virus infection.

Prognosis

The prognosis for children with viral hepatitis depends on etiology, as well as the child's age and underlying health status, at the time of infection. For HAV infection, the outcome is generally good, with an uneventful recovery. Infants and children infected with HBV, on the other hand, are at high risk of becoming chronic carriers, especially if infected at a young age. Approximately 25% of carriers develop chronic, active hepatitis, which often progresses to cirrhosis. In addition, the risk of developing hepatocellular carcinoma is 12 to 300 times higher in these patients compared with the rest of the population.

Chronic hepatitis also occurs with HCV infection, though it is unknown whether chronic infection and subsequent complications are higher for neonates. Autoimmune complications such as arthritis, serum sickness, and erythema multiforme are common with chronic disease. Approximately 70% of patients with acute HCV infection later develop chronic hepatitis, and 10% to 20% progress to cirrhosis and hepatic failure. Hepatocellular carcinoma has also been described in a small proportion of patients.

Likewise, complications of hepatitis D, such as cirrhosis and portal hypertension, are not uncommon. They occur more frequently than with hepatitis B alone and progress more rapidly. Infection with HEV does not result in a chronic condition. Fatal hepatitis A is a rare occurrence. The overall mortality associated with HBV, HCV, and HEV is also low (approximately 1%–2%), though HEV can be fatal in 20% of infected pregnant women. For hepatitis D, mortality is more variable, ranging from 2% to 20%. Figures increase to 30% for HBV with coinfection with hepatitis D.

CASE RESOLUTION

In the case study, the teen has a classic presentation of viral hepatitis despite no clear history of exposure, such as travel to an endemic area. Statistics point to probable infection with hepatitis A, and exposure possibly occurred at the fast-food restaurant. Because he does not appear to be dehydrated or seriously ill, he can be managed as an outpatient. Serologic testing for hepatitis A, B, and C should be performed, in addition to liver function tests (LFTs) and coagulation studies. The parents should be informed of the probable diagnosis, and if confirmed as hepatitis A, all household contacts should receive hepatitis A vaccine or prophylaxis with Ig. They should also be educated on the infectivity of the disease and counseled about supportive therapy. Public health officials should be consulted for management of other individuals who were possibly exposed. The boy should have limited physical activity while symptomatic and should be scheduled for a follow-up visit in a few days for repeat LFTs and coagulation tests. The prognosis is good.

Selected References

Advisory Committee on Immunization Practices; Fiore AE, Wasley A, Bell BP. Prevention of hepatitis A through active or passive immunization: recommendations of the Advisory Committee on Immunization Practices (ACIP). *MMWR Recomm Rep.* 2006;55(RR-7):1–23

American Academy of Pediatrics. Hepatitis A. In: Pickering LK, Baker CJ, Kimberlin DW, Long SS, eds. *Red Book: 2012 Report of the Committee on Infectious Diseases.* 29th ed. Elk Grove Village, IL: American Academy of Pediatrics; 2012:361–369

American Academy of Pediatrics. Hepatitis B. In: Pickering LK, Baker CJ, Kimberlin DW, Long SS, eds. *Red Book: 2012 Report of the Committee on Infectious Diseases.* 29th ed. Elk Grove Village, IL: American Academy of Pediatrics; 2012:369–390

American Academy of Pediatrics. Hepatitis C. In: Pickering LK, Baker CJ, Kimberlin DW, Long SS, eds. *Red Book: 2012 Report of the Committee on Infectious Diseases.* 29th ed. Elk Grove Village, IL: American Academy of Pediatrics; 2012:391–395

Buggs AM. Viral hepatitis. http://emedicine.medscape.com/article/775507-overview. Updated August 23, 2012. Accessed March 12, 2014

Centers for Disease Control and Prevention. Viral hepatitis statistics & surveillance. http://www.cdc.gov/HEPATITIS/Statistics/index.htm. Accessed March 12, 2014

Curry MP, Chopra S. Acute viral hepatitis. In: Mandell GL, Bennett JE, Dolin R, eds. *Mandell, Douglas, and Bennett's Principles and Practice of Infectious Diseases.* 7th ed. Philadelphia, PA: Elsevier; 2010:1577–1592

Kim WR. The burden of hepatitis C in the United States. *Hepatology.* 2002;36(5 Suppl 1):S30–S34

Mast EE, Weinbaum CM, Fiore AE, et al. A comprehensive immunization strategy to eliminate transmission of hepatitis B virus infection in the United States: recommendations of the Advisory Committee on Immunization Practices (ACIP) part II: immunization of adults. *MMWR Recomm Rep.* 2006;55(RR-16):1–33

Tovo PA, Lazier L, Versace A. Hepatitis B virus and hepatitis C virus infections in children. *Curr Opin Infect Dis.* 2005;18(3):261–266

Neurologic Disorders

CHAPTER 119

Hypotonia

Kenneth R. Huff, MD

CASE STUDY

A 6-month-old girl is brought to the office because she does not reach for her toys anymore. The pregnancy was full term, but the mother remembers that the fetal kicking was less than with an older brother. Delivery was uncomplicated, and the newborn fed well from birth. The girl began to show visual attention at 2 to 3 weeks, smiled socially at 1 month, and pushed up while prone at 2 months. Although she turned over at 4 months, she has not done this in the last month. She no longer reaches up to the mobile over her crib.

On examination, the girl lies quietly on the table and watches the examiner intently. Her growth parameters, including head circumference, are normal. After she has been undressed, it is apparent that she "seesaw" breathes (ie, abdomen rises with inspiration) and has a "frog-leg" posture (batrachian position). Her cranial nerve examination is normal except for head-turning strength. When she is pulled to a sitting position, her head lags far behind and her arms are straight at the elbows. She cannot raise her arms off the table. When a rattle is placed in her hands, she manipulates the toy, which she regards from the corner of her eye. Her deep tendon reflexes are absent, but her pain sensation is intact.

Questions

1. How is the level of nervous system involvement determined in infants with hypotonia?
2. What is the significance of a loss of developmental milestones or abilities?
3. When are genetic tests appropriate for children with hypotonia?
4. How are clinical management issues related to prognosis?

Infants with decreased tone are referred to as hypotonic or "floppy." Hypotonia is most simply defined as lower than normal resistance to passive motion across a joint but is also suggested by abnormal posture. Although the lack of resistance may have other components (eg, connective tissue abnormalities suggested by an unusual range of joint mobility and hyperelastic skin, features of Ehlers-Danlos syndrome, features of Down syndrome), muscle strength is a key component. Tone can be used as a surrogate indicator of strength in infants who cannot cooperate with resistance testing. Weakness can also be inferred from functional observations and the inability to sustain limbs against gravity or the lack of a withdrawal response of a limb to a painful stimulus. Identification of the level of the nervous system affected (eg, upper motor neurons, spinal cord, anterior horn cell, peripheral nerve components, myoneural junction, muscle fibers) is most important in determining the etiology of hypotonia in infants and children. Only after this localization is the likely pathology defined in most cases.

Epidemiology

Hypotonia is not unusual in neonates, and non-neuromuscular causes of hypotonia are more common than neuromuscular conditions. Non-neuromuscular causes include hypoxic-ischemic encephalopathy and brain lesions related to premature birth, such as intraventricular hemorrhage and periventricular leukomalacia. Genetic abnormalities also are frequently present shortly after birth. Spinal muscular atrophy (SMA) is a common progressive genetic condition with an incidence similar to cystic fibrosis, about 1 in 5,000. Duchenne muscular dystrophy, presenting at age 2 to 5 years, is the most common neuromuscular condition in childhood, with an incidence of 1 in 1,700 to 1 in 3,500 male births. The Duchenne gene has been found to spontaneously mutate in approximately 50% of the cases. Among non–genetically acquired disorders, the incidence of acute postinfectious polyneuritis or Guillain-Barré syndrome is 2 to 8 per 100,000.

Clinical Presentation

Hypotonia in infants often presents as an unusual posture of the infant, diminished resistance to passive movements of limbs or trunk, or an excessive range of joint mobility. Hypotonic infants have delayed motor milestones, decreased movements, and poor head and trunk control (Figure 119-1). Older children may have decreased ability to resist with strength testing of individual muscle groups as well as impaired functional strength in sitting, standing, walking, climbing, or running (D_x Box). Swaybacked posture in standing may indicate hip girdle or proximal weakness. Pointed toes in the supine position may indicate an upper motor cause.

Pathophysiology

Tone is a product of connective tissue structural elements, including ligaments, tendons, and joint capsules; muscle fiber number and integrity; and nerve fiber input to muscle. Nerve input to the muscle includes the number and myelination of axon fibers,

Figure 119-1. Hypotonic infant being pulled into sitting position. Arms are completely extended, head control is poor, and legs are abducted at the hip.

 Hypotonia

- Decreased resistance to passive movement of a joint
- Muscular weakness in older children
- Etiologic diagnosis related to the nervous system level of the lesion

trophic factors from the nerve, and frequency of action potentials depolarizing the muscle membrane. The control of tone through the anterior horn cell is complex and involves more than just corticospinal tract (upper motor unit) but also other descending tract influences. Lesions of the neuromuscular apparatus (lower motor unit), which includes muscle, nerve, nerve sheaths, and anterior horn cell, can most directly decrease tone, but lesions of any of the other structures at many levels of the nervous system can also affect tone. The final common pathway of upper or lower motor unit modification of tone is through the gamma loop (fusimotor) system. Gamma motor neurons within the anterior horn of the spinal cord innervate the contractile muscle portions on each end of the intrafusal fiber and enhance the sensitivity of the sensory endings to stretch, which in turn transmit signals back to the alpha motoneurons in the anterior horn innervating the rest of the muscle. Different levels of the central nervous system (CNS) (motor cortex, thalamus, basal ganglia, vestibular nuclei, reticular formation, and cerebellum) can modify tone through their effect on the gamma motor neuron.

The nature of the lesion at different levels of the nervous system may be quite variable. For example, ultrastructural abnormalities occur in congenital myopathies, including those related to respiratory chain defects; anterior horn cell apoptosis occurs in SMA and may also occur with ischemic insults; stripping of myelin by macrophages occurs with acute postinfectious polyneuritis; and muscle voltage-gated channels are involved in periodic paralyses.

Differential Diagnosis

Distinguishing clinical features in determining the level of the lesion in the nervous system include pattern of weakness, activity of deep tendon reflexes, presence of fasciculations or sensory loss, cerebrospinal fluid findings, serum muscle enzyme levels, **electromyography (EMG)** pattern, nerve conduction studies, and histologic appearance or assays of the muscle or nerve biopsy. It is useful when assessing the hypotonic child to separate first upper motor neuron or brain causes from neuromuscular causes (Table 119-1). The former include perinatal hypoxia-ischemia, intracranial hemorrhage, and cerebral dysgenesis. These problems may present with hypotonia in infancy but later are evident as a static encephalopathy. A child with a CNS cause may have a below-normal level or range of attention and may lack age-appropriate social skills. Seizures or hemiparesis also signify a likely CNS cause. Fine motor coordination, quality and repertoire of movements, and language may be affected in an older child. The deep tendon reflexes may be brisk or easily elicited. The Babinski reflex may be dorsiflexor. In infants, fisting of the hands, scissoring of the extended legs on vertical suspension, and movement through postural reflexes such as the asymmetric tonic neck reflex are clues to an upper motor neuron process. In a patient with an upper motor neuron lesion, serum muscle enzymes, EMG, nerve conduction, and muscle biopsy would all be normal if assessed. However, a child with one of the neuromuscular causes (including congenital myopathy, SMA, muscular dystrophy, and acute

Table 119-1. Differential Diagnosis of Infantile Hypotonia	
Level	**Specific Lesion**
Cerebral hemisphere	Static encephalopathy related to perinatal or prenatal insults
	Dysgenesis (eg, Down syndrome)
	Degenerative conditions (eg, storage disease)
Spinal cord	Traumatic transection
	Dysraphism or other malformation
Anterior horn cell	Spinal muscular atrophy
	Enterovirus myelitis
Peripheral nerve	Leukodystrophy
	Type III hereditary sensorimotor neuropathy
	Acute polyneuritis (rarely occurs in infancy)
Myoneural junction	Myasthenia gravis
	Toxin (botulism or Mycin antibiotic)
	Hypermagnesemia
Muscle	Congenital structural myopathy
	Congenital myotonic dystrophy
	Congenital muscular dystrophy
	Mitochondrial myopathy
Systemic	Amino and organic acidopathies, hypercalcemia, renal acidosis, rickets, celiac disease, hypothyroidism, collagen disease, congenital heart disease

postinfectious polyneuritis) for the hypotonia that doesn't also involve brain or facial nerves or muscles, may have an interested and visually attentive facial appearance. This may be the case even in the presence of severe weakness that allows only sparse or nearly absent limb movements. Deep tendon reflexes may be difficult to elicit or absent in many of these neuromuscular lesions.

Older children may display a different pattern of weakness that gives a clue to the level of involvement. If the weakness is preferentially in upper extremity extensor and lower extremity knee flexor, ankle dorsiflexor, and ankle evertor muscle groups, the lesion may involve the upper motor neuron. Static bilateral hemiparesis may suggest severe hypoxemic-ischemic insult; diplegia may suggest periventricular leukomalacia in a former prematurely delivered infant. This differential weakness from CNS causes may be present and contribute to hypotonia for a long period before spasticity intervenes and increases tone. However, if the weakness involves agonist and antagonist muscles equally across a limb joint, it probably represents a neuromuscular process. It should also be remembered that hypotonia can result from disorders with combined lesions in levels above the lower motor neuron and in the motor unit. Examples include Krabbe disease, glycogen storage disease type 2 (Pompe disease), and hypoxic-ischemic insults involving the upper motor neuron and anterior horn cell.

Evaluation

A methodical assessment using clinical and laboratory features in children to localize the lesion to a level of the nervous systems can help anatomically narrow a wide differential diagnosis (Table 119-2).

History

Particular areas of the history are especially important (Questions Box). Strength of fetal movements relative to other pregnancies and ischemic, toxic, metabolic, or infectious fetal exposures should be ascertained. Relatively decreased fetal movements may signify an early degenerative condition. Polyhydramnios can signal prenatal weakness in swallowing. Birth events should be investigated for sources of possible insults to the neonatal nervous system, such as prematurity or birth asphyxia. The physician should determine whether any of the child's developmental skills have been lost. Any associated loss of tone or strength could signify a progressive

Questions

Hypotonia

- Were the fetal movements of the child abnormal or less than those of previous pregnancies?
- Was the pregnancy full term? Was the delivery complicated?
- Does the mother, any siblings, or other family members suffer from a similar weakness?
- Has the child lost any developmental skills? Is the problem getting worse?

condition rather than a static problem as would occur with a birth injury. The acuity of the developing weakness also is an important clue in differential diagnosis. Rapid-onset hypotonia accompanied by constipation, poor feeding, and other bulbar involvement may suggest botulism. Acute losses of tone and strength may also occur with enteroviral poliomyelitis, Guillain-Barré syndrome, myasthenia, and myositis. Relapsing-remitting courses of hypotonia may be seen with myasthenia, metabolic myopathies including mitochondrial disorders, and periodic paralysis in the older child. Recent hiking may suggest tick paralysis. A parallel deterioration in intellectual functions might point to a leukodystrophy, storage disorder, or other degenerative disorders, including one of the several types of Leigh disease, particularly if ataxia, brain stem symptoms, and respiratory dysfunction subsequently develop.

In addition, family history should be determined. The presence of weakness or hypotonia in other family members or prior unexplained neonatal or childhood deaths in the family may indicate a genetic or maternal basis for the patient's hypotonia.

Physical Examination

Dysmorphic features should be noted in developmentally delayed children with hypotonia because they may suggest cerebral dysgenesis as part of a multiple malformation syndrome or a chromosomal anomaly (eg, the characteristic stigmata of Down syndrome) in some instances, or neuromuscular conditions (eg, hypoplastic mandible, high-arched palate, thin ribs with deformed rib cage, pectus excavatum) in other instances. Poor feeding with small male genitalia in the neonate may suggest Prader-Willi syndrome. A large tongue with decreased growth parameters may point to

Clinical Feature	Cerebrum	Spinal Cord	Anterior Horn Cell	Neuromuscular Junction	Muscle
Alertness	Decreased	Normal	Normal	Normal	Normal
Cry	Decreased	Normal	Normal/weak	Weak	Normal/weak
Eye movements	Sometimes abnormal	Normal	Normal	Abnormal	Normal
Tongue fasciculations	Absent	Absent	Present	Absent	Absent
Muscle bulk	Normal	Normal	Decreased	Normal	Decreased
Deep tendon reflexes	Normal/increased	Decreased/increased	Absent	Normal	Normal/decreased

Table 119-2. Approach to the Diagnosis of Hypotonia — Anatomic Site

hypothyroidism. Hepatomegaly may be seen with Niemann disease and cerebrohepatorenal (Zellweger) syndrome. Signs of brain dysfunction, such as lethargy, unresponsiveness to the environment, and lack of social skills, should be noted. The neonate who acutely develops signs like those of sepsis along with generalized hypotonia may have an inborn error of metabolism that is decompensating and requires emergent intervention. Age-appropriate cognitive abilities should be assessed as a measure of cerebral function. This assessment may range from primarily observation of visual attention in very young infants to evaluation of language and academic skills in older children. Cranial nerve examination with regard to eye movements, facial strength, and presence of tongue fasciculations is important, especially in differential diagnosis of many neuromuscular conditions. Ocular muscle involvement may be part of mitochondrial myopathies, myotubular myopathy, and myotonic dystrophy. Blindness and hyperacusis responses may suggest Tay-Sachs disease. Deafness may be part of a mitochondrial disorder. Facial muscle involvement is common in some congenital myopathies and myotonic dystrophy but not a part of SMA. Sucking and swallowing difficulty is a feature of SMA, congenital myotonic dystrophy, myotubular and nemaline myopathies, neonatal myasthenia, and Prader-Willi syndrome, in addition to birth asphyxia.

Tone and strength should be examined carefully in the awake infant in trunk and limbs with the head in midline. Passive pronation, supination, flexion, extension, and gentle shaking of hands and feet can demonstrate hypotonia, as can the traction maneuver for head control, horizontal prone suspension for trunk tone, scarf sign and axillary suspension for shoulder girdle tone, and popliteal angle for lower extremity tone. In premature neonates there is normally a caudal-rostral progression of tone development, particularly flexor tone, correlated with age up to 40 weeks' term. Individual joint movements should be observed and agonist-antagonist strengths should be tested bilaterally to look for asymmetries and focal discrepancies. There may be a paucity of spontaneous limb movements, and breathing may be paradoxical with chest lowering and stomach rising due to primarily diaphragmatic strength. Severe respiratory compromise along with profound hypotonia may be features of neonatal spinal cord injury as well as congenital myopathies. A loss of pain sensation (evidenced by facial grimace following a painful stimulation) below the neck would suggest the former cause rather than the latter. The plantar response should be elicited in older children. The presence of contractures is common in congenital muscular dystrophy and congenital myotonic dystrophy. Some infants present with multiple joint contractures (arthrogryposis) sustained with intrauterine anterior horn cell damage. The older child may have developed scoliosis from gravity effects on a weak spine. Important clues are the absence of deep tendon reflexes in neuropathies and the presence of percussion myotonia in myotonic dystrophy. Sensory testing is important in suspected neuropathies, including hereditary motor sensory neuropathies, radiculopathies, and myelopathies. The responses to be observed are latency, limb movement quality (more than stereotyped triple flexion), facial grimace and cry, and

habituation. In the case of a hypotonic neonate, the mother may also need to be examined for the presence of signs of myotonic dystrophy or myasthenia gravis.

Observation rather than formal individual muscle testing is often easier and more revealing, particularly in infants and preschool-aged children. Useful activities to observe include walking, running, climbing stairs or stepping onto a stool, lying on the floor and coming to a standing position unassisted, smiling, closing the eyes tightly, and speaking. The ambulatory child may have a waddling gait from hip girdle weakness, genu recurvatum from quadriceps weakness, or talipes planus from foot weakness. Arising from a prone position on the floor, the child may demonstrate the Gower sign by first getting to the hands and knees, then walking the feet forward to the hands, and finally "walking" the hands up the trunk to gain an upright position, rather than quickly rising from squatting without using the hands.

Laboratory Tests

Evaluation of the hypotonic depressed neonate should include an evaluation for infection (complete blood cell count and appropriate cultures) as well as an assessment of pH, blood gas, glucose, electrolytes, liver function tests, ammonia, amino acids in the blood, and sugars, organic acids, and ketones in the urine. Spinal fluid examination is sometimes helpful if there is an increase in white cells related to possible infection or inflammation or if there is an increased level of protein as seen in immune, storage, or necrotizing CNS conditions.

Screening blood or plasma tests can also be important for diagnosis of severe neonatal hypotonia, which can be a result of inborn errors of metabolism, such as peroxisomal disorders, glycine encephalopathy, pyruvate dehydrogenase deficiency or other congenital lactic acidoses, organic acidemias, fatty acid oxidation disorders, maple syrup urine disease, molybdenum cofactor deficiency, vitamin D–dependent rickets type 1, magnesium toxicity, creatine metabolism disorders, and hyperammonemic encephalopathies. **Serum creatine phosphokinase (CPK),** a screen for muscle fiber necrosis, should be requested when the history suggests a degenerative condition or examination indicates the cause of hypotonia is in the neuromuscular unit. Creatine phosphokinase is 10 to 100 times higher than normal in children with muscular dystrophy, and it may also be mildly elevated in female carriers of the mutant dystrophin gene in their first 3 decades of life. The serum CPK level may be less markedly elevated in children with inflammatory myopathies, such as dermatomyositis and polymyositis, and to some extent following muscle trauma.

One purpose of laboratory tests in children with neuromuscular conditions is to confirm the level of the nervous system involved (Table 119-3). Useful information about the presence of neuropathic, myopathic, and neuromuscular junction disorders can be obtained from the nerve conduction velocity and EMG. Demyelinating neuropathies slow **nerve conduction** or produce signs of a segmental conduction block. If the problem is a motor neuropathy, an axonal neuropathy may have depressed amplitude of the nerve action

Table 119-3. Laboratory Tests Useful in the Diagnosis of Hypotonia Caused by Neuromuscular Lesions

Test	Anatomic Site		
	Anterior Horn Cell	Neuromuscular Junction	Muscle
Muscle enzymes	Normal	Normal	Normal/increased
Neostigmine test	Normal	Abnormal	Normal
Electromyography	Neuropathic	Decremental/incremental	Myopathic
Muscle biopsy	Group atrophy	Normal	Myopathic

potential or fibrillation potentials on EMG. In some myopathies, small amplitude potentials and myotonia may be seen on EMG. Decremental response to stimulation and other abnormalities are evident with myasthenia gravis and neuromuscular junction blockade caused by the botulinum toxin. An intramuscular (IM) neostigmine test can confirm diagnosis of myasthenia gravis in children with easy fatigability by history or on examination. Some neuromuscular conditions are associated with cardiomyopathies and, therefore, the electrocardiogram and echocardiogram can help in diagnosis as well as bring to light potentially critical problems needing acute intervention, such as heart conduction block.

When properly handled, **muscle biopsy** gives useful diagnostic information about neuromuscular disorders that may cause hypotonia. A large portion of the tissue should be frozen for histochemical studies. Histochemistry can differentiate neuropathic changes from myopathic changes related to fiber-type specificities as well as disclose structural abnormalities pointing to dystrophy, glycogen storage disease, or congenital myopathy such as nemaline bodies, central cores, or amphinuclei. Histochemical stains can also give information about metabolic myopathic disorders, and immunohistochemical stains can establish marker evidence for specific diagnoses. Another portion of the muscle should be fixed in glutaraldehyde for electron microscopy to determine if ultrastructural abnormalities, such as those seen in mitochondrial myopathies, are present. Tissue can be subjected to other specific expression analyses such as dystrophin protein levels, glycolytic enzyme activity, cytochrome-c oxidase and other respiratory chain enzyme complex assays, free and acyl carnitine levels, or fatty acid transport and beta oxidation assays to confirm a diagnosis.

Metabolic and molecular genetic studies can sometimes be done on blood or urine samples, such as thyroid functions if clinical suspicion of hypothyroidism persists, white blood cell enzymatic assays, very long-chain fatty acid profiles for peroxisomal disorders including neonatal adrenoleukodystrophy, lysosomal enzyme screens such as acid maltase for glycogen storage disease type 2, plasma amino acid levels, and urine organic acid levels. Cytogenetic analysis may be useful when Down syndrome or other chromosomal aberrations are suspected, and DNA methylation analysis is done when Prader-Willi

syndrome is suspected as a cause of non-paralytic hypotonia. When examination and screening laboratory tests have narrowed the diagnostic possibilities to a level of the nervous system, molecular techniques, including use of specific nucleic acid probes, comparative genomic hybridization, copy number variance, and exon sequencing screens, can sometimes be used to help make specific diagnoses for genetic disorders (eg, Duchenne or other X-linked muscular dystrophies, myotonic dystrophies, mitochondrial cytopathies, SMA). Often these blood tests have eliminated the need for painful electromyography or muscle biopsy.

Imaging Studies

A brain magnetic resonance imaging (MRI) scan is diagnostically helpful in at least 4 situations: when deficits in mental status, cognitive function, or attention are apparent in children with hypotonia; when neurologic examination suggests an upper motor neuron component to the weakness or hypotonia, such as active deep tendon reflexes or persistent ankle clonus; when a progressive congenital muscular dystrophy or a mitochondrial cytopathy such as Leigh disease is suggested by myopathic and CNS signs; and when children have hypotonia as part of a multiorgan dysgenesis, such as with a chromosomal aberration, because of the high likelihood of a brain component to the dysgenesis. A computed tomography scan is rarely helpful. A muscle MRI scan can be useful in selecting a muscle for biopsy in cases of suspected inflammatory myopathy.

Management

Specific management depends on diagnosis but ranges from supportive respiratory measures and anti-inflammatory therapies to physical and orthopedic therapy to improve function. Sometimes the potential for partial or full recovery is an important factor in determining the goals in clinical management and therapy for children with neuromuscular conditions. An infant with a congenital myopathy may gradually increase in strength and should, therefore, receive intensive supportive care, including long-term ventilatory support and gastrostomy feeding. On the other hand, the family of an infant with a rapidly degenerative terminal condition, such as the severe infantile type of Werdnig-Hoffmann anterior horn cell disease, may elect not to undertake respiratory support after they understand the course of the disease and lack of curative therapy. Such families usually continue to benefit from the ongoing information provided by the physician and support of paramedical personnel and lay groups, and affected children can benefit from palliative therapies and hospice care.

Children with profound weakness easily succumb to respiratory infections and have difficulty with recovery from anesthesia; therefore, they require vigilance on the parent's or caregiver's part and early intervention because they may need intense **respiratory support.** Children with long-term neuromuscular weakness can sometimes benefit from **orthopedic** procedures for scoliosis stabilization to prevent respiratory compromise.

Children with acquired acute hypotonic weakness (Box 119-1) may require therapies more directed at the underlying

Box 119-1. Specific Etiologies of Hypotonia Caused by Acute Generalized Weaknesses

- Acute postinfectious polyradiculoneuritis (Guillain-Barré syndrome)
- Postinfectious myositis
- Enteroviral poliomyelitis
- Acute myasthenia gravis
- Infantile botulism
- Tick paralysis
- Periodic paralysis (hyperkalemic, hypokalemic, and normokalemic)
- Metabolic myopathy

pathophysiological process. Acute postinfectious polyneuritis and variants requires careful, frequent monitoring of respiratory status and artificial ventilation when significant loss of vital capacity has occurred. In addition, children should be considered for **plasmapheresis** or intravenous immunoglobulin (IVIG), particularly for small children when their condition rapidly worsens early in the course of the disorder. Specific antisera are used for botulinum intoxication. Removal of the tick from the skin results in recovery from tick paralysis in 1 to 2 days. Dysimmune myasthenia can be treated with anticholinesterase medication, IVIG, or thymectomy when it is resistant to immunosuppressive medication. In addition to more acute disorders, chronic relapsing polyneuritis and myositis can be treated effectively with various anti-inflammatory agents, including prednisone and immunoglobulin, during periods of exacerbation. Suspected metabolic disorders can be managed with focused metabolic therapy, such as eliminating a toxic nutrient from feeding; using a high-energy alternative nutrient (glucose or fatty acids); treating hyperammonemia with benzoate, phenylbutyrate, or arginine or using dialysis when the ammonia level becomes dangerously high; administering insulin to control hyperglycemia; reducing periods of catabolism during an infection; and supplementing vitamin cofactors and carnitine. Metabolic myopathies are sometimes empirically treated with thiamine, riboflavin, nicotinamide, coenzyme Q10, biotin, l-carnitine, succinate, vitamin C or K, and medium-chain triglyceride oil. Use of these therapies in some cases may be based on tissue analysis.

Treatment and care of children with muscular dystrophy is presently directed individually toward maintaining mobility and preventing contractures through physical therapy, bivalved casts, braces, and surgical repair to improve limb function by joint stabilization or equalizing of muscle strengths across joints. **Physical and occupational therapy** can accelerate recovery after procedures and maximize function. Inactivity generally increases disability. Many new hardware technologies (eg, long leg braces, electric wheelchairs, battery-operated ventilators, noninvasive positive-pressure ventilation for some cases of respiratory insufficiency) have allowed affected children to overcome previously insurmountable disabilities. Adjunctive corticosteroid therapy is useful in children with Duchenne muscular dystrophy, but temporary beneficial effects must be weighed against steroid toxicity. Presently, new therapies for

providing dystrophin expression are under active investigation, including "exon skipping" promoting drugs and dystrophin gene fragment-carrying viral vectors.

Prognosis

Spinal muscular atrophy type 1 generally progresses to death over a couple of years, and Duchenne muscular dystrophy generally progresses to full-time artificial ventilation over 15 to 20 years. However, the course of many genetic conditions can be quite variable and related to different alleles at the disease gene locus or different positions of a critical base pair substitution or deletion. Other loci may also have a modifying effect on disease gene expression or the pathophysiology of the disease. For example, SMA and dystrophinopathies have genes that have multiple abnormal modes of expression with widely different prognostic implications for disease course.

The weakness of congenital myopathies, however, usually slowly improves. Acquired toxin and immune-mediated conditions such as infant botulism and Guillain-Barré syndrome generally have a good outcome (up to 85%), although long-term supportive measures may be necessary.

CASE RESOLUTION

The 6-month-old girl in the case study was judged to have hypotonia caused by a neuromuscular condition, in part because of her alert appearance and absent deep tendon reflexes. Neuropathic abnormalities on electromyography and muscle biopsy were also present. A blood test for the survival motor neuron genes did not detect any normal sequences, confirming the diagnosis of spinal muscular atrophy type 1. The family received genetic counseling, became involved in a support group, and eventually reached a decision to forego intubation when respiratory failure overtakes their daughter. The physician coordinated hospice services for the family.

Selected References

Dubowitz V. *Muscle Disorders in Childhood.* 2nd ed. Philadelphia, PA: WB Saunders; 1995

Huff K. Approach to the child with weakness or paralysis. In: Osborne L, DeWitt T, First L, Zenel J, eds. *Pediatrics.* Philadelphia, PA: Elsevier; 2006

Leonard JV, Morris AA. Diagnosis and early management of inborn errors of metabolism presenting around the time of birth. *Acta Paediatr.* 2006;95(1): 6–14

Pena-Garza JE. The hypotonic infant. In: *Fenichel's Clinical Pediatric Neurology: A Signs and Symptoms Approach.* 7th ed. New York, NY: Elsevier Saunders; 2013: 147–169

Sarnat H, Menkes J. Diseases of the motor unit. In: Menkes J, Sarnat H, Maria B, eds. *Child Neurology.* Philadelphia, PA: Lippincott; 2006

Swaiman K. Muscular tone and gait disturbances. In: Swaiman K, Ashwal S, Ferriero D, eds. *Pediatric Neurology Principals and Practice.* 4th ed. Philadelphia, PA: Elsevier; 2006

Volpe J. Neonatal hypotonia. In: Jones HR, Devivo D, Darras B, eds. *Neuromuscular Disorders in Childhood and Adolescence.* Philadelphia, PA: Butterworth Heinemann; 2003

CHAPTER 120

Headaches

Kenneth R. Huff, MD

CASE STUDY

A 12-year-old girl is brought in with a history of headaches. Although she has been sent home from school twice in the last 6 weeks, she has experienced headaches for at least a year. The last episode, 1 week ago, was typical. The headache began as a dull feeling over both eyes, radiated up to the top of her head, and eventually became pounding. She had no preliminary visual symptoms or other warning signs prior to the head pain. The episode began during an afternoon class after she had been outside on a hot, sunny day for physical education. The headache worsened after she walked home from school. Once she got home, she went to her room, drew the curtains, and lay down on her bed. She experienced some nausea and loss of appetite but no vomiting. She did not get up for dinner. She denied diplopia, vertigo, ataxia, or limb weakness, and her speech was observed to be articulate and coherent. She took two 80-mg children's acetaminophen tablets without

significant relief but eventually fell asleep. The following morning she felt fine.

Between headaches, her behavior has not changed, and she has continued to make above-average grades. She has not experienced any major changes in her home environment. When initially questioned, her mother denied having migraines, but she admits to needing to lie down because of headaches about once a month. A detailed neurologic examination of the girl is completely normal.

Questions

1. What are the major classes of headache?
2. How do the symptoms help differentiate the classes?
3. How does family history influence the etiology and help in management of the headache?
4. What is the appropriate treatment for the problem headache?

Headaches, which are very common in adolescents and older children, frequently prompt parents to bring their children to the physician's attention. The physician must differentiate headaches that are symptomatic of a progressive intracranial process from those that may possibly be intermittently disabling but do not necessitate surgery. The cornerstone of this determination is obtaining key historical information and determining whether there are abnormalities on examination of the nervous system. Decisions about management strategies are most influenced by etiology and the effect headaches are having on the child's life.

Epidemiology

The contribution of "symptomatic" headaches (those related to tumors, vascular abnormalities, or meningitis) to the overall prevalence of headache is relatively small. Chronic recurrent headaches in children that are not related to a self-limited condition are frequently lumped together as migraine, which includes classic and common migraine. The prevalence of migraine that comes to a physician's attention is about 3% to 10% for all children, but as many as 75% of all children and 85% of adolescents admit to having experienced a headache in the last year. Although initial headache symptoms begin most often between ages 6 and 12 years, many patients come to medical attention for the first time during adolescence, especially girls whose headache prevalence at that age is double that of boys. Headaches are also commonly associated with trauma, acute

intercurrent infection, or other systemic illness. A multigenerational family history of "sick headaches" is a frequent finding in the child with migraine. This history must be specifically elicited by the physician, however, because its significance is often discounted by parents.

Clinical Presentation

Parents must interpret the nature and severity of their child's experience and symptoms, which may be difficult, especially in younger children. Younger children more rarely complain of head pain but more commonly complain of stomachache or present with nausea or vomiting. Later, as the child grows older, the same episodic setting and behavior are associated with a headache complaint. The episodic syndromes of cyclic vomiting and abdominal migraine are related presentations to childhood migraine. Other younger children present with similarly related benign paroxysmal vertigo. Adolescents, on the other hand, may report persistent, dull, aching, or pounding head pain, which can recur daily. As opposed to headaches increasing in intensity or frequency and associated with neurologic signs, which may suggest an intracranial mass lesion, migraine episodes may be relatively stable in frequency over many weeks or months, accompanied by a normal neurologic and ophthalmologic examination, and similar to that experienced by other family members (D$_x$ Box). Classic migraine, which is relatively unusual in children, is distinguished from common migraine by the presence of an

Dx Headaches (Migraine)

- Head pain, often pounding in character, over the eyes, at the vertex, or in the occipital region
- Pain frequently accompanied by nausea, anorexia, photophobia, or phonophobia
- Pain sometimes preceded by visual symptoms such as scotomas
- Frequent presence of trigger factors
- Family history of headaches (often)

aura of specific sensory symptoms that precede the headache. Both types of headache may be associated with lethargy, irritability, slowness of movement and response, concentration problems, intolerance of intense sound or light, and loss of appetite.

Pathophysiology

Pain fibers are carried in the trigeminal nerves from the scalp, skull, meninges, and vessel walls within the brain. Traction on these fibers or inflammation at the endings produces the pain that is associated with mass lesions or meningeal inflammation. The usual distinction between migraine and tension headache pathophysiology is more difficult to make in the child and may involve the types of factors that trigger headaches at different ages (Box 120-1). Several different mechanisms involving one or more environmental or internal factors trigger headaches in genetically predisposed individuals. A drop in hormones may trigger menstrual migraines, for example. The rare condition, familial hemiplegic migraine, has been related to mutations in 3 different genes so far, illustrating a very specific predisposition. The "migraine generator" probably resides in the brain stem and has input to the trigeminal nucleus, which innervates intracranial blood vessels. "Cortical spreading depression of Leão," believed to be the electrophysiologic correlate of the migraine aura, also activates trigeminal afferents. The pathogenic neurotransmitter at the vascular nerve endings is likely serotonergic (perhaps released intravascularly from platelet stores), precipitating a cascade of local cytokines, substance P, calcitonin gene-related peptide (CGRP), and histamine in and around the vessel walls, leading in turn to changes in vascular permeability and local swelling. The relative roles of genetic susceptibility and environmental trigger agents

Box 120-1. Triggers of Migraine

- Glare, dazzle, bright sunlight, or fluorescent lighting
- Physical exertion, fatigue, lack of sleep, hunger
- Change in ambient temperature or humidity
- Allergic reactions, pungent odors
- Certain foods, alcoholic beverages, and cold foods or beverages
- Anxiety, stress, and worry
- Head trauma
- Menstruation and oral contraceptives
- Refractive errors (rare)

are subjects of ongoing investigation, from molecular aspects to the use of animal models.

Differential Diagnosis

Acute Headaches

Emergent causes should be considered if headaches have an abrupt onset, develop rapidly, or are especially severe or if children describe them as a "thunderclap" or "the worst of my life." **Intracranial hemorrhage** from a ruptured aneurysm or an arteriovenous malformation or, rarely, as a secondary effect of hypertension is foremost on the list of such causes. If children have a condition that may potentially lead to stroke, such as coagulopathy, hemoglobinopathy, or heart disease, the stroke may become hemorrhagic and produce such an acute, severe headache.

Nonhemorrhagic meningeal irritation, such as the inflammation produced by bacterial or viral meningitis, may also cause acute headaches. These conditions may render patients confused and lethargic while still conscious and are often associated with fever. Both types of meningeal irritation produce nuchal rigidity and Kernig and Brudzinski signs.

Chronic Progressive Headaches

Children with brain tumors, brain abscesses, or a block in cerebrospinal fluid (CSF) flow producing hydrocephalus frequently have a "crescendo" history, usually less than 6 months long, of increasing severity or frequency of headaches. The headache may be consistently localized to one side or the occipital area, or it may awaken the patient from sleep, presumably related to relative shift in intracranial traction forces due to gravity and the horizontal position. Interestingly, many children with brain tumors do not complain of a localized headache and may present with persistent vomiting without headache as a prominent symptom. Idiopathic intracranial hypertension (IIH) most often presents with headaches of recent onset and associated papilledema. Intracranial venous sinus obstruction, hypervitaminosis A, steroid withdrawal, tetracycline treatment, and obesity have all been related etiologically.

Chronic Recurrent Headaches

The pain of **migraine headaches,** the most common chronic headache type, is throbbing in character, and if headaches are severe, patients avoid intense sensory stimuli or physical activity. Episodes may last 30 minutes to 2 days but often resolve with a period of sleep. Nausea or dizziness, anorexia, and visual blurring are often associated. The pain may be severe enough to curtail activities, or the child may participate under duress, particularly at school. Classic migraine is migraine headache preceded by 10 to 20 minutes of a sensory phenomenon, usually lights or visual patterns.

Sinus infection may be a cause of chronically recurring or acute headaches, especially if the pain is facial in additional to cranial. Symptoms of chronic nasal congestion, allergies, and postnasal drip may be associated with sinus headaches. Children with asthma also have recurring headaches possibly triggered by sinus involvement, generalized cytokine release, or other aspects of asthmatic pathophysiology such as smooth muscle reactivity and medication side effect susceptibility.

Other types of headaches may recur without progression. **Chronic daily headaches** (more than 15 headache days per month) in some cases may be "transformed migraine" or "rebound headache" due to abortive medication overuse. Adolescents may have frequently recurring headaches triggered by irregular lifestyles such as not exercising enough, eating regularly, or getting adequate sleep, if they are susceptible individuals. The symptomatology in some individuals is more consistent with **tension headaches** characterized by a feeling of a tightening band around the head rather than a throbbing pain, an occurrence late in the day, and an association with anxiety, depression, or a stressful environment. There is overlap in this group with migraineurs in symptoms and response to therapy. **Posttraumatic headaches** may recur with gradually decreasing severity for several months following concussion.

Cluster headaches are very different than the other types discussed and are associated with unilateral lancinating pain, tearing, nasal stuffiness, and nighttime pacing and are unusual in children.

Evaluation

History

Information should be obtained from patients, parents, and other caregivers concerning when headaches first began; the quality, intensity, and location of headaches; as well as other associated symptoms before and during headaches (Questions Box). Duration, clinical course, and conditions that evoke, intensify, or alleviate the pain are

also important. It is useful to have children describe a typical episode (perhaps the most recent), including the circumstances of when and where the headache began and how it affected activities at the time. The degree to which the headache problem affects the child's lifestyle strongly influences the management plan for chronic recurrent headaches.

Physical Examination

Blood pressure should be noted even though primary hypertension is an unusual cause of headaches in children. Growth abnormalities and neurocutaneous findings may be relevant. A thorough neurologic examination is needed to determine if findings suggest an emergent problem, such as meningitis, or a potential neurosurgical condition, such as intracranial hemorrhage or brain tumor. Examination should assess for the presence of sinus tenderness, nuchal rigidity, funduscopic abnormalities such as papilledema or hemorrhages, signs of trauma, and any focal neurologic signs. A brain tumor or other space-occupying lesion may present with ataxia and cranial nerve signs for a posterior fossa lesion, loss of visual fields or hypothalamic dysfunction (endocrine abnormalities) for a suprasellar or third ventricular region lesion, and hemiparesis, hemisensory deficit, or language dysfunction for a cerebral hemispheric lesion. Personality changes or developmental regression should be especially noted. Increased intracranial pressure (ICP) may lead to papilledema, loss of upward gaze, general hypertonicity, leg weakness, positive Babinski sign, spastic gait, loss of continence, or confusion or stupor owing to blockage of CSF by the tumor.

Rarely, children in the midst of a migraine headache may display confusion, aphasia, unilateral numbness, or, less commonly, weakness, hemianopsia, or sensory distortion ("Alice in Wonderland" syndrome). In these circumstances, diagnosis of complications of a migraine syndrome is reached only after diagnostic tests have eliminated other acute encephalopathies.

Laboratory Tests

If stiff neck is present and focal or lateralized neurologic signs are absent, an immediate CSF examination is indicated to diagnose the cause of meningeal inflammation. When hemorrhagic fluid is encountered, it is often useful to centrifuge a specimen to check for xanthochromia and to count cells in a subsequent sample to differentiate a traumatic spinal tap from subarachnoid hemorrhage. If papilledema is present and imaging studies are normal, a lumbar puncture should be done to measure CSF pressure.

A sleep study may be indicated if there is a history of obstructive snoring or recurrent sleep disruption.

Imaging Studies

Recent trauma, persistent vomiting, depressed alertness, crescendo or change in pattern, and even recent onset of headaches all may be indications for an immediate head magnetic resonance imaging (MRI) or computed tomography (CT) scan. The risk of missing an anatomic diagnosis should be weighed against the risk of anesthesia for the study and perhaps false reassurance from an inadequate study.

Questions

Headaches

- Where is the child, what time of day is it, and what is the child doing when a typical headache or the last recalled headache begins?
- Where is the pain located? How severe is the pain? How long does the pain last?
- Is nausea, vomiting, or photophobia associated with the headache?
- What does the child do after getting the headache? Does the episode require cessation of activities?
- Does the child take any medication for the pain? If so, was it successful? What else, if anything, allows the child to feel better?
- How long ago did the first headache occur? Are headaches becoming more frequent or severe?
- Have headaches ever awakened the child at night?
- Have there been any changes in speech, vision, gait, or personality or any loss of skills or abilities between headaches?
- Does the child have any warning symptoms before the pain? Does unilateral visual loss, weakness or numbness, diplopia, confusion, or loss of consciousness occur with the headache?
- How often does the child miss school because of a headache?
- Do other members of the family have headaches? Do they ever need to lie down or take medicine for these headaches?

Such decisions are also influenced by the reliability and ease of communication with the child's caregivers. The yield of imaging is low in the absence of neurologic signs. If signs or symptoms of increased ICP are apparent, a CT or an MRI scan must be obtained to help diagnose etiology of the headaches. New focal or general neurologic signs also indicate the need for a CT or an MRI scan. Cerebral angiography may be necessary in rare cases to locate a focal source of subarachnoid hemorrhage, and a magnetic resonance venogram may assist in diagnosing dural sinus thrombosis. Head imaging studies are also helpful with the diagnosis of chronic or recurrent sinus headaches and Chiari type 1 malformation.

Management

The presence of progressive symptoms, abnormal neurologic signs, or a hemorrhage or space-occupying lesion on an imaging study usually necessitates a neurologic or neurosurgical consultation. It may be necessary to urgently initiate measures for managing increased ICP. In the absence of a mass, increased ICP related to IIH also requires treatment. A serious sequela of IIH is eventual loss of vision if pressure is not relieved. This complication can be monitored with field testing and optical coherence tomography. Therapies include CSF withdrawal, diuretics such as acetazolamide, and surgical CSF diversion.

If a careful assessment has revealed no acute or progressive conditions, pain is not severe, frequency is low, duration is short, and effect on lifestyle or daily activities is minimal, the appropriate management is often just **reassurance.** Frequently, parental anxiety about a potential mass or hemorrhage far outweighs the morbidity produced by the headache symptom itself. Sometimes placing the child's headache problem in context with the parent's or other family member's headaches will help with reassurance, and sometimes in milder cases, non-pharmacologic or nonprescription medication strategies can be agreed on as a management plan. Education and sometimes a headache diary or log helps patients and their families take control and own their own problem (discern triggers and track intervention efficacy), particularly when they can correlate headaches with inadequate exercise, skipping meals, and inadequate sleep.

However, it may be apparent that the headaches have produced significant discomfort or disruption of activities or lifestyle for the child and more than reassurance is needed (Table 120-1). Interventions,

Table 120-1. Drugs Useful in Childhood Headaches	
Abortive (Symptomatic)	
Acetaminophen, PO	325–975 mg every 4 h (15 mg/kg/dose) (max: 5 doses/24 h)
Ibuprofen, PO	200–800 mg every 6 h (10 mg/kg/dose) (max: 40 mg/kg/24 h)
Naproxen, PO	5–7 mg/kg/dose every 8–12 h (max: 15 mg/kg/24 h [age >2 y])
Sumatriptan, SC, IN, or PO	6 mg SC or 5–20 mg IN or 25–100 mg PO (may repeat after 1 h SC, 2 h IN and PO) (max: 2 doses/24 h)
Ergotamine, PR	¼ rectal suppository (2 mg), repeat ¼ suppository every 30 min as needed (max: 4 mg/d [older children and adolescents])
Rizatriptan, PO	5–10 mg orally disintegrating or regular tablets (may repeat after 2 h) (max: 3 doses/24 h)
Isometheptene mucate with dichloralphenazone and acetaminophen, PO	1–2 caps at onset (may repeat every 1 h to 3–5 caps/d)
Dihydroergotamine, IN or IV	4 mg IN (1 spray each nostril, repeat once after 15 min) or 0.25–1 mg at onset and 1 mg/h $\times$ 2 (max: 6 mg/wk [older children and adolescents])
Dexamethasone, IV Prochlorperazine, IV	4–16 mg single dose (0.25 mg/kg) or rapidly tapering every 6 h 5–10 mg single dose (older children and adolescents) 0.1–0.15 mg/kg/dose (younger children)
Prophylactic	
Propranolol	10–40 mg 2–4 times/d (max: 40–80 mg/24 h if ≤35 kg)
	120–160 mg/24 h if >35 kg; no more than 320 mg/24 h)
Cyproheptadine	1–4 mg 2–4 times/d (0.25–0.5 mg/kg/24 h) (max: 16 mg/24 h)
Amitriptyline	10–75 mg at bedtime (max: 150 mg/24 h [older children and adolescents])
Verapamil	40 mg every 8 h (age 1–5 y); 40–80 mg every 8 h (age >5 y) (max: 240 mg/24 h)
Valproic acid	10–15 mg/kg/d initial, 30–60 mg/kg/d maintenance, divided twice/d or every day if ER (max: 60 mg/kg/d [follow clinical signs of toxicity and serum level])
Topiramate	50–200 mg/d divided twice/d after ramping from 25 mg twice/d over a few weeks
Fluoxetine	10 mg every morning initial (max: 40 mg/d)

Abbreviations: ER, extended release; IN, intranasally; IV, intravenously; PO, orally; PR, rectally; SC, subcutaneously.

nevertheless, should always weigh side effects against effectiveness of treatment and the possibility of medication overuse headache if the symptomatic treatment is taken more frequently than twice a week. A goal is a reduction in headache frequency, severity, duration, or disability with improved quality of life. The initial trial should usually be **acetaminophen or nonsteroidal anti-inflammatory drugs if these have not already failed. Symptomatic treatment** should be taken as soon after the onset of prodromal or headache symptoms as possible. If children are allowed medication at school and are able to lie down for 30 minutes, many can finish the school day. Naproxen is beneficial particularly if there is head or neck muscle tenderness, and indomethacin if there is unilateral continuous pain with autonomic symptoms (hemicrania continua). Headaches in adolescents are sometimes helped by **isometheptene mucate.** For severe, recurrent headaches, serotonin 1b/1d receptor agonists (triptans) are useful. **Sumatriptan and other triptans, which lower CGRP levels,** have relatively tolerable but occasionally anxiety-provoking side effects, and patients need to be informed about them as with any new medication. Sumatriptan in combination with naproxen may have increased efficacy over each individually. Dihydroergotamine, zolmitriptan, or sumatriptan given intranasally are also effective abortive treatments in vomiting patients and work faster than tablets, but they may have a disagreeable taste if they should enter the posterior oropharynx. Very severe refractory headaches may respond to intravenous (IV) diphenhydramine, ketorolac, or prochlorperazine (Compazine) or IV **dihydroergotamine** or **dexamethasone along with a bolus of IV fluids.**

The decision to begin a **prophylactic medication** should be based on the frequency and severity of headaches. Medication overuse headaches often benefit solely from abstinence for 1 to 2 weeks. Anticonvulsants such as **valproic acid and topiramate** have been found to be successful anti-migraine agents. The β-blockers, including **propranolol,** have demonstrated efficacy as prophylactic agents, and the antihistamine **cyproheptadine** has been successful in many younger patients. **Amitriptyline** and nortriptyline are effective preventive treatments in older children and adolescents; a single bedtime dose should be used at first. Amitriptyline can be combined with propranolol if necessary. Calcium channel blockers such as **verapamil, N-methyl-d-aspartate receptor agonist memantine,** and selective serotonin reuptake inhibitors (SSRIs) such as **fluoxetine (if care is taken to monitor for serotonin syndrome if a triptan and an SSRI are used together)** may also be useful in older children and adolescents. Riboflavin, magnesium, and botulinum toxin injections have had isolated success. A 2- to 4-week trial is necessary before concluding the initial treatment using any of the prophylactic medications has been ineffective.

Chronic daily headaches may be successfully treated with education, use of prophylactic medication, avoidance of analgesics because of rebound potential, and assistance for children working their way back into a functional daily routine. Healthy lifestyle changes have been very beneficial, particularly in adolescents, but biofeedback-assisted relaxation training, guided imagery, hypnosis, meditation, and acupuncture have had to overcome problems of limited availability and high cost. If severe environmental stressors or psychologic trauma is present as an ongoing headache trigger, patients may benefit from psychotherapy.

Prognosis

Many children with headaches have a good prognosis and do not require ongoing intervention after families are reassured of the benign nature of the problem. For other children, symptomatic medications are frequently effective. Prophylactic medication is necessary in a few cases. Headaches with psychiatric comorbidity have a less good prognosis. For patients receiving prophylactic therapy, periodic withdrawal of the medication should be attempted to establish that it is still necessary. Pediatric patients frequently experience remission of their headaches by late adolescence, and, by adulthood, the incidence of headaches has decreased, particularly for males.

CASE RESOLUTION

In the case study, the child's symptoms and circumstances of the headache suggest a diagnosis of migraine. No laboratory tests or imaging studies are necessary. The girl is begun on amitriptyline and instructed to keep a calendar of headache occurrences. She has 2 headaches in the first 2 weeks, which are aborted effectively with ibuprofen. Following these episodes, she has no further recurrences, and the amitriptyline is withdrawn successfully after 3 months.

Selected References

Ball AK, Clarke CE. Idiopathic intracranial hypertension. *Lancet Neurol.* 2006;5(5):433–442

El-Chammas K, Keyes J, Thompson N, Vijayakumar J, Becher D, Jackson JL. Pharmacologic treatment of pediatric headaches: a meta-analysis. *JAMA Pediatr.* 2013;167(3):250–258

Landy S. Migraine throughout the life cycle: treatment through the ages. *Neurology.* 2004;62(5 Suppl 2):S2–S8

Lewis D. Headaches in infants and children. In: Swaiman K, Ashwal S, Ferriero D, eds. *Pediatric Neurology Principals and Practice.* Philadelphia, PA: Elsevier; 2006

Mack KJ. An approach to children with chronic daily headache. *Dev Med Child Neurol.* 2006;48(12):997–1000

Rothner AD. Pediatric headaches. *Semin Pediatr Neurol.* 2001;8:1–51

CHAPTER 121

Tics

Kenneth R. Huff, MD

CASE STUDY

An 8-year-old boy has unusual recurring behaviors that began 2 to 3 months ago. He stretches his neck or raises his eyebrows suddenly several times a day. Sometimes he is able to suppress these actions. The boy's parents report that in the last 2 years he has displayed several repetitive behaviors, including blinking, grimacing, rubbing his chin on his left shoulder, making a "gulping" sound, and sniffing. Originally they thought the sniffing was related to hay fever, but the boy has no other allergic symptoms. He does not use profane words. In conversations, he sometimes repeats the last phrase of a sentence that was just uttered by himself or someone else. In addition, he must touch each light switch in the hallway every time he leaves his room, and he must retie his shoelaces several times until they are exactly the same length. Although his schoolwork has not deteriorated, he has always had trouble completing tasks and finishing homework. His teacher and his best friend have asked about his strange

behavior. His mother has a "psychological" problem with her son's gulping sounds (ie, they recur in her own mind), and she recalls that her father had a habit of frequently looking over one shoulder for no apparent reason.

Although during examination the boy does not exhibit any unusual behaviors, he raises his eyebrows twice and places his hand over his crotch several times while his parents are interviewed. Except for mild fine motor incoordination, the neurologic examination is normal.

Questions

1. What are the characteristics of tics?
2. What are the social implications of tics?
3. Should pharmacologic treatments be part of the management of tic disorders?
4. What other problems are associated with the tic disorder that also should receive intervention?

Tics are brief, abrupt, non-purposeful movements or utterances. They occur in a background of normal activity and are repetitive and involuntary but can be suppressed. Tourette syndrome is the most common etiology of tics in children. It is defined by multiple types of tics displayed over time, including motor tics and vocal tics. Tourette syndrome most frequently manifests solely as a non-disabling movement disorder but may also be associated with other neurobehavioral problems, which may include attention-deficit/hyperactivity disorder (ADHD), obsessive-compulsive disorder, mood and rage disorders, anxiety, and personality and conduct difficulties that may be more disabling than the tics.

Epidemiology

Tics are relatively common in children but often go unrecognized as a movement disorder. The onset of tics associated with Tourette syndrome is generally between 5 and 12 years of age but can be as late as 21 years of age. The prevalence of tics is 5 times higher in males than females. By various estimates, Tourette syndrome prevalence is between 0.1% and 3%, but many cases of Tourette syndrome are familial (some features occur in a parent in up to 25% of cases), and family members may have had symptoms so mild that they never sought medical attention. The risk of Tourette syndrome in a sibling is about 8%. Tics are more common in male family members, but other family members may have only non-tic manifestations of the

syndrome, such as obsessive-compulsive symptoms occurring most often in females.

Clinical Presentation

Children with tics display sudden repetitive movements of the face, neck, shoulders, or hands in the context of normal behaviors, and normal behaviors are sometimes used to mask the tics. Sometimes tics can be suppressed when they would be embarrassing or during a time of intense physical activity, concentration, or performance, but they also may be worsened by stress or strong emotional feelings. Tics associated with Tourette syndrome will vary in their manifestations over periods of weeks to months. Some examples of tics are blinking, eye rolling, grimacing, neck stretching, head turning or shaking, shoulder shrugging, stomach tensing, and wrist flicking. Many affected children describe a brief premonitory sensation, which is an indescribable, uncomfortable feeling that is subsequently relieved by the motor tic. Tics may bizarrely mimic normal, sometimes complex, movements or postures or involve a series of orchestrated simple movements, such as sequential finger flexing, wrist bending, and arm stretching. Tics may include sudden repetitive sounds from the vocal apparatus (D_x Box), which may be produced by a sudden movement of air or saliva within the larynx or pharynx or a clicking of the tongue or teeth. Sounds may include throat clearing, sniffing, grunting, squeaking, sucking, or blowing. In addition,

Dx Tics

- Sudden, brief uncontrolled movements
- Repetitive sounds from the vocal apparatus
- Behaviors occurring in the context of or mimicking normal behaviors but having no purpose

children with Tourette syndrome may also have socially inappropriate words or gestures or repeat a new word or phrase or one they have just said or heard.

Children with Tourette syndrome may have learning problems, including easy distractibility and inability to finish schoolwork. They also may have intrusive or repetitive thoughts, unfounded fears, or ritualistic actions that may involve touching, cleanliness or neatness, counting and exactness, symmetry or evenness, or irrational checking. Sleep disturbances are not unusual.

Classifications of tics according to the nature of the action can be helpful in understanding apparently widely different movements as being part of the same disorder because of ultimately shared central nervous system chemistry or circuitry (Box 121-1). Clonic tics are brief and dystonic tics are more sustained movements. In addition to simple tics, patients may rarely have other unusual behaviors (complex tics) including echopraxia (repetitive gestures), copropraxia (obscene gestures), and coprographia (obscene writing). Unusual speech patterns include irrelevant or nonsense words, palinphrasia (repeating one's own words), echolalia (repeating another's words), and coprolalia (obscene speech). Diagnosis is often delayed because of misunderstandings about the common and uncommon manifestations of Tourette syndrome (Box 121-2).

Pathophysiology

Tics are thought to be generated from a functional abnormality in deep brain nuclei that might include the striate nuclei, globus pall-

Box 121-1. Types of Tics Seen in Children With Tourette Syndrome

Simple Tics
- Clonic
- Dystonic

Complex Tics
- Series of different or similar simple tics
- More complicated coordinated movement
- Copropraxia and coprographia

Vocal Tics
- Oropharyngeal, nasopharyngeal, or laryngeal sounds
- Consonants or syllables
- Meaningless or nonsense words or phrases
- Coprolalia
- Palinphrasia and echolalia

Box 121-2. Misconceptions in Diagnosing Tourette Syndrome

- Attributing the unusual tic symptom to attention-getting or emotionally based behavior
- Diagnosing the episodic behavior as a seizure on the basis of inadequate historical information
- Attributing a vocal tic to an upper airway, sinus, or allergic condition
- Attributing an ocular tic to an ophthalmologic problem
- Requiring tics to be observed in the office before making the diagnosis
- Waiting for coprolalia to be present before making the diagnosis
- Assuming severe tics are necessary for the diagnosis, or assuming mild tics are a normal developmental phase

idus, subthalamic nuclei, and substantia nigra. The prefrontal cortex, thalamus, and limbic systems may also be involved.

Dopaminergic neurotransmission within these structures is likely to be part of the abnormal function because of one class of medication (stimulants) worsening the symptoms and another class (dopamine antagonists) effective as a treatment. In patients with Tourette syndrome, the cerebrospinal fluid contains low baseline levels of homovanillic acid, a dopamine metabolite, which could result, as has been hypothesized, from a hypersensitive dopamine receptor. In addition, amphetamines and methylphenidate increase dopamine release, and in some instances, these agents precipitate tic symptoms. Haloperidol, an effective tic-suppressing medication, blocks dopamine receptors and, therefore, may block a potentially hypersensitive Tourette dopamine receptor. The observation of a good clinical response with relatively low doses of dopamine blockers such as haloperidol and the finding of increased homovanillic acid levels due to receptor desensitization long after disappearance of the drug support this hypothesis. The physiology is undoubtedly more complex, as medications involving other transmitters are also effective. Rare genetic causes of Tourette syndrome are mutations in the gene SLITRK1 and the gene for histidine decarboxylase. The latter enzyme converts histidine to histamine in histamine neurons and influences dendritic growth in the basal ganglia. It is unknown how either of these genes cause symptoms.

An observed association of the sudden onset or exacerbation of obsessive-compulsive or tic symptoms with preceding group A streptococcal infections of the pharynx has been termed PANDAS (*pediatric autoimmune neuropsychiatric disease associated with streptococcus*). It is intriguing that a clear relationship has been known for some time between the same bacteria and another movement problem, Sydenham chorea, but the evidence for causality or any role of the bacteria or of related autoimmunity is conflicting and unconfirmed by large studies involving Tourette syndrome or obsessive-compulsive disorder; therefore, routine screening or prophylaxis has not been recommended when these diagnoses or PANDAS are being considered.

Differential Diagnosis

The duration, frequency, and appearance of the movement and circumstances of occurrence of tics help distinguish them from several other episodic movement disorders. Myoclonus is a lightning-like, non-suppressible jerk of a small group of muscles, and chorea involves nearly constant, small amplitude movements of the fingers, hands, and feet that are often accompanied by grimacing movements of the face. Tremor is an oscillatory movement of an extremity or the head. Hemiballismus is an uncontrollable episodic throwing movement of an extremity. Hyperekplexia is a hyperactive startle response provoked by touch or sudden noise. Torticollis, or neck writhing, may be paroxysmal but is generally part of a benign transient disorder or a chronic degenerative disorder, such as familial dystonia. Paroxysmal kinesigenic choreoathetosis, an unusual episodic condition precipitated by a sudden movement, is characterized by a twisted trunk and limb posture lasting a few seconds (longer than tics, generally) and not accompanied by loss of consciousness. Hypnagogic jerks and bruxism are persistent normal variant behaviors that occur in sleep.

Other repetitive behaviors are sometimes confused with tics. Compulsions are complex actions that are done against one's will or better judgment. Stereotypies are persistent repetitive senseless movements. Perseverative behaviors are continued activity after the cause for it has ceased. Self-injurious behaviors are usually biting or banging of a body part during periods of agitation. Addictive behaviors occur with psychologic dependence due to a reward system. Habits are fixed practices established by repetition. Mannerisms are stereotyped movements or habits peculiar to an individual and part of that individual's personality. Anger outbursts are sudden emotion-generated behaviors occurring with relatively little provocation.

Tic disorders are sometimes divided into 3 groups: **simple transient tics,** which are monomorphic (always the same appearance over a period of months), last fewer than 12 months, and may be caused by particular environmental situations or psychological states; **chronic tics,** which last longer than 12 months but are of a single type; and the **tics of Tourette syndrome** (Box 121-3). However, all 3 types of tic disorders are sometimes found in the same family. Tics can also be seen in Huntington disease, neuroacanthosis, Sydenham chorea, infectious encephalitis, carbon monoxide poisoning, stroke, schizophrenia, head trauma, static developmental encephalopathies, and drug reactions, particularly stimulants, anticonvulsants, and antipsychotics.

Evaluation

History

A thorough history should be taken when evaluating children with potential tic disorders. The physician should find out as much as possible about the duration, circumstances of occurrence, and frequency of the movements (Questions Box). Parents may imitate the behavior or, if possible, bring in a video recording of the child's behavior. This may give the physician more telling information than verbal descriptions. The physician should suggest an array of tic behaviors because the parent may not be aware that these behaviors could be tics.

Physical Examination

Frequently, tics are not seen by the physician when observing the child during the examination because the child is able to suppress them, but the physician might be able to observe the child unobtrusively while still in the waiting room or during the course of the parent interview. As part of the examination, a screen of cognitive abilities and fine-motor coordination should be included because of the comorbidity of ADHD, learning disabilities, and associated fine motor dysmaturity.

Laboratory Tests

There are no definitive diagnostic or supportive laboratory tests for tics generally or Tourette syndrome specifically. Children with atypical or ambiguous movement disorders should be screened for potential metabolic abnormalities, including routine determinations of calcium, magnesium, glucose, liver function enzymes, and ceruloplasmin levels (for Wilson disease). Thyroid function tests may also be requested if there are other signs or symptoms of thyroid dysfunction.

Imaging Studies

Research evaluations of patients with Tourette syndrome have demonstrated volumetric increases in primarily right frontal white matter and the anterior parts of the corpus callosum and decreases in the caudate nuclei in magnetic resonance imaging (MRI) studies, reduced right basal ganglia activity in single-photon emission computed tomography studies, and increased right caudate and frontal cortex activity in functional MRI studies during tic suppression. These imaging modalities have not yet proven clinically useful in the care of individual patients, however.

Box 121-3. Conditions Necessary for Diagnosis of Tourette Syndrome

- Multiple motor and vocal tics variably manifested over time
- Tics present for at least 1 year
- Onset of tics before 21 years of age
- Tics not caused by another known condition or substance

Questions

Tics

- How long and how often has the child been displaying the unusual behaviors?
- In what circumstances do the unusual behaviors occur? For example, do the behaviors occur when the child is eating or sleeping, engrossed in an activity, or excited? Or do they occur when attention is on the child or after a startle or other triggering behavior?
- Can the parents or other caregivers imitate or show a video recording of the child's unusual behavior?
- Can the child suppress the behavior?
- Does the child have an uncomfortable premonitory sensation just before the motor tic that is relieved by the tic?
- Is the child having difficulty at school (cognitively or socially)?

Management

Goals of management should include reduction in the frequency of tics during critical circumstances with a minimum of medication side effects and attention to other coexisting learning or behavioral disabilities. Before physicians prescribe drug treatment, they must consider the severity of the tic disorder; the local pain it might be producing from muscle, tendon, or joint stress; and its potential for production of psychosocial disability including family, peer, and school relationships. Some children do not need medication for the movement disorder, and they and their families can be reassured by an understanding of the problem. Other children may experience bullying, recess altercations, or incorrect teacher judgments. Successfully treated patients may also experience remission of their disorder for weeks or months, during which they can reduce or discontinue their medications. Several classes of drugs are useful in the treatment of tic disorders. A medication for mild cases because of its fair efficacy but good side-effect profile and convenience is clonidine, an α_2-adrenergic agonist which is available in a tablet, or the **Catapres** transdermal skin patch. Dosage is titrated by effective tablet strength or size and strength of the patch. Guanfacine, an oral formulation in the same class, is also effective. The most direct therapy for the tics but producing more sedative side effects are dopamine blockers, such as pimozide and fluphenazine, and the dopamine-depleting tetrabenazine. An electrocardiogram is recommended before beginning these medications because they have been associated with long QT syndrome, and concomitant use of inhibitors of CYP3A liver metabolism is not recommended. **Haloperidol** has been used in divided doses starting as low as 0.5 mg/day up to 2 to 6 mg/day but has a small risk of tardive dyskinesia. Atypical antipsychotics, particularly risperidone, have also been effective with less sedation or potential for extrapyramidal side effects but more conducive to weight gain and glucose intolerance. With any of these medications, children should begin with a low dose, which is then titrated up to efficacy or the development of intolerable side effects. **Botulinum toxin type A** injections may be useful for isolated persistent tics involving muscles that are needle accessible. Habit reversal training has a growing body of supportive evidence of efficacy, including a controlled, single blinded trial, but involves a considerable time commitment of child and parents and an expense possibly not covered by insurance.

Treatment for children with Tourette syndrome should be multimodal and prioritize, address, and monitor all problematic aspects of the syndrome (Box 121-4). Children with Tourette syndrome should also be assessed for learning disabilities, including ADHD. Interventions may include organizational aids, homework time management, reduction in potential environmental distractions, and more **individualized instruction. Pharmacologic therapy** may include clonidine, a tricyclic antidepressant, atomoxetine, or a stimulant. Long-acting methylphenidate or mixed amphetamine salt preparations are not necessarily contraindicated in children with Tourette syndrome; these drugs do not worsen tics in all patients. Although much less frequently, children with Tourette syndrome are

Box 121-4. Therapies Useful in Tourette Syndrome

Tics
- Clonidine (Catapres transdermal patch): α_2-adrenergic agonist
- Risperidone (low dose): serotonin dopamine receptor antagonist
- Haloperidol (low dose): dopamine receptor blocker
- Pimozide (Orap): dopamine receptor blocker
- Fluphenazine: dopamine receptor blocker
- Guanfacine (Tenex): α_2-adrenergic agonist
- Habit reversal training

Attention-Deficit/Hyperactivity Disorder and Learning Disability
- Clonidine (Catapres transdermal patch): α_2-adrenergic agonist
- Methylphenidate: if tics are not worsened
- Atomoxetine: norepinephrine transporter inhibitor
- Desipramine: tricyclic antidepressant
- Education interventions: individualized or small-group instruction

Obsessive-Compulsive Disorder
- Fluoxetine (Prozac): serotonin uptake inhibitor (non-tricyclic)
- Clomipramine (Anafranil): tricyclic antidepressant

Depression and Adjustment Problems
- Psychotherapy (individual and family)
- Imipramine: tricyclic antidepressant
- Support group

also susceptible to obsessive-compulsive symptoms. **Fluoxetine, sertraline,** and **clomipramine** are useful for this comorbidity.

In its severe form, Tourette syndrome may be socially devastating and provoke secondary frustrations, low self-esteem, depression, and other emotional problems as well as the primary psycho-behavioral difficulties that may be part of the syndrome. Children with Tourette syndrome and their families frequently benefit from **lay educational materials** about the syndrome, **support groups** composed of other families that have children with the syndrome, and local chapters of the National Tourette Syndrome Association (www.tsa-usa.org). Referral for psychologic or psychiatric counseling for patients and their families may also be necessary, however.

Prognosis

The prognosis in most children with tics is good. Less than 20% of adults and older children who were symptomatic in grade school still continue to manifest clinically significant tic symptoms. Some symptomatic children, however, have ongoing problems with a productive educational experience or developing appropriate peer relationships. Therefore, according to the severity of these issues early in childhood, the physician must individualize the management strategy to achieve a favorable prognosis later when educational and social problems may be harder to reverse. Because the movements may change or even remit over long periods, the psychologic adjustments become very important in the long-term prognosis.

CASE RESOLUTION

The boy in the case study is diagnosed as having Tourette syndrome. After a discussion with his family about the syndrome, he is treated with Catapres patches. A questionnaire is sent to his teacher concerning attention-deficit/hyperactivity disorder symptoms at school. At a 6-week follow-up visit, he has fewer tics and is doing better in school (classroom situation of 15 students for most of the day).

Selected References

Coffey BJ, Shechter RL. Treatment of co-morbid obsessive compulsive disorder, mood, and anxiety disorders. *Adv Neurol*. 2006;99:208–221

Dale RC. Post-streptococcal autoimmune disorders of the central nervous system. *Dev Med Child Neurol*. 2005;47(11):785–791

Denckla MB. Attention-deficit hyperactivity disorder (ADHD) comorbidity: a case for "pure" Tourette syndrome? *J Child Neurol*. 2006;21(8):701–703

Erenberg G. The relationship between Tourette syndrome, attention deficit hyperactivity disorder, and stimulant medication: a critical review. *Semin Pediatr Neurol*. 2006;12:217–221

Huff K. Approach to the child with movement disorders. In: Osborn L, Dewitt T, First L, Zenel J, eds. *Pediatrics*. Philadelphia, PA: Elsevier; 2005:770–777

Jankovic J, Kurlan R. Tourette syndrome: evolving concepts. *Mov Disord*. 2011; 26(6):1149–1156

Knight T, Steeves T, Day L, Lowerison M, Jette N, Pringsheim T. Prevalence of tic disorders: a systematic review and meta-analysis. *Pediatr Neurol*. 2012;47(2): 77–90

Kurlan R. Clinical practice. Tourette's syndrome. *N Engl J Med*. 2010;363(24): 2332–2338

Leckman JF, Bloch MH, Scahill L, King RA. Tourette syndrome: the self under siege. *J Child Neurol*. 2006;21(8):642–649

Leckman JF, King RA, Gilbert DL, et al. Streptococcal upper respiratory tract infections and exacerbations of tic and obsessive-compulsive symptoms: a prospective longitudinal study. *J Am Acad Child Adolesc Psychiatry*. 2011;50(2): 108–118

Piacentini JC, Chang SW. Behavioral treatments for tic suppression: habit reversal training. *Adv Neurol*. 2006;99:227–233

Robertson MM. Tourette syndrome, associated conditions and the complexities of treatment. *Brain*. 2000;123(Pt 3):425–462

Singer HS, Gilbert DL, Wolf DS, Mink JW, Kurlan R. Moving from PANDAS to CANS. *J Pediatr*. 2012;160(5):725–731

Snider LA, Swedo SE. PANDAS: current status and directions for research. *Mol Psychiatry*. 2004;9(10):900–907

Zinner SH, Mink JW. Movement disorders I: tics and stereopathies. *Pediatr Rev*. 2010;31(6):223–233

Dermatologic Disorders

CHAPTER 122

Acne

Monica Sifuentes, MD

CASE STUDY

A 15-year-old male comes to your office for a preparticipation sports physical evaluation. He is healthy and has no questions, complaints, or concerns.

The adolescent is well developed and well nourished, with normal vital signs, including blood pressure. The physical examination is entirely normal except for the skin. Multiple closed comedones (whiteheads) are noted along the hairline. Erythematous papules and pustules are present across the forehead and over both cheeks. Scattered open comedones (blackheads) are located over the nose and cheeks as well. The chest and back are clear, with no lesions.

Questions

1. What is the pathogenesis of acne vulgaris?
2. What are some contributing factors in the development of acne?
3. What are the different types of acne lesions?
4. What management options are available for the treatment of mild, moderate, and severe acne in adolescents?
5. What are the indications for the use of isotretinoin?
6. What is the prognosis for adolescent patients with acne?

Acne vulgaris is a common condition that most frequently occurs in adolescents. The spectrum of disease varies among individuals and is caused by a variety of factors. Regardless of the etiology and extent of acne, the disease can be devastating to adolescents physically and psychologically. Primary care physicians should, therefore, acknowledge acne as a chronic medical problem, even when patients do not initially appear concerned about it, and treat the condition early and aggressively to prevent permanent sequelae such as scarring.

Epidemiology

Most cases of acne that require treatment occur in individuals 9 to 24 years of age, although the condition can also affect neonates, young infants, and older adults. Boys and girls are equally affected, but the condition is usually more severe in males and typically lasts longer in females. Certain individuals may be genetically susceptible to acne. White teens are more likely to have acne than African American and Asian teens. Certain cultural practices, such as the use of oil-based hair care products by some African Americans, also can lead to a specific pattern of lesions along the forehead and temporal areas (pomade acne). Estimates indicate that more than 85% of adolescents in the United States are affected by acne and that more than $1 billion is spent annually on acne treatments. And although acne is generally believed to be a pubertal event, a fair number of young adults continue to manifest lesions after 25 years of age.

Several factors contribute to the development of acne-like eruptions. Internal agents include endogenous hormones (eg, androgens, progesterone) and specific drugs (eg, progestin-only contraceptives, isoniazid, phenytoin, corticosteroids, anabolic steroids, lithium-containing compounds). External agents include skin bacteria, especially *Propionibacterium acnes,* industrial chemicals (eg, petroleum, animal and vegetable oils), oil- or wax-containing cosmetics, greasy sunscreen or suntan preparations, overzealous facial cleansing, and local skin occlusion from sports gear such as headbands, shoulder pads, helmets, or chin straps. Excessive perspiration and emotional stress also can aggravate acne. Peri-menstrual exacerbations are common. Specific foods such as chocolate, caffeine-containing soda, pizza, and french fries have not been shown to directly cause or worsen acne, although emerging research suggests that diets with high-glycemic indices may contribute to inflammation and the development of lesions.

Clinical Presentation

The lesions of acne vulgaris primarily affect the face, especially the cheeks, forehead, and chin; the chest; the back; and the shoulders. Lesions can be non-inflamed or inflamed (D_x Box). Non-inflamed lesions, or comedones, can be opened or closed to the environment.

Dx Acne

- Occurs predominantly during puberty.
- Lesions are more severe in males.
- Located on face, chest, back, and shoulders.
- Non-inflamed, open comedones (blackheads) or closed comedones (whiteheads).
- Inflamed papules or pustules.
- Nodules, cysts, or scarring may be present.
- Possible exacerbation premenstrually, related to stress or other environmental factors.

Closed comedones (whiteheads) are small, flesh-colored bumps with no surrounding erythema, and open comedones (blackheads) are small, dome-shaped papules with a dilated orifice that contains central, dark material. Inflamed lesions are typically erythematous papules, pustules, or nodules and may be more cystic in appearance.

Lesions are generally concentrated in the centrofacial areas or "T-zone" early in the course of acne. The T-zone includes the forehead, nose, and chin areas, which are rich in sebaceous glands. Over time, lesions can develop in other areas of the body, such as the neck, chest, shoulders, and back.

Pathophysiology

Although the exact etiology of acne remains unclear, the pathogenesis of acne involves 4 specific interrelated processes that occur within the pilosebaceous unit.

1. Abnormal follicular keratinization. The earliest change in the formation of acne occurs in the horny cells that line the sebaceous follicle. A disturbance in the differentiation of these cells leads to excessive shedding of the cells into the lumen. Impaction of the follicle occurs as these horny cells stick together.

2. Overproduction of sebum. The sebaceous gland is highly responsive to hormonal stimulation, namely gonadal and adrenal androgens. With the rise in androgens during puberty, hypertrophy of the sebaceous gland occurs, and the production of sebum is increased. The flow of sebum is obstructed by the above follicular hyperkeratosis, resulting in retention of all material.

3. Proliferation of *P acnes.* The overproduction of sebum in acne provides a ripe environment for the proliferation of *P acnes,* an anaerobic diphtheroid that, along with *Staphylococcus epidermidis* and *Pityrosporum ovale,* is part of the microflora of the sebaceous follicle. In addition, *P acnes* possess a lipase that hydrolyzes sebum triglycerides into free fatty acids. These acids irritate the follicular wall and cause inflammation.

4. Immune response and inflammation. The expulsion of sebum into the dermal layer of the skin occurs as a result of the rupture of the pilosebaceous follicle. This initiates an inflammatory process and the formation of inflammatory lesions such as pustules and cysts. In addition, *P acnes* produce biologically active extracellular materials, which increase the permeability of the follicular epithelium. The bacterium also produces chemotactic factors that are responsible for the migration of inflammatory cells to the area.

These processes can lead to a number of noninflammatory and inflammatory lesions (Table 122-1). Comedones are early noninflammatory lesions made up of sebum, horny cells, and bacteria. They can be closed or open. A **closed comedo,** or **whitehead,** is a dilated plugged sebaceous follicle that is closed to the surface of the skin. An **open comedo,** or **blackhead,** occurs as a result of dilatation of the follicular orifice at the surface of the skin and open communication with the outside environment. The dark color at the surface of the skin, however, is not dirt and may be from a number of processes, such as melanin deposition in the horny cells, interference with the transmission of light through compacted

Table 122-1. Classification of Acne

Category	Physical Findings
Grade 1 (mild)	Noninflammatory acne → open and closed comedones Closed comedones then lead to any of the next 3 levels of inflammatory acne.
Grade 2 (mild inflammatory)	Early inflammatory acne → presence of comedones and scattered superficial papules/pustules (obstructed follicles)
Grade 3 (moderate inflammatory)	Moderate, localized inflammatory acne → comedones and pustules or larger, more inflamed papules (increased number of lesions)
Grade 4 (severe inflammatory)	Severe, more generalized inflammatory acne → cystic, nodular lesions (extensive involvement; may have scarring)

epithelial cells, or oxidation of keratinous material and certain lipids in sebum.

Pustules and **papules** are inflammatory lesions. Pustules lie in the superficial epidermal layer of the skin, and papules occur in the lower dermal layer. Because of their deeper location, papules are often accompanied by a more severe inflammatory reaction, and scarring may result. **Nodules** or **cysts** are suppurative inflammatory lesions located deep within the dermis. Associated with the most severe form of acne, nodules are the result of deep pustules that rupture and then become lined with epithelium. When nodules are present, significant scarring can be a major problem.

Evaluation

History

The primary historical issues to explore in patients with acne vulgaris are medical and psychologic (Questions Box). From a medical standpoint, practitioners should determine how long the acne has been present and if the condition has ever been treated. Psychologic aspects should include questions to assess the patient's overall self-esteem. Expectations about treatment and recovery also should be assessed at the initial visit before therapy is begun. A general review of systems is important to exclude symptoms associated with androgen excess such as hirsutism, deepened voice, and irregular menses.

Physical Examination

The physical examination should focus on the primary sites of acne—face, chest, back, and shoulders—although the entire skin should be inspected closely at the first visit. Individual lesions should be checked for signs of inflammation (erythema) and infection at each follow-up visit. Their distribution also should be recorded along with their response to treatment. The presence or absence of scarring should be assessed as a measure of the severity of acne and a predictor of outcome. Young women with irregular menses and obesity should be examined for hirsutism, which might indicate excessive adrenal or ovarian androgen production as a contributor to the development of acne.

Acne

Questions

Medical Aspects

- How long has the adolescent had lesions?
- Has the adolescent ever received treatment for acne?
  — How long did treatment continue?
  — What treatment methods were used?
  — For what reasons was the therapy discontinued?
- Is the adolescent currently using any treatment products?
  — Do the lesions seem to be getting better or worse?
- If the acne has never been treated, is treatment desired?
- Do any activities, medications, or environmental agents seem to exacerbate the lesions?
- Does the adolescent have a family history of acne with or without scarring?
- Is the adolescent taking any medications?
- Does the adolescent have any other medical conditions?

Psychologic Aspects

- Is the adolescent bothered by the lesions?
- Is the adolescent embarrassed about his or her appearance? If so, does this embarrassment prevent the adolescent from participating in certain activities?
- Is the adolescent ever ridiculed by his or her peers because of the acne?

For Postpubertal Females

- Does the acne worsen prior to menses?
- Are menses regular?
- Is there any evidence of hirsutism? Deepening of her voice? Male pattern baldness?
- Is the adolescent sexually active?
- Is she using any hormonal contraception?
- Does she desire oral contraception?
- Is there a family history of thromboembolic events?

Laboratory Tests

In general, no laboratory studies are needed at the time of the initial evaluation or during the treatment of mild to moderate acne. If there is a history of irregular menses, obesity, and evidence of hirsutism or virilization in the adolescent female, free testosterone, early morning cortisol and 17-hydroxyprogesterone, and serum dehydroepiandrosterone sulfate levels are indicated to differentiate between the various causes of hyperandrogenism. In the case of severe acne when isotretinoin is indicated, several pretreatment studies are necessary. A complete blood cell count, liver function tests, and a fasting lipid profile are recommended. In addition, a pregnancy test must be performed prior to and within 2 weeks of starting isotretinoin in female adolescents. These studies should be obtained in consultation with a dermatologist, who is generally responsible for prescribing isotretinoin through the iPLEDGE program (see Isotretinoin Therapy).

Management

The general management of acne begins with counseling and should include patient education on the pathophysiology of the condition to dispel any myths about its etiology and treatment. In addition, the patient's motivation should be assessed to better individualize therapy. Realistic expectations of duration of therapy, medication-related side effects, and likely outcome of treatment should be reviewed with the teenager and parent to maximize adherence and efficacy. Parental involvement is particularly important in cases of severe acne.

All adolescents with acne should follow these general recommendations:

1. Wash skin with a mild soap-free cleanser and water once or twice daily. Antibacterial washes, other than benzoyl peroxide (BP), have not been shown to be useful. Frequent or excessive washing and scrubbing will not improve acne and may only irritate the skin further.
2. Use cosmetics and moisturizers sparingly or switch to oil-free products that indicate they are noncomedogenic.
3. Avoid picking at lesions and excessive scrubbing, especially with abrasive cleansers. Traumatizing acne lesions will contribute to scar formation.
4. Note that dietary modifications generally are not indicated, although a low-fat, low-glycemic diet has been shown in recent studies to improve acne lesions.
5. Use sunscreen daily; most acne medications are photosensitizing and restrict ultraviolet therapy.
6. Follow the prescribed regimen carefully (Table 122-2), manage medication-related side effects, and understand that long-term treatment is often required.

The specific therapies prescribed depend on the severity and duration of the acne, the type of lesions, and the patient's ability to comply with the proposed treatment regimen. The patient's skin type should be taken into consideration when selecting the appropriate vehicle for the active ingredient, such as a cream, gel, lotion, solution, or ointment. Oily skin types tend to respond better to gels or solutions, whereas creams, lotions, and ointments are better for dry

Table 122-2. Treatment of Acne	
Classification	*Recommended Treatment Regimen*
Grade 1 (mild)	BP 2.5%–5% every other day and/or topical retinoid at bedtime. May increase to daily, if no response and side effects tolerated
Grade 2 (mild inflammatory)	BP or topical retinoid as above plus topical antibiotics once or twice a day if inflammation present, or topical combination product (BP combined with antibiotic) or topical retinoid at bedtime
Grade 3 (moderate inflammatory)	BP in the morning and topical retinoid at bedtime plus oral antibiotic
Grade 4 (severe inflammatory)	Treatment for grade 3 acne plus referral to a dermatologist for consideration for treatment with isotretinoin

Abbreviation: BP, benzoyl peroxide.
Courtesy of Victor C. Strasburger, MD.

skin. The most effective regimens include topical products such as BP, retinoic acid, and antibiotics; systemic antimicrobials; hormonal agents; and isotretinoin. Most often, however, combination therapy is used and subsequently modified according to the patient's response and adherence to the initial treatment regimen. Physicians should remember to discuss with the adolescent that the acne often looks worse before it gets better and that treatment is long-term. Medications only control the acne but do not cure it. The only exception to this is isotretinoin. Noticeable improvement of acne from any treatment regimen usually takes at least 4 to 8 weeks.

Topical Therapy

Several topical products are available for the treatment of acne. **Benzoyl peroxide** is bactericidal for *P acnes* and acts as a comedolytic and anti-inflammatory agent as well. It should be considered as the first line of therapy for the management of comedonal and mild inflammatory acne. Although over-the-counter products are available, the more effective gel preparations are preferable and available by prescription. The lowest concentration possible should be used initially (eg, 2.5% or 5% concentration). Higher concentrations may be used in cases in which the trunk or back are involved; however, increasing the concentration does not necessarily increase its efficacy and may just result in more irritation. In the case of back involvement, a BP wash may be effective.

Therapy should be initiated gradually, especially if used in combination with retinoic acid, because BP is inherently irritating and drying. Initially, a thin application should be used once a day every other day, and the frequency should be increased as tolerated. Allergic contact dermatitis manifested by erythema with pruritic small papules and vesicles rarely develops, but if it does, treatment must be discontinued immediately. A non-acnegenic, noncomedogenic sunscreen is recommended as well to protect against the photosensitivity associated with BP usage.

Tretinoin or retinoic acid (eg, Retin-A, Retin-A Micro, Avita, Atralin) is the mainstay of therapy for noninflammatory or comedonal acne. This vitamin A derivative reduces microcomedo formation by normalizing follicular keratinization and decreasing the adhesiveness of horny cells shed into the follicular lumen. It also has some anti-inflammatory effects. It is available by prescription as a gel, cream, or liquid in several different concentrations. Microsphere technology is less irritating and allows the medication to be delivered slowly at higher concentrations. It seems to be as effective as the older formulations.

Like BP, retinoic acid can be very irritating and may cause some erythema, peeling, stinging or burning, and dryness, which are thought to be dose-dependent. Therefore, therapy should be initiated cautiously with a cream or gel, which is less potent and drying than the liquid preparation. To further reduce irritation, patients should be instructed to wash with a mild soap-free cleanser no more than 2 times a day and to wait at least 20 to 30 minutes for the skin to dry completely before applying the product. Physicians often recommend that patients apply retinoic acid before bedtime rather than in the mornings, which tend to be more hectic for the average

teenager. A small, pea-sized dot of tretinoin should be used each time and divided into 3 smaller dots on the skin before rubbing a thin film gently to most of the face, concentrating on the affected areas but also applying it to some of the less affected skin. Patients also should be cautioned against excessive sun exposure while using retinoic acid because this agent lowers the sunburn threshold. Combined daily treatment with BP is warranted in cases of mild inflammatory acne; however, because BP inactivates tretinoin, the 2 drugs cannot be applied simultaneously. Most clinicians recommend BP in the morning and tretinoin at night.

Adapalene (Differin) and tazarotene (Tazorac) are 2 relatively new third-generation topical retinoids that have been used in the treatment of acne. Adapalene is less irritating and has been shown to be more photostable than tretinoin; however, it is not approved for children younger than 12 years. It is available in an alcohol-free gel, cream, or lotion and can be used in fixed combination with BP. Tazarotene, originally created for the treatment of psoriasis, is the most effective of the topical retinoids but is more expensive and irritating than the other retinoids, and there are concerns about its teratogenicity (pregnancy category X). It is therefore not widely prescribed for the treatment of acne.

Azelaic acid (Azelex), a naturally occurring derivative from wheat, has antibacterial and anti-keratinizing activity. It inhibits the growth of *P acnes* and has an antiproliferative effect on keratinocytes. Although less potent than tretinoin, azelaic acid may be useful in patients with mild to moderate inflammatory and comedonal acne who cannot tolerate topical tretinoin or BP because it seems to be less irritating. Pruritus, burning, stinging, tingling, and erythema have been reported, however. It is available by prescription as a 20% cream and should be applied once or twice daily.

Antibiotic Therapy

Topical as well as systemic antibiotics can be used in the treatment of mild to moderate inflammatory acne. The choice of which to use usually depends on the extent of skin involvement and severity of inflammation. **Topical antibiotics** are often useful in patients with mild inflammatory lesions that are unresponsive to BP or retinoic acid alone. Such antibiotics act by inhibiting the growth of *P acnes* and reducing the number of comedones, papules, and pustules. Erythromycin and clindamycin are available as topical preparations. The **erythromycin gel** is most popular; the recommended dosage is twice daily. Allergic reactions from topical formulations rarely occur. Compared with systemic antibiotics, topical preparations have fewer systemic side effects because of decreased absorption. Topical antibiotics alone are not recommended as monotherapy because resistance generally develops with prolonged use and the therapeutic response can take a while. Erythromycin and clindamycin are available in fixed combination with BP and are very effective against *P acnes*. Although combination preparations are generally more costly, adherence is improved with their usage. Over-the-counter BP and topical erythromycin or clindamycin can be used simultaneously to reduce the cost.

Systemic oral antibiotics are the mainstay of therapy in patients with nodular or cystic inflammatory acne and in patients who have not responded to topical antibiotics or who have inflamed lesions involving the trunk as well as the face. However, systemic agents have not been shown to be effective with comedonal acne and are not US Food and Drug Administration (FDA) approved for the treatment of acne, with the exception of extended-release minocycline. The success of oral antimicrobial therapy relates to the suppression of *P acnes* and the inhibition of bacterial lipases. As a result, free fatty acids and other by-products are reduced, thereby decreasing inflammation.

Tetracycline and its derivatives (**doxycycline and minocycline**) are the preferred first-line oral antibiotics for the treatment of moderate to severe inflammatory acne and should be used in combination with a topical regimen that includes BP. Alternatives such as clindamycin, trimethoprim-sulfamethoxazole, and azithromycin may be used in select patients but generally are not used. Other systemic antibiotics such as erythromycin have been used in the past; however, antibiotic resistance is now a problem. In addition, clindamycin is used much less frequently because of its associated side effects like pseudomembranous colitis. Doxycycline and minocycline are particularly beneficial when lesions fail to respond to tetracycline. However, tetracycline and doxycycline are not recommended in children younger than 8 years or in pregnant females. The most common side effects include candida vaginitis, especially in females who also take oral contraceptives (OCPs); gastrointestinal (GI) disturbances; and photosensitivity. Phototoxicity and pill esophagitis occur most commonly with oral doxycycline; therefore, patients must be instructed to use sunscreen liberally and remain upright for at least 1 hour after ingestion of the medication. Significant potential adverse effects associated with tetracycline, doxycycline, and minocycline are reviewed in detail in the excellent reference by Eichenfield et al. The ultimate goal of oral antibiotic therapy is use of the minimum dose to control lesions and minimize side effects. Most patients require prolonged or frequent intermittent courses of oral antibiotics, however, before remission occurs. In general, the dose of the antibiotic and the dosing interval should not be reduced before a significant clinical effect is seen, which may take 6 to 8 weeks. Once new inflammatory lesions have stopped emerging, the dose of the oral antibiotic may be gradually tapered within 1 to 2 months and topical antibiotic treatment may be substituted.

Hormonal Therapy

Hormonal therapy is indicated as second-line therapy in menstruating females with moderate to severe acne who are unresponsive to other forms of treatment and who are candidates for isotretinoin or as adjunctive therapy in sexually active teens with inflammatory acne who want to prevent pregnancy. Oral contraceptives antagonize the action of circulating androgens by increasing the production of sex-binding globulin, which decreases biologically active free testosterone. In addition, there is decreased androgen production by the ovaries through feedback inhibition of pituitary gonadotropin secretion. Although clinical improvement in inflammatory lesions has been reported with many combination OCPs, only 3 are currently approved by the FDA specifically for the treatment of acne:

ethinyl estradiol (35 μg) and the progestin norgestimate (Ortho Tri-Cyclen), ethinyl estradiol (20 μg/30 μg/35 μg)/norethindrone (Estrostep), and ethinyl estradiol (20 μg)/drospirenone (Yaz). The use of very low dose OCPs in young adolescents remains controversial because it is unclear if 20 μg ethinyl estradiol is sufficient for bone mass accrual and the lower age limit to initiate use is unknown. Given these concerns, experts recommend not prescribing OCPs for the treatment of acne unassociated with endocrine pathology until 1 year after menarche. A family history of thromboembolic events also must be ruled out before OCPs are prescribed. In general, OCPs must be taken for 3 to 4 months before any improvement is seen, with relapses occurring if treatment is discontinued. Maximum effects are usually seen by 6 months.

Specific endocrine disorders, such as polycystic ovarian syndrome and metabolic syndrome, also may exacerbate acne and should be investigated in female adolescents with a history of oligomenorrhea, hirsutism, obesity, and insulin resistance. In these cases, hormonal therapy will treat the hyperandrogenism as well as the accompanying acne by decreasing adrenal androgen production.

Systemic Therapy

Because sebaceous glands are androgen-dependent, antiandrogens such as spironolactone can reduce sebum production and therefore improve acne. However, this therapy is generally reserved for adult females. Doses range from 100 to 200 mg/day; however, lower doses may also be effective. Several months of spironolactone therapy are needed for maximum benefit, with prolonged therapy often required. Gynecomastia occurs not infrequently. Agranulocytosis is a rare complication.

Isotretinoin Therapy

Isotretinoin (Accutane, Claravis, Sotret, Amnesteem), a systemic oral analog of vitamin A, is currently the most effective treatment available for severe nodulocystic acne that is resistant to conventional therapy. This agent is also useful in patients with a propensity for scarring. It influences all aspects of acne formation: sebum secretion, follicular keratinization, and inflammatory responses. For patients with severe forms of inflammatory acne, isotretinoin has been hailed as a miracle drug despite its many side effects.

Given the numerous potentially serious adverse effects of the drug, referral to a dermatologist is strongly recommended for patients who require isotretinoin therapy. The most significant and well known of these adverse effects is teratogenicity. Common side effects and toxicities include dryness and chapping of the skin and mucous membranes, musculoskeletal effects (myalgia), GI issues, neurologic problems, and hematologic abnormalities. Isotretinoin can also elevate triglyceride levels, particularly in patients with diabetes mellitus, obesity, alcohol abuse, and familial hyperlipidemia. Serious adverse events have been attributed to isotretinoin use, including major depressive disorder and suicide ideation; however, studies do not currently support a causative association, despite the addition of black box warnings by the FDA. However, given the high likelihood of depressive symptoms in an adolescent with recalcitrant acne, clinicians are advised to be aware of the coexistence of a mental health disorder when prescribing isotretinoin and are urged to monitor patients closely for a psychiatric referral if indicated. Refer to the reference by Eichenfield et al for a complete discussion of this controversial topic with consensus recommendations regarding oral isotretinoin therapy.

To minimize fetal exposure to isotretinoin, a mandated distribution program called iPLEDGE was implemented by the FDA in 2007 to register all patients receiving isotretinoin along with physicians and pharmacies prescribing the medication and manufacturers of the drug. This computer-based risk management program ensures monthly monitoring of the pregnancy status in females of childbearing age and includes specific educational materials as well as policies and procedures that must be read and signed by the prescribing physician. In addition, informed consent is required of all patients for whom the medication is being prescribed. Two forms of birth control for female patients and documentation of a negative pregnancy test also are required prior to dispensing of the medication. An identifying qualification sticker must be affixed to all isotretinoin prescriptions indicating the prescribing physician is appropriately registered with the FDA distribution program. Monthly follow-up by the prescribing dermatologist is mandatory.

Prognosis

Fortunately, most uncomplicated cases of acne (approximately 90%) resolve by the third decade of life. For those individuals with nodulocystic lesions, however, unwanted long-term effects of inflammatory acne such as significant scarring may continue to be a problem. Therefore, early and aggressive treatment is imperative.

CASE RESOLUTION

In the case study, the adolescent should be offered treatment for his mild to moderate comedonal and inflammatory acne. This may include benzoyl peroxide, retinoic acid (Retin-A), and topical antibiotics. The common side effects of the medications (eg, dry skin, peeling) should be reviewed, and the teen should be instructed to use a noncomedogenic sunscreen. A follow-up appointment should be arranged after 4 to 6 weeks to assess adherence to and tolerance of the prescribed treatment regimen and to address any questions or concerns.

Selected References

Basak SA, Zaenglein AL. Acne and its management. *Pediatr Rev.* 2013;34(11):479–497

Eichenfield LF, Krakowski AC, Piggott C, et al. Evidence-based recommendations for the diagnosis and treatment of pediatric acne. *Pediatrics.* 2013;131(Suppl 3):S163–S186

Goldsmith LA, Bolognia JL, Callen JP, et al. American Academy of Dermatology Consensus Conference on safe and optimal use of isotretinoin: summary and recommendations. *J Am Acad Dermatol.* 2004;50(6):900–906

Koblenzer CS. The emotional impact of chronic and disabling skin disease: a psychoanalytic perspective. *Dermatol Clin.* 2005;23(4):619–627

Krowchuk DP. Managing adolescent acne: a guide for pediatricians. *Pediatr Rev.* 2005;26(7):250–261

National Campaign to Control Acne. Secaucus, NJ: Thomas Professional Postgraduate Services; 2003

Paller AS, Mancini AJ. Disorders of the sebaceous and sweat glands. *Hurwitz Clinical Pediatric Dermatology: A Textbook of Skin Disorders of Childhood and Adolescence.* 3rd ed. Philadelphia, PA: WB Saunders; 2006:185–195

Sawni A, Singh A. Complementary, holistic and integrative medicine: acne. *Pediatr Rev.* 2013;34(2):91–93

Smith JA. The impact of skin disease on the quality of life in adolescents. *Adolesc Med.* 2001;12(2):343–353

Szczepaniak D, Treadwell PA. Acne therapy in primary care: comprehensive review of current evidence-based interventions and treatments. *Adolesc Med State Art Rev.* 2011;22(1):77–96

Tom WL, Friedlander SF. Acne through the ages: case-based observations through childhood and adolescence. *Clin Pediatr (Phila).* 2008;47(7):639–651

Yan AC. Current concepts in acne management. *Adolesc Med Clin.* 2006;17(3):613–637

Zaenglein AL, Thiboutot DM. Expert committee recommendations for acne management. *Pediatrics.* 2006;118(3):1188–1199

CHAPTER 123

Disorders of the Hair and Scalp

Ki-Young Yoo, MD; Kathy K. Langevin, MD, MPH; and Noah Craft, MD, PhD

CASE STUDY

A 6-year-old girl presents with a 1-month history of a swelling on the right side of her scalp that is associated with hair loss. She has previously been in good health, and she has no history of fever. On examination, she is afebrile, has normal vital signs, and appears well. An area of non-tender, boggy swelling 2 × 2 cm with associated alopecia is apparent over the scalp in the right temporal area. Small pustular lesions are scattered over the involved area. Generalized scaling of the scalp and occipital adenopathy are evident.

Questions

1. What are the common causes of circumscribed hair loss in children?
2. What are the common causes of diffuse hair loss in children?
3. What are the common causes of scalp scaling in children?
4. What features distinguish tinea capitis from alopecia areata?
5. What is the treatment for tinea capitis? Is there a role for topical antifungal agents?

Disorders of the scalp may be congenital or acquired during childhood or adolescence. Conditions may be further classified according to the presence or absence of hair loss (alopecia), whether the hair loss is diffuse or circumscribed, and whether the hair loss results in scarring of the scalp.

Epidemiology

Acquired circumscribed hair loss is more commonly seen than diffuse hair loss. Most cases of acquired circumscribed hair loss result from tinea capitis, alopecia areata, or trauma due to traction or trichotillomania.

Tinea capitis is a fungal infection of the scalp most often caused by the dermatophytes *Microsporum canis* or *Trichophyton tonsurans*. *Trichophyton tonsurans* accounts for most cases in the United States, but in a given geographic area, the etiologic fungus may change over time. Tinea capitis, which is less common in infants and postpubertal adolescents, is seen primarily in school-aged children between the ages of 3 and 7 years. Prevalence is estimated to be between 3% and 13% in the pediatric population. Boys are affected more often than girls with *M canis,* though both are affected equally in epidemics caused by *T tonsurans*. African American and Latin American children are more vulnerable to infection. Human-to-human transmission is more common with *T tonsurans,* an anthropophilic fungus. Children who handle dogs or cats, which harbor *M canis,* a zoophilic fungus, are susceptible to infection. Carriers are most commonly adults exposed to affected children, and carriers are considered contagious. Up to 60% of affected children are asymptomatic. Tinea capitis can result in localized patches of hair loss and in scarring if the infection becomes inflammatory.

Alopecia areata is believed to be an organ-specific autoimmune disorder with a prevalence of 0.1% to 0.2%, occurring equally in males and females. Family history is positive in 10% to 50% of affected patients. Although alopecia areata may develop at any age, it is rare before the age of 1 year, and 40% to 50% of cases of alopecia areata develop before the age of 21 years. It may be seen in association with atopic dermatitis, Down syndrome, and other autoimmune diseases.

Trichotillomania, or compulsive pulling at the hair, may be seen in association with other impulse disorders such as thumb sucking and nail biting (see Chapter 53). It results in hair loss caused by self-induced trauma. Usually, scalp hair is involved, but eyebrows or eyelash hair may also be affected. Although trichotillomania may be seen at any age, onset is usually between the ages of 5 and 12 years. It is more commonly seen in girls and women rather than boys and men and in children rather than adults. **Traction alopecia** is more commonly seen in females whose hair-grooming practices result in excessive tension and trauma to the hair.

Clinical Presentation

Children may present with specific complaints, including localized baldness, pruritus, scaling, or inflammation (D$_x$ Box). Occasionally, lymphadenopathy, particularly in the occipital area, is the major presenting symptom.

Pathophysiology

An understanding of the physiology of the normal hair growth cycle helps in the evaluation of hair and scalp disorders. The scalp of an average human being contains about 100,000 hairs. Individuals with blonde hair generally have 10% more hairs and those with red hair

Dx Disorders of the Hair and Scalp

- Circumscribed or generalized hair loss (alopecia)
- Scaling
- Pruritus
- Erythema of the scalp
- Localized or generalized swelling of the scalp
- Occipital adenopathy

have 10% less. Healthy terminal hair grows an average of 0.3 mm per day or approximately 1 cm per month.

The hair follicle is responsible for most disturbances of hair growth because the hair shaft itself is a nonliving structure. Normal hair growth is a cyclic process composed of 3 stages. The anagen phase, the period of active hair growth, lasts for an average of 3 years (range: 2–6 years). Normally, about 85% to 90% of scalp hair is in this phase at any one time. The catagen phase, the transition period, lasts for about 10 to 14 days. The telogen phase, the final resting phase, lasts for about 3 to 4 months. About 13% of scalp hairs are in this phase at one time. The average individual loses about 100 to 150 telogen hairs per day. The normal hair cycle results in replacement of each scalp hair every 3 to 5 years.

Tinea capitis is a communicable infection and can be acquired via interpersonal contact, contact with infected animals, and fomites. There are 3 patterns of hair invasion. In endothrix infections (eg, *T tonsurans*), the fungus produces chains of spores within the hair shaft. In ectothrix infections (eg, *M canis*), spores are present around the exterior of the hair shaft. Favus, the most severe form of tinea capitis, demonstrates hyphae and air spaces within the hair shaft. This is usually caused by *Trichophyton schoenleinii*, a less common etiologic organism. Although dermatophytes have a relatively short incubation period (up to 3 weeks), they are viable in fomites for months. Subcutaneous invasion in conjunction with an exaggerated host response can result in kerion.

Alopecia areata is thought to be caused by aberrant expression of class 1 human leukocyte antigens on early anagen follicles, resulting in T lymphocyte recognition of these normally immune hairs. There follows an immunologic attack causing premature transition to the telogen stage. The hairs then break easily at the surface of the scalp. The hairs at the margins of alopecia are easily plucked and they have an "exclamation mark" appearance with the proximal end thinner than the distal end.

Differential Diagnosis

While some hair disorders can be easily recognized clinically, the differential diagnosis can be challenging at times. Familiarity with the appearance of these conditions is critical. The Internet can be valuable in providing access to images of many dermatologic conditions. Some sites, such as VisualDx (www.visualdx.com), display pictorial representations and allow for searching by features such as hair loss patterns, symptoms, exposures, skin color, scalp location, age, immune status, and many other factors.

Scalp Disorders Without Associated Hair Loss

These conditions are divided into those disorders seen most often in neonates and young infants and those seen more frequently in children and adolescents (Box 123-1). **Caput succedaneum,** a generalized edema involving the soft tissues of the scalp, and **cephalhematoma,** a subperiosteal hematoma, are 2 of the most common lesions of the scalp that occur during the neonatal period. A cephalhematoma does not extend beyond the suture lines of the affected bone, which distinguishes it from caput succedaneum. Both conditions result from birth trauma and generally resolve spontaneously within a few weeks to months without further complications.

Other neonatal scalp conditions include infections such as **scalp abscess** and **human herpesvirus infection**. Scalp abscess occurs most commonly as a complication of scalp electrode placement and has an incidence of 0.4% to 4.5%. The infectious agents are usually flora of the cervix and vagina. Management depends on the severity of the infection (eg, associated cellulitis, signs of systemic involvement). Although most cases are self-limited, the abscess can be complicated by intracranial infection. Human herpesvirus infections of the scalp are not uncommon in neonates; 85% of neonatal human herpesvirus infections occur at time of delivery and the scalp usually has the longest contact with the cervix, one of the sites for transmission of infection. Herpes lesions are typically vesicular, but petechial, purpuric, or bullous lesions may also be apparent. Skin lesions typically develop at 1 week of life but may be present at birth or develop as late as 3 weeks later.

Atopic dermatitis and **seborrheic dermatitis** are the 2 most common diagnoses of scalp scaling among infants and children younger than 10 years. **Seborrheic dermatitis** is a red, scaly eruption that occurs mainly on the scalp (otherwise known as cradle cap), face, and postauricular and intertriginous areas (see Chapter 125). It is often seen in infants and children younger than 2 years. Additionally, the scale, often termed *dandruff* in children 2 to 10 years,

---

Box 123-1. Common Disorders of the Scalp Without Associated Hair Loss

Neonatal Period and Early Infancy
- Birth trauma to the scalp (eg, caput succedaneum, cephalhematoma)
- Scalp abscess (at fetal scalp electrode site)
- Herpes simplex infection
- Cradle cap/seborrheic dermatitis
- Atopic dermatitis[a]
- Scabies

Childhood and Adolescence
- Seborrheic dermatitis[a]
- Atopic dermatitis[a]
- Head lice (pediculosis capitis)
- Psoriasis[a]

[a]May occur with or without associated hair loss.

is usually associated with seborrheic dermatitis, and this is seen more in African American children. Unlike atopic dermatitis, seborrheic dermatitis is generally non-pruritic. Occasionally, the inflammatory process is severe enough to result in diffuse hair loss. Psoriasis and Langerhans cell histiocytosis presenting on the scalp can mimic seborrheic dermatitis. Skin biopsy may be required for definitive diagnosis. It is often seen in conjunction with adenopathy of the head and neck without associated tinea infection.

Atopic dermatitis on the scalp is also characterized by erythema and scaling of the scalp, and it can overlap with seborrheic dermatitis. Atopic dermatitis on the scalp can be associated with significant pruritus with rubbing and scratching that result in the secondary effects of crusting and lichenification. Severe atopic and seborrheic dermatitis, as well as psoriasis, can result in **tinea amiantacea** (not a fungal infection), which usually presents as localized, thick, adherent, and white or gray scale.

Head lice (pediculosis capitis) is an extremely common childhood infestation that affects girls more often than boys and is most common in children aged 3 to 11 years. Lice are spread by direct contact with infected individuals or infested clothing, combs, or other hair accessories. Pruritus is the primary symptom along with erythema and scaling, with secondary impetigo being common. The viable ova or nits may be visible as small, oval, tan to brown specks found most commonly in the hair above the ears and the nape of the neck. Hatched eggs are clear to white. Generally, only the ova closest to the scalp are viable. They are difficult to remove.

Scabies, a pruritic infestation commonly seen in children, generally does not affect the scalp, except in infants, the elderly, and the immunocompromised. On the scalp of infants, 2- to 3-mm erythematous papules are seen, with overlying excoriations and, often, secondary bacterial infection.

Scalp Disorders Associated With Hair Loss

Box 123-2 lists the common scalp disorders associated with hair loss. When evaluating hair loss in children, it is important to determine whether the loss is diffuse or circumscribed.

Nevus sebaceus is a congenital lesion that mainly occurs on the face and scalp, occurring in about 3 of 1,000 neonates. These lesions are characteristically hairless. In addition, they are usually solitary, well-circumscribed plaques on the scalp, yellow-orange in color, and ovoid to linear in shape. Nevus sebaceus can be associated with a small risk of malignant transformation, namely basal cell carcinoma, at a rate of less than 1% before the age of 18 years. Other growths within nevus sebaceus may also occur at a rate of approximately 1%. Therefore, regular monitoring or consideration of excision should be part of the management. Because of the relatively low risk and low metastatic potential, it is reasonable to postpone excision until later in life. **Aplasia cutis congenita** is a congenital skin defect with localized areas of epidermal, dermal, or subcutaneous tissue loss. Lesions can occur anywhere on the body, but most are found along the midline of the scalp. At birth, the lesions usually appear as punched out, round or oval defects that may have an overlying thin, glistening membrane. Erosion, ulceration, or a scar due to healing

---

Box 123-2. Common Disorders of the Scalp With Associated Hair Loss

Circumscribed Hair Loss

Congenital
- Aplasia cutis congenita
- Nevus sebaceus
- Epidermal nevus

Acquired
- Tinea capitis
- Alopecia areata
- Traction alopecia
- Trichotillomania
- Discoid lupus erythematosus
- Secondary syphilis
- Human herpesvirus
- Lichen planus

Diffuse Alopecia

Congenital
- Congenital hypothyroidism
- Hair shaft defects (eg, Menkes syndrome, monilethrix)
- Ectodermal dysplasia and other genetic syndromes

Acquired
- Seborrheic dermatitis
- Psoriasis
- Telogen effluvium
- Anagen effluvium (secondary to toxins or chemicals)
- Endocrine (eg, diabetes mellitus)
- Hypothyroidism-hypoparathyroidism-hypopituitarism
- Medication-induced (isotretinoin)
- Androgenic alopecia (eg, male pattern baldness)
- Loose anagen syndrome

Other
- Nutritional (eg, acrodermatitis enteropathica, malnutrition, iron deficiency, rickets)
- Systemic lupus erythematosus

---

in utero can also be seen. A "hair collar" may surround the lesion. Aplasia cutis congenita is a result of many possible etiologies, and it can be an isolated defect or in association with other congenital defects such as cleft lip or palate, syndactyly, or multiple other anomalies. Small defects generally heal well, whereas larger defects may require surgical excision and eventual skin grafting. Preoperative imaging studies may be required for extensive, severe cases.

Tinea capitis, a fungal infection of the scalp, is one of the most common causes of acquired hair loss in children. This condition is characterized by patchy alopecia with broken-off hairs and scaling of the scalp. *Trichophyton tonsurans* infection sometimes appears as a series of black dots within the affected area because of the presence of fragmented hairs. The diagnosis can be difficult in children with diffuse scalp scaling or a diffuse pustular eruption without significant alopecia. Occasionally, an intense hypersensitivity response may result in a boggy swelling of the scalp known as a **kerion.** The surface of the kerion may be smooth or covered with small pustules, mimicking a bacterial infection. Uncomplicated tinea capitis leaves no scars, but kerion or favus may result in permanent, scarring hair loss.

Alopecia areata, which frequently leads to hair loss, is characterized by well-defined areas of complete hair loss without associated scaling, irritation, or inflammation of the scalp. Hairs at the periphery of bald patches can usually be easily plucked. The most common presentation is that of one or more round or oval bald patches. A less common subtype is the ophiasis pattern, in which hair loss is present in a band along the periphery of the temporal and occipital scalp. Associated nail defects, including nail pitting (most common) and ridging, may be seen. Occasionally, alopecia totalis (loss of all scalp hair) or alopecia universalis (loss of all body and scalp hair) may result.

Common traumatic causes of alopecia in children are traction alopecia and trichotillomania. **Traction alopecia** often occurs along the margins of the hairline secondary to having the hair pulled back in tight ponytails or braids. Short, broken hairs and follicular papules may be seen. Chronic, prolonged traction can result in permanent, scarring alopecia. **Trichotillomania** is a self-induced form of traction alopecia in which children twist or pull out their hair either consciously or subconsciously (see Chapter 53). Hair pulling is generally believed to occur in a younger population and usually resolves with minimal or no intervention needed. Trichotillomania is now classified in *Diagnostic and Statistical Manual of Mental Disorders, Fifth Edition,* in the habit and impulse disorders category. Hair is generally plucked in a wavelike fashion across the scalp or centrifugally from a starting point. The occiput is generally spared. Trichotillomania may mimic other types of alopecia, but the diagnosis can usually be made on the basis of the bizarre patterns of hair loss with hairs broken at differing lengths. Children occasionally eat the hairs as they are pulled out, resulting in the formation of a **trichobezoar** (hair ball) in the stomach.

Discoid lupus erythematosus, lichen planus, and **secondary syphilis** are uncommon causes of localized hair loss from the scalp in children. The patches of alopecia in discoid lupus erythematosus often appear hypopigmented with hyperpigmentation at the periphery. Because adnexal structures are involved in discoid lupus, scarring alopecia is commonly seen. Lichen planus, an idiopathic inflammatory disease of skin and mucous membranes, can result in scarring and non-scarring alopecia. Secondary syphilis lesions appear as "moth-eaten" patches of alopecia that are non-scarring.

A variety of structural defects, endocrine and metabolic disorders, and toxins may be associated with diffuse loss of scalp hair (see Box 123-2). **Intrinsic structural defects of the hair** may cause hairs to break, thus resulting in failure of hair growth. In some forms of **ectodermal dysplasia,** the number of hair follicles is reduced or the follicles are altogether absent, giving the appearance of sparse or thinning hair. Many of the ectodermal dysplasias have abnormalities of the teeth, nails, and sweat glands. **Monilethrix** is an autosomal-dominant condition that can appear in isolation or in association with other anomalies. Microscopic evaluation of hairs shows a "beads on a string" appearance due to alternating nodes and internodes resulting in fractures between the nodes. Pili torti can be seen in several syndromes, including **Menkes disease (kinky hair syndrome).** Affected patients have twisted hair leading to premature breakage and, thus, chronically short hair. There is often baldness at sites of friction.

Telogen effluvium is a common cause of diffuse hair loss that may occur 2 to 4 months after a variety of events, including pregnancy, discontinuation of oral contraceptives, severe febrile illness, medications, severe diets, or significant emotional stress. Hair loss results from the abrupt conversion of numerous scalp hairs from the anagen (growth) phase to the telogen (resting) phase. Loss of more than 150 hairs per day is considered abnormal. Patients may complain of losing several hundred hairs a day, but the occurrence of clinically significant baldness is rare. Estimates indicate that individuals must lose about 25% of their hair before thinning becomes clinically apparent. The hair loss may continue for several weeks, but complete regrowth usually occurs within 6 to 12 months. **Anagen effluvium** results in the loss of growing hairs due to a sudden cessation of the growing phase. It occurs most commonly after systemic chemotherapy.

Loose anagen syndrome is a disorder in which the anagen hair follicle is anchored improperly, resulting in easy, painless plucking of the hairs. This can result in patchy diffuse hair loss or focal areas of alopecia. This is a familial condition, with fair-haired females more commonly affected. Often, these children will not need a haircut through early childhood. The hair is expected to spontaneously become normal by the teenage years without treatment.

Evaluation

History

The age of the child guides the differential diagnosis because some lesions are more common at one age than another. See the Questions Box to review pertinent history that may be helpful in diagnosis.

Physical Examination

The scalp should be examined to see if the hair loss is diffuse or circumscribed and whether scalp hairs can be plucked easily. Signs of irritation, inflammation, or scaling of the scalp should also be noted, as well as the presence of adenopathy, nail changes, or hair loss elsewhere on the body.

Wood light examination of the scalp for fungus is helpful if positive. A negative examination does not rule out the possibility of fungal infection, however, because *T tonsurans,* the most common cause of tinea capitis in the United States, does not fluoresce. *Microsporum canis* fluoresces yellow-green under the Wood light.

Laboratory Tests

Laboratory assessment is useful in some cases. If fungal infection is suspected, a potassium hydroxide examination should be performed

Questions

Disorders of the Hair and Scalp

- Is the child losing any hair?
- If so, is the child losing hair from all over the scalp or only from localized areas on the scalp?
- Has the child lost any body hair (eg, eyebrows, eyelashes) in addition to the scalp hair?
- How long has the child been losing hair?
- Is the scalp pruritic or scaling?
- Have the parents noticed the child twisting or pulling the hair?
- Is the child's hair often in ponytails or braids?
- Has there recently been any significant stress in the child's life?
- Do any pets live in the home?
- Is the child taking any medications?
- Is anyone else in the home or anyone in close contact with the child having similar symptoms?

by the primary care physician. Scales and broken hairs can be obtained from involved areas by brushing, scraping (eg, with a No. 15 scalpel blade), plucking, or rubbing a moistened 4″ × 4″ gauze over affected areas and then removing broken hairs and scale from the gauze with forceps. The scrapings should be placed on a glass slide, dissolved in potassium hydroxide solution, heated gently, and examined under the microscope. Hyphae and spores within the hair shaft (eg, *T tonsurans* infection) or surrounding the hair shaft (eg, *M canis* infection) should be noted.

In addition to microscopic examination, fungal cultures are recommended in all cases of suspected tinea capitis. Brushings using a moistened sterile cotton swab or a sterile brush as used in Papanicolaou tests will yield the most reliable results. Hair or scalp scrapings are inoculated onto Sabouraud agar or dermatophyte test medium (DTM). Within 5 to 14 days, a distinctive growth seen on the Sabouraud agar or a color change from yellow to red in the DTM confirms the diagnosis. A negative potassium hydroxide examination and fungal culture, in addition to a lack of inflammation and scaling, may be required for differentiating trichotillomania or alopecia areata from tinea capitis.

The diagnosis of telogen effluvium is usually suggested by the history and counting the number of hairs lost each day. If the diagnosis is in question, the patient may be referred to a dermatologist for examination of the involved hair roots via biopsy and determination of the anagen-telogen ratio, which is usually about 85:15. A telogen count of more than 25% is considered to be diagnostic of telogen effluvium. The ratio of anagen to telogen hairs is normal in trichotillomania.

A more extensive laboratory workup may be required if the hair loss is persistent or the history or physical examination is suggestive of systemic disease (see Box 123-2). Studies that may be considered include liver function tests, thyroid function studies, a serum VDRL test, antinuclear antibodies, and serum electrolytes.

Management

Management depends on the diagnosis. Herpetic infection in a newborn requires immediate attention and systemic antiviral therapy because the risk of systemic infection is significant. Scalp electrodes and vacuum-assisted vaginal deliveries should be avoided in neonates with mothers known to have human herpesvirus infections because these can increase the rate of infection transmission. Currently, cesarean delivery remains the standard of care, though most cases of herpes simplex in neonates are in those born to mothers without known infection at time of delivery.

Children suspected of nevus sebaceus should be referred to a dermatologist. Excision may be considered, not only because of the risk, albeit low, of secondary neoplastic changes but also because these lesions can become more prominent and warty in appearance and friable during puberty and adulthood.

Seborrheic dermatitis can persist into the pubertal years, contrary to previously held belief. Cradle cap, which refers to seborrheic dermatitis seen during infancy, can be treated with simple skin care measures such as bathing and the use of moisturizing emollients. Gentle shampoos, low-potency corticosteroids, and, if needed, 2% ketoconazole cream can resolve most cases. Past infancy, seborrheic dermatitis may be treated with **shampoos containing tar, zinc pyrithione, ketoconazole, or selenium** in rotation. Topical, mild corticosteroid solutions can be used if pruritus is significant.

Head lice may be treated with **pyrethrin products,** such as permethrin 1% cream rinse (Nix) or the prescription 5% cream typically used for scabies. Other medications, such as malathion and ivermectin, can also be effective. All topical medications should be used twice, 1 week apart, regardless of package insert information. A fine-toothed comb or tweezers may be required after rinsing to remove the ova or nits of head lice. Other alternative treatments have been unsubstantiated, such as using mayonnaise or petroleum jelly. Heat, such as that associated with blow-drying the hair, also kills a large percentage of the lice.

Permethrin 5% cream is the preferred scabicide. It should be applied from head to toe in infants and children younger than 2 years and from neck to toe for those older than 2 years, for 8 to 12 hours, washed off, and repeated in 1 week. Permethrin 5% cream can be used in infants as young as 2 months and pregnant women. For these patients, sulfur 6% ointment can also be used. For scabies and lice, the treatment of fomites is also important. Clothing, bed linens, and towels should be washed in hot water and machine-dried in high heat. Fomites that cannot be laundered should be sealed in plastic for 48 to 72 hours.

Oral griseofulvin administered for at least 6 to 12 weeks has been the long-held treatment of choice for **tinea capitis.** Although griseofulvin can have many side effects, including gastrointestinal disturbances, hepatotoxicity, and leukopenia, it is generally well tolerated by children and is available in suspension form. Hematologic, renal, and liver function studies can be monitored in children on high doses or prolonged treatment. Higher dosing is occasionally required due to increasing resistance. Care should be made to use proper dosing when using micronized (20–25 mg/kg) or ultra-micronized (10–15 mg/kg) griseofulvin. Newer antifungal agents are also being used with great success, often for shorter durations than griseofulvin, which can increase compliance. **Itraconazole** can be given as continuous or pulse therapy and is available as a solution. **Fluconazole,** also available as solution, is usually administered for 3 to 6 weeks or at a higher dose once weekly for 8 to 12 weeks. **Terbinafine,** available in tablets or granules, has been effective at shorter treatment times than griseofulvin. Monitoring of blood cell counts and liver and renal function are recommended monthly before and during treatment. Ketoconazole is contraindicated because of its potential for adverse effects, especially in light of other available agents. Generally, longer courses of treatment are needed for *M canis* infection. Topical antifungal agents are not effective on the scalp for treatment of tinea capitis because the hair follicle must be penetrated, requiring the use of systemic therapy. Twice-a-week shampooing with ketoconazole or selenium sulfide shampoos has been shown to reduce carriage of spores and reduce infectivity. A course of oral **prednisone** may be required in conjunction with an oral antifungal if a kerion is present to minimize discomfort and permanent, scarring hair loss. Children with kerion are often misdiagnosed as having a bacterial infection of the scalp and treated with oral antibiotics. However, the pustules in kerion are generally sterile, and even when secondary bacterial infection is present (ie, about 30%–50% of patients), antibiotics do not alter the course of the condition.

Children believed to have alopecia areata should be referred to a dermatologist immediately. Therapy for **alopecia areata** consists of **topical and intralesional corticosteroids,** topical anthralin, or minoxidil. Topical immunotherapy with a sensitizer such as squaric acid has also been used for the treatment of extensive alopecia areata. Occasionally, oral steroids can be tried for extensive or rapidly progressing disease. Many psychosocial factors should be considered when treating children with this condition. Children with severe forms of the disease may benefit psychologically from wearing a wig. The National Alopecia Areata Foundation (www.naaf.org) is available as a support group for affected children and their families.

Prognosis

Common disorders of the scalp, such as seborrheic dermatitis, head lice, and tinea capitis, generally respond well to treatment and rarely result in long-term sequelae. The course and prognosis of alopecia areata are quite variable and may be difficult to predict. Generally, prognosis for regrowth is good if hair loss has occurred in only a few patches. Prognosis is usually poorer with younger age at onset, positive family history, nail involvement, and an ophiasis (band-like) pattern of hair loss. It is important to pursue further workup if a

condition does not respond to therapy because it is critical that a condition such as Langerhans cell histiocytosis, a mimicker of seborrheic dermatitis, not be missed. Many of the hair disorders are a result of syndromes that will not respond to therapy; thus, education for patients and their families is important.

CASE RESOLUTION

The child presented in the case study exhibits physical findings of a kerion. Diagnosis can be made clinically on the basis of the appearance of the lesion. The diagnosis is established by microscopic evidence of hyphae and culture confirmation. Treatment with oral antifungals and possibly oral steroids should be initiated. Carriers should also be identified and treated. The child should be examined in 4 weeks to ascertain the response to therapy and check for any adverse reactions.

Selected References

Burkhart CN, Burkhart CG, Morrell DS. Infestations. In: Bolognia JL, Jorizzo JL, Schaffer JV, eds. *Dermatology.* Elsevier Saunders; 2012:1423–1429

Chosidow O. Clinical practices. Scabies. *N Engl J Med.* 2006;354(16):1718–1727

Harrison S, Sinclair R. Optimal management of hair loss (alopecia) in children. *Am J Clin Dermatol.* 2003;4(11):757–770

Honig PJ, Caputo GL, Leyden JJ, McGinley K, Selbst SM, McGravey AR. Treatment of kerions. *Pediatr Dermatol.* 1994;11(1):69–71

Kakourou T, Uksal U; European Society for Pediatric Dermatology. Guidelines for the management of tinea capitis in children. *Pediatr Dermatol.* 2010;27(3):226–228

Koot RW, Reedijk B, Tan WF, De Sonnaville-De Roy Van Zuide. Neonatal brain abscess: complication of fetal monitoring. *Obstet Gynecol.* 1999;93(5 Pt 2):857

McCalmont TH. Adnexal neoplasms. In: Bolognia JL, Jorizzo JL, Schaffer JV, eds. *Dermatology.* Elsevier Saunders; 2012:1830–1831

Möhrenschlager M, Seidl HP, Ring J, Abeck D. Pediatric tinea capitis: recognition and management. *Am J Clin Dermatol.* 2005;6(4):203–213

Nield LS, Keri JE, Kamat D. Alopecia in the general pediatric clinic: who to treat, who to refer. *Clin Pediatr (Phila).* 2006;45(7):605–612

Rosen H, Schmidt B, Lam HP, Meara JG, Labow BI. Management of nevus sebaceus and the risk of Basal cell carcinoma: an 18-year review. *Pediatr Dermatol.* 2009;26(6):676–681

Sperling LC, Sinclair RD, El Shabrawi-Caelen L. Alopecias. In: Bolognia JL, Jorizzo JL, Schaffer JV, eds. *Dermatology.* Elsevier Saunders; 2012:1093–1114

Sybert VP, Zonana J. Ectodermal dysplasias. In: Bolognia JL, Jorizzo JL, Rapini RP, eds. *Dermatology.* St Louis, MO: Mosby; 2003:906–913

Weiner EJ, McIntosh MS, Joseph MM, Maraga N, Davis PG. Neonatal scalp abscess: is it a benign disease? *J Emerg Med.* 2011;40(5):e97–e101

Williams JV, Eichenfield LF, Burke BL, Barnes-Eley M, Friedlander SF. Prevalence of scalp scaling in prepubertal children. *Pediatrics.* 2005;115(1):e1–e6

CHAPTER 124

Diaper Dermatitis

Ki-Young Yoo, MD; Kathy K. Langevin, MD, MPH; and Noah Craft, MD, PhD

CASE STUDY

A 6-month-old boy has a 3-day history of a rash in the diaper area. The mother has been applying cornstarch, but the rash has gotten worse and has spread to the inner thighs and abdomen. The infant has no history of fever, upper respiratory tract symptoms, vomiting, or diarrhea. He was seen in the emergency department 1 week ago for acute gastroenteritis, which has since resolved. On examination, a poorly demarcated, shiny, erythematous rash is noted over the convex surface of the buttocks, lower abdomen, and genitalia, with relative sparing of the intertriginous creases. The rest of the physical examination is within normal limits.

Questions

1. What are the common causes of rashes in the diaper area (diaper dermatitis)?
2. What are the features that distinguish one type of diaper dermatitis from another?
3. What systemic diseases may present with diaper dermatitis?
4. What are some common treatments for diaper dermatitis?

Diaper dermatitis is used to describe a wide variety of skin disorders that present with a rash in the area covered by the diaper. The most familiar form of diaper rash, irritant contact diaper dermatitis, is one of the most common skin disorders of infants and young children. Other infectious and inflammatory processes in the diaper area can also result in dermatitis. Successful management requires making the correct diagnosis and identifying the etiology and associated factors.

Epidemiology

Diaper dermatitis is the most common dermatologic disorder in infancy, with a peak incidence at 9 to 12 months of age, though some reports have shown a high incidence in the first month of life. Prevalence in infants is estimated at anywhere from 7% to 35%. This disorder is not limited to infants and small children but to any individual who wears diapers, though the incidence in adults is unknown.

Clinical Presentation

Diaper dermatitis primarily affects the skin of the buttocks, gluteal cleft, lower abdomen, genitalia, perineum, and proximal thighs. **Irritant contact dermatitis,** the most common type of diaper dermatitis, appears as scaly erythematous papules and plaques or poorly demarcated, glistening erythema over the convex surfaces, with relative sparing of the intertriginous folds (Figure 124-1A). Candidal infection is another common form of diaper dermatitis and is characterized by a beefy red, sharply demarcated plaque with white scale at the border or small, satellite papules and pustules along the margins. Candidal infections may be primarily concentrated within the skin folds (D$_x$ Box) (Figure 124-1B). Other etiologic causes of

Dx Diaper Dermatitis

- Urinary or fecal incontinence requiring diaper wearing
- Erythematous rash over anogenital region
- Associated gastroenteritis, antibiotic therapy, or oral thrush

diaper dermatitis can be challenging to distinguish from one another but can usually be differentiated by their distribution and response to therapy.

Pathophysiology

Many factors are involved in the pathophysiology of irritant diaper dermatitis. Prolonged contact with moisture, urine, feces, or irritating chemicals plays an important role in the initiation of these disorders. Friction generated as the infant tries to move around may further aggravate the condition and lead to maceration of the skin. Secondary infection, most often with *Candida albicans,* may be seen in many cases.

The cause of irritant diaper dermatitis is multifactorial, with prolonged exposure to moisture resulting in fragile skin and a compromised protective barrier, leading to increased irritant penetration and potential growth of microorganisms. Fecal enzymes (proteases, lipases, and urease) also weaken this barrier. Friction from a diaper can easily abrade this fragile skin. Diapers clearly play a role in this disorder; societies in which diapers are not worn do not see this condition. Ammonia produced by bacterial breakdown of urea is no longer believed to be the causative factor in cases of irritant diaper dermatitis.

Figure 124-1. Diaper dermatitis. A, Diaper dermatitis secondary to irritant contact. Convex surface areas are affected. B, Diaper dermatitis secondary to *Candida*. Intertriginous areas are affected, and satellite lesions are present.

Differential Diagnosis

While most cases of diaper dermatitis can be easily recognized clinically, the differential diagnosis can be challenging at times or when the condition fails to respond to therapy. Familiarity with the difference in appearance of these conditions is critical. The Internet can be valuable by providing access to images of many dermatologic conditions. Some sites, such as VisualDx (www.visualdx.com), display a pictorial representation and allow for searching by features such as rash morphologies, symptoms, exposures, skin color, body location, and many other factors.

Diaper dermatitis is a general term to refer to a rash that occurs in the area covered by the diaper. Therefore, a specific diagnosis based on the etiology of the diaper dermatitis is important. The differential diagnosis of diaper dermatitis is presented in Box 124-1.

Irritant contact dermatitis, the most common cause of diaper dermatitis, is most prominent on the skin of the buttocks, perineum, lower abdomen, and proximal thighs. The skin of the creases is relatively unaffected. Exposure to proteolytic enzymes and irritant chemicals in the face of excessive heat or moisture is believed to lead to this condition. Friction with the diaper at sites of contact may aggravate it. Such a rash is poorly demarcated and can give the skin a glistening, red appearance.

Box 124-1. Differential Diagnosis of Diaper Dermatitis

Most Common Causes
- Irritant contact dermatitis
- Candidiasis
- Seborrheic dermatitis

Less Common Causes
- Allergic contact dermatitis
- Impetigo
- Perianal streptococcal or staphylococcal disease
- Atopic dermatitis
- Psoriasis
- Zinc deficiency, including acrodermatitis enteropathica
- Biotin deficiency
- Langerhans cell histiocytosis
- Congenital syphilis

Granuloma gluteale infantum is a possible complication of irritant diaper dermatitis, presenting with violaceous nodules and plaques on the buttocks, vulva, scrotum, and perineum. Though alarming in appearance, these are benign and will resolve once the dermatitis is cleared, though scarring can result. The development of granuloma gluteale infantum does not necessarily correlate with the severity of the preexisting irritant dermatitis. **Jacquet erosive dermatitis** is another potential complication in which the irritant dermatitis is severe. This form is characterized by small, well-demarcated erosions or ulcers that can also feature elevated borders. With chronic irritant dermatitis, children may develop **perianal pseudoverrucous papules and nodules,** which are small bumps characterized by a flat-topped, moist, smooth, shiny surface. All 3—granuloma gluteale infantum, Jacquet erosive dermatitis, and perianal pseudoverrucous papules and nodules—are considered to be less common manifestations of irritant contact dermatitis.

Candidiasis, due to infection with *C albicans,* typically begins in the creases (intertriginous areas) and then spreads to other surfaces. Sometimes associated with oral thrush, candidiasis is also a common sequela of systemic antibiotic therapy. The rash appears as bright, beefy red plaques with sharp, raised borders and many small satellite papules, vesicles, and pustules along its margins, often with desquamation. *Candida albicans* can be a cause of secondary infection of already inflamed skin as well as a primary causative factor in some cases of diaper dermatitis. Recurrent candidal diaper dermatitis can be associated with candidal colonization of the gut and oral cavity.

Seborrheic diaper dermatitis, like candidal diaper dermatitis, also primarily affects the intertriginous areas of the groin. The rash has a characteristic salmon-colored appearance with soft, yellowish scale. Satellite lesions can be seen. Seborrheic dermatitis of the face, scalp (including postauricular areas), neck, trunk, and proximal extremities is usually seen in association with seborrheic dermatitis of the diaper area.

Allergic contact dermatitis is a less common cause of diaper dermatitis but should be considered in patients who do not respond to standard therapeutic interventions. Allergens can be from the chemical makeup of the diaper itself or from topical preparations such as soaps, emollients, and baby wipes that are applied to the diaper area. For example, rubber additives such as mercaptobenzothiazole found in the elastics of disposable diapers have been shown to cause allergic diaper dermatitis on the hips and outer buttocks, a distribution reminiscent of a cowboy's gun holster; hence, the nickname "Lucky Luke" dermatitis. Other allergens to consider are emulsifiers in topical preparations, fragrances, disperse dye, and preservatives.

Bacterial infections can cause diaper dermatitis. **Impetigo,** especially bullous impetigo, is a not uncommon eruption in the diaper area. Bullous impetigo is caused by *Staphylococcus aureus* and is toxin-mediated. The rash presents as vesicles that may enlarge into 3- to 5-cm bullae that easily rupture, leaving superficial erosions with thick, honey-colored crusts. There can be associated systemic symptoms of fever and diarrhea. Perianal bacterial disease can result from group A beta-hemolytic streptococcus or *S aureus.* Classically, perianal streptococcal dermatitis manifests as well-demarcated, bright red, tender patches. Rectal bleeding and painful defecation may also be noted.

Congenital syphilis can present with diaper dermatitis findings in 30% to 60% of those born with this infection. Initially, there is usually a bright erythematous morbilliform eruption that fades to a coppery color, often with scaling. Pustules can develop later. Buttocks, face, extremities, palms, and soles are generally affected.

Diaper rashes that appear to persist despite seemingly adequate therapy should raise suspicion for other systemic diseases. Though less common, these include psoriasis, atopic dermatitis, zinc deficiency, biotin deficiency, and Langerhans cell histiocytosis. **Psoriasis** may occur anywhere on the body, but lesions typically occur on the scalp, face, elbows, and knees. In infants, generally between 2 to 8 months of age, psoriasis may involve the diaper area. Lesions elsewhere on the body are typically well-circumscribed, erythematous plaques with a thick, silvery scale. However, psoriatic lesions in the diaper area may be difficult to differentiate from seborrheic dermatitis or candidal infection. Plaques are brightly erythematous and sharply demarcated but without obvious scale given the moisture from the occluded diaper area. Skin biopsy, family history of psoriasis, or nail involvement may help confirm the diagnosis.

Atopic dermatitis typically spares the diaper area, even in infants who have lesions elsewhere on the body. The relative sparing of the diaper area is perhaps a result of the increased moisture of the skin in this area. (See Chapter 125 for a discussion of atopic dermatitis.)

Zinc deficiency can cause dermatitis in a characteristic periorificial distribution (mouth, nose, ears, eyes, and anogenital area) and distal extremities. Zinc deficiency may result from an inherited defect called acrodermatitis enteropathica or develop secondary to insufficient intake or malabsorption, such as in patients with cystic fibrosis. **Acrodermatitis enteropathica** is a rare, autosomally recessive inherited disorder with mutations in *SLC39A* resulting in defective zinc transporters in the small intestine. In breastfed infants, the disease becomes manifest shortly after weaning, whereas in bottle-fed infants, signs and symptoms appear days to weeks after birth. Afflicted infants are irritable and listless and present with diarrhea, failure to thrive, and skin lesions in the previously mentioned distribution featuring erythematous bullous and pustular lesions as well as dry, red, scaly plaques. Candidal and *S aureus* superinfection can occur. Treatment consists of oral zinc supplementation. Biotin deficiency, as well as several other nutritional deficiencies, can present with identical skin findings, and treatment is with supplementation of the deficient nutrient.

Langerhans cell histiocytosis refers to a group of disorders characterized by proliferation of macrophages, a progenitor cell in the bone marrow. Members of this group include Letterer-Siwe and Hand-Schüller-Christian diseases, eosinophilic granuloma, and congenital self-healing reticulohistiocytosis. Skin lesions may involve the scalp and flexural areas of the perineum, axilla, and neck. The lesions appear as small, pink to tan scaling papules and pustules that can coalesce; associated purpura or ulceration may be apparent in the inguinal crease with secondary impetiginization (honey-colored crusting caused by *S aureus* superinfection). The rash is most often confused with that of seborrheic dermatitis. Diagnosis can be confirmed by skin biopsy.

Evaluation

History

A thorough history should be obtained (Questions Box). Candidal diaper dermatitis should be suspected if oral antibiotic therapy has recently been used.

Physical Examination

On physical examination, the presence of skin lesions elsewhere on the body should be noted. This is particularly important in the case of a persistent, resistant, or recurrent diaper rash in which generalized skin disorders such as psoriasis must be considered. The distribution of the rash within the diaper area itself may provide clues to the diagnosis. Candidal and seborrheic dermatitis occur primarily in the creases, whereas irritant contact dermatitis usually affects the

---

Questions

Diaper Dermatitis

- When did the rash begin?
- Does the rash resolve and then recur?
- Is the rash pruritic?
- Is the infant feeding and sleeping? Is he or she irritable?
- Have any home remedies or previous treatments been used? Which ones?
- Does the infant have a family history of atopic dermatitis or psoriasis?
- Is the infant taking antibiotics now or has the infant used them recently?
- What type of diapers is used?
- How frequently are the diapers changed?

convex areas of the skin with relative sparing of the intertriginous areas. Streptococcal disease manifests primarily as marked perianal erythema.

Laboratory Tests

Although the diagnosis of candidal diaper dermatitis is usually evident clinically, microscopic examination of skin scrapings with potassium hydroxide may be performed to establish the diagnosis. Typically, budding yeast with hyphae or pseudohypha is seen. The diagnosis of perianal streptococcal disease or bullous impetigo may be confirmed by bacterial cultures from the perianal area or bullous lesions, respectively. Biopsies may be warranted for recalcitrant diaper dermatitis. Other laboratory studies may be carried out to investigate for suspected nutritional deficiencies.

Management

The mainstay of therapy for irritant diaper dermatitis is prevention, requiring **good hygiene,** which involves keeping the diaper area clean and dry. Gentle but thorough cleansing of the diaper area is necessary when stool is present and can be done with water alone or water and mild soap. The area should then be patted dry and allowed to air-dry completely if possible or dry with the use of cotton balls. Cleansing frequently with harsh soaps or scrubbing too vigorously can further irritate skin that is already damaged and inflamed.

In addition, the diaper should be **changed frequently.** The diaper area should be exposed to as much air as reasonably possible (eg, by allowing the infant to sleep without a diaper). Cloth and regular disposable diapers are not as effective as superabsorbent gel diapers in decreasing moisture. Although **dusting powders** such as cornstarch or talc minimize friction and talc does not enhance the growth of yeast on skin, concern about pulmonary effects from inhalation precludes their routine use even in the absence of any skin inflammation. **Moisture-resistant barrier ointments or creams** such as zinc oxide or petrolatum are very helpful in reducing irritation. The role of hygiene in all forms of diaper dermatitis cannot be overemphasized. Topical application of medicated creams and ointments is not effective in the presence of poor hygiene.

Irritant contact dermatitis usually responds to previously described hygienic measures and the application of barrier ointments and low-potency **topical corticosteroids,** such as 0.5% or 1% hydrocortisone ointment or cream. Seborrheic dermatitis usually resolves spontaneously but can also be treated with low-potency topical corticosteroids. Candidal diaper dermatitis responds to **topical antifungal creams** such as nystatin, miconazole, or clotrimazole. In addition, a low-potency corticosteroid may be required if inflammation is severe. Oral antifungal therapy is usually not indicated, though may be needed in cases of recurrent candidiasis. Oral antibiotic therapy usually clears perianal streptococcal or staphylococcal disease,

but the relapse rate is high. The topical antibiotic mupirocin may be used to treat bullous impetigo only if the lesions are superficial, few, and isolated. Oral antibiotics (eg, cephalexin, clindamycin) may be required for more extensive bacterial infections. Combination topical medications containing a corticosteroid and an antifungal should not be recommended routinely because they usually contain high-potency corticosteroids. When topical steroids and antifungals are used in conjunction with barrier ointment, the medication should be applied before the barrier ointment.

When the more common causes of diaper dermatitis, such as irritant contact dermatitis, *Candida,* or seborrheic dermatitis, do not respond to conventional therapy, further workup must be initiated because there may be an underlying systemic disease manifesting as diaper dermatitis; some of these can be life-threatening.

Prognosis

Although recurrence of diaper dermatitis is common, the usual varieties respond well to measures aimed at keeping the diaper area clean and dry and medicated creams.

CASE RESOLUTION

The infant presented in the case study has irritant contact dermatitis. He has a recent history of gastroenteritis, and stool is known to be particularly irritating to the skin. Treatment includes keeping the diaper area clean and dry with frequent diaper changes, use of superabsorbent diapers, and fastidious toilet habits, as well as topical application of a low-potency corticosteroid ointment or cream and a barrier ointment such as zinc oxide after bathing.

Selected References

Heath C, Desai N, Silverberg NB. Recent microbiological shifts in perianal bacterial dermatitis: *Staphylococcus aureus* predominance. *Pediatr Dermatol.* 2009;26(6):696–700

Paller AS, Mancini AJ. *Hurwitz.* 3rd ed. Elsevier Saunders; 2011:21-23

Robson KJ, Maughan JA, Purcell SD, Petersen MJ, Haefner HK, Lowe L. Erosive papulonodular dermatosis associated with topical benzocaine: a report of two cases and evidence and granuloma gluteale, pseudoverrucous papules, and Jacquet's erosive dermatitis are a disease spectrum. *J Am Acad Dermatol.* 2006;55(5 Suppl):S74–S80

Scheinfeld N. Diaper dermatitis: a review and brief survey of eruptions of the diaper area. *Am J Clin Dermatol.* 2005;6(5):273–281

Smith WJ, Jacob SE. The role of allergic contact dermatitis in diaper dermatitis. *Pediatr Dermatol.* 2009;26(3):369–370

Ward DB, Fleischer AB Jr, Feldman SR, Krowchuk DP. Characterization of diaper dermatitis in the United States. *Arch Pediatr Adolesc Med.* 2000;154(9):943–946

CHAPTER 125

Papulosquamous Eruptions

Ki-Young Yoo, MD; Kathy K. Langevin, MD, MPH; and Noah Craft, MD, PhD

CASE STUDY

A 6-month-old girl presents with an erythematous, confluent, slightly raised and scaly rash on the cheeks. The extremities are also covered with a fine papular rash. The infant has had some scaling behind the ears and on the scalp since early infancy, but the symptoms have recently increased. The mother has been applying baby oil to the scalp to relieve the scaliness. Except for some intermittent rhinorrhea, the infant has otherwise been well. Immunizations are deficient; she received only the first set when she was 2 months old. The family history is positive for bronchitis. The infant's weight is at the 75th percentile and height is at the 50th percentile. Vital signs are normal. The physical examination is normal except for the presence of the rash.

Questions

1. What are the characteristics of papulosquamous eruptions?
2. What are the common conditions associated with papulosquamous eruptions in children?
3. What are the appropriate treatments for common papulosquamous eruptions?
4. When should children with papulosquamous eruptions be referred to a dermatologist?

Rashes, a common problem in children, can be classified in ways that help to establish a diagnostic approach. First, rashes are assessed in terms of appearance: macular (flat), papular (raised), squamous (scaly), vesicular (fluid-filled), or bullous (large, fluid-filled). Next, the extent of the rash is determined. Rashes may be described as generalized or localized. Location is also important. The site of a localized rash may be consistent with certain diagnoses (eg, diaper dermatitis). Pruritus is an important distinguishing feature. Other systemic symptoms must also be taken into consideration. Rashes may be a primary skin condition or a manifestation of an underlying infection or reaction to a precipitating agent.

Papulosquamous eruptions, the subject of this chapter, are rashes characterized by scaly papules and plaques. Eczema is a broad group of skin disorders characterized clinically by scale and histologically by spongiosis and makes up a large component of the papulosquamous disorders. The etiology of many papulosquamous eruptions is unknown, and the clinical appearance of lesions is the reason they are classified together.

Epidemiology

Although a large number of conditions may cause papulosquamous eruptions in children, a select number of diagnoses account for most problems. One of the most common types of papulosquamous eruptions in children is atopic dermatitis. Atopic dermatitis has become increasingly more common, and the prevalence in school-aged children in the United States is estimated to be between 10% to 20%. Positive family history is often elicited. The severity of atopic dermatitis generally improves with age; however, lifelong dry, itchy skin, in varying degrees of severity, is not uncommon. Seborrheic dermatitis is another common papulosquamous rash seen in the pediatric population. Although most commonly described in infants younger than 3 or 4 months, it can occur in all pediatric age groups. It is estimated to have a prevalence of up to 5%, encompassing pediatric and adult populations.

Scabies occurs worldwide and is frequently encountered in general pediatric and dermatologic settings. The prevalence is much greater in developing countries and in situations in which populations are forced into close proximity (eg, during wars, incarcerated individuals). Family members and close contacts are at greatest risk of infection.

Clinical Presentation

Papulosquamous eruptions consist of skin-colored to erythematous, scaly papules and plaques that may involve the face, trunk, or extremities. The lesions can be pruritic, and scratching may lead to crusting or secondary infection. Sometimes multiple family members are affected (D_x Box). Chronicity and repeated manipulation may lead to lichenification (thickening) of involved skin.

Papulosquamous Eruptions

- Raised, scaly papules and plaques
- Pruritus
- Afebrile, unless secondary infection is present
- Personal or family history of allergies
- Intertriginous rash

Pathophysiology

The pathophysiology of atopic dermatitis has not been definitively established. Recent evidence suggests that mutations in the filaggrin gene, which is important for skin barrier function, may play a large role in atopic dermatitis. It is also important to keep in mind that atopic dermatitis is a multifactorial disease with variable expression, influenced by environmental factors. Inheritance of this disease is associated with atopy, made up of the triad of atopic dermatitis, allergic rhinitis, and asthma. The disorder is attributed largely to skin barrier function; however, immune dysfunction and reactivity of nerves and blood vessels may also be involved. Initially, the disease is characterized by Th1 cytokine predominance, but later in chronic disease, there is activation of the Th2 immune pathway with a resultant synthesis of cytokines, including IL-4 and IL-5, causing elevated immunoglobulin (Ig) E levels, eosinophilia, and diminished cell-mediated immunity. Elevated IgE is reported in up to 80% of patients with atopic dermatitis.

Like atopic dermatitis, the etiology of seborrheic dermatitis remains unclear. There is believed to be an association with the yeast *Pityrosporum ovale (Malassezia ovalis)*, though whether this organism is causative has not been established. It is widely accepted that this yeast has some role in seborrheic dermatitis, which is further substantiated by the improvement of this skin condition with antifungal agents. Individuals with seborrheic dermatitis that is severe or extensive may have some sort of immune dysfunction, as in uncontrolled HIV and AIDS.

The inflammatory response in scabies is triggered by an infestation with a mite, *Sarcoptes scabiei*. The adult female burrows under the skin and lays 60 to 90 eggs. After 2 weeks, the eggs become adults. Affected individuals may be asymptomatic on first exposure. Up to 2 to 6 weeks after infestation, the host's immune system becomes sensitized to mites or scybala (mite feces), resulting in systemic pruritus and rash. In most individuals, the rash associated with scabies is an allergic phenomenon and does not represent mites at each eruptive papule on the body.

Differential Diagnosis

While many papulosquamous eruptions are easily distinguishable clinically, the differential diagnosis can be challenging at times. Familiarity with the appearance of these conditions and their differentiating features is critical. The Internet can be valuable by providing access to images of many dermatologic conditions. Some sites, such as VisualDx (www.visualdx.com), display pictorial representations and allow for searching by features such as rash morphologies, symptoms, exposures, skin color, body location, age, immune status, and many other factors.

Conditions that present as papulosquamous eruptions in children include atopic dermatitis, seborrheic dermatitis, contact dermatitis, psoriasis, pityriasis rosea, lichen planus, lichen striatus, scabies, and fungal infections of the skin.

Eczema is a general term that is used to denote a type of papulosquamous eruption. The most common eczematous conditions seen in children are atopic eczema or dermatitis, seborrheic dermatitis, and contact dermatitis. **Atopic dermatitis** is a disorder of infancy and childhood and may persist into adulthood. More than half of affected individuals are symptomatic by 1 year, and 90% of cases have their onset by 5 years of age. The area of involvement changes with age. In infancy, the face, scalp, and extensor surfaces are involved, often areas where the infant can relieve itching by rubbing, and the diaper area is often spared (Figure 125-1A). By childhood, the more typical pattern seen in adulthood becomes prominent, with involvement of the neck and antecubital and popliteal fossae. Adults tend to have greater extremity involvement, along with the head and neck. Clinically, xerosis (dry skin), erythema, and a pruritic papular eruption are apparent. Scratching and rubbing lead to crusting, weeping, and eventually, lichenification. Changes in color, including hypopigmentation and hyperpigmentation, may also occur. Hypopigmented areas with fine scale that are usually noted on the face are called pityriasis alba (considered to be the mildest form of atopic dermatitis). Xeroderma, or dry skin, is a frequent coexisting condition. Ichthyosis vulgaris,

Figure 125-1. Typical distribution of papulosquamous eruptions in children. A, Atopic dermatitis: usually located on cheeks, creases of elbows, and knees. B, Seborrheic dermatitis: usually located on scalp, behind ears, thigh creases, and eyebrows. C, Scabies: usually located on axillae, webs of fingers and toes, and intra-gluteal area.

characterized by dirty-appearing excessive scaling and hyper-linear palms, is seen in half of patients affected with atopic dermatitis. Lesions around mucosa (Morgan folds in the infraorbital fold under the eye and cheilitis around the mouth) may also be seen. Symptoms of other atopic conditions, such as allergic rhinitis, asthma, or food-related allergies, will occur in many of these patients.

Seborrheic dermatitis, which frequently develops during the first 3 months of life, is characterized by scaly papules or confluent scaly plaques, particularly of the scalp. Scalp eruptions in infancy are referred to as cradle cap. Seborrheic dermatitis has a predilection for areas with a high density of sebaceous glands, such as the scalp, face, ears, presternal chest, penis, and intertriginous areas, including the folds of the diaper region (Figure 125-1B). The red or pink papules and plaques may have a greasy quality. Secondary infections may occur with *Candida,* particularly in the intertriginous areas. Seborrheic dermatitis is usually not exceedingly pruritic, and this feature can be used to distinguish between it and atopic dermatitis. The intertriginous involvement and the onset shortly after birth also differentiate these 2 types of dermatitis. Severe seborrheic dermatitis can be associated with an immune deficiency.

Irritant or allergic contact dermatitis occurs when individuals come into physical contact with an irritant or a specific allergen, respectively. Irritant dermatitis is caused by direct cytotoxic effect, while allergic contact dermatitis is a delayed type 4 hypersensitivity response to an allergen. Although their etiologies are different, they typically have a similar clinical appearance. Individuals usually develop well-defined erythematous vesicles, papules, or plaques, often with scale, and can have oozing and subsequent lichenification. Diaper dermatitis is one of the most common types of irritant dermatitis in the pediatric population (see Chapter 124). Rhus dermatitis (poison ivy/oak) and nickel allergy are 2 common types of allergic contact dermatitis seen in older children and adolescents. It remains controversial whether atopic dermatitis is a risk factor for allergic contact dermatitis. However, children with atopic dermatitis may have more exposure to sensitizers, in conjunction with a damaged epithelial barrier, putting them at risk.

Plaque-type psoriasis, a chronic papulosquamous skin condition manifested most commonly as well-defined erythematous papules and plaques with silvery scale, is a not uncommon disease of childhood. About 40% of adult patients with psoriasis report having the disease in childhood. It most commonly affects the scalp in the pediatric population as well as the face and intertriginous areas. Infrequently, a young infant may develop psoriasis in the diaper area. Guttate psoriasis features smaller scaly papules and is usually precipitated by group A streptococci infection in the pharynx or perianal area. Pruritus is variable but not prominent. Classically, psoriatic lesions can develop at sites of trauma (scratches and cuts), known as the Koebner phenomenon.

Pityriasis rosea is a self-limited papulosquamous eruption that is frequently seen in adolescents. The lesions tend to be round or ovoid and classically have a symmetric distribution on the trunk extending downward from the midline at a 45-degree angle. Classically, there is a larger "herald patch" preceding the eruption by a few days to weeks. It should be duly noted that the classic presentation is not always present—many patients cannot recall a herald patch and the pattern over the trunk is commonly haphazard. It is generally self-limited and resolves in 1 to 2 months. It is pruritic in about one-quarter of those affected. The etiology is unknown, although some evidence suggests an association with human herpesvirus 6 or 7 infection.

Lichen planus is an uncommon papulosquamous eruption in the pediatric population. It is characterized by pruritic, polygonal, pink to purplish flat-topped papules, sometimes with an overlying network of delicate white lines called Wickham striae. Etiology is also unknown, though hepatitis C, as well as other viruses, can occasionally be associated. Flexor surfaces are usually affected and these lesions can koebnerize.

Lichen striatus is an asymptomatic eruption consisting of flat-topped papules that are skin colored to slightly hyperpigmented. The lesions develop along the Blaschko lines and may be arranged in a curvilinear distribution. This eruption spontaneously resolves over months to years. It is most commonly seen between 9 months to 9 years of age. The etiology is unknown.

Scabies may resemble atopic or seborrheic dermatitis in infants and young children. The lesions may be papules, pustules, or vesicles. The characteristic burrow, which is only 3- to 10-mm long, is often difficult to appreciate unless certain diagnostic maneuvers are undertaken. The lesions are most often noted on the skin of the hands and feet, including the palms and soles in infants and young children. Intertriginous areas, such as the intra-gluteal region, groin, and finger webs, are commonly infected (Figure 125-1C). In infants, the face and head may be involved. Scratching and secondary infection may alter the appearance of the rash. Reddish-brown nodules may be characteristic of more chronic infection. In institutionalized or immunosuppressed individuals, extensive mite infection can occur, resulting in thick, greasy-appearing, yellowish scale and crusts over the extremities and trunk, a condition referred to as *crusted scabies.*

Fungal infections (eg, tinea corporis, tinea pedis) commonly appear as papulosquamous eruptions. The lesions usually assume a characteristic morphology, with scaly papules grouped in a circle or coalesced into a plaque with central clearing.

Evaluation

History

A thorough history should be obtained (Questions Box). The presence of a rash in other family members suggests a contagious condition such as scabies or a familial disorder such as atopic dermatitis or psoriasis. An onset in the first few weeks of life is consistent with seborrheic dermatitis. It is important to determine if any medications have been used because these may modify the appearance of the rash. In addition, certain medications can cause a rash themselves, though these tend to be more morbilliform in appearance (see Chapter 126). Pruritus should be noted. Asking about lesions developing at sites of previous trauma can aid in diagnosing eruptions that koebnerize, such as psoriasis and lichen planus.

Papulosquamous Eruptions

- How long has the child had the rash?
- What did the rash look like when it first appeared?
- Are other family members affected?
- Have any medications been used to treat the rash or any been given prior to the onset of the rash?
- Is pruritus present?
- Does the child have any other symptoms such as wheezing or rhinorrhea?
- Does the child have a history of any contact between the affected skin and any irritating substance?
- Has the child been febrile?

Physical Examination

The physical examination helps define the exact nature of the eruption and its distribution, which is often the clue to its etiology. The entire body should be examined, and particular attention should be paid to the intra-gluteal region and web spaces between fingers and toes. Certain rashes have characteristic appearances. For example, a circular cluster of scaly papules with central clearing signifies tinea corporis, whereas the presence of a herald patch preceding a more generalized eruption can suggest pityriasis rosea. The presence of burrows characterizes scabies. Burrows appear as a 3- to 10-mm grayish-white line (only about 1 mm wide). Vesicles, pustules, and nodules may also be present in scabies.

It is important to distinguish if any secondary lesions, such as linear excoriations, are present. Secondary infections are also important to diagnose and treat because they can complicate many of the papulosquamous eruptions.

Associated cutaneous features can also aid in diagnosis. Hyperlinear palms, keratosis pilaris (erythematous 1- to 2-mm folliculocentric papules often on lateral upper arms, anterior thighs, and cheeks), and perioral or periocular lichenified papules are often seen in children with atopic dermatitis.

Overall health, including height and weight, should be assessed. Failure to thrive in conjunction with eczematous skin changes should raise suspicion for an immunodeficiency.

Laboratory Tests

Certain diagnostic tests may help clarify the etiology of certain papulosquamous eruptions. In children with atopic dermatitis, approximately 30% may have coexisting food allergies and 70% may have coexisting respiratory allergies. Food allergies tend to develop during early infancy, whereas respiratory allergies may develop during childhood. While it is important to identify food (and later on, environmental) allergies via skin or radioallergosorbent/ImmunoCAP testing, which measures allergen-specific IgE (Chapter 83), parents must understand that food allergies **infrequently** cause or exacerbate atopic dermatitis. Based on misperceptions on the role of food allergies in atopic dermatitis, parents may, on their own, institute dietary restrictions for their child, which often results in gross undertreatment of the skin itself and may even lead to dangerous levels of malnutrition. Therefore, proper referral and counseling are especially important in infants who have atopic dermatitis and food allergies. Patch testing may identify allergens causing contact dermatitis. Serologic IgE may or may not be elevated in children with atopic dermatitis.

The burrow of the mite that causes scabies may not be readily apparent. Scrapings with mineral oil are most commonly done today to help identify the mite, eggs, or feces (scybala)—any of these are diagnostic. Multiple burrows or web spaces are scraped. Scrapings of skin also assist in diagnosing candidal or tinea infections. These scrapings should be mixed with 10% to 20% potassium hydroxide, which facilitates the dissolution of epithelial debris and allows for identification of the spores or hyphae.

If a secondary bacterial infection is suspected, cultures of the skin are indicated. Most papulosquamous eruptions are diagnosed clinically and no other specific diagnostic tests, short of a skin biopsy, assist in the diagnosis.

Management

Management is determined by the diagnosis.

Management of atopic dermatitis hinges on skin barrier function and the reduction of dryness and irritation with **vigilant skin care.** There has been debate whether frequent short baths daily versus bathing infrequently is more beneficial. It is most crucial that these patients bathe for short times only, applying cleansers only to the face, groin, and other soiled areas. The cleanser should be soap-free or the soap should be nonirritating, nondrying, and perfume- and dye-free. The skin should be patted dry after bathing with immediate application of emollient or medication. Thick emollients, such as petroleum jelly or other greasy ointments, are preferable. For school-aged children, using greasier emollients at night under pajamas and thinner emollients during the day may increase compliance. Avoiding scratchy clothing such as wool can be helpful, as can humidifiers in the winter to prevent excessive environmental dryness. Humidifiers should be cleaned regularly to prevent mold buildup, and a cool mist is considered safer to prevent burns.

Topical steroids are used to treat various papulosquamous eruptions, especially during flares. These are the mainstay of therapy designed to minimize inflammation. The agents usually prescribed in cases of atopic as well as seborrheic dermatitis are triamcinolone 0.025% or 0.1% and hydrocortisone 1% creams or ointments. Though ointment vehicles allow for better penetration and, often, less irritation, they are often disliked for their greasy texture, minimizing their usefulness because they are not applied regularly. The weaker topical steroids (eg, hydrocortisone) should be used for the face and groin and the higher strengths (eg, triamcinolone) in areas of thicker skin. Chronic use should be discouraged to avoid skin atrophy. Parents can be educated on applying the medication to the appropriate areas for 1 to 2 weeks for flares, with maintenance use on weekends or a few days per week. Sometimes brief courses of systemic steroids may be needed during more severe exacerbations, but if a patient is requiring oral steroids regularly, a referral to a dermatologist may be needed to consider other treatments such as systemic immunomodulators or ultraviolet (UV) therapy, both used for atopic dermatitis and psoriasis. Oral steroids may be required for rhus contact dermatitis, one of the more common forms of allergic contact dermatitis, and should be given for 2 to 3 weeks to prevent flaring.

For scaly scalp psoriasis, seborrheic dermatitis, and atopic dermatitis, several treatments can be used. For pruritus and inflammation, a topical steroid in gel, liquid, oil, or foam vehicle can be applied. Mineral or baby oil can help loosen scale, which can be washed out using a gentle shampoo or antiseborrheic shampoo. It should be massaged gently onto the scalp and allowed to sit for several minutes before rinsing.

Tacrolimus and pimecrolimus are topical calcineurin inhibitors, which can be used as **steroid-sparing agents,** most often in mild cases of atopic dermatitis, seborrheic dermatitis, and inverse (intertriginous) psoriasis. As of January 2006, a black box warning was placed on these 2 medications because of theoretical risks of skin cancer and lymphoma among patients using these drugs. The warning was based on the risk in transplant patients who are on systemic calcineurin inhibitors. No evidence exists that topical calcineurin inhibitors are associated with increased risk for developing skin cancer and lymphoma. Thus, dermatologists, allergists, and immunologists prescribe these medications in conjunction with topical steroids for their patients. As stand-alone agents, they are not as effective as steroids for more severe cases and are substantially more expensive.

In psoriasis, topical steroids are often used in conjunction with **calcipotriene** ointment or cream. **Tar** and **anthralin** are still used today as adjunctive topical treatments, though they are falling out of favor due to their messy quality and more favorable alternatives.

Antihistamines may play a role in reducing pruritus, especially at bedtime, due to their sedating effect. Hydroxyzine and diphenhydramine work well in the evenings. For daytime, fexofenadine, cetirizine, or loratadine are less-sedating choices. Regular use of antihistamines during a flare can help to break the itch-scratch cycle often observed in children with atopic dermatitis. The other conditions can have variable degrees of pruritus for which antihistamines can be useful. Clipping fingernails decreases the risk of skin trauma after scratching.

Antibiotics are indicated if secondary infection is present. The most common pathogen involved is *Staphylococcus aureus*. Staphylococcal antigens also exacerbate the inflammation of atopic dermatitis. Treatment with antistaphylococcal systemic antibiotics such as cephalosporins may be needed for more widespread secondary infections. Topical antibiotics such as mupirocin may be used in localized secondary infections. Streptococcal-associated guttate psoriasis should also be treated with appropriate antibiotics.

Seborrheic dermatitis is generally treated with a combination of products including topical keratolytics, corticosteroids, and antifungals (see also Chapter 123). The seborrheic dermatitis of infancy can be treated with topical shampoos containing selenium sulfide and gentle sloughing of the scaly lesions using a soft brush or cloth. Topical calcineurin inhibitors have anti-inflammatory properties without skin atrophy side effects but are generally reserved for periorbital or recalcitrant cases owing to the cost of the medications.

Atopic dermatitis can be complicated by infection with herpes simplex (eczema herpeticum), in which case treatment should be initiated with **acyclovir.** Involvement of the periorbital skin or nasal tip is concerning for eye involvement and warrants an ophthalmologic consult. If involvement is severe, the patient may need to be hospitalized for intravenous antiviral therapy. Children with atopic dermatitis are also prone to viral infections resulting in warts and molluscum contagiosum; these should be managed accordingly.

Coinfection with *Candida,* which occurs with seborrheic dermatitis and psoriasis, requires the use of topical medications such as **nystatin, clotrimazole, or miconazole.** Antifungal shampoos may also help in reducing the scaling due to fungal agents such as *Pityrosporum*. Tinea corporis responds to topical antifungal agents. Tinea capitis will require systemic antifungals (see Chapter 123).

The treatment for pityriasis rosea remains controversial, especially because it is a self-resolving condition. There are several studies demonstrating effectiveness of **acyclovir**, **erythromycin**, or **UV therapy** to speed recovery.

There are several medications used to treat scabies. The current preferred product is 5% **permethrin** cream. It is approved for infants 2 months or older, although its safety and efficacy has been reported in a 23-day-old. It should be applied from head to toe in infants and from neck to toe in small children and adults, left on for 8 to 12 hours, then rinsed off. **Lindane,** which has been used for more than 50 years and previously used worldwide, is a 1% cream. Because of concern about the percutaneous absorption of lindane and its potential neurotoxicity, it is no longer widely used and is not available in some areas. Oral **ivermectin** is also a successful scabicide. A single dose of 200 µg/kg, repeated in 1 week, can be used in children weighing more than 15 kg and women who are not pregnant or breastfeeding. All scabicides should be re-administered 7 days after initial treatment. The effective elimination of scabies necessitates that all affected household members be treated simultaneously and that bed linens and clothing be washed in hot water. Patients should be warned that the pruritus of scabies often takes several weeks to subside and can be treated supportively with steroids and antihistamines.

Prognosis

In general, the prognosis for children with papulosquamous eruptions is excellent with appropriate management, which is contingent on accurate diagnosis. Atopic and seborrheic dermatitis tend to improve as children get older. However, chronic problems such as hand dermatitis, which can be exacerbated by occupational exposures, can become a significant problem in patients with atopic dermatitis. Children with significant atopic dermatitis should be counseled against careers with frequent wet work, such as hairdressers, hospital workers, or food service. It is also critical to counsel families that maintaining atopic dermatitis with the prevention of flares is the primary goal and is more important than having perfect skin. Families of children with severe atopic dermatitis can have difficulty in maintaining a good quality of life for these patients, and the entire family structure can suffer as chronic care can be challenging. Children with atopic dermatitis frequently face remissions and exacerbations, particularly associated with seasonal changes. Prevention and maintenance must be stressed. It is advisable that patients with recalcitrant eczema have further workup with an allergist to eliminate triggers.

Many of these eruptions, such as lichen striatus and pityriasis rosea, are self-limited and only need symptomatic treatment. Psoriasis has a more chronic course, and early diagnosis and treatment can help to reduce disease severity and progression. Chronic disease such as atopic dermatitis and psoriasis can be psychologically challenging for children because they can often be ridiculed at school and excluded from activities for unfounded fears of contagiousness. Teachers may need to be educated as well and emotional and psychologic support provided for these children.

Scabies and tinea will improve with appropriate management and education to prevent recurrence.

CASE RESOLUTION

The infant's presentation in the case study is characteristic of seborrheic dermatitis. The baby experienced the onset of symptoms as a young infant (most atopic patients develop symptoms after 2 months of age). Seborrheic dermatitis can often affect the head and face of young patients. Xerosis is also apparent.

The most important discussion with the mother should be on good skin care. The mother should be advised that although she may use the baby oil to loosen the scale on the scalp, she should shampoo afterward with a mild antiseborrheic shampoo to prevent buildup. A mild topical steroid, such as hydrocortisone 1% ointment, may also be recommended, though chronic use should be dissuaded. If skin scrapings reveal secondary infection with *Candida,* an antifungal cream should be added to the regimen; if a secondary bacterial infection is suspected, a culture should be taken and treatment with topical or systemic antibiotics initiated. Short baths with a mild cleanser and regular application of emollients are critical.

The mother should also be educated on potential flares with vaccinations and infections, as well as with climate changes. It is important that the infant catch up on her vaccinations, but cautioning the mother about a potential flare can prevent distress.

Selected References

Bieber T, Bussman C. Atopic Dermatitis. In: Bolognia JL, Jorizzo JL, Schaffer JV, eds. *Dermatology.* Elsevier Saunders; 2012:203-217

Clayton TH, Wilkinson SM, Rawcliffe C, Pollock B, Clark SM. Allergic contact dermatitis in children: should pattern of dermatitis determine referral? A retrospective study of 500 children tested between 1995 and 2004 in one U.K. centre. *Br J Dermatol.* 2006;154(1):114–117

Eichenfield LF, Friedlander SF. Coping with chronic dermatitis. *Contemp Pediatr.* 1998;15:53–66

Gupta AK, Bluhm R, Cooper EA, Summerbell RC, Baltra R. Seborrheic dermatitis. *Dermatol Clin.* 2003;21(3):401–412

Lewkowicz D, Gottlieb AB. Pediatric psoriasis and psoriatic arthritis. *Dermatol Ther.* 2004;17(5):364–375

Nelson JS, Stone MS. Update on selected viral exanthems. *Curr Opin Pediatr.* 2000;12(4):359–364

Peterson CM, Eichenfield LF. Scabies. *Pediatr Ann.* 1996;25(2):97–100

Sidbury R, Poorsattar S. Pediatric atopic dermatitis: should we treat it differently? *Dermatol Ther.* 2006;19(2):83–90

Williams JV, Eichenfield LF, Burke BL, Barnes-Eley M, Friedlander SF. Prevalence of scalp scaling in prepubertal children. *Pediatrics.* 2005;115(1):e1–e6

CHAPTER 126

Morbilliform Rashes

Kathy K. Langevin, MD, MPH, and Noah Craft, MD, PhD

CASE STUDY

A 10-month-old girl is brought to the office with a history of rhinorrhea, cough, and fever for 3 days prior to the onset of a confluent, erythematous rash. The rash started on her face. She has been irritable, and her eyes are red and teary. Her immunizations include 3 sets of diphtheria, tetanus, and acellular pertussis; polio; rotavirus; *Haemophilus influenzae* type b; conjugated pneumococcal; and hepatitis B vaccines. No one at home is ill. The girl was seen in the emergency department 2 weeks earlier because she caught her finger in a car door. On physical examination, the girl's temperature is 102.2°F (39°C). A confluent eruption of erythematous macules and papules is evident on the face, trunk, and extremities. Rhinorrhea and conjunctivitis are also present.

Questions

1. What are the common causes of febrile macular/papular or morbilliform rashes in children?
2. What features distinguish one disease from another?
3. How does a child's nutritional status affect his or her reaction to certain exanthem-inducing viruses?
4. What are the public health considerations concerning viral exanthems in children?

Exanthems are skin findings resulting from an underlying disease, most often caused by a viral infection. In children, these exanthems are most commonly macular, papular, or mixed. The rash of measles is described as morbilliform, and this adjective is used to describe similar-appearing eruptions of macules and papules. Frequently, these rashes are seen in conjunction with fever, and additional symptoms include myalgia, rhinorrhea, conjunctivitis, headache, gastrointestinal (GI) complaints, and lymphadenopathy. The exanthems of various underlying viruses can also be seasonal. Although many of the common childhood illnesses of the past are now prevented by immunizations, not all segments of the population are adequately immunized. In addition, some children are not eligible for immunization because of their young age. Allergic reactions to medications, particularly antibiotics, may also result in similar eruptions and can be accompanied by symptoms of low-grade fever and pruritus. Differentiating viral exanthems from allergic reactions may be difficult in febrile children who have been empirically started on antimicrobial agents.

Epidemiology

In most children, viruses that cause exanthems produce mild disease without significant morbidity or long-term sequelae. Of greater concern to the public health is the risk of potential spread through the population. Morbilliform eruptions are a common presenting complaint, particularly in certain age groups and at certain times of the year.

Measles, also known as rubeola, is caused by an RNA virus and has markedly decreased in the United States since the live vaccine was introduced in 1963. It is transmitted by direct contact with infectious droplets or by airborne spread. In temperate climates, it is most frequently seen in the winter and spring. In the pre-vaccine era, measles was a significant cause of morbidity and mortality. Periodic resurgences have occurred, particularly among unimmunized preschoolers, older adolescents, and young adults. In addition, young infants are also at risk because of decreased levels of passively transferred maternal immunity related to lack of maternal natural infection or immunization. Vaccine-related immunity apparently wanes more rapidly in mothers than does naturally acquired immunity. Because of the increased number of cases in preschoolers and children with primary vaccine failure who received the vaccine appropriately, a 2-dose recommendation by the American Academy of Pediatrics was implemented in 1989, although there continue to be cases each year. Measles is no longer endemic in the United States but continues to be imported. The incubation period of measles is about 10 days. Individuals are infectious from about 3 to 5 days before the onset of rash until 4 days following its appearance.

Rubella is also caused by an RNA virus and is no longer considered endemic in the United States, with rare cases reported annually. Sporadic outbreaks are reported, generally in foreign-born or under-immunized persons, and the last confirmed endemic case in the Americas was diagnosed in Argentina in 2009. However, about 5% to 10% of US individuals older than 5 years are considered to be susceptible. Peak incidence is in the late winter to spring, and it is likely transmitted via direct or droplet contact from nasopharyngeal secretions. Though generally a mild disease, its most serious manifestation is congenital rubella syndrome, which may develop in the offspring of infected pregnant women, with the greatest risk of congenital defects during the first trimester. The incubation period is 14 to 23 days.

Erythema infectiosum, also called fifth disease, is most commonly seen in school-aged children during late winter to early spring. Most adults have antibodies indicating previous infection. The disease is caused by an acute infection with parvovirus B19, a DNA virus, and spread through respiratory secretions, percutaneous exposure to blood or blood products, and vertical transmission from mother to fetus. The incubation period is generally 4 to 14 days but may be up to 21 days.

Exanthem subitum, also known as roseola infantum, generally affects children from 6 months to 2 years of age, as maternal antibodies are protective until the age of 6 months. The illness is due to infection with human herpesvirus (HHV) 6 or 7, although HHV-6b, a DNA virus, is most commonly the etiologic agent. The virus is shed in the saliva, even among healthy, previously infected individuals. Almost all children are seropositive for HHV-6b by the age of 4. Reactivation is possible, though not common, and there is no seasonal pattern. The incubation period for HHV-6 is likely 5 to 15 days and is unknown for HHV-7.

Enteroviruses are the most common cause of exanthems in the summer and fall. They are all RNA viruses of the picornavirus group and include coxsackieviruses (groups A and B), echoviruses, and enteroviruses. Infection is spread through fecal-oral and respiratory routes as well as via fomites. There is also vertical transmission. Infection is more common in young children and people with poor hygiene. The incubation period is usually 3 to 6 days.

Kawasaki disease, an acute self-limited vasculitis, is of uncertain etiology, although an infectious cause is suspected due to epidemics occurring usually in the winter and spring. Most patients are between 6 months and 5 years of age. Males outnumber females by a ratio of 1.5:1. The incidence of the disorder among Asians is higher than in other populations, suggesting genetic factors play a role. Incubation period is unknown.

Gianotti-Crosti syndrome, also known as papular acrodermatitis of childhood, has historically been associated with hepatitis B infection. In the United States, it is believed to be a host response to multiple viral infections including, but not limited to, hepatitis B, Epstein-Barr virus (EBV), parvovirus B19, HHV-6, and the enteroviruses. It is seen most frequently in children 1 to 6 years of age.

Scarlet fever is a cutaneous reaction to several pyrogenic exotoxins produced by group A streptococcus (GAS). It is transmitted through respiratory secretions. Scarlet fever is usually seen in young children between 1 to 10 years with pharyngitis. It occurs most commonly in cooler climates during the late fall, winter, and early spring. The incubation period is 2 to 5 days.

Rocky Mountain spotted fever (RMSF) is caused by *Rickettsia rickettsii*, an intracellular organism. Infection is transmitted by the bite of *Ixodes* ticks, which are reservoirs and vectors of the organism. It can be seen throughout the United States, with most cases seen in the southern states. Children of any age are at risk, with those 5 to 9 years of age and those not recalling a tick bite, an occurrence

in about half of pediatric cases, having the greatest mortality. Highest incidence of infection is seen between April and September. The incubation period lasts from 2 to 14 days.

Clinical Presentation

Morbilliform eruptions may involve the face, trunk, or extremities. The eruption is usually erythematous, and the lesions are flat or slightly raised. Occasionally, lesions within the mouth, referred to as enanthema, are evident. Most children are febrile (D_x Box) and may have other symptomatic complaints.

Pathophysiology

The mechanism for development of a rash is variable. In some cases, the rash is the reaction of the body to infection or to the presence of a toxin. In general, the sequence involves exposure to an infectious agent and then acquisition of the agent, most commonly through droplet infection or fecal-oral contamination. The agent, usually a virus, then replicates, perhaps in the reticuloendothelial system. Lymph nodes enlarge, reflecting the involvement of the reticuloendothelial system. Associated viremia may be present.

In Kawasaki disease, vasculitis affects multiple organ systems. Various cytokines and autoantibodies play a role in the inflammatory response. In a toxin-mediated rash (eg, scarlet fever), previous exposure to the toxin is believed to sensitize the individual.

Differential Diagnosis

While many exanthems can be easily recognized clinically, the decreased frequency of many of these usual childhood diseases means that physicians encounter these conditions less frequently than in the past. Familiarity with the appearance of these conditions is critical to diagnosis. The Internet can be valuable by providing access to images of many dermatologic conditions. Some sites such, as VisualDx (accessible at www.visualdx.com), display pictorial representations and allow for searching by features such as rash morphologies, symptoms, exposures, skin color, body location, age, immune status, and many other factors.

Morbilliform exanthems are associated with several infectious diseases, such as measles, rubella, erythema infectiosum, roseola, enterovirus infections, Gianotti-Crosti syndrome, Kawasaki disease, scarlet fever, and RMSF. Drugs can also cause eruptions similar to those caused by the aforementioned diseases.

Dx Morbilliform Rashes

- Macular, papular, or combined rash
- Fever
- Enanthema (lesions in the mouth)
- Lymphadenopathy
- Respiratory symptoms
- Gastrointestinal symptoms

The rash associated with **measles** is preceded by the 3 Cs of cough, coryza, and conjunctivitis in addition to fever, which last for several days before the eruption of the exanthem. Lesions on the buccal mucosa, called Koplik spots, are well-circumscribed white-gray papules (Figure 126-1) that appear during the prodrome and resolve after 3 to 4 days. This enanthema, though rare, is pathognomonic for measles. The measles rash itself usually begins on the head, particularly behind the ears and around the margin of the scalp, then spreads cephalocaudally. After 2 to 3 days, the eruption becomes confluent and copper-colored, fades in the order it appeared, and then may desquamate. The greatest morbidity and mortality are seen in immunocompromised and malnourished individuals. Complications include secondary bacterial infection, pneumonia and encephalitis.

Rubella produces a relatively minor illness in children, although adults, particularly women, may experience painful arthritis. Up to half of infections are asymptomatic. There can be a prodrome of fever, headache, conjunctivitis, and upper respiratory symptoms. The eruption consists of fine erythematous macules and papules that become near confluent, starting on the face and progressing caudally to the trunk, resolving after 3 days. Lymphadenopathy, particularly of the postauricular or suboccipital nodes, is characteristic of the disease. Forschheimer spots are pinpoint rose-colored macules that can develop on the soft palate in patients with this infection. Congenital rubella syndrome results in multisystem anomalies that can follow maternal infection and is part of the TORCH congenital infections (*t*oxoplasmosis, *o*ther agents [hepatitis B, coxsackievirus, syphilis, varicella-zoster virus, HIV, parvovirus B19], *r*ubella, *c*ytomegalovirus, *h*erpes simplex).

Erythema infectiosum (EI) is characterized by a distinctive eruption that may be preceded by mild prodromal symptoms including low-grade fever, headache, myalgia, and malaise.

Eruption generally occurs 7 to 10 days after the prodrome. The facial rash consists of erythematous patches on the cheeks with sparing of the nasal bridge and periorbital areas. This "slapped-cheek" appearance generally fades after several days and is considered the first stage of the illness. In the second stage, the extremities may develop a lacy reticulated rash of macules and papules 1 to 4 days later that can be pruritic. Palm and sole involvement is rare. This usually lasts about a week but may have recurrences over several weeks in the third stage, with triggers such as activity, sunlight, emotional stress, and hot baths. Most children are only mildly ill and may attend school, but children with underlying hematologic disorders may experience aplastic crises because of the affinity of parvovirus B19 for developing red blood cells. Immunocompromised children are also at risk for chronic anemia. Pregnant females may transmit this infection to their fetuses, which can result in fetal hydrops, growth retardation, anemia, isolated pleural and pericardial effusions, high-output congestive failure, and fetal loss. Adults with parvovirus infection frequently develop arthritis, although only 10% of children experience this symptom. Neurologic disturbances including encephalitis and neuropathies may follow parvovirus infection, though this is rare. **Papular-purpuric gloves-and-socks syndrome (PPGSS)** is a self-limited acute eruption linked to parvovirus B19 infection. It occurs usually in the spring and summer, characterized by often-pruritic edema and erythema and progressing to purpuric macules and papules with a sharp line of demarcation at the wrists and ankles. A nonspecific enanthema of petechiae and erosions can occur. Symptoms of myalgia, lymphadenopathy, anorexia, and fatigue may follow the rash. The exanthem generally resolves after 1 to 2 weeks with no residual sequelae.

Exanthem subitum (roseola infantum) usually causes a fairly mild illness in children, although there can be associated complications. Defervescence usually accompanies the rash, which consists of fine, non-pruritic, blanchable, pink macules or papules with a surrounding halo that generally appear first on the trunk and then spread centrifugally. Some may develop an enanthema consisting of erythematous papules on the soft palate and uvula called Nagayama spots. Periorbital edema can also be seen. On average, the rash evolves over 12 hours and usually resolves by 2 days. Infants may appear sickest during the prodromal phase, when fever is high (temperature often ≥103°F [39.5°C]), and infants are irritable as a result. Fever generally lasts 3 to 5 days and can be accompanied by upper respiratory symptoms and lymphadenopathy. Seizures during the febrile period can occur in up to 15% of primary infections. Workup to rule out sepsis is often warranted.

Skin eruptions associated with **enterovirus infections** are highly variable. They may be distinct and characteristic, such as hand-foot-and-mouth disease, most commonly associated with coxsackievirus A16 and enterovirus 71 (see Chapter 127). However, many of the enteroviral exanthems are less distinctive and have a generalized morbilliform appearance. Neurologic complications associated with enteroviral infections include aseptic meningitis and encephalitis and have been reported in infections with coxsackievirus B and enterovirus 71. Other systems affected by enteroviral infections

Figure 126-1. Koplik spots.

include respiratory, GI, ophthalmic, and cardiac. In a 2011–2012 North American outbreak due to coxsackievirus A6, affected individuals had distinctive skin findings mimicking eczema herpeticum (discussed in Chapter 127), as well as Gianotti-Crosti syndrome–like rash and petechial or purpuric eruptions.

The rash of **Kawasaki disease** is also highly variable; it may be morbilliform, urticarial, or scarlatiniform or resemble erythema multiforme. During the first week of illness, there may be desquamation of the perineum. The diagnosis of Kawasaki disease requires fever (generally temperature >39°C [lasting at least 5 days]) and 4 out of the following 5 following findings: bilateral non-purulent conjunctivitis; changes in the oropharyngeal mucosa including fissured lips, oral erythema, and strawberry tongue; changes in the extremities such as erythema/edema or desquamation; cervical lymphadenopathy with one node measuring at least 1.5 cm in diameter; and the exanthem described previously. Irritability, arthralgia, abdominal pain, and diarrhea are not uncommon. Incomplete Kawasaki disease can be diagnosed when only 2 of the additional criteria are met; thus, the practitioner should consider this diagnosis when persistent high fever and only 2 or 3 of these symptoms are present. The major complication of Kawasaki disease is coronary artery abnormalities, and males and those younger than 12 months are at increased risk.

The exanthem of **Gianotti-Crosti syndrome** consists of monomorphic, pink- to skin-colored, usually non-pruritic papules on the face, buttocks, and extremities, with sparing of the trunk. There is often a prodrome of fever and upper respiratory symptoms with associated generalized lymphadenopathy and hepatosplenomegaly. The exanthem fades after 2 to 3 weeks but can last up to several months.

Scarlet fever is primarily a disease of childhood. Onset is marked by sudden high fever, headache, vomiting, malaise, and sore throat. Within 12 to 48 hours, erythema develops on the neck, chest, and axillae. The rash quickly becomes generalized to a sandpaper-like rash of fine red papules on an erythematous background. Linear accentuation in the axillary, antecubital, and inguinal folds is known as Pastia lines. The face is flushed, except around the mouth (circumoral pallor). There is pharyngeal injection with exudate developing after a few days. The tongue is initially white with prominent red papillae (Figure 126-2), known as strawberry tongue. As the scarlet fever rash resolves, desquamation begins in 7 to 10 days, lasting up to 6 weeks.

The rash of **RMSF** begins as blanchable pink macules or papules that evolve into petechial or purpuric non-blanching lesions. They begin on the wrists and spread centripetally. The palms and soles are almost always involved. Exanthem is preceded by symptoms of fever, headache, and malaise. Gastrointestinal symptoms such as nausea, vomiting, and diarrhea can be present. The rash generally develops 2 to 3 days after the prodrome.

Morbilliform rashes are the most common type of cutaneous **drug eruption.** The most common culprits include sulfonamides, penicillins, cephalosporins, and anticonvulsants. They generally begin as erythematous macules and papules on the trunk that spread to the extremities symmetrically. There is usually concurrent

Figure 126-2. Strawberry tongue.

eosinophilia. Pruritus and low-grade fever can also be present, often confounding the diagnosis. Although most drug rashes begin 1 to 2 weeks after starting a drug, an eruption may develop after a drug has been discontinued. After stopping the offending medication, the rash usually resolves over 1 to 2 weeks, but some show improvement even if the offending medication is continued. The underlying pathogenesis of many of these drug rashes continues to be unclear; however, recent studies found that levels of a soluble fatty acid synthetase ligand were increased in patients with drug-induced morbilliform eruptions, as well as in those with toxic epidermal necrolysis, but negative in those with viral exanthems.

Infection with **EBV** is associated with rash in young children and in adolescents on antibiotics, usually ampicillin or amoxicillin. Eruption is morbilliform, and the lesions may be erythematous or copper-colored. Fever, upper respiratory symptoms, lymphadenopathy, hepatosplenomegaly, and facial and peripheral edema, including unilateral periorbital edema, may be noted. The rash is likely due to an immunologic interaction between the infectious agent and the drug.

Evaluation

History

A thorough history should be obtained (Questions Box).

Physical Examination

The focus of the physical examination is to help define the characteristics of the eruption such as location, extent, and degree of coalescence. The presence of any associated physical findings, such as fever, lymphadenopathy, enanthema, desquamation, rhinorrhea, conjunctivitis, organomegaly, or central nervous system (CNS) symptomatology, should be determined.

Morbilliform Rashes — **Questions**

- What does the rash look like? Has a similar rash occurred before?
- What symptoms, if any, are associated with the rash or occurred before the onset of rash?
- How long has the child had these symptoms?
- Is the child taking any medications (antibiotics)?
- Does the child have any ill contacts?
- What is the child's immunization status?

Laboratory Tests

Laboratory assessment may be helpful in certain conditions, although most of these diagnoses are made clinically. Serologic testing is most valuable for defining a community outbreak of a specific disease such as measles. In most viral exanthems, the results of serologic studies are not available until the condition has resolved and the patient has recovered. Tests may include acute and convalescent titers for specific viruses. Alternatively, immunoglobulin M levels of antibodies against certain infections may be used to document that the infection was recent. Repeat testing may be needed for partially immunized individuals. Polymerase chain reaction may also be useful. Isolating the virus can confirm the diagnosis but is often difficult to obtain. Because neutropenia and lymphocytosis characterize many viral illnesses, such findings are not helpful in differentiating specific causal agents. Lymphocytosis, with characteristically atypical lymphocytes, distinguishes EBV infection. Although a heterophil antibody test is usually positive in older children and adolescents, it may be nonreactive in young children, where infection is documented by specific EBV serology.

Pregnant women with suspected parvovirus B19 infection should have IgM and IgG levels drawn. If infection is confirmed, serial ultrasounds should be performed to monitor for symptoms of hydrops fetalis. Confirming diagnosis of rubella in a pregnant woman is also important because of the potential risk of congenital rubella syndrome.

Kawasaki disease is associated with elevation in markers of inflammation, including leukocytosis, thrombocytosis, elevated erythrocyte sedimentation rate, and C-reactive protein, though no test is diagnostic. Sterile pyuria is noted in 70% of the cases. Scarlet fever is characterized by leukocytosis. Eosinophilia can also be seen after a few weeks in up to 20% of patients. Laboratory confirmation, via rapid streptococcal test or throat culture, should be done to confirm that the pharyngitis is due to GAS, not a virus. If pharyngitis has resolved, serologic studies such as antistreptolysin O provide evidence of the recent infection.

A 4-fold or greater change in titer between acute and convalescent serum as determined by indirect immunofluorescent antibody assay is diagnostic for RMSF. Many patients will have thrombocytopenia, leukopenia, anemia, and hyponatremia. In general, any child presenting with headache, fever, and possible exposure to tick bite should be evaluated for this disease.

Imaging Studies

An echocardiogram to check for evidence of coronary artery aneurysm is a mandated part of the evaluation in Kawasaki disease during the acute phase and with serial repeat examinations, more frequently and earlier in those at high risk.

Management

Management of most viral exanthems is supportive and symptomatic. Hydration is critical because GI complaints of diarrhea are often associated. Antihistamines should be used for symptoms of pruritus in addition to regular use of emollients. Painful oral lesions can be treated with topical analgesics. In cases in which complications such as encephalitis or pneumonia develop, hospitalization is indicated. Spread of infection, such as measles, to susceptible contacts can be reduced through the use of vaccine within 72 hours of exposure or immunoglobulin within 6 days. Measles vaccine should be administered after the immunoglobulin in children who have been exposed, with the time interval dependent on dose received and age of the child. The measles, mumps, rubella vaccine is administered for the 2-dose vaccine series to children at 12 to 15 months of age and again at 4 to 6 years. Measles, mumps, rubella, varicella (MMRV) is available for children 12 months to 12 years of age in the United States, although there is greater risk for febrile seizures with MMRV vaccine. HIV infection is not a contraindication to measles vaccination, unless severely immunocompromised, but MMRV should not be administered to these individuals. Currently, administration of vitamin A is recommended to all children with measles regardless of their country of residence. Antibiotic therapy should be initiated if bacterial coinfection is suspected but should not be started empirically. The management of Kawasaki disease includes the administration of intravenous immunoglobulin (IVIG) and aspirin, which should be started within 10 days of onset of fever. The current recommendation is to administer a single dose at 2 g/kg given as an infusion over 10 to 12 hours. Periodic echocardiograms are also required in these patients with close monitoring by a cardiologist.

If there is a concern for hepatitis in patients with Gianotti-Crosti syndrome, workup should be initiated.

Control measures are important because most morbilliform exanthems are due to infectious agents. Children with postnatal rubella should be kept from school or child care facilities for 1 week after onset of rash. Those with congenital rubella syndrome are considered contagious for 1 year, and caregivers must be educated. Females receiving rubella vaccine should not become pregnant for 28 days following vaccination. Hand hygiene is an important control measure that should be used to minimize spread of many of these viruses.

Vigilant education about the importance of immunizations is vital to reducing the effect of diseases such as measles and rubella. Although the number of cases in the United States is low, importation of these viruses from other countries mandates continued widespread vaccination. In addition, parental concerns of potential adverse reactions due to vaccinations have led to vaccine refusal by some.

Pregnant women infected with parvovirus B19 with ultrasound suggestive of hydrops fetalis should be referred to a tertiary care facility because intrauterine blood transfusions have proven successful. Routine exclusion of pregnant women from the workplace where erythema infectiosum has been identified is not recommended because the virus is transmitted before the onset of rash and, thus, exclusion is unlikely to be effective. Patients with aplastic crisis and chronic parvovirus infection may be contagious for extended periods and require longer periods of precautions. In addition, patients with PPGSS are considered infectious when clinical symptoms of their eruption are present. Patients with aplastic crises may need transfusions, and IVIG has been used successfully in immunocompromised patients with chronic infection. However, most cases of EI do not require absence from school or treatment beyond supportive care.

Intravenous immunoglobulin and high-dose aspirin continue to be first-line treatment to decrease the risk of coronary artery aneurysms in patients with Kawasaki disease. Aspirin should be continued indefinitely in patients in whom coronary abnormalities do develop.

The goal of therapy in scarlet fever is to prevent acute rheumatic fever by initiating antibiotics within 9 days from the onset of symptoms. It is unclear if treatment can prevent the onset of poststreptococcal glomerulonephritis.

Treatment with doxycycline is the drug of choice in patients of any age for infection with *R rickettsia* and should be started as soon as RMSF is suspected. Penicillin is the drug of choice. Erythromycin can be used in patients allergic to penicillin.

Prognosis

The prognosis for most morbilliform rashes of childhood is generally good, with full resolution of symptoms unless children are very young, have congenital disease, have an underlying condition, or develop long-term complications. In some young infants, viruses that cause exanthems may produce severe complications such as pneumonia and encephalitis. Subacute sclerosing panencephalitis is a late-onset, rare, and serious degenerative CNS disease that occurs as a complication of wild-type measles infection. Some patients with roseola may develop chronic neurologic sequelae, but most cases are benign. The prognosis for Kawasaki disease is usually favorable with appropriate management. Up to 25% of untreated children and a fraction of those who have been treated may develop coronary artery aneurysms, sometimes with symptoms remaining silent for years, thus requiring vigilance during the acute phase. Kawasaki disease is the leading cause of acquired heart disease in children in the United States. In patients with severe infection with RMSF, long-term neurologic complications can be seen.

CASE RESOLUTION

The infant in the case study has the classic symptoms of measles. Normally such a young infant would not yet have received immunization against measles because the first dose is administered at 12 to 15 months of age with the second dose at 4 to 6 years of age. Immunoglobulin will likely not modify the disease in this patient because her rash is near confluent, suggesting exposure more than 6 days ago. She should be evaluated for evidence of complications, including pneumonia. Unimmunized household contacts, as well as pregnant women and other contacts younger than 1 year, should receive immunoglobulin. Treatment is supportive.

Selected References

American Academy of Pediatrics. *Red Book: 2012 Report of the Committee on Infectious Diseases.* 29th ed. Pickering LK, Baker CJ, Kimberlin DW, Long SS, eds. Elk Grove Village, IL: American Academy of Pediatrics; 2012

Gerding R. Kawasaki disease: a review. *J Pediatr Health Care.* 2011;25(6): 379–387

Mathes EF, Oza V, Frieden IJ, et al. "Eczema coxsackium" and unusual cutaneous findings in a enterovirus outbreak. *Pediatrics.* 2013;132(1):e149–e157

McLean HQ, Fiebelkorn AP, Temte JL, Wallace GS; Centers for Disease Control and Prevention. Prevention of measles, rubella, congenital rubella syndrome, and mumps, 2103: summary recommendations of the Advisory Committee on Immunization Practices (ACIP). *MMWR Recomm Rep.* 2013;62(RR-04):1–34

Meissner HC, Strebel PM, Orenstein WA. Measles vaccines and the potential for worldwide eradication of measles. *Pediatrics.* 2004;114(4):1065–1069

Paller AS, Mancini AJ, eds. *Hurwitz Clinical Pediatric Dermatology.* 4th ed. Edinburgh, Scotland: Elsevier Saunders; 2011

Pinna GS, Kafetzis DA, Tselkas OI, Skevaki CL. Kawasaki disease: an overview. *Curr Opin Infect Dis.* 2008;21(3):263–270

Romano A, Demoly P. Recent advances in the diagnosis of drug allergy. *Curr Opin Allergy Clin Immunol.* 2007;7(4):299–303

Stur K, Karlhofer FM, Stingl G. Soluble FAS ligand: a discriminating feature between drug-induced skin eruptions and viral exanthemas. *J Invest Dermatol.* 2007;127(4):802–807

CHAPTER 127

Vesicular Exanthems

Kathy K. Langevin, MD, MPH, and Noah Craft, MD, PhD

CASE STUDY

A 2-year-old boy is evaluated for a 2-day history of fever (temperature: 103.1°F [39.5°C]), runny nose, decreased appetite, and a rash over the abdomen. The boy has had no previous known exposures to chickenpox (varicella) and no history of varicella vaccination. He attends child care daily. No one at home is ill. The boy is currently taking no medications except for acetaminophen for fever, and he has no history of dermatologic problems. On physical examination, the heart rate is 120 beats/min, the respiratory rate is 20 breaths/min, and the temperature is 100.4°F (38.0°C). The toddler's overall appearance is nontoxic. The skin examination is significant for a few scattered erythematous vesicular lesions over the abdomen and one erythematous papule on the back. The rest of the examination is normal.

Questions

1. What are the most likely causes of vesicular exanthems in febrile children?
2. How can types of vesicular rashes be differentiated on the basis of patient history?
3. What are the key historical questions to ask?
4. What is the natural course of varicella?
5. What treatment options are available for children with varicella? What options are available for other vesicular exanthems?

Exanthems are generalized, erythematous rashes that are caused by an underlying disease. They are most frequently caused by viral or bacterial infections, though they can also be caused by noninfectious etiologies. Infectious eruptions are most commonly morbilliform in the pediatric population, but they can have variable manifestations, including vesicular, bullous, petechial, and purpuric eruptions. Vesicles are elevated, fluid-filled lesions that measure 1 cm or less in diameter. Bullae are quite similar, only larger in size. Vesicles often lose their initial morphology quickly because they can break spontaneously or coalesce into bullae. They can arise de novo or from macules or papules. Vesicles may be discrete, grouped, generalized, or linear, depending on their etiology, and their specific distribution is often helpful in formulating a differential diagnosis.

Epidemiology

Epidemiologic factors can help differentiate infectious from noninfectious etiologies. Patient age, season of the year, presence or absence of similar cases in the community, and regular attendance at child care or school, which may contribute to exposure, should all be considered. Gender and ethnicity are usually less informative but can help distinguish certain diseases causing exanthems.

Primary human herpesvirus 3, also called varicella-zoster virus, or chickenpox, is one of the most common vesicular exanthems seen in childhood. Males and females are equally affected. Most reported cases in the pre-vaccine era were in children younger than 10 years. Since universal vaccination has been implemented, children aged 10 to 14 years are becoming the group with the greatest incidence of infection, though still less than during the pre-vaccine period. It is primarily transmitted person to person by airborne spread of aerosolized viral particles from vesicles of infected persons. It may also be transmitted through respiratory secretions and vertically from mother to fetus. It is extremely infectious, with almost all susceptible household contacts becoming infected. The incubation period ranges from 10 to 21 days (usually 14–16) after exposure but can be longer if varicella-zoster immune globulin is administered. Neonates born to mothers with active infection around the time of delivery can develop varicella 2 to 16 days after birth. Patients are considered contagious from 1 to 2 days before onset of cutaneous lesions until all are crusted over.

Human herpesvirus 1 and 2, also called herpes simplex virus, is a DNA virus, with human herpesvirus 1 and 2 affecting most adults worldwide. Historically, human herpesvirus 1 infections generally occurred outside the genital area and human herpesvirus 2 within the anogenital area. Now, either virus can be found in both areas. Neonatal infection is generally acquired at delivery from an infected mother who is often unaware of her infection. Herpes herpesvirus 1 is typically transmitted by direct contact with oral secretions or lesions and human herpesvirus 2 from direct contact with infected genital secretions. Shedding of viral particles can occur in the absence of active infection. The incubation for human herpesvirus infection beyond the neonatal period is 2 days to 2 weeks. Most affected neonates will have signs of clinical infection in the first month of life.

Hand-foot-and-mouth disease and herpangina are caused by enteroviral infections. Hand-foot-and-mouth disease is most commonly caused by infection with coxsackievirus A16 or enterovirus 71. These enteroviral infections occur most commonly in summer and early fall. The usual incubation period for most enteroviruses is between 3 to 6 days.

Bullous impetigo is a less common form of impetigo than the non-bullous forms. Bullous impetigo is most frequently seen in the summer and is transmitted by direct person-to-person contact, possibly via fomites as well. It is usually caused by *Staphylococcus aureus* and is a localized reaction to exfoliative toxin released by the bacteria. It affects mostly neonates, infants, and younger children.

Infections caused by scabies or fungi can cause vesicular eruptions as well. Scabies is transmitted during prolonged close contact with an infested individual. Scabies has an incubation period of 4 to 6 weeks in patients without previous exposure. Reexposed patients develop symptoms a few days after repeat exposure. Tinea pedis is a common infection worldwide, though less so in children. It is acquired via contact with infected skin scales and in damp areas where the fungi reside. Tinea capitis, a common fungal infection in children (see Chapter 123), does not result in a vesicular rash, but like tinea pedis, can result in a dermatophytid or id reaction that is vesicular. The incubation period of fungal infections is unknown.

Dyshidrotic eczema is a disease that can occur in children with chronic eczematous dermatitis or atopic dermatitis but can occur in non-atopic children as well. Rhus dermatitis is the prototypical allergic contact dermatitis, which develops about 1 to 3 days after exposure to plants such as poison ivy, poison oak, and poison sumac. Linear papules and vesicles are seen at points of contact between the plant antigen and the skin.

Clinical Presentation

Vesicular exanthems are eruptions of distinctive lesions that are raised and fluid-filled (D_x Box). They may be located anywhere on the child's body and, depending on the etiology, may or may not be pruritic. Other symptoms that may accompany such rashes include fever, upper respiratory symptoms, and gastrointestinal and central nervous system (CNS) involvement.

Pathophysiology

Vesicles and bullae arise from a cleavage at various levels of the skin within the epidermis (intraepidermal) or at the epidermal-dermal junction (subepidermal). Sometimes the 2 types of lesions can be differentiated based on the amount of pressure required to collapse the lesion, especially if the lesion is a large bulla. In addition, the thickness of the wall of a bulla can be estimated by its translucency or flaccidity. A biopsy of the lesion, however, is the only way to

reliably differentiate between the 2 areas of separation, though this will not necessarily provide the diagnosis. Specific changes occur in the epidermis depending on the etiology of the vesicular exanthem. For example, with certain viral infections such as human herpesvirus, varicella, and herpes zoster, a "ballooning degeneration" of epidermal cells occurs.

In bullous impetigo, the vesicles and bullae are caused by staphylococcal exfoliative toxin, which cause the keratinocytes in the granular layer of the epidermis to split apart. There are no bacteria seen within the blister cavity and a few inflammatory cells can be present.

The rash caused by scabies infestation is the result of a hypersensitivity reaction to the proteins of the parasite. In vesicular lesions, there is spongiosis, or intercellular edema, in the epidermis caused by the mite, which can result in a vesicle. Spongiosis also leads to vesicle formation in dyshidrotic eczema (pompholyx), though the pathogenesis of this disease is not known. *Dyshidrotic* is a misnomer because this disease is not related to sweat gland dysfunction or occlusion. Spongiosis is also present in id reactions and allergic contact dermatitis.

Differential Diagnosis

While many vesicular eruptions are easily distinguishable clinically, the differential diagnosis can be challenging at times. Familiarity with the appearance of these conditions and their differentiating features is critical. The Internet can be valuable by providing access to images of many dermatologic conditions. Some sites, such as VisualDx (www.visualdx.com), display pictorial representations and allow for searching by features such as rash morphology, symptoms, exposures, skin color, body location, age, immune status, and many other factors.

Primary human herpesvirus 3 infection (chickenpox) usually consists of hundreds of vesicles, existing in various stages of resolution. Lesions progress from erythematous macules and papules to vesicles and, eventually, to pustules that then crust and heal normally without scarring unless secondarily infected and deeply inflamed. Characteristically, the vesicle has been described as a "dewdrop on a rose petal." Associated prodrome includes malaise and mild fever and is usually present. Symptoms tend to be more severe in infants and older patients. Since universal vaccine implementation, breakthrough cases have become more common and have a milder clinical presentation. Fetal infection during the first or early second trimester can result in fetal demise or in congenital varicella syndrome, consisting of limb hypoplasia, cutaneous scarring, ophthalmic abnormalities, and CNS defects. Infection acquired from 5 days antepartum to 2 days postpartum can also be fatal because of the absence of protective maternal antibodies. Bullous varicella can result when *S aureus* infects the vesicles of chickenpox, with greater chance for scarring.

Herpes zoster, a reactivation of a latent infection with human herpesvirus 3, can also cause a vesicular rash. The virus, which rests dormant in neuronal cells, travels along the nerves when reactivated

Dx **Vesicular Exanthems**

- Raised, fluid-filled vesicles on the skin
- Lesions may be pruritic
- Possible associated fever, upper respiratory infection symptoms, myalgia
- History of affected contacts
- Lesions on mucous membranes

and becomes released into the skin. It is generally a disease of older people, though children can be affected. In zoster, the lesions are grouped unilaterally in the distribution of 1 to 3 sensory dermatomes. It can be quite painful, and postherpetic neuralgia can last for months. In immunocompromised patients, the rash of zoster can become disseminated.

Disseminated, CNS, or SEM (skin, eyes, and/or mouth) human herpesvirus infection in an infant is usually caused by human herpesvirus 2, very severe, and often accompanied by skin findings. In children and adolescents, human herpesvirus 1 gingivostomatitis and perioral vesicles are the most common clinical findings and can also be asymptomatic. A prodrome of paresthesia with recurrent infection is not uncommon. There can also be an ulcerative enanthema. Human herpesvirus 1 and 2 persist for life in the sensory ganglia and, when reactivated, result in single or grouped vesicles, often on the vermilion border with an erythematous base. Triggers include stress, ultraviolet exposure, and fever.

Hand-foot-and-mouth disease is associated with a brief, mild prodrome of fever, malaise, and mouth pain. The exanthem consists of erythematous macules and papules with a central gray vesicle. Generally, the volar surfaces of the hands and feet, as well as the buttocks, tend to be involved. In a recent North American 2011–2012 epidemic, infection with coxsackievirus A6 resulted in hand-foot-and-mouth disease with more extensive areas of cutaneous involvement, more protean morphologies, as well as localization to areas of active dermatitis, termed "eczema coxsackium." The concomitant enanthema is seen on the tongue, buccal mucosa, palate, uvula, and anterior tonsillar pillars. In herpangina, patients acutely develop fever, malaise, headache, and neck pain. There is a painful enanthema of small grayish-white vesicles on the soft palate, uvula, buccal mucosa, pharynx, and tonsils. These ulcerate with a surrounding red halo.

Impetigo is the most common bacterial skin infection in children. In bullous impetigo, there can be associated fever, weakness, and diarrhea, though there are often no systemic symptoms. Small vesicles enlarge rapidly into flaccid bullae that easily rupture. These lesions can be generalized and can arise from normal-appearing skin.

Parasites such as the tiny mite *Sarcoptes scabiei* can cause an intensely pruritic, generally papular eruption, though vesicular lesions can occur. Commonly, secondary excoriations are seen (see Chapter 125). In older children and adults, interdigital folds, flexor wrists, waistline, trunk, and genital area are more commonly affected. A linear burrow is pathognomonic but often difficult to identify clinically. Patients younger than 2 years have involvement predominantly of the head, neck, palms, and soles. In this age group, the eruption is more likely to be vesicular (Box 127-1). Arthropod bites can also result in isolated and scattered vesicles.

Fungal pathogens that cause tinea pedis include *Trichophyton rubrum, Trichophyton mentagrophytes, Trichophyton tonsurans,* and *Epidermophyton floccosum*. Infection can directly cause a scaly or vesicular rash or can result in a hypersensitivity reaction to the fungi, presenting as vesicles on the palms, soles, sides of the fingers, and occasionally on the extremities and trunk. *T mentagrophytes* can

---

Box 127-1. Common Causes of Acute Vesicular Exanthems

Infectious

Viral
- Human herpesvirus 3
- Human herpesvirus 1 and 2
- Enterovirus

Bacterial
- *Staphylococcus aureus*

Fungal
- *Trichophyton rubrum*
- *Trichophyton mentagrophytes*
- *Trichophyton tonsurans*
- *Microsporum canis*
- *Epidermophyton floccosum*

Infestations
- Scabies *(Sarcoptes scabiei)*
- Arthropod bites

Noninfectious
- Allergic contact dermatitis
- Dyshidrotic eczema
- Id reaction

---

cause vesicles and bullae on the medial foot. It can be associated with an id reaction, in which deep-seated pruritic vesicles develop secondary to tinea infection elsewhere. An id reaction, most commonly on the hands, face, and trunk, can also result from tinea capitis, usually caused by *T tonsurans* and *Microsporum canis.*

The clinical appearance of dyshidrotic eczema can be identical to that of an id reaction or fungal infection and consists of "tapioca," pearl-like, deep-seated vesicles frequently on the palms and soles as well as the lateral sides of the fingers that are extremely pruritic. Secondary impetiginization (bacterial superinfection) is common. Cases can be acute and recurrent, as well as chronic.

A delayed type 4 hypersensitivity reaction secondary to contact with plants of the genus *Toxicodendron* is a common cause of allergic contact dermatitis. The main allergen in these plants is a catechol. Rhus dermatitis causes a classic linear vesicular rash (see Chapter 125). Contact with other allergenic substances may also produce a vesicular rash and such substances include nickel, rubber compounds, fragrances, and preservatives in cosmetics.

The differential diagnosis of acute vesicular exanthems can also be organized according to the distribution of the lesions. Distinctive locations as well as specific patterns are important to consider in each individual case. The presence or absence of fever can assist in developing the appropriate differential (Figure 127-1). Epidemiologic, as well as historic, information may suggest the diagnosis. For example, known exposure to human herpesvirus 3 (chickenpox) 10 to 21 days prior to a vesicular eruption facilitates diagnosis of this disease. A history of hiking, camping, or other outdoor activities suggests possible contact with poison ivy or poison oak.

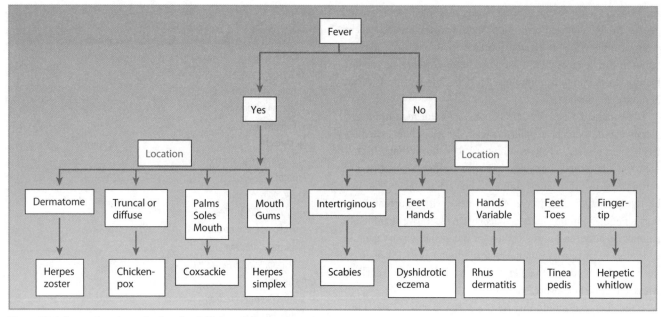

Figure 127-1. Approach to the evaluation of vesicular eruptions.

In addition, the presence of a specific prodrome can often be elicited with primary or recurrent herpes simplex. Pain on swallowing often occurs with enteroviral infection. A history of similar lesions lessens the likelihood of acute primary infection and suggests a chronic condition such as the recurrent disorder pompholyx (dyshidrotic eczema).

Evaluation

History

A thorough history should be obtained (Questions Box). Practitioners must inquire about the current state of general health, as well as the specific details about the eruption.

Questions

Vesicular Exanthems

- How long has the child had the rash? Where is it located?
- Does the child have associated symptoms such as fever, runny nose, cough, or sore throat?
- Does the child have nonspecific symptoms such as decreased appetite?
- If the child has any symptoms accompanying the rash, did these develop at the same time as the rash?
- Is there any reason to suspect that the patient is relatively immunocompromised from chronic steroid use, chemotherapy, or an acquired immunodeficiency?
- Does the child have a history of similar lesions?
- Does anyone else in the family have a similar rash?
- Has the child been camping or hiking in the woods?
- Are there pregnant contacts?

Physical Examination

Although the physical examination focuses on the skin, other aspects of the examination are helpful diagnostically. Vital signs should be taken to verify the presence or absence of fever. The oropharynx should be examined closely for any lesions on the tongue, gingiva, buccal mucosa, palate, anterior tonsillar pillars, and posterior pharynx. The lips should also be examined for any evidence of vesicular lesions that may occur with a primary or recurrent herpes simplex infection.

Patients should be completely unclothed to permit a thorough examination of the skin. The distribution of the lesions should be noted. Physicians should determine whether the vesicles are grouped in a particular dermatomal distribution, as with zoster (shingles), or more generally distributed and in various stages of development, as with varicella. A linear distribution may suggest contact with poison ivy or poison oak. Physicians should also note the following: Do the lesions include or exclude the palms and soles? Are the buttocks involved? Are the lesions concentrated on one specific part of the body, such as the feet and toes or the hands? Are the sizes of the lesions uniform? If not, are other larger bullous-like lesions present in addition to vesicles?

It is also helpful, if at all possible, to examine the skin of family members for similar lesions.

Laboratory Tests

Few, if any, laboratory studies are usually needed in healthy children with vesicular eruptions because the diagnosis is often made clinically. A Tzanck test showing multinucleated giant cells that contain intranuclear viral inclusions may be useful in making a preliminary diagnosis of herpes simplex or varicella. Direct fluorescent antibody and polymerase chain reaction are rapid and sensitive methods to diagnose varicella. Culture and polymerase chain reaction should be obtained for diagnosis of neonatal herpes simplex infection.

Definitive confirmation of scabies can be made by microscopic examination of skin scrapings from suspicious lesions. The presence of the adult mite or ova, larvae, nymphs, or feces (scybala) is diagnostic. For children with suspected tinea pedis, a skin scraping mixed with potassium hydroxide can be performed and examined under the microscope. Fungal cultures can also be taken.

Management

The mainstay of treatment for most vesicular eruptions is parent and child education as well as reassurance. For example, most varicella, herpes simplex, gingivostomatitis, hand-foot-and-mouth disease, and herpangina infections are self-limited and no treatment except parental reassurance and education on adequate hydration is necessary. These diseases can, however, be quite serious, as the recent epidemic of enterovirus 71 in Asia did result in death in severe cases. Any neonate with lesions suggestive of herpes simplex should also be worked up and treated aggressively because sequelae can be devastating. Depending on the etiology of the vesicular rash, children who are immunocompromised, such as those with HIV or AIDS, and patients who are receiving chemotherapeutic agents or systemic corticosteroids may require specific intervention.

Topical agents such as calamine lotion, oatmeal soaks, or Aveeno baths should be used in children with intense pruritus or multiple lesions. Topical products, which are potentially sensitizing (eg, diphenhydramine-containing agents) should be used cautiously and discontinued if the condition is not improving. Cool, wet compresses with plain water or aluminum acetate (Burow solution) can be quite soothing in cases of rhus dermatitis, scabies, or tinea pedis.

Antipyretics (acetaminophen) may be used to treat otherwise healthy children with varicella. Aspirin-containing medications should be avoided in children with varicella because of the association with Reye syndrome. Oral analgesics may also be indicated for symptomatic relief of pain associated with herpetic gingivostomatitis or enterovirus mouth lesions.

Oral antihistamines (diphenhydramine or hydroxyzine) may be used in children with varicella or scabies for treatment of pruritus. These drugs are also helpful in allergic contact dermatitis (rhus dermatitis) and dyshidrotic eczema. Though the sedating antihistamines are generally more effective, non-sedating antihistamines can also be used in the daytime, particularly for the more chronic dyshidrotic eczema.

Steroids may be effective in the control of some vesicular rashes; however, the practitioner must first be certain the lesions are not secondary to varicella or herpes simplex. In certain cases, steroids may be used in infectious diseases, such as eczema herpeticum, but in conjunction with antiviral therapy and under close monitoring. Topical steroids can be used for outbreaks of vesicles of dyshidrotic eczema, reserving oral steroids for severe outbreaks. In severe cases of rhus dermatitis, a course of systemic steroids, such as prednisone, 1 to 2 mg/kg/d, may be warranted and generally requires at least 2 to 3 weeks of therapy. Topical steroids can also be used to treat an id reaction, as well as treating the underlying cause of the reaction. Use of an oral histamine2 blocker such as ranitidine or famotidine can help prevent gastritis as a complication of oral prednisone.

Oral acyclovir or valacyclovir is not recommended routinely for the treatment of uncomplicated varicella in otherwise healthy children but should be considered when the risk of developing moderate to severe disease is increased. Acyclovir or valacyclovir should be considered in unvaccinated patients older than 12 years; those with chronic cutaneous or pulmonary disorders; those receiving chronic or short, intermittent courses of corticosteroids (systemic or aerosolized); or those receiving salicylates long term. It can also be considered for secondary household cases who may suffer more severe disease. Intravenous (IV) acyclovir or oral valacyclovir, initiated within 24 hours of rash development, is recommended for patients who are immunocompromised. Oral acyclovir or valacyclovir may be warranted in pregnant women with varicella in their second or third trimester, with IV acyclovir for pregnant women with more serious complications. Acyclovir is most effective if initiated within the first 24 hours of the exanthem, though the effects on symptoms may be minimal. Varicella-zoster immune globulin may help modify the course of the disease.

Additional recommendations for children with varicella include keeping fingernails short in young children to prevent superinfection of lesions from scratching. Children should drink plenty of fluids to avoid dehydration. Patients are considered contagious from 1 to 2 days prior to the onset of the rash until the lesions are all dried and crusted (usually 5–7 days after the rash develops), at which time they may return to school. In children with persistent or recurrent fever, secondary complications should be considered, such as bacterial superinfection with *S aureus* or group A beta-hemolytic *Streptococcus*. A rare association between primary varicella injection and invasive group A beta-hemolytic streptococcal infection resulting in streptococcal toxic shock syndrome and necrotizing fasciitis has been recognized.

Since 2006, the recommendation has been for 2 doses of varicella vaccine because immunity appears to wane with only one dose and sporadic outbreaks occur. Incidence of human herpesvirus 3 infection has decreased significantly since this implementation, with 98% effectiveness with 2 doses versus 86% for one in one post-licensure study. Recipients of 2 doses are less likely to have breakthrough disease or zoster.

Intravenous acyclovir is the treatment of choice for neonates with herpes simplex infection. Primary genital infections should be treated with oral acyclovir or valacyclovir. Children with recurrent, frequent (>6/y) outbreaks of herpes simplex may benefit from suppressive therapy with one of these agents. Herpetic whitlow is a herpes simplex infection on the fingertip, usually as a result of direct autoinoculation from oral or genital lesions. Treatment is not required, though it may help with pain and faster healing. Herpes gladiatorum and herpes rugbiaforum are cutaneous herpes simplex infections on the skin of wrestlers and rugby players, respectively.

While they do not require treatment with antiviral agents such as acyclovir, athletes should not be engaged in person-to-person contact when herpes lesions are present. Eczema herpeticum is a herpes simplex infection in children with underlying atopic dermatitis or other chronic skin disease that results in rapidly progressive widespread vesicles in areas of active underlying disease that then erode and crust. There can be significant fever and irritability, and severe infection may warrant hospitalization for treatment with IV acyclovir.

Localized bullous impetigo in otherwise healthy patients can be treated with topical mupirocin 2% or retapamulin 1% ointments. More widespread or complicated infections require **oral antistaphylococcal therapy** with agents such as amoxicillin and clavulanate (Augmentin), erythromycin, or cephalexin (Keflex). Recurrent disease should warrant workup for carriage and treatment if needed. Local knowledge of methicillin-resistant *S aureus* rates and bacterial cultures should be considered. For the treatment of tinea pedis, topical **antifungal agents** in powder, cream, or ointment formulations can be effective when applied twice daily until clear. Discomfort can be alleviated with cool water or Burow solution soaks. Tinea pedis can be difficult to control. Its treatment is centered on meticulous foot hygiene. Because careful foot care is often not a priority for most patients, complete eradication is not realistic. Patients should be instructed to wash their feet and change their socks when they return from school, dry their feet completely, avoid occlusive shoes, and wear open-air shoes or sandals whenever possible. Topical antiperspirants may be needed (aluminum chloride). Cotton socks are recommended. In severe or refractory cases, an oral antifungal preparation such as griseofulvin, terbinafine, or itraconazole may be prescribed for an extended period. Tinea capitis also requires oral antifungal therapy (see Chapter 123). For the treatment of scabies, see Chapter 125.

Prognosis

Overall, the prognosis for vesicular exanthems caused by infection is good, with most children recovering in 1 to 2 weeks, depending on the etiology. Secondary infections can occur with varicella, however, and should be suspected in children with persistent or recurrent fever. Additional complications in patients who are not immunosuppressed include bacterial superinfection of the skin, pneumonia, CNS involvement, Reye syndrome, glomerulonephritis, and arthritis. Complications from herpes simplex infections include conjunctivitis, keratitis, and encephalitis.

Secondary infections with skin flora can be a complication of any of these skin conditions because denuded lesions allow for superinfection. In addition, many of these rashes can be pruritic, resulting in open, excoriated skin.

CASE RESOLUTION

In the case presented, the toddler has a classic presentation of primary varicella (chickenpox). Management should include symptomatic treatment with acetaminophen and antihistamines, along with topical preparations such as calamine lotion and oatmeal baths. The parent should be instructed on the natural course of this infection and be informed that the infection is highly contagious. In addition, symptoms indicating possible complications, such as persistent or recurrent fever, circumferential redness or swelling of the lesions, and shortness of breath, should be reviewed with the parents.

Selected References

American Academy of Pediatrics Committee on Infectious Diseases. *Red Book: 2012 Report of the Committee on Infectious Diseases.* Pickering LK, ed. 29th ed. Elk Grove Village, IL: American Academy of Pediatrics; 2012

Chayavichitsilp P, Buckwalter JV, Krakowski AC, Friedlander SF. Herpes simplex. *Pediatr Rev.* 2009;30(4):119–130

Gershon AA. Varicella-zoster virus infections. *Pediatr Rev.* 2008;29(1):5–11

Mancini AJ, Shani-Adir A. Other viral diseases. In: Bolognia JL, Jorizzo JL, Rapini RP, eds. *Dermatology.* St Louis, MO: Mosby; 2008:1219–1222

Mathes EF, Oza V, Frieden IJ, et al. "Eczema coxsackium" and unusual cutaneous findings in an enterovirus outbreak. *Pediatrics.* 2013;132(1):e149–e157

Paller AS, Mancini AJ, eds. *Hurwitz Clinical Pediatric Dermatology.* Edinburgh, Scotland: Elsevier; 2011:370

Yang LP, Keam SJ. Spotlight on retapamulin in impetigo and other uncomplicated superficial skin infections. *Am J Clin Dermatol.* 2008;9(6):411–413

SECTION XII

The New Morbidity

CHAPTER 128

Autism Spectrum Disorders

Robin Steinberg-Epstein, MD

CASE STUDY

The mother of 18-month-old twin boys is concerned because one twin is not talking as much as his twin sibling. They are both very active. She feels that even though the child is quiet, he is very smart. He likes to figure out how things work. He seems very sensitive to sounds and covers his ears around loud noises. He loves music and even knows which CD his favorite song is on. He will play with his sibling but doesn't seem interested in other children.

In your office, both boys are very active. It is difficult to get an adequate examination because this child is screaming the whole time. While both children have stranger anxiety, the twin about whom the mother is concerned seems to have extreme stranger anxiety. He otherwise appears well.

Questions

1. What is autism spectrum disorder (ASD)?
2. How does ASD differ from language delay?
3. How do you evaluate a child for ASD?
4. Where can a clinician refer a patient with an ASD?
5. What types of treatment are available?
6. Should a child suspected of having an ASD receive further immunizations?

Autism spectrum disorder (ASD) is characterized by impairments in social communication and social interaction as well as restrictive and repetitive behaviors or interests. According to the new *Diagnostic and Statistical Manual of Mental Disorders, 5th Edition, Text Revision,* a person with an ASD must display persistent communication, interaction, and behavioral challenges across multiple contexts. These disturbances must be present early on but may not be apparent until social demand exceeds the limitation. It must cause significant degrees of impairment (Box 128-1) and cannot be caused by cognitive impairment.

This new term, ASD, includes the previous terminology of autistic disorder, Asperger syndrome, and pervasive developmental disorder–not otherwise specified but no longer includes Rett syndrome. While criteria differ somewhat, all of these disorders had in common an impairment in social communication and repetitive or unusual interests of varying degrees. These disorders require similar management and treatment, and there is some subjectivity in assessing the level of impairment. Therefore, a single term—ASD—best incorporates all those who are significantly affected by its symptomatology.

Epidemiology

As recently as 1999, the prevalence of ASD was thought to be 1 in 2,500. More recent numbers from the Centers for Disease Control and Prevention (2012) cite 1 in 88 children. This amounts to 2 million Americans. The incidence is rising by almost 15% a year. Boys are affected approximately 4 times as often as girls, which equates to 1 in every 70 boys. However, affected girls are often more impaired.

Autism is considered the fastest-growing developmental disability. This increase is, in part, the result of an understanding of a broader phenotype.

Clinical Presentation

Autism spectrum disorder is truly a spectrum of social communication deficits. While there is a certain set of behaviors that defines the disorder, any child may have any combination of the symptoms that lead to the same result—severe and incapacitating social deficits. Furthermore, the challenges that face this population are more than just developmental delays; their behaviors are aberrant and odd.

Many children with an ASD have difficulty with eye contact and body posture. Even those who have some eye contact often do not use their eyes to convey a social message. They may look out of the corner of their eyes, focus only on the lips of the speaker, or only look infrequently. In other words, they may make eye contact but at the wrong time. They may talk to you with their bodies facing away from you. They may not gesture to help clarify intention.

While some children have limited communication, some offer too much information. They may be quick to talk to you about things they are interested in but are not able to talk to you about your interests. They seem socially insensitive. As younger children, they are often entertained by their own interests for long periods. Some have limited need for relationships, yet others desire interaction but do not understand how to initiate or maintain interactions. While many of these children are nonverbal, some repeat or echo what they hear from movies, television, or nearby conversation. Others seem able

---

Box 128-1. *Diagnostic and Statistical Manual of Mental Disorders (DSM-5)*
Diagnostic Criteria for Autism Spectrum Disorder

A. Persistent deficits in social communication and social interactions across multiple contexts, as manifested by the following, currently or by history (examples are illustrative, not exhaustive):

1. Deficits in social-emotional reciprocity, ranging, for example, from abnormal social approach and failure of normal back-and-forth conversation; to reduced sharing of interests, emotions, or affect; to failure to initiate or respond to social interactions.

2. Deficits in nonverbal communicative behaviors used for social interaction, ranging, for example, from poorly integrated verbal and nonverbal communication; to abnormalities in eye contact and body language or deficits in understanding and use of gestures; to a total lack of facial expressions and nonverbal communication.

3. Deficits in developing, maintaining, and understanding relationships, ranging, for example, from difficulties adjusting behavior to suit various social contexts; to difficulties in sharing imaginative play or in making friends; to absence of interest in peers.

Specify current severity:

Severity is based on social communication impairments and restricted, repetitive patterns of behavior.

B. Restricted, repetitive patterns of behavior, interests, or activities, as manifested by at least two of the following, currently or by history (examples are illustrative, not exhaustive):

1. Stereotyped or repetitive motor movements, use of objects, or speech (eg, simple motor stereotypies, lining up toys or flipping objects, echolalia, idiosyncratic phrases).

2. Insistence on sameness, inflexible adherence to routines, or ritualized patterns of verbal or nonverbal behavior (eg, extreme distress at small changes, difficulties with transitions, rigid thinking patterns, greeting rituals, need to take same route or eat same food every day).

3. Highly restricted, fixated interests that are abnormal in intensity or focus (eg, strong attachment to or preoccupation with unusual objects, excessively circumscribed or perseverative interests).

4. Hyper- or hyporeactivity to sensory input or unusual interest in sensory aspects of the environment (eg, apparent indifference to pain/temperature, adverse response to specific sounds or textures, excessive smelling or touching of objects, visual fascination with lights or movement.)

Specify current severity:

Severity is based on social communication impairments and restricted, repetitive patterns of behavior

C. Symptoms must be present in the early developmental period (but may not become fully manifest until social demands exceed limited capacities, or may be masked by learned strategies in later life).

D. Symptoms cause clinically significant impairment in social, occupational, or other important areas of current functioning.

E. These disturbances are not better explained by intellectual disability (intellectual developmental disorder) or global developmental delay. Intellectual disability and autism spectrum disorder frequently co-occur; to make comorbid diagnoses of autism spectrum disorder and intellectual disability, social communication should be below that expected for general developmental level.

Note: Individuals with a well-established DSM-IV diagnosis of autistic disorder, Asperger's disorder, or pervasive developmental disorder not otherwise specified should be given the diagnosis of autism spectrum disorder. Individuals who have marked deficits in social communication, but whose symptoms do not otherwise meet criteria for autism spectrum disorder, should be evaluated for social (pragmatic) communication disorder.

Specify if:

With or without accompanying intellectual impairment

With or without accompanying language impairment

Associated with a known medical or genetic condition or environmental factor

Associated with another neurodevelopmental, mental, or behavioral disorder

With catatonia

Reprinted with permission from American Psychiatric Association. *Diagnostic and Statistical Manual of Mental Disorders.* 5th ed. Washington, DC: American Psychiatric Association; 2013.

---

to converse but have trouble with social banter. It is important not to be deceived by a child who interacts or hugs but only on his own terms.

Children with an ASD often have a fascination with patterns. The pattern may be in the form of household routines or within a particular subject area. This may manifest in an obsession for sameness and resistance to change or an obsessive need to know everything about a particular topic. Many know all there is to know about such favorite topics as Thomas the Tank Engine or dinosaurs from the Jurassic period but cannot answer a question such as, "How are you?" or "What is your name?" They may be upset by a road detour or a furniture rearrangement. Some of these children, out of an incredible ability to recognize patterns, will be able to read as early as 2 years of age, even though they are unable to speak functionally and cannot comprehend what they read.

A significant portion of children have difficulty with sensory processing. This takes the form of problems with smells, tastes, sounds, sights, and touch. This symptom may be manifest in the need to taste everything, including nonfood items; covering ears in loud situations; or an inability to tolerate tags in clothing.

There is a huge variation in cognitive ability. The severity of ASD is independent of cognitive ability. While a significant portion of those with ASD have intellectual disabilities, many are of normal intelligence and even gifted.

Parents often raise behavioral concerns. It is important to recognize red flags and behaviors that demand further evaluation (boxes 128-2 and 128-3). In other words, there are certain classic symptoms, but be mindful of the child who is just unable to connect with others. Clinicians should rely on their own instincts. Inconsistent symptoms are the hallmark of this disorder. Some parents of children with an ASD describe a phenomenon whereby the children are developing normally until 12 to 15 months of age and then suddenly lose skills or stop progressing. This is particularly concerning.

Pathophysiology

There are numerous proposed etiologic possibilities for the origins of ASD, from the inbreeding of computer "whizzes" to exposure to microwaves. However, no consistent explanation or pattern has emerged. We do know that the structure of the brain is different, but why?

Up to 10% of those with an ASD have another medical condition (Box 128-4) that might have led to this disorder. However, this leaves 90% without an etiology.

Genetics seem to play a role in the development of ASD. There is a risk of the disorder among siblings of up to 20%, which is more than 20 times the risk in the normal population. Family members are more likely to exhibit social deficits, anxiety, or depression than

---

Box 128-3. Absolute Indications for Referrals
• Not babbling or gesturing (pointing, waving) by 12 months.
• No single words by 16 months.
• Absence of 2-word non-echolalic phrases by 24 months.
• *Any* loss of *any* language or social skills at *any* age requires immediate evaluation.

From Filipek PA, Accardo PJ, Baranek GT, et al. The screening and diagnosis of autism spectrum disorders. *J Autism Dev Disord.* 1999;29(6):439–484, with permission.

Box 128-4. Medical Conditions Associated With Autism Spectrum Disorder
• Epilepsy
• Fragile X syndrome
• Tuberous sclerosis
• Prader-Willi syndrome
• Visual or auditory impairment syndrome
• Down (trisomy 21) syndrome
• Cerebral palsy
• Neurofibromatosis
• Congenital rubella

---

are family members who do not have a relative with the disorder. Several candidate chromosomes have been suggested as being associated with this disorder, but no one loci is responsible for this disorder.

It is also important to realize that up to 30% of children with an ASD have abnormalities on electroencephalogram (EEG). This may point to the structural abnormalities in an autistic brain but does not seem to account for the disease itself. The epileptiform changes should be evaluated by a neurologist to determine if medication is indicated.

Several environmental markers have also been suggested as being linked to ASD, but none has proved credible. Major epidemiologic studies within the United States and internationally have examined the roles of vaccinations, diet, and thimerosal preservative in the development of this disorder. None of these studies has found proof to support these theories. Children with an ASD should receive routine health maintenance, including all recommended immunizations. There are noted associations such as older paternal age, prematurity, and jaundice.

Differential Diagnosis

Very few entities present with impairment in the same 2 domains as those that are affected by ASD. There are a limited number of disorders that mimic ASD (Box 128-5). On the other hand, there are several disorders that commonly occur with ASD (Box 128-6) that, if not identified, will make treatment more difficult.

Box 128-2. Red Flags (Common Aberrant Behaviors Associated With Autism Spectrum Disorder)
• Decreased eye contact (common but *not* universal)
• Only wants to be cuddled on his or her terms
• Areas of unusual knowledge—recognizes entire alphabet by 2 years of age, all types of dinosaurs by 4 years, names of all Thomas trains, interest in fans or spinning items
• More interested in how things work than with playing
• Unusual sensitivities—oversensitive to hearing, bright lights, shirt tags, new foods, new places
• Smelling or licking nonfood items
• Repeating words instead of answering questions or answering off topic
• Difficulty interacting with other children
• Plays amongst children, not with them
• Resistance to change, "very independent"
• "In his/her own world"
• Lines things up
• Unusual hand movements or jumping when emotional
• Things have to be a certain way
• Odd tone of voice (prosody)
• Increased pain tolerance

Box 128-5. Disorders That May Mimic Autism Spectrum Disorder

- Hearing impairment
- Global developmental delay
- Tourette syndrome and comorbidities
- Selective mutism
- Reactive attachment disorder
- Lead ingestion
- Sensorimotor integration dysfunction
- Severe auditory processing/language deficit
- Severe anxiety
- Severe attention-deficit/hyperactivity disorder
- Brain trauma
- Childhood-onset schizophrenia

Box 128-6. Disorders That Can Occur With Autism Spectrum Disorder

- Tuberous sclerosis
- Congenital blindness
- Global developmental delay
- Chromosomal abnormalities (eg, Down syndrome, fragile X syndrome, Prader-Willi syndrome)
- Phenylketonuria
- Epilepsy
- Elevated lead level
- Congenital infections
- Brain trauma
- Bipolar disorder
- Neurofibromatosis
- Congenital profound hearing loss
- Tourette syndrome
- Landau-Kleffner syndrome
- Inborn errors of metabolism
- Anemia
- In utero exposure to drugs/alcohol
- Depression/anxiety
- Attention-deficit/hyperactivity disorder

Evaluation

There is not one diagnostic test, blood or otherwise, that will confirm the diagnosis of ASD. Diagnosis is based on history and interaction with the child.

History

Regular developmental surveillance and screening should be part of every well-child evaluation, especially between ages 9 and 30 months. The American Academy of Pediatrics recently recommended adding a 30-month visit for developmental screening in an attempt to capture atypical development to target for early intervention. Special attention should be given to a child who has a sibling with an ASD or a child whose parent or caregiver has expressed concern. Several standardized screening tools can be used, including the Parents' Evaluation of Developmental Status, Ages & Stages Questionnaires, and the BRIGANCE. The Modified Checklist for Autism in Toddlers, Revised, is another excellent screening tool (moderate sensitivity and high specificity) to identify developmental and social competency skills which, when deficient, may be associated with ASD. These screening tools are quick and easy and can be filled out by the parent in the waiting area or with minor assistance from office personnel.

Once you suspect that a child has a developmental difference, it is important to gather as much information as possible. Thorough birth and medical histories are important in helping to understand if early experiences may predispose this child to any deficits. For example, there is a higher risk among children born prematurely. Monozygotic and dizygotic twins have high concordance. Older fathers or infertility treatments may have a role.

Family history is also important because ASD is presumed to have a genetic contribution. Furthermore, it may help to consider other etiologies. Family structure will help to determine if abuse, neglect, or maternal depression play any role in the child's delay. However, ASD is *not* caused by poor parenting.

Developmental history is the most important part of the history. It is important to probe all 4 areas of development: fine motor, gross motor, language, and social development (see Chapter 29). Again, it is expected that the most significant delays are in language and social interaction, but delays may be seen in all components of development. Additionally, probing for abnormal behaviors specific to ASD helps distinguish this disorder from others. See the Questions Box for some suggestions that may help elicit information relevant to a diagnosis of ASD in a toddler, but adjust the history depending on the age of the child. Always include early language milestones. Be aware that children with an ASD tend to have splinter skills, which are skills that may be normal or above developmental level for age. Don't let these skills distract from probing areas of suspected delay.

Finally, parents and physicians often fall victim to common myths and excuses about development (Box 128-7) because it is not easy for many parents to discuss or admit delays. These myths, while they sound plausible, are not substantiated and only serve to further delay onset of intervention.

Physical Examination

A thorough physical examination with special attention directed to the growth parameters, neurologic examination, dysmorphic features, and neurocutaneous stigmata are essential to a complete evaluation. Height, weight, and head circumference should be plotted. Keep in mind that 25% of children with an ASD have a head circumference greater than the 97th percentile. That is not to say that everyone with a large head has an ASD, only that it is an associated feature. Of course, in utero infections may predispose to a small occipitofrontal circumference, but both have developmental implications for ASD.

Detecting subtle physical signs, such as clinodactyly, simian crease, or a high-arched palate, while not diagnostic, are somewhat helpful in raising suspicion for neurodevelopmental delays. A Wood

Autism Spectrum Disorder

Questions

Questions to Ask Parents

- Does your child seem to hear you? Did your child have a hearing test in the neonatal period?
- Does your child make noises? If so, what kind?
- When did your child say his or her first word after "mama" and "dada"? Does your child have 2-word phrases?
- Are there any other behaviors that concern you?
- Can your chlid scribble? Has your child lost any skills? Does your child line things up?
- When did your child first walk? What does your child like to play with?
- Do tags on the back of clothes bother your child?
- Is your child interested in other children? What does your child do if he or she sees another child in a park?
- When do you first remember your child pointing with one finger?
- Does your child play peekaboo? Will your child try to engage you?
- Does your child talk into a play phone?
- Does your child eat a variety of foods?
- Does your child turn when you call him or her?

Questions to Ask Yourself as the Clinician

- Are there any complicating historical factors that may predispose this child to a developmental problem?
- Is this merely personality variation, or does this represent delays and aberrant behavior?
- Is this a language delay, or is there concern about more social or odd behaviors?
- What should be done to evaluate?
- What types of intervention would be helpful?

Box 128-7. Common Excuses for Unusual Behaviors

1. We speak 2 languages at home. (By age 3 years in a bilingual home, language should follow a normal progression. Social and unusual behaviors should always follow a normal trajectory.)
2. He is a boy. (This is accounted for in the range of normal.)
3. She is a twin. (If one twin has an ASD, the other twin has a great risk of having an ASD or being delayed.)
4. He is the first child. (There is no evidence that firstborns speak late.)
5. She is the baby. (There is no evidence that children born last speak late.)
6. He is having a bad day.
7. She watches too much television. (Neglect can lead to delays, but these children still need intervention.)

These are *not* reasons to delay evaluation!

---

lamp evaluation may be helpful in uncovering neurocutaneous stigmata.

A series of dysmorphic features, like a thin upper lip, flat philtrum, and upturned nose, might suggest a syndrome such as fetal alcohol syndrome. Hypotonia is a common finding among children with an ASD but might suggest an inborn error of metabolism. One must also check reflexes because degenerative disorders, such as muscular dystrophy, can present with language delay.

One of the most useful examinations in the office is to simply have a conversation with an older child or to play with a younger child. Bring out bubbles and engage in a popping game. Watch the child's eyes and his or her interaction with you and the parent. Pretend the otoscope is a phone that rings, pick it up, talk briefly, and pass it to the child. Watch the child's response. Does he or she play with you, just with the bubbles, or neither? Does the child display repetitive flapping when excited?

Laboratory Tests

No single laboratory or radiologic evaluation will make the diagnosis. However, some tests are helpful to rule out comorbid conditions. If the child has not had an audiologic evaluation, this is step one. However, do not wait for audiology results before referring the patient for help. From a medical perspective, a tiered approach to the workup is often helpful. The first tier would include laboratory studies such as a chromosomal microarray (comparative genomic hybridization) and a DNA test for fragile X. In those with global developmental delay or regression (or when indicated), consider a lead level, carnitine profile, plasma homocysteine levels, serum amino acids, urine organic acids, thyroid evaluation, and vision evaluation. Consider ammonia, lactate, and pyruvate on those with a severe presentation. An EEG would be appropriate if concerns of seizures are present. Check the results of the newborn screen. The yield of this evaluation is anticipated to be low (approximately 7%) but, if positive, may aid in the diagnosis of a specific comorbidity.

Tier 2 would include an evaluation aimed toward specific rare diseases. Some consideration might be given to chromosomal 15 methylation, methyl CpG binding protein 2 (in males and females), phosphatase and tensin homolog deleted on chromosome 10, fibroblast karyotype if pigmentary abnormalities are noted, sterol profile, guanidinoacetate urine analysis (only in males), or other associated genetic evaluations. Current literature would suggest that evaluations for ASD yield an etiology 15% of the time.

Imaging Studies

If there is a history of regression, microcephaly, or the presence of focal findings suggestive of central nervous system malformations, consider magnetic resonance imaging; otherwise, it is considered low yield. Children with regression, more significant involvement, or behavior suspicious of a seizure should receive an EEG. While positron emission tomography and single-photon emission computed tomography scans will show abnormalities, they are not considered specific enough for diagnosis or to direct care. There are no present indications for their use in an individual child with an ASD; they are used primarily in the research setting.

Management

Making the diagnosis is sometimes challenging, but early diagnosis is critical in changing ultimate outcomes. Early diagnosis and intervention can reduce cost of lifelong care by two-thirds.

For children younger than 3 years, refer to the local governmental agency. In most states, there exists a government-sponsored early intervention program for children 0 to 3 years of age. This agency is responsible for the evaluation and behavioral, educational, and therapeutic interventions for children with suspected delays. This should lead to a comprehensive diagnostic evaluation and placement in an intensive intervention program. Therefore, once a hearing test has been completed, a referral to such an agency is the next step. It takes, on average, 6 months from the time a child is seen in a physician's office to when those services are obtained. Therefore, it is important to identify children before age 2½ years. Furthermore, private insurance in many states will be responsible for these services as a primary or secondary source. Make those referrals!

For children older than 3 years, the responsibility belongs to the local school system, medical insurance, and government-sponsored agency in children with moderate to severe impairments. Even though a child is not yet of school age, the child's local school district is responsible for the evaluation and interventions necessary to appropriately remediate this child. However, clinicians should check with local resources to ensure that such a system exists in the respective state. Be aware that between ages 3 and 21 years, each child is entitled to a free and appropriate education guaranteed under the federal mandate known as the Individuals with Disabilities Education Act. This program should be comprehensive and individualized to each child's needs. After a thorough assessment, the school will meet with parents to develop an Individualized Education Plan.

Most children with an ASD require at least speech and language services, occupational therapy, and social skills training. Many require a one-on-one aide in a mainstream class, and others benefit from special education services in the form of pullout or a special day class. Augmentation can be created privately. Some states have mandated that medical insurance support these additional, yet necessary, services, but in others it is the sole responsibility of the parent.

Interventions

Autism spectrum disorder is a neurologic condition that can improve with intensive **multimodality interventions.** This improvement is slow. There are no quick solutions, magic medications, or diets to "cure" ASD. Behaviors like impulsive aggression, repetition, resistance to change, and obsession are frequently targeted by systematic interventions. Furthermore, some basic social learning behaviors can be shaped with different types of intervention. There are a number of different techniques (Box 128-8) based on different psychologic principles that may be used to help improve the difficulties associated with ASD. The best studied therapy is known as applied behavior analysis (ABA). A child's behavior is scrutinized by a trained behaviorist. Goals and trials are developed to slowly shape appropriate responses. The parent is then taught the skills necessary for the desired outcome.

Speech and language services are also a vital component of intervention. The initial goal is to help establish communication. In

---

> ### Box 128-8. Techniques Used for Treatment of Autism Spectrum Disorders
>
> **Floortime**
>
> This intervention uses personal relationships and play in the child's area of interest to draw the child through increasingly complex developmental tasks.
>
> **Applied Behavior Analysis**
>
> Applied behavior analysis strives to achieve pre-learning skills such as eye contact, imitation, sitting, and following simple directions using the principles of conditioning and behavioral psychology. In a one-on-one fashion, a child is trained to respond in a predetermined way using a specific curriculum and reinforcers.
>
> **Behavior Analysis**
>
> This method uses close study of behaviors, determining antecedent triggers and consequences, such as a tantrum. The goal is to substitute acceptable responses, such as using words, and increases rewards for substituted behaviors.
>
> **Pivotal Response Treatment**
>
> This strategy uses principles of behavior analysis but also uses the child's interests and internal drives to motivate. The hope is to generalize the skills from a therapy room to a variety of environments. Children with an autism spectrum disorder (ASD) often have difficulty performing the same previously mastered skill in a new setting.
>
> **Picture Exchange Communication System**
>
> This system uses pictures that the nonverbal child can use to show a caregiver what he or she wants.
>
> **Treatment and Education of Autistic and Related Communication Handicapped Children**
>
> This is a complete program that incorporates the child into a large ASD community. The goal is toward autonomy and uses many methods based on cognitive therapeutic principles.
>
> **Social Stories**
>
> These are often used as a complementary strategy. These stories describe in detail basic social skills in different scenarios.

---

higher-functioning children who already have established language, this service is vital for the establishment and development of prosocial language—eye contact, inferences, understanding jokes, and the more subtle aspects of language. Social skills groups are often used to teach appropriate social responses in a semi-naturalistic environment.

Occupational therapy is often necessary to help with fine motor skills and the processing of sensory information. This can be helpful in easing transitions. There is not a great deal of research to support its use for sensory concerns, but it is a widely accepted premise that sensory exposure helps children who have an oversensitive or under-sensitive sensory system.

Special education in the form of an aide, classroom pullout, or special day class is often necessary to help with commonly associated learning difficulties. Children with an ASD can have a full array of learning difficulties. Commonly associated learning difficulties are in reading comprehension, written expression, specific math disability, and auditory comprehension.

Under the law, these services should occur in the least restrictive and most appropriate environment.

Pharmacotherapy

The mainstay for treatment of ASD remains behavioral. Medications do not seem to help the core symptoms of ASD. However, almost 2 of 3 of these children receive medications for behaviors that, despite intensive behavioral intervention, continue to obstruct progress or become dangerous.

Only 2 drugs are US Food and Drug Administration–approved for use in this population; risperidone and aripiprazole are approved for the agitation associated with this disorder. On the other hand, there are many other targeted behaviors for which medications are used. The choice to use medication is not a simple one. It should be directed toward the emotion or psychologic function causing the symptom. The most common medications include selective serotonin reuptake inhibitors and stimulants. However, research and clinical experience tells us that children with an ASD are more sensitive to side effects and at lower doses. Therefore, the choice and direction of medication management in this population is often best guided by a developmental-behavioral pediatrician, neurologist, or child psychiatrist (see Chapter 130).

Alternative Treatments

A variety of alternative treatments have been suggested. Secretin injections, dietary restrictions, chelation, high-dose vitamins, antifungals, and neuron injections are just some of the interventions considered in this realm. Some of these methods reported anecdotal improvement; others are dangerous and have resulted in death. None of these methods is considered traditional or the standard of care because there are minimal empiric data to support their use.

Prognosis

Many children show dramatic improvements with early intervention. Unfortunately, others show minimal improvement. Therefore, all children need intensive interventions. Some prognostic indicators such as IQ, early and intensive interventions, and a supportive family bode well. Obtaining an accurate IQ is often challenging. The major determinant of ultimate outcome seems to be progress in a comprehensive, early intervention program for 2 years, prior to age 5 years. Having little or no language by age 6 is a poor prognostic indicator. Therefore, the goal remains focused on early identification, intensive treatment, and advocacy for children to receive such interventions with ongoing support.

Intensive early intervention programs have only been available since about 1995. Children with an ASD have now moved into the mainstream. In spite of receiving early intervention, these children continue to have problems with transitions, more complex social interactions, and higher-level organization tasks. Therefore,

physicians must continue to advocate for and support these families through the years.

Many adults with an ASD also continue to require significant support. They may require sheltered living and work environments, safety monitoring, ongoing medical support, and, depending on severity, institutionalization.

Another significant portion of children with an ASD attend college, get married, and have children. This portion is difficult to quantify because these numbers are changing very rapidly and the true number of children with this disorder has yet to be realized.

CASE RESOLUTION

The child described in the case study was evaluated by a developmental-behavioral pediatrician and the local governmental agency, where he received a comprehensive assessment by a multidisciplinary team. The diagnosis was confirmed and his brother was also noted to have a language delay. They were both placed into an early intervention program. The primary patient was placed in a one-on-one structured teaching environment for 4 months. After significant improvement, he was moved to a therapeutic preschool setting that emphasized generalization of his newly acquired skills, speech therapy, occupational therapy, and social skills. His brother received speech therapy 2 times a week. Both are due to start a regular kindergarten class in the fall with ongoing speech and social support. The primary patient has been placed on a stimulant medication to control hyperactivity and problems with attention.

Selected References

Aman MG. Treatment planning for patients with autism spectrum disorders. *J Clin Psychiatry.* 2005;66(Suppl 10):38–45

American Academy of Pediatrics Council on Children With Disabilities, Section on Developmental Behavioral Pediatrics, Bright Futures Steering Committee, Medical Home Initiatives for Children With Special Needs Project Advisory Committee. Identifying infants and young children with developmental disorders in the medical home: an algorithm for developmental surveillance and screening. *Pediatrics.* 2006;118(1):405–420

American Psychiatric Association. *Diagnostic and Statistical Manual of Mental Disorders.* 5th ed. Text rev. Washington, DC: American Psychiatric Association; 2013

Autism and Developmental Disabilities Monitoring Network Surveillance Year 2002 Principal Investigators; Centers for Disease Control and Prevention. Prevalence of autism spectrum disorders—Autism and Developmental Disabilities Monitoring Network, 14 sites, United States, 2002. *MMWR Surveill Summ.* 2007;56(1):12–28

Autism and Developmental Disabilities Monitoring Network Surveillance Year 2008 Principal Investigators; Centers for Disease Control and Prevention. Prevalence of autism spectrum disorders—Autism and Developmental Disabilities Monitoring Network, 14 sites, United States, 2008. *MMWR Surveill Summ.* 2012;61(3):1–19

Autism Society. http://www.autism-society.org. Accessed March 13, 2014

Barbaresi WJ, Katusic SK, Voigt RG. Autism: a review of the state of the science for pediatric primary health care clinicians. *Arch Pediatr Adolesc Med.* 2006; 160(11):1167–1175

Courchesne E, Carper R, Akshoomoff N. Evidence of brain overgrowth in the first year of life in autism. *JAMA.* 2003;290(3):337–344

Filipek PA, Accardo PJ, Baranek GT, et al. The screening of autism spectrum disorders. *J Autism Dev Disord.* 1999;29(6):439–484

Järbrink K, Knapp M. The economic impact of autism in Britain. *Autism.* 2001;5(1):7–22

Madsen KM, Hviid A, Vestergaard M, et al. A population-based study of measles, mumps, and rubella vaccination and autism. *N Engl J Med.* 2002;347(19): 1477–1482

Richardson AJ, Montgomery P. The Oxford-Durham study: a randomized, controlled trial of dietary supplementation with fatty acids in children with developmental coordination disorder. *Pediatrics.* 2005;115(5):1360–1366

Van Naarden Braun K, Pettygrove S, Daniels J, et al. Evaluation of a methodology for a collaborative multiple source surveillance network for autism spectrum disorders—Autism and Developmental Disabilities Monitoring Network, 14 sites, United States, 2002. *MMWR Surveill Summ.* 2007;56(1):29–40

CHAPTER 129

Attention-Deficit/ Hyperactivity Disorder

Andrew J. Barnes, MD, MPH, and Iris Wagman Borowsky, MD, PhD

CASE STUDY

Cody, a 10-year-old boy, has visited a primary care clinic annually for well-child care, seeing different pediatricians each time. After failing all subjects during the first half of fourth grade, his teacher asks his mother to see if Cody's doctor can do anything to help him at school. When the appointment is made, the clinic obtains standardized attention-deficit/hyperactivity disorder (ADHD)-specific behavioral rating scales from Cody's parents and teachers. Prior to the visit, the pediatrician reviews these rating scales and Cody's medical history. She discovers that at Cody's 6-year well-child visit, a colleague documented, "Likely has ADHD, medication is indicated." The medical records indicate that the family deferred starting stimulant medication and were told to follow up as needed. There is no further mention of ADHD. Cody also has a history of several urgent care and emergency department visits for minor unintentional injuries.

Questions

1. What are the primary symptoms of ADHD? What other conditions should be considered in the differential diagnosis of ADHD?
2. What other psychiatric disorders or neurodevelopmental disabilities commonly coexist with or mimic ADHD?
3. What is the appropriate evaluation of children with suspected ADHD?
4. What treatment modalities are useful in the management of ADHD?
5. What is the role of primary care in the long-term management of ADHD?

Clinicians should initiate a thorough evaluation for attention-deficit/ hyperactivity disorder (ADHD) in any child aged 4 to 18 years who exhibits social, academic, or behavioral problems associated with inattention, impulsivity, and hyperactivity. Three kinds of ADHD are described in the *Diagnostic and Statistical Manual of Mental Disorders, Fifth Edition (DSM-5)*: (1) predominantly inattentive presentation, (2) predominantly hyperactive/impulsive presentation, and (3) combined hyperactive-inattentive presentation. Most children and adolescents with the disorder exhibit symptoms of the combined type. Growing evidence suggests that differentiating such subtypes has little bearing on prognosis or treatment.

The diagnosis of ADHD is based solely on clinical judgment, requiring documentation of sufficiently impairing criteria from the inattentive and/or hyperactive/impulsive *DSM-5* domains (Box 129-1). Some symptoms of ADHD must be present before 12 years of age, and several symptoms must persist in at least 2 major contexts of the child's life (eg, home and school) for at least 6 months. These symptoms must be more frequent and severe than those typically seen in someone of the same developmental age and must impair the child's developmental competence, learning, or social interactions. The symptoms should not be better explained by another condition (eg, anxiety). If impairing symptoms occur at

sub-diagnostic levels or are associated with a *DSM-5* exclusionary condition, a diagnosis of ADHD, not otherwise specified, should be made. Treatment, however, is symptomatic and not specific to subtype.

Transient behavioral variations, challenging temperamental features, and problem-level ADHD-like symptoms that are not frankly disordered or sufficiently impairing are better classified using the framework of *DSM-Primary Care (DSM-PC)* instead of *DSM-5* (eg, "Hyperactive/Impulsive Developmental Variation—Middle Childhood: The child plays active games for long periods. The child may occasionally do things impulsively, particularly when excited"). One advantage of the *DSM-PC* is that it takes into account specific environmental and psychosocial contexts, stressors, and developmental factors that influence children's behavior.

Epidemiology

Attention-deficit/hyperactivity disorder is the most common neurobehavioral disorder in children. An estimated 4% to 12% of school-aged children have ADHD, and there is a 3:1 predominance of boys in community samples. Over the past 2 decades, ADHD diagnoses have increased; it remains unclear whether this represents a true increase in incidence, secular changes in diagnostic criteria and

Box 129-1. *DSM-5* Criteria for Attention-Deficit/Hyperactivity Disorder	
Diagnostic Criteria for ADHD	

A. Either 1 or 2

  1) For children up to age 16, at least 6 of the following symptoms of **inattention,** or at least 5 for adolescents 17 and older and adults, have persisted for at least 6 months to a degree that is maladaptive and inappropriate for developmental level:

  Inattention

    a) Often fails to give close attention to details or makes careless mistakes in schoolwork, at work, or with other activities

    b) Often has difficulty holding attention on tasks or play activities

    c) Often does not seem to listen when spoken to directly

    d) Often does not follow through on instructions and fails to finish schoolwork, chores, or duties in the workplace (eg, loses focus, side-tracked)

    e) Often has trouble organizing tasks and activities

    f) Often avoids, dislikes, or is reluctant to engage in tasks that require sustained mental effort (such as schoolwork or homework)

    g) Often loses things necessary for tasks and activities (eg, school materials, pencils, books, tools, wallets, keys, paperwork, eyeglasses, mobile telephones)

    h) Is often easily distracted

    i) Is often forgetful in daily activities

  2) For children up to age 16, at least 6 of the following symptoms of **hyperactivity-impulsivity,** or at least 5 for adolescents 17 and older

and adults, have persisted for at least 6 months to a degree that is maladaptive and inappropriate for developmental level:

Hyperactivity

  a) Often fidgets with or taps hands or feet, or squirms in seat

  b) Often leaves seat in situations when remaining seated is expected

  c) Often runs about or climbs excessively in situations where it is not appropriate (in adolescents or adults, may be limited to feeling restless)

  d) Often unable to play or take part in leisure activities quietly

  e) Is often "on the go" acting as if "driven by a motor"

  f) Often talks excessively

Impulsivity

  g) Often blurts out an answer before a question has been completed

  h) Often has difficulty awaiting turn

  i) Often interrupts or intrudes on others (eg, butts into conversations or games)

B. Some hyperactive-impulsive or inattentive symptoms that caused impairment were present before 12 years of age.

C. Several symptoms are present in 2 or more settings (eg, at home, school, or work; with friends or relatives; in other activities).

D. There is clear evidence that the symptoms interfere with, or reduce the quality of, social, school, or work functioning.

E. The symptoms do not occur exclusively during the course of schizophrenia or another psychotic disorder and are not better explained by another mental disorder (eg, mood disorder, anxiety disorder, dissociative disorder, or a personality disorder).

Abbreviations: ADHD, attention-deficit/hyperactivity disorder; *DSM-5, Diagnostic and Statistical Manual of Mental Disorders, Fifth Edition.*

Reprinted with permission from American Psychiatric Association. *Diagnostic and Statistical Manual of Mental Disorders.* 5th ed. Washington, DC: American Psychiatric Association; 2013.

practices, sociocultural bias, or effects of unspecified environmental factors.

Clinical Presentation

Children with ADHD have problems with selective attention and mental stamina for non-rewarding or non-preferred activities. They often make careless mistakes or fail to pay attention to details. They may be easily distracted and have difficulty starting tasks and concentrating on tasks long enough to complete them. Stopping a preferred activity can also be problematic, and caregivers often note that their children with ADHD overfocus or "get lost" in their favorite activities, such as video games, drawing, or reading. Difficulties following instructions and organizing tasks and activities are also characteristic of ADHD. Poor impulse control manifests as difficulty waiting one's turn, frequently blurting out responses at inappropriate times, and interrupting or intruding on others. Symptoms of hyperactivity include fidgetiness, excessive talking at inappropriate times, difficulty remaining seated or playing quietly, and subjective feelings of restlessness or impatience in older children and adolescents. Difficulties with social relationships and low frustration tolerance are also commonly seen in children with ADHD.

Pathophysiology

The etiology of ADHD is unknown. Interacting genetic, prenatal/perinatal, environmental/psychosocial, and neurologic factors all play a role. Family studies indicate that first-degree relatives of children with ADHD have a risk of ADHD that is 5 times greater than the risk in the general population. In addition, measures of behavior and attention are more alike in monozygotic twins than in same-gender dizygotic twins. The most widely confirmed gene association with ADHD is the 7-repeat allele of the D_4 dopamine receptor gene that, while found in about 30% of the general population, is found in 50% to 60% of those with ADHD. Prenatal and perinatal risk factors that have been associated with ADHD include in utero exposure to alcohol or cigarettes; extreme prematurity; brain injury or stroke; and severe early deprivation, neglect, and maltreatment.

Attention-deficit/hyperactivity disorder is currently conceptualized as a chronic neurodevelopmental-behavioral condition. Patients with frontal lobe lesions have long been known to exhibit severe and intractable inattention, hyperactivity, behavioral disinhibition, and impulsivity. Recent neurodevelopmental research suggests that ADHD is associated with developmental differences in specific frontal and prefrontal regions of the brain involved in executive functions, including organizing, planning, sequencing, selective attention, impulse inhibition, the ability to stick to a plan yet change it as needed (set maintenance), the ability to self-talk through internal rules, and working memory. A number of recent studies, some longitudinal, show delayed maturation (myelination) and abnormal activation/inactivation of critical prefrontal circuits and fronto-striatal reward-motivation circuits in children and adolescents with ADHD compared with controls. Dopamine and norepinephrine are involved in neurotransmission within these brain pathways, and the prefrontal cortex is rich in catecholamine receptors. Psychostimulants can improve ADHD symptoms by increasing the availability of these neurotransmitters in the brain, thus improving efficiency in attention and motivation circuits. Stimulants seem to primarily increase activity in key areas of the striatum, such as the ventral tegmental area, in turn activating the prefrontal cortex and executive functions.

Differential Diagnosis

The symptoms of ADHD can be seen in a variety of other conditions (Box 129-2). Sensory deficits, especially hearing impairment, can imitate attention deficits. Attention-deficit/hyperactivity disorder symptoms are often a component of autism spectrum disorders (ASDs) and other neurodevelopmental conditions, such as neurofibromatosis, co-occurring with typical features of the respective diagnoses, such as impaired social communication in children with ASDs. Lead and other heavy metals have dose-related detrimental effects on behavior and development; likewise, chronic iron deficiency can result in or mimic ADHD. Seizure disorders, such as petit mal (absence) or partial complex seizures, may cause altered attention or behavioral changes that can mimic ADHD. Other neurologic disorders that can present with symptoms of ADHD include Wilson disease and adrenoleukodystrophy; however, focal and often progressive neurologic deficits of acute-to-subacute onset are the hallmarks of these rare conditions, as opposed to the more soft and static neurologic signs of ADHD. Certain medications, such as high-dose corticosteroids, phenobarbital, and theophylline, may cause ADHD-like mental status effects, as can recreational drugs of abuse, including inhalants and marijuana. Hyperthyroidism can cause the hyperactive symptoms of ADHD, but other signs of increased metabolism, such as elevated heart rate, tremors, or weight loss, should be apparent. Exposure to alcohol or drugs in utero has been associated with subtle difficulties with learning and attention as the child develops. Congenital infections, central nervous system infections in early childhood, and traumatic brain injuries may produce behaviors similar to those seen in ADHD. Sleep disorders, especially sleep apnea, can cause severe behavioral problems that often resolve after definitive treatment of the underlying sleep condition. Severe or chronic psychosocial-environmental stressors, such as bullying, marital discord, unemployment, poverty, homelessness, trauma/maltreatment, substance abuse, and ineffective parenting (eg, overly permissive, overly harsh), can also masquerade as, co-occur with, or exacerbate ADHD.

Box 129-2. Differential Diagnosis of Attention-Deficit/Hyperactivity Disorder

- Developmental delay
- Learning disability
- Language disorder
- Sleep disorder/apnea
- Sensory deficiencies (eg, hearing or vision impairment)
- Autism spectrum disorders
- Seizure disorder
- Neurogenetic syndromes (eg, neurofibromatosis type 1)
- White matter disorders
- Iron deficiency
- Environmental toxins (lead)
- Side effects of medication (eg, phenobarbital)
- Hyperthyroidism
- Congenital infection
- In utero exposure to drugs or alcohol
- Previous brain insult (eg stroke, trauma, infection)
- Family or social stresses
- Ineffective parenting
- Psychiatric disorders
  —Conduct disorder
  —Oppositional disorder
  —Anxiety disorders
  —Affective disorders (depression, bipolar illness)
  —Personality disorders (aggression, antisocial behavior)
  —Substance abuse

Children with ADHD have an increased prevalence of co-occurring pathology, which can magnify or overshadow the core symptoms of the disorder. These include oppositional defiant disorder (35%), conduct disorder (26%), depressive disorders (18%), anxiety disorders (26%), Tourette syndrome and tics, sleep disorders (especially insomnia), developmental coordination disorder, speech and language disorders, and specific learning disabilities, such as dyslexia and dyscalculia. In adolescents and young adults, aggression, delinquency, and other antisocial behaviors, as well as substance abuse, are often seen together with untreated or undertreated ADHD. Children with ADHD and co-occurring conditions are served well by primary care clinicians working within a multidisciplinary context, which may include developmental-behavioral or neurodevelopmental pediatricians, child and adolescent psychiatrists, child neurologists, psychologists, or therapists.

Evaluation

Children and adolescents with symptoms of inattention, hyperactivity, academic or social underachievement, or impulsivity should be evaluated first by a primary care clinician, ideally one with whom the child has enjoyed continuity of care, rapport, and a strong therapeutic alliance. A complete evaluation of this nature is best accomplished with plenty of time for face-to-face review of records and a comprehensive history and examination; 90 to 120 minutes is a suggested minimum amount of time to do this effectively and correctly, usually necessitating several appointments spaced apart by days or weeks.

History

The diagnostic evaluation of ADHD should begin with multiple informants (caregiver[s], child, sibling[s]) giving a comprehensive medical history that includes details of the child's problem behaviors, antecedents, and outcomes and consequences (Questions Box). The clinician should find out how these informants perceive and handle the child's behavioral problems and, in turn, how the child responds. Social/family stresses and the home-school environment should be described and evaluated and school reports and report cards reviewed. Interviewing the child alone provides an opportunity to better understand his or her thoughts, feelings, insight, judgment, self-image, and developmental status; however, children generally have poor insight into their ADHD symptoms and are generally not considered reliable informants for *DSM* ADHD symptoms. Interviewing caregivers alone and talking with teachers over the phone before or after the visit can be very helpful and alleviate some of the burden on the child of what is often initially a problem-oriented discussion about him or her. The clinician should inquire about the child's difficulties, developmental strengths and competencies, adaptive strategies, stress management skills, self-regulation, protective factors, and adjustment. Other important information includes developmental history (and academic history for older children), family history, and sleep and diet history.

Historical information should cover all *DSM* criteria (see Box 129-1). Parents and teachers may report the child's behaviors using an ADHD-specific questionnaire or rating scale (eg, National Initiative for Children's Healthcare Quality Vanderbilt assessment scales), which can be found in the American Academy of Pediatrics (AAP) *Caring for Children With ADHD: A Resource Toolkit for Clinicians.* Non–ADHD-specific developmental screening tools do not replace this type of comprehensive ADHD assessment because their sensitivity and specificity for ADHD are inadequate. For younger children (aged 4–7 years), few validated screening tools exist (eg, Conners Comprehensive Behavior Rating Scales; ADHD Rating Scales–IV). Questionnaires can suggest a diagnosis but are not sufficient; only clinical interview and observation can definitively confirm or rule out ADHD.

The clinician should evaluate for coexisting conditions that would warrant further investigation. This is where broad screening tools, such as the Child Behavior Checklist; Behavior Assessment System for Children, 2nd Edition; Strengths & Difficulties Questionnaires; or Pediatric Symptom Checklist, can be useful. For example, frequent sadness or isolation would suggest depression, and persistent negative, hostile, and defiant behavior toward authority would suggest oppositional defiant disorder. The AAP toolkit for clinicians includes a scale specific to ADHD behaviors and a broader scale for possible coexisting conditions.

Physical Examination

The child's weight, height, and head circumference should be plotted on a growth curve and the pattern of growth evaluated; pubertal status should be recorded. Children should be examined for congenital anomalies, syndromic stigmata, or dysmorphic features, such as fetal alcohol facies or café au lait skin macules. A musculoskeletal evaluation should be done to document bulk, strength, tone, gait, station, and fine and gross motor coordination; a neurologic examination should include assessment of the cranial nerves, sensation including hearing and vision, balance and proprioception, and repetitive movements, tics, or tremors. The psychiatric and behavioral status examination should include an assessment of the child's mental status, affect, mood, insight, judgment, social-emotional reciprocity, joint attention, speech/language and communication, memory, fund of knowledge, and thought content and processes.

Observing the child's behavior during the office visit is crucial, with the caveat that many children with ADHD do not appear grossly hyperactive or inattentive in the office. Interaction between the child and his or her parents should be observed and documented nevertheless. The clinician should note how the child does with complex parental and examiner instructions, directives, and questions and how parents deal with any misbehavior. Does the child cooperate and comply with the examination, and does he or she seem motivated to change? How well does the child relate to adults? The

---

Questions

Screening for Attention-Deficit/ Hyperactivity Disorder

- History of presenting complaint (from multiple informants)
  - What concerns do you have about the child's development, behavior, or learning?
  - How is the child doing in school academically and socially?
  - Is the child happy in school?
  - Has the child been held back in any grade, suspended, dropped out, or considered dropping out?
  - How often does the child have problems completing home chores, class work, or homework?
  - How often does the child have major problems controlling his or her behavior at home, in school, or with friends?
  - How often is behavior management, self-regulation, or discipline difficult at home or school?
  - What are the antecedents and consequences for problem behaviors at home and school? What discipline techniques have been tried and what effects did each have?
- Perinatal, developmental, academic, and medical history
- Psychologic history and previous treatments
- Social and environmental history
- Family history (focused especially on immediate family attention-deficit/hyperactivity disorder, school problems, developmental delays, conduct problems, and cardiac, musculoskeletal, neurologic, or psychiatric conditions)

clinician should watch the child play (eg, draw, play with toys) and note the child's organization of activities, attention span, distractibility, and motor activity.

Laboratory Tests

Diagnostic tests, such as specific neuropsychologic or psychiatric metrics (eg, IQ tests), are not indicated for initial ADHD evaluations and should be guided by selected findings on the history and physical examination. Psychometric testing or standardized school district tests may show that a discrepancy exists between the child's raw abilities (IQ) and academic progress in one or more areas (achievement scores or grades); in this case, a referral for psychoeducational testing to rule out specific learning disabilities is indicated. Referral for further evaluation of speech, hearing, and vision should also be done as indicated. Blood tests, such as hematocrit, lead level, and thyroid hormone, likewise, are only indicated if there are relevant signs or symptoms. Additionally, computerized continuous performance tasks designed to measure vigilance or distractibility have low sensitivity and specificity and fail to adequately differentiate children with ADHD from controls.

Brain imaging (eg, magnetic resonance imaging, positron emission tomography) currently has no role in the evaluation of ADHD. Despite their utility in population-level studies, such measures cannot yet accurately differentiate between the brains of individuals with and without ADHD. An electroencephalogram or neurologic consultation is indicated only if absence or partial complex seizures are suspected by history or physical examination.

Management

Treatment of ADHD must be multimodal, continuous, and longitudinal, recognizing that ADHD is a chronic condition. Because of its chronicity, ADHD is a special health care need that should be managed within a medical home model. Frequent follow-up (at least quarterly) and consistent management is the key to sustaining the benefits of behavioral and pharmacologic treatments for ADHD. Family education should emphasize the strengths of children and families and address parental concerns; clinicians should also foster a close working relationship between families and their children's school systems. Families should be aware that children with untreated or undertreated ADHD often experience functional impairments in academic achievement, self-esteem, social skills, peer status, and family relationships; more unintentional injuries; and above-average emergency department use. The clinician can ease parents' guilt by explaining the neurodevelopmental basis of ADHD and assuring that ADHD is not the result of insufficient parenting. Children who discover that their problems are not their fault may feel that a heavy burden has been lifted from their shoulders. However, parents and children may find it difficult to accept that the child has a chronic disorder. Support groups and parent training through organizations such as Children and Adults with ADHD (www.chadd.org) may be helpful for families. Clinicians should work together with the child, family, and school personnel to specify appropriate target outcomes. They should then monitor the child for target behaviors and adverse effects. If target outcomes are not met, the clinician should reevaluate the initial diagnosis, use of available treatments, adherence to the plan, and potential for coexisting conditions.

Behavior Management

For preschoolers with ADHD, behavior management should be the first-line treatment for ADHD. Behavioral treatment may also be effective for older children, particularly those with anxiety or disruptive or oppositional problems. The goals of behavior management are to modify the child's physical and social environment at home and school to influence positive behavioral change. Behavioral modification techniques include rewards for the target outcome behaviors (eg, verbal praise hugs; points or stars on a chart that can be traded for material objects or a desired activity, such as a game or special time with a parent) and punishments for unacceptable behaviors (eg, time-out, loss of a privilege, extra chores, reduction in allowance). Acceptable and unacceptable behaviors should be clearly defined and measurable, and rewards and punishments should be spelled out in a contract drawn up with the child. The strongest behavioral interventions follow immediately after a behavior (eg, immediate praise when a child follows a command after the first time it was given). If rewards or punishments are used over time, parents and teachers must be creative in periodically varying the rewards and penalties. Management of overactive children who have difficulty focusing attention, following rules, and controlling impulses can be challenging for parents and teachers. The best results come from praising and reinforcing positive behaviors and ignoring negative behaviors unless they are dangerous or intolerable. Using praising and ignoring in combination can be very successful. Parent commands should be clear and countable (eg, "You need to go upstairs to brush your teeth before the egg timer goes off in 3 minutes"). Because children with ADHD can have difficulty carrying out multistep commands, it is best to set them up for success by giving clear, doable, single-step commands. Behavior management in combination with medication management can be extremely effective. Potential benefits of behavioral therapy when used concurrently with medication include improved scores on some academic measures, improved behavior, and decreased anxiety symptoms. Interventions such as play therapy, psychotherapy, and cognitive therapy have no documented efficacy in managing core ADHD symptoms but may be indicated for common co-occurring conditions such as anxiety, conduct disorder, and depression. Approaches that target executive function training and cognitive-emotional self-regulation may be useful adjuncts as well.

Educational Interventions

The pediatrician can improve the child's educational experience by contacting the child's teachers and even attending school conferences and special education meetings. While most children with ADHD can be managed in the regular classroom, special education in a smaller, more focused setting may be indicated for behavioral or academic difficulties.

Teachers can use specific strategies to help children with ADHD focus their attention and follow directions in the classroom (Box 129-3). Behavioral therapy should be integrated into the classroom, focusing on a child's strengths and minimizing stigma. Teachers and caregivers who are most successful in working with children with ADHD are able to set firm limits and discipline children without anger or frustration, while at the same time remaining flexible enough to recognize when a change in tactics or even "rolling with it" is necessary. Caregivers of children with ADHD can request needed classroom accommodations through Section 504 of the Americans with Disabilities Act of 1990, and children whose ADHD symptoms lead to significant learning deficits may qualify for an Individual Education Plan through the Individuals with Disabilities Educational Act. A letter from a primary care clinician documenting a child's health impairments, developmental risks, and academic limitations attributable to ADHD can go a long way in helping to ease this process for families and schools. Preschool-aged children with ADHD should be referred to early intervention services in their school district to see if they qualify for educational services that would help prepare them for kindergarten entry.

Because children with ADHD are easily provoked into misbehavior and are prone to clashes with peers, they can also benefit from closer supervision in unstructured school areas such as the playground, cafeteria, halls, and bus. Programs designed to improve social competence and peer relationships (eg, group social skills training, therapeutic recreational activities) may also be helpful.

Pharmacotherapy

Research has shown that psychostimulant medication with and without behavioral therapy is efficacious in reducing the core symptoms of ADHD. Furthermore, there is some evidence that these effects translate into an increased ability to follow rules, improved classroom behavior, and improved relationships with peers and parents; effects on higher-order executive functions are less predictably attained. Effects of stimulant medication on learning are not well-studied. Caution should be used when treating children younger than 5 years or weighing less than 20 kg with stimulant medication because many pharmaceutical stimulant preparations have narrower therapeutic windows and more adverse effects on a per-kilogram basis for children of smaller stature. However, for preschoolers without access to behavioral treatment or with frequent dangerous impulsive behaviors, methylphenidate has been well-studied in randomized controlled trials and can be considered first-line treatment if the benefits are thought to outweigh the risks.

Psychostimulants are the most commonly used agents for ADHD and by far the most evidence-based. Currently available stimulants include short-acting (3–6 hours), intermediate-acting (6–8 hours), and long-acting (10–12+ hours) formulations of methylphenidate and amphetamines (Box 129-4). Studies have found few, if any, differences between the efficacy of methylphenidate and amphetamine, but some children will respond better to, or have fewer side effects with, one or the other.

Box 129-3. Strategies for Managing Children With Attention-Deficit/Hyperactivity Disorder in the Classroom

- Seat children where distractions are minimized and teachers can see how and when children are paying attention.
- Cue children discretely or nonverbally to remind them to refocus their attention.
- Give clear, succinct, 1- to 2-step directions, and repeat them frequently and patiently.
- Break up work periods by allowing children to get up and move around (eg, handing out papers, cleaning blackboard).

Box 129-4. Stimulant Medications

Methylphenidate
- Short (Ritalin, Methylin, Focalin)
- Intermediate (Ritalin SR, Metadate ER, Methylin ER)
- Extended release (Concerta, Metadate CD, Ritalin LA, Focalin XR, liquid [Quillivant] and transdermal [Daytrana])

Amphetamine
- Short (Dexedrine, Dextrostat, Desoxyn)
- Intermediate (Adderall, Dexedrine Spansule)
- Extended release (Adderall XR, Vyvanse)

Stimulants affect behaviors within 30 to 60 minutes and affect attention (eg, for a school subject like math) within 1.5 hours after administration. There is little evidence of tolerance to stimulants over time, but short-term tolerance occurs so that blood levels must increase during the day to maintain efficacy. Long-acting stimulants eliminate the need to take medication at school and may persist during after-school homework time. A transdermal delivery system and liquid formulations are available for some stimulants.

The most common side effects of stimulant medications are decreased appetite, stomachaches, headaches, delayed sleep onset, and jitteriness, occurring in 4% to 10% of children. Less common effects include severe emotional lability/sadness or agitation, transient rebound irritability or hyperactivity (as the medication wears off), delusions or mania, and hallucinations (especially somatic creepy-crawly feelings). Transient motor tics may occur while on the medication (or an existing chronic tic or Tourette syndrome exacerbated or unmasked). At higher doses, stimulants can negatively influence height velocity and may slightly decrease predicted adult height. While dosing of stimulant medication is based on individual variation in response, researchers have found that children generally do better on a maximized tolerable dose of stimulant medications, which is body-weight dependent, rather than the lowest dose that shows a clinical effect. The best stimulant dose for an individual child is thus the dose that produces near-complete symptom remission while producing acceptable side effects (eg, appetite suppression is usually tolerable, whereas growth suppression is not). For this reason, it is recommended that clinicians do a controlled open-label titration trial of multiple dosages of a single agent using a systematic method. For example, one might use either long-acting methylphenidate in 18-, 36-, and 54-mg dosages or long-acting amphetamine in 10-, 20-, and 30-mg dosages in 1-week blocks, with teacher- and parent-completed *DSM*-based rating scales (eg, NICHQ Vanderbilt assessment scales) at the end of each week. The clinician can then use these scales to develop a medication management plan with the family. Published guidelines and algorithms, such as those from the AAP, can aid the clinician in this regard.

Once the medication dosage is stable and helpful, often after 2 to 4 visits over 1 to 2 months, follow-up should occur at least every 3 to 4 months, with particular attention to emerging developmental competencies, self-mastery, and improvement in targeted goal behaviors. Such visits should minimally include an interim history, weight, height, blood pressure, and scales of clinical response from caregivers and teachers.

If a particular stimulant does not produce symptom remission at all or only does so with severe or intolerable adverse effects, the clinician should systematically try 1 or 2 other stimulants because 70% to 80% of children can achieve complete remission of symptoms in this manner. If 2 or 3 psychostimulants are not effective or produce unacceptable or intolerable side effects, other medications can be used. Atomoxetine (Strattera) is a non-stimulant medication that selectively inhibits the norepinephrine transporter. Atomoxetine is approved for children older than 6 years, has once-daily dosing, should be titrated to an effective weight-based dose, and often takes 1 to 6 weeks to produce effects; adverse effects can include gastrointestinal upset and mood irritability. α_2-agonists such as clonidine (Catapres, Kapvay) and guanfacine (Tenex, Intuniv) are often useful as adjuncts for children with poorly controlled hyperactivity/impulsivity or comorbid tics, although few children with ADHD achieve adequate symptom remission on α_2-agonist monotherapy. Tricyclic antidepressants, selective serotonin reuptake inhibitors, or bupropion can have positive effects on ADHD symptoms for some children, although again, they are rarely used as monotherapy and are typically fourth-line agents. Pemoline (Cylert) is generally not used because of the potential for fatal hepatotoxicity. Modafinil, mood stabilizers, antiepileptics, and atypical antipsychotics are generally not indicated in the treatment of ADHD in the primary care setting.

Complementary and alternative medicines, such as vitamins, dietary restrictions, and occupational therapy or sensory integration, are used by 54% of parents, but only 11% discuss these with their child's clinician. Primary care practitioners are challenged to help families safely navigate the limited evidence available on such therapies' risks and benefits. For example, melatonin is safe and often helpful for comorbid sleep disorders prevalent in children with ADHD, and eliminating artificial colors from the diet may help children sensitive to effects on their activity level. There is no evidence, or negative evidence, for some popular holistic approaches, such as behavioral optometry or the Feingold elimination diet. Finally, while there may be neurobehavioral toxicity associated with low doses of

various environmental toxins, particularly in young children, pediatricians are encouraged to emphasize primary prevention; there is no role for chelation in this context.

Prognosis

Attention-deficit/hyperactivity disorder is a chronic condition, persisting into adolescence and adulthood in about two-thirds of affected children. Overall, adults who had untreated or undertreated childhood ADHD complete less schooling, hold lower-ranking occupations, have lower self-esteem and more social-skill deficits, and exhibit more antisocial behavior and alcohol and drug abuse. However, ADHD does not preclude attaining high educational and vocational goals, and some adults who had childhood ADHD may no longer meet full *DSM* criteria. Hyperactivity usually greatly diminishes or resolves in high school or early adulthood; some young adults experience a bothersome sense of inner restlessness. Attention problems and impulsivity may continue or worsen, to varying degrees. Adults with ADHD may choose occupations that match their strengths and minimize limitations (eg, on-the-road salesperson vs desk-job accountant). While some adults with ADHD choose to continue medication, others may function well without medication.

CASE RESOLUTION

Cody's primary care clinic reorganized its system of care to leverage the core concepts of the **medical home** to improve care for children with chronic conditions, including attention-deficit/hyperactivity disorder (ADHD). One of the clinic's nurses, Karen, has been trained to coordinate referrals to behavioral health and other specialists as indicated, communicate and coordinate care with schools and community services, and monitor adherence and response to treatments.

During Cody's visit, the pediatrician confirms the diagnosis of ADHD and probable comorbid anxiety using AAP clinical practice guidelines and standardized criteria. She educates Cody and his family about multimodal evidence-based interventions for these conditions and introduces the family to Karen and the medical home model of care. Karen follows up with the family by phone 1 week later as planned and learns that they are reluctant to start Cody on any medicine. She guides Cody's parents to voice their preferences and cultural perspectives on possible interventions and then assists them in making another appointment with the same pediatrician, ensuring continuity of care. At the next visit, the pediatrician uses motivational interviewing to help the family find agreement on a watchful waiting approach with close, continuous school and home follow-up by Karen and at least quarterly visits with the same pediatrician. One month later, following a behavioral crisis at school, Cody's parents request an urgent appointment with same-day access. The pediatrician reviews recent parent and teacher behavioral rating scales at the point of care (gathered by Karen the prior week) and reiterates the available first-line treatment options. The family agrees to pursue an open titration trial of stimulant medication for ADHD symptoms and referral to a therapist for evaluation and possible treatment of the anxiety symptoms. Another clinic visit is scheduled in 1 month, while Karen follows up weekly with parents, teachers, and therapists.

Selected References

American Academy of Pediatrics Subcommittee on Attention-Deficit/Hyperactivity Disorder, Steering Committee on Quality Improvement and Management. ADHD: clinical practice guideline for the diagnosis, evaluation, and treatment of attention-deficit/hyperactivity disorder in children and adolescents. *Pediatrics.* 2011;128(5): 1007–1022

American Academy of Pediatrics Task Force on Coding for Mental Health in Children. *The Classification of Child and Adolescent Mental Diagnoses in Primary Care: Diagnostic and Statistical Manual for Primary Care (DSM-PC) Child and Adolescent Version.* Elk Grove Village, IL: American Academy of Pediatrics; 1996

American Psychiatric Association. *Diagnostic and Statistical Manual of Mental Disorders.* 5th ed. Washington, DC: American Psychiatric Association; 2013

August GJ, Winters KC, Realmuto GM, Fahnhorst T, Botzet A, Lee S. Prospective study of adolescent drug use among community samples of ADHD and non-ADHD participants. *J Am Acad Child Adolesc Psychiatry.* 2006;45(7):824–832

Barkley RA. Major life activity and health outcomes associated with attention-deficit/hyperactivity disorder. *J Clin Psychiatry.* 2002;63(suppl 12):10–15

Molina BS, Hinshaw SP, Swanson JM, et al. The MTA at 8 years: prospective follow-up of children treated for combined-type ADHD in a multisite study. *J Am Acad Child Adolesc Psychiatry.* 2009;48(5):484–500

National Center for Education in Maternal and Child Health. *Bright Futures in Practice: Mental Health—Volume II, Tool Kit.* http://www.brightfutures.org/ mentalhealth/pdf/tools.html. Accessed December 13, 2013

Pliszka S; American Academy of Child and Adolescent Psychiatry Work Group on Quality Issues. Practice parameter for the assessment and treatment of children and adolescents with attention-deficit/hyperactivity disorder. *J Am Acad Child Adolesc Psychiatry.* 2007;46(7):894–921

Pliszka SR, Crismon ML, Hughes CW, et al. The Texas Children's Medication Algorithm Project: revision of the algorithm for pharmacotherapy of attention-deficit/hyperactivity disorder. *J Am Acad Child Adolesc Psychiatry.* 2006;45(6): 642–657

Rojas NL, Chan E. Old and new controversies in the alternative treatment of attention-deficit hyperactivity disorder. *Ment Retard Dev Diabil Res Rev.* 2005; 11(2):116–130

Swanson JM, Kraemer HC, Hinshaw SP, et al. Clinical relevance of the primary findings of the MTA: success rates based on severity of ADHD and ODD symptoms at the end of treatment. *J Am Acad Child Adolesc Psychiatry.* 2001; 40(2):168–179

WETA. LD OnLine. http://www.ldonline.org. Accessed December 13, 2013

CHAPTER 130

Psychopharmacology in Children

Robin Steinberg-Epstein, MD, and Kenneth W. Steinhoff, MD

CASE STUDY

An 8-year-old girl has been diagnosed with high-functioning autism spectrum disorder. The local developmental-behavioral pediatrician has recommended treating her anxiety and inattention with atomoxetine. The girl's mom is very hesitant. She trusts you and wants your opinion.

Questions

1. How does one assess the safety and appropriateness of psychotropic medications?
2. What kind of blood tests are used to maximize safe administration and how often are they performed?
3. What is the evidence that psychotropic medications are overprescribed?
4. What are the usual side effects of commonly used psychotropic medications?

Psychopharmacologic agents are now used with greater frequency in the pediatric population. Approximately 50% of children and adolescents will, at some point before age 18 years, meet criteria for a psychiatric diagnosis. Almost a quarter of children will have substantial impairment as a result of those symptoms. Unlike antibiotics or other medications used in children, psychopharmacologic agents are used daily and for extended periods. Furthermore, it is important to recognize that there is a dearth of evidence-based information supporting the use of many medications in children, including psychotropic medications. Therefore, most of these medications are used in an **off-label** fashion. The medical community must then rely on published data (often in adult subjects), clinical experience, and expert consensus to guide medication choice, dose, and management. This often provokes parental anxiety and sparks numerous concerns from families who don't understand that the US Food and Drug Administration (FDA) label limits the claims a manufacturer can make but does not limit a clinician's use of medications. Furthermore, families are often anxious because clinicians rely almost exclusively on history and structured behavioral observation, which is the most important "test" for most of these disorders. Unfortunately, there is a national shortage of pediatric subspecialists trained to choose, monitor, and manage these medications for children. It is, therefore, necessary for pediatricians to be familiar with the various medication classes and the controversies facing families of affected children.

Pediatricians need to understand the principles guiding the use of these medications and become familiar with some of the more frequently used psychopharmacologic agents. The most used classes of medication in children include **stimulants, selective norepinephrine reuptake inhibitors (SNRIs), selective serotonin reuptake inhibitors (SSRIs),** and **atypical neuroleptics,** also known as **serotonin-dopamine antagonists (SDAs).** This information can also be useful in helping families navigate this confusing maze.

The decision to use psychopharmacologic agents should not be made without considerable thought. Medication should be an integral part of a comprehensive treatment program that addresses the academic, behavioral, medical, and developmental needs of the child. The decision to place a child on any agent should be based on significant dysfunction as well as discussion and full disclosure of potential risks and benefits with the parents and child. Rating scales should be employed and target symptoms identified as a means of monitoring medication benefit. A medication trial, once undertaken, should be carefully monitored, methodically addressing adverse events and effectiveness. It is generally best to change one agent or dose at a time, followed by structured observation (eg, rating scale[s]) to determine the effect of the change. Therefore, one usually begins with **monotherapy,** optimizes the dose, and assesses risks and benefits before developing a more complex regimen. Such a trial necessitates frequent visits and discussion with the administering physician. Given current scientific information and clinical experience, the use of psychopharmacologic agents in young children (<5 years) should be reserved for extraordinary circumstances.

It should come as no surprise that children are not little adults. Pharmacokinetics in children is affected by increased rates of metabolism in their relatively larger livers, a faster glomerular filtration, and variable fatty tissues. Some children, therefore, require a larger dose than those used for adults. Conversely, perhaps due to size, fat distribution, and other explanations, a much smaller, and seemingly ineffective, dose may be enough. There is little correlation between blood level and treatment response for most agents. Furthermore, some medications have a duration of effects that well exceed their **half-life** (atomoxetine), but for others (eg, stimulants), their effect diminishes despite having a significant blood level. Additionally, for most agents (eg, stimulants, SDAs), there is no correlation with milligrams per kilogram. Frequent clinical monitoring and communication with parents and family are vital to understanding medication benefit and adherence.

Psychostimulants

Psychostimulants (see Chapter 129) are the most studied psychotropic medications used in pediatrics. These medications are used to treat the hyperactivity, inattention, and impulsivity seen with **attention-deficit/hyperactivity disorder (ADHD)** and disturbances of attention seen in other disorders (eg, **autism spectrum disorder [ASD], traumatic brain injury, depression).** Stimulants are also used in the treatment of **narcolepsy.** Over the past decade, many new delivery systems have been developed with differing durations of action, which help to cater to the specific lifestyle needs of the patient. Much work has been done to determine optimal blood level delivery leading to the most consistent effect. Overall, the duration of action and clinical efficacy are more relevant than the blood level in this class of medication.

The mechanism of action of psychostimulants is to increase **dopamine** and **norepinephrine** in the synapse. Overall, this enhances activity in the **prefrontal cortex** of the brain responsible for attention, focus, and **executive function** (organization and planning).

There is substantial evidence in multisite, double-blind, placebo-controlled studies (eg, Multimodal Treatment Study of Children With Attention-Deficit/Hyperactivity Disorder) to support the first-line use of these medications in the treatment of school-aged children and adolescents with ADHD. There is evolving evidence (Preschool Attention-Deficit/Hyperactivity Disorder Treatment Study) to support the use of these drugs in preschoolers. There is a growing body of evidence to support their use in ASD, albeit at lower doses and with a lower threshold for side effects.

Parents have a variety of concerns related to stimulants, much of which is propagated by the media; however, not treating ADHD results in significant comorbidities and risks for negative outcomes. Nonetheless, several areas of controversy exist and often become a primary focus for hesitant parents. Understanding the facts can help to demystify these medications for parents. For example, a risk of substance abuse has long been linked with stimulant medication. There is a substantial body of evidence to show that the use of stimulant medication does **not** lead to an increased risk of later substance abuse. In fact, it is the untreated ADHD, linked with the development of maladaptive behaviors, that places adolescents at a higher risk of substance abuse. The hypothesis is that treatment of ADHD with stimulant medication will actually reduce substance abuse and

a whole host of other potential negative outcomes, such as early tobacco use, undesired pregnancy, and motor vehicle crashes. More long-term studies will be needed to clarify this issue.

Another frequently raised concern includes the association between stimulants and an increase in sudden unexpected deaths. This would obviously raise discomfort for any parent. However, scrutiny over these statistics by the FDA actually revealed a lower incidence of sudden unexpected deaths in those on stimulants compared with the unmedicated population. Those who died tended to have an underlying cardiac defect. This led to the FDA recommendation (2006) that those persons with **preexisting cardiac conditions** not use stimulants and those families with a history of cardiac structural defects or sudden unexpected death receive an echocardiogram and cardiac clearance prior to starting medication.

Height suppression has also historically been raised as a concern with these medications. Numerous studies have tried to answer this question. A recent longitudinal study (over 10 years) supports an initial growth suppression emphasized in the first 3 years that appears to resolve over the remaining 7. Parents can be further reassured that if there is height suppression, it seems to be minimal, in the range of 1.5 cm. It is better to have a high school graduate who is slightly shorter than a taller dropout. Finally, parents believe that their children will be "zombies" on medication. Children who are overmedicated can appear glassy-eyed and overly passive, but good communication and interaction between families and doctors will quickly alleviate this problem. Additional information about these medications may be found in Chapter 129.

Selective Norepinephrine Reuptake Inhibitors

The SNRIs presently include one medication that is frequently used in children: **atomoxetine** (Strattera). Atomoxetine is used in the treatment of ADHD and for the **inattention** and **anxiety** associated with ASD.

The mechanism of action for atomoxetine is to block the reuptake of norepinephrine in the synapse. This may have a direct effect on enhancing the signal-to-noise ratio in the brain and may also ultimately lead to an increase in dopamine in the prefrontal cortex of the brain. Unlike stimulant medications, atomoxetine avoids the nucleus accumbens so that it has no abuse liability.

Atomoxetine was originally studied as an antidepressant, but early investigation did not yield robust antidepressant effects. Marketed as providing "continuous symptom relief," a careful duration of action study shows little effect on core ADHD symptoms after 9 hours, but some possible other small effects (compliance) may last slightly longer. Its attractiveness stems from its identity as an FDA-approved **non-stimulant.** Although usually less effective than stimulants, it has a different side-effect profile and may show slight mood benefits.

Research shows that this medication, which is FDA approved for ADHD, is effective in treating symptoms of this disorder for a given individual but in groups of people is not as effective as stimulant medications. Atomoxetine generally has a 60% response rate (measured by 25% reduction in ADHD ratings) compared with a 70% to 80% response (measured by 30% reduction in ADHD ratings) found in stimulant medications. Furthermore, 3 different head-to-head studies with stimulants have demonstrated atomoxetine as less effective on average; however, some individual patients do well with this medication. It should especially be considered in cases of stimulant failure (poor tolerance or poor effect of a trial on a methylphenidate preparation and a trial on an amphetamine preparation), worries about substance use and diversion, exacerbation of tic disorder with stimulants, and the presence of comorbid anxiety or ASD.

This medication is not without **side effects,** which are very similar to traditional stimulants with the added concerns of drowsiness, dizziness, and cough. Furthermore, atomoxetine carries a warning citing a slightly increased risk of suicidal thought similar to SSRIs. It is not associated with tic exacerbation. Response to this medicine is more like that of an antidepressant in that it may take 4 to 6 weeks to see the full effect of a particular dose. The dosage range is 0.5 mg/kg to 1.8 mg/kg. Those on the autism spectrum tend to respond at lower doses and with a lower threshold for adverse side effects.

There have been a few reports of a serious **idiosyncratic reaction** suggesting liver failure. These patients were on FDA-approved doses of atomoxetine for several months. They had vomiting, jaundice, and elevated liver enzymes. These findings resolved off medication and returned with reexposure to the drug. This led to an FDA warning to consider potential liver failure in a vomiting patient on atomoxetine.

In consideration of stimulants and SNRIs, the American Academy of Pediatrics and American Academy of Child and Adolescent Psychiatry recommend stimulants and SNRIs as first-line treatments for ADHD. There is no indication that blood or urine tests need to be monitored for either class of medication. Improvement, adverse event, and adherence monitoring using rating scales should occur regularly—at least every 3 months (once dose and agent have been optimized).

Parents often want to know if these medications can be used intermittently and stopped as soon as possible. Stimulants and SNRIs have their best results when administered 7 days a week and without large breaks. Longitudinal studies suggest that while some symptoms may resolve over time, significant impairment from even a small number of symptoms persists into adulthood for 60% to 70%

of those diagnosed with ADHD. Therefore, many people may continue on medication for a number of years. To assess for continued benefit, a break from medication should be attempted annually. It is beneficial to re-optimize doses and agents throughout treatment. As children grow larger, they often need higher doses. However, as compensatory mechanisms develop and some symptoms subside, some patients may require less medication. "Holidays" from medications have no established intrinsic value on their own and should only be recommended for children with significant medication side effects such as substantial weight loss. If a parent is requesting a **drug holiday,** it is a signal that the parent may need to review the value of the medication. A discussion should ensue as to whether the parent and child continue to see benefit, the patient is having troubling side effects, or the medication at any dose is not helpful with concerning symptoms. Consider that atomoxetine, once stopped, needs time to rebuild in the system.

Selective Serotonin Reuptake Inhibitors

Selected serotonin reuptake inhibitors (Table 130-1) are frequently used in children and adolescents to treat a variety of depression- and anxiety-based symptoms (Box 130-1). Similar to SNRIs, SSRIs block presynaptic reuptake of serotonin after it is released into the synapse, thereby enhancing serotonin activity in the synapse. Empirical evidence has established their benefit in the treatment of depressive and anxiety disorders.

Medication is not a substitute for therapeutic support. As a matter of fact, most clinical guidelines recommend psychotherapy as first-line treatment for most anxiety and depressive disorders in children. Biologic intervention should only be undertaken if psychotherapy progress is minimal or impairment severe. **Obsessive-compulsive disorder** (OCD) is a unique anxiety disorder that typically requires

---

Box 130-1. Disorders Treated by Selective Serotonin Reuptake Inhibitors	
• Depression	• Selective mutism
• Obsessive-compulsive disorder	• Post-traumatic stress disorder
• Generalized anxiety disorder	• Autism spectrum disorder
• Separation anxiety disorder	• Bulimia
• Panic disorder	

Table 130-1. Selective Serotonin Reuptake Inhibitors						
Generic	*Product*	*FDA Pediatric Approval*	*Suggested Pediatric Dose, mg*	*Half-life*	*Time Steady State, days*
Fluoxetine	Prozac	Depression/OCD	2.5–60	4–6 d	28–35
Sertraline	Zoloft	OCD	12.5–200	26 h	5–7
Fluvoxamine	Luvox	OCD	12.5–100 bid	15 h	5–7
Paroxetine	Paxil	None	5–30	21 h	5–10
Citalopram	Celexa	None	5–40	36 h	7
Escitalopram	Lexapro	Depression	2.5–20	27–32 h	7

Abbreviations: bid, twice a day; FDA, US Food and Drug Administration; OCD, obsessive-compulsive disorder.

higher doses of SSRIs but is also responsive to a specific form of cognitive-behavioral therapy that includes exposure response prevention.

Medications are chosen based on side-effect profile and half-life. Due to a significant placebo effect and a lack of multiple, large, highly powered studies in children, only a few have any FDA approval in children (see Table 130-1). There are numerous studies that may not meet strict scientific criteria but taken together with vast clinical experience and consensus imply reasonably well-tolerated and beneficial effects of these medications. Studies have consistently found SSRIs to be more effective and safer than tricyclic antidepressants as a treatment for depression.

These drugs are metabolized via the liver through the **cytochrome P450 system.** There are individual enzyme variations that lead to variable metabolism of any of the many medications that travel through these pathways. Overwhelming this system may lead to inhibition and buildup of medications or facilitated rapid metabolism of others. Thus, monitoring of all medications metabolized via this pathway is necessary. Reduced metabolism of SSRIs may lead to **serotonin syndrome,** a relatively rare response to a flood of serotonin, presenting with confusion, hypomania, restlessness, diaphoresis, shivering, tremor, hyperreflexia, and diarrhea. This syndrome often goes unrecognized and these patients may find their way to a pediatrician's office or emergency department (ED). Occasionally, the combination of an SSRI with an atypical antipsychotic or stimulant may precipitate such a response.

Many children with anxiety or depression go on to experience intermittent exacerbations throughout life. This does not mean that they should stay on these medications forever. Present recommendations support an initial 6- to 12-month treatment period with the SSRI that provided response. If the symptoms return after discontinuation, the next trial should last 2 years. Finally, if the symptoms again return, this suggests longer-term treatment. Occasionally, symptoms will not respond the next time the same agent is used.

Selective serotonin reuptake inhibitors are generally well tolerated with mild transient side effects such as gastrointestinal symptoms, headache, increased motor activity, or insomnia. One needs to monitor for less common side effects like disinhibition, a phenomenon of increased impulsive behaviors in association with SSRIs that is usually dose related. Those with ASDs are particularly susceptible to this response.

There are no specific recommendations on dose other than to start low and go slow. Typically, effects may be seen between 1 and 4 weeks. The value of increasing the dose (except in the case of OCD) versus continuing on at the same dose versus changing agents is not clear until a patient has been treated for at least a month. See suggested dosage ranges in Table 130-1.

A withdrawal phenomenon can occur, especially if SSRIs are discontinued suddenly. This risk is inversely proportional to the half-life. For example, paroxetine, with its short half-life, tends to be associated with a far greater risk of withdrawal symptoms than something with a longer half-life, such as fluoxetine. This "syndrome" may present as flu-like symptoms, including vomiting, diarrhea, and body aches. Simply re-administering the skipped dose and tapering off over a week or two alleviates symptomatology.

Again, controversy follows these medications. In 2004, the FDA created a black box warning advising that children and adolescents on SSRIs should be monitored for worsening depression, agitation, and suicidality, particularly in the early stages of treatment. This warning came out of an FDA meta-analysis showing an increased risk of suicidal ideation in depressed teens soon after starting the medications. No completed suicides occurred. This prompted an FDA recommendation to see children placed on SSRIs weekly for a month, then bimonthly for a month, then monthly, and, ultimately, at longer regular intervals. This expectation was felt to be impractical for clinicians in practice. Therefore, these recommendations have recently been relaxed to incorporate physician judgment. It is advised to monitor each individual patient carefully, but the potential for benefit usually outweighs the risks. These concerns should not detract from the importance of these medications.

The FDA warning led to a decrease in prescriptions of SSRIs, which resulted in the first increase in the suicide rate since the FDA SSRI approval. The FDA warnings should serve only to increase awareness, not be a contraindication. An increase in suicidality has not been noted in adolescents with isolated anxiety or ASD. Selective serotonin reuptake inhibitors serve a vital role in helping children paralyzed by anxiety, obsession, and depression to lead more normal lives.

Atypical Antipsychotics (Serotonergic Dopamine Antagonists)

Atypical antipsychotics or **second-generation antipsychotics** (Table 130-2), also known as **SDAs,** are medications with dopamine D2 and serotonin 5-hydroxytryptamine type 2 antagonism. These newer medications offer a lower risk of **extrapyramidal side effects** like **dystonia; akathisia,** a feeling of restlessness; tremor; tardive dyskinesia; and hyperprolactinemia compared with conventional antipsychotics. However, these medications carry significant cardio-metabolic risks.

Table 130-2. Serotonin-Dopamine Antagonists (Atypical Antipsychotics)

Generic	Product	FDA Pediatric Approval	Dose
Risperidone	Risperdal	Agitation with ASD, schizophrenia, mania, and bipolar disorder	0.25–10 mg/d
Olanzapine	Zyprexa	Bipolar mania and schizophrenia	2.5–20 mg/d
Quetiapine	Seroquel	Bipolar mania	12.5–250 mg bid
Ziprasidone	Geodon	None	20–120 mg/d
Aripiprazole	Abilify	Agitation with ASD, schizophrenia, mania, and bipolar disorder	0.5–30 mg/d

Abbreviations: ASD, autism spectrum disorder; bid, twice a day; FDA, US Food and Drug Administration.

Although initially billed as a safer alternative to traditional antipsychotics, some have suggested that these newer medications merely substitute one set of severe side effects for another. These medications offer benefits for severe behaviors that are not responsive to other intervention.

While often used off-label, these medications are incorporated into best practice clinical guidelines for psychotic depression, schizophrenia, bipolar disorder, oppositional defiant disorder, conduct disorder, agitation in intellectual disability, Tourette syndrome, stuttering, and ASD. The only diagnoses for which an atypical antipsychotic has pediatric approval are schizophrenia, bipolar disorder, mania, and agitation associated with ASD. Therefore, while these medications often lack enough empiric evidence to be validated for all the indications mentioned, clinical consensus by experts recommend judicious use in treating children with serious mental illness after other forms of intervention have failed or in cases of severe psychosis or aggression. These medications should not be used to promote weight gain, as a sedative or sleep aid, or as a treatment for ADHD.

Medications are chosen based on clinical experience and side-effect profile. These medications are not innocuous; they must be used with full disclosure to parents. The most common side effects are listed in Box 130-2. The severity of some of the side effects deserves discussion. The SDAs, with the possible exception of aripiprazole, have caused significant increases in weight, glucose, and lipids and decreases in sensitivity to insulin, otherwise known as *metabolic syndrome.*

There have been transient elevations of **prolactin** among recipients of these medications. The clinical significance of this increase is unclear. Weight gain frequently accompanies these medications and must be monitored. Long QT syndrome on electrocardiogram (ECG) is rarely noted and has not been associated with death but remains a clinical concern.

Risperidone is the best studied medication of its class for children. However, the studies on which its FDA approvals hinged exposed side effects, most notably weight gain. Therefore, anticipatory counseling on diet management is routinely recommended. Another important finding indicated that a small but significant number of children with agitation and ASD were successfully able to stop treatment after 6 months, suggesting that a trial off medication may be warranted in those patients with agitation and ASD successfully treated for 6 months.

Neuroleptic malignant syndrome is a rare, potentially life-threatening complication of neuroleptics that is extremely unlikely with the newer generation of medication. However, because of its lethality and potential presentation to a pediatric office or ED, this entity should be mentioned. Neuroleptic malignant syndrome is characterized by hyperthermia, autonomic instability, diaphoresis, lead pipe rigidity, increased creatine phosphokinase due to rhabdomyolysis, and delirium. It may occur at any point during treatment with these medications.

There is no set agreement on appropriate monitoring of these medications in children. Most conservative suggestions include following body mass index (BMI) at each visit, after 6 weeks, and again each 9 to 12 months, and checking complete blood cell count, a comprehensive chemistry including liver function tests, triiodothyronine, thyroxine, HbA_{1c}, prolactin, fasting glucose, and lipid levels, especially in children who are overweight or families with a history of diabetes mellitus. An ECG prior to starting medications, 1 month after baseline, and biannually are only necessary for children on ziprasidone to monitor the QT interval. Children are often sent to the primary care physician to obtain these tests and monitor BMI.

As with any medication, psychotropic agents are sometimes incorrectly prescribed. By and large, however, psychopharmacologic agents are still underused in the treatment of many disorders. Hopefully, new and ongoing research will help physicians recognize mental illness in children and substantiate and refine the use of such medications in their care.

Careful thought and discussion of target symptoms as well as side effects will help physicians choose the best medication and treatment plan. It will also prepare parents to observe the positive and negative responses to medication.

While this chapter goes into significant detail on side effects, it is critical to understand that the diseases being treated are often incapacitating. Informed consent and parent and child involvement are vital in medication choice. Pediatricians have an extremely influential voice in supporting compliance. Therefore, knowledgeable guidance is crucial in helping parents make an uncomfortable and difficult decision that may ultimately lead to dramatic improvements in quality of life.

Box 130-2. Serotonin-Dopamine Antagonists: Potential Side Effects	
• Weight gain	• Dry mouth
• Sedation	• Headache
• Dizziness	• Increased liver function tests
• Hypotension	• Decreased triiodothyronine, thyroxine
• Long QT syndrome	
• Metabolic syndrome (hyperglycemia and increased lipids)	• Extrapyramidal side effects
	• Akathisia (sense of restlessness)
• Constipation	• Cataracts (in dogs)

CASE RESOLUTION

You empathize with the mother over this decision but are able to explain that this medication is a reasonable and safe one to try. The patient starts the medication and experiences some nausea in the first few days. With your reassurance, this resolves. Her mother calls a few weeks later to thank you for your advice and to let you know that while her daughter still has difficulties from the autism spectrum disorder, she seems to be somewhat less anxious and is functioning better at school.

Selected References

American Academy of Pediatrics Subcommittee on Attention-Deficit/Hyperactivity Disorder, Steering Committee on Quality Improvement and Management. ADHD: clinical practice guideline for the diagnosis and treatment of attention-deficit/hyperactivity disorder in children and adolescents. *Pediatrics.* 2011;128(5): 1007–1022

Autism and Developmental Disabilities Monitoring Network Surveillance Year 2006 Principal Investigators; Centers for Disease Control and Prevention. Prevalence of autism spectrum disorders—Autism and Developmental Disabilities Monitoring Network, United States, 2006. *MMWR Surveill Summ.* 2009;58(10): 1–20

Biederman J, Spencer TJ, Monuteaux MC, Faraone SV. A naturalistic 10-year prospective study of height and weight in children with attention-deficit hyperactivity disorder grown up: sex and treatment effects. *J Pediatr.* 2010;157(4): 635–640

Correll CU, Kratochvil CJ, March JS. Developments in pediatric psychopharmacology: focus on stimulants, antidepressants, and antipsychotics. *J Clin Psychiatry.* 2011;72(5):655–670

Filipek PA, Steinberg-Epstein R, Book TM. Intervention for autism spectrum disorders. *NeuroRx.* 2006;3(2):207–216

Greenhill L, Kollins S, Abikoff H, et al. Efficacy and safety of immediate-release methylphenidate treatment for preschoolers with ADHD. *J Am Acad Child Adolesc Psychiatry.* 2006;45(11):1284–1293

Hammad TA, Laughren T, Racoosin J. Suicidality in pediatric patients treated with antidepressant drugs. *Arch Gen Psychiatry.* 2006;63(3):332–339

March J, Silva S, Petrycki S, et al. Fluoxetine, cognitive-behavioral therapy, and their combination for adolescents with depression: Treatment for Adolescents With Depression Study (TADS) randomized controlled trial. *JAMA.* 2004;292(7): 807–820

McCracken JT, McGough J, Shah B, et al. Risperidone in children with autism and serious behavior problems. *N Engl J Med.* 2002;347(5):314–321

Merikangas KR, He JP, Burstein M, et al. Lifetime prevalence of mental disorders in US adolescents: results from the National Comorbidity Survey Replication—Adolescent Supplement (NCS-A). *J Am Acad Child Adolesc Psychiatry.* 2010; 49(10):980–989

MTA Cooperative Group. A 14-month randomized clinical trial of treatment strategies for attention-deficit/hyperactivity disorder. Multimodal Treatment Study of Children with ADHD. *Arch Gen Psychiatry.* 1999;56(12):1073–1086

National Autism Center. http://www.nationalautismcenter.org. Accessed March 13, 2014

Pediatric OCD Treatment Study (POTS) Team. Cognitive-behavior therapy, sertraline, and their combination for children and adolescents with obsessive-compulsive disorder: the Pediatric OCD Treatment Study (POTS) randomized controlled trial. *JAMA.* 2004;292(16):1969–1976

Pliszka S; AACAP Work Group on Quality Issues. Practice parameters for the assessment and treatment of children and adolescents with attention-deficit/hyperactivity disorder. *J Am Acad Child Adolesc Psychiatry.* 2007;46(7): 894–921

Sadock B, Sadock V. *Kaplan and Sadock's Synopsis of Psychiatry.* 9th ed. Philadelphia, PA: Lippincott Williams & Wilkins; 2003

Steinberg-Epstein R, Book T, Wigal SB. Controversies surrounding pediatric psychopharmacology. *Adv Pediatr.* 2011;58(1):153–179

US Food and Drug Administration Center for Drug Evaluation and Research Psychopharmacologic Drugs Advisory Committee. Sparlon (Provigil/Modafinil) Cephalon Inc. NDA 20-717 (S-109). http://www.fda.gov/ohrms/dockets/ac/06/slides/2006-4212S1-01-01-FDAMannheim.ppt. Created March 23, 2006. Accessed March 13, 2014

Walkup JT, Albano AM, Piacentini J, et al. Cognitive-behavioral therapy, sertraline, or a combination in childhood anxiety. *N Engl J Med.* 2008;359(26): 2753–2766

Wigal T, Wigal S, Shanklin A, Kapelinski A, Steinberg-Epstein R. ADHD in preschoolers: a diagnosis or just a "phase"? *Consult Pediatr.* 2008;(suppl):S2–S8

CHAPTER 131

Physical Abuse

Melissa K. Egge, MD, and Sara T. Stewart, MD

CASE STUDY

A 6-month-old boy arrives at the emergency department after becoming limp and nonresponsive at home. The mother states that her son was fine when she left him in the care of her boyfriend before going to the store for cigarettes. When she returned 1 hour later, he was asleep, but then he seized and stopped breathing. The infant is being ventilated by bag-valve-mask ventilation. On examination, the infant is pale and limp. His heart rate is 50 beats/min and blood pressure is 130/80 mm Hg. There are no external signs of injury.

Questions

1. What are the major lethal injuries associated with physical abuse of children?
2. What are the types of injuries seen in physically abused children?
3. What are the presenting signs in children with head injuries?
4. What are the legal obligations of physicians in the area of child abuse?

Physical child abuse was first described in the pediatric literature in 1962 by Kempe et al in their classic paper on the **battered child syndrome.** Child abuse or maltreatment takes many forms, including physical abuse, **failure to thrive** (Chapter 133), **sexual abuse** (Chapter 132), **emotional abuse, prenatal exposure to substances** such as drugs and alcohol (Chapter 135), and **pediatric condition falsification (also referred to as medical child abuse),** a complex disorder previously known as Munchausen syndrome by proxy in which parents confabulate or create a medical condition in their children.

The nature and extent of inflicted injuries are variable and may include **bruises, burns, fractures, lacerations, internal hemorrhage,** and **ruptures.** Physicians must be aware of the legal obligations related to the suspicion of child abuse. They must assess the nature of the injuries, initiate appropriate medical therapy, and determine if the history offered is consistent with the medical findings.

Epidemiology

It is estimated that the rate of childhood victimization in the United States is 10 per 1,000 and that approximately 15% to 20% of these children suffer some form of physical abuse. Certain factors are associated with physical abuse. Most victims are young children; two-thirds are younger than 3 years and one-third are younger than 6 months. Caring for young children is frequently demanding, so crying infants and toilet-training toddlers are particularly at risk for abuse. Factors such as **lower socioeconomic class, substance abuse, poor parenting skills,** and **domestic violence** place children at increased risk for abuse.

Clinical Presentation

Children who have been physically abused present with injuries that range from non-severe to lethal (D_x Box). Visible bruises, bites, and burns may be noted. Children may also have symptoms related to fractures, such as crying or refusal to walk or move an extremity. More severely injured children may present with seizures, apnea, shock, or cardiopulmonary arrest.

Pathophysiology

Injuries in children who experience physical abuse are the result of direct trauma inflicted on the children. Abusive parents often have unrealistic expectations of their children, leading to frustration and abuse when the child does not meet the expectations. Parents who have often been victims of abuse themselves know only corporal punishment as a disciplinary modality. These parents often exhibit poor impulse control; they do not intend to harm their children but desire to alter their children's behavior. As a result, sometimes the outcome is unexpected.

Physical Abuse

- Bruises
- Bites
- Burns
- Fractures
- Intracranial hemorrhage
- Intra-abdominal hemorrhage
- Apparent life-threatening event
- Retinal hemorrhage
- History that changes
- Injuries not explained by history

Head injuries, the most deadly form of abuse, may result from a direct blow to the head or from rotational head movement (eg, shaking). Classically, a crying infant is vigorously shaken and suffers **diffuse axonal injury** or **intracranial hemorrhage.** In particular, subdural hemorrhage may occur from shearing of the bridging veins. The infant may also become apneic during or after the trauma. Seizures, cerebral edema, hypoxic brain injury, and retinal hemorrhages may also occur. Such injuries are frequently associated with a fatal outcome or long-term damage to the central nervous system.

Abdominal trauma is the second most common cause of fatal child abuse and is typically due to a direct blow to the abdomen. Skeletal fractures result from multiple different types of traumatic forces to the bones. Rib fractures are most classically associated with the head trauma of shaking and are due to compression of the ribs by the hands that are holding the infant or child.

Differential Diagnosis

When evaluating children with physical injuries, the major differentiation is the distinguishing of injuries that are **abusive or inflicted** from those that are **accidental.** Practitioners should be suspicious of changing histories, histories that are inconsistent with the injuries sustained, and histories that do not match the developmental capabilities of the child. Unwitnessed injuries in young children, particularly pre-ambulatory infants, should also be suspect.

Bruises, burns, and fractures may be abusive or accidental. Normal ambulatory children commonly sustain bruises over bony prominences such as the forehead, elbows, and shins with unintentional, accidental trauma. Bruises over soft areas such as the cheeks or the pinnae of the ear, as well as bruises on protected areas such as the inner thighs or neck, are more suggestive of inflicted trauma. Injuries to the oral mucosa may result from efforts at forced feeding or occlusion of the mouth in an effort to silence crying. **Retinal hemorrhages** in infants most often result from abusive head trauma, such as shaking. They may also be due to other medical conditions that can usually be discerned from the history and physical examination and by consultation with an ophthalmologist. Ideally, a pediatric ophthalmologist performs indirect retinal examination of dilated eyes within 24 hours of the patient's admission (Box 131-1).

Children may be intentionally burned by being immersed in hot water or having hot objects such as irons or cigarettes held against them. Children who are immersed in hot water develop circumferential burns that may envelop an entire extremity. Such a burn is usually in a glove or stocking pattern or in a doughnut pattern on the buttocks. These burns are distinct from splash or spill burns, which take on an irregular drip pattern. In distinguishing inflicted from accidental burns, a scene investigation is often helpful to measure the water temperature in the home water heater and determine the length of time required to reach that temperature in the location of the alleged incident. Families should be advised to set their water heaters to 120°F to prevent accidental scald injuries.

Long bone fractures (especially humerus and femur) should be suspect, particularly in preverbal or pre-ambulatory children. Certain fractures, such as **classic metaphyseal lesions** and **rib, sternum,** and **scapula fractures** are highly suggestive of inflicted trauma.

Numerous medical conditions may mimic abuse. Bullous impetigo may resemble burns. A coagulopathy may lead to multiple bruises. Leukemia, thrombocytopenia, and aplastic anemia are also associated with bruising. Osteogenesis imperfecta or rickets may result in multiple fractures. Bone cysts and osteoporosis due to inactivity from multiple causes (eg, cerebral palsy, paralysis, meningomyelocele) may predispose to the development of pathologic fractures.

Evaluation

Children who present with injuries need to be evaluated with a careful history and complete physical examination. Infants with altered mental status, apnea, or seizures should be evaluated in a similar manner because their symptoms may be secondary to intracranial injury.

History

The history should focus on an explanation for the medical findings (Questions Box) and, in infants and toddlers, a thorough developmental history should be included. Children should be interviewed alone if they are of an appropriate age. Physicians should determine

Box 131-1. Causes of Mild Retinal Hemorrhages	
• Abusive head trauma	• Hyponatremia or hypernatremia
• Unintentional head trauma	• Vasculitis
• Birth trauma	• Papilledema
• Retinopathy of prematurity	• Hypertension
• Blood dyscrasia	• Cytomegalovirus retinitis
• Leukemia/lymphoma	• High-altitude illness
• Meningitis/sepsis	• Carbon monoxide toxicity
• Extracorporeal membrane oxygenation	• Osteogenesis imperfecta
	• Glutaric aciduria

Questions

Physical Abuse

- What caused the injury?
- Was the child healthy until the injury occurred?
- Has the child sustained similar injuries in the past?
- Is there a family history of any conditions that would account for easy bruising or fragility of the bones (eg, von Willebrand disease, osteogenesis imperfecta)?
- Is the child developmentally normal? What are the child's motor skills?
- Who was with the child when the injury occurred?
- What was done immediately after the injury? Was medical care sought?

if other risk factors, such as domestic violence or substance abuse, are present.

Physical Examination

A child's state of hygiene and growth parameters should be noted, and the physical examination should be comprehensive. The location, color, and size of bruises, abrasions, lacerations, or other skin trauma should be recorded. Dating of bruises cannot be done because the degradation rate of hemoglobin, and therefore the rate of color change, varies according to the depth and extent of the bruise and by the child's health and nutritional status. Large blue-gray spots, which occur commonly on the back and buttocks in darker-skinned children, are termed *mongolian spots* or *congenital dermal melanocytosis*. These should not be mistaken for bruises.

Medical practitioners should also note any skin findings that resemble characteristic patterns of inflicted skin trauma, such as slap marks to the face or gag marks around the mouth. Pinch marks can also be seen on the genitalia of a toilet-training toddler. Belts, cords, and blunt objects may leave patterned marks on the skin after a child is hit with the object. Bite marks are composed of indentations, bruises, or breaks in the skin that reflect the configuration of teeth that is unique to the perpetrator (Figure 131-1). Inflicted burns may also assume a characteristic pattern depending on the mechanism of injury (Figure 131-2).

The extremities, skull, and rib cage should be carefully examined to detect the presence of skeletal trauma. Findings such as decreased range of movement, tenderness, swelling, redness, or bruising may be associated with an underlying bone fracture. These findings are not always present, however, particularly if the fracture is in its healing stages.

Practitioners should be aware that infants with head or abdominal injuries may also present with no external signs of trauma. Those with head injury may have seizures, apnea, vomiting, increased crying, or altered mental status, often with no explanation as to the etiology. The retina should be evaluated for hemorrhages in these children. Children with abdominal injuries may present in shock or with symptoms such as vomiting, abdominal pain, or distention. They may have a rigid abdomen with guarding and decreased bowel sounds. Inflicted abdominal injuries may include hematomas of the bowel wall, bowel perforations, or trauma to the liver, spleen, pancreas, or kidneys.

Laboratory Tests

Children who present with bruises should have a hematologic assessment with a complete blood cell count (CBC) and differential (including a platelet count), a prothrombin time, and a partial thromboplastin time. Cultures from lesions may help differentiate infection from burn injury.

Children with fractures should be assessed with a chemistry panel (including blood urea nitrogen and creatinine) and calcium, phosphorus, and alkaline phosphatase levels.

Children with suspected abdominal trauma should be evaluated with a CBC, urinalysis, liver function studies, amylase, and lipase. These studies may demonstrate anemia secondary to hemorrhage, hematuria from renal injury, or elevated liver or pancreatic enzymes due to solid or hollow viscus organ trauma (see Chapter 65).

Imaging Studies

Children younger than 2 years who are suspected victims of physical abuse are at the highest risk of having an inflicted skeletal fracture. For this reason, this group of patients should be evaluated with a radiographic skeletal survey to identify any acute or healing fractures that may be present. Bone scintigraphy is also useful in detecting occult fractures and may be useful in conjunction with the skeletal survey. Follow-up skeletal survey (excluding the skull radiograph) in 2 weeks can also be useful to assess for fractures that were not noted at the time of the initial films.

If there is concern that children have suffered non-accidental head trauma, they should be evaluated with a computed tomography (CT) scan and magnetic resonance imaging. The combination of these modalities is particularly helpful in dating intracranial bleeding (see Chapter 67).

Abdominal radiographs may demonstrate air-fluid levels from dysmotility, distended loops of bowel, or free air under the diaphragm. Abdominal and pelvic CT scans with intravenous contrast may show bowel or solid organ disruption or hemorrhage.

Belt buckle | Looped cord | Coat hanger

Knuckles | Bite | Hand

Figure 131-1. Patterned bruises associated with inflicted trauma.

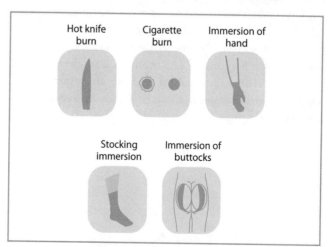

Figure 131-2. Patterned burns associated with inflicted trauma.

Management

The management of children who are suspected victims of abuse focuses on medical stabilization, careful and thorough documentation of medical findings, and psychosocial investigation. Injuries should be treated in the appropriate manner. Children with extensive internal injuries frequently require admission to an intensive care unit. Consultation with appropriate surgical specialists in neurosurgery, orthopedics, or general surgery should be obtained.

The psychosocial assessment of the family often requires the expertise of a social worker. Further assessment may require an in-home evaluation such as that conducted by law enforcement or child protective services. All 50 states require that physicians who suspect child abuse report these suspicions to appropriate agencies. Physicians do not have to be certain of the abuse.

These mandated agencies pursue the investigation and provide supportive family services as needed. Children may be removed from their homes and placed in foster homes to ensure their safety. Cases of suspected abuse are usually evaluated in court to determine the safety of the children's environment, ability of parents to care for their children, and criminal culpability of suspected perpetrators. Physicians may be expected to offer testimony in such hearings.

Prognosis

The prognosis is variable. Some children succumb to inflicted injuries before coming to medical attention, and others sustain permanent neurologic damage. Even in cases in which the physical well-being of children is ensured, their mental and emotional well-being is often significantly affected, requiring intensive and ongoing mental health care.

Recent longitudinal studies in adults have shown a link between adverse childhood experiences and health problems in adulthood.

Prevention

Practitioners should preemptively discuss with families those developmental stages that are at higher risk for parental frustration and subsequent child abuse, including infant colic, toddler potty training, and tantrums. Infant crying is the most common trigger for abusive head injury. Pediatricians may offer guidance in handling these difficult situations and should assess the parents' coping skills with such behaviors when they arise. Pediatricians should also inquire about stressors particular to each family, such as unemployment, mental health issues, social isolation, and intimate partner violence. Support systems for the family should be identified and positive attributes praised.

CASE RESOLUTION

The case study describes a classic case of abusive head trauma. The infant was left alone with an individual with limited parenting skills. The infant has evidence of increased intracranial pressure and may have traumatic axonal injury or intracranial hemorrhage. The infant is intubated, given anticonvulsants, and admitted to a pediatric intensive care unit. Consultation with neurosurgery, ophthalmology, and social services is obtained. Appropriate imaging studies and skeletal surveys are performed when the infant is sufficiently stabilized, and the child is ultimately diagnosed with subdural hemorrhage, retinal hemorrhages, and rib fractures.

Selected References

American Academy of Pediatrics. *Child Abuse: Medical Diagnosis & Management.* Reece RM, Christian C, eds. 3rd ed. Elk Grove Village, IL: American Academy of Pediatrics; 2009

Christian CW, Block R; American Academy of Pediatrics Committee on Child Abuse and Neglect. Abusive head trauma in infants and children. *Pediatrics.* 2009;123(5):1409–1411

Egge MK, Berkowitz CD. Controversies in the evaluation of young children with fractures. *Adv Pediatr.* 2010;57(1):63–83

Flaherty EG, Stirling J; American Academy of Pediatrics Committee on Child Abuse and Neglect. The pediatrician's role in child maltreatment prevention. *Pediatrics.* 2010;126(4):833–841

Leetch AN, Woolridge D. Emergency department evaluation of child abuse. *Emerg Med Clin North Am.* 2013;31(3):853–873

Legano L, McHugh MT, Palusci VJ. Child abuse and neglect. *Curr Probl Pediatr Adolesc Health Care.* 2009;39(2):31.e1–31.e26

Levin AV. Retinal hemorrhages: advances in understanding. *Pediatr Clin North Am.* 2009;56(2):333–344

Offiah A, van Rijn RR, Perez-Rossello JM, Kleinman PK. Skeletal imaging of child abuse (non-accidental injury). *Pediatr Radiol.* 2009;39(5):461–470

Preer G, Sorrentino D, Newton AW. Child abuse pediatrics: prevention, evaluation, and treatment. *Curr Opin Pediatr.* 2012;24(2):266–273

Shipman K, Taussig H. Mental health treatment of child abuse and neglect: the promise of evidence-based practice. *Pediatr Clin North Am.* 2009;56(2):417–428

Stirling J, American Academy of Pediatrics Committee on Child Abuse and Neglect and Section on Adoption and Foster Care; Amaya-Jackson L, American Academy of Child and Adolescent Psychiatry, National Center for Child Traumatic Stress. Understanding the behavioral and emotional consequences of child abuse. *Pediatrics.* 2008;122(3):667–673

Swerdlin A, Berkowitz C, Craft N. Cutaneous signs of child abuse. *J Am Acad Dermatol.* 2007;57(3):371–392

CHAPTER 132

Sexual Abuse

Sara T. Stewart, MD

CASE STUDY

A 4-year-old girl is brought to the emergency department with the complaint of vaginal itching and discharge. Her past health has been good, and she has no medical problems. She lives with her biological parents and her 2-year-old brother.

On physical examination, the vital signs are normal and the child is well except that the genital area is swollen and erythematous and a green vaginal discharge is present. The girl is interviewed briefly but denies that anyone has touched her. The mother states that she has never left her daughter unattended and is angered by the questions.

Questions

1. What are the anogenital findings in prepubescent and postpubescent children who may have experienced sexual abuse?
2. What behavioral problems are common in children who have been sexually abused?
3. What are the pitfalls in disclosure interviews of children who have been sexually abused?
4. What is the significance of sexually transmitted infections in children who have been sexually abused?

Child sexual abuse is the involvement of children and adolescents in sexual activity that they cannot consent to because of their age and developmental level. An age disparity exists between the victims, who are younger, and the perpetrators, who are older. The intent of the abuse is the **sexual gratification** of the older individuals, and the abusive incident(s) may or may not include physical contact. Sexual abuse may include acts of **oral, genital,** or **anal** contact by or to a child and may involve acts such as **exhibitionism** or involvement in **pornography.** It is differentiated from "sexual play" by the difference in the developmental levels of the participants and the coerciveness of the behavior.

Sexual abuse has been recognized with increasing frequency since the 1980s, in part because medical knowledge about the anogenital anatomy in molested and non-molested prepubescent children has expanded. Technical advances have altered the manner in which these children are evaluated. In particular, the colposcope, with its potential for magnification and photographic or videotape documentation, has been valuable. Parental awareness and school-based programs have led to increased disclosures about abuse as well as a greater willingness on the part of adults to believe these disclosures.

Patient interviews are another key component of the assessment process that has been shaped by continued research in the field. Non-leading, open-ended questions are asked by interviewers as few times as possible, and when available, these questions are asked by specialized forensic interviewers.

Epidemiology

In 2011, an estimated 680,000 children were victims of child maltreatment in the United States, and approximately 10% of these are victims of sexual abuse. Exact figures on the prevalence of child sexual abuse are not readily available because they depend on reports of a condition that may not come to medical attention for many years. Anonymous surveys indicate that about 20% to 25% of women and 10% to 15% of men have been sexually abused before reaching adulthood.

Victims of sexual abuse come from all socioeconomic and ethnic groups. Girls experience sexual abuse at a rate 5 times that of boys. Some investigators believe that the statistics for boys are falsely low because boys are generally reluctant to disclose their abuse. Men are more commonly the perpetrators than women, and at least 20% of perpetrators are adolescents. Frequently, the sexual abuse has been occurring for several years. Perpetrators are usually known by the victims, and recent national data showed that 37% of perpetrators were biological parents, 23% were nonbiological parents, and 40% were other individuals. The mean time from onset of abuse to disclosure is 3 years. Sometimes children are not ready to disclose but the abuse is discovered accidentally because the victims develop symptoms, such as vaginal discharge or functional complaints.

Clinical Presentation

Most cases of child sexual abuse come to the attention of authorities after the child **discloses** the abuse. There may or may not be associated physical or behavioral complaints. Physical symptoms in the anogenital area may include **bleeding, pain, swelling, dysuria, vaginal discharge,** or **difficulty stooling.** More often, however, children have no specific anogenital symptoms. Instead, they have nonspecific complaints such as headache, abdominal pain, or vague systemic symptoms such as fatigue (D_x Box).

Behavioral changes may also be noted as these children respond to the stress of their victimization and their environments. These

Child Sexual Abuse

- Anogenital erythema
- Anogenital bleeding
- Genital discharge
- Anogenital scarring
- Behavioral symptoms (eg, encopresis, enuresis)
- Disclosure of abuse
- Somatic complaints (eg, abdominal pain, headache)
- Sexually transmitted infections
- Sexualized behavior
- Pregnancy (adolescents)
- Delinquency, promiscuity (adolescents)

Box 132-1. Conditions Mistaken for Sexual Abuse	
Genital	*Anal*
• Accidental trauma	• Inflammatory bowel disease
• Lichen sclerosus et atrophicus	• Hemorrhoids
• Urethral prolapse	• Anal abscess associated with neutropenia
• Labial adhesions	• Perirectal abscess
• Congenital malformations	• Perianal streptococcal infection
• Hemangioma	

changes may include **sleep disturbances, hyperactivity, enuresis, encopresis, decreased appetite,** and **depression.** Sexually abused adolescents may manifest **school failure, delinquency**, and **suicide** attempts. Children may also respond with sexual behavior or sexual knowledge that is considered to be inappropriate or excessive for age.

Psychophysiology

Children suffer sexual abuse after becoming **entrapped.** They may be enticed with promises of rewards or presents or may be made to feel special or grown up by being allowed to engage in adult behavior. Some children do not regard the sexual experiences as threatening but rather as a means by which they can obtain the love they crave. Only when they grow older do they realize that these sexual relationships were not normal or appropriate.

Other children are **coerced** into sexual activity with threats of physical harm. Once they have acquiesced, they are maintained in the relationship with threats of reprisal if they disclose the abuse. Children feel guilty and responsible for what has happened. This sense of responsibility for family disruption is often perpetuated by the legal system, which may remove the children from their families or place the offending family member in custody.

Lastly, some children enter into sexual relationships out of **curiosity.** They too become entrapped, particularly because they were initially willing to participate.

As a child reacts to an abusive experience, it is common to feel a need for secrecy. As a result, disclosures of abuse are often delayed, and when they do occur, the child often provides the information incrementally over time. Children may also recant their disclosures about abuse; such recantations are not considered to reliably indicate that the abuse did not occur.

Differential Diagnosis

A number of medical conditions that involve the anogenital area may be mistaken for acute or chronic changes due to sexual abuse (Box 132-1).

Children may sustain accidental blunt or **penetrating** injuries to the genital area. The most common of these are **straddle injuries** that occur from falls. Pain and bleeding are the most common symptoms with these injuries, and the labia majora, labia minora, or periurethral areas are typically affected. The hymen is unaffected.

Genital bleeding is also a frequent complaint in girls with **urethral prolapse,** a condition that is reported most often in prepubescent African American girls between 4 and 8 years of age. These girls have a protuberant mass extruding from the urethra. The condition is of uncertain etiology but it is not related to abuse.

Lichen sclerosus et atrophicus is a less common dermatologic condition that can also be confused with the sequelae of sexual abuse. In this condition, there is typically atrophic, hypopigmented skin in a figure-8 configuration in the anogenital area with associated macules, papules, and hemorrhagic blisters. The skin changes may be misinterpreted as scarring from prior abuse and because the atrophic skin is easily traumatized, findings may also be confused with recent abuse. One factor that may differentiate this condition from injuries related to sexual abuse is that the hymen is unaffected in lichen sclerosis et atrophicus.

Labial adhesions occur most commonly in toddlers and may be confused with scarring from prior sexual abuse. The adhesions develop as the result of inflammation in the genital area of a prepubertal (hypoestrogenic) female. There can be multiple causes of the inflammation, including poor hygiene, recurrent vulvovaginitis, and trauma. The presence of labial adhesions is not a specific indicator of past sexual abuse.

Congenital malformations may also affect the anogenital area. **Failure of midline fusion** along the median raphe can have the appearance of denuded skin and may be confused with an abrasion or superficial laceration of the area. This failure of fusion is a congenital finding, however, and there is no bleeding as with a traumatic injury. Other congenital malformations include hemangiomas that may bleed and be mistaken for traumatized tissue. These hemangiomas are most often noted in infants and children younger than 2 to 3 years, and they usually regress with time.

Medical conditions may also affect the perianal area and may be mistaken for abuse. **Crohn disease** may lead to fissures, fistulas, perirectal abscesses, or tags. In general, Crohn disease affects older children and produces other symptoms such as fever, weight loss, and stooling problems, or extraintestinal symptomatology. Perirectal abscesses may occur in patients with neutropenia, sometimes as the presenting complaint of leukemia. Hemorrhoids occur rarely in children, and their presence should raise concern about intraabdominal venous congestion.

Box 132-2. Conditions Associated With Vaginal Discharge	
• Gonorrhea	• Shigellosis
• *Chlamydia*	• Group A beta-hemolytic streptococcus infection
• *Trichomonas*	• Vaginal foreign body
• Bacterial vaginosis	
• Candidiasis	

Box 132-3. Problems Reported in Children Who Have Been Sexually Abused	
• Enuresis	• Sleep disturbances
• Encopresis	• Suicide
• Sexualized behavior	• School failure
• Pseudo-maturity	• Delinquency (adolescents)
• Vaginal discharge	• Promiscuity (adolescents)

Conditions causing **vaginal discharge** (Box 132-2) may be related to sexual abuse, particularly if they are secondary to sexually transmitted infections (STIs) such as **gonorrhea** or *Chlamydia* infection. Other agents, including *Candida, Shigella,* and **group A beta-hemolytic streptococci,** may produce similar symptoms, yet not be sexually acquired. The streptococci may produce a painful erythematous rash in the perianal area, which is frequently misdiagnosed as secondary to trauma or sexual abuse.

Evaluation

The extent and urgency of the evaluation is in part dependent on whether the allegations involve an acute abusive episode or one that occurred in the past. An acute abusive episode (one that has occurred within the previous 72 hours) warrants an immediate assessment for evidence that may otherwise be lost within hours.

History

When a child presents with a physical finding, statement, or behavior that raises the concern of possible sexual abuse, it is important for the examiner to ask carefully thought-out, non-leading questions to determine whether the level of suspicion has been reached such that the examiner is mandated to report the concern to a child protective services agency. Beyond that, an attempt should be made to minimize the number of times that the child is questioned about the abuse-related incidents. It is also important to establish sufficient medical history to address any pressing clinical issues. Such a history should include a review of systems, menstrual history, sexual activity history, past incidents of abuse, and any prior genital trauma or medical procedures of the anogenital area. A psychosocial history should also be obtained, as behavioral problems, depression, anxiety, suicidality, homicidality, and other issues requiring mental health expertise are common in children who have been sexually abused (Box 132-3).

Because most victims of sexual abuse have a normal physical examination, the history is often of primary importance in the case. As a result, the child must also be interviewed by someone with professional expertise in the areas of interviewing and child sexual abuse. This individual may be a physician or a social worker, psychologist, rape counselor, or specialized detective or district attorney. The interview should be structured to include open-ended questions such as, "Can you tell me what happened?" (Questions Box). Interview tools such as drawings may be used but are best left to experts with experience in these controversial modalities. Statements that children make should be recorded in the medical record as close to verbatim as possible.

Child Sexual Abuse **Questions**

- Can you tell me what happened?
- Has anything like this happened before? If so, what happened the first time?
- Who did this to you?
- Has anyone else done this to you?
- How often has this happened?
- Where were other people (eg, your mother) when this happened?
- Did you tell anyone? Who? What did they do?

Physical Examination

It is helpful for the examiner to be familiar with the normal **anogenital** anatomy of prepubescent children. The anatomy of boys remains constant throughout childhood, except for the increase in size of the penis and testes and the appearance of pubic hair during adolescence. Figure 132-1 shows the normal anogenital anatomy of girls, which changes from infancy through adolescence. All girls are born with a hymen, which is thick and full and covers the hymenal orifice in newborns. As maternal hormones regress, the hymen becomes thinner and more translucent, frequently taking on an annular or crescentic configuration. When puberty begins, the hymen once again becomes thickened, scalloped, and full. Careful examination of the hymen may involve positioning a child in not only the supine frog-leg position

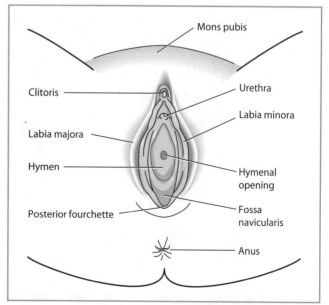

Figure 132-1. Normal anogenital anatomy of prepubescent girls.

but also the prone knee-chest position (Figure 132-2). For a variety of reasons, there are frequently no genital abnormalities noted on examination in victims of sexual abuse. Penetration of the hymen in postpubertal adolescents may result in stretching without tearing of the tissue, and in prepubescent children, hymenal transections may heal with little residual evidence of the trauma. Many types of abuse (eg, orogenital contact, fondling) commonly leave no visible findings. The medical examiner must therefore realize that a normal anogenital examination does not preclude sexual abuse.

In cases of acute molestation, evidence of injury may be readily apparent, particularly if the examination is performed with the assistance of magnification such as **colposcopy** or enhancing agents such as toluidine blue O, which is preferentially taken up by exposed endothelium. Injuries that may be noted include **ecchymoses, petechiae, active bleeding, abrasions,** and **lacerations.** Those caused by penile penetration commonly involve the hymen in the 6-o'clock position and the area of the posterior fourchette (see Figure 132-1).

The evaluation of children who have been molested in the past or on a chronic basis is more problematic. Many injuries heal with little residual scarring. Scarring that does occur may appear as a notch or concavity in the contour of the hymenal edge. The pattern of blood vessels may also be interrupted, and areas of increased or decreased vascularity may be apparent. Sometimes a marked reduction in the amount of hymenal tissue is present in an area of prior trauma.

Male genitalia are less often injured by sexual abuse. More often the injuries seen in prepubescent boys, as well as in some girls, involve changes in the perianal area. The incidence of these changes in all children who have been sodomized is unknown but is believed to be low. When changes do occur, they may appear as scars, tags, or irregularities in perianal rugae and anal tone.

Laboratory Tests

When the molestation has occurred within 72 hours of the examination and the mechanism of injury could have resulted in deposition of body fluids on the child, **forensic evidence** should be collected as required by law enforcement. This evidence usually involves samples of vaginal washings and dried secretions, which are evaluated for the presence of DNA in an effort to identify the perpetrator. Clothing that was worn at the time of the assault should also be submitted because it is frequently positive for DNA evidence. **Forensic packages,** which are referred to as **rape kits** and are distributed by law enforcement agencies, have specific instructions concerning the appropriate collection of samples.

Studies indicate that 1% to 5% of children who were sexually abused acquire an **STI** as a result of the abuse. Because of this, testing for STIs is typically targeted toward any child with a history of genital, oral, or anal penetration; a sibling with an STI; an assailant with a history of an infection; or a child, sibling, or assailant with signs or symptoms of an STI. If testing is indicated, cultures should be obtained from the involved body areas (eg, vagina or urethra, rectum, throat). At a minimum, a child with genital discharge should be evaluated for *Neisseria gonorrhoeae, Chlamydia trachomatis,* and *Trichomonas vaginalis.* The presence of these infections in a prepubertal child, in the absence of perinatal transmission, is indicative of prior close genital contact. Most frequently this is due to sexual abuse. It is impossible to determine the etiology of vaginal discharge based only on its clinical characteristics.

All tests for STIs in prepubertal children should be evaluated in a reliable laboratory because of the legal implications of venereal infections in young children. Culture is considered to be the gold standard for diagnosing gonorrhea and *Chlamydia* in this setting because of its high specificity. While newer nucleic acid amplification tests (NAATs) may have higher sensitivity in some settings, there are limited data on their use in prepubertal children, so they should not be used as the sole method of evaluation. A positive NAAT should be confirmed by culture or by a second nucleic acid test targeting a different DNA sequence. Nucleic acid amplification tests should not be used to test for gonorrhea and *Chlamydia* in extragenital sites.

Testing for HIV, syphilis, hepatitis B, and hepatitis C should be performed if signs or symptoms of the diagnosis are present, another

Figure 132-2. Various positions for an anogenital examination in a prepubescent girl. A, Seated on the mother's lap. **B,** Supine, frog-leg position. **C,** Prone, knee-chest position.

STI is detected, the perpetrator is known to be infected, or the patient or family wishes to undergo the testing. Genital warts can be diagnosed clinically, and any lesions suspicious for human herpesvirus 1 or 2 should be cultured and typed. While culture remains the gold standard for diagnosing human herpesvirus infection, serologies for human herpesvirus type-specific glycoprotein G antigens may be helpful if culture is not available. Lastly, pregnancy testing should be considered in any postpubertal girl.

Management

The management of children who have been sexually abused has 3 major components.

1. Any medical problem sustained as a result of the abuse, such as traumatic injuries, must be addressed. In addition, STIs should be managed (Table 132-1). See Chapter 101 for a more extensive discussion of STIs in adolescents. Adolescents who have been the victims of an acute assault should be offered pregnancy counseling, STI prophylaxis, and emergency contraception as medically indicated.

2. The emotional well-being of patients must be ensured. In cases of acute assault, crisis intervention is mandatory. If children have been the victims of chronic or prior sexual abuse, referral to appropriate counseling services should be done.

3. The physician must report the incident of sexual assault or abuse to the appropriate agencies, as mandated by the laws of the

locality in which the physician practices. The physician may be required to testify in court about particular findings and whether abuse occurred. Testifying may be intimidating. It is helpful for the physician to review the medical records ahead of time and to discuss this information with the attorney who issues the subpoena to the physician.

Prognosis

Several factors influence the prognosis in cases of child sexual abuse, including the relationship of the perpetrator to the child, chronicity of the abuse, support following the disclosure, and preexisting psychosocial conditions. Physical injuries are usually nonexistent or minor, and healing occurs with minimal residual evidence. In most cases, psychologic counseling is indicated. Such counseling is beneficial, and emotional recovery is not only possible but likely to occur in a supportive environment.

Studies of **adverse childhood experiences** have shown that child sexual abuse is associated with an increased risk of medical, psychologic, and social problems in adulthood.

CASE RESOLUTION

In the case study presented at the beginning of this chapter, the mother claims that no one has access to her child, but the girl's symptoms strongly suggest an infection with *Neisseria gonorrhoeae*. Secrecy about abuse is very common. The child and mother should be interviewed by a skilled person. Cultures for gonorrhea should be carefully collected and sent to the most reliable laboratory. Antibiotic therapy may be initiated if the child is symptomatic. The case may be referred immediately to social services and law enforcement agencies if there is a disclosure. Alternatively, if the child denies the abuse, the referral may be deferred pending laboratory confirmation of the diagnosis.

Table 132-1. Management of Sexually Transmitted Infections in Children		
Infection	**Medication**	**Dose**
Neisseria gonorrhoeae	Ceftriaxone	250 mg IM × 1 dose
	Cefixime (age >8 y, weight ≥45 kg)	400 mg po × 1 dose
Chlamydia	Azithromycin	20 mg/kg po × 1 dose (max: 1 g)
	Erythromycin (weight <45 kg)	50 mg/kg/d divided qid × 14 d
	Doxycycline (age >8 y, weight ≥45 kg)	100 mg po bid × 7 d
Genital herpes	Acyclovir	1,200 mg/d divided tid × 7–10 d (max: 80 mg/kg/d)
Trichomonas	Metronidazole	15 mg/kg/d divided tid × 7 d OR 2 g oi × 1 dose (weight ≥45 kg)
Bacterial vaginosis	Metronidazole	15 mg/kg/d divided tid × 7 d OR 2 g po × 1 dose (weight ≥45 kg)
Syphilis	Benzathine penicillin	50,000 U/kg, single IM dose (max: 2.4 million U)

Abbreviations: bid, twice a day; IM, intramuscularly; po, orally; qid, 4 times a day; tid, 3 times a day.

Selected References

Adams JA. Medical evaluation of suspected child sexual abuse: 2011 update. *J Child Sex Abus*. 2011;20(5):588–605

Bechtel K. Sexual abuse and sexually transmitted infections in children and adolescents. *Curr Opin Pediatr*. 2010;22(1):94–99

Fortin K, Jenny C. Sexual abuse. *Pediatr Rev*. 2012;33(1):19–32

Hammerschlag MR, Guillén CD. Medical and legal implications of testing for sexually transmitted infections in children. *Clin Microbiol Rev*. 2010;23(3):493–506

Jenny C, Crawford-Jakubiak JE; American Academy of Pediatrics Committee on Child Abuse and Neglect. The evaluation of children in the primary care setting when sexual abuse is suspected. *Pediatrics*. 2013;132(2):e558–e567

Kaufman M; American Academy of Pediatrics Committee on Adolescence. Care of the adolescent sexual assault victim. *Pediatrics*. 2008;122(2):462–470

Perepletchikova F, Kaufman J. Emotional and behavioral sequelae of childhood maltreatment. *Curr Opin Pediatr*. 2010;22(5):610–615

Werner J, Werner MC. Child sexual abuse in clinical and forensic psychiatry: a review of recent literature. *Curr Opin Psychiatry*. 2008;21(5):499–504

Workowski KA, Berman S; Centers for Disease Control and Prevention. Sexually transmitted diseases treatment guidelines, 2010. *MMWR Recomm Rep*. 2010;59(RR-12):1–110

CHAPTER 133

Failure to Thrive

Carol D. Berkowitz, MD

CASE STUDY

A 2-year-old girl is brought to the office because of her small size. She was born at term but weighed only 2,200 g (<fifth percentile) and measured 43 cm (<fifth percentile). The mother is a 30-year-old gravida 5, para 4, aborta 1 who smoked during pregnancy but denies using alcohol or drugs. She received prenatal care for only 2 weeks prior to delivery, and she claims to have felt well.

The child's physical health has been good. She is reported to be normal developmentally but speaks only 4 to 5 single words. She has not yet started toilet training.

The family history for medical problems, including allergies, diabetes, and cardiac and renal disease, is negative. The mother is 5 feet (152 cm) tall, and the father is 5 feet, 4 inches (163 cm) tall. The girl has 3 siblings, aged 5 years, 4 years, and 3 years, who are all normal. The father is no longer in the household. The mother is not employed outside of the home, and she receives public assistance. She states that frequently there is not enough food in the home, although she receives food stamps.

On physical examination, the girl is below the fifth percentile in height and weight. Although she is very active, she does not use any understandable words. The rest of the examination is normal.

Questions

1. What are the key prenatal factors that affect the growth of children?
2. How can caloric adequacy of a diet be assessed?
3. How do parental measurements affect their children's stature?
4. What are the behavioral characteristics of infants with environmental failure to thrive (FTT)?
5. What are some strategies to increase caloric intake of infants and children?
6. What, if any, laboratory studies should be routinely obtained when evaluating children for FTT?

Failure to thrive (FTT) can be defined as the failure of children to grow and develop at an appropriate rate. The term is most often applied to infants and toddlers younger than 3 years. Failure to thrive is not a disease or even a diagnosis but represents a sign that a child's size or rate of growth is below the expected. The term FTT first appeared in the pediatric literature in 1933 and was used for children whose growth impairment related to a suboptimal environment. Prior to 1933, the condition was referred to as **cease to thrive.** The terms **growth deficiency, growth impairment, undernutrition,** and **inadequate growth** are sometimes used interchangeably. Historically, FTT has been divided into 2 distinct categories, **organic** and **nonorganic.** In organic FTT, an underlying **medical problem,** such as cystic fibrosis or congenital heart disease (CHD), is believed to contribute to the failure to grow at an appropriate rate. In nonorganic FTT, also referred to as **environmental deprivation,** inadequate growth is attributed to lack of nourishment and a non-nurturing home environment. Some clinicians use the term FTT exclusively to mean environmentally related growth impairment. It is important to recognize that many children with growth problems have organic and environmental components, a condition sometimes referred to as *multifactorial* or *mixed* FTT.

The diagnosis of FTT is entertained when the growth parameters of children as plotted on a standardized curve are below the fifth percentile in height or weight. Children who are above the fifth percentile may also be diagnosed with FTT if the rate of growth has decelerated and 2 major percentiles (eg, decreased from the 75th percentile down to the 10th percentile) have been crossed within 6 months (D$_x$ Box). Studies have shown, however, that between birth and 6 months of age, approximately 39% of healthy infants crossed 2 major percentiles on the weight-for-age curve (up or down), as did up to 15% of children between 6 and 24 months of age. Similar trends were noted for length. Physicians should, however, carefully track these infants to be certain that such changes are related to the child's genetic disposition and not an environmental or medical problem.

The challenge for the physician caring for the child with FTT is to determine the etiology of the problem, which may not be readily apparent. Nonspecific, nondirected laboratory tests are not helpful

Dx Failure to Thrive

- Weight below fifth percentile
- Height below fifth percentile
- Weight for height below fifth percentile
- Rate of growth lower than expected
- Delayed developmental milestones
- Disturbed interactional skills

because their yield is low and their cost is high. The evaluation of small, underweight children requires a careful history and physical examination as well as an assessment of mother-infant interactions. A home visit helps because it permits evaluation of the mother-infant relationship in a more natural setting and an assessment of the family's economic and food resources.

Epidemiology

The prevalence of FTT varies in different segments of the population. **Poverty** puts children at risk for **undernutrition,** and 12% of Medicaid recipients are below the third percentile in weight. **Child neglect** can lead to FTT but is not a necessary component; approximately 60% of cases of child abuse are reported for child neglect. Several other factors may contribute to variations in growth. All of these are not the result of a pathologic process but may reflect variations in individual genetic potential.

Environmentally related FTT may occur in different family settings. In some families, an **acute depressive episode** in the mother is the key component (see Chapter 21). Family living conditions are good, and the educational background of the mother is adequate. The depressive episode may be related to a loss that occurred during the pregnancy or shortly after delivery or to perinatal mood and anxiety disorders, a group of mental health conditions associated with pregnancy and delivery and manifested after birth. In these cases, the mother is too depressed, withdrawn, or preoccupied to interact effectively with her children. The condition may affect 25% to 30% of mothers. In other families, **financial resources** are marginal. The mother may be **chronically depressed** and the father involved in alcohol or substance abuse. Domestic violence frequently occurs (see Chapter 142). Spacing between children is fewer than 18 months, and the number of children is often the same as the age of the oldest child. The mother is too overwhelmed to meet the needs of all the children. A third type of family also involves a mother who is depressed and has experienced losses, usually of a chronic nature. Her financial and educational backgrounds are adequate, but she views one of her children (the one who now presents with FTT) as bad or evil and the source of all her problems. As a result, an individual child is singled out, and the neglect is intentional.

Clinical Presentation

Children with FTT present with **low weight, short stature, poor appetite,** or **failure to gain weight or grow taller.** Sometimes parents may express concern; at other times, teachers may detect children's growth problems. Some children with FTT are diagnosed during a health maintenance visit or when they are being evaluated for another medical problem, such as a febrile illness. Following a child longitudinally will give the physician a better sense of the child's growth pattern and a clue to the etiology of observed growth impairments. When nutrition is suboptimal, weight tends to decrease first, followed by length and, ultimately, head circumference.

Box 133-1. Factors Affecting Calories Available for Growth	
Insufficient Intake	**Increased Loss**
• Poverty	• Malabsorption
• Inadequate access to food	**Increased Needs**
• Improper formula preparation	• Congenital heart disease
• Eating difficulties	• Chronic lung disease
• Vomiting	

Pathophysiology

The common pathway for the development of FTT in organic and nonorganic cases is **insufficient calories** to sustain growth (Box 133-1). Caloric intake may be inadequate for several reasons. Some factors are societal, specifically poverty and inadequate access to food. Other factors may involve increased caloric needs. Certain chronic conditions are characterized by increased caloric expenditure (eg, some forms of chronic lung disease) or increased loss of ingested food (eg, diarrhea, malabsorption syndromes).

In environmentally related FTT, a disturbed mother-infant interaction is believed to contribute to reduced caloric intake and any associated gastrointestinal symptoms (ie, vomiting). Although various disturbances in mother–FTT infant dyads have been described, maternal depression is the most common maternal feature noted in environmentally related FTT. Infants withdraw after unsuccessful attempts to interact with nonresponsive mothers, and infants become apathetic and disinterested in food. Alternatively, overactive mothers, some of whom have an untreated bipolar (manic-depressive) disorder, are out of synchrony with their infants. The infants become agitated, especially during feedings, and cannot feed and frequently vomit. These infants, who may interact with persons other than their mothers, usually do well in other environments.

Older children with long-standing environmental deprivation have **disturbed hypothalamic-pituitary functioning.** The etiology of this dysfunction is uncertain but has been attributed to sleep disturbances with an effect on levels of growth hormone.

Differential Diagnosis

The growth of children with FTT may be impaired with regard to weight, height, head circumference, or any combination of growth parameters. If weight is the only abnormal parameter, inadequate caloric intake, excess caloric loss, or increased caloric expenditure is probably the major problem. If height is reduced and weight is appropriate or high for height, the diagnosis may be short stature rather than FTT. Small head circumference in the face of low growth parameters suggests a central nervous system (CNS) basis for the growth delay. It is important to determine if children's skills are developmentally appropriate when determining the etiology of FTT. Affect and interactional skills should also be noted. Environmentally deprived infants are apathetic and noninteractive. They appear hypertonic and may be diagnosed with cerebral palsy or have features suggestive of infantile autism spectrum disorder, but their symptoms resolve with a change in surroundings.

The most common causes of short stature include **familial short stature** and **constitutional delay.** Children with familial short stature are small because the parents are short. Except for a deceleration in growth, which usually occurs between the ages of 6 and 18 months, children with constitutional delay appear healthy. They have a delayed bone age that is comparable to their height age (the age when their height is at the 50th percentile), however. In children with familial short stature or constitutional delay, growth parameters at birth are usually normal.

Children with low growth parameters at birth may have been premature or experienced **intrauterine growth restriction (IUGR).** Most studies support the notion that well premature infants exhibit catchup growth (head circumference by 18 months, weight by 24 months, and height by 40 months). Ill preterm infants may not demonstrate such **catch-up growth** because of increased caloric needs related to residual medical problems (eg, bronchopulmonary dysplasia) or impaired nutritional intake resulting from certain conditions (eg, cerebral palsy). Overall, 15% of infants who are classified as IUGR or **small for gestational age (SGA)** do not exhibit catch-up growth. There is significant evidence now that IUGR may be associated with insulin resistance and subsequent propensity to obesity and metabolic syndrome. Disturbances in leptin, ghrelin, and adiponectin have also been described. This recent finding has significant implications for the management of these infants vis-à-vis their nutritional intake. It is postulated that some individuals are "programmed" to be slighter and smaller, and nutritional interventions to achieve a more average weight have deleterious effects down the line.

Children who are **SGA** may have suffered any of several in utero insults that affect postnatal growth, including exposure to cigarettes, alcohol, and illicit drugs. In addition, maternal infection with such diseases as rubella may result in a congenital infection in infants with subsequent growth impairment.

A number of other conditions may lead to disturbed growth, including endocrine disorders, skeletal dysplasia, food allergies, and malabsorption. These conditions occur less frequently and are usually more readily apparent as children undergo evaluation for the growth problem.

Evaluation

History

Careful questioning about certain topics provides clues to diagnosis in about 95% of cases. The physician should learn about the pregnancy and delivery, children's medical and dietary history, and family history.

It is important to obtain a history of the pregnancy and delivery (Questions Box: Pregnancy and Delivery). The infant's birth weight and gestational age are key pieces of information. Low birth weight is said to account for 20% to 40% of short children from low-income families. It is helpful to confirm that the neonatal screen for genetic and metabolic diseases was normal. Recurrent spontaneous

Questions

Pregnancy and Delivery

- Was the pregnancy planned?
- How did the mother feel when she learned that she was pregnant?
- Was the baby wanted?
- Was prenatal care obtained?
- How many times has the mother been pregnant?
- Is there a history of abortions (spontaneous or therapeutic)?
- How much alcohol did the mother drink during the pregnancy, if at all?
- How much did the mother smoke during the pregnancy, if at all?
- How much did the mother use drugs (prescribed or illicit) during the pregnancy, if at all? If so, which drugs did she use?
- Did the mother take any medications during the pregnancy?
- Did the mother have any rashes or illnesses during the pregnancy?
- Has the mother felt depressed, sad, or hopeless?
- Has the mother felt little interest or pleasure in doing things?
- Was the baby term or premature?
- How much did the infant weigh at birth?

abortions suggest that mothers may have an underlying problem such as a balanced chromosomal translocation that leads to fetal wastage. Mothers who have experienced repeated losses may have difficulty bonding with subsequent babies. The physician should determine whether mothers used cigarettes, alcohol, or drugs during the pregnancy by asking mothers questions beginning with the phrase, "How much?" Any medications taken by the mother may affect the subsequent growth of the infant.

A review of children's medical history may also provide a clue to the etiology of FTT (Questions Box: Medical and Family History). It is essential that the physician obtain as many of the previous growth parameters as possible to determine whether children are small but growing at a normal rate or if their rate of growth is too slow. Previous illnesses should be assessed because these events may interrupt growth temporarily. Certain complaints may indicate underlying organic disorders, and recurrent infections raise the possibility of a congenital or acquired immune disorder, including infection with HIV. A history of easy fatigability may be a clue to CHD. Although most children with CHD grow normally, growth problems may occur

Questions

Medical and Family History

- Is the child's growth rate normal or slow?
- Has the child had any previous illnesses (eg, gastroenteritis, recurrent pneumonia)?
- Does the child tire easily?
- Is the child taking any medications, and if so, for how long?
- How tall are the parents?
- Are there any medical problems that run in the family?

with congestive heart failure, some forms of cyanotic heart disease, and complex atrial septal defects, especially if associated with pulmonary hypertension. A history of diarrhea may suggest an underlying gastrointestinal disorder with subsequent malabsorption. Children with urinary incontinence may have renal disease that interferes with their growth. The presence of seizures may be a sign of a CNS problem that makes it difficult to obtain adequate nutrition. Some children with seizures are heavily medicated and are too sleepy to eat.

It is important to query whether children are on any medications. The chronic use of some medications such as corticosteroids and certain stimulants used to manage attention-deficit/hyperactivity disorder have been associated with decelerated linear growth in some children.

A family history as well as a **social history** is important to obtain. Determination of parental heights, which is best accomplished by measuring the parents, is critical. This is particularly important in children with short stature. Specific **mid-parental height curves** allow the physician to determine if a child's height is appropriate given parental stature.

A nutritional assessment is an essential part of the history. The physician or another member of the health care team, such as a dietitian, can perform this assessment. The dietary history can be determined by using a **24-hour recall** of children's intake during the previous day or a prospective **3-day diary** in which parents record the kinds and quantities of foods their children eat. This nutritional information can be used to find ways to alter children's diet to ensure adequate and balanced meals.

Physical Examination

The essential component of the physical examination is determination of growth parameters. Calculation of the **body mass index** (BMI = weight [kg]/height [m]^2) is useful in children older than 2 years. Children with a low BMI are suffering from undernutrition; short children with a normal BMI are not. Infants and children younger than 2 years should be plotted on a weight-for-length curve to determine their degree of undernutrition or overnutrition. The World Health Organization has developed and distributed growth curves for children up to 24 months of age. These curves, felt to reflect optimal rather than average growth, having been developed from a longitudinal study of healthy breastfed infants, can be accessed at www.cdc.gov/mmwr/preview/mmwrhtml/rr5909a1.htm. Measuring arm circumference and triceps skinfold thickness is also useful and provides information about body composition that is not obtained by height and weight. Children should be evaluated for dysmorphic features (eg, limb-length discrepancies in Silver-Russell syndrome). It is important to remember that children with Down syndrome grow at different rates than other children, and separate standardized curves for assessing these children are available (see Chapter 39). Separate curves are also available for children with Turner and Williams syndromes. The presence of one major congenital anomaly or 2 minor anomalies suggests the existence of other anomalies. The incidence of growth hormone deficiency is reportedly higher in

children with cleft lip and palate. Children with heart murmurs may have FTT related to CHD or to a syndrome such as Williams syndrome, in which the heart disease is but one feature.

Infants with environmentally related FTT exhibit certain **behavioral characteristics** that are easy to recognize. They refrain from making eye contact and exhibit **gaze** avoidance. Infants are not cuddly and do not like being held. When held, they may arch their backs in an effort to avoid the holder. Their muscles seem tense, and they are often considered to be hypertonic. These children may also exhibit specific disabilities, including oromotor dyspraxia and sensory-motor disorder, and they may demonstrate food texture aversion or difficulty with chewing and swallowing (**sensory food aversion).** Children with neurologic disabilities often exhibit difficulties with oral skills. Children who have negative early experience with eating may have what has been termed *posttraumatic feeding disorder.*

Psychosocial Assessment

The evaluation of children with FTT and their families entails a detailed psychosocial assessment to determine what environmental factors may be affecting children's growth. Such an assessment is helpful even if the FTT has an organic basis because chronic disease affects family functioning. This evaluation can be carried out by a primary care physician, social worker, or psychologist. The key is to query the caregiver about living conditions, adequacy of food supply, and economic resources.

Laboratory Tests

Routine laboratory tests appropriate for any pediatric health maintenance visit should be obtained in children with FTT if these studies have not been performed recently. Such tests include hemoglobin, lead level (screening as determined by risk factors and geographic area), and urinalysis. Other laboratory tests should be determined by the findings on history and physical examination. For instance, stool for ova and parasites should be obtained in a child with diarrhea who has immigrated from or spent time visiting a developing country. There is no recommended uniform diagnostic evaluation for FTT. Evaluation for endocrinopathies, such as hypothyroidism or growth hormone deficiency, should be carried out in children whose bone age is less than their height age or who have symptoms of these disorders. Genetic consultation or chromosomal assessment should be performed in children with dysmorphic features or in families with a history of fetal wastage.

Imaging Studies

Radiographs to determine bone age are useful in children with short stature that is not related to parental heights. Children with constitutional delay have a bone age that is consistent with their height age.

Management

Any recognized underlying medical problem (eg, nephrogenic diabetes insipidus) should be managed appropriately. Children with

IUGR who are not demonstrating catch-up growth may be candidates for growth hormone therapy. Consultation with pediatric endocrinology is warranted.

Adequate Caloric Intake

Ensuring that children receive appropriate caloric intake is essential. The caloric intake, which averages 120 to 150 cal/kg/day for most infants, should be based on children's ideal rather than actual weight (see Chapter 25). For infants on formula, the physician should review the exact preparation of formula with the mother. Overly diluted formula results in an unusually large intake volume with a lack of weight gain. For infants who are breastfed, the physician should observe a feeding session to be certain that mothers have an adequate milk supply and infants are able to suck and swallow appropriately (see Chapter 26). Infants should be weighed before and after feeding. Some infants with FTT have neurologic problems that prevent them from sucking and swallowing consistently without becoming fatigued.

Children who are slow feeders may require **formula concentration** (Table 133-1). These infants may also receive added calories in the form of Polycose (glucose polymer) or oil such as medium-chain triglycerides mixed in the milk. Older children may be placed on supplemental feedings such as PediaSure or instant breakfast drinks, prepared with whole milk. These drinks are a less expensive form of nutritional supplementation than PediaSure and are well tolerated. Up to 24 oz/day of the breakfast drinks can be consumed and are given in addition to, not in place of, a balanced diet.

One food supplement that has been used globally to treat severe acute malnutrition is Plumpy'Nut, a peanut-based paste with sugar, vegetable fat, and skimmed milk and enriched with vitamins and minerals. It is not used in the United States.

Mothers should be advised that many children preferentially tolerate 6 small meals a day rather than 3 large ones. In addition, parents should be told that access to non-nutritional foods such as cookies adversely affects children's appetites. Excess consumption of fruit juices should also be limited because it decreases the intake of other foods and may induce diarrhea. The physician should inform parents about foods that can be added to children's diets to increase caloric intake, including powdered milk, cheese, sour cream, avocado, and peanut butter. Often, children have a few favorite foods. Although food variety is appealing to adults, many children prefer a small number of nutritious foods. They should be allowed to consume these foods freely.

Children with neurologic disorders and associated problems with chewing and swallowing may need chronic gavage feeding or to be fed through a gastric feeding tube.

Parenting Issues

Some parents need more help with appropriate child-rearing practices than the physician can provide. They should enroll in parenting programs that address multiple aspects of the parenting process. Mothers with substance abuse problems may need to participate in drug treatment programs. Other caregivers may need individual counseling for depression or emotional problems. A nurturing father has an important role in caring for an infant, particularly if a mother is experiencing postpartum depression.

In some middle-class families, mealtime has evolved into a battle of control. Some children find that food is supplied in a manner more conducive to its consumption at school rather than at home. Parents should be counseled about avoiding conflicts about meals with children because the children win simply by closing their mouths. Parents should be encouraged to allow toddlers independence around mealtime. Eating in front of the television, however, should be discouraged.

Families may also require supplementary services to ensure that food supplies are adequate and financial resources are sufficient. Such services include Supplemental Nutrition Assistance Program (formerly food stamps); Special Supplemental Nutrition Program for Women, Infants, and Children; and Temporary Assistance for Needy Families.

Regardless of the individual needs of the family, it is critical that the physician craft a therapeutic alliance with the child's caregivers.

Home Visitation

Home visitation services provide useful diagnostic information and help parents implement advice. Such information may include lack of access to running water, overcrowding, and inadequate food resources. Home visitation may be available in the community through the use of public health nurses or private visiting nurse agencies. These nurses should interact with the primary care physician so that families' compliance with treatment recommendations can be determined.

Child Protective Services

Involvement by **child protective services** (CPS) may be necessary if parents are unable to comply with medical recommendations, children do not grow, or there is intentional neglect on the part of families. In some families with children with FTT, the home environment is not safe for children and they require placement elsewhere. Families in which one child is singled out as "bad" and is intentionally

Table 133-1. Concentration of Infant Formula to Increase Caloric Intake		
Concentrated Infant Formula (13-oz can)		
Formula (oz)	*Water (oz)*	*Calories (cal/oz)*
13	13	20
13	10	23
13	8	25
Powdered Formula		
Formula (scoops)	*Water (oz)*	*Calories (cal/oz)*
1	2	20
5	8	25

neglected need immediate referral to CPS, and some families over-whelmed by multiple problems, including parental substance abuse, also need such a referral (see Epidemiology on page 874).

Hospitalization

Hospitalization is occasionally necessary if infants with FTT are severely malnourished and food must be given in a controlled environment. Concern about refeeding syndrome can be addressed in the inpatient setting. In addition, these infants may have intercurrent illnesses that require inpatient care. Also, health care professionals may determine that the home environment is unsafe and that no other placement, such as foster care, is available.

Children with organic or environmentally related FTT usually gain weight in the hospital. Thus, the hospitalization of children with FTT simply to demonstrate appropriate weight gain in a different environment is considered neither appropriate nor cost-effective. Some insurance companies will not pay hospitals for inpatient management of children with FTT. Additionally, some children with environmentally related FTT do not gain weight in the hospital because they are subjected to many diagnostic tests that interfere with nutritional intake (eg, receiving nothing orally while awaiting the procedure), and they acquire nosocomial infections.

Prognosis

Many children with FTT respond dramatically to change in diet or environment. Improvement in affect and cognitive functioning frequently follows nutritional improvement. These children grow and achieve and maintain normal stature. With early intervention, cognitive abilities also can be fully realized. Even when intervention has been delayed, catch-up growth and development are expected, although 25% to 30% may have weight and occasionally height below the fifth percentile. Continued monitoring for residual psychosocial or neurodevelopmental disabilities is appropriate even after growth has normalized. School performance and cognitive outcome in children who have experienced FTT are poorer than in children who have not experienced FTT. It is unclear if this association is related to early iron deficiency anemia, lack of calories or other micronutrient deficiencies, or psycho-environmental deficits.

CASE RESOLUTION

In the case study presented, the full-term child had a low birth weight, which suggests intrauterine growth restriction. Although the mother reports using no alcohol or drugs, such denial is not uncommon. The child's growth pattern should be determined to see if the rate of growth has changed recently, and body mass index should be calculated to check for undernutrition and short stature. A mid-parental height curve should be used to determine if the child's short stature is related to the parents' short stature. Intervention should involve mobilizing resources for the child and family to ensure adequate food and financial and emotional support.

Selected References

Berkowitz CD. Failure to thrive: a comprehensive approach. *Fam Pract Recertification.* 2004;26:41–59

Black MM, Dubowitz H, Krishnakumar A, Starr RH Jr. Early intervention and recovery among children with failure to thrive: follow-up at age 8. *Pediatrics.* 2007;120(1):59–69

Block RW, Krebs NF; American Academy of Pediatrics Committee on Child Abuse and Neglect and Committee on Nutrition. Failure to thrive as a manifestation of child neglect. *Pediatrics.* 2005;116(5):1234–1237

Cook JT, Frank DA, Berkowitz C, et al. Food insecurity is associated with adverse health outcomes among human infants and toddlers. *J Nutr.* 2004;134(6):1432–1438

Drotar D, ed. *New Direction in Failure to Thrive: Research and Clinical Practice.* New York, NY: Plenum Press; 1985

Frank DA, Blenner S, Wilbur MB, Black MM, Drotar D. Failure to thrive. In: Reece RM, Christian CW, eds. *Child Abuse: Medical Diagnosis & Management.* 3rd ed. Elk Grove Village, IL: American Academy of Pediatrics; 2009:465–511

Gahagan S. Failure to thrive: a consequence of undernutrition. *Pediatr Rev.* 2006;27(1):e1–e11

Graham EA. Economic, racial, and cultural influences on the growth and maturation of children. *Pediatr Rev.* 2005;26(8):290–294

Jaffe AC. Failure to thrive: current clinical concepts. *Pediatr Rev.* 2011;32(3):100–108

Mei Z, Grummer-Strawn LM, Thompson D, Dietz WH. Shifts in percentiles of growth during early childhood: analysis of longitudinal data from the California Child Health and Development Study. *Pediatrics.* 2004;113(6):e617–e627

Oates RK, Kempe RS. Growth failure in infants. In: Helfer ME, Kempe RS, Krugman RD, eds. *The Battered Child.* 5th ed. Chicago, IL: The University of Chicago Press; 1997:374–391

Vitiello B. Understanding the risk of using medications for attention deficit hyperactivity disorder with respect to physical growth and cardiovascular function. *Child Adolesc Psychiatr Clin N Am.* 2008;17(2):459–474

CHAPTER 134

Fetal Alcohol Syndrome

Melissa K. Egge, MD

CASE STUDY

A 6-year-old boy is brought into the clinic by his maternal aunt who expresses concerns about her nephew's behavior that are echoed by his kindergarten teacher. The teacher has reported that the child has a limited attention span and is often disruptive in class. The child's growth parameters have remained at the third percentile since birth. He has a smooth philtrum, thin upper lip, and short palpebral fissures.

Questions

1. What are the diagnostic criteria outlined by the Centers for Disease Control and Prevention for fetal alcohol syndrome (FAS)?
2. What is the differential diagnosis of the facial characteristics of FAS?
3. What typical behavioral and learning problems do children with FAS experience?
4. What therapeutic interventions are appropriate to recommend for children with FAS?

Fetal alcohol syndrome (FAS) refers to a clinical diagnosis that requires careful evaluation by an experienced clinician to recognize the physical, behavioral, and cognitive abnormalities in an affected child. Diagnosis may be made at birth, but the condition is often not diagnosed until school age. Fetal alcohol syndrome has been recognized in the medical literature for decades and in historical literature for centuries; however, fine-tuning the criteria for diagnosis has been an ongoing process. Although several groups have created guidelines to help analyze children with FAS, in 2004, the Centers for Disease Control and Prevention (CDC) published broad-based criteria (Box 134-1) that are helpful for a number of reasons. First, they educate clinicians and caregivers about the wide spectrum of phenotypes that manifest after prenatal alcohol exposure. Second, using the most recent CDC criteria for FAS, the greatest number of potentially affected children is captured in the hopes that earlier intervention with a wider scope of services may be provided. Criteria must be met in all 3 categories of facial features, growth problems, and central nervous system (CNS) abnormalities. For cases in which FAS is suspected but diagnostic criteria are incompletely met, the term *fetal alcohol spectrum disorders* (FASDs) may be used to couch the findings, especially when maternal alcohol exposure is confirmed. The next step will be establishing criteria for FASDs. However, at this time, the term is not intended for diagnostic purposes but rather a descriptor of recognized phenotypes along a spectrum leading up to FAS.

Part of the difficulty in delineating a phenotype for alcohol exposure is that the degree of exposure is variable during embryogenesis (and organogenesis): quantity ingested, concomitant drug exposures, malnutrition, and individual genetic responses to exposure. This wide variability in degree of exposure and individual response leads to a multitude of clinical presentations.

Box 134-1. Centers for Disease Control and Prevention Diagnostic Criteria for Fetal Alcohol Syndrome

Requires all 3 of the following:

1. Facial features—all 3 required
   a. Palpebral fissure length—10th percentile for age/race
   b. Smooth philtrum rank 4–5
   c. Thin upper lip rank 4–5
2. Growth parameters—at least 1 required at any age (not height for weight)
   a. Height ≤10th percentile
   b. Weight ≤10th percentile
3. Central nervous system abnormalities—at least 1 of the following
   a. Structural—1 required
      i. Head circumference ≤10th for age, sex
      ii. Brain abnormality by imaging
   b. Neurologic
      i. Seizures
      ii. Measured delay in motor skills
      iii. Abnormal neurologic examination not attributed to another condition
   c. Functional—1 required
      i. Cognitive delay or global developmental delay (<3rd percentile)
      ii. Deficits in ≥3 functional domains (<16th percentile)
         1. Cognitive
         2. Executive function
         3. Motor function (fine or gross)
         4. Attention-deficit/hyperactivity disorder symptoms
         5. Deficits in social skills
         6. Other (eg, sensory, memory, language)

Adapted from Bertrand J, Floyd RL, Weber MK, et al. *Fetal Alcohol Syndrome: Guidelines for Referral and Diagnosis.* Atlanta, GA: Centers for Disease and Prevention; 2004

Epidemiology

Prenatal alcohol exposure is much more common than the number of diagnosed cases of FAS. It has been estimated by surveys of women of childbearing age that approximately 15% engage in regular consumption of alcohol and 2% are binge drinkers. Although estimates of children affected by FAS vary by region and population, an estimated 1 in 1,000 live births would meet criteria for diagnosis. The estimate jumps 10-fold when certain high-risk groups are the focus. Approximately 1 in 100 children in foster care and nearly that many (3–9/1,000) Native American children meet criteria for diagnosis of FAS. If one includes children who meet some but not all FAS criteria, the prevalence is 1 in 100 or greater.

Pathophysiology

Alcohol is a teratogen, and like other teratogens its effect on the developing fetus depends on several factors, many of which are difficult to record. While it is important to ask about the timing, quantity, and pattern of prenatal alcohol exposure, it is often difficult to obtain an accurate history. In addition, due to genetic differences in women's abilities to metabolize ethanol by alcohol dehydrogenase, each baby receives a unique "dose" during gestation. Also individualized is each woman's nutritional intake and use of other drugs or medications. Alcohol acts as a toxin to cause damage and apoptosis to neurons in the fetal brain. Alcohol also inhibits proper migration, development, and functioning of cells during embryogenesis, contributing to structural anomalies in multiple organ systems, such as the kidney, heart, and brain.

Clinical Presentation

Signs and symptoms of FAS may be recognized at birth or not until later in childhood. At birth, a neonate may present with asymmetric intrauterine growth restriction, small for gestational age, head circumference disproportionately smaller than the body, or appropriate for gestational age. A variety of birth defects have been associated with fetal alcohol exposure, and many of these have been demonstrated in animal models. Newborns may exhibit signs of withdrawal from alcohol or concomitant drug exposure. With time, the infant may demonstrate failure to thrive or poor weight gain due to poor nursing. Alcohol-exposed infants also present with nonspecific symptoms of irritability and dysregulated sleep patterns. In toddlerhood, developmental delays may be recognized by a caregiver or during developmental screening questions by a primary care physician. As children approach school age, teachers may report behavioral concerns and poor school performance. Concerns such as distractibility, hyperactivity, and difficulty processing multistep directions may be raised in school. In addition, children may exhibit signs of fine motor delay, such as difficulty tying shoes or fastening buttons. Deficits in visual-spatial and math concepts are common for children with fetal alcohol exposure. Age-appropriate social skills are lacking in affected children, who often fail to develop street smarts. They take the blame, succumb to peer pressure, and are oblivious to social norms. Approaching the teen years, the classic facies may become less distinctive. As teenagers mature, their cognitive and behavioral weaknesses predispose them to mental health issues such as depression, anxiety, and problems with substance abuse.

Diagnosis

Facial Dysmorphia

There are 3 classic facial features required for the diagnosis of FAS. The characteristics are typical of midface hypoplasia and include short palpebral fissures, smooth philtrum, and thin upper lip. Other facial characteristics, such as epicanthal folds and flat nasal bridge, may be present but are not required for diagnosis. To accurately measure the palpebral fissures, the child should look directly up while the distance between the endocanthion and the exocanthion is measured. Palpebral fissure length (PFL) must be less than 2 standard deviations below the mean for a diagnosis of FAS.

There are lip-philtrum guides created by the University of Washington for whites and for African Americans accounting for ethnic differences in contour of lips (Figure 134-1). The images are ranked 1 through 5, with 5 representing the most affected phenotype: thinnest lip and smoothest philtrum. When the child is not white or African American, a best approximate is used. To properly use the lip-philtrum guides, the child's face should be relaxed, or the lip and philtrum will appear thinner and smoother. The clinician should evaluate the child's face within a specific horizontal planar view to avoid the illusion of a thinner lip. There are guidelines on how to use the images published on the University of Washington FAS Web site at http://depts.washington.edu/fasdpn.

Growth Problems

The criteria for deficiencies in growth may involve the child's weight or length or both at any time. With the CDC criteria, one may qualify to meet criteria for growth problems based on birth or postnatal measurements. The child's weight or length must be less than or equal to the 10th percentile for age and sex. It is important, however, to evaluate other organic and environmental etiologies of short stature or poor weight gain, such as poor nutrition. Considerations for small head circumference are accounted for in the CNS abnormalities.

Central Nervous System Abnormalities

The criteria for neurologic problems may be met several ways as children manifest an array of cognitive, behavioral, and developmental deficits. Criteria for structural abnormalities are met by a head circumference at the 10th percentile or lower at any age or 3% or less when the child's weight and height are less than 10%. An experienced neuroradiologist may detect an abnormally small cranial structure, such as the cerebellum or corpus callosum, on magnetic resonance imaging. Manifestations of structural abnormalities include seizure activity not attributed to another cause or other focal deficits. Other functional CNS abnormalities may not be recognized until the child enters school and is compared with peers.

Lip-Philtrum Guide 1   Lip-Philtrum Guide 2

Figure 134-1. **Lip philtrum guidelines for whites and African Americans. (Reproduced with permission from Susan Astley.)**

Table 134-1. Syndromes With Facies Resembling Fetal Alcohol Syndrome			
Syndrome	Long or Smooth Philtrum	Thin Upper Lip	Small Palpebral Fissures
de Lange	X	X	
Aarskog	X		
Williams	X		X
Dubowitz			X
Toluene embryopathy	X	X	X
Brachmann-de Lange	X		
Fetal hydantoin			
Noonan			
Fetal valproate	X	X	
Maternal phenylketonuria	X	X	X
Floating-Harbor	X		
Opitz	X		X

History

A confirmed history of maternal alcohol consumption is not required for diagnosis, according to the CDC guidelines, but should be documented if available. A detailed developmental history is important to document, including feedback from teachers or child care providers.

Physical Examination

As detailed previously, measurement of the PFL and ranking of the child's philtrum and upper lip should be documented. Current and previous height, weight, and head circumferences should be plotted on an appropriate growth chart. Also, any additional physical features may be recorded to support diagnosis.

Diagnostic Studies

Imaging studies to screen for cranial malformations are not currently recommended unless the child is experiencing some focal neurologic deficits or seizure activity. Similarly, targeted imaging of other organ systems is warranted when there are signs of an abnormality (eg, murmur would warrant an echocardiogram).

Consultation with a geneticist may be appropriate to rule out other disorders with similar phenotype (Box 134-2).

Management

Once a diagnosis related to alcohol exposure is suspected by a clinician, the referral process should begin. A dysmorphologist or experienced clinician may do the detailed measurements of the PFL and rank the facial features. Depending on local resources, a multidisciplinary team evaluation is ideal. A child psychologist or developmentalist can assess age-appropriate skills and need for therapeutic

Differential Diagnosis

The hazards of using a "gestalt approach" to diagnosing FAS can lead to inappropriate stigmatizing labels and missed opportunity to diagnose another genetic disorder, which may carry a different prognosis. Several syndromes share facial features of FAS (Table 134-1). Fetal alcohol syndrome should be considered a diagnosis of exclusion when in utero alcohol exposure cannot be confirmed.

Evaluation

It is important that appropriately trained professionals assess the child for each component of diagnosis, but initial data should be gathered prior to referral.

Box 134-2. Physical Findings and Malformations Associated With Prenatal Alcohol Exposure

Cardiac
- Atrial or ventricular septal defects, aberrant great vessels, and tetralogy of Fallot

Skeletal/Extremity
- Shortened fifth digits, clinodactyly (curved fifth digit), radioulnar synostosis, Klippel-Feil syndrome, flexion contractures, hemivertebrae, camptodactyly (flexion contracture of digit), scoliosis, short metacarpals, short/webbed neck, hockey stick palmar crease

Renal
- Aplastic, dysplastic, hypoplastic kidneys
- Ureteral duplications, hydronephrosis, horseshoe kidneys

Ocular
- Strabismus, refractive problems secondary to small globes, ptosis
- Retinal vascular anomalies

Auditory
- Conductive hearing loss, neurosensory hearing loss

Skin
- Hemangiomas, hypoplastic nails

Genitourinary
- Hypoplastic labia majora

Facial features that are common but not required for diagnosis
- "Railroad track" ears
- Epicanthal folds
- Flat nasal bridge
- Cleft lip

---

intervention. Only validated instruments should be used to test developmental capabilities. When delays are detected, referral to appropriate therapies should be initiated through early intervention services. An Individual Education Plan may be requested of the school by a caregiver who retains the child's educational rights. Public schools may provide occupational, physical, and speech therapies and social skills training. A psychiatrist may select therapies and medications particular to a child's unique mental health needs (see chapters 129 and 130). Social workers are integral to providing support and additional resources to the family. As teens approach adulthood, referrals to vocational training and programs to transition young adults to independent living are important.

Prognosis

Unfortunately, many of the neurotoxic effects of alcohol on the developing fetus have lasting sequelae. Early interventions may improve but not correct cognitive deficits and associated mental health issues of aging children and adults with FAS. The mental health disorders are thought to be the result of adverse childhood experiences (eg, ridicule, harassment, failures) related to a child's behavioral and cognitive deficits. Some of the mental health disorders include oppositional defiant disorder, conduct disorder, depression, adjustment disorders, anxiety disorders, substance abuse, and sleep disorders. Unfortunately, many adults with FAS have failed to finish high school and become unemployed or incarcerated. A fraction of adults with FAS will require assisted living arrangements.

CASE RESOLUTION

This child meets diagnostic criteria for fetal alcohol syndrome. It is recommended to the caregiver that she initiate obtaining "educational rights" over her nephew so she can request an Individual Education Plan from his school's administration. An assessment for attention-deficit/hyperactivity disorder (ADHD), such as the Conners, National Initiative for Children's Healthcare Quality Vanderbilt, or another standardized measure for ADHD, should be given to the caregiver and teacher to each evaluate the child. Prescription for stimulant medications may be warranted in conjunction with behavioral therapy. Depending on local resources, the caregiver and child may be referred for psychotherapy, including parent-child interactive therapy in which his aunt may be coached on how to deal with his behaviors in the most positive, effective manner.

Selected References

American Academy of Pediatrics Committee on Substance Abuse and Committee on Children With Disabilities. Fetal alcohol syndrome and alcohol-related neurodevelopmental disorders. *Pediatrics*. 2000;106(2):358–361

Bertrand J, Floyd RL, Weber MK, et al. *Fetal Alcohol Syndrome: Guidelines for Referral and Diagnosis*. Atlanta, GA: Centers for Disease and Prevention; 2004

Bonthius DJ, Olson HC, Thomas JD. Proceedings of the 2006 annual meeting of the Fetal Alcohol Spectrum Disorders Study Group. *Alcohol*. 2006;40(1):61–65

Goodlett CR. Fetal alcohol spectrum disorders: new perspectives on diagnosis and intervention. *Alcohol*. 2010;44(7–8):579–582

Riley EP, McGee CL. Fetal alcohol spectrum disorders: an overview with emphasis on changes in brain and behavior. *Exp Biol Med (Maywood)*. 2005;230(6):357–365

University of Washington Center on Human Development & Disability. FAS Diagnostic & Prevention Network. http://depts.washington.edu/fasdpn. Accessed December 16, 2013

CHAPTER 135

Newborns of Substance-Abusing Mothers

Sara T. Stewart, MD

CASE STUDY

A neonate is born by emergency cesarean delivery because of abruptio placentae. The mother is a 29-year-old gravida 6, para 4, aborta 2 with a history of crack cocaine and heroin abuse during pregnancy. The newborn is 36 weeks' gestation with a birth weight of 2,400 g and length of 43 cm. Physical examination is normal. The newborn does well for the first 10 hours but then develops jitteriness with irritability, diarrhea, sweating, and poor feeding. A urine toxicology test on the newborn and mother are positive for cocaine.

Questions

1. What complications affect neonates secondary to maternal substance abuse during pregnancy?
2. What withdrawal symptoms do newborns experience as a result of maternal substance abuse during pregnancy?
3. What typical behavioral and learning problems are found in newborns, infants, and children whose mothers abused illicit substances during pregnancy?
4. What are the appropriate management strategies for neonates who have experienced in utero drug exposure?

Maternal substance abuse during pregnancy places neonates at risk for a number of medical, psychosocial, and developmental problems. The particular problems experienced by newborns depend on the drug (or drugs) to which they have been exposed; many have been exposed to multiple drugs in addition to cigarettes and alcohol. The long-lasting effects of alcohol exposure are well established, but the effects of newer drugs are less well defined. Illicit drugs change in their popularity, form of use, and availability at different points in time.

The environment into which children are born also affects their health and development. Environments in which substance abuse is common are frequently suboptimal for normal growth and development because of the effect of substance abuse on parenting; fragmentation of families; domestic violence; incarceration of significant family members; illnesses, including HIV infection; limited financial resources; homelessness or substandard housing; unemployment; child abuse and neglect; and limited access to health care. Because of these environmental issues, many drug-exposed neonates are cared for by foster parents or non-parental family members. These factors also make it difficult to determine, in a given newborn, which problems are caused by the drug exposure versus accompanying environmental conditions. This differentiation is of less significance to the physician than the researcher or epidemiologist because the physician will care for the problems that drug-exposed newborns manifest regardless of etiology.

Epidemiology

Approximately 10% of women between the ages of 15 and 44 years report having used illicit substances in the past month. While data collected via maternal self-report are typically an underestimate of prevalence, one national survey reported that 5.2% of women used illicit substances while pregnant. The highest rate of use was among pregnant adolescents aged 15 to 17 years—22% reported illicit drug use in the past month. The same survey also found that 12% of women reported drinking alcohol and 16% reported smoking cigarettes while pregnant. Meconium analysis has demonstrated not only extensive differences in the prevalence of in utero drug exposure among hospitals but has also shown differences in the substances of choice in different geographic areas. While polysubstance abuse is the most common clinical scenario in all communities, national data on the primary drug of choice for pregnant teens admitted for substance abuse treatment have shown changes over the past 15 years. Primary alcohol abuse has decreased by 50%, primary cocaine abuse has decreased by 66%, primary methamphetamine abuse has increased by 4.4%, and primary marijuana abuse has increased by 2.4%.

Clinical Presentation

Many of the different substances that women use while pregnant can result in similar sequelae in the newborn, infant, or child. In utero growth restriction, irritability, disordered eating or sleeping, and hypertonicity may be seen in newborns and infants. Older children may have developmental delays, symptoms of attention-deficit/hyperactivity disorder (ADHD), learning disabilities, or behavioral difficulties such as oppositional or impulsive behavior. Newborns that have been prenatally exposed to opiates such as heroin or methadone may manifest symptoms of neonatal abstinence syndrome (drug withdrawal), including respiratory, gastrointestinal (GI), or nervous system effects such as apnea, tachypnea, emesis, diarrhea, irritability, hypertonicity, tremors, seizures, temperature instability, and sneezing. Symptoms often occur within 72 hours of birth, but because of the long half-life of methadone, symptoms of methadone withdrawal may take up to 5 days to develop.

Alcohol and cocaine have been associated with birth defects as well. Abnormalities such as absent limbs, cardiac defects, genitourinary anomalies, ocular anomalies, and microcephaly have been reported with cocaine exposure. Alcohol has been associated with a spectrum of effects, termed fetal alcohol spectrum disorders (FASDs). (See Chapter 134.) Within this spectrum, a subset of patients fit the well-defined criteria for a diagnosis of fetal alcohol syndrome (FAS), including facial dysmorphology, growth deficiency, and neurodevelopmental abnormality. The presence of the following 3 sentinel features in the facial dysmorphology is the most sensitive and specific diagnostic finding for FAS: a flat philtrum, thin upper lip, and short palpebral fissures. The spectrum of neurodevelopmental problems includes diagnoses such as microcephaly and seizures, as well as many types of developmental, cognitive, and behavioral difficulties. Also included within FASD is a category for alcohol-related birth defects, which includes anomalies such as congenital heart defects, skeletal deformities, renal anomalies, hearing loss, ophthalmologic abnormalities, and cleft lip and palate.

Pathophysiology

Drugs used by pregnant women may affect newborns in 3 different ways: the drugs may be addictive and result in symptoms of withdrawal during the neonatal period; they may be toxic and lead to impaired functioning and neurodevelopmental problems; and they may be teratogenic and cause congenital anomalies and a dysmorphic appearance. The ultimate effects of the drugs are a complex interaction of environmental and genetic influences that are variable depending on the timing of the prenatal exposure. Differences in maternal metabolism of drugs lead to differences in fetal exposure to toxins, and genetically determined differences in fetal susceptibility to the toxins lead to a spectrum of effects in exposed neonates. During gestation, the effects of drug exposure also vary depending on the timing of exposure. Each organ has a unique period of susceptibility as it forms during the first trimester. Prenatal substance exposure during this period is more likely to result in organ malformation. The second and third trimesters primarily involve organ growth, cell differentiation, and functional maturation of organs, so exposure during this period is more likely to result in growth abnormalities or functional difficulties. The specific effects of the different substances on the developing fetus can be understood in terms of their biochemical properties.

In utero exposure to opiates such as heroin and methadone results in physiological addiction. These drugs bind to opiate receptor sites in the brain and GI tract. When the drugs are no longer present after birth, the newborn experiences withdrawal. Animal models have also found that prenatal exposure to opiates can lead to decreased density of cortical neurons and decreased development of neurons.

Cocaine and its metabolites cross the placenta and concentrate in amniotic fluid. Cocaine is toxic and teratogenic, and it interferes with 3 neurotransmitter pathways in the brain.

- Cocaine blocks the reuptake of norepinephrine. This is associated with tachycardia, hypertension, diaphoresis, and an increased incidence of preterm labor. Diffuse vasoconstriction may affect the placenta and lead to anomalies such as placental infarcts or abruptio placentae. The fetus may also be affected by the vasoconstriction and its resultant hypoperfusion and ischemia and may develop anomalies such as atresia of the GI tract, stroke, or absent limbs.

- Cocaine decreases the reuptake of dopamine. This effect is apparent in cocaine-using mothers who have decreased appetite and subsequent poor nutrition during pregnancy. Stereotypical behavior, hyperactivity, euphoria, confidence, and heightened sexuality may be associated with sexual promiscuity and increased risk of acquiring HIV and sexually transmitted infections (STIs).

- Cocaine decreases serotonin reuptake, leading to decreased sleep. The sleep cycle of cocaine-exposed neonates is often disrupted.

Methamphetamine is commonly manufactured from ephedrine or pseudoephedrine and has greater central nervous system (CNS) penetration than its metabolite, amphetamine. It has direct toxic effects on the CNS and causes increased release and decreased reuptake of dopamine, norepinephrine, and serotonin. These neurotransmitter alterations result in symptoms that are similar to those described for cocaine. There are limited published data on the incidence of teratogenesis as a result of in utero methamphetamine exposure, but recent data show that exposed newborns are at risk of being born small for gestational age.

Direct effects of methamphetamine use are dose- and frequency-dependent in the adult user. It has been shown to have cardiovascular, pulmonary, renal, and hepatic toxicity. Higher dose and increased frequency have also been associated with psychosis and toxicity to subcortical structures. More recent data have noted subcortical white matter and gray matter changes in prenatally exposed children.

Reports have documented the occurrence of withdrawal symptoms within days after birth in alcohol-exposed neonates, but more common effects of prenatal alcohol exposure are direct cellular toxicity and teratogenesis. The specific mechanism by which alcohol and its metabolites damage fetal tissues is unknown, but it has been shown to affect CNS neuronal migration and synaptogenesis. For a given level of alcohol intake, the precise level of fetal exposure to metabolites is likely to vary among women, depending on maternal genetic makeup and the resulting variability in alcohol metabolism. Timing of the exposure during different periods of development can also lead to different teratogenic effects on the fetus. Exposure during the first trimester may affect organogenesis or craniofacial development;

exposure in the second and third trimesters can cause poor growth and neurotoxicity. Maternal alcohol use may also be associated with poor nutrition, resulting in poor delivery of nutrients to the fetus.

Phencyclidine (PCP) has sympathomimetic effects, including increases in blood pressure, heart rate, respiratory rate, deep tendon reflexes, and tone. In addition, PCP has cholinergic effects, causing sweating, flushing, drooling, and pupillary constriction. Neonates exposed to PCP in utero do not exhibit these symptoms but display neurologic and developmental disorganization.

Differential Diagnosis

Major differential diagnoses relate to the symptomatology produced by the abused substance or substances (D_x Box). Neonates exposed to addictive substances, most commonly opiates such as methadone and heroin, may present with symptoms of withdrawal (Box 135-1). Irritability and jitteriness may be symptoms of drug withdrawal or direct drug neurotoxicity but may also be caused by hypoglycemia, hypocalcemia, hypomagnesemia, and sepsis. Seizures occur in 1% to 3% of heroin-exposed neonates, and the differential diagnosis for neonatal seizures includes intracranial hemorrhage, hypoxic-ischemic encephalopathy, CNS infection, CNS malformation, and metabolic disorders. Gastrointestinal symptoms such as vomiting or diarrhea may be confused with reflux, formula intolerance, obstruction, or infectious gastroenteritis.

Dysmorphic appearance may also be the result of alcohol or drug exposure. Fetal alcohol syndrome is the most clearly defined dysmorphic syndrome related to maternal substance abuse during pregnancy. In making such a diagnosis, other genetic disorders that may have overlapping findings should be considered as well.

Failure to thrive (FTT) may be a presenting complaint in newborns, infants, or children with a history of in utero drug or alcohol exposure. (See Chapter 133 for a discussion of the differential diagnosis of FTT.) It is important to consider maternal substance abuse in all patients who have been diagnosed with FTT, particularly if they were born small for gestational age.

Older children may present with a wide range of neurodevelopmental and behavioral problems. Common behavioral complaints include impulsivity, inattention, hyperactivity, and antisocial behavior. While many of these symptoms have been correlated with prenatal drug exposure, postnatal environmental factors such as continued parental substance abuse, violence, inconsistent or poor parenting, and foster care placement are also significant contributors. As a result, it may be difficult to clearly determine the precise etiology of developmental and behavioral problems in a child exposed to drugs or alcohol.

Maternal substance abuse should be considered in all neonates who present with STIs such as syphilis, hepatitis B, hepatitis C, and HIV.

Evaluation

History

The possibility of maternal substance abuse should be considered in the face of certain maternal risk factors, including the absence of prenatal care, evidence of poor maternal nutrition, poor maternal weight gain, presence of STIs, symptoms of acute intoxication, abruptio placentae, precipitous delivery, and a history of domestic violence.

Newborns who manifest symptoms of withdrawal should be evaluated for the possibility of maternal substance abuse. This assessment involves an appropriate history as well as a toxicologic evaluation. Mothers disclose their drug history to varying extents, depending on the circumstances of the interview. If mothers are concerned about the health and well-being of their newborns and do not fear legal repercussions, they are more likely to discuss their drug use. An appropriate drug history should be obtained in a nonjudgmental manner (Questions Box). Studies have shown that the use of a structured questionnaire rather than a cursory

---

Dx | Newborns of Substance-Abusing Mothers

- Symptoms of withdrawal (See Box 135-1.)
- Congenital anomalies
- Developmental delay and behavioral disorders
- Growth retardation
- Sexually transmitted infections

Box 135-1. Symptoms of Neonatal Abstinence Syndrome	
• Irritability	• Vomiting
• Jitteriness	• Diarrhea
• Tremors	• Apnea
• Hypertonicity	• Tachypnea
• Seizures	• Sweating
• Mottling	• Poor feeding
• Temperature instability	• Sleeping difficulties

Questions | Newborns of Substance-Abusing Mothers

- Did the mother use any substances such as alcohol, cigarettes, marijuana, or prescription and illicit drugs during the pregnancy?
- Has she ever used these substances? Is she currently using these substances?
- If so, how much? How frequently? By what route? To what extent is she trying to abstain?
- Is the mother at risk for sexually transmitted infections? Has she ever been tested?
- Did the mother have prenatal care? When did the care start?
- What is the status of other children in the family?
- Does the father abuse alcohol or drugs?

interview increases the incidence of reported substance abuse by 3- to 5-fold.

Physical Examination

Newborns should be assessed for common complications related to maternal substance abuse. They should undergo a full physical examination to check for the presence of any malformations. Growth measurements should be noted, and physicians should determine if evidence of growth impairment or microcephaly is present. Premature neonates should be monitored for problems related to prematurity, such as intraventricular hemorrhage and necrotizing enterocolitis. Assessment for signs of neonatal abstinence syndrome should be done in the days after birth (see Box 135-1). Neurologic and developmental status should be assessed and monitored at each visit. Abnormalities such as hypertonicity, coarse tremors, and extensor leg posture are frequently noted in the newborn period, and disturbances in fine and gross motor coordination may persist through the toddler years.

Laboratory Tests

In addition to obtaining a toxicologic history, screening for drugs should also be performed. The legal guidelines for screening mothers for drugs vary in different localities. In general, if clinical symptoms indicate a need, neonates can be screened on medical grounds without specific parental consent because the information obtained is important in the care of the newborn. Screening of the mother's urine without her consent is more problematic, however, because of the potential legal implications of a positive test result.

Testing is most commonly performed on urine samples, which are typically able to detect an exposure within the prior 3 days. It is important to realize that a negative screening test result does not rule out the possibility of exposure within this window of time, however, as a drug's metabolite may be present but not to the level of the test's detection threshold. Newer tests include meconium analysis, which is more sensitive and specific than urine and is able to detect exposures in the second and third trimesters. Recent data indicate, however, that its greatest sensitivity lies with exposures beyond 24 weeks' gestation. Analysis of newborn hair samples can also detect exposures occurring during the third trimester. At present, there is limited ability to determine precisely when an exposure occurred during gestation, other than according to the broad detection windows discussed here in conjunction with maternal self-reporting on the timing of drug use.

Most screening tests of urine, meconium, and hair samples use immunoassay techniques, which are inexpensive and sensitive but not very specific. False-positive results may be obtained for multiple illicit substances. Common scenarios include a positive amphetamine screen result in a patient who has taken over-the-counter medication containing ephedrine or pseudoephedrine, or a positive opiate screen result in a patient who is using cough medicine with dextromethorphan. For this reason, and because of the potential legal implications of a positive result in this setting, it is strongly recommended that positive immunoassay results be confirmed with further testing of the sample via gas chromatography or mass spectrometry.

Further evaluation in the neonatal period should include an evaluation for the presence of STIs, particularly HIV, hepatitis B, hepatitis C, and syphilis.

Imaging Studies

There is no routine imaging recommended based solely on a history of in utero substance exposure. Instead, imaging should be directed by symptomatology. For example, newborns with a heart murmur and history of prenatal alcohol exposure warrant a cardiac evaluation and possible echocardiography. Also, newborns with prenatal drug exposure and abnormal neurologic examinations should have a thorough neurologic evaluation, which may include neuroimaging.

Management

In the neonatal period, the management of newborns exposed to drugs requires attention to associated conditions such as prematurity, in utero growth restriction, and in utero infection with STIs.

Irritability and crying may occur from withdrawal or as the result of drug toxicity on the CNS. These newborns may respond to swaddling, a soothing voice, or a quiet environment as a means to reduce the symptoms. Some exposed newborns may have slow or disordered feeding and may require evaluation by an occupational therapist or nutritionist as well.

The assessment of a newborn's withdrawal symptoms is typically done using a standardized scoring tool to assist in the documentation of symptom severity. Once scores reach a threshold level, pharmacologic treatment may be required. For opiate-exposed neonates, treatment is with an opiate such as methadone or diluted tincture of opium. Phenobarbital is also commonly used in cases of polydrug exposure. Diazepam is useful for symptoms related to alcohol withdrawal or rapidly reverse symptoms of opioid withdrawal. Problems with using diazepam relate to the presence of sodium benzoate in the preparation, which can displace bilirubin from albumin. Medications should be tapered over time, allowing infants to outgrow the dosage.

Social service is also a key component of management. In many jurisdictions, child protective services must be notified of positive toxicologic test results on newborns or their mothers. Likewise, newborns who display symptoms of neonatal drug withdrawal may also have to be reported to these agencies. These agencies are generally responsible for performing a home assessment and determining the adequacy of the home environment. In some cases, newborns may be assigned to foster homes, and parents may be ordered to participate in drug treatment programs and parenting classes.

After the newborn period, the focus of management is on the provision of **well-child care** and **developmental monitoring.** Attention should be paid to physical growth and administration of immunizations. If a sensory impairment or neurodevelopmental delay is apparent, children should be referred to appropriate community agencies. Federal programs that operate under the Individuals with

Disabilities Education Act provide interventional services for disabled and at-risk children 6 years and younger.

Symptoms of ADHD or other behavioral problems in older children may require intervention, with recommendation for specific school programs as well as pharmacologic treatment. Regular assessments of school performance should be obtained from children's teachers. Standardized neurodevelopmental tests should be administered at periodic intervals to ensure appropriate progress.

Prognosis

Many neonates, particularly those exposed to alcohol in utero, suffer long-term sequelae and disability. Most commonly, these effects are subtle but can have far-reaching effects for the newborn. Remedial educational programs help but do not cure problems. Recent studies have shown that for children who were exposed to drugs, the environment in which they are raised is a significant factor affecting their ultimate outcome. A stable, nurturing environment minimizes the many adverse effects of prenatal drug exposure and promotes normal neurodevelopment by enforcing the acquisition of skills and knowledge.

CASE RESOLUTION

The case study presented highlights typical features of the neonate who was exposed to drugs. Management includes testing for hepatitis B, hepatitis C, syphilis, and HIV and administering medication such as phenobarbital if irritability does not respond to swaddling or other measures. The situation should be reported to child protective services to ensure an assessment of the neonate's home environment.

Selected References

Bandstra ES, Morrow CE, Mansoor E, Accornero VH. Prenatal drug exposure: infant and toddler outcomes. *J Addic Dis.* 2010;29(2):245–258

Behnke M, Smith VC; American Academy of Pediatrics Committee on Substance Abuse and Committee on Fetus and Newborn. Prenatal substance abuse: short- and long-term effects on the exposed fetus. *Pediatrics.* 2013;131(3):e1009–e1024

Cotten SW. Drug testing in the neonate. *Clin Lab Med.* 2012;32(3):449–466

Hudak ML, Tan RC; American Academy of Pediatrics Committee on Drugs and Committee on Fetus and Newborn. Neonatal drug withdrawal. *Pediatrics.* 2012;129(2):e540–e560

Jansson LM, Velez M. Neonatal abstinence syndrome. *Curr Opin Pediatr.* 2012;24(2):252–258

Jansson LM, Velez ML. Infants of drug-dependent mothers. *Pediatr Rev.* 2011;32(1):5–13

Lester BM, Lagasse LL. Children of addicted women. *J Addict Dis.* 2010;29(2):259–276

Nguyen D, Smith LM, Lagasse LL, et al. Intrauterine growth of infants exposed to prenatal methamphetamine: results from the infant development, environment, and lifestyle study. *J Pediatr.* 2010;157(2):337–339

Substance Abuse and Mental Health Services Administration. Results from the 2010 National Survey on Drug Use and Health: Summary of National Findings. NSDUH Series H-41, HHS Publication No. (SMA) 11-4658. Rockville, MD: Substance Abuse and Mental Health Services Administration; 2011. http://oas.samhsa.gov/nsduhLatest.htm. Accessed October 21, 2013

University of Washington Center on Human Development and Disability. FAS Diagnostic & Prevention Network. http://depts.washington.edu/fasdpn. Accessed October 21, 2013

CHAPTER 136

Substance Abuse

Monica Sifuentes, MD

CASE STUDY

A 17-year-old male is brought to your office by his father with a chief complaint of chronic cough. You have followed this patient and his siblings for several years and know the family quite well. The father appears very concerned about "this cough that just won't go away." The adolescent is not concerned about the cough, however, and reports no associated symptoms such as fever, sore throat, chest pain, or sinus pain. You ask the father to step out of the room for the rest of the interview and the physical examination.

On further questioning, the patient reports that he smokes a few cigarettes a day and has tried marijuana as well as cocaine. He denies regular use of these substances but reports exposure to these drugs at parties and when he hangs out with "certain friends." The adolescent is now in the 11th grade, attends school regularly, and thinks school is "OK." His grades are average to above average, but he thinks he might fail history this semester. Although he used to play baseball, he dropped out last year. He hopes to get a part-time job at a local fast-food restaurant this summer if his parents let him. Currently he is sexually active and uses condoms occasionally. He denies suicidal ideation and exposure to any firearms.

On physical examination, he appears well developed and well nourished with an occasional dry cough. He is afebrile, and his respiratory rate, heart rate, and blood pressure are normal. Pertinent findings on examination include slight conjunctival injection bilaterally and mild erythema of the posterior pharynx. No tonsillar hypertrophy is apparent. The rest of the examination is within normal limits.

Questions

1. What are the most common manifestations of substance use and abuse in adolescents?
2. What are the risk factors associated with substance abuse in adolescents?
3. What other conditions must be considered when evaluating adolescents with a history of chronic substance abuse?
4. What laboratory evaluations, if any, should be considered in adolescents with suspected substance use or abuse?
5. What are the specific consequences, if any, of short-term and long-term use or abuse of substances such as alcohol, marijuana, cocaine, opiates, and hallucinogens?

Primary care practitioners are in a unique position to educate patients, particularly young teenagers, about substance use and abuse through primary prevention and anticipatory guidance. Opportunities for education include health maintenance visits, the preparticipation sports physical evaluation, and encounters for an acute injury or illness. More importantly, given their long-standing relationship with families, primary care practitioners can identify and treat a substance abuse problem as it develops and assist patients and their families with appropriate referrals and local resources.

Ideally, all preteens and adolescent patients should be questioned and counseled about the use of illicit drugs, alcohol, and tobacco at each health maintenance visit (see chapters 6 and 35). Unfortunately, this occurs inconsistently because most health care professionals often feel uncomfortable opening Pandora's box or simply do not have the resources to intervene. Time constraints, unfamiliar billing codes, and difficulty maintaining confidentiality for sensitive services in a busy office or clinic make screening for substance use a major challenge. Primary care practitioners thus lose a valuable opportunity to adequately assess adolescents for substance abuse and provide them with the necessary guidance to ensure their future health, safety, and well-being.

Substance use can be defined as the use of or experimentation with illicit drugs, alcohol, or tobacco. Illicit drugs include marijuana; cocaine; amphetamines; hallucinogens such as lysergic acid diethylamide (LSD), mescaline, and psilocybin, which is found in *Psilocybe mexicana* mushrooms; opiates; and phencyclidine (PCP). **Substance abuse** refers to the chronic use of mind-altering drugs in spite of adverse effects. **Addiction**, a chronic relapsing disorder, is the term applied to compulsive and continued use of a substance in the face of these adverse consequences. Because addiction is neurologically based, the substance may produce physical dependence or symptoms of withdrawal when it is discontinued.

Epidemiology

Current Trends and Prevalence Rates

A wide range of substances are currently being used by adolescents in the United States. Alcohol, tobacco, and marijuana are clearly the more common and most popular substances and serve as gateway drugs to more serious drug use. Several surveys tracking adolescent substance use and abuse are conducted annually in the United States to identify the magnitude of high-risk behavior among 8th to 12th graders. The 3 most well-known of these surveys are Monitoring the Future, administered annually to 8th, 10th, and 12th graders by the University of Michigan for the National Institute on Drug Abuse; the Youth Risk Behavior Surveillance System (YRBSS) survey, conducted biannually by the Centers for Disease Control and Prevention (CDC) of students in grades 9 through 12; and the National Household Survey on Drug Abuse and Health, a computer-assisted interview of residents 12 years and older conducted in the home. It is important to remember that most statistics do not include the estimated 15% to 20% of students who drop out of high school before their senior year.

In a recent survey of graduating high school seniors (2011 YRBSS), approximately 70% admitted to **alcohol** use at some time during their life. Almost 40% of students reported drinking alcohol during the month preceding the survey, and 3% to 5% admitted that they used alcohol daily. Binge drinking has probably contributed most to the overall morbidity and mortality associated with alcohol use in adolescents and young adults. Among high school seniors in the class of 2011, almost one-third reported having 5 or more drinks in a row at least once during the previous 2 weeks. Although **tobacco** use among adolescents decreased from 1999 to 2011, data from the CDC reveal that approximately 20% of teenagers nationwide still report current cigarette use. Eight percent of adolescents smoked half a pack or more of cigarettes per day in 2011 compared with 11% in 2005 and 19% in 1977. Among students nationwide who smoked cigarettes and are younger than 18 years, 14% report buying them themselves in a store (eg, convenience store, supermarket, discount store) or gas station. Nationwide, current smokeless tobacco use (eg, chewing tobacco, snuff, dip) and cigar or cigarillo use is 8% and 13%, respectively. As expected, its use is much higher among males than females.

Marijuana is the most commonly used illicit psychoactive substance. In 1993, 35% of high school seniors reported ever having used marijuana; in 1997, this figure increased to more than 50%. Current estimates from the 2011 YRBSS report this figure to be approximately 40%, with nearly 25% reporting marijuana use one or more times during the month preceding the survey. Daily use of marijuana has been reported in 5% of high school seniors.

The use of other substances among adolescents had generally taken a downward trend in the late 1980s and early 1990s; however, figures are increasing again. This is known in the substance abuse literature as "generational forgetting," as adverse effects of specific drugs fade over the years. Reportedly, approximately 9% of high school graduates in 1997 tried cocaine, with approximately 4% having used it in the previous month. These figures remained essentially unchanged until 2007, when its use declined and is currently at an historical low of 2.6% among 12th-graders. The 1991 prevalence rate for LSD usage was 5%, and its use also remained stable over in the next 10 years until 2001, when it increased to 8% and became more widespread than cocaine use among high school students. According to the 2011 YRBSS survey, 14% of 12th-grade males nationwide tried LSD or another hallucinogenic drug. Lifetime amphetamine use among 12th-graders was 4% in 2011 and ranged from 2.3% to almost 8% across state surveys. In addition, nationwide ecstasy use was reported as approximately 8%.

Concurrently, the reported use of over-the-counter (OTC) nonprescription stimulants that contain caffeine has increased, with popular energy drinks now sold in many convenience stores and supermarkets. Other substances used to "get high," such as inhalants (eg, aerosol spray paints, hair sprays, paint thinners, whipped cream containers), are often used by younger students (preteens) and unfortunately can be found in many garages and basements. Although decreased from 1997, 14% of adolescents continue to report sniffing or inhaling substances to become intoxicated in 2011. Dextromethorphan also has become popular as an OTC product abused by adolescents secondary to its hallucinogenic effects and easy accessibility in cough syrups. Studies confirm an increasing trend in its abuse, particularly in teens younger than 18 years.

The nonmedical use and abuse of prescription drugs such as Oxycontin, Percocet, Vicodin, Adderall, Ritalin, and Xanax has increased more than most illicit drugs in the past 2 decades. Many teens report the ease at which prescription drugs can be obtained, leading to continued abuse and future dependence as an adult. In 2011, nonmedical prescription drug use was reported by 20% of teenagers one or more times during their life. Certain prescription drugs, namely opioids, stimulants, sleeping pills, and anxiolytics, now represent the third most widely abused substance in adolescents after alcohol and marijuana.

Although not considered an illicit substance by some, anabolic steroids are abused by some adolescents, mostly males, to increase muscle size and strength. In 1997, approximately 3% admitted to using them at some time in their lives. More recently, studies indicate as many as 5.5% of high school students participating in sports use anabolic steroids (6.6% males, 3.9% females). The 2011 nationwide figure per the CDC is almost 4%; however, these figures vary across state and local surveys from 2% to 7%.

Demographics

In general, adolescent males use illicit drugs more than females do, with a few exceptions. Males are more likely to use anabolic steroids, but females reportedly use amphetamines, barbiturates, tranquilizers, and OTC diet pills more than their male counterparts. In addition, although annual prevalence rates for overall alcohol use show little gender difference, adolescent males have a higher rate of heavy or binge drinking. Tobacco usage is essentially the same for both genders, except for smokeless tobacco and cigars, where males predominate.

Non–college-bound adolescents are more likely to use illicit substances than their college-bound counterparts, and these adolescents are also more likely to use drugs more frequently. There is no difference, however, between the 2 groups in the rates of ever having tried illicit substances. Binge drinking also continues to escalate among older adolescents and young adults attending college. The specific influence of parental education, socioeconomic status, and race or ethnicity on the use and abuse of illicit substances is difficult to determine because many other factors, such as genetics and the environment, contribute to drug use and addiction.

Risk Factors and Behaviors

Although alcohol and tobacco are considered licit or lawful drugs, it is illegal for minors to purchase and use alcohol and tobacco in the United States. Their use, however, often begins during adolescence, including during the preteen years. The strongest predictor of drug use by youth is having friends who use drugs (alcohol, tobacco, or other substances) regularly. In addition, it has been shown that the more risk factors identified, the greater the risk of substance abuse in the teenager.

Several factors are important precursors (risk factors) to drug use during adolescence. These include association with drug-using peers; attitudinal factors, such as favorable attitudes toward drug use in the family; low religiosity; poor school performance or academic failure, often beginning in the late elementary years; young age of initiation of alcohol or drug use; presence of a conduct disorder; environmental factors, such as the prevalence of drug use in a given community; family history of alcoholism or drug use; poor parenting practices; high levels of conflict within the family; minimal bonding between parents and children; and early and persistent problem behaviors during childhood, such as untreated attention-deficit/hyperactivity disorder (ADHD).

It is well documented in the literature that early age of onset of alcohol and tobacco use is predictive for the use of other drugs, a greater variety of drugs, and more potent agents. Additionally, the use of alcohol at an early age is associated with future alcohol-related problems such as lifetime alcohol dependence and abuse. The early initiation of alcohol also results in greater sexual risk-taking behavior during adolescence (ie, unprotected sexual intercourse, exposure to multiple sexual partners, being drunk or high during sexual intercourse, and increased risk of pregnancy) as well as academic problems and delinquent behavior later in adolescence. Long-term effects during young adulthood include difficulties with employment, criminal and aggressive behavior, and continued substance abuse.

The role of the media and technology in adolescent alcohol and tobacco use has been the subject of much discussion over the last 10 years. A number of studies have confirmed that exposure to television and movie smoking is one of the key factors that prompt teens to smoke and that preteens whose parents forbid them from viewing R-rated movies are less likely to begin smoking or drinking. One prospective study revealed that exposure to R-rated movies or having a television in the bedroom significantly increased the risk of initiating smoking for white teenagers. Additionally, watching more movie depictions of alcohol use is strongly predictive of drinking onset and binge drinking in adolescents in the United States. Advertising also contributes to the depiction of alcohol and tobacco use as normative activities. In fact, it has been reported that advertising may be responsible for up to 30% of adolescent alcohol and tobacco use.

Clinical Presentation

Adolescents who are involved in alcohol or drug use may present to the physician in several different ways. Illicit substance use might be uncovered during the routine interview for an annual health maintenance visit, preparticipation sports physical evaluation, or urgent care appointment. Alternatively, the adolescent might have physical complaints including chronic cough, persistent allergies, chest pain, and fatigue. Chronic conditions such as asthma may continue to worsen despite appropriate therapy in the adolescent smoking tobacco or marijuana.

Abdominal tenderness may be noted on physical examination and found to be associated with gastritis, hepatitis, or pancreatitis. The adolescent also recently may have been in a motor vehicle crash or involved in other trauma, or their parents may complain of the teen's frequent mood swings, irritability, or erratic sleep patterns.

Pathophysiology

Although several theories have been proposed to explain why casual substance use develops into abuse and addiction in some adolescents and not others, the most critical factor seems to be the presence of underlying psychopathology. Adolescents who have untreated major depressive disorders, ADHD, or schizophrenia, for example, may use mood-altering substances to treat unpleasant feelings of dysphoria and low self-esteem. Initially used as a temporary measure, this method of self-medication increases the likelihood of chronic substance abuse.

It is well known that genetic influences also play a role in adult use and abuse of alcohol; however, less evidence exists for adolescent drug use. What is known is that families and parental attitudes play a significant role in the development of alcohol and other drug use in teens. Permissive attitudes toward alcohol and drug use by parents or guardians and parental or older sibling drug use predict greater drug and alcohol use in the adolescent.

Differential Diagnosis

The differential diagnosis for symptoms and behaviors associated with substance abuse includes underlying psychiatric disorders. Affective, antisocial, and conduct disorders as well as ADHD can be the primary or secondary condition in adolescents who are abusing drugs. Like adults, adolescents may be using illicit drugs to self-medicate. The pharmacology and toxicity of the illicit substances most commonly used by adolescents are summarized in Table 136-1.

Evaluation

History

The interview should be conducted in a private, quiet area to minimize interruptions. If parents or guardians have accompanied the adolescent, they should be politely asked to leave the room after they have had an opportunity to express their concerns and after issues of confidentiality are addressed in the presence of both parties. This helps to avoid future uncomfortable moments when parents return and ask what was disclosed in their absence. After parents have left the room, issues addressing confidentiality and privacy should be reviewed once again with the patient. Special circumstances, such as a disclosure of sexual or physical abuse or possible suicide

Table 136-1. Pharmacology and Toxicity of Substances Commonly Used by Adolescents

Substance	Pharmacology	Effects	Toxicity
Nicotine	Potent psychoactive drug, acting on receptors in CNS to produce effects: stimulation, relaxation, focused attention		**Non-tolerant individuals** Weakness, nausea, vomiting Feeling unwell
Marijuana	Active ingredient (Δ^9-tetrahydro-cannabinol) rapidly absorbed into bloodstream from inhaled smoke	**Low dose** Euphoria, relaxation, time distortion, auditory and visual enhancement **High dose/toxic** Mood fluctuations, hallucinations, paranoia, psychosis	**Acute** Panic attacks, psychosis (rare) **Chronic** Short-term memory impairment, amotivational syndrome, reduced sperm counts
Alcohol	Causes nerve cell membranes to expand and become more "fluid"—interfering with neuronal conduction Interference of neurotransmitters	**Mild** Disinhibition, euphoria, mild impaired coordination, mild sedation **Moderate** Increased sedation, slurred speech, ataxia	**Severe** Confusion, stupor, coma, respiratory depression
Cocaine	Increased release and decreased reuptake of biogenic amines causing CNS and peripheral nervous system stimulation Local anesthesia Vasoconstriction	Produces a sense of well-being and heightened awareness, decrease in social inhibition, intense euphoria	Delirium, confusion, paranoia, hypertension, tachycardia, hyperpyrexia, mydriasis
Stimulants Amphetamines Crystal methamphetamine Ecstasy	CNS stimulation (sympathomimetic)	Heightened awareness Restlessness and agitation, decreased appetite Low doses increase ability to concentrate.	Hypertension, hyperthermia, seizures, stroke, coma, arrhythmias
Hallucinogens LSD Mescaline Mushrooms	Inhibits release of serotonin	Distortions of reality—perceptual alterations, synesthesia common (eg, "hearing" smells)	Paranoia, flashbacks, psychosis, depression
PCP	Dissociative anesthetic with analgesic, stimulant, depressant, and hallucinogenic properties	Dissociative anesthetic Dose-dependent euphoria, dysphoria, perceptual distortion	Psychoses; aggressive, violent behavior; depression; seizures, rhabdomyolysis
Opiates Opium Heroin Methadone	Binds to opioid receptors in CNS, causing CNS depression	Sedative analgesics Euphoria followed by sedation, somnolence	Respiratory depression, CNS depression, miosis, bradycardia, hypotension, arrhythmia, seizures, rhabdomyolysis
Sedatives Benzodiazepines Barbiturates	CNS depression, binds to specific receptor that potentiates GABA	Sedation Anxiety reduction	Similar to opioid intoxication
Anabolic steroids	Bind to androgen receptors at cellular level, stimulate production of RNA and protein synthesis	Euphoria Increased irritability and aggressiveness Induction of mental changes at high doses	Psychosis
Inhalants	CNS stimulation and excitement, progressing to depression	Euphoria, hallucinations, psychosis	Respiratory depression, arrhythmia, seizures, sudden sniffing death syndrome (sudden death secondary to arrhythmia)

Abbreviations: CNS, central nervous system; GABA, γ-aminobutyric acid; LSD, lysergic acid diethylamide; PCP, phencyclidine.

Data from Schwartz B, Alderman EM. Substances of abuse. *Pediatr Rev.* 1997;18(6):204–215, and Joffe A, Blythe MJ, eds. Mental health, psychotropic medications, and substance abuse. *Adolesc Med.* 2003;14:455–466.

ideation or homicidal intent, that dictate that confidentiality be broken also should be discussed with the teen (see Chapter 6).

The interview should then proceed in a casual, non-pressured, non-judgmental fashion. Initial inquiries should cover less-threatening general topics such as school, home life, and outside activities, including activities with friends. **HEADDSSS** (*h*ome environment, *e*mployment and education, *a*ctivities, *d*iet, *d*rugs, *s*afety, *s*exual activity/sexuality [including a history of sexual abuse or assault], *s*uicide/depression) allows for a thorough review of the essential components of the psychosocial history (see Chapter 6). Another interview tool, **SSHADESS** (*s*trengths, *s*chool, *h*ome, *a*ctivities, *d*rugs/substance abuse, *e*motion/depression, *s*exuality, *s*afety), has been developed to emphasize and review positive components in an adolescent's life in addition to his or her high-risk behavior.

Some practitioners prefer to use questionnaires to obtain this background information. A questionnaire is given to patients to fill out while they are waiting to be seen, and responses are reviewed privately during the actual visit. Some questionnaires address only issues related to substance abuse (Box 136-1), while others are more general but also include questions about alcohol, tobacco, and drugs (Box 136-2). Controversy exists about the role of such questionnaires, primarily concerning the truthfulness of answers, because parents may be with teenagers as they are attempting to complete the form.

More specific questions related to the use of alcohol and tobacco as well as illicit substances should be asked after general subjects have been discussed (Questions Box). If adolescents seem wary of

---

Box 136-1. Questionnaire Items Relevant to Substance Abuse

		Y	N
1.	Do you smoke cigarettes?	Y___	N___
2.	Do you smoke marijuana?	Y___	N___
3.	Do you often feel "bummed out," down, or depressed?	Y___	N___
4.	Do you ever use drugs or alcohol to feel better?	Y___	N___
5.	Do you ever use drugs or alcohol when you are alone?	Y___	N___
6.	Do your friends get drunk or get high at parties?	Y___	N___
7.	Do you get drunk or get high at parties?	Y___	N___
8.	Do your friends ever get drunk or get high at rock concerts?	Y___	N___
9.	Do you ever get drunk or get high at rock concerts?	Y___	N___
10.	Have your school grades gone down recently?	Y___	N___
11.	Have you flunked any subjects recently?	Y___	N___
12.	Have you had recent problems with your coaches or advisers at school?	Y___	N___
13.	Do you feel that friends or parents just do not seem to understand you?	Y___	N___

From American Academy of Pediatrics. *Substance Abuse: A Guide for Professionals.* Schonberg SK, ed. Elk Grove Village, IL: American Academy of Pediatrics; 1988.

Box 136-2. Rapid Assessment for Adolescent Preventive Services

1. In the past 12 months, have you tried to lose weight by taking diet pills or laxatives, making yourself vomit (throw up) after eating, or starving yourself?
2. Do you eat some fruits and vegetables every day?
3. Are you active after school or on weekends (walking, running, dancing, swimming, biking, playing sports) for at least 1 hour, on at least 3 or more days each week?
4. Do you always wear a lap/seat belt when you are driving or riding in a car, truck, or van?
5. Do you always wear a helmet when you are biking, rollerblading, skateboarding, motorcycling, snowmobiling, skiing, or snowboarding?
6. During the past month, have you been threatened, teased, or hurt by someone (on the Internet, by text, or in person) or has anyone made you feel sad, unsafe, or afraid?
7. Has anyone ever abused you physically (hit, slapped, kicked), emotionally (threatened or made you feel afraid), or forced you to have sex or be involved in sexual activities when you didn't want to?
8. Have you ever carried a weapon (gun, knife, club, other) to protect yourself?
9. In the past 3 months, have you smoked cigarettes or any other form of tobacco (cigars, black and mild, hookah, other) or chewed/used smokeless tobacco?
10. In the past 12 months, have you driven a car drunk, high, or while texting or ridden in a car with a driver who was?
11. In the past 3 months, have you drunk more than a few sips of alcohol (beer, wine coolers, liquor, other)?
12. In the past 3 months, have you smoked marijuana, used other street drugs, steroids, or sniffed inhalants ("huffed" household products)?
13. In the past 3 months, have you used someone else's prescription (from a doctor or other health provider) or any nonprescription (from a store) drugs to sleep, stay awake, concentrate, calm down, or get high?
14. Have you ever had any type of sex (vaginal, anal, or oral sex)?
15. Have you ever been attracted to the same sex (girl to girl/guy to guy) or do you feel that you are gay, lesbian, or bisexual?
16. If you have had sex, do you always use a method to prevent sexually transmitted infections and pregnancy (condoms, female barriers, other)?
17. During the past month, did you often feel sad or down as though you had nothing to look forward to?
18. Do you have any serious problems or worries at home or at school?
19. In the past 12 months, have you seriously thought about killing yourself, tried to kill yourself, or have you purposely cut, burned, or otherwise hurt yourself?
20. Do you have at least one adult in your life who you can talk to about any problems or worries?
21. When you are angry, do you do things that get you in trouble?

Reproduced with permission from Possibilities for Change, ©2006, The Regents of the University of Michigan, Version 5 (2014). Further reproduction or use is not permitted. For authorized use of RAAPS survey, visit www.raaps.org.

Adolescent Substance Abuse   **Questions**

- Do any of the adolescent's friends drink alcohol, smoke marijuana or tobacco, or use any other drugs?
- What drugs, including alcohol and tobacco, are currently being used by the adolescent? For how long and how frequently?
- In what environments does the adolescent use these substances?
- Has the adolescent ever blacked out or been arrested while under the influence of drugs or alcohol?
- Has drug or alcohol use ever interfered with school, work, or other social activities?
- Has drug or alcohol use adversely affected relationships with family, friends, or romantic partners?
- Has the patient ever had sexual encounters while under the influence of drugs or alcohol?
- Does the adolescent ever use drugs or alcohol to feel better or to forget why he or she feels sad?
- Do the adolescent's parents use alcohol, tobacco, or illicit drugs?

Box 136-3. The CRAFFT Questions: A Brief Screening Test for Adolescent Substance Abuse[a]

C   Have you ever ridden in a CAR driven by someone who was "high" or had been using alcohol or drugs?

R   Do you ever use alcohol or drugs to RELAX, feel better about yourself, or fit in?

A   Do you ever use alcohol or drugs while you are by yourself (ALONE)?

F   Do you ever FORGET things you did while using alcohol or drugs?

F   Do your FAMILY or FRIENDS ever tell you that you should cut down on your drinking or drug use?

T   Have you ever gotten into TROUBLE while you were using alcohol or drugs?

[a]Two or more "yes" answers suggest that the adolescent may have a significant problem with abuse or dependence and warrants an additional assessment.

From Knight JR, Sherritt L, Shrier LA, Harris SK, Chang G. Validity of the CRAFFT substance abuse screening test among adolescent clinic patients. *Arch Pediatr Adolesc Med.* 2002;156(6):607–614. © John R. Knight, MD, Boston Children's Hospital, 2014. All rights reserved. Reproduced with permission. For more information, contact cesar©childrens.harvard.edu.

---

answering these questions, it may be helpful to initially inquire about their friends. Questions should be phrased with the assumption that the responses will be affirmative (eg, "How many beers do your friends drink in a week? And you, do you drink the same amount?"). It is hoped that this less-threatening approach invites more honest answers. An assessment of the risk of suicidal behavior is also indicated.

Because many clinicians do not have unlimited time to interview adolescents and obtain all of the details at one visit, another approach has been developed to efficiently screen for drug and alcohol problems using 3 questions: During the past 12 months, have you smoked marijuana or hashish? Have you drank any alcohol? Have you used anything else to get high? If adolescents answer "no" to all 3 questions, they should still be asked if they have ridden in a car with a driver who was high or had been using alcohol or drugs. Additional screening is recommended for any teenager who answers "yes" to any of the 3 initial screening questions. Six questions, known as the **CRAFFT screen**, are then reviewed with the adolescent to further identify drug and alcohol risk or problems (Box 136-3). The teen receives 1 point for each "yes" answer; a total score of 2 or more indicates a positive screen and high risk for a substance use disorder. It also indicates the need for additional follow-up as well as referral to a mental health professional or program. The validity of this brief, developmentally appropriate tool for screening adolescents has been reported in the literature and is well supported by experts in the field of adolescent and addiction medicine for use by primary care practitioners.

Physical Examination

Positive findings on physical examination are rare, especially in adolescents who use alcohol or other substances only occasionally. In adolescents with a history of chronic substance abuse, however, certain physical findings may be present.

All vital signs should be reviewed. Tachycardia and hypertension occur primarily with acute intoxication with cocaine or stimulants such as amphetamines. The current weight also should be recorded and compared with previous values, and any significant weight loss should be noted. The skin should be examined closely for track marks, skin abscesses, or cellulitis, especially if patients admit to using drugs intravenously. Findings consistent with hepatitis (hepatomegaly and jaundice) may be present in these individuals. The presence of diffuse adenopathy, thrush, leukoplakia, seborrheic dermatitis, or parotitis should raise the suspicion of HIV infection. A nonspecific maculopapular rash also may be seen during the acute viremic phase of an HIV infection. Upper respiratory symptoms such as chronic nasal congestion, long-lasting "colds" and "allergies," and epistaxis can occur with chronic inhalation of cocaine. Signs of nasal congestion, septal perforation, and wheezing may be noted on examination. In addition, smoking crack cocaine can cause chronic cough, hemoptysis, and chest pain. Smoking marijuana over long periods can result in similar findings. Gynecomastia can be seen with use of anabolic steroids, marijuana, amphetamines, and heroin. In the adolescent female using anabolic steroids, there may be signs of virilization, such as a deep voice, hirsutism, and male pattern baldness. The detailed neurologic evaluation is probably the most important part of the examination. Any abnormalities in memory, cognitive functioning, or affect should be noted. Chronic marijuana use is sometimes accompanied by an amotivational syndrome.

Acute intoxication with some drugs such as cocaine may lead to delirium, confusion, paranoia, seizures, hypertension, tachycardia, arrhythmias, mydriasis, and hyperpyrexia. Acute PCP intoxication produces abnormal neurologic signs, tachycardia, and hypertension. Findings such as central nervous system and respiratory depression, miosis, and cardiovascular effects (eg, pulmonary edema, orthostatic hypotension) are consistent with opiate overdose. However, signs and symptoms of acute intoxication are generally seen in the emergency department setting rather than in the primary care physician's office or clinic.

Laboratory Tests

Routine drug screening in the evaluation of possible substance abuse is not recommended and generally not indicated. Specific laboratory studies should be performed only in those patients who are known substance abusers and enrolled in a drug treatment program to monitor for abstinence, who are required by court order, or with an acute presentation of altered mental status, intoxication, or abnormal neurologic findings, such as may be seen in an emergency department setting. In the office setting, these symptoms are frequently absent, and urine or serum studies to "check" for drug use are not warranted or useful.

If these tests are performed, they require the adolescent's consent. The results should not be shared with anyone other than the patient, unless the patient gives permission or the substance found is the cause of an acute medical condition. According to the American Academy of Pediatrics (AAP) and the Society for Adolescent Health and Medicine, obtaining a urine drug test without the consent of the adolescent undermines the physician-adolescent relationship and the development of a meaningful, trusting relationship at this critical time in the patient's life. Drug testing should not be performed simply to allay parental anxiety or confirm suspicions about possible substance abuse for a parent, teacher, or athletic coach.

If urine is obtained for drug testing, it is critical that it is not contaminated or diluted and that the practitioner be familiar with the particular laboratory performing the drug test as well as the reported sensitivity and specificity of each test. Urine testing is available to detect marijuana and its metabolites, cocaine, amphetamines, PCP, opiates, barbiturates, and benzodiazepines. Blood levels can be obtained for alcohol, marijuana, cocaine, amphetamines, barbiturates, and benzodiazepines. Although salivary or urinary concentrations of cotinine and nicotine concentrations can also be performed, these measurements are primarily used in research studies.

Testing for specific inhalants is not routinely done. The deleterious effects of these substances on the hematologic, liver, and renal systems can be evaluated by performing a complete blood cell count, liver function tests, prothrombin time and partial thromboplastin time, and blood urea nitrogen and creatinine, but results are generally nonspecific.

Management

One of several approaches to the problem of substance use and abuse can be chosen depending on the adolescent's degree of risk-taking behavior and drug involvement (experimentation, limited use, problematic use, abuse, or addiction/dependence), the practitioner's relationship with the adolescent and family, the adolescent's desire to change behavior, and the family's awareness of the problem. The reader is referred to the excellent and informative 2011 policy statement, "Substance Use Screening, Brief Intervention, and Referral to Treatment for Pediatricians," by the AAP Committee on Substance Abuse for a more detailed discussion.

Anticipatory Guidance

If preteens (middle school students) or adolescents and their peers are not participating in any high-risk behaviors, including tobacco, alcohol, or drug use (ie, the answers to all 3 CRAFFT screening questions are "no"), pediatricians should provide patients with age-appropriate anticipatory guidance. This should include advice and information on safety issues, consequences of alcohol and tobacco use, and exposures to illicit and prescription drugs. Adolescents should be praised for making smart choices and encouraged to continue their current behavior but should be invited to return to the office if they have any questions or problems. This may be particularly helpful for patients whose daily environment exposes them to high-risk situations for alcohol and drug use. The pediatrician should encourage an open dialogue about substance abuse between adolescents and their parents to assist teenagers in developing strategies for drug avoidance.

Early Intervention

Primary care practitioners should provide early intervention guidance to preteens and adolescents who have begun or are engaging in occasional high-risk behavior and are considered at moderate risk of having substance use–associated problems. These are patients who have started using alcohol or drugs and score 0 or 1 on the CRAFFT screen. Such use implies only occasional or casual use of illicit substances by patients or peers. This scenario is the most challenging because many adolescents, as well as their parents, perceive occasional alcohol or drug use as "experimental" or a phase of "normal teen behavior" and therefore may trivialize any advice given by the pediatrician. Interventional guidance involves clear advice to stop alcohol and other drug use and a discussion of potential risks created by the adolescent's current behavior. For example, individuals who drink alcohol or smoke marijuana at parties have an increased risk of involvement in a motor vehicle crash afterward as the driver or passenger. Another common scenario involves alcohol intoxication and poor judgment with regard to sexual behavior. All teens should be made aware of the possible consequences of their unsafe behavior, especially if their occasional drug use has progressed to more regular use in risky situations. Further, they should receive educational counseling about the unhealthy effects of alcohol use as a teen (eg, alcohol's deleterious effects on developing brain cells). Experts also recommend including strength-based counseling to recognize the positive qualities of the adolescent.

Specialized Programs

Preteens or adolescents who are routinely using drugs but are clearly motivated to stop can often be managed by primary care physicians alone or collaboratively with child and adolescent mental health specialists. Teenagers who began using illicit substances at an older age, have a fairly good relationship with their families, have supportive relationships with friends who do not use drugs, and who continue to do well in school and participate in other outside activities are more likely to be successful. Practitioners initially should identify the problem and establish whether adolescents desire to change their behavior. Then, after obtaining consent from the patient, practitioners should meet with families, develop an appropriate strategy for treatment intervention, and follow the adolescents periodically in the office. Timely and consistent reinforcement by the primary care physician is necessary, especially in the beginning of treatment. Referral to outpatient programs, such as Alcoholics Anonymous, Alateen, or Narcotics Anonymous, also may be indicated. Appropriate community resources for the teenager and family should be reviewed.

Mental Health or Treatment Programs

Referral to a mental health or addiction specialist or a specialized treatment program (eg, drug detoxification center) is indicated for adolescents who display clear signs of dangerous behavior and continue to use drugs despite office treatment by the primary care practitioner and adverse effects on their daily lives and relationships. Adolescents who are using intravenous drugs, combining sedative drugs, or consuming large quantities of alcohol also warrant immediate intervention. In addition, those teenagers who are suspected to have a concomitant psychologic or psychiatric condition should be referred immediately for psychiatric evaluation. Other criteria for specialty treatment programs include a long history of drug abuse, a serious life-threatening event in conjunction with substance abuse (eg, attempted suicide, motor vehicle crash), familial strife, or persistent involvement with a drug-dependent crowd. Primary care practitioners should become familiar with local inpatient programs and residential substance abuse treatment facilities in their community and partner with mental health and addiction specialists to provide the patient and family with optimal services. Although the selection of a program may be influenced by financial resources and insurance coverage options, it is very important to select an appropriate one for the adolescent and family. Guidelines exist to aid practitioners in the selection process for public and private facilities. These guidelines include total abstinence, appropriate professionals with expertise in drug addiction, familial involvement in the program, family therapy, and appropriate outpatient follow-up. Regardless of the final deposition of the patient, it is important for the primary care practitioner to remain involved with the family while making these difficult decisions and support their experience throughout the recovery process.

Prevention Programs

Prevention programs have been developed to assist and influence the decisions young people make about the use of illicit substances. Current programs focus on multiple aspects of the lives of children and adolescents. Programs may involve individual decision-making, self-esteem, and basic education about drugs. They frequently emphasize communication skills, family values and dynamics, parenting skills, and positive peer associations. Structured curricula also have been created for use in the schools, and community outreach programs have been organized by groups such as local police departments. The actual effectiveness of each type of program is a subject of controversy, but they are all aimed at somehow preventing the initial or continued use of illicit substances in children and preteens.

For an excellent resource and guide for parents and professionals, refer to *Reaching Teens: Strength-Based Communication Strategies to Build Resilience and Support Healthy Adolescent Development*, edited by Kenneth R. Ginsburg, MD, MSEd, FAAP, FSAHM, and Sara B. Kinsman, MD, PhD.

Prognosis

It is difficult to assess the outcome for adolescents who undergo treatment for substance abuse because definitions of success vary. For some teenagers, success implies periods of sobriety; for others, it means complete abstinence; and for still others, it is abstinence in addition to recovery from other contributing problems. Specific outcome data that are available, however, reveal that abstinence rates are positively correlated with regular attendance in a support group and parental participation in these groups. In addition, general success rates range from 15% to 45%, depending on short- or long-term assessments. As expected, there is a lifetime potential for relapse among all adolescents with a history of substance abuse.

CASE RESOLUTION

In the case presented at the beginning of this chapter, the adolescent is at high risk for continued substance abuse given his drug-using friends, tobacco use, possible school failure, and recent change in extracurricular activities (ie, dropping out of baseball). The findings on physical examination also are consistent with his smoking history. The physician should review these risk factors with the teenager in private and acknowledge the difficulty in removing one's self from such an environment. The adolescent's motivation to change his behavior should be assessed, and referrals to special intervention programs can be discussed. Regardless of the outcome, the physician should continue to see the teenager at an agreed-on interval to monitor his ability to quit smoking and high-risk behavior.

Selected References

Adger H, Saha S. Alcohol use disorders in adolescents. *Pediatr Rev.* 2013;34(3):103–114

American Academy of Pediatrics. *Reaching Teens: Strength-Based Communication Strategies to Build Resilience and Support Healthy Adolescent Development.* Ginsburg KR, Kinsman SB, eds. Elk Grove Village, IL: American Academy of Pediatrics; 2014

American Academy of Pediatrics Committee on Substance Abuse. Alcohol use by youth and adolescents: a pediatric concern. *Pediatrics.* 2010;125(5):1078–1087

American Academy of Pediatrics Committee on Substance Abuse. Substance use screening, brief intervention, and referral to treatment for pediatricians. *Pediatrics.* 2011;128(5):e1330–e1340

American Academy of Pediatrics Committee on Substance Abuse. Testing for drugs of abuse in children and adolescents. *Pediatrics.* 1996;98(2):305–307

American Academy of Pediatrics Committee on Substance Abuse and Council on School Health. Testing for drugs of abuse in children and adolescents: addendum—testing in schools and at home. *Pediatrics.* 2007;119(3):627–630

American Academy of Pediatrics Council on School Health and Committee on Substance Abuse. The role of schools in combating illicit substance abuse. *Pediatrics* 2007;120(6):1379–1384

Anderson SL, Schaechter J, Brosco JP. Adolescent patients and their confidentiality: staying within legal bounds. *Contemp Pediatr.* 2005;22:54–64

Blankson KL, Thompson AM, Ahrendt DM, Patrick V. Energy drinks: what teenagers (and their doctors) should know. *Pediatr Rev.* 2013;34(2):55–62

Bryner JK, Wang UK, Hui JW, Bedodo M, MacDougall C, Anderson IB. Dextromethorphan abuse in adolescence: an increasing trend: 1999–2004. *Arch Pediatr Adolesc Med.* 2006;160(12):1217–1222

Dandoy C, Gereige RS. Performance-enhancing drugs. *Pediatr Rev.* 2012;33(6):265–272

Eaton DK, Kann L, Kinchen S, et al. Youth risk behavior surveillance—United States, 2011. *MMWR Surveill Summ.* 2012;61(4):1–162

Frankowski BL, Leader IC, Duncan PM. Strength-based interviewing. *Adolesc Med State Art Rev.* 2009;20(1):22–40

Frese WA, Eiden K. Opioids: nonmedical use and abuse in older children. *Pediatr Rev.* 2011;32(4):e44–e52

Gray KM, Upadhyaya HP, Deas D, Brady KT. Advances in diagnosis of adolescent substance abuse. *Adolesc Med Clin.* 2006;17(2):411–425

Heyman RB. Screening for substance abuse in the office setting: a developmental approach. *Adolesc Med State Art Rev.* 2009;20(1):9–21

Hollman D, Alderman E. Substance abuse counseling. *Pediatr Rev.* 2007;28(9):355–357

Knight JR, Sherritt L, Shrier LA, Harris SK, Chang G. Validity of the CRAFFT substance abuse screening test among adolescent clinic patients. *Arch Pediatr Adolesc Med.* 2002;156(6):607–614

Kulig JW; American Academy of Pediatrics Committee on Substance Abuse. Tobacco, alcohol, and other drugs: the role of the pediatrician in prevention, identification, and management of substance abuse. *Pediatrics.* 2005;115(3):816–821

Levy S, Knight JR. Helping adolescents to stop using drugs: role of the primary care clinician. *Adolesc Med.* 2008;19:83–98

Rimsza ME, Moses KS. Substance abuse on the college campus. *Pediatr Clin North Am.* 2005;52(1):307–319

Rogers PD, Copley L. The nonmedical use of prescription drugs by adolescents. *Adolesc Med State Art Rev.* 2009;20(1):1–8

Sanchez-Samper X, Knight JR. Drug abuse by adolescents: general considerations. *Pediatr Rev.* 2009;30(3):83–93

Strasburger VC; American Academy of Pediatrics Council on Communications and Media. Children, adolescents, substance abuse, and the media. *Pediatrics.* 2010;126(4):791–799

CHAPTER 137

Eating Disorders

Monica Sifuentes, MD

CASE STUDY

A 16-year-old female is brought to the office by her mother because she feels that her daughter is too thin and appears tired. The mother complains that her daughter does not eat much at dinner and always says she is not hungry. Recently, the girl bought diet pills that were advertised in a teen magazine. The teen claims that she hasn't taken the pills, so she doesn't understand why her mother is so upset. She says she feels fine and considers herself healthy because she has recently become a vegetarian.

The girl is a 10th-grade student at a local public school and attends classes regularly, although her friends are occasionally truant. She is involved in the drill team, swim team, and student council. She has many friends who have "nicer" figures than she does. Neither she nor her friends smoke tobacco or use drugs, but they occasionally drink beer at parties. The girl is not sexually active and denies a history of abuse. Her menstrual periods are irregular; the last one was approximately 3 months ago.

She currently lives with her mother, father, and 2 younger siblings. Although things are "OK" at home, she thinks her parents are too strict and don't trust her. They have just begun to allow her to date, but she dislikes that she has a curfew.

Her physical examination is significant for a thin physique and normal vital signs. On the growth chart, her weight is at the 15th percentile and her height at the 75th percentile, giving her a body mass index of 17 (10th percentile). The remainder of her physical examination is unremarkable.

Questions

1. What are the common characteristics of disordered eating in adolescents?
2. What are the important historical points to include when interviewing patients with suspected eating disorders? Which teens are considered at risk?
3. How is the diagnosis of anorexia nervosa (AN) and bulimia nervosa (BN) made?
4. What is the treatment plan for adolescents with eating disorders?
5. What are the medical complications of AN and BN?
6. What is the prognosis for these conditions? How can primary care practitioners help improve the outcome?

Eating disorders are complex problems that are sometimes difficult to diagnose based on strict *Diagnostic and Statistical Manual of Mental Disorders, Fifth Edition,* criteria (Box 137-1). Adolescents may have partial or atypical presentations, a history of anorexia nervosa (AN) and bulimia nervosa (BN), or an underlying affective component that confuses the issue. They may not display a blatant refusal to eat but may instead exhibit subtle characteristics of disordered eating: constant dieting, obsession with a certain physical exercise, or irregular menstruation. In addition, preoccupation with physical appearance and weight is not uncommon or necessarily pathologic in today's Western society. The fashion industry and media promote the idea that thinness and beauty are interrelated. Thus, typical adolescents who long to be accepted by peers and who are learning to develop a sense of independence and control are prime targets for the development of eating disorders. The primary care physician is in a unique position to recognize individuals at risk, appropriately screen those teenagers with specific behaviors, and provide early intervention to prevent the development of a full-blown eating disorder (Box 137-2). The overall goal is to decrease the lifelong medical and psychologic morbidity and mortality associated with this condition in adolescents.

Epidemiology

In general, eating disorders are most common among white females and in more affluent communities. Although they occur in many other settings, in previous years they were nearly unheard of in lower socioeconomic groups, among ethnic minorities, or in children younger than 12 years. Today they can be seen in all ethnic, cultural, and social backgrounds in the United States as well as in other developed countries. In addition, males make up an estimated 5% to 10% of all patients with eating disorders.

Although dieting behavior among adolescents and young adults is not uncommon, true AN has a prevalence of approximately 0.5% to 1% in these individuals. Estimates have ranged from 1% to 10% in high-risk groups such as upper- and middle-class white females. Less than 5% of these cases are males, with a female-male ratio of 9:1. The age of onset historically was reported to occur during middle adolescence (age 14–16 years). However, it has become increasingly more common for school-aged children and younger teens to be dissatisfied with their weight and concerned with body image. Studies of middle-income elementary school girls have reported significant body and weight dissatisfaction. Skipping meals and

---

Box 137-1. Diagnostic Criteria for Anorexia Nervosa and Bulimia Nervosa

Anorexia Nervosa

A. Restriction of energy intake relative to requirements, leading to a significantly low body weight in the context of age, sex, developmental trajectory, and physical health

B. Intense fear of gaining weight or becoming fat, or persistent behavior that interferes with weight gain, even though at a significantly low weight

C. Disturbance in the way in which one's body weight or shape is experienced, undue influence of body weight or shape on self-evaluation, or persistent lack of recognition of the seriousness of the current low body weight

Bulimia Nervosa

A. Recurrent episodes of binge eating, characterized by both of the following:
   (1) Eating, in a discrete period, an amount of food that is definitely larger than most people would consume under similar circumstances and in a similar period
   (2) A sense of lack of control over eating during the episode

B. Recurrent inappropriate compensatory behavior to prevent weight gain (self-induced vomiting; misuse of laxatives, diuretics, or other medications), fasting, or excessive exercise.

C. Criteria A and B both occur on average at least once a week for 3 months.

D. Self-evaluation is unduly influenced by body shape and weight.

E. The disturbance does not occur exclusively during episodes of anorexia nervosa.

Adapted and reproduced with permission from American Psychiatric Association. *Diagnostic and Statistical Manual of Mental Disorders.* 5th ed. Washington, DC: American Psychiatric Association; 2013.

Box 137-2. *Diagnostic and Statistical Manual for Primary Care Child and Adolescent Version* **Diagnostic Criteria: Dieting/Body Image Problem**

- Dieting and voluntary food restrictions that result in weight loss or failure to gain weight as expected during growth, but behaviors not intense enough to qualify for diagnosis of anorexia nervosa.
- Individual becomes obsessed with the pursuit of thinness and develops fears of gaining weight.
- Consistent disturbance in body perception; denies dieting or weight loss is a problem.

Adapted from American Academy of Pediatrics. *The Classification of Child and Adolescent Mental Diagnoses in Primary Care: Diagnostic and Statistical Manual for Primary Care (DSM-PC) Child and Adolescent Version.* Wolraich ML, ed. Elk Grove Village, IL: American Academy of Pediatrics; 1996.

Variants of eating disorders, which do not meet full diagnostic criteria but cause significant distress or impairment in social, occupational, or other important areas of functioning (eating disorder not otherwise specified), are not uncommon in preteens and adolescents. Exact numbers are uncertain because many of these patients remain "under the radar" and the consequences of their eating behaviors are not fully recognized. Additionally, more than half of junior high and high school girls have dieted at some time, many repeatedly.

Clinical Presentation

Patients with eating disorders may present with general complaints related to weight loss such as fatigue or syncope. They also may exhibit minimal weight gain according to standard growth charts or a delay in the onset of puberty or progression of pubertal development. More importantly, many adolescents also may present with primary or secondary amenorrhea noted incidentally during an annual health maintenance or sports physical examination. Sometimes an underlying psychiatric condition, such as obsessive-compulsive disorder (OCD), is the grounds for the medical referral. Occasionally, patients with undiagnosed eating disorders are hospitalized because of complications related to their condition, such as electrolyte disturbances associated with diuretic use, hematemesis from induced vomiting, or syncope from hypovolemia. Finally, the preteen or adolescent may be referred to the primary care physician by concerned parents, well-intentioned friends, informed coaches, or astute school personnel who notice significant weight loss.

Pathophysiology

Anorexia Nervosa

Although several risk factors predispose individuals to the development of AN, this condition has no single cause (Box 137-3). Longitudinal studies clearly point to a significant role of inappropriate dieting behavior in the pathogenesis of an eating disorder. However, because not all dieters develop an eating disorder, other significant

desserts, fasting, and vomiting were all reported specifically to lose weight. Unfortunately, the goal for many of these young girls is not to be of normal weight but to be underweight.

The prevalence of BN is approximately 1% to 4%, although some studies report that as many as 8% of adolescents and college women and 0.4% of men are bulimic. The age of onset tends to be later than for AN, with symptoms beginning during late adolescence (age 17–20 years) and young adulthood. Females outnumber males by a factor of 5. Several behavioral and affective disorders have been associated with the development of AN and BN. These include comorbid psychiatric conditions such as depressive, bipolar, and anxiety disorders; alcoholism and substance abuse; other addictive behaviors (eg, laxative abuse); poor impulse control; and obsessive-compulsive personality. Girls who are obese or experience early puberty also are at increased risk for developing an eating disorder, with symptoms starting in the context of dieting. A past history of sexual abuse may be present among patients with eating disorders. In addition, suicidal behavior (attempts) is more likely in individuals with BN, as are reports of an increased incidence of family members with substance abuse and dependence disorders. In general, eating disorders occur more frequently in patients with a family history of eating and mood disorders as well as obesity.

Box 137-3. Risk Factors for the Development of an Eating Disorder

- Family history of an eating disorder or obesity
- Affective illness or alcoholism in a first-degree relative
- Specific activities/sports: ballet, gymnastics, modeling, running, wrestling
- Personality characteristics (eg, perfectionism)
- Parental eating behavior and weight
- Low self-esteem
- Physical or sexual abuse
- Body image dissatisfaction
- History of excessive dieting, frequently skipped meals, compulsive exercise

Adapted from Rome ES, Ammerman S, Rosen DS, et al. Children and adolescents with eating disorders: the state of the art. *Pediatrics*. 2003;111(1):e98–e108

---

contributing factors must be involved. Current theory suggests that a complex relationship exists among multiple factors and that genetic-environmental interactions, along with the adolescent's personal experiences (epigenetics) and individual personality traits, contribute to the etiology of AN.

Biological Factors

It has been postulated that the normal increase in adipose tissue with the onset of puberty creates a special problem for some females. An eating disorder may develop as an attempt to control or combat this normal pubertal weight gain with the initiation of dieting behavior. Preexisting hypothalamic dysfunction also has been implicated as a contributing factor to AN. In addition, changes in neurotransmitter levels have been shown to occur with initial vomiting or dieting. These changes may lead to specific psychiatric symptoms that may perpetuate disordered eating. However, recent data with neuroimaging studies have shown that most of the physiological disturbances resolve with normalization of the patient's body weight. In addition, a premorbid disturbance in the neurotransmitter serotonin has been speculated to be a risk factor for the development of AN and BN. Serotonin controls appetite by creating a sensation of fullness or satiety. In addition, it is known to have an effect on sexual and social behavior, mood, and stress responses. Although further studies are needed to confirm the exact role of this hormone in the development of an eating disorder, it has been shown that decreases in this brain neurotransmitter have been associated with impulsivity, aggression, and depression.

Leptin, a circulating hormone produced in adipose tissue, also seems to have a significant role in mediating the neuroendocrine effects of AN. Decreased concentrations of leptin are seen with reduced body fat stores as a result of decreased caloric intake and energy deficits. Paradoxically, leptin levels also appear to contribute to physical hyperactivity (compulsive exercise, restlessness), which is often seen in patients with AN despite their inadequate metabolic intake.

Genetic Factors

A genetic predisposition to anorexia has been shown in studies of monozygotic twins. The incidence of the disorder is increased in sisters and other female relatives of patients with AN.

Personal Characteristics

In general, patients with anorexia are described as obsessive-compulsive personality types, perfectionists, and overachievers, particularly in academics and sports. They also display low self-esteem and high anxiety levels despite their perceived successes by others. They are the "model daughters" who have never caused any previous problems given their compliant, self-sacrificing, dutiful, nonassertive nature.

There is an increased association between AN and major depression as well, and many studies of women have shown that first-degree relatives of patients with AN have higher rates of depression than the general population. However, many depressive symptoms in patients with AN improve with the restoration of body weight. Therefore, some of these clinical features of depression also may be secondary to the adolescent's state of severe malnutrition or starvation.

Familial Influences

Researchers have noted that certain family dynamics may serve to initiate and perpetuate AN, although it is no longer believed that family dysfunction is the main cause of disordered eating. Typically, however, the family is overprotective and rigid, with the mother often enmeshed in her daughter's life. Conflict resolution tends to be poor, and an inability to express feelings within the family is often evident. Diagnosis of an eating disorder often causes additional stress in the family, thus contributing to more difficulties in their relationships. Multiple case-control studies have shown there is a higher rate of AN and BN in relatives of patients with eating disorders. This may be due to inheritance patterns of personality traits as well as comorbid mood and anxiety disorders.

Social/Environmental Pressures

The media and post-industrialized, high-income societal standards are believed to play a role in setting the stage for the development of an eating disorder. Affluent communities are especially at risk if thinness, food, eating, and obsessive exercise become the prime focus of daily activity. In addition, young women become caught in what has been labeled a "slender trap" in which thinness is equivalent to attractiveness and success. Food restriction or purging is a means of attaining thinness. An inability to maintain thinness equals failure. Role models in the media, such as fashion models and actresses, also serve as ideals by which young people create their physical standards.

Other Influences

Involvement in particular extracurricular activities that promote thinness, such as ballet, gymnastics, figure skating, and running, may contribute to the development of AN in females. For male athletes, such influences include participation in sports such as wrestling, crew, or long-distance running, in which maintaining a given weight is important and dieting is used to achieve that weight. Chronic medical conditions, such as diabetes mellitus or inflammatory bowel disease (IBD), also may contribute to the development of an eating disorder.

Bulimia Nervosa

Several theories have been proposed to explain the etiology of BN, but similar to AN, no single etiology has been confirmed. Most likely, multiple factors contribute to the development of this eating disorder, and it is the complex interaction between these factors at a particular developmental point in an older adolescent's life that leads to this condition.

Biological, psychologic, familial, and societal influences are thought to contribute to the development of BN in older teenagers and young adults. Among other issues, adolescent and parental obesity are risk factors for BN, as are early menarche, early sexual experiences, and a history of childhood sexual or physical abuse that occurs in conjunction with a comorbid psychiatric condition. More importantly, dieting has been documented as an important risk factor in this age group.

Familial dysfunction and high levels of conflict also have been associated with BN. Unlike with AN, conflict might be discussed openly but negatively within the family, and there may be an inadequate expression of emotions that may lead to a lack of parental warmth and concern. Thus, the relationship between the parent and teenager is distant rather than enmeshed. The adolescent generally has a low level of self-esteem, high impulsivity, and body image dissatisfaction. Additionally, parents and relatives have a high rate of affective and eating disorders as well as alcoholism.

Differential Diagnosis

It is important to differentiate AN from BN, although occasionally this distinction may be difficult to make if patients display behavior consistent with both conditions. In addition, approximately 50% to 60% of patients with eating disorders have associated comorbid psychiatric disorders. Major affective disorders to consider include depression, bipolar disorder, and OCD. Anxiety disorders and substance abuse also are commonly seen, although the latter is more strongly associated with BN.

Other diagnoses to consider when evaluating patients for AN include IBD, malabsorption, celiac disease, diabetes mellitus, malignancies, Addison disease, hyperthyroidism or hypothyroidism, hypopituitarism, tumors of the central nervous system (CNS), and chronic substance abuse, particularly with amphetamines and crack cocaine. Superior mesenteric artery syndrome is another important condition to consider in the differential diagnosis; however, it also can be a consequence of an eating disorder, specifically AN.

Evaluation

History

A complete medical history including a detailed review of systems should be obtained from all adolescents with suspected eating disorders to rule out the multiple other conditions in the differential diagnosis of weight loss. The primary care physician then should interview the patient alone and focus on establishing the diagnosis of disordered eating by addressing more specific issues related to

changes in food preferences (eg, vegetarian, vegan, low-fat diet), eating behaviors, dieting, calorie counting, weight history, exercise routine, and body image concerns (Questions Box). (See Steinegger and Katzman in Selected References for a detailed discussion of interviewing techniques to use in patients with a suspected eating disorder.) The severity of the medical and nutritional aspects of the condition should be determined initially, followed by a thorough psychosocial evaluation. Inquiries should focus on symptoms associated with complications of eating disorders, such as dysphagia secondary to esophagitis from recurrent vomiting, constipation from fluid restriction, or muscle weakness associated with emetine toxicity from chronic ipecac use. Although rarely seen by the primary care physician at the initial visit when the diagnosis of an eating disorder is made, recognition of serious medical complications is paramount to determining the direction and urgency of further care.

Questions

Eating Disorders

- Have there been any changes in the adolescent's weight? What is the most and least the adolescent has ever weighed? When did these weights occur and for how long?
- How does the adolescent feel about how he or she looks? Is there anything he or she would like to change? How long has he or she been feeling this way?
- How much does the adolescent want to weigh?
- How often does the adolescent weigh himself or herself?
- What is a typical day of eating like, including eating times, types of foods, beverages, amount consumed, and portion size?
- What did he or she eat yesterday (24-hour dietary recall)?
- Does the adolescent have any food restrictions? Is the teenager a vegetarian? Does he or she count calories? Binge eat?
- Does the adolescent hide or throw away food?
- How does the adolescent and his or her friends handle weight control?
- What does the adolescent do when he or she feels "fat"? Does the adolescent vomit to lose weight? How often does this occur? Triggers?
- Has the adolescent or any of his or her friends ever used diuretics, diet pills, ipecac, enemas, or laxatives to lose weight or compensate for overeating?
- Does the adolescent exercise? If so, what type and how often? Is he or she stressed if a workout is missed?
- In what sports or dance activities, if any, does the adolescent participate?
- For females, are menstrual periods regular? Last menstrual period? Age at menarche?
- Does the adolescent have any other symptoms associated with complications of eating disorders?
- Does the adolescent have any depressive symptoms, such as sleeping problems or fatigue, that can accompany eating disorders?

For Patients With Bulimia Nervosa
- When do binges occur?
- What are the precipitating factors?
- What happens specifically during a typical episode?
- Does the adolescent use drugs or alcohol?
- Is there a history of depression or attempted suicide? Sexual or physical abuse?

Interviewing an adolescent with an eating disorder can be quite challenging; however, a thorough psychosocial assessment should be performed after a discussion about confidentiality has occurred with the adolescent and his or her parents. The **HEADDSSS** format (home environment, employment and education, activities, diet, drugs, safety, sexual activity/sexuality, suicide/depression) is useful to direct the psychosocial interview from general topics to more sensitive ones (see Chapter 6). Particular attention should be paid to the adolescent's overall functioning at home, with friends, and at school; the presence of other comorbid psychiatric disorders such as depression or anxiety; and a history of suicidal ideation or sexual/physical abuse. Out-of-control behavior as a result of substance abuse also should be assessed. The use of psychological testing/questionnaires to assess cognition and depression may be beneficial, depending on the comfort level of the primary care practitioner with these tools. Otherwise, immediate consultation with a mental health professional is warranted.

A detailed menstrual history also must be obtained from females because secondary amenorrhea is frequently present in patients as an early sign of AN secondary to decreased body fat. Primary amenorrhea in the context of pubertal delay also can occur with AN. With BN, menses may be irregular or absent. A family history of eating disorders, substance abuse, or psychiatric disease should be reviewed with the teenager and confirmed by the parent or guardian.

A dietary history should be obtained from the adolescent as well as the parents or guardian independently and should focus on any dietary restrictions or aversions. This may be difficult initially because the patient often does not believe he or she has a problem with food. A 24-hour dietary recall can be an important place to begin the assessment.

Physical Examination

In both conditions, the patient should undress, wearing only underwear, for the physical examination. This prevents any bulky clothes from hiding the true body habitus. The current height and weight should be plotted on a growth chart and the body mass index calculated (weight [kg]/height [m^2]). Delayed growth or short stature should be noted because it can occur with severe malnutrition as well as other systemic conditions. Vital signs, including blood pressure, should be recorded and compared with previous measurements. Evidence of cardiovascular instability can be manifested by tachycardia, bradycardia, or orthostatic hypotension. The patient also may be hypothermic as a result of his or her overall malnutrition. The general appearance and affect of the patient must be noted. Adolescents with full-blown AN are often emaciated with an obvious loss of subcutaneous tissue and may appear apathetic or anxious or have a flat affect. Patients with BN may be mildly obese or of normal weight with a full-appearing facies secondary to parotid and submaxillary swelling, a complication of frequent purging. In most cases, however, the teen appears "normal" at the initial visit.

Characteristic physical findings in patients with **AN** are consistent with a "state of hibernation." Hypothermia, orthostatic hypotension, bradycardia, and lanugo (downy hair) on the arms and back

are seen. The palms and soles may be yellow secondary to hypercarotenemia, and pigmentation of the chest and abdomen may be increased as a result of malnutrition. Thinning or loss of pubic and scalp hair as well as dry or pale skin also may be seen. The breasts should be examined carefully for sexual maturity rating (SMR) (Tanner staging) as well as galactorrhea. The presence of galactorrhea, along with a history of amenorrhea, warrants further investigation for a prolactinoma. Of note, patients with AN may have interrupted or delayed pubertal development. A cardiac murmur must be noted and further evaluated because one-third of patients with anorexia have mitral valve prolapse. The abdomen should be palpated for tenderness or masses and may be scaphoid in appearance. Bowel sounds are often decreased in patients with anorexia, and stool may be palpated secondary to constipation. The presence of pubic hair (genital SMR) also should be noted. A rectal examination should be performed for any evidence of bloody stool, which is a finding consistent with IBD, or evidence of rectal prolapse. The extremities should be evaluated for coldness, mottling, or edema. They should also be palpated for tenderness because fractures may be present due to loss of bone mineralization. Finally, a complete neurologic examination, including a mental status evaluation and funduscopic examination, should be performed to exclude any signs of a CNS lesion or endocrine disorder.

In patients with **BN,** specific physical findings, if any, are often associated with dehydration and electrolyte imbalances that occur as a result of chronic vomiting or laxative abuse. Vital signs should be reviewed for tachycardia, sinus bradycardia, and orthostatic hypotension; their presence indicates hemodynamic instability. The patient also may be hypothermic. The skin should be inspected on the dorsum of the hand over the knuckles for scratches, scars, or calluses from self-induced vomiting (Russell sign). Periorbital petechiae and subconjunctival hemorrhages also may be seen as a result of recurrent or severe retching. The oropharynx should be inspected for dental caries, enamel erosion, or discoloration as well as for parotid hypertrophy. In addition, palatal scratches or mouth sores can be seen. The abdomen should be palpated for epigastric tenderness, fullness, or mid-abdominal pain. Positive findings may be the result of esophagitis, gastritis, or pancreatitis.

From a musculoskeletal standpoint, any muscle weakness or cramping should be appreciated and may indicate an electrolyte abnormality. Edema of the extremities may be seen in laxative abusers and should be noted.

Laboratory Tests

Box 137-4 lists the laboratory studies necessary in the evaluation of patients with **AN.** A complete blood cell count may be helpful because leukopenia, anemia, and, rarely, thrombocytopenia can be found with this disorder. Electrolytes (sodium, potassium, chloride, and carbon dioxide) and blood urea nitrogen are important, especially if patients use diuretics, laxatives, or ipecac. Serum magnesium, calcium, and phosphorous must be monitored, especially in the refeeding phase of treatment. The erythrocyte sedimentation rate may be low with anorexia and high with IBD or some other

---

**Box 137-4. Initial Laboratory Assessment
for a Patient With an Eating Disorder**

Anorexia Nervosa
- Complete blood cell count, erythrocyte sedimentation rate
- Serum electrolytes (Na, K, Cl, CO_2)
- Blood urea nitrogen/creatinine
- Serum glucose
- Serum calcium, phosphorous, magnesium, zinc
- Serum protein, albumin, cholesterol
- Liver function tests
- Endocrine laboratory tests (perform in patients with amenorrhea)
  — Urine pregnancy
  — Follicle-stimulating hormone
  — Luteinizing hormone
  — Estradiol
  — Thyroid function: thyroid-stimulating hormone/T_4/T_3
  — Prolactin
- Urine pH and urinalysis
- Electrocardiogram

Bulimia Nervosa
- Serum electrolytes (Na, K, Cl, CO_2)
- Serum glucose
- Serum calcium, phosphorous, magnesium, zinc
- Blood urea nitrogen/creatinine
- Serum amylase
- Urine pH and urinalysis
- Electrocardiogram

---

inflammatory process. Normal liver function tests aid in excluding other causes of weight loss. A normal serum amylase and lipase rule out other etiologies for recurrent vomiting such as pancreatitis. Serum tissue transglutaminase and immunoglobulin A levels can be obtained if there are concerns for celiac disease. Other urine and serum tests help differentiate an endocrine disorder from AN, especially in patients with primary or secondary amenorrhea (see Box 137-4). An electrocardiogram (ECG) allows practitioners to diagnose QTc prolongation, heart block, and arrhythmias. In addition, an ECG is indicated in patients with electrolyte abnormalities or with a history of significant purging or weight loss.

Laboratory abnormalities in **BN** reflect the type and extent of purging behavior of adolescents with this diagnosis. Box 137-4 summarizes the necessary laboratory studies for patients with BN.

Radiographic imaging studies, such as computed tomography of the head or magnetic resonance imaging of the brain, are indicated if the diagnosis of an eating disorder is uncertain or the neurologic examination is abnormal. Bone density studies, such as a dual-energy x-ray absorptiometry scan, are not performed routinely except in adolescents with sustained amenorrhea for 6 months or more. An upper and lower gastrointestinal series may be warranted in patients with esophageal complaints or if IBD is a strong

consideration. The performance of other procedures, however, should be based on the individual case.

Management

It is the role of primary care practitioners to recognize when inappropriate dieting and weight loss become an obsession for adolescents and when abnormal and unhealthy behaviors develop for maintenance of obvious malnutrition. When treating patients with eating disorders, physicians must first establish trust; in doing so, patients should be reassured that physicians are not attempting to remove all control by trying to make the adolescent "fat." The goal is to create a therapeutic alliance among the physician, adolescent, and family to restore and maintain the patient's health and well-being. Depending on the severity of symptoms and the comfort level of the physician in monitoring the early medical, nutritional, and psychologic issues, the adolescent may be followed by the primary care physician in conjunction with a registered dietitian, family therapist, and mental health professional (psychologist or psychiatrist). Early in the treatment course, the primary physician must be willing to follow the patient frequently (as often as once or twice a week if necessary). If the physician wishes to refer the patient to an experienced multidisciplinary team of specialists, it is important that the primary physician remain informed and involved in the care of the teenager.

A consensus must be reached among the adolescent, pediatrician, and mental health professional on the minimum acceptable weight given the patient's age, height, pubertal stage, premorbid weight, and previous growth trajectory. This should be done with the assistance of a registered dietitian who is experienced in working with children and teenagers with eating disorders. Unlike with adults, weight restoration in the adolescent also must take into account the requirements for normal pubertal growth. An agreement that describes goals of treatment and maintenance of health should then be established between the adolescent and all members of the treatment team. Weight gain must be the initial priority, especially in adolescents with AN, as long as the patient is otherwise medically stable and does not require inpatient hospitalization. Details about this nutritional regimen, which includes a stepwise increase in daily caloric intake, amounts of protein to be ingested, daily fat intake, vitamins and mineral requirements, and treatment goal weights, should be developed by the dietitian and reviewed with the adolescent and his or her family in conjunction with mental health support and close medical follow-up. Early nutritional rehabilitation and timely medical stabilization are essential to correct the cognitive deficits associated with disordered eating, especially severe restrictive AN.

Family and individual counseling is an important part of the overall therapeutic plan. Patients with disordered eating often try to hide or minimize their illness and generally have difficulty with their abnormal eating behavior and patterns and degree of weight loss. Parents, too, may be in denial or simply unaware of the extent of their teenager's condition. The primary care physician must work cooperatively with mental health colleagues to provide the necessary psychologic and psychiatric services for the patient. Although extremely difficult, patients must begin to acknowledge their behaviors and accept the need for assistance before effective mental health intervention can occur. This also allows adolescents to assert themselves and remain in control. Support groups may be beneficial and frequently are an important component of a day-treatment program (day hospitalization, partial hospitalization) for those adolescents with eating disorders who require more intensive outpatient care but not an inpatient hospitalization or residential program. Day-treatment programs are generally less costly and may be more accessible than traditional hospital-based programs.

Pharmacotherapy with agents such as selective serotonin reuptake inhibitors are generally not prescribed in adolescents with AN except to treat comorbid conditions like depressive and anxiety disorders. Several studies have shown, however, that these same medications can be effective in patients with BN by decreasing binge eating and purging behaviors. Serotonin or norepinephrine reuptake inhibitors are also an option.

Numerous studies have shown that eating disorders are best treated by an interdisciplinary professional team experienced in the care of children, adolescents, and young adults with eating disorders. This team generally consists of the primary care physician, an adolescent medicine specialist with expertise in caring for patients with eating disorders, a psychologist or psychiatrist, a registered dietician, and a social worker. Ideally, the team is available to offer inpatient and outpatient services, although most mild to moderately ill teens are managed in an outpatient setting. Criteria for inpatient admission should be established by the team and reviewed with patients and their families at the onset of therapy.

Medical complications of eating disorders are well established (Box 137-5). Inpatient treatment is required for less than 75% ideal body weight for age, gender, and stature; continued weight loss despite intensive outpatient treatment; or a history of rapid weight loss. Refusal to eat and body fat less than 10% also are criteria for hospital admission. Other indications include cardiovascular compromise, such as bradycardia (<50 beats/min during the day or <40 beats/min at nighttime), orthostatic hypotension (changes in blood pressure >10 mm Hg, or pulse >20 beats/min), or altered mental status; evidence of persistent hypothermia (<35.6°C [96.08°F]); suicidality (ideation, plan, or attempt) or out-of-control behavior; intractable vomiting; electrolyte disturbances or uncompensated acid-base abnormalities (serum potassium <3.2 mEq/L or serum chloride <88 mEq/L); hematemesis; and significant dehydration as evidenced by systolic blood pressure lower than 90 mm Hg or syncope. Cardiac arrhythmias, including prolonged QTc, also require inpatient monitoring. Rarely does confirmation of the diagnosis warrant an inpatient stay. The goal of hospitalization is to correct medical complications, document appropriate weight gain, and establish healthy and safe eating habits. Hospital admission also has been shown to improve the long-term prognosis of children and adolescents with eating disorders.

Box 137-5. Medical Complications of Eating Disorders

Associated With Purging Behavior

- Fluid and electrolyte imbalances (from laxative abuse and vomiting)
- Irreversible cardiac muscle damage (from ipecac toxicity)
- Esophagitis, dental erosions, Mallory-Weiss tears (from chronic vomiting)
- Renal stones (from dehydration)
- Amenorrhea, hypoestrogenemia, osteopenia (from decreased body mass index [BMI])

Associated With Caloric-Restrictive Behavior and Weight Loss

- Electrocardiogram abnormalities: low voltage, sinus bradycardia, sinus tachycardia, segment depression (from electrolyte abnormalities), prolonged QTc
- Cardiac arrhythmias, including supraventricular beats and ventricular tachycardia, with or without exercise
- Mitral valve prolapse
- Pericardial effusion
- Delayed gastric emptying, slow gastrointestinal motility, constipation, bloating, fullness, abnormal liver function tests (from fatty infiltration of the liver)
- Increased blood urea nitrogen, increased risk of renal stones, total body depletion of sodium and potassium
- Refeeding syndrome (from extracellular shifts of phosphorous)
- Leukopenia, anemia, thrombocytopenia
- Amenorrhea, hypoestrogenism, osteopenia (from decreased BMI)
- Growth retardation, pubertal delay
- Cognitive deficits
- Cortical atrophy, seizures

Modified from Rosen DS; American Academy of Pediatrics Committee on Adolescence. Identification and management of eating disorders in children and adolescents. *Pediatrics.* 2010;126(6):1240–1253, and Goldstein MA, Dechant EJ, Beresin EV. Eating disorders. *Pediatr Rev.* 2011;32(12):508–521

Prognosis

Overall, the outcome for patients with eating disorders is variable, with the recovery of some patients after minimal intervention and the development of more chronic problems in others. Binge eating, for example, may replace food restriction. Most studies report the prognosis as more favorable if the patient's condition is identified early and treated rapidly and aggressively. Predictors of poor outcome for AN include very low body weight at the time of initial treatment, long duration of illness, a concomitant personality disorder, a dysfunctional parent-child relationship, and a compulsion to exercise. For BN, factors found to be predictive of poor outcome include longer duration of illness at presentation, severity of eating pathology and frequency of vomiting, premorbid obesity, associated comorbid disorders such as personality disorder or substance abuse, and suicidal behavior. A family history of alcoholism also has been reported as a poor prognostic factor for BN.

The mortality rate for adolescents with AN is approximately 2%. Higher numbers were reported in the past when adult and adolescent data were combined. Exact figures for BN have not been determined, although it has been quoted as being similar to that of AN. The most common cause of death in both disorders is suicide. Medical causes are often due to cardiac arrhythmias from electrolyte abnormalities.

CASE RESOLUTION

In the case study presented at the beginning of this chapter, the girl does not meet the strict criteria for the diagnosis of anorexia nervosa, but her preoccupation with dieting in the context of continued weight loss is worrisome. Concerns about her eating and dieting behaviors should be discussed with the teenager and her family. The patient and her family should be strongly encouraged to seek treatment. She should be referred to a mental health professional and registered dietician with experience in the treatment of eating disorders for further evaluation. The emphasis should be on the teen's overall health. She should be followed frequently until her weight and eating behaviors have reached the mutually agreed-on goal among all professionals involved in her care, after which she should continue to be seen at regular intervals.

Selected References

American Academy of Pediatrics Committee on Sports Medicine and Fitness. Medical concerns in the female athlete. *Pediatrics.* 2000;106(3):610–613

American Academy of Pediatrics Committee on Sports Medicine and Fitness. Promotion of healthy weight-control practices in young athletes. *Pediatrics.* 2005;116(6):1557–1564

American Academy of Pediatrics Section on Endocrinology. Bone densitometry in children and adolescents. *Pediatrics.* 2011;127(1):189–194

Butryn ML, Wadden TA. Treatment of overweight in children and adolescents: does dieting increase the risk of eating disorders? *Int J Eat Disord.* 2005;37(4):285–293

Fisher M. Treatment of eating disorders in children, adolescents, and young adults. *Pediatr Rev.* 2006;27(1):5–16

Fisher M, Golden NH, Jacobson MC, eds. The spectrum of disordered eating: anorexia nervosa, bulimia nervosa, and obesity. *Adolesc Med.* 2003;14:1–173

Fortune RS, Kaplan DW. Leg swelling in a patient with anorexia nervosa. *Adolesc Med State Art Rev.* 2012;23(2):266–270

Goldstein MA, Dechant EJ, Beresin EV. Eating disorders. *Pediatr Rev.* 2011;32(12):508–521

Katzman DK. Medical complications in adolescents with anorexia nervosa: a review of the literature. *Int J Eat Disord.* 2005;37(Suppl):S52–S59

Levine RL. Endocrine aspects of eating disorders in adolescents. *Adolesc Med.* 2002;13(1):129–143

Phillips EL, Pratt HD. Eating disorders in college. *Pediatr Clin North Am.* 2005;52(1):85–96

Rome ES, Ammerman S, Rosen DS, et al. Children and adolescents with eating disorders: the state of the art. *Pediatrics.* 2003;111(1):e98–e108

Rosen DS; American Academy of Pediatrics Committee on Adolescence. Identification and management of eating disorders in children and adolescents. *Pediatrics.* 2010;126(6):1240–1253

Sim LA, Lebow J, Billings M. Eating disorders in adolescents with a history of obesity. *Pediatrics.* 2013;132(4):e1026–e1030

Steinegger C, Katzman DK. Interviewing the adolescent with an eating disorder. *Adolesc Med.* 2008;19:18–40

CHAPTER 138

Body Modification: Tattooing and Body Piercing

Monica Sifuentes, MD

CASE STUDY

A 16-year-old girl comes to your office for her annual physical examination. Although previously healthy, the mother is concerned that her daughter seems irritable and unwilling to participate in recent family events. The adolescent is currently in 10th grade at a local public school, gets As and Bs in most subjects, is a member of the volleyball team, and has just begun working at a movie theater part-time. Both of her parents are employed and the adolescent gets along well with her 19-year-old sister, who is currently in college, and her 14-year-old brother. She has many friends in the neighborhood as well as at school.

You interview the adolescent alone and learn that she occasionally smokes marijuana, has tried cocaine on one occasion, and attends parties where many people are drinking alcohol. She has been sexually active in the past but is not currently. She denies depression and describes her mood as generally happy, except when she is forced to spend what she believes is excessive time with her family instead of friends.

On physical examination, the adolescent's height and weight are in the 50th percentile for age. Her body mass index is 21. Vital signs are normal. You note a small tattoo at her right hip area. The girl's mother is unaware of its presence, according to the teen. She obtained it a few months prior while visiting her sister in college.

Questions

1. What is the epidemiology of body modification in adolescents and young adults?
2. What is the motivation for obtaining tattoos and body piercing in this age group, and is there an association with high-risk behavior?
3. What techniques are used to place tattoos and perform body piercing?
4. What adverse consequences can be seen following body modification, and what should be done to treat them?
5. How can the primary care physician assist an adolescent to make a safe and healthy decision about body modification?

Body modification is the practice of permanently altering one's appearance and historically has been practiced in many cultures for thousands of years. This includes tattooing, body piercing, scarification, and branding. Although much less common than tattooing and body piercing, scarification is the use of various techniques to produce scars on the skin. It is described as a more "intense" form of body modification and has been reported to be more appealing to darker-pigmented individuals or those seeking a more dramatic result. The practice of body modification should be differentiated from cutting, which is a disorder of self-mutilation that can be seen in adolescents suffering from anxiety, depression, or abuse and is beyond the scope of this discussion (see Chapter 53).

Although in the past, body modification has been associated primarily with the disenfranchised, such as criminals, gang members, or psychiatric patients, it is now considered mainstream among individuals aged 16 to 25 years in our society. **Body art** is seen in most clinical settings serving youth and young adults as well as in middle schools and high schools and on college campuses. Additionally, it is not uncommon to encounter a teenager with multiple tattoos and body piercings or to evaluate an adolescent for a possible complication of the procedure. Whether described as a rite of passage, expression of their own individuality, or desire to join a particular peer group, obtaining a tattoo or body piercing has become a widespread experience during adolescence and young adulthood and therefore should be added to the primary care physician's list of issues to review during the routine health maintenance visit.

Epidemiology

It was previously estimated that 13% to 25% of the general population had a tattoo in the United States. However, because tattooing has grown in popularity and become a fast-growing retail business, these figures are probably a gross underestimation. Surveys conducted in outpatient clinics and on high school and college campuses confirm that more than 10% to 15% of teens aged 12 to 18 years have a tattoo. In one particular study of more than 2,000 US high school students, 55% expressed interest in obtaining a tattoo regardless of its permanence or the students' academic success in school. In addition, it has been reported in the literature that half of new tattoos are obtained by women and that many are obtained while in college. In fact, surveys conducted in the last 10 years reveal that approximately 20% to 25% of college students have a tattoo.

Body piercings are more common in adolescents and young adults than tattoos, and some experts speculate that this may be because the procedure is not permanent, allowing the individual to remove the jewelry at any time. In one study among college students, 45% had undergone body piercing and 22% had tattoos with and without piercings. Other studies that include younger adolescents attending an outpatient adolescent clinic report approximately 27% of teens with body piercing and 13% with a tattoo. Most studies also confirm that females are more likely to obtain a piercing than males, although male athletes are more likely to obtain a tattoo than their nonathlete counterparts.

The motivation for obtaining body art also has been reviewed in the literature, with most studies confirming adolescents' search for uniqueness and desire to enhance their independence and self-identity. For some teenagers, it is seen as a form of decoration, an opportunity to be creative, or it fulfills a desire for peer acceptance and can solidify group membership. This has been documented by studies that show that friends or peers provide the strongest influence for youth pursuing body art. Tattoos in particular can be seen as a quest to permanently document a relationship with an individual or group. Despite popular belief, studies do not confirm that most adolescents obtain a tattoo or body piercing impulsively while under the influence of illicit drugs or alcohol. In fact, many older teens and young adults report taking quite a while to decide whether to obtain a tattoo or piercing.

Parental involvement and permission to have a tattoo placed or body piercing performed are variable for many teenagers. In most cases, parents are not consulted prior to the procedure, although in many states parental consent is required by law, and tattooing of minors is prohibited. However, current legislation is not consistently enforced, and in many states, tattooing and body piercing have different regulations.

Clinical Presentation

Tattoos can be found on any area of the body and, depending on the talent of the artist and the desire of the client, can be simple and one color or very elaborate with many colors. In general, amateur tattoos (those performed by a nonspecialist or friend) are less intricate and are considered more risky because they are often not performed under ideal circumstances, following antiseptic techniques, or with conventional pigments and applicators. Unconventional pigments include charcoal, india ink, and mascara. Pencils, pens, sewing needles, and other sharp objects, including guitar strings, may be used to apply the dye for a self-administered or amateur tattoo.

The most common site for piercing is high on the pinna of the ear. Regular lobular ear piercings are not generally included in the context of body modification because they occur commonly at any age. Other body sites that are pierced include the tragus of the ear,

eyebrows, tongue, nose, nasal septum, cheek, lip, navel, and nipples. Intimate or genital piercings also can be seen in males and females. The foreskin, penis, scrotum, clitoris, perineum, and labia are all common areas for intimate piercings. Although specific data by gender are not available, it is reported that more men than women tend to obtain genital piercings.

Technique, Application, and Safety Standards

Tattoos

The process for applying a professional or commercial tattoo is fairly standardized, although different tattoo parlors may have their own individual practices. In general, the client selects a design from flash sheets in the shop or an individualized design by the artist, and the tattoo is stenciled or drawn on clean-shaved skin. The skin is then cleansed again with an antiseptic solution, and petroleum jelly is placed on the site. Most professionals in the United States use an electric tattoo gun, which is similar to a dental drill, that holds one or several needles in a needle bar that is dipped in ink and then will puncture the skin a few millimeters deep, up to several thousand times a minute. Of note, in Europe, small amounts of ink are applied directly to the skin and the needle is used to push the ink into the skin. Regardless of which method is used, the pigment reaches the level of the dermis via the solid bore needle(s), while blood and serosanguineous fluid are wiped away as tattoo placement continues. When the tattoo is completed or the session is finished, an antibiotic ointment is applied, and a bandage is placed over the site.

The client is instructed to remove the dressing in 24 hours and to keep the area moist with an antibiotic ointment. Additionally, clients may place Keri Lotion or vitamin E oil over the healing tattoo several times a day. The area should be cleansed with a mild soap and patted dry (not rubbed). If aftercare instructions are followed carefully, most tattoos heal in approximately 1 to 2 weeks. Swimming, however, is discouraged for 3 to 4 weeks.

Ideally, the application process uses inks that are poured into one-time–use disposable containers and sterile needles that are disposed of after each client. However, although the tattoo ink pigments are subject to US Food and Drug Administration regulation, the tattooing process itself and the use of the inks are not regulated. In addition, certain pigments may not be approved for intradermal use and have been known to contain lead, mercury, or arsenic.

The practice of universal precautions is required by state and local regulatory agencies and advocated by specific educational groups such as the Alliance of Professional Tattooists (APT), a nonprofit organization established in 1992 to promote standards for professional and associate tattooists and develop guidelines for consumers to evaluate the safety of individual tattooing establishments. The organization also sponsors regular educational seminars for the artist on the prevention of disease transmission in tattooing. Membership in APT is voluntary and requires that the professional tattooist participate in a health and safety seminar and have at least 3 years of full-time experience at a consistent location. Despite this organization's efforts and standards, however, specific areas of concern about the tattoo industry remain, including unlicensed tattoo artists and establishments, the presence of unregulated ingredients in the pigments, inconsistent cleaning of equipment between clients, an inability to reliably sterilize all parts of the equipment despite good efforts, and infrequent inspections of tattoo parlors by regulatory agencies.

Body Piercing

The process for body piercing is generally less complicated than tattooing and depends, in part, on the site to be pierced. The client chooses the jewelry and body part to be pierced, the area is cleaned with a topical antiseptic, and a large hollow needle is brought through the skin. The jewelry is then brought through the hole following the needle and sealed with a bead, bar, or metal disc. Because the procedure is relatively quick, topical anesthetics are generally not required.

While earlobe piercings are relatively straightforward, they are commonly performed using a "piercing gun" at a local mall, cosmetic shop, or kiosk. Because the stud is driven through the earlobe via the gun rather than through a hollow tube manually, the tissue ends up torn or crushed rather than pierced. Additional concerns about the piercing gun include inconsistent and informal training of personnel, an inability to sterilize all parts of the gun, and embedded earrings and ear backs. The gun cannot be adjusted for the thickness of other tissues, so although it is a popular method for earring placement, this tool is not recommended for sites other than the earlobe.

The immediate aftercare of piercing varies by the site pierced. For example, local skin discoloration and a non-malodorous serous exudate can occur with piercings of the nares or navel. Tongue or lip piercings have been associated with significant swelling for several days following the procedure. In addition, a yellow-white fluid secretion can occur that can mimic an infection to the unfamiliar examiner. Clients with oral piercings are generally instructed to dissolve ice in their mouths immediately post-piercing to help with pain and swelling, treat further discomfort with a nonsteroidal anti-inflammatory agent, and elevate the head when sleeping.

Healing times greatly vary depending on the body site. In general, sites with greater vascularity and exposure, such as the face and tongue, tend to heal faster than those through cartilage, which is poorly vascularized. Areas of the body that are subject to movement also have slower healing times. For example, the tongue may take 1 to 2 months to heal, the nasal septum 1 to $1^{1}/_{2}$ months, the nostril 2 to 3 months, and the tragus of the ear 2 to 4 months. High-ear piercings through the cartilage also can take 2 to 4 months to heal. Navel piercings have the longest healing time (up to 9 to 12 months) because of friction and moisture from clothing and often are associated with the most complications.

As with tattooing, not all states have regulations and safety standards in place for body piercing, and if they do exist, local governing bodies do not consistently enforce them. Universal precautions should be strictly practiced, and the adolescent needs to be familiar with these guidelines as well as know how to find a reputable piercer prior to obtaining body art.

Because no formal training programs exist for piercers, many learn by video or apprenticeship. In general, practitioners in studios have completed an apprenticeship and have more training than those in cosmetic shops, malls, or ear-piercing kiosks. They also are more experienced in piercing sites other than the ears and may be members of the Association of Professional Piercers (APP). Established in 1994, the APP is a nonprofit organization dedicated to the education, health, and safety of body piercing for the public. It has developed self-regulatory policies for the industry, standards for membership in the organization, and annual conferences on health and safety issues. Membership includes at least 1 year of piercing experience, documented training in blood-borne pathogens and cardiopulmonary resuscitation, and certification in first aid. Members also must show photographic proof of a medical-grade autoclave in the piercing studio and send in spore test results from the autoclave. To help document this, a detailed video of the studio is required along with copies of all aftercare education given to clients. Once this process is completed, the member receives a certificate to mount in the studio.

Current legislation addressing minors and piercing is regulated by individual states; in some states, such as California, there is an exclusion of ear piercing performed with piercing guns from the definition of body piercing. With regard to minors, the APP requires that the parent or legal guardian as well as the minor show proof of identification prior to signing the consent form for body piercing. In addition, nipple or genital piercings are not performed on anyone younger than 18 years.

Evaluation

History

All teenagers should be interviewed alone, after their parent or legal guardian has had an opportunity to discuss their concerns with the primary care physician (see Chapter 6). A visible tattoo or body piercing allows the primary care physician to inquire about the circumstances surrounding the body art at the beginning of the interview in contrast to body art noted in an inconspicuous area of the body during the physical examination. Whether parental consent was obtained prior to the procedure should be addressed directly because this issue could be a basis for current as well as future familial conflict. The type of facility where the tattoo or piercing was obtained should be reviewed, along with whether the adolescent recalls if universal precautions were followed. A general review of systems should be performed to exclude systemic conditions such as viral hepatitis as well as any other complications related to obtaining the tattoo or piercing. Specific questions about the area of the body that has been pierced also should be reviewed (Questions Box). For example, the teenager with a tongue piercing should be asked if he or she has problems with mastication, swallowing, loss of taste or movement, or permanent numbness.

Tattoo and Body Piercing

Questions

- When was the tattoo or body piercing placed?
- Did the teenager obtain the parent or legal guardian's consent prior to getting the tattoo or piercing?
- Is the adolescent satisfied with the tattoo or piercing?
- Was the tattoo or body piercing placed by a professional or by a friend or relative?
- Where was the studio located? Was it licensed? Was it clean "like a medical facility"?
- Did the tattooist or piercer wash his or her hands before gloving? Use new disposable gloves? Open all equipment in front of the teen?
- For tattoos, did the tattooist remove a sterile needle and tube set from a new envelope? Did he or she pour new ink in a new disposable container?
- For body piercing, did the piercer use individually wrapped sterile needles? Did he or she use a piercing gun?
- Did the teen receive aftercare education, including written material?

It has been reported that amateur or self-administered tattoos are associated with increased psychosocial problems including substance abuse at a younger age, hard drug use, lower academic achievement (ie, grades), and a greater number of tattoos overall.

Other studies have shown, however, that not all adolescents and young adults with tattoos or body piercing engage in high-risk behavior (Box 138-1). Successful academic achievement and close family support have been reported in tattooed and non-tattooed college students. Despite the fact that they are permanent, more than 50% of academically successful high school students with consistently good grades have reported an interest in tattoos.

Whether body art is seen as an expression of individuality, rebellious behavior, or succumbing to peer pressure, the presence of a tattoo or body piercing on an adolescent probably warrants an in-depth psychosocial assessment for risk-taking behavior and possible exposure to a viral infection such as hepatitis C.

Physical Examination

The routine physical examination in most adolescents with a tattoo or body piercing is completely normal unless there has been a past complication with the tattoo or piercing or there is a current problem. Poor aftercare and hygiene can prolong healing time in body piercings. In addition, smoking can delay the healing time associated with oral piercings. If the teen has recently had a tongue piercing performed, a larger barbell will be seen through the tongue. Larger barbells initially are placed with tongue piercing to accommodate the swelling associated with the procedure. Later, the barbell is replaced with a shorter rod.

Infectious and noninfectious complications from tattoos and body piercings can be seen and are listed in Box 138-2. While local infection occurs in only approximately 5% of tattoos, infectious complications have been reported in as many as 30% of body piercings.

Box 138-1. The Association Between Body Modification and High-Risk Behavior in Teens

Numerous studies have been conducted to explore the association between high-risk behavior and body modification in adolescents. To date, while there are no definitive answers, research has shown

- Adolescents with tattoos or body piercings were more likely to have engaged in risk-taking behaviors and at greater degrees of involvement than those without either. Risk-taking behaviors included disordered eating behavior, gateway drug use (cigarettes, alcohol, and marijuana), hard drug use (cocaine, crystal methamphetamine, and ecstasy), sexual activity, and suicide. Additionally, violence was associated with males having tattoos and with females having body piercings. Gateway drug use was associated with younger age of tattooing and body piercing. (Carroll ST, Riffenburgh RH, Roberts TA, Myhre EB. Tattoos and body piercings as indicators of adolescent risk-taking behaviors. *Pediatrics.* 2002;109[6]:1021–1027)
- Adolescents with body modification had 3.1-times greater odds of problem substance use compared with those without body modification. (Brooks TL, Woods ER, Knight JR, Shrier LA. Body modification and substance use in adolescents: is there a link? *J Adolesc Health.* 2003;32[1]:44–49)
- Tattooing was significantly associated with older age, living in a single-parent household, and lower socioeconomic status. There also was greater involvement in sexual intercourse, higher levels of substance abuse in themselves as well as their peers, increased violent behaviors, and school problems. (Roberts TA, Ryan SA. Tattooing and high-risk behavior in adolescents. *Pediatrics.* 2002;110[6]:1058–1063)
- A correlation was found between body piercing in teens and increased rate of sexual intercourse, smoking, marijuana use, school truancy, running away, suicidal ideation or attempts, and peer substance use. (Armstrong ML, Roberts AE, Owen DC, Koch JR. Contemporary college students and body piercing. *J Adolesc Health.* 2004;35[1]:58–61)

Acute signs of infection include erythema, warmth, swelling, and pain at the site, in addition to drainage in some cases. Rarely, a fluctuant, fluid-filled mass is seen if an abscess has developed.

Because some of the noninfectious complications can be related to the type of metal found in the jewelry, knowledge of this specific information is useful with body piercing. Only jewelry made from surgical stainless steel, titanium, solid 14- or 18-karat (k) gold, or solid platinum should be used in healed piercings to avoid allergic dermatitis. Certain metals such as nickel, cobalt, and chromium have been associated with the development of contact dermatitis in sensitive individuals. However, initially, during the healing phase of piercings, surgical steel and 14-k gold jewelry should be avoided because it may contain trace amounts of nickel. Permanent makeup also has been reported to cause severe allergic contact dermatitis that can take from months to years to completely heal. The reported reactions included tenderness, itching, and "bumps" at the site of the permanent makeup application. Hypersensitivities to dyes or pigments from a professional tattoo also can appear as an erythematous outline of the original work. This can occur with temporary

Box 138-2. Complications of Tattoos and Body Piercing: Infectious and Noninfectious	
Tattooing Complications	*Body Piercing Complications*
Infectious	**Noninfectious**
Bacterial etiologies	*Body jewelry, in general*
• Local skin infections	• Artifact on radiographs
— Superficial pyodermas	*High-ear piercing*
— *Staphylococcus aureus*	• Pinna deformity
• Systemic infections	*Tongue piercing*
— Syphilis	• Airway obstruction
— *Mycobacterium tuberculosis*	• Chipped/cracked teeth
— *Mycobacterium leprae*	• Interference with mastication/swallowing
— Chancroid	• Permanent numbness
— Tetanus	• Articulation disorders
— Endocarditis	• Loss of taste/movement
Viral etiologies	• Oral mucosa inflammation
• Human papillomavirus	*Lip piercing*
• Hepatitis B and C	• Injury to salivary ducts
• HIV	• Aspiration of jewelry
Noninfectious	*Navel piercing*
• Hypersensitivity to dyes or pigments	• Allergic dermatitis
• Allergic granulomas	*Nipple piercing*
• Malignant melanoma and basal cell carcinoma at tattoo site	• Trauma/avulsion of nipple
• Keloid formation	*Genital piercing*
• Swelling and burning during magnetic resonance imaging	• Tissue inflammation in sexual partner
Body Piercing Complications	• Scarring
Infectious	• Interruption of urinary flow (in males)
Bacterial etiologies	
• *S aureus*	
• *Pseudomonas aeruginosa*	
• Group A beta-hemolytic streptococcus	
— Cellulitis	
— Septic arthritis	
— Acute glomerulonephritis	
— Erysipelas	
— Endocarditis	
• *M tuberculosis*	
• *Clostridium tetani*	
Viral etiologies	
• Hepatitis B and C	
• HIV	

tattoos from henna, which is approved as a hair dye and not for use on the skin. Its use has been associated with severe contact dermatitis, especially if an additive containing phenylenediamine is mixed with the henna to give the normal red-brown paste an additional black-and-blue color.

Keloids and hypertrophic scars can appear as a flesh-colored mass at the area of the tattoo or piercing and differ in their timing and resolution. A hypertrophic scar generally appears within 6 weeks of the tattooing or piercing, is confined to the margins of the wound, and has a tendency to regress spontaneously. In contrast, a keloid may present as long as 1 year after the initial wound, often grows beyond the border of the wound, and persists. Keloids are seen primarily in African American and Asian patients and can cause an itching or burning sensation that may prompt referral for removal.

Laboratory

In general, laboratory studies are not necessary if the adolescent is not engaged in high-risk behavior and is certain that universal precautions were followed when the tattoo or piercing was placed. In most cases, however, the teen may be uncertain or not remember the details. If this is the case, a serum test for viral hepatitis B and C should be obtained because it has been reported that hepatitis C virus is found in approximately 30% of people with tattoos compared with 3.5% of people without them. Additionally, an antibody test for HIV should be sent as it continues to be a major public health concern with regard to the industry. However, there have been no definitive documented cases of HIV transmission from tattooing or body piercing in the literature to date.

A serum test for syphilis also should be sent because, unlike HIV, transmission of this and other sexually transmitted infections has been reported from tattooing or piercing, although rare.

If there is evidence of abscess formation such as what may be seen with perichondritis, a specimen of the purulent fluid should be obtained and sent for culture and antimicrobial sensitivities.

Management

Although not ordinarily requested by most adolescents, tattoo removal or modification is available for the patient that no longer wants his or her tattoo or is unhappy with its current appearance. Recent studies have examined the motivation for tattoo removal after a duration of at least 10 years. Reasons for removal are varied and include embarrassment, a need to disassociate from the past, improved self-esteem, being tired of the tattoo, and negative social remarks about the tattoo. Interestingly, professional employment or job advancement was not consistently cited as a common reason for removal.

In the past, tattoo removal was very difficult, and only about 70% of tattoos could be completely cleared because of impurities in tattoo pigments, different ink densities and depths, and the presence of certain metals in the dyes. Newer technology aimed at the development of a selective type of laser targeted at specific color pigments (selective photothermolysis) is now available and has become very effective at removing several ink colors. However, none is 100% successful at removing all evidence of the tattoo, and in most cases, immediate lightening of the skin occurs with subsequent hypopigmentation. Hyperpigmentation, allergic reactions, and scarring due to thermal burn injury may also occur after laser treatment. Although these complications are usually transient, they can be permanent, so the patient must be aware of the risks associated with each process. The cost for tattoo removal is not negligible; while the cost for tattoo placement might be $50 to $100, it can cost more than $1,000 for its removal. Other, less popular techniques for tattoo removal include dermabrasion (less desirable secondary to infection concerns), salabrasion (use of a salt solution to abrade the skin), scarification, and surgical removal (with or without the use of tissue expanders). Camouflaging also can be performed: a new pattern is made using skin-toned pigments or the tattoo is modified and made into another one. For instance, the name of a person can be incorporated into a new tattoo of an animal or object. Certain nonprofit organizations also offer tattoo removal to ex-gang members as a part of their employment and educational services.

Although it seems counterintuitive, removal of jewelry is not recommended if a piercing appears infected. The concern is that, without a wick or surgical drain, any potential space left at the site when the jewelry is removed could result in the development of an abscess. Instead, the adolescent should be instructed to leave the jewelry in place to allow drainage of the wound, use warm compresses, and clean the area with an antimicrobial soap and water. The use of topical antibiotic ointments is controversial because they can be occlusive and contribute to delayed healing.

Oral antibiotic coverage against skin staphylococcal and streptococcal species should be administered if the tattoo or piercing appears superficially infected and other measures have not been effective. More aggressive treatment is required if the piercing site involves the cartilage such as with high-ear piercings. Auricular infections can occur even after the use of strict antiseptic techniques and may appear a few weeks after the initial piercing. The cartilaginous helical area of the ear is particularly prone to infection because it is poorly vascularized and takes a long time to heal. Additional antimicrobial coverage against *Pseudomonas aeruginosa* is essential in these cases, along with diligent follow-up to monitor the initial response to oral antibiotic therapy. Currently, oral fluoroquinolones offer good anti-pseudomonal as well as anti-staphylococcal coverage and penetrate cartilage well. Inpatient hospitalization for intravenous antimicrobial therapy and subsequent drainage of the site may be required for moderate or unresponsive infections. Early recognition of perichondritis and its appropriate treatment are essential to prevent the development of a persistent infection as well as to minimize a permanent auricular deformity. In addition, timely consultation with a plastic surgeon or otolaryngologist early in the course of the suspected infection is recommended for early incision and drainage of a perichondral abscess, appropriate wound care, and possible reconstruction of any disfigurement.

Role of the Primary Care Physician

For the adolescent who has not yet obtained a tattoo or piercing or who already has one and is contemplating the placement of another, education is essential. The practitioner should inquire where the adolescent plans to have the procedure performed and educate them on what key questions to ask and how to find a reputable studio. Additional information such as the APT (www.safe-tattoos.com) and APP (www.safepiercing.org) Web sites should be shared with the teenager, and written materials that contain safety guidelines should be given to the adolescent at the visit. Teenagers are often reluctant to ask their health care professionals for information about obtaining tattoos and piercings and almost never contact them if they believe they may have a complication associated with tattooing or piercing. Instead, they tend to ask their peers or contact the establishment where the tattoo or piercing was initially placed. Primary care physicians should be a nonjudgmental resource during health maintenance visits to ensure the adolescent's continued health and safety. Additionally, the appearance of an uncommon medical condition such as unexplained hepatitis, endocarditis, or toxic shock in the adolescent patient warrants careful consideration of a possible complication related to tattooing or body piercing.

Prognosis

Most teens experience no adverse effects from body modification. Complications, while uncommon with the placement of a professional tattoo but more common with body piercing, are usually amenable to medical management. Risk-taking behavior that may occur in conjunction with body modification may carry long-term sequelae.

CASE RESOLUTION

Because the presence of one tattoo puts this adolescent at risk for obtaining another, the primary care physician should review safety guidelines for obtaining a tattoo and body piercing with the adolescent and offer the teenager educational material or Web site references to reinforce the discussion. The immunization status of the teenager also should be checked, with particular attention to tetanus and hepatitis A and B. Additionally, while alone with the teenager, the physician should review concern about the adolescent's current high-risk behavior and its possible consequences. It also may be worthwhile to begin a discussion with the teen about telling her parents about the tattoo before they find out inadvertently.

Selected References

Alliance of Professional Tattooists. http://www.safe-tattoos.com. Accessed April 14, 2014

Armstrong ML, Caliendo C, Roberts AE. Genital piercings: what is known and what people with genital piercings tell us. *Urol Nurs.* 2006;26(3):173–179

Armstrong ML, Roberts AE, Owen DC, Koch JR. Contemporary college students and body piercing. *J Adolesc Health.* 2004;35(1):58–61

Association of Professional Piercers. http://www.safepiercing.org. Accessed April 14, 2014

Beers MS, Meires J, Loriz L. Body piercing: coming to a patient near you. *Nurs Pract.* 2007;32(2):55–60

Braverman PK. Body art: piercing, tattooing, and scarification. *Adolesc Med Clin.* 2006;17(3):505–519

Brooks TL, Woods ER, Knight JR, Shrier LA. Body modification and substance use in adolescents: is there a link? *J Adolesc Health.* 2003;32(1):44–49

Carroll ST, Riffenburgh RH, Roberts TA, Myhre EB. Tattoos and body piercings as indicators of adolescent risk-taking behaviors. *Pediatrics.* 2002;109(6):1021–1027

Desai NA, Smith ML. Body art in adolescents: paint, piercings, and perils. *Adolesc Med State Art Rev.* 2011;22(1):97–118

Larzo MR, Poe SG. Adverse consequences of tattoos and body piercings. *Pediatr Ann.* 2006;35(3):187–192

Laumann AE, Derick AJ. Tattoos and body piercing in the United States: a national data set. *J Am Acad Dermatol.* 2006;55(3):413–421

Meltzer DI. Complications of body piercing. *Am Fam Physician.* 2005;72(10):2029–2034

Messahel A, Musgrove B. Infective complications of tattooing and skin piercing. *J Infect Public Health.* 2009;2(1):7–13

More DR, Seidel JS, Bryan PA. Ear-piercing techniques as a cause of auricular chondritis. *Pediatr Emerg Care.* 1999;15(3):189–192

Nicoletti A. Perspectives on pediatric and adolescent gynecology from the allied health care professional. Teens, tattoos and body piercing. *J Pediatr Adolesc Gynecol.* 2004;17(3):215–216

Roberts TA, Ryan SA. Tattooing and high-risk behavior in adolescents. *Pediatrics.* 2002;110(6):1058–1063

Stewart GM, Thorp A, Brown L. Perichondritis—a complication of high ear piercing. *Pediatr Emerg Care.* 2006;22(12):804–806

Straetemans M, Katz LM, Belson M. Adverse reactions after permanent-makeup procedures. *N Engl J Med.* 2007;356(26):2753

Tohme RA, Holmberg SD. Transmission of hepatitis C virus infection through tattooing and piercing: a critical review. *Clin Infect Dis.* 2012;54(8):1167–1178

CHAPTER 139

Childhood Obesity

H. Mollie Greves Grow, MD, MPH

CASE STUDY

A 10-year-old girl is brought to the office by her mother to discuss concerns about the child's weight, which is 59 kg (130 lb). Her height is 140 cm (55 in), giving her a body mass index of 30 kg/m^2 (>95th percentile for age). The rest of the physical examination, including vital signs, is normal. The mother, who also is overweight, says she doesn't want her daughter to "end up like me." The patient says she gets teased at school for being "fat." The history reveals that this patient is an only child who lives with her single mother in low-income housing in a large urban city. The mother works the day shift as a nurse's aide at a nearby nursing home. Because the mother is often tired, meals are simple and frequently consist of prepackaged foods such as pastries for breakfast and frozen dinners for supper. At school, the girl buys her lunch, which usually includes whole milk, a processed entrée, and a dessert. After school, the girl goes home, where she watches television and snacks on chips and soda until her mother arrives home from work. The mother does not allow her daughter to play outside because the neighborhood is unsafe.

Questions

1. How is obesity defined and measured, and what are some pitfalls in measurement?
2. How do genetic susceptibility and environment interact to influence a person's risk for obesity?
3. What are the complications of obesity?
4. What is the role of primary care physicians in addressing childhood obesity?
5. How can obesity be treated?

Childhood obesity is of significant concern because children who are overweight are more likely to become overweight adults and are at increased risk for multiple chronic conditions. In addition, being obese carries a tremendous psychosocial toll for affected adults and children, as it remains one of the most stigmatized conditions. Children who are obese are often shunned by peers at school, feel isolated, and have fewer friends, while adolescents who are obese complete less schooling, go on to have lower household incomes, and are more likely to live in poverty than their non-obese counterparts. The primary care physician is usually the first (and frequently only) resource available to help patients and their families in screening, diagnosing, discussing, and treating childhood obesity.

Defining obesity presents certain challenges. Ideally, a measure of obesity would correlate with adiposity and predict morbidity and mortality. Body mass index (BMI) (weight in kilograms/height in meters^2) is the best and most widely used surrogate measure for obesity but does not completely correlate with adiposity for all individuals. Standards for adults have established a BMI of 25 or greater as overweight and 30 or greater as obese, based on increased risk of morbidity and mortality above these levels. While BMI is the current preferred method for assessing degree of obesity in children, other criteria are also used (D$_x$ Box). Experts classify children at the 85th to 95th percentile of BMI for age as **overweight** and those greater than the 95th percentile of BMI for age as **obese.** Because BMI is not a direct measure of adiposity, it is important to recognize that children who meet the BMI criteria for overweight and obesity will not all have adverse health effects of their weight status. A general helpful rule of thumb is that the higher the BMI rises above the 95th percentile, the greater

 Obesity

- Body mass index >95th percentile for age (≥85 percentile is considered overweight).
- Weight-for-height >95th percentile.
- Greater than 120% of ideal body weight for height and age.
- Greater than 99th percentile is considered severe obesity.

likelihood of adverse health effects. For BMI greater than the 99th percentile, which is associated with the most comorbidities, switching to a BMI number, like adults, is often used. The BMI changes as children grow older because of changes in their proportion of bone mass and lean-to-fat tissue composition. After about 1 year of age, BMI-for-age values begin to decline and continue to do so during the preschool years until the BMI reaches a minimum around 5 to 6 years of age, before rising throughout the remainder of childhood, into adolescence and adulthood. This phenomenon of increasing BMI after the nadir in the preschool years is referred to as **adiposity rebound.** Early adiposity rebound (age <4.8 years) is a predictor of later obesity and can be used clinically to identify children at risk.

Epidemiology

The prevalence of obesity is on the rise in developed countries. Between 1980 and 2000, the percentage of overweight children and adolescents in the United States tripled, reaching 17.1% in 2003–2004. Since then, no significant increases have been seen overall among the US youth population, except for increases in the highest BMI group (>97th percentile). Hispanics, African Americans, and Native Americans are disproportionately affected. People with lower education and those in poverty are also at highest risk. Prevention and treatment of obesity is important to avoid health risks that affect the individual and are costly to society as a whole. In the United States, the overall spending associated with overweight and obesity was $93 billion in 2002 dollars, half of which was publicly financed through Medicare or Medicaid.

Clinical Presentation

Children who are obese usually present to the physician in 1 of 2 ways. The parents or the child may come in concerned that the child is overweight. The physician must then consider the growth parameters and BMI for age to make an appropriate determination of the child's overweight status. The more common presentation is when parents do not recognize that their child is overweight and in fact may believe that being big is a sign of health. The lack of awareness of their child's risk may particularly affect parents during the time of the adiposity nadir (ie, the preschool and early school-age years when children are most lean), when early intervention to improve energy balance might yield the most benefit. Measurement of the child's height and weight and determination of BMI for age is important at all ages to identify children who are overweight or obese or gaining weight more rapidly than expected; it is especially critical during early childhood when outward appearances may be most unreliable. Seeing change in percentiles is particularly helpful to differentiate children who may be healthy and grow steadily along a higher BMI curve, such as those 5% at the 95th percentile who are naturally in the high BMI range but are not actually overfat.

Pathophysiology

Our understanding of the pathophysiology of obesity continues to evolve. Certain neurohormones affect appetite, satiety, and the balance between fat storage and energy production. In the end, obesity results when energy intake exceeds expenditure. The storage of excess calories was an advantage to our ancestors who faced intermittent food shortage; however, this predisposition to store excess calories has contributed to increasing rates of obesity in our current setting in which the environment provides ubiquitous highly palatable, high-calorie, convenient foods and limited opportunities for physical activity.

It is known from studies of twins and others that susceptibility to obesity is influenced substantially by **genetics.** Yet the magnitude of recent increases in obesity rates suggests the genetic susceptibility interacts with an **obesogenic environment** that facilitates unhealthy behaviors. National surveys indicate that Americans are consuming more calories now than they were 35 years ago. This trend is most related to increasingly widespread and easily available calorically dense foods in larger portions than ever before. A smaller but also important contribution of the population weight gain comes from less physical activity and more sedentary lifestyles. The

reasons for this are myriad and include changes in transportation patterns, shifts in the workforce to less manual jobs, and automation of household work. Children have decreased opportunities for activity owing to safety concerns; parental work habits; the availability of television, computers, and other electronic toys; and reduced availability of physical education in school and after-school programs.

Differential Diagnosis

Most children who present to physicians with excess weight have primary obesity resulting from an imbalance of caloric intake and activity levels. Only a small proportion of children who are overweight will have an organic cause, although many parents may initially inquire about an organic etiology. A thorough history including review of systems, physical examination, and evaluation of growth parameters will help differentiate primary from organic obesity in most cases. While children with primary obesity tend to have normal or increased height for age, children with an organic etiology, such as hypothyroidism, are typically shorter than normal or have a delayed rate of linear growth. Certain genetic syndromes, such as Prader-Willi syndrome, pseudohypoparathyroidism, Bardet-Biedl syndrome, and Laurence-Moon syndrome, are associated with obesity. However, children with these syndromes have other findings, such as developmental delay, dysmorphic features, and short stature, that are usually identifiable during the physical examination. While there may not be an organic cause of weight gain initially, there is evidence that weight gain can be exacerbated by acquired diagnoses, such as sleep apnea, that develop as complications of obesity.

Evaluation

History

The history should include the age of the child, parental weight, and lifestyle information (Questions Box). Knowledge of a child's birth weight and gestational age may be helpful. Full-term babies weighing more than 9 pounds are at increased risk of obesity. Prematurity is also a risk factor for subsequent obesity, possibly related to early metabolic effects of rapid catch-up weight gain after birth. Exclusive formula feeding may be a risk factor for obesity, whereas breastfeeding has been found to be somewhat protective against obesity in epidemiologic observational studies. A diet history, such as the 24-hour recall method or, alternatively, use of screening questions filled out by the parent in the waiting room, can be helpful to understand the dietary factors contributing to the child's overweight status as well as to identify areas for potential change. In addition, a history of signs or symptoms of complications of obesity should be elicited. For example, a teen may complain of hip or knee pain suggestive of slipped capital femoral epiphyses (SCFE). There may be a history of snoring, or apneic pauses followed by gasping for breath during sleep, and daytime sleepiness indicating sleep-disordered breathing and necessitating further evaluation for obstructive sleep apnea (OSA). A history of irregular menstrual periods is useful in evaluation for polycystic ovary syndrome (PCOS). A mental health history, including depression and anxiety symptoms, disordered eating, and history of bullying, is important to obtain. The family history, especially familial obesity, diabetes, hypertension, and early cardiac death, gives clues to the risk of obesity complications. Finally, a social history, including family social stressors, substance use, poverty, and food insecurity, is important to gauge the child's risks and the family's need for support to address obesity concerns.

Physical Examination

The accurate measurement of height and weight using appropriate equipment and plotting growth parameters on a BMI chart should be essential components of every well-child visit. For children 2 years and older, the revised 2000 growth curves (developed by the US National Center for Health Statistics) enable the physician and other health care professionals to evaluate BMI for age relative to other children of the same gender. Prior to age 2 years, the World Health Organization weight-for-length curves should be used to assess proportional growth. Both sets of growth curves are available at www.cdc.gov/growthcharts. Children should also be examined for any dysmorphic features suggestive of an underlying genetic syndrome.

The physician should assess for potential complications of obesity when examining a child who is overweight. While many complications of obesity do not manifest until adulthood, children who are overweight are at risk for a number of conditions, including hypertension, hyperlipidemia, type 2 diabetes, nonalcoholic fatty liver disease, OSA, and orthopedic problems such as Blount disease and SCFE. Blood pressure should be accurately measured with an appropriate-sized cuff (larger cuffs are needed for youth who are overweight) and compared with age-based standards. The skin should be examined for striae and acanthosis nigricans, the velvety pigmented lesion commonly found on the neck or axilla, which is associated with insulin resistance in children who are overweight. Skin findings of hirsutism and acne in obese adolescent girls may indicate the presence of PCOS. The musculoskeletal examination should assess joint alignment and range of motion for Blount disease (severe tibial bowing), SCFE, or other degenerative joint diseases. Tanner stage should be assessed for evidence of premature puberty.

Laboratory Tests

One-third to one-half of obese children will have evidence of **metabolic syndrome,** a cluster of traits that include hyperinsulinemia, obesity, hypertension, and hyperlipidemia. The higher the BMI for age is, the greater the risk that the child or teen will have metabolic complications. Laboratory studies to evaluate for potential complications of obesity are recommended starting at age 10 years, or before if there are specific concerns such as severe obesity (ie, >99th percentile BMI for age) or a strong family history of type 2 diabetes or hyperlipidemia. Children aged 10 years and older with a BMI above the 95th percentile (and for those >85th percentile with family or other risk factors) are recommended to have fasting glucose and a fasting lipid panel. Some experts also recommend screening for fatty liver disease with an alanine transaminase. The fasting glucose or the hemoglobin A_{1c}

Questions

Obesity

- Open-ended questions to engage lifestyle and family changes rather than targeting the child include
  - What concerns do you have about the child's health? How do you feel about the child's weight?
  - How has the current weight affected the child's life (eg, teasing, difficulty exercising or with sleep)?
  - What are you and your family already doing to support healthy eating and activity?
- Specific probes to learn more about the child's usual daily activities and home environment include
  - Who cares for the child during the day? (Home-based child care provided by grandparents or other family members is associated with increased risk of overweight.)
  - How often does the child get to be physically active (eg, recess, physical education class, after school, on weekends)?
  - Where are opportunities to add more activity (eg, to or from school, on weekends, playing sports or recreation, with parents)?
  - How much time does the child spend watching television, playing video games, or using the computer? What are family guidelines for screen time? What media devices are in the child's bedroom?
  - On a typical day, starting first thing in the morning, what does the child eat?
  - How often does your family eat meals together? How often do you eat fast food or go out to eat?
  - Who does the shopping and food preparation? Do they worry about food running out before they can get more?
  - How often does the child drink soda or juice drinks? How often does the child drink milk and water?
  - What time does the child go to sleep and wake up? Is child rested during the day?
- Questions to set a mutual agenda include
  - What are some things you and your family would like to change for healthier eating and activity?
  - Who might support you and your family in making changes?
- Some additional questions for older children/adolescents include
  - Has the child/teen tried to lose weight before? How?
  - Is the child/teen depressed?
  - Has the child/teen participated in fad dieting? Fasting? Laxative use? Diuretic use?
  - Has the child/teen used drugs to lose weight (illicit, over the counter, or prescription)?
  - Has the child/teen used nutritional supplements for weight loss?
  - Has the child/teen ever binged? Purged?
  - Does the child/teen use tobacco? Alcohol?

---

can help screen for diabetes or prediabetes. These tests should be repeated if results are abnormal to confirm diagnosis. Higher rates of nutritional deficiencies reported among overweight youth include vitamin D, calcium, and iron, so screening for these should be considered based on dietary history and other risk factors.

If a genetic condition is suspected, an evaluation by a geneticist is indicated for high-resolution karyotype and other genetic tests, as directed by the suspected syndrome. For rare cases in which an underlying endocrinologic disorder is suspected, thyroid function studies or cortisol levels may be considered.

Children with a history of sleep-disordered breathing should be referred for a sleep study.

Imaging Studies

Radiologic studies are indicated when orthopedic complications of obesity such as Blount disease or SCFE are suspected. An echocardiogram for evaluation of ventricular hypertrophy is a consideration in children with long-standing hypertension (left ventricle may be affected) or OSA (right ventricle may be affected).

Management

Because not all children who are obese will go on to be obese adults, a **staged approach** is now recommended in treating childhood obesity. The pediatrician's first task is to help prevent obesity through identifying risk and using patient-directed counseling to promote healthy target behaviors (and avoid unhealthy ones). Risk is largely determined by the child's age and history of parental obesity; however, race/ethnicity may also play a role. Obese children younger than 3 years without obese parents are at low risk for future obesity. These children should be monitored but, for the most part, do not require intervention. Between the ages of 3 and 5 years, parental obesity substantially increases the risk of a child becoming an obese adult. The chance of adult obesity in an obese preschooler with at least one obese parent is above 60%. In older children, the child's own obesity is an increasingly important predictor of adult obesity, regardless of whether the parents are obese. The probability that an overweight child older than 6 years will be obese as an adult is 50%, regardless of parental obesity status. Children determined to be at high risk for future obesity require close surveillance and intervention by the physician.

Once a child has been identified as overweight, the **recommended stages of obesity treatment** are

- Stage 1: *Prevention plus:* Initial treatment in the primary care office focuses on behavioral strategies for eating and activity changes to address causes of energy imbalance.
- Stage 2 (if no improvement within 3–6 months after stage 1): *Structured weight management* involving specific targeted goal behaviors for eating, activity, and reducing sedentary time; should include self-monitoring in the office or another setting for individual or group treatment.
- Stage 3 (if no improvement within 3–6 months after stage 2): *Comprehensive multidisciplinary management* in pediatric weight management center or equivalent program.
- Stage 4 (for patients with BMI >99th percentile or more severe comorbidities): *Tertiary care intervention* in a tertiary care facility that oversees more targeted medical weight loss and may offer surgical approaches.

The core of child obesity treatment focuses on behavior and lifestyle modification, the aims of which are to reduce BMI through sustainable and appropriate healthy eating and physical activities that do not lead to disordered eating or inappropriate body image.

Throughout assessment and management of obesity, primary care physicians need to help families recognize the importance of physical fitness and overall health, not just body size, and that the whole family needs to be involved. In addition, physicians should monitor children and teens for inappropriate focus on weight or engaging in unhealthy weight loss practices including laxative abuse, induced vomiting, and fasting (see Chapter 124).

The initial weight change goal in caring for the prepubertal child who is overweight is slowing weight gain or maintaining weight during normal linear growth. If more advanced treatment is indicated, the goal may move to weight loss, but not more than 1 pound per month is recommended for children aged 2 to 5 years. Youth aged 12 to 18 years (or postpubertal) may start at any of the 4 treatment stages, depending on severity and readiness to change. Initial treatment goals for the older age group may be slowed weight gain or weight loss, with weight loss not more than 2 pounds per month above age 5 years recommended. As a quaternary intervention, surgical treatments for obesity are available for teenagers in some centers, but due to cost, complications, and side effects, they are reserved only for those with extreme obesity already resulting in health problems.

Physicians can feel most successful and efficacious in managing obesity if they tailor recommendations for the individual child and family and access available community resources. **Motivational interviewing** techniques (Box 139-1) can be helpful in determining and promoting a family's readiness to make changes to address weight concerns. For families who are less ready, the physician's role can be more focused on understanding values and current barriers, ordering appropriate testing to help families assess risk, checking back in frequently, and providing encouragement while respecting autonomy. For more ready families, the physician's role moves into actively eliciting from the patient and parent what they consider to be important and feasible lifestyle changes and how they want to go about reaching their goals.

Given the difficulty of modifying behaviors related to food and activity, patients and their families require ongoing support and attention from their primary care physician and additional clinical and community resources as they attempt to integrate and maintain healthy habits in their lives. Engaging with the family to elicit solutions and brainstorm solutions to barriers is more likely to yield positive results than blanket advice or recommendations. Even well-intentioned clinical recommendations are unlikely to be implemented if they are inconsistent with a patient's and family's values, culture, and resources. For example, a child's participation in an after-school sports program may not be a realistic option if a family cannot afford the fees or transportation to and from the program is not available; instead, a school-based after-school program or an evening or weekend class at a community center with the parent might be an option.

In preventing and treating childhood obesity, physicians must also recognize the gaps between knowledge and behavior; understanding that good nutrition and physical activity are important does not necessarily translate into healthy eating or regular exercise. For example, a parent may know to limit fat and sugar but may still buy a lot of processed foods because of convenience or price or not knowing how to prepare healthier foods. Alternatively, some families may have food insecurity or periods with inadequate food that may lead to overeating inexpensive, energy-dense foods. These families should be connected with nutrition assistance programs (eg, Women, Infants, and Children Supplemental Nutrition Assistance Program [WIC] [formerly known as food stamps]). Most families need additional education on appropriate serving sizes, healthful food preparation, interpreting food labels, and making healthy food choices among the many mixed nutrition messages in the media. Given time limitations to provide this kind of support in primary care office visits, referral to a dietitian or nutrition classes through WIC can be an initial step in providing the education and planning needed for families to change eating habits. Dietitians can be particularly useful for motivated families in providing ideas to plan healthful daily meals and snacks.

Because the options for actively treating childhood obesity are still somewhat limited in the primary care setting, it is critically important for physicians to be aware of what treatment programs are available in the local area and take full advantage of these. Successful, evidence-based programs are now increasingly available to help children attain a healthier weight. To date, the most efficacious programs are moderate-intensity, family-based behavioral treatment, generally of 3 to 12 months' duration. Physicians can play an active role in referring to structured treatment programs by being a knowledgeable source of information and helping families learn about and become interested in these programs. Families often need support and encouragement from a trusted provider to participate. If structured overweight treatment programs are not available in the local area, the physician can recommend and refer to structured physical activity programs, such as those at local YMCAs or community centers, that can help patients improve physical fitness and lower metabolic risks related to obesity, even if not leading to weight loss per se.

A basic set of guidelines that physicians can use to help families move toward a healthier lifestyle is included in Box 139-2. Items on this list are evidence based from the standpoint that families who have

---

Box 139-1. Brief Motivational Interviewing Approach to Child Obesity Management

Goal: Through nonjudgmental questions and reflective listening, elicit a realistic plan for addressing child's weight/health consistent with family's values and goals.

Use: Basic motivational interviewing skills or OARS

- O: Open-ended questions (eg, those starting with "How," "What," or "Tell me about . . .")
- A: Affirmations (eg, "You are already doing a good job with . . .")
- R: Reflections (eg, "It sounds like you would like some help with changing . . .")
- S: Summaries (eg, "Let me see if I can summarize our discussion and plans between now and the next visit . . .")

Steps: Basic approach in 15 minutes

1. Assess body mass index (BMI), inform parent/patient, elicit response.
   "Your child's BMI (his or her balance of weight to height) is in a range where we start to be concerned about extra weight causing health problems. What concerns, if any, do you have about your child's weight?"
2. Set agenda: Assess what parent/patient have already done, their goals for change, and possible target behaviors.
   See Questions Box.
3. Assess motivation and confidence to make the changes.
   "On a scale of 1 to 10, with 10 being highest, how important are the changes we have talked about for you? Why are you an X [number they chose] and not a Y ?"
4. Ask about ways to implement the parent/patient's plans/goals.
   "Who can help you with your plans? What will help you be successful? How have you been able to make a change in the past?"
5. Summarize: Review plans (including follow-up), express confidence in the family, offer further help.
   "Let's summarize our discussion today. You have planned to ____, and this is important to you because ____ . You will get some help from ____ to be successful. This sounds like a plan that can work. I know you can do it if you set your mind to it. I suggest we meet again in one month to check in. I look forward to hearing about how well you are doing. At that time we can discuss other ways I might be able to help, like a referral to a nutritionist or an exercise program."

Box 139-2. Ten Guidelines to Help Families Toward a Healthier Lifestyle

1. Learn about the child's and family's usual diet and activity pattern so you can elicit ideas about helpful changes they are interested in and capable of making.
2. Promote simple 5210 guidelines for healthy living: 5 fruits and vegetables a day, 2 hours or less of screen time, 1 hour or more of physical activity, and 0 sugar-sweetened beverages per day.
3. Encourage intake of more "natural" foods such as fruits and vegetables (fresh or frozen). Limit processed and prepackaged foods and snacks (which have added sugar and fat kids don't need) by keeping them out of the house as much as possible.
4. Set family guidelines on recreational screen time with a goal of less than 2 hours a day including television, video games, and computers. Keep televisions out of children's and teens' bedrooms (easier to do if physicians help educate about not putting them there in the first place).
5. Promote "fitness over fatness": Incorporate physical activity into the child's and family's daily routine with a goal of 60 minutes per day. Find sports or activities that the child enjoys and can master.
6. Teach healthy beverages for all ages: Milk and water is all we need. For children older than 1 to 2 years, change to 1% or fat-free milk. Limit milk to 16 to 20 oz per day after the first year of life. If parents serve juice, limit to less than 4 oz per day for toddlers and 6 oz for older children. Limit soda to special occasions (eg, birthday).
7. Limit eating out, especially at fast-food restaurants.
8. Have regular family meals cooked at home.
9. Encourage appropriate portion sizes for family members based on need (teach parents to respond to hunger cues when children are infants and toddlers).
10. Promote healthy sleep, including regular bedtimes and adequate sleep (10–11 hours for school-aged children; 8–9 hours for teenagers).

implemented these generally have children with healthier weight. Some involve fairly simple changes, such as reducing intake of sugar-sweetened beverages or switching to lower-fat milk. Other suggestions may require more knowledge or motivation to implement successfully. Many Web sites provide excellent educational resources for families, including the US Department of Agriculture ChooseMyPlate.gov (www.choosemyplate.gov) and *Dietary Guidelines for Americans,* which is published every 5 years (www.health.gov/dietaryguidelines); Nemours KidsHealth (www.kidshealth.org); and the Let's Move! campaign initiated by First Lady Michelle Obama (www.letsmove.gov).

Given the complexity of managing obesity, more clinical tools and additional training for pediatric professionals are becoming available, including the American Academy of Pediatrics (AAP) Section on Obesity and Institute for Healthy Childhood Weight (www.aap.org/obesity) and *We Can!* resources from the National Institutes of Health National Heart, Lung, and Blood Institute (www.nhlbi.nih.gov/health/public/heart/obesity/wecan).

Prevention

Prevention of obesity is the best option for reversing the growing epidemic of obesity and obesity-related comorbidities. Prevention of obesity should be a priority for all physicians who care for children and should focus on 3 broad areas: (1) anticipatory guidance starting in infancy on healthful eating, adequate sleep, minimizing screen time, and providing access to regular physical activity with an emphasis on promoting overall health; (2) early intervention for families whose children are at higher risk for developing obesity; and (3) advocacy for public health measures to increase opportunities for healthful eating and regular physical activity within our communities. Pediatricians can take an active role to improve obesity trends in supporting changes in school and child care institutions, communities, and national policies (see resources available through the AAP at www.aap.org/obesity).

Prognosis

Without intervention, the average American life expectancy is currently projected to decrease because of the increasing incidence of diseases associated with obesity, such as diabetes. Poor diet and sedentary lifestyles rival smoking as a preventable cause of premature death. Obese children who remain obese into adulthood are at greatly increased risk for all of the complications of obesity. However, there is hopeful evidence that early intervention at the family and community levels can change this trajectory. Pediatricians continue to improve rates of BMI screening and referral; those who have had training in obesity management are even more likely to implement current recommendations. Globally, more physicians and organizations are taking an active role in preventing and treating childhood obesity, and treatment options continue to evolve and improve. The fact that current childhood obesity rates in the United States have begun to stabilize may be a positive sign for the future.

CASE RESOLUTION

The case study describes a girl who is obese. She is at substantial risk for remaining obese into adulthood based on her present weight and her mother's history of obesity, as well as social and economic risk factors. Working with a dietitian, the mother and daughter learn about simple changes for healthy diets. They begin to plan meals and snacks that include fruits and vegetables and can be prepared in advance. The daughter starts making her own lunch each night before school. The mother changes her grocery shopping: She buys 1% milk instead of whole milk and stops buying as many cookies, chips, and soda, except as an occasional treat. A social worker helps find an after-school program at the nearby YMCA. The patient starts attending and, with some special attention from the coach, finds she enjoys basketball and would like to try out for the school team next year. The mother wants to exercise more, so she and her daughter plan after-dinner walks around the track at the local high school.

Over the next 6 months, you follow mother and daughter closely. The most recent growth parameters show that the girl has maintained her weight at 59 kg but has grown 5 cm to 145 cm, giving her a body mass index of 28. The mother has lost 5 lb during this period, and both are excited about continuing their new lifestyle.

Selected References

American Academy of Pediatrics Committee on Nutrition. Prevention of pediatric overweight and obesity. *Pediatrics.* 2003;112(2):424–430

American Academy of Pediatrics Council on Sports Medicine and Fitness and Council on School Health. Active healthy living: prevention of childhood obesity through increased physical activity. *Pediatrics.* 2006;117(5):1834–1842

Barlow SE; Expert Committee. Expert Committee recommendations regarding the prevention, assessment, and treatment of child and adolescent overweight and obesity: a summary report. *Pediatrics.* 2007;120(Suppl 4):S164–S192

Daniels SR, Arnett DK, Eckel RH, et al. Overweight in children and adolescents: pathophysiology, consequence, prevention, and treatment. *Circulation.* 2005; 111(15):1999–2012

Dietz W, Lee J, Wechsler H, Malepati S, Sherry B. Health plans' role in preventing overweight in children and adolescents. *Health Aff (Millwood).* 2007;26(2): 430–440

Freedman DS, Mei Z, Srinivasan SR, Berenson GS, Dietz WH. Cardiovascular risk factors and excess adiposity among overweight children and adolescents: the Bogalusa Heart Study. *J Pediatr.* 2007;150(1):12–17

Halfon N, Larson K, Slusser W. Associations between obesity and comorbid mental health, developmental, and physical health conditions in a nationally representative sample of US children aged 10 to 17. *Acad Pediatr.* 2013;13(1):6–13

Institute of Medicine Committee on Prevention of Obesity in Children and Youth. *Preventing Childhood Obesity: Health in the Balance.* Washington, DC: National Academy of Sciences; 2004

Klein JD, Sesselberg TS, Johnson MS, et al. Adoption of body mass index guidelines for screening and counseling in pediatric practice. *Pediatrics.* 2010;125(2): 265–272

Ogden CL, Carroll MD, Kit BK, Flegal KM. Prevalence of obesity and trends in body mass index among US children and adolescents, 1999-2010. *JAMA.* 2012; 307(5):483–490

Whitlock EP, O'Connor EA, Williams SB, Beil TL, Lutz KW. Effectiveness of weight management interventions in children: a targeted systematic review for the USPSTF. *Pediatrics.* 2010;125(2):e396–e418

CHAPTER 140

Divorce

Carol D. Berkowitz, MD

CASE STUDY

A 7-year-old girl who has been your patient for 5 years is brought in by her mother with abdominal pain that occurs on a daily basis and is not associated with any other symptoms. The pain is periumbilical. In obtaining the history, you learn that the father has moved out of the home and the parents are planning a divorce. The mother believes that her daughter's symptoms may relate to the impending divorce, and she wants to know what else to expect.

Questions

1. What are the problems faced by children whose parents are undergoing divorce?
2. What are the age-related reactions of children in families undergoing divorce?
3. What are the custodial issues and arrangements following divorce?
4. What is the role of pediatricians in counseling families undergoing divorce?
5. What anticipatory guidance can be offered about custody and remarriage?
6. How can pediatricians help stepfamilies adjust?

Divorce represents the **"death"** of a marriage and in some ways may be more devastating for children than the death of a parent. When a parent dies, that parent becomes idealized in the mind of children, but when parents divorce, the noncustodial parent is often devalued. In fact, each parent is frequently devalued by the other. For children, parents are no longer the idealized figures that they once were. The challenge for pediatricians is to maintain a neutral position. This may be particularly difficult because much of the contact has been with one parent rather than the other, usually the mother.

Pediatricians play a specific role in managing children going through parental divorce because other resources are few. **Extended families** are no longer as available to provide help. Religious institutions have often failed to assume a counseling role in this area; some religions view divorce unfavorably. Most families do not seek out mental health services unless problems are overwhelming. Therefore, it is important for pediatricians to become involved in anticipatory guidance of families undergoing divorce. This guidance focuses on preparing children and families for times ahead. In addition, pediatricians serve as child advocates. The parents themselves are so consumed by their emotional turmoil that they are often not available or are not even aware of the stress and trauma their children are experiencing. Pediatricians should be aware of the effect of the divorce on children and their subsequent psychologic development. In addition, pediatricians can help as new families form, assisting the transition of caregivers into the role of stepparents.

Epidemiology

Divorce affects nearly 50% of marriages, although the rate recently has decreased to closer to 40%, attributed in part to the decrease in the marriage rate. **Ethnic differences** exist; 38% of European American children's parents, compared with 75% of African American children's parents, divorce prior to the children's 18th birthday. The National Vital Statistics System reported 877,000 provisional divorces and annulments for 2011, a figure that is lower than the actual number of cases because California, Georgia, Hawaii, Louisiana, and Minnesota do not report their data. Divorce usually occurs in the first 14 years of marriage (mean: 7.8 years). Approximately 1 million children per year are affected by divorce. Nearly one-third of all children live in households in which parents are divorced or remarried. Children between the ages of 3 and 8 years are the major age group affected. Children involved with parental divorce take 2½ to 3 years to regain their equilibrium and master a sense of control. Divorce usually results in a decline of **economic resources** to mothers and children. In the first year after divorce, income is reduced to 58% of the pre-divorce level. Even after 5 years, income for mothers and children is only 94% of the pre-divorce amount; for intact couples, income has risen to 130% during that period. Decreased income is often associated with multiple moves to more affordable housing along with change in schools and loss of friends. More affordable neighborhoods may not provide the same resources and environment to which the children were previously accustomed.

Types of custody include **single parent, joint, joint legal,** and **joint physical,** in which parents have physical access to the child with equal frequency. **Bird's-nest custody** is joint custody in which children remain in the home and parents take turns moving in and out. Many states now allow for joint custody, which is associated with higher levels of involvement by the biological father, increased child support payments, and greater paternal satisfaction. Issues of **remarriage** and **step-siblings** are also important. Eighty percent of divorced men and 75% of divorced women remarry, and 40% of these remarriages end in divorce. As a result of the high rate of remarriage, 1 in 3 children in the United States has a stepparent. Eighty-six percent of stepfamilies include the biological mother and a stepfather. Children in stepfamilies often have to readjust to differing roles in differing households and differing relationships between their biological parents, stepparents, biological siblings, and step-siblings.

Psychophysiology

The experience that children have following parental divorce is influenced by many factors. When the divorce is contentious and the children are exposed to hostility between their parents, such high levels of stress can result in physiological changes, including elevated levels of cortisol, which can be associated with sleep disturbances, anxiety, irritability, and weight change.

The individual child's **temperament** and **personality also affect their adjustment to parental divorce.** An easygoing child with strong self-esteem and a positive outlook fairs better than a child with a difficult temperament and less positive personality traits. The reaction to divorce also depends, to a large extent, on the age of the child (Table 140-1). In general, children do not have the cognitive ability to understand the meaning of divorce until they are 9 or 10 years of age. The experience is also different for children without siblings ("onlies"). Not only do they lack brothers or sisters with which to commiserate, they may also experience parental overconcern, manifested by being asked repeatedly how they are feeling and how they are doing. Studies have demonstrated that the negative effect of parental divorce on adolescent academic performance is mitigated by increased sibship size.

Children up to the age of 2 years experience **sleeping** and **feeding disturbances,** as well as spitting up and clinginess. Between the ages of 2½ and 4 years, children usually manifest **regressive behavior.** They become needy and dependent, and their behavior is characterized by irritability, whining, crying, fearfulness, increased separation anxiety, and sleep problems. Aggression and regression, particularly in the area of toilet training, may develop. One-third of children in this age group continue to exhibit regressive behavior 1 year after divorce.

Children between the ages of 3½ and 5 years often show more aggressive patterns of behavior with hitting, biting, and temper tantrums. Regressive behavior may also be seen. Young children feel particularly responsible for their parents' divorce (ie, the parents are divorcing the child). At this point in development, children experience what Piaget has referred to as an egocentric way of thinking. Self-blame, decreased self-esteem, and a high level of fantasy, particularly about parental reunion, are apparent. Approximately 1 year after divorce, 65% of these children still show decreased levels of functioning. Preschoolers may repetitively ask the same questions as a way to process and assimilate the information. Such questioning should be met with patience and reassurance.

Children who are 5 to 6 years of age are often **depressed** and may exhibit immature behavior. Girls in this age group seem to handle a divorce more poorly than boys. Two-thirds of girls are less well-adjusted 1 year after the divorce, as opposed to only about one-fourth of boys. These children seem moody and daydream. They may also be whiny and have temper tantrums.

Children between the age of 6 years and adolescence seem to experience profound disequilibrium, with feelings of shame, anger, and loneliness. This anger may be manifested by antisocial behavior. Older children also talk about an overwhelming feeling of sadness and grief. Their somatic complaints include headache, abdominal pain, and an increase in symptoms of preexisting medical conditions such as asthma. Sometimes the somatic complaints of children, particularly those in the school-aged group, are attributed by one parent to the poor living conditions at the other parent's household.

It is important for physicians to anticipate that 50% of children involved in parental divorce show a deterioration in their school performance. Therefore, the school should be notified about the divorce and changes in family structure. Decreased school performance is attributed to decreased ability to concentrate, sadness, and depression.

Parental divorce is particularly difficult for adolescents, who describe it as "extraordinarily painful." They may exhibit externalizing (eg, risk taking, alcohol use) and internalizing (eg, anxiety, depression) behavior. The experience is worse for younger adolescents. During the first stages of divorce, they experience a personal sense of abandonment and a loss of parental love. Older adolescents are concerned about their future potential as marital partners. They also feel anxious about financial security, especially money for college. **De-idealization** of both parents is precipitous. Adolescent girls do better than boys early on, but this reverses with time. This pattern is referred to as a **sleeper effect** or **delayed effect,** with girls subsequently feeling rejected and unattractive as they reinterpret their parents' divorce with their additional maturation. Divorce during adolescence sometimes leads to **precocious sexual activity** or risk- or thrill-seeking behavior. Studies suggest that paternal involvement following the divorce reduces the risk of alcohol abuse. Adolescents from divorced families are more likely to experience teenaged parenthood. Adolescent girls from divorced families are less likely to succeed academically than girls from families in which there has not been a divorce. In addition, adolescents may turn to alcohol or drug use to help cope with the stress of parental divorce. Boys may engage in illegal activities such as burglary.

Table 140-1. Children's Reaction to Divorce	
Age	*Symptoms*
2½–4 y	Regressive behavior
3½–5 y	Aggressive behavior
5–6 y	Whiny, immature behavior
6 y–adolescence	• Disequilibrium • Depression • Somatic complaints • Poor school performance

Differential Diagnosis

Children who present with complaints including headache, abdominal pain, enuresis, and poor school performance should always be assessed for environmental factors that may be contributing to their symptomatology. When evaluating a child with suspected **somatic complaints,** it is appropriate to consider organic etiologies.

Many parents who are undergoing a divorce do not appreciate the effect the divorce is having on their children. They are often caught up in their own personal feelings and are not aware of their children's symptomatology. In addition, divorcing parents actually experience a deterioration in their physical and mental well-being, and divorced mothers have an increased rate of illness.

Parents engaged in custody disputes may express concerns that their child is maltreated by the other parent. These concerns may include allegations of sexual abuse, which may require a referral to a child advocacy center (see Chapter 132).

Evaluation

The focus of the evaluation should be on the interviewing process. Determination of the full extent of the effect of home factors on children's symptomatology may take several visits. It is not appropriate to pursue extensive laboratory tests without first adequately determining what changes are occurring within the household.

History

The medical evaluation of children experiencing a parental divorce should include a review of the medical history and a discussion with the child of factors of change (Questions Box). This may help open up a discussion that reveals that the parents are in the process of divorce or that the father has moved out of the household. Specific parental concerns related to child maltreatment should be noted in detail.

Physical Examination

Any symptom or specific complaint, such as headache or abdominal pain, should also be addressed (see chapters 116 and 120). Depression and the risk for suicide should also be evaluated (see Chapter 144). A complete physical examination is usually warranted because children who are experiencing stress may also develop stress-related medical problems. If there are concerns about the genital findings, a careful anogenital examination is indicated.

Laboratory Tests

Some simple baseline laboratory studies may be warranted, particularly in children who have complaints such as abdominal pain or enuresis. These tests may include a complete blood cell count or urinalysis.

Management

Management of children whose family is undergoing divorce is complex. In addition to treating any somatic complaints that may be related to the divorce, physicians play a key role in anticipatory guidance. Children need to understand that they didn't cause the divorce and that they will not be able to "cure" it. Physician involvement before parents actually separate helps. Initially, physicians should advise parents about how to talk to children and what to expect in terms of their reaction. It is important for parents to tell children that they are separating from one another and not from the children. As stated previously, parents undergoing a divorce are in so much turmoil that they themselves may not see their children's problems. In addition, their parenting skills may suffer, and routine procedures such as meals and bedtime may become disrupted, sporadic, and irregular.

Box 140-1 summarizes advice given to parents when talking with their children. **Who, when, how, where,** and **what** to tell should be discussed. Generally, children should be told of impending divorce by both parents with support from the extended family. Unfortunately, studies report that 80% of preschoolers were told by one parent.

When to tell depends on children's ages. Younger children should be told a few days before the actual separation. Older children should be told at least several weeks before. Practitioners should advise parents about **how** to tell. Displays of emotion are permissible. Parents should be encouraged to show their emotions but not to the extent that they appear overwhelmed or uncontrollable.

Questions

Divorce

- Is there anything different about the child's house now?
- Who lives in the house?
- How are things going between the parents?
- Has the child shown any regressive or aggressive behaviors?
- Has the child been eating and sleeping normally?
- How is the child doing in school?

Box 140-1. Talking to Children About Divorce

Who
- Who tells? Both parents
- Who is told? Children, physicians, teachers, neighbors

When
- Before either parent leaves
- Age-dependent
- Older children: weeks ahead
- Younger children: days ahead

How
- Calmly, with emotional control

Where
- Privately, in the home

What
- Stress that children are not to blame; that the divorce is between parents, not between parents and children; it is the parents who cannot get along.
- Explain expected living arrangements.

Who to tell includes not only the children but also the neighbors and the school, so that the feeling of shame or secrecy is less. **What** to tell involves freeing the children of any blame for the divorce and answering their questions.

It is important for physicians not to become involved in custody disputes, but if they are asked to give an opinion, they should try to evaluate the parenting skills of both parents. In the past, custody was given to the mother in 90% of cases, but this is now decreasing. Questions that physicians should ask themselves when advising about custody include the following: What are the emotional ties between parents and children? Do children indicate a preference for one parent? Children may be overwhelmed by feelings of loyalty and be torn if asked to choose one parent over the other, which makes this a difficult problem. What is the capacity of each parent to provide emotional and physical support for children? It is important to consider a need for continuity, and it is vital to keep conditions as close as possible to the pre-divorce situation. Children should not have to move. Living arrangements need to be reassessed on a periodic basis. Pediatricians may also refer parents to community programs that may involve didactic sessions well as parent groups. One such program, New Beginnings, has been shown to improve mother-child relationships and decrease internalizing behavior in children and externalizing behavior in adolescents.

Physicians should be aware of factors that support joint custody. Joint custody tends to maintain a parent-child attachment, and children experience less of a sense of loss. They have more cognitive and social stimulation. Joint custody relieves the burden of single parenthood, and parents who have joint custody are less likely to use children as bargaining tools. Parents themselves are freer to enter into different relationships and are less emotionally dependent on their children. Although physicians should not become involved in monetary issues, concerns related to payment, insurance coverage, and cost of medical care are appropriate to discuss. Practitioners should consider involving noncustodial parents in children's health care. Such parents could be notified if medical problems occur.

Pediatricians may also be helpful in counseling noncustodial parents about interacting with children. Unfortunately, contact with noncustodial parents may decrease rapidly following a divorce. While 25% of children have weekly visits with their noncustodial father, 20% of children see their father only several times a year or not at all. In general, visitation should reflect previous relationships as closely as possible. Noncustodial parents should be advised not to become camp counselors who focus on fun and games but to be influential figures who help children meet the challenges of normal living, such as completing homework and doing chores and tasks. It is also important for noncustodial parents to be consistent. If a meeting is planned, the parents must show up. Although the parents are no longer married, they can still be co-parents rather than rivals. Noncustodial parents should be encouraged to participate in school and sports activities. Multiple modalities, such as e-mail and texting, can facilitate more frequent communication.

Custodial parents may attribute children's somatic complaints to poor care while under visitation with noncustodial parents. Allegations related to abuse, most often sexual abuse, may also arise. These allegations should be taken seriously. An appropriate medical and psychologic evaluation is necessary (see Chapter 132). The most difficult situations involve allegations of sexual abuse of preverbal children, in which conclusions may be contingent on the physical findings, which are usually inconclusive.

Issues related to parental dating and remarriage should be addressed at an early stage. Parents should be advised that pediatricians may be a resource in helping families readjust. Remarriage is often a difficult time for children because they experience feelings of rejection secondary to displacement by stepparents. Grandparents may also be a source of support.

Remarriage may result in a family involving same-sex parents. Many children with gay or lesbian parents have undergone the divorce of their heterosexual parents. Marriage between same-sex parents has been legalized in an increasing number of states. The 2010 US Census report identified 131,729 married same-sex households. Children may, however, move to families with same-sex parents who are not married. The same report noted 514,735 same-sex unmarried partner households. Studies show that children raised by same-sex parents function similarly to those in heterosexual families.

The pediatrician can also serve as a resource for stepparents. Although stepparents do not have legal rights to consent for medical care of their stepchildren, they should become familiar with the children's medical history. Stepparents grow into their parenting role, and it takes 2 to 7 years for families to become blended. The pediatrician can help families adjust by recommending books or giving referrals to organizations such as the National Stepfamily Resource Center (www.stepfamilies.info).

Prognosis

The prognosis for children undergoing a parental divorce depends, in part, on the degree of dysfunction that existed in the family before separation and the ability of the children to communicate their concerns. It takes most children 2 to 3 years to adjust to parental divorce and 3 to 5 years to adjust to a remarriage. Supportive intervention by family, friends, and physicians is key to facilitating the necessary adjustment. For adolescents, a positive belief about parental divorce is a major predictor of their adjustment. Family resilience and hardiness as well as family communication are associated with a good adjustment. Being a child of divorced and remarried parents has been likened to having dual citizenship. The experience is rewarding if the countries are not at war with one another.

CASE RESOLUTION

The case study reflects that functional somatic complaints are not uncommon, especially in school-aged children of divorced parents. The mother and her daughter should be advised about how stressful divorce is for children. A careful medical examination may reassure the mother and daughter about the child's physical well-being. Issues related to custody, financial responsibility, and the need for consistency should all be addressed. In addition, the pediatrician should refer the family to outside agencies, if necessary.

Selected References

American Academy of Pediatrics Committee on Psychosocial Aspects of Child and Family Health. Coparent or second-parent adoption by same-sex parents. *Pediatrics*. 2002;109(2):339–340

Bryner CL Jr. Children of divorce. *J Am Board Fam Pract*. 2001;14(3):201–210

Cohen GJ; American Academy of Pediatrics Committee on Psychosocial Aspects of Child and Family Health. Helping children and families deal with divorce and separation. *Pediatrics*. 2002;110(5):1019–1023

Hetherington EM. Divorce and the adjustment of children. *Pediatr Rev*. 2005; 26(5):163–169

Kleinsorge C, Covitz LM. Impact of divorce on children: developmental considerations. *Pediatr Rev*. 2012;33(4):147–155

McClain DB, Wolchik SA, Winslow E, Tein JY, Sandler IN, Millsap RE. Developmental cascade effects of the New Beginnings Program on adolescent adaptation outcomes. *Dev Psychopathol*. 2010;22(4):771–784

Perrin EC, Siegel BS; American Academy of Pediatrics Committee on Psychosocial Aspects of Child and Family Health. Promoting the well-being of children whose parents are gay or lesbian. *Pediatrics*. 2013;131(4):e1374–e1383

Shin SH, Choi H, Kim MJ, Kim YH. Comparing adolescents' adjustment and family resilience in divorced families depending on the types of primary caregiver. *J Clin Nurs*. 2010;19(11–12):1695–1706

Storksen I, Roysamb E, Moum T, Tambs K. Adolescents with a childhood experience of parental divorce: a longitudinal study of mental health and adjustment. *J Adolesc*. 2005;28(6):725–739

Tomcikova Z, Madarasova Geckova A, Reijneveld SA, van Dijk JP. Parental divorce, adolescents' feelings toward parents and drunkenness in adolescents. *Eur Addict Res*. 2011;17(3):113–118

Vélez CE, Wolchik SA, Tein JY, Sandler I. Protecting children from the consequences of divorce: a longitudinal study of the effects of parenting on children's coping processes. *Child Dev*. 2011;82(1):244–257

Books for Parents

Clapp G. *Divorce and New Beginnings: A Complete Guide to Recovery, Solo Parenting, Co-Parenting, and Stepfamilies*. Hoboken, NJ: John Wiley & Sons; 2000

Garon RJ. *Talking to Your Children about Separation and Divorce: A Handbook for Parents*. Columbia, MD: National Family Resiliency Center, Inc; 1999

Book for Teens

Ricci I. *Mom's House, Dad's House for Kids: Feeling at Home in One Home or Two*. New York, NY: Simon & Schuster; 2006

CHAPTER 141

School-Related Violence

Catherine A. DeRidder, MD

CASE STUDY

A mother brings in her 9-year-old son, Alex, complaining of recurrent abdominal pain. His pain has become so severe that Alex misses school frequently. He denies any vomiting or diarrhea. His weight has been stable over the last 6 months. Alex's mother reports that lately he seems more withdrawn and passive. He used to be engaged in his schoolwork but now, with his frequent absences, has lost interest in school. His mother says he is often anxious or nervous about new situations.

Questions

1. How does school-related violence affect children's health and well-being?
2. What is the relationship between bullying and adult criminal behavior?
3. What is cyberbullying?
4. What children are at risk for being bullied or for becoming a bully?
5. What can pediatricians do to help address violence in the school, home, and communities?

Violence is defined as an act of aggression that can be **physical, sexual,** or **psychologic.** Its form, level of severity, and frequency are affected by biological, individual, clinical, intrapersonal, situational, and sociocultural factors. Categorization of violence is also dependent on the relationship of the perpetrator and victim, as well as their ages. **Intimate partner violence (IPV)** occurs among individuals in an established relationship; **child abuse** predominantly occurs between an adult and a minor; and **bullying** is usually between peers. From a developmental perspective, bullying may be the earliest form of violence instigated by children and can progress to IPV, **criminal delinquency, suicide,** or **homicide** in adolescence and adulthood. While violence may be considered a social issue, it affects the physical and mental health of all of those involved. The primary care physician has unique opportunities to prevent violence and identify those potentially at risk.

Prevalence and Risk Factors

Suicide and homicide represent the most lethal forms of violence. Suicide and homicide are responsible for approximately one-fourth of deaths among persons aged 10 to 24 years in the United States. Approximately 3 million youths are at risk for suicide, with 37% of at-risk individuals attempting to kill themselves (see Chapter 144). In 2010, suicide was the third leading cause of death among 15- to 24-year-olds, and over the last 20 years it has increased 100% among 10- to 14-year-olds. It is estimated that approximately 12 youths die each day in the United States from suicide. Homicide is also increasing among children and adolescents. According to the Centers for Disease Control and Prevention, homicide is the fourth leading cause of death for youths 10 to 14 years of age and the second leading cause of death for 15- to 19-year-olds in the United States.

In 2007, more than 500,000 individuals younger than 24 years were treated in emergency departments for injuries sustained because of violence. In 2011, nationwide surveys of high school students noted that 12% reported being in a physical fight one or more times in the 12 preceding months on school property. Five percent reported carrying a weapon such as a gun, knife, or club on one or more of the 30 days preceding the survey. Furthermore, 6% of students reported not going to school on one or more days in the 30 days preceding the survey because they felt unsafe at school or on their way to and from school. Bullying was found to be much more prevalent, with 20% reporting being bullied on school property and 16% reporting being bullied electronically.

In a 2001 national survey of sixth- to 10th-grade students, approximately 30% reported moderate or frequent involvement in bullying; this could include being the bully, the victim, or both (known as the *bully-victim*). Those who reported being a bully or victim were more likely to carry weapons to school as well as to be involved in frequent fights. Bullying itself is most common in the middle school years. Boys are more likely than girls to be involved in bullying. Boys tend to participate in physical and verbal bullying, while girls use more verbal and relational bullying, such as rumors and social exclusion.

Risk factors associated with bullying are complex and involve the individual, family, peers, and community (Box 141-1). Demonstrated risk factors associated with violent behavior include exposure to violence as a witness or victim, childhood aggression, and **antisocial behavior, substance abuse, depressed mood,** and **hyperactivity.** Protective factors include academic achievement and parent-family connectedness. Victims of bullying are more likely to be children who are considered different from their peers, eg, children who are obese, who have a developmental delay or learning disability, or who are lesbian, gay, bisexual, transgender, or questioning (LGBTQ).

Box 141-1. Risk Factors Associated With Bullying

Victim	Bully
Individual Risk Factors[a]	**Individual Risk Factors[a]**
• Physical traits different from peers, especially obesity	• Poor academic achievement
• Chronic illnesses	• Behavioral or emotional problems
• Behavioral or emotional problems	• Involvement with drugs, alcohol, or tobacco
• Sexual orientation (LGBTQ)	• Criminal involvement
• Physical or learning disabilities	**Family Risk Factors**
Family Risk Factors	• Abuse (physical, sexual, or psychologic)
• Abuse (physical, sexual, or psychologic)	• Witness to violence
• Witness to violence	• Poor family functioning
• Poor family functioning	**Social Environment Risk Factors**
Social Environment Risk Factors	• Association with delinquent peers/peer pressure
• Social rejection by peers	• Socioeconomic disadvantage
• Socioeconomic disadvantage	• Low commitment to school and school failure
• Low commitment to school and school failure	• Inner-city upbringing
• Inner-city upbringing	

Abbreviation: LGBTQ, lesbian, gay, bisexual, transgender, questioning.

[a]Adapted with permission from Waseem M, Ryan M, Foster CB, Peterson J. Assessment and management of bullied children in the emergency department. *Pediatr Emerg Care.* 2013;29(3):389–398.

Bullying

Tragic mass killing events, especially those at schools, coupled with reports of the perpetrators being victims or bullies during childhood, has raised the awareness of the seriousness of bullying as an early form of violence. Unfortunately, many parents, teachers, and health care professionals still see bullying as a normal behavior of children.

Bullying is defined as repeated acts of verbal or physical intimidation, coercion, and aggression An imbalance of power exists with the more powerful attacking the less powerful, whether because of physical size or social power. Bullying occurs in an environment that supports the behavior. Participants include the bully, the victim, and the bystander. The bully is often an aggressive individual who uses violence to dominate others. In contrast with common perception, bullies do not have poor self-esteem but rather have a strong desire to control others. The victim may be more passive and anxious. This individual is often less secure than his or her peers and may be lonely, playing alone at school. When the victim is attacked by a bully, he or she usually withdraws rather than retaliates. A minority of youth may be classified as a bully-victim or a provocative victim. These individuals are anxious and aggressive; while they are primarily victims of bullying, they may provoke the bully.

There are different forms of bullying. Direct bullying includes physical or verbal bullying. Physical bullying can involve hitting or kicking, while verbal bullying can involve spreading rumors and social exclusion. Cyberbullying is a new form of bullying that can include bullying via e-mail, social networks, or texting. The bully who uses cyberbullying can remain anonymous and send aggressive messages to a large number of people.

Bullying predominantly occurs in unstructured school environments, such as during recess, at lunch, on the way to or from school, in hallways, or on the bus. Children often do not report bullying to adults for fear of and retaliation by the bully and the concern of disbelief by the adult. Studies demonstrate that adults underestimate the prevalence of bullying events compared with student reports.

Consequences of Bullying

Bullying affects the physical and mental health of all of those involved. Fear and anxiety about the school environment is most common. Other clinical signs of bullying can include bed-wetting, headaches, sleeping problems, abdominal pain, poor appetite, and feelings of tension or tiredness. This can progress to avoidance of school, low self-esteem, depression, and suicide.

A dose-response relationship has been seen between those who are only bullied at one time point compared with children who are chronically bullied. Strong associations in adolescence and early adulthood have been made between bullying and suicide and murder. The child who was victimized may react later in life with self-destructive acts or lethal retaliation.

Six percent of adults in the United States report a lifetime history of bullying. In adulthood, higher rates of depression and poor self-esteem are seen among individuals with a history of being bullied.

A cohort study of 1,420 individuals aged 9 to 26 years in western North Carolina found that victims of bullying and bully-victims had significantly higher likelihood of poor health, wealth, and social-relationship outcomes compared with children who were not bullied. Pure bullies were not at increased risk for adverse outcomes as an adult when other environmental factors and childhood psychiatric disorders were controlled.

Many of the recent killing sprees in the United States were committed by individuals who as children felt they were victimized. A review of 37 mass school shootings found more than two-thirds of perpetrators felt they had been persecuted, bullied, threatened, or attacked; often, they were acting out of revenge.

Other studies have found that those who were bullies in middle school had at least one criminal conviction by age 24 years, and 35% to 40% had 3 or more convictions by 24 years of age compared with 10% among control boys who not involved in bullying. Longitudinal studies report that bullies and bully-victims go on to more criminal activity than their counterparts. One study of Finnish boys reported 9% being bullies in childhood. These same individuals accounted for 33% of criminal activity in the study. Bullies were more likely to commit occasional infractions, while bully-victims were more likely to commit repeated offenses.

Bystanders are also affected because bullying distracts from the learning environment. Furthermore, they develop strategies to avoid being bullied, including avoiding the restroom and staying home. One study reported that 1 in 5 secondary schoolchildren avoid restrooms out of fear at school. Another study stated that 7% of eighth graders stay home at least 1 day a month out of fear of other students.

Role of the Primary Care Physician: Assessment

Childhood bullying is a complex abusive behavior with demonstrated serious consequences. Physicians are poised to identify at-risk individuals, screen for psychiatric comorbidities associated with bullying, counsel families, and advocate for school-based interventions. Because bullies or victims commonly will not identify themselves as such, physicians need a systematic approach to screen for this early form of violence. Integrating screening during anticipatory guidance may be optimal for toddlers and school-aged children, while assessing risk factors at well- and acute-care visits may be needed for adolescents.

Multiple instruments have been used in a research setting for identifying bullying or associated internalizing or externalizing symptoms, but they have not been widely implemented in the primary care setting. Screening younger patients requires conversations with the child and family members. The American Academy of Pediatrics developed Connected Kids: Safe, Strong, Secure, which can be integrated into Bright Futures for well-child care visits. This violence prevention program focuses on screening for risk, preventive education, and links to counseling and treatment resources. When talking directly with adolescents, the use of the psychosocial interview **HEADSSS** (*h*ome environment, *e*ducation and employment, *a*ctivities, *d*rugs, *s*exual activity/sexuality, *s*uicide/depression/self-image, *s*afety) may be useful in screening for high-risk behaviors and risk factors for violence (see Chapter 6).

When questioning a family about bullying, keep in mind that children will often not tell their parents that bullying occurred. When parents are told about bullying, they may consider the situation as being normal behavior for young people and dismiss the event.

Once bullying involvement is suspected, follow-up questions can then be asked to further characterize the involvement and obtain more details (Box 141-2).

Role of the Primary Care Physician: Prevention

Prevention efforts need to focus on the individual, family, and community. In early childhood, parents can model for children appropriate social interaction, how to resolve conflict, and how to manage frustration and anger. School-wide bullying prevention programs are effective and should be advocated. The Olweus program focuses on caregivers and schools showing positive interest in students, setting firm limits for unacceptable behavior, using consistent nonphysical consequences when rules are broken, and acting as positive role models to ultimately change social and behavioral norms. For older children and adolescents, identifying psychiatric symptoms and providing the appropriate intervention may prevent more serious violent behavior. At the individual level, physicians and parents can counsel children who are bullies or victims about appropriate behaviors (Box 141-3).

In a randomized controlled study, Borowsky and colleagues demonstrated the effectiveness of identifying at-risk youth aged 7 to 15 years in a primary care setting and providing a **family-level intervention** to reduce violent behavior and injuries among youth. Families who received the telephone-based intervention focusing on positive parenting reported decreased parent-reported bullying, physical fighting, fight-related injuries requiring medical care, and child-reported victimization by bullying.

The US Department of Health and Human Services developed a resource kit on bullying, which is available at www.stopbullying.gov. Printed resources are available for parents and teachers. The PACER Center National Bullying Prevention Center at www.pacer.org/bullying also has digital-based resources for parents, educators, teens, and youth. Specifically for LGBTQ youth, the Gay, Lesbian & Straight Education Network is available at www.glsen.org and the It Gets Better Project can be found at www.itgetsbetter.org.

The National Suicide Prevention Lifeline is available at www.suicidepreventionlifeline.org or can be reached at 1-800-273-TALK (8255) or by texting ANSWER to 839863. This lifeline provides 24-hour crisis counseling and mental health resources.

Box 141-2. Questions to Assess Bullying Involvement	
Bully	**Victim**
1. How often do you bully others?	1. How often are you bullied?
2. How long have you bullied others?	2. How long have you been bullied?
3. Where do you bully others?	3. Where are you bullied?
Eg, school, sports, home, neighborhood	
4. a) How do you bully others?	4. a) How are you bullied?
Eg, hitting, insults, gossiping, text messaging, social networks	
4. b) How do you think the kids you bully feel?	4. b) How do you feel when you are bullied?

Adapted with permission from Lamb J, Pepler DJ, Craig W. Approach to bullying and victimization. *Can Fam Physician*. 2009;55(4):356–360.

Box 141-3. The Physician's Role in Counseling Bullies and Victims

- Be vigilant for signs and symptoms of bullying and other psychosocial trauma and distress in children and adolescents.
- Increase awareness of the social and mental health consequences of bullying and other aggressive behaviors.
- Screen for psychiatric comorbidities in at-risk youth, and provide appropriate referrals for treatment for affected youth.
- Counsel affected youth and their families on effective intervention programs and coping strategies.
- Advocate for family, school, and community programs and services for victims and perpetrators for bullying and other forms of violence and aggression.

Box 141-4. Individual-Level Prevention Strategies

Advice for Victims of Bullying
- Resist reacting to the bully; hold your frustration and anger.
- Walk away from the situation; ignore the bullying.
- Avoid retaliation or bullying back.
- Tell an adult.
- Talk about the bullying event with your family.
- Each bullying situation should be assessed individually.
- Use a buddy system at school and traveling to and from school.
- Develop friendships by joining social organizations.

Management of Bullies
- Reinforce that bullying is a serious problem.
- Set limits and provide consequences for acts of aggression.
- Emphasize tolerance for people's differences; everyone deserves respect.
- Determine whether friends are also involved in bullying; seek a group intervention.
- Provide positive reinforcement for appropriate behavior.
- Work closely with school teachers and staff on behavior modification.
- Emphasize that it's the behavior that is not acceptable.

Physicians are a vital component of youth violence prevention (Box 141-4). Prevention begins early in a child's development by providing positive reinforcement of appropriate pro-social behavior. Bullying is an early form of aggression. Bullying may seem harmless, but longitudinal studies as well as analysis of mass school shootings demonstrate the large effect aggression early in life can have on the future well-being of children, adolescents, and adults. Successful interventions require cooperation by parents, teachers, students, and health care professionals.

CASE RESOLUTION

Victims of bullying often present with psychosomatic symptoms, such as headache or abdominal pain. Once organic etiologies have been ruled out, further questioning should focus on psychosocial stresses. Alex's abdominal pain is worse in the morning before going to school. When asked specifically about bullying, Alex states that a few of his classmates tease him and rough him up each day on his way to school. In the last few weeks, they are text messaging him about how they are going to haze him the next day. Alex has not told anyone about the experience because he thought he would be viewed as a coward. Alex shares that he would rather avoid going to school than face potential bullying.

The physician needs to assure Alex that it is not his fault that he is a victim of bullying. Prevention should include interventions at the individual, family, and school level. Alex should walk away from the conflict when possible and not feel uncomfortable about reporting the event to school staff. He may want to find a friend with whom he can walk to school. His family needs to understand that bullying is not a normal kid behavior. He should be encouraged to talk about bullying events and work with his family to identify solutions. The school should be notified about the event and encouraged to promote a non-bullying school environment.

Selected References

American Academy of Pediatrics Committee on Injury, Violence, and Poison Prevention. Role of the pediatrician in youth violence prevention. *Pediatrics.* 2009;124(1):393–402

Borowsky IW, Mozayeny S, Stuenkel K, Ireland M. Effects of a primary care-based intervention on violent behavior and injury in children. *Pediatrics.* 2004;114(4):e392–e399

Duke NN, Pettingell SL, McMorris BJ, Borowsky IW. Adolescent violence perpetration: associations with multiple types of adverse childhood experiences. *Pediatrics.* 2010;125(4):e778–e786

Fekkes M, Pijpers FI, Fredriks AM, Vogels T, Verloove-Vanhorick SP. Do bullied children get ill, or do ill children get bullied? A prospective cohort study on the relationship between bullying and health-related symptoms. *Pediatrics.* 2006;117(5):1568–1574

Nansel TR, Overpeck MD, Haynie DL, Ruan WJ, Scheidt PC. Relationships between bullying and violence among US youth. *Arch Pediatr Adolesc Med.* 2003;157(4):348–353

Puhl RM, Peterson JL, Luedicke J. Weight-based victimization: bullying experiences of weight loss treatment-seeking youth. *Pediatrics.* 2013;131(1):e1–e9

Robinson JP, Espelage DL, Rivers I. Developmental trends in peer victimization and emotional distress in LGB and heterosexual youth. *Pediatrics.* 2013;131(3):423–430

Sourander A, Jensen P, Rönning JA, et al. Childhood bullies and victims and their risk of criminality in late adolescence: the Finnish From a Boy to a Man study. *Arch Pediatr Adolesc Med.* 2007;161(6):546–552

Wang J, Iannotti RJ, Nansel TR. School bullying among adolescents in the United States: physical, verbal, relational, and cyber. *J Adolesc Health.* 2009;45(4):368–375

Wolke D, Copeland WE, Angold A, Costello EJ. Impact of bullying in childhood on adult health, wealth, crime, and social outcomes. *Psychol Sci.* 2013;24(10):1958–1970

CHAPTER 142

Intimate Partner Violence

Sara T. Stewart, MD

CASE STUDY

A 6-year-old boy is brought in by his mother for an annual well-child visit. He sits quietly as his mother reports no significant medical history. His medical records reflect that at his last visit he was talkative, doing well in school, and enjoyed playing baseball. As you speak with his mother, she seems reticent and does not spontaneously offer information. You determine that the boy's school performance has declined significantly over the past year and that he no longer wants to play baseball.

On physical examination, the boy has linear ecchymoses over his buttocks, and you notice bilateral areas of bruising on his mother's upper arms. When you ask about the marks, she becomes tearful. You ask her if she would like to speak privately with you.

Questions

1. How often do child abuse and intimate partner violence (IPV) co-occur?
2. What are potential strategies to screen for IPV?
3. What are common clinical presentations of victims of IPV and children exposed to IPV?
4. What are the long-term consequences of IPV on children?
5. What are key factors to take into account when determining the degree and immediacy of danger to a victim of IPV?

Intimate partner violence (IPV) has been defined as a pattern of assaultive and coercive behaviors that may include repeated battering and injury, sexual assault, progressive social isolation, deprivation, and intimidation. It is perpetrated by an individual who is or was involved in an intimate relationship with an adult or adolescent and whose intent is to establish control over the other partner. It is not only associated with negative physical and mental health outcomes for the victim but is also associated with negative mental health outcomes for children in the home. Childhood exposure to IPV is considered to have occurred when a child sees, hears, or observes the effects of verbal or physical assaults between partners. Intimate partner violence is also associated with the occurrence of child abuse in the home.

Epidemiology

Intimate partner violence affects both sexes and occurs in all ethnic, socioeconomic, sexual orientation, and religious groups. Approximately 2 to 4 million women and 500,000 to 1 million men report victimization annually in the United States. In 2007, 14% of homicides nationwide were the result of IPV, and the majority of these victims were female. While both men and women fall victim to IPV, women are more likely to sustain life-threatening injuries, leading to an increasing disparity between victimization rates with increased severity of physical assault. The financial cost of IPV to society has been estimated at $8.3 billion, including medical and mental health costs as well as the indirect cost of lost productivity. In total, victims lose millions of days of paid work time annually.

While there is no uniform profile of a victim or perpetrator of IPV, risk factors for victimization include a personal history of maltreatment as a child, adolescent or young adult age, disparity of status (eg, educational, professional) between partners, and high level of dependence of one partner on another. Batterers have also been found to frequently have a history of emotional or physical maltreatment as a child, a history of substance abuse, very low levels of self-esteem, and difficulty identifying and expressing emotion.

Between 3 and 15 million children are exposed to IPV in their homes annually, and these children are at risk of victimization themselves. They are almost 5 times more likely than unexposed children to sustain physical abuse and 2.5 times more likely to be victims of sexual abuse.

Clinical Presentation

Adult victims of IPV may present for medical care for themselves or may present for care of their children for issues related to the violence. Approximately one-third of victims injured in an assault by a partner seek medical care for their injuries. While these injuries vary in severity, skin injuries are most common. Injury can occur on any part of the body; however, injury to the head, neck, and face has been particularly associated with IPV.

Many victims present to primary care physicians and emergency departments, and only a fraction are correctly identified as suffering from IPV. A recent report noted that only 28% of abused women who sought care frequently (at least 7 times) were ever identified as victims of IPV. Barriers to diagnosis are patient and physician based. Patients may not disclose the abuse because of fears of social, financial, or legal repercussions; concerns for safety based on prior threats from the abuser; feeling ashamed at being a victim; and inability to

Box 142-1. Signs and Symptoms of Childhood Exposure to Intimate Partner Violence

- Depression
- Anxiety
- Somatization
- Attention-deficit/hyperactivity disorder
- Aggression
- Developmental delay
- Low self-esteem
- Hypervigilance
- Poor academic performance or truancy
- Antisocial or delinquent behaviors

trust that others can help. They fail to appreciate that violence frequently escalates. Often they fear an investigation by child protective services and that they may lose custody of their children in the process. They may fabricate a story such as a fall to explain their injuries, thereby discouraging the physician from further inquiry. Even in the absence of a story, physicians may avoid inquiring about the injuries, citing time constraints and lack of knowledge to effectively respond if a disclosure is made.

Parents may also seek care for their children who manifest effects of the trauma, altered stress physiology, and disrupted caregiver attachment (Box 142-1). Children exposed to IPV are more likely than their peers to be anxious, fearful, and hypervigilant and have difficulty with aggression and peer relationships. Adolescents are more likely to have school failure, substance abuse difficulties, high-risk sexual behaviors, and violent dating relationships. As they move to adulthood, these children are at higher risk for mental health disorders and substance abuse. In fact, the Adverse Childhood Experiences Study enumerates multiple negative overall physical and mental health consequences in adults exposed to IPV as children.

Pathophysiology

The prevalent dynamic in relationships with IPV is the need for one partner to dominate or have power over the other. Often, this characteristic is interpreted as devotion early in a relationship, but an abuser eventually isolates the victim socially and financially. Ultimately, the violence includes a physical or sexual component as well as a psychologic one. The psychologic component, which typically precedes any physical violence, includes threats, humiliation, and intimidation and can be the most difficult to treat.

The cycle of violence between intimate partners is chronic and cyclical in nature with 3 phases. The first is the tension-building phase when the abuser uses verbal, emotional, and physical threats. Next is the violent episode, which includes some combination of physical, sexual, emotional, and psychologic assault. The final phase is the honeymoon phase, when the abuser apologizes and assures the victim that it will not happen again, and re-bonding occurs. These phases escalate over time as the violence becomes more frequent and more severe and the honeymoon phase shortens. At least 50%

of women who suffer sexual IPV report multiple rapes, and two-thirds of men and women with physical violence report multiple episodes of assault as well. The violence can also continue after the relationship has ended, and this most commonly manifests as stalking of the victim by the abuser. The violence also becomes intergenerational, as children exposed to IPV are at increased risk for victimization and perpetration of violence in their future intimate relationships.

There are particular circumstances that place IPV victims at even higher risk of harm. Threats from the perpetrator to harm or kill the victim or another person, the use of drugs or alcohol at the time of the violent episode, and the use of a weapon are all associated with an increased risk of injury. Approximately 4% to 8% of women report having experienced IPV during a pregnancy, though the reason for this increased incidence during this vulnerable period is unclear. It has been hypothesized that this is a time of increased stress as well as a time when a woman's attention may be diverted from her partner. Victims are also at increased risk of injury or death at the time they report the abuse or attempt to leave the relationship. In comparison with the systems in place for children, there are no protective service agencies with mandates to protect these adult victims, and as a result, disclosure of IPV may not occur unless the victim feels that she or he has a plan for escape.

Differential Diagnosis

Adult or adolescent victims of IPV often present with vague complaints, and women who have been abused are 3 times more likely than women who have not been abused to present with gynecologic complaints, such as recurrent sexually transmitted infections, vaginal bleeding, or chronic pelvic pain. These victims may also present with nonspecific symptoms of sleeping difficulties, appetite changes, weight loss, chronic pain, or syncope. They are 3 times more likely to experience depression and 4 times more likely to experience post-traumatic stress disorder (PTSD) than non-abused women and may present to their physician with symptoms of anxiety or following a suicide attempt. Other complaints reflect conditions associated with stress, such as irritable bowel syndrome, headaches, or temporomandibular joint disorder. Pregnant victims may present with vaginal bleeding, preterm labor, placental abruption, or fetal distress. The most common adverse birth outcome attributed to IPV during pregnancy is low birth weight of the neonate.

Mental health manifestations of childhood exposure to IPV may vary depending on the developmental stage of the child; however, these children may present with developmental delay, low self-esteem, symptoms of PTSD and hypervigilance, poor academic performance or truancy, or antisocial behavior. Exposed children also have significantly more internalizing (eg, depression, anxiety, somatization) and externalizing (eg, attention-deficit/hyperactivity disorder, aggression) disorders than nonexposed children.

There is limited research on the short-term effects of IPV on the physical health of children. Some studies have shown a higher incidence of asthma, failure to thrive, and malnutrition. Children in the home may also sustain direct trauma, whether as the result of being held in a parent's arms during an episode of violence or an effort to intervene and protect a parent during a violent episode. The children may also be direct targets of the violence and present with head, skin, skeletal, or abdominal findings caused by physical abuse (see Chapter 131).

Evaluation

History

Many victims of IPV do not freely offer information about the violence occurring in their relationships, even if they present with overt injuries. Screening for IPV in medical settings is cited as the optimal approach and is an area of continued research. Proposed approaches in the primary care or emergency department environment have included universal screening of all women and targeted screening of women with high-risk signs and risk factors. While there are proponents of each of these approaches, a 2013 US Preventive Services Task Force statement recommended that clinicians screen all women of childbearing age. Universal screening may detect increased numbers of cases of IPV and open the door to effective intervention, but the question remains as to whether there have ultimately been improved social, physical, or mental health outcomes with this approach. Critics of universal screening argue that forcing the issue before a woman is psychologically and logistically ready to leave the situation may put her at increased risk of harm and decreased likelihood of success. The universal screening approach has also not typically addressed the population of male victims of IPV.

Alternatively, targeted screening is performed in some medical settings on patients who present with risk factors for IPV (Box 142-2). Studies have shown that self-administered, written screening tools are more sensitive and are preferred by victims over verbal questioning. Such written screening tools have been validated for use in clinical settings and are available from the Centers for Disease Control and Prevention at www.cdc.gov/NCIPC/pub-res/images/IPVandSVscreening.pdf.

Because IPV has been shown to have a direct effect on the health and well-being of children in the home, the pediatric medical setting is one potential site for IPV screening to occur. Targeted

screening practices may focus on families of children with anxiety, depression, or somatization or when child abuse is suspected. Surveys of mothers generally support IPV screening in the pediatric office setting, and women who have been abused are more likely to seek medical care for their children than for themselves. Sensitivity to whether children should witness discussions of positive screening questions is necessary, as older children may react to or repeat portions of an overheard conversation, ultimately placing the victim, their mother, at higher risk of harm.

Physical Examination

Caregiver Injuries

Although blunt trauma from a hand or fist is the most common scenario for the abused partner, IPV can result in injuries from blunt force or penetrating trauma. Injury can occur on any part of a victim's body; however, studies have shown that trauma to the head, neck, and face is most specific for IPV as the etiology compared with other traumatic events. Findings may also include bruising of the bilateral upper arms from being grabbed and patterned injury from being hit with an object. Strangulation may result in bruising or abrasions on the neck, facial petechiae, or subconjunctival hemorrhage.

Child Injuries

Children in the home where IPV is occurring are at increased risk of physical abuse, and a complete unclothed physical examination should be performed to look for evidence of skin, head, skeletal, or abdominal trauma. Accidental injuries typically result in cutaneous bruises over bony prominences, such as knees and elbows, anterior shins, and the forehead. Unusual areas for accidental injury include the neck, ears, cheeks, medial thighs, and genital area. If physical abuse is suspected, additional radiographic imaging and an ophthalmologic examination may be indicated (see Chapter 131).

Management

The response to any disclosure of IPV should be supportive and focus on a safety assessment to determine the severity and immediacy of danger (Box 142-3). This should include an assessment of the pattern of escalating violence, availability of weapons to the abuser, and comfort level of the victim to return home. More imminent danger necessitates the creation of an emergent safety plan, and social work

---

Box 142-2. Risk Factors for Intimate Partner Violence

- History of childhood abuse
- Adolescent or young adult age
- Disparity in professional or educational status of partners
- Geographic or cultural isolation
- Dependency on partner due to chronic illness or disability
- Pregnancy
- Depression
- Anxiety
- Frequent physical injury
- Substance abuse
- Poor compliance with medical care

Box 142-3. Components of Safety Assessment

- Is the violence escalating?
- How severe has the violence been in the past?
- Is the victim comfortable returning home?
- Is child abuse occurring?
- Are weapons available to the perpetrator?
- Does the perpetrator have substance abuse issues or a mental health disorder?
- Does the victim have a social support network?

colleagues or professionals from an IPV shelter, hotline, or advocacy organization can assist with this. It is important to remain sensitive to the fact that leaving an abusive home is disruptive to the daily lives of the adult and child victims and may be a difficult step to take.

If immediate safety is of less concern, a victim may opt to take more time in creating a safety plan for leaving. This may include things such as collecting money, car keys, house keys, and important documents; asking neighbors to contact police if violence is overheard in the home; establishing a code that the victim can use to communicate to others that violence is occurring and understanding what will be done if the code is used; and disarming or removing weapons from the home.

While all states require that medical professionals report cases of suspected child abuse and neglect to child protective agencies, there is variability in the mandated reporting statutes for IPV and child exposure to IPV. State statutes fall into the following general categories with respect to IPV: requirement to report injuries caused by weapons, requirement to report injuries resulting from a crime, requirement to report IPV, and no mandatory reporting law. For those states with no mandatory reporting requirement, factors that may influence a physician's decision to report may include the potential for danger, the caregiver's ability to plan for safety, a victim's level of connection to family or community support, and the degree of suspicion that a child's exposure to IPV constitutes emotional abuse. Online resources such as the *Compendium of State Statutes and Policies on Domestic Violence and Health Care,* published by the Family Violence Prevention Fund in 2010, can assist with the determination of local state laws on mandatory reporting of IPV. Any suspicion of child abuse should be reported to child protective services, regardless of whether IPV is being reported as well. If child abuse and IPV are co-occurring, it is important to note this in the child abuse report so that appropriate measures can be taken in the child protection response.

Prognosis

Direct victimization from IPV and childhood exposure to IPV are associated with increased risk of adult morbidities. Women who have experienced interpersonal violence are at risk for depression, anxiety, and PTSD and are 15 times more likely to abuse alcohol and 9 times more likely to abuse drugs. Childhood exposure to IPV is associated with an increased risk of adult morbidities, including substance abuse disorders, obesity, physical inactivity, depression, and suicide attempts. This is of particular concern because of the limited availability and often limited recognition of the importance of mental health resources in addressing the psychologic effect of IPV.

For those women who do disclose the abuse and are referred to advocacy programs, preliminary data indicate that intensive programs may have a beneficial effect on reducing physical violence for several years. For other intervention strategies, the research is often limited and does not yet provide sound evidence of positive effects on physical, emotional, and quality-of-life outcomes. Further research is necessary to determine what components of the programs and what intensity and time frame of involvement are most beneficial in different clinical scenarios.

Although many IPV shelters and advocacy organizations have legal assistance available to victims, most victims do not obtain temporary restraining orders. Of those who do, approximately two-thirds have the orders violated by the abuser. Most cases are not prosecuted, and for those cases that do progress in the legal system, courts often struggle with how to address the IPV issues in the child custody and family treatment plans. While there are multiple models of treatment programs for perpetrators of IPV, there is evidence of only a small reduction in the likelihood of repeat violence. Further research is necessary to modify treatment approaches to reduce this recidivism.

Prevention

Prevention efforts may be primary, secondary, or tertiary. In this setting, primary prevention includes attempts to change social norms of violence and acts at the level of the individual, relationship, or community. Current efforts in that regard include attempts to break the generational cycle by studying and supporting resilience factors in those who do not perpetuate violence after childhood exposure, the development of safe dating programs to reduce adolescent dating violence, the creation of peer empowerment programs for adolescents and young adults to enhance their ability to identify and intervene in IPV that they witness, and the development of family-based interventions to enhance nonviolent communication skills.

Secondary prevention includes early detection of IPV, and a significant amount of research is underway on screening practices in the medical setting. Tertiary prevention is the attempt to prevent death and disability in families in which IPV occurs.

Sound research on IPV prevention is still a work in progress. Much of the current research has had methodological challenges, and many prevention strategies are not yet validated by sound evidence of benefit. Also, traditional thinking has been that most abusers are male and most victims are female, and prevention programs were built on this premise. Recent data, however, suggest that females also instigate IPV, so the subtleties of the patterns of violence of men versus women and how best to prevent them is a new area for growth and understanding.

CASE RESOLUTION

When alone with you, the mother reports that the boy's bruising occurred after her boyfriend hit him with a belt and that her marks occurred when the boyfriend was drunk and angry about the dinner she had prepared. She has contemplated leaving the relationship but is financially dependent on him and pregnant with his child. He has threatened to harm her son if she leaves. She is currently afraid to return home but is not sure what to do.

You contact a social worker who assists in referring the mother and child to an intimate partner violence (IPV) shelter and an IPV advocacy group. The social worker and the agencies work on an immediate safety plan while the mother and child wait in the office. As a mandated reporter of child abuse, you contact the child abuse hotline. The social worker assists you with the requirements in your state to report IPV or childhood exposure to IPV. The mother should be advised that a child abuse report was initiated, and child protective authorities should also be made aware that IPV and child abuse are co-occurring in this family.

Selected References

Bair-Merritt MH. Intimate partner violence. *Pediatr Rev.* 2010;31(4):145–150

Casanueva C, Martin SL, Runyan DK. Repeated reports for child maltreatment among intimate partner violence victims: findings from the National Survey of Child and Adolescent Well-Being. *Child Abuse Negl.* 2009;33(2):84–93

Durborow N, Lizdas KC, O'Flaherty A, Marjavi A. *Compendium of State Statutes and Policies on Domestic Violence and Health Care.* San Francisco, CA: Family Violence Prevention Fund; 2010. http://www.acf.hhs.gov/programs/fysb/resource/state-compendium-fv. Accessed December 17, 2013

Lamers-Winkelman F, Willemen AM, Visser M. Adverse childhood experiences of referred children exposed to intimate partner violence: consequences for their wellbeing. *Child Abuse Negl* 2012;36(2):166–179

Moyer VA; US Preventive Services Task Force. Screening for intimate partner violence and abuse of elderly and vulnerable adults: U.S. Preventive Services Task Force recommendation statement. *Ann Intern Med.* 2013;158(6):478–486

Rabin RF, Jennings JM, Campbell JC, Bair-Merritt MH. Intimate partner violence screening tools: a systematic review. *Am J Prev Med.* 2009;36(5):439–445

Ramsay J, Carter Y, Davidson L, et al. Advocacy interventions to reduce or eliminate violence and promote the physical and psychosocial well-being of women who experience intimate partner abuse. *Cochrane Database Syst Rev.* 2009;(3): CD005043

Rhodes KV, Kothari CL, Dichter M, Cerulli C, Wiley J, Marcus S. Intimate partner violence identification and response: time for a change in strategy. *J Gen Intern Med.* 2011;26(8):894–899

Thackeray JD, Hibbard R, Dowd MD; American Academy of Pediatrics Committee on Child Abuse and Neglect and Committee on Injury, Violence, and Poison Prevention. Intimate partner violence: the role of the pediatrician. *Pediatrics.* 2010;125(5):1094–1100

Toohey JS. Domestic violence and rape. *Med Clin North Am.* 2008;92(5): 1239–1252

CHAPTER 143

Disaster Preparedness

Katherine E. Remick, MD, and Timothy K. Ruttan, MD

CASE STUDY

A family comes in for a well-child visit with their 9-month-old daughter, who has complex congenital heart disease, and their 7-year-old son. The mother is concerned after a recent tornado in the next town resulted in prolonged power outages and what the family might do in this situation. The daughter needs daily breathing treatments and often requires oxygen at night-time. She is on multiple medications and a special formula. All of her specialty doctors are at the children's hospital, which is more than an hour from their house. She is also concerned because her husband has a seizure disorder that requires medication. She asks whether the family should stay together in a disaster or separate to get her daughter to the children's hospital.

Questions

1. How should families prepare for disasters, particularly natural ones known to occur in their area?
2. What should be included in disaster preparedness kits? How should medications for all family members be included?
3. When should families consider getting a generator?
4. How can families notify the utility company that they need to be flagged for priority return of service during a power outage?
5. What is the role of the local hospital and emergency medical services when families have children with special health care and critical medical needs?
6. What should the pediatrician recommend to families about children's immunization records and important medical history?
7. How do you assess for the effect of traumatic events on children and their families?

Disaster preparedness has become increasingly relevant to children and their families. While natural disasters, war, and pandemic infections have always threatened human populations, increasing population density, global warming, international trade, and terrorist threats have heightened our awareness of disasters and the need for preparedness. In the past, disaster planning was managed primarily by federal programs. The combination of a growing need, the availability of resources, and the recognition of inherently delayed response times makes disaster preparedness important, not just on state and national levels, but also for families and local communities. Recent major disasters, whether human-induced events such as the 2001 terrorist attacks in New York, NY, or natural events such as the 2011 Japanese tsunami and resulting nuclear disaster, demonstrate the vulnerability of communities and the need for extensive local preparation. In the first hours to days following a disaster, community response is vital to well-being. While state and federal systems are an essential component of disaster preparedness, there can be significant delays in the delivery of resources. Communities need to be prepared to play a greater role than was anticipated in the past. As frontline health care providers and advocates for children, pediatricians have a particular responsibility to maintain a baseline understanding of chemical, biological, and radioactive exposures as well as emerging pandemic infections to provide guidance to families in the event of such disasters.

In addition to disasters, incidents in which local emergency medical services (EMS) are overwhelmed by the number and severity of casualties, termed *mass casualty incidents* (MCIs), also have the potential to overwhelm community resources. These may include catastrophic events such as mass transit accidents, multiple-shooting victims, and hazardous materials spills. All patients must be quickly triaged, treated, and transported. Typically, local government will facilitate the initial response in accordance with emergency preparedness policies and procedures. This may include coordinating efforts with surrounding communities as per regional preparedness plans along with additional assistance as needed from state government. A public health emergency is declared only when an event exceeds the ability of local, regional, and state resources to provide routine care as the result of any incident that poses substantial risk of human fatalities or long-term disabilities. Preparedness experts suggest looking at public health emergencies from what is called an **all-hazards approach.** This approach focuses on the key elements that are needed to ensure that routine care can be provided during any type of disaster or MCI. Specific scenarios that occur rarely, such as chemical or radiation exposure, will require access to specialized resources that may be impractical to stockpile or are limited in availability. From a practical view, it is more effective to have the essential resources that are needed across all types of disasters.

In contemplating disaster response, the pediatrician should understand the concept of multiple phases of disasters and the importance of advocating for children at each of these steps. The main elements are planning, rescue, recovery, and mitigation. *Planning* includes training and education as well as identifying specific local risks. For example, some communities might need to anticipate hurricanes, while others would be more concerned about earthquakes. This is one of the key areas for pediatricians to intervene with families to develop disaster plans as well as to interact with the local disaster response community to improve the capacity to care for children. *Rescue* is the actual steps taken during a disaster, and this is typically what receives the most attention in the media and public. *Recovery* is the process that begins immediately after the disaster occurs—often simultaneously with the rescue phase—in which the community works toward returning to normal routines. This is also the phase during which mental health problems will begin to emerge. *Mitigation* is an often overlooked phase in which individuals and the community learn from the response to the disaster to prevent future occurrences or improve on the response to decrease the effect of future disasters.

Multiple factors make children more vulnerable than adults during a disaster. In the United States, children make up approximately 25% of the population. Younger children, especially, are reliant on others for food, shelter, and, importantly, psychologic support. Their unique nutritional needs put them at risk for malnutrition. In addition, their immune systems are often less mature. In a setting of physical stress and unreliable sanitation, children are at greater risk of infection. Moreover, decreased fluid reserves make children more susceptible to blood loss or dehydration from agents that cause diarrhea and vomiting. In a setting of blasts or falls, children are at increased risk of traumatic brain injury due to their large head to body ratio. Their more pliable skeleton also makes internal organ injury more likely. Furthermore, children are at increased risk for exposure from chemical, biological, and radiation disasters because of their unique physiology. Infants and children have higher minute ventilation, resulting in increased inhalation of aerosolized agents. Their smaller height increases their exposure to high–vapor density agents, which are in higher concentrations closer to the ground. Also, the skin of infants and children is more permeable due to less keratinization. Finally, they have a larger surface area to body mass ratio. As a result, exposed children receive a higher dose of transdermally absorbed toxins than adults exposed under identical circumstances. This larger surface area to body mass ratio also complicates treatment because children are at higher risk of hypothermia during the decontamination process. Finally, the psychologic effect of being separated from family and experiencing other disaster-related trauma can be devastating in the short and long term.

Unfortunately, many disaster response teams lack pediatric training, protocols, and equipment. Recently, various public health and disaster organizations have lobbied for states to mandate disaster preparedness regulations for children. Specifically, many states lack basic emergency preparedness regulations for schools and child care facilities. The developmental vulnerabilities of infants, toddlers, and young children make them physically less able to escape a disaster scene as well as cognitively less able to recognize the need to flee and follow directions from authorities. Children with special health care needs because of physical or cognitive disabilities require specific attention. Pediatricians can assist schools and child care centers in developing disaster preparedness plans. All child care facilities should have a plan in place that addresses all-hazards safety, medical needs, evacuation and transportation, and reunification with families. The idea of family-centered care that seeks to keep family units together even as care is needed for individual members is important for the immediate physical health and long-term mental health of children during and after disasters.

Pediatricians' Role With Families

Pediatricians serve as a resource to families to prepare for disasters in advance. Disaster preparedness can be incorporated into primary care pediatricians' anticipatory guidance with families. Pediatricians should consider assessing a family's level of readiness for a disaster and then tailor their anticipatory guidance accordingly. It is important for families to realize that everyone is susceptible to some type of disaster, and pediatricians need to ensure that families understand the importance of preparation as well as the special needs of children during a disaster. The US Federal Emergency Management Agency (FEMA) now offers a free smartphone application (http://www.fema.gov/smartphone-app) that includes specific information on various types of natural disasters, how to build a disaster kit, resources for victims of disasters, and a disaster reporting feature. Families should prepare an emergency kit that provides up to 3 days of basic essentials, including food, water, and clothing. Families need to include formula and diapers for newborns and infants and any daily medications for all family members. Copies of immunization and general medical information can be useful as well as pictures of family members in case the family unit is separated. Parents need to be prepared to handle non-emergent problems because formal medical care may be limited to the seriously ill and injured during a disaster. If a family needs acute medical care, children may have to be treated in adult facilities; alternatively, for the family unit to remain together, adults within the family may need to be treated in pediatric facilities. The more information families can provide about any medical conditions requiring attention, the easier it will be to receive appropriate care in a disaster.

Families of children with special needs are especially vulnerable following a disaster because access to routine medical care may not be available. Experience in Japan during the 2011 earthquake showed higher mortality among children with special needs as well as increased hospitalizations for children who are technology dependent. Common supplies such as a feeding tube or catheters may be in short supply or unavailable during a disaster. Families should not only have a sufficient supply of medication, but they should have a surplus of necessary medical equipment and nutritional supplements. Families with a child on a ventilator or who is oxygen dependent should notify local utilities to flag their address for priority status during power outages. They should consider the risks and benefits of backup battery units as well as having a backup generator in the house. These families would also benefit by notifying their local EMS agency and hospital of their child's medical needs. Some EMS systems keep a registry of children with special needs. In addition, the

American Academy of Pediatrics (AAP) and American College of Emergency Physicians offer an **emergency information form (EIF)** that can be completed with the pediatrician and should be part of the emergency preparedness kit. The EIF contains information on diagnoses, procedures, medications, common presenting problems, and suggested medical management. (See Selected References on page 942.) Families can also contact the National Organization on Disability (www.nod.org) or Family Voices (www.familyvoices.org) for more detailed information on preparing for a disaster with a child who has special needs. Some communities have developed systems in which posters are disseminated that are to be placed in the window specifying if any occupant may require special services from EMS should a disaster or terrorist attack occur.

During the recovery phase after a disaster, children and adolescents may develop chronic medical problems as a result of injuries sustained during the event. Such problems need to be addressed case by case by the pediatrician. Beyond physical injuries, all disasters have a psychologic effect on children. Multiple studies of various types of disasters demonstrate the increase in mental health symptoms among children and adolescents exposed to a disaster. This is true even if a family is not directly affected by the disaster but is exposed to the event within the community, on the television, or through the Internet and social media. Children may present with somatic complaints such as headaches and stomachaches, or they may not want to participate in their normal activities. Long-term effects include depression, anxiety, aggression, and substance abuse. Age-appropriate discussions should be encouraged along with validation of the child's concerns while assuring their individual safety. Post-traumatic stress disorder should be considered in the differential diagnosis of patients with persistent symptoms that are not responding to family support. Families and health care professionals can obtain further information through the AAP (www.aap.org) and the Substance Abuse and Mental Health Services Administration (www.samhsa.gov).

Pediatricians' Role in the Community

As part of the planning phase of disaster response, pediatricians can participate in the development of a community-wide disaster preparedness plan (eg, identifying emergency meeting locations) as well as surveillance to identify potential disasters. Many state and regional disaster preparedness plans are tailored for an adult population and may not consider the special needs of children. From an operational standpoint, it is more effective to have one plan that can take into consideration the needs of multiple vulnerable populations rather than have separate disaster preparedness plans for each population. Pediatricians can serve as consultants about local preparation and provide guidance about the unique medical, nutritional, and psychologic needs of children. For example, increased staffing needs should be anticipated when caring for younger children and infants. Depending on availability of human milk, newborns and infants may require formula and a sterile water supply. The food needs of young children will differ from adults. Stockpiling of medications for biological, chemical, or radiation disasters also needs to take into consideration

dosing differences for children compared with adults. Suspensions of medications will need to be available in addition to pill forms. Furthermore, many recommended antidotes and treatments are not approved for use in the pediatric population, and policies on the risks and benefits of their use in disasters should be established.

Ideally, children should remain with their caregiver as part of family-centered disaster care. If this is not possible, a child advocate needs to be with the child at all times, although the nature of disaster response may make this challenging if not planned in advance. Additionally, incorporation of child life specialists and techniques for distraction during medical procedures should be encouraged. Children may not respond well to new environments and disaster protocols. The simple process of decontamination can be devastating to a young child without the presence of a parent. A child may have concerns about being sprayed with water or refuse to disrobe in front of strangers, which may affect the success of decontamination for children and adolescents. It is assumed that adults will comply with protocols, but such compliance is less predictable in a pediatric population. Children may be afraid of strangers or simply wander off before triage is complete. Nonmedical personnel or bystanders may be called on to assist with supervising ambulatory children.

Emergency medical services systems are charged with the initial and rapid triage of all victims. Various well-known triage algorithms are available, including Sort, Assess, Lifesaving Interventions, Treatment/Transport (SALT) and Simple Triage and Rapid Assessment (START). Common to all is the rapid sorting of patients based on ability to ambulate followed by assessment of respiratory status, circulation/perfusion, and motor skills. While multiple triage tools exist, the physiologic parameters and mental status assessments used in adult-based algorithms may not be suitable for children of all ages. Triage systems need to take into account physiological differences of children as well as their psychologic response to strangers. For example, young children may not be able to communicate their complaint, and because their vital signs are normally different from those of adults, medical personnel accustomed to working with adults may misinterpret physical findings and over-triage children. JumpSTART is a widely recognized pediatric-specific disaster triage tool that parallels START. However, it fails to capture children who are dependent on technology or those with special health care needs. Whether or not a triage tool is readily available, clinical decision-making can be relied on to help sort and triage victims in a disaster. When possible, families should be triaged together with the most critical patient.

Facility-based issues must also be addressed in regional disaster preparedness plans. These include providing for increased staffing in adult facilities caring for children as well as the need for those facilities to stockpile pediatric supplies. Similarly, parents may be triaged with their children, so pediatric facilities should be prepared to manage adult victims. In addition, facilities need to plan for children arriving without a caregiver and establish an identification system that allows children to be reunited with their families. This was a significant problem for children displaced during Hurricane Katrina. Strategies to address this include using digital cameras to photograph children on arrival with their original clothing as a way to facilitate reuniting families.

Pediatricians' Role in Disaster Surveillance and Management

Pediatricians function as key public health workers. Their knowledge and diligence aids in local and regional surveillance for potential chemical, biological, and radiation disasters. Families may seek care from their pediatrician rather than an emergency department for early symptoms during and after a disaster. Although it is beyond the scope of this chapter to provide details about signs and symptoms following every type of disaster, the following section highlights important concepts in identifying and treating patients with exposures to chemical and biological agents as well as radiation.

Chemical exposures usually result in immediate symptoms and require special protection for emergency personnel as well as decontamination for the victims. These exposures can occur from terrorism as well as the more common source of industrial accidents. Organophosphates include insecticides, herbicides, and nerve gases that inhibit the enzyme acetylcholinesterase. This results in the accumulation of acetylcholine and excessive cholinergic stimulation at muscarinic and nicotinic receptors. Symptoms include the muscarinic SLUDGE toxidrome (increased *s*alivation, *l*acrimation, *u*rination, *g*astric *d*istress, and *e*mesis) as well as the MTWHF nicotinic toxidrome (*m*ydriasis, *t*achycardia, *w*eakness, *h*ypertension, and *f*asciculation). The nerve gas sarin was used in the 1995 Tokyo subway attack. Vesicant exposure leads to irreversible damage to mucous membranes, skin, and the respiratory system that occurs soon after exposure. Agents include mustard and lewisite. Cyanide is another common chemical agent, known for its bitter almond taste. Cyanide inhibits cellular metabolism and causes rapid hypotension, coma, seizures, and death. Agents other than nerve agents usually do not result in severe mortality but rather incapacitate the victim. Many other chemical agents from industrial accidents can cause a variety of skin and pulmonary symptoms.

Biological agents include bacteria, viruses, and preformed toxins. These agents may be easy to disperse and can affect large populations. Unlike chemical exposures, the onset of symptoms is delayed by hours to days, and symptoms are more difficult to distinguish from common ailments. Secondary transmission of the infection is also of concern with some agents. Management of biological disaster requires detailed surveillance and containment of exposed populations.

Although there are too many biological agents to discuss in any detail in this brief chapter, a few of particular relevance for disaster planning are mentioned here. **Anthrax,** from *Bacillus anthracis,* is a gram-positive sporulating rod. When used as a bioterrorism agent in its inhaled form, victims present with severe influenza-like symptoms with an associated high fatality rate. Fever and dyspnea associated with a widened mediastinum are common and may progress to shock. Ciprofloxacin and doxycycline are recommended for prophylaxis and treatment among adults. Despite the bone and cartilage risks that generally restrict its use to healthy children, ciprofloxacin is approved by the US Food and Drug Administration (FDA) for use in children with

inhalational anthrax exposure. Doxycycline should generally be avoided in children younger than 8 years, although it may be considered on a case-by-case basis. Clinicians need to consider consulting with experts to assist in assessing the risks and benefits associated with using these medications. Among the viruses, variola, more commonly known as **smallpox,** is an agent of concern. After its global eradication in 1980, children were no longer immunized, leaving all children and most adults susceptible to the virus. Similar to varicella, it presents with vesicles with umbilicated centers but is associated with a higher mortality rate of 3% to 30% among non-immunized individuals. Exposure to the potent **botulinal toxin** results in cranial nerve disturbances, descending paralysis, and respiratory distress. **Ricin,** derived from the castor bean, is another potent toxin. Inhalation results in fever, cough, and pulmonary edema, often resulting in death within days. Ingestion presents with severe vomiting and diarrhea, resulting in hypovolemic shock. For a complete list of biological agents, presenting symptoms, and potential treatment or prophylaxis, clinicians should consult the Centers for Disease Control and Prevention.

Radiation exposure may occur as a result of damage to a facility that contains nuclear material, detonation of a nuclear weapon, or dispersal of nuclear material by a radioactive dispersal device. Ionizing radiation presents the greatest health risk because of its high-frequency energy. It causes chromosomal breaks in cells that can cause long-term damage and increased risk of cancer. There are 5 types of ionizing radiation that have specific characteristics, behaviors, and toxicities: alpha particles, beta particles, gamma rays, x-rays, and neutrons. Alpha particles have limited ability to penetrate but when inhaled or ingested can cause internal damage. Beta particles are most commonly found in a medical setting, and they have greater penetration than alpha particles. Beta particles can cause skin damage as well as damage when ingested. Gamma rays and x-rays are part of the electromagnetic spectrum. Gamma rays are high energy and cause significant damage. This type of radiation would be seen after a nuclear detonation or from radioactive materials. Much less common are neutrons, which can actually induce radioactivity. Exposure to radiation is classified as external, internal, whole body, and partial body. The effects of radiation can directly damage the target tissue, or the effects can be indirect due to free radicals created by the radiation. Tissue sensitivity is based on the cellular rate of division and level of differentiation. The most sensitive to least is as follows: lymphoid>gastrointestinal>reproductive>dermal>bone marrow>nervous system. The severity of exposure is also dependent on the dose of radiation, type of radiation, and age of victim.

Radiation exposure is quantified by the amount of energy absorbed (**rad,** for radiation absorbed dose) and the relative biological effectiveness of doses (RBE) based on the type of ionizing radiation. The rem is the product of the rad and RBE. Under the International System of Units, the rad and rem are being replaced by the gray (1 Gy = 100 rad) and sievert (1 Sv = 100 rem). Typically, doses for common radiation exposures are given in millisieverts (1 mSv = 0.001 Sv). Radiation exposure from common radiographic procedures can range from 0.1 mSv for a chest radiograph to 2 to 20 mSv for a computed tomography scan.

Symptoms associated with radiation exposure depend on the total exposure. Nausea and vomiting can present with exposures of 0.75 to 1 Gy and lymphoid and bone marrow suppression with exposures of 1 to 6 Gy. The mean lethal dose, the radiation dose for which half of the population is expected to die within 60 days, is 4 Gy. Long-term effects of radiation include increased incidence of cancer and psychologic distress. Evacuation is the ideal intervention to decrease exposure, but this may not be feasible in a timely fashion in highly populated areas.

Seeking shelter can greatly decrease the level of exposure, with large cement structures providing the best protection. The use of potassium iodide is effective in exposures to radioactive iodine, which is associated with nuclear power facilities. It can be dispensed in a pill and suspension form. Dosage is based on level of radiation exposure and the age of the patient, and clinicians should consult the FDA (www.fda.gov) or the Nuclear Regulatory Commission (www.nrc.gov) to determine the appropriate dosage of potassium iodide depending on the level of radiation exposure. For individuals seeking medical care, containment and decontamination are essential. Removal of clothing and washing the skin with warm water is very effective. Supportive medical care is essential in managing patients with radiation exposure. Radiation results in significant immune suppression, neutropenia, and lymphocytopenia, which last for weeks and need close monitoring. Clinicians should be aggressive in managing infections and consider treatments to increase bone marrow regeneration. Expert consultation in radiation sickness would be prudent.

In addition to caring for patients, pediatricians need to take into consideration the well-being of their family as well as that of office staff. During a disaster, office staff may not be able to come to work. For those able to report to work, extra supplies of food and water need to be available in case staff are not able to return to their homes. An office disaster plan should be implemented with emergency contacts and preparation for the staff's basic needs. Basic medical supplies should be available to care for patients during a disaster. Depending on the type and severity of the disaster, access to the office facility may be prohibited. Plans for backing up of patient medical records should be implemented as well as alternative sites in which medical services can be delivered.

Clinicians need to review their medical liability policies addressing the provision of care in a disaster situation. Most policies only provide coverage of care that is provided in the office setting. Good Samaritan laws vary in each state about what level of protection is provided to the health care professional. The AAP recommends that during a disaster situation, pediatricians who volunteer do so under the auspices of an official disaster agency or recognized relief organization to ensure the greatest protection from liability.

Conclusion

Pediatricians have a vital role in pre-disaster, disaster, and post-disaster management on the local, regional, state, and national level, not only as a medical service professional but also as an advocate for the special needs of children and their families. The essential components of disaster management are to provide for all basic human requirements, reduce an individual's vulnerability to disasters, and, once a disaster has occurred, reduce the exposure risk. Pediatricians can educate and assist families in preparing for disasters. In addition, they can guide communities in their disaster preparedness planning to accommodate the particular vulnerabilities of children. As with other health care professionals, pediatricians can also contribute to the essential medical and public health workforce during a disaster. Pediatricians can access the most current guidelines and recommendations through multiple professional and governmental resources. It is imperative for the practitioner to have easy access to phone numbers and Web sites specific to pediatric disaster preparedness and response for the relevant local, state, and federal agencies.

Online Resources

American Academy of Pediatrics. Children and disasters: disaster preparedness to meet children's needs. http://www.aap.org/disasters. Accessed December 17, 2013

American College of Emergency Physicians. Clinical & practice management: EMS and disaster preparedness. http://www.acep.org/disaster. Accessed December 17, 2013

Centers for Disease Control and Prevention. Emergency preparedness and response: caring for children in a disaster. http://emergency.cdc.gov/children. Accessed December 17, 2013

Family Voices. Disasters and emergencies: keeping children and youth safe. http://www.familyvoices.org/work/caring?id=0004. Accessed December 17, 2013

National Safety Council. Emergency preparedness. http://www.nsc.org/safety_home/emergencypreparedness/Pages/EmergencyPreparedness.aspx. Accessed December 17, 2013

US Department of Health and Human Services Assistant Secretary for Preparedness and Response. Pediatric preparedness for healthcare coalitions. http://www.phe.gov/Preparedness/planning/abc/Pages/webinar-resources-130620.aspx. Presented June 20, 2013. Accessed December 17, 2013

CASE RESOLUTION

The family is relieved to discuss the importance of preparing for a disaster. They now have an idea of what is involved in disaster preparation and feel less vulnerable. They plan to create and store an emergency kit with a 3-day supply of food, water, and medications as well as a first aid kit. In addition, they will refer to the US Federal Emergency Management Agency application for further recommendations. Together with their pediatrician, they complete an emergency information form for the kit. In the event of a disaster, they plan to stay together. The mother also shares her plan to consider purchasing a backup generator and to call their local utility company to identify their house as a priority during a power failure. Prior to leaving, the mother shares that her son has been sleeping less since the tornado and does not want to go to school because he is afraid of being away from the family. The pediatrician encourages the family to discuss his fears while ensuring his safety. Having the son participate in making the emergency kit and creating a family plan may help. A follow-up visit is scheduled to reassess his symptoms and decide if further intervention is needed.

Selected References

American Academy of Pediatrics. *Pediatric Terrorism and Disaster Preparedness: A Resource for Pediatricians.* Foltin GL, Schonfeld DJ, Shannon MW, eds. Rockville, MD: Agency for Healthcare Research and Quality; 2006. AHRQ Publication No. 06(07)-0056. http://archive.ahrq.gov/research/pedprep. Accessed December 17, 2013

American Academy of Pediatrics Committee on Pediatric Emergency Medicine, Committee on Medical Liability, and Task Force on Terrorism. The pediatrician and disaster preparedness. *Pediatrics.* 2006;117(2):560–565

American Academy of Pediatrics Committee on Pediatric Emergency Medicine and Council on Clinical Information Technology, American College of Emergency Physicians Pediatric Emergency Medical Committee. Emergency information forms and emergency preparedness for children with special health care needs. *Pediatrics.* 2010;125(4):829–837

Baker LR, Cormier LA. Disaster preparedness and families of children with special needs: a geographic comparison. *J Community Health.* 2013;38(1):106–112

Cicero MX, Baum CR. Pediatric disaster preparedness: best planning for the worst-case scenario. *Pediatr Emerg Care.* 2008;24(7):478–481

Gausche-Hill M. Pediatric disaster preparedness: are we really prepared? *J Trauma.* 2009;67(2 Suppl):S73–S76

Hagan JF; American Academy of Pediatrics Committee on Psychosocial Aspects of Child and Family Health and Task Force on Terrorism. Psychosocial implications of disaster or terrorism on children: a guide for the pediatrician. *Pediatrics.* 2005;116(3):787–795

Markenson D, Reynolds S; American Academy of Pediatrics Committee on Pediatric Emergency Medicine and Task Force on Terrorism. The pediatrician and disaster preparedness. *Pediatrics.* 2006;117(2):e340–e362

Nakayama T, Tanaka S, Uematsu M, et al. Effect of a blackout in pediatric patients with home medical devices during the 2011 eastern Japan earthquake. *Brain Dev.* 2014;36(2):143–147

Olympia RP, Rivera R, Heverley S, Anyanwu U, Gregorits M. Natural disasters and mass-casualty events affecting children and families: a description of emergency preparedness and the role of the primary care physician. *Clin Pediatr (Phila).* 2010;49(7):686–698

Sakashita K, Matthews WJ, Yamamoto LG. Disaster preparedness for technology and electricity-dependent children and youth with special health care needs. *Clin Pediatr (Phila).* 2013;52(6):549–556

Tanaka S. Issues in the support and disaster preparedness of severely disabled children in affected areas. *Brain Dev.* 2013;35(3):209–213

CHAPTER 144

Adolescent Depression and Suicide

Monica Sifuentes, MD, and Robin Steinberg-Epstein, MD

CASE STUDY

A 15-year-old girl is brought to your office by her mother with the chief complaint of easy fatigability. The mother is concerned because her daughter is always tired, although several other physicians have told her that the girl is healthy. The adolescent, who states no complaints or concerns, appears very shy. She is currently in the 10th grade, likes school, receives average grades, and speaks English and Spanish. The mother, a single parent, moved to the United States from El Salvador approximately 2 years ago with her 2 daughters. They are currently living with relatives in a 2-bedroom apartment. The mother is employed as a housekeeper, and the patient and her sister help their mother clean homes on weekends. During the week they make dinner for the rest of the family as a means of contributing to the rent. When you speak to the girl alone, she acknowledges she has a few friends at school and adamantly denies any drug, alcohol, or tobacco use. She has never been sexually active and reports no history of sexual

or physical abuse. The girl's physical examination is entirely normal, although her affect appears somewhat flat.

Questions

1. What is the significance of nonspecific symptoms, such as fatigue, during adolescence?
2. What factors contribute to depression in adolescents?
3. What are the classic signs and symptoms of depression in adolescents?
4. What are some important historical points to cover when interviewing adolescents with suspected depression?
5. How is the risk of suicide assessed in adolescent patients?
6. How should suicidal behavior (ie, suicide attempts) be managed in adolescents?

Depression has been identified as one of the multiple risk factors that predispose adolescents to suicide. However, not all teenagers who try to take their own life are depressed and, conversely, not all depressed adolescents attempt suicide. This distinction is important to keep in mind when evaluating adolescents for depression or suicidal behavior. Early identification of risk factors in the susceptible adolescent along with early intervention for those with depressive symptoms will hopefully benefit the teenager at risk for suicide and allow the primary care pediatrician to provide the first line of intervention for the adolescent patient experiencing emotional distress.

Epidemiology

Depression

The exact prevalence of depression in adolescents is difficult to determine because depression is an illness and a symptom. However, it is considered one of the main psychiatric conditions affecting children, along with anxiety. Depressive symptoms have been reported in as many as 50% of girls and 40% of boys in the 14- to 15-year age group. The overall prevalence of depression as an illness is approximately 5%; mild depression is reported in 13% to 28% of teens, moderate

depression in 7%, and severe depression in 1.3%. Depression occurs more commonly in adolescents than in prepubertal children and is more frequent in females than males after puberty.

Several risk factors contribute to the development of depressive disorders in adolescents (Box 144-1). Certain psychiatric conditions also are associated with depression, including anxiety disorders, eating disorders, substance abuse, conduct disorders, and borderline personality disorders.

Suicide and Suicidal Behavior

Suicide is the third-leading cause of death in the United States in individuals 10 to 24 years of age; only motor vehicle crashes and homicides result in more deaths in young people. In 1960, the annual suicide rate in this age group was 5.2 per 100,000; by 1990, it had more than doubled to the highest recorded level of 13.2 per 100,000. By 2007, the rate had decreased to 6.7 per 100,000, in part because of the use of selective serotonin reuptake inhibitor (SSRI) antidepressants, the first of which came out in 1990. This amounts to more than 4,000 completed suicides in adolescents 15 to 24 years old in 2007. It has been stated that for every suicide that is completed successfully, 50 to 100 suicides are attempted.

Box 144-1. Risk Factors Associated With Depressive Disorders in Adolescents

- Family history of psychiatric illness (eg, parent with an affective condition, another family member with a bipolar or recurrent unipolar disorder)
- Age at onset of depression in the affected parent (the earlier the age of onset, the greater the likelihood of depression in the children)
- Exposure to an unexpected suicide attempt/completion in the school or community
- History of environmental trauma (eg, sexual or physical abuse, loss of a loved one)
- Chronic illness
- Certain medications (eg, propranolol, phenobarbital, prednisone)

Box 144-2. Risk Factors Associated With Suicide in Adolescents

- History of a previous suicide attempt (most important)
- Male gender
- Preexisting psychiatric condition (depressive/bipolar disorder, conduct disorder, post-traumatic stress disorder)
- Alcohol and illicit substance abuse or dependence
- Psychologic characteristics such as aggression, impulsivity, and hopelessness or severe anger
- Family history of psychiatric disorders, especially depression, substance abuse, and suicidal behavior
- Family disruption or stressful life event, including violence, divorce, or the death of a loved one
- Impaired parent-child relationship
- Exposure to an unexpected suicide attempt/completion in the school or community
- Chronic debilitating illness
- Anxiety about sexual identity (homosexuality or bisexuality)
- History of physical/sexual abuse or exposure to violence
- Availability of firearms in the home
- Living outside the home (homelessness or in corrections facility or group home)

According to the 2011 Youth Risk Behavior Survey of the Centers for Disease Control and Prevention, 15.8% of all students in grades 9 to 12 nationwide had seriously considered attempting suicide during the previous 12 months. Approximately 13% of students had made specific suicide plans, more than 50% of students with suicide plans reported attempting to take their lives, and 2.4% of the individuals who attempted suicide required medical attention. Rates also differ by race and ethnicity, with African American teenagers having lower suicide rates than white youth, and African American females having the lowest suicide rate of all adolescents. American Indian/Alaska Native males have the highest suicide rate among this age group.

Several risk factors associated with adolescent suicide have been identified (Box 144-2). Although adolescent females are more likely to attempt suicide than males (22% vs 12%), males are more likely to succeed (boys-girls ratio of 4:1). This fact may result from the lethality of the methods, such as firearms or hanging, that males usually choose. While females are more likely to ingest pills, the role of firearms is increasing. The availability of firearms and alcohol, which varies from state to state, greatly contributes to the occurrence of suicide. Up to 45% of individuals who have committed suicide show some evidence of intoxication at the time of death. Although most suicide attempts are impulsive, studies have shown that adolescents often have communicated their suicidal intent or ideation to someone before the attempt. Fifty percent of adolescents who attempt suicide have sought medical care within the preceding month and 25% within the preceding week. In contrast, only one-third have received previous mental health care.

Clinical Presentation

Depressed or suicidal adolescents may visit physicians for a variety of clinical reasons, but rarely do they seek professional assistance for feeling "depressed." Adolescents have a difficult time accurately understanding their emotions. A depressed teen often presents as irritable, argumentative, or angry rather than sad. Teens may exhibit diminished interest or pleasure in activities or relationships and changes in cognitive functioning (eg, concentration), sleep, appetite, or energy, which lead to impairments in multiple areas of daily living. They may

also present with seemingly non-emergent complaints and a flat affect or with multiple somatic concerns and an anxious appearance. Additionally, the teen may have frequent visits to the primary care practitioner's office for acute conditions that on first glance seem unrelated but later indicate possible substance abuse or a mood disorder. Some adolescents are accompanied by a family member or friend, which initially may make the teen reticent to discuss psychosocial issues with the physician. According to the *Diagnostic and Statistical Manual of Mental Disorders, Fifth Edition, Text Revision,* major depressive disorder (MDD) is diagnosed when at least 5 out of 9 listed symptoms or signs occur for at least 2 weeks. At least one symptom must be sadness or loss of interest for most of every day and there has to be a significant change in function. Changes can be manifested by poor academic performance, school attendance issues (including truancy and disruptive behaviors), and difficulties with peer and familial relationships (see Box 144-1). There is also the introduction of a new mood disorder, disruptive mood dysregulation disorder, which is an important differential to consider in the evaluation of depression.

Pathophysiology

The exact neurobiological etiology of depression remains elusive. It is believed to involve impaired serotonin and norepinephrine transmission in critical areas of the brain, most notably the frontal lobes. Like other complex psychiatric conditions, the etiology of depression seems to be multifactorial, with a strong genetic and psychosocial/environmental basis. The **genetic basis** of depression is suggested by statistics that indicate, for instance, that 25% of children who take their own lives have a family member or close relative who has committed suicide. Similarly, a family history of major depression is a significant risk factor for the development of depression in children. Studies suggest the incomplete penetrance of a dominant gene as a possible etiology for this finding. Regardless of the exact mechanism, genetic influences can increase the adolescent's vulnerability for depression. Specific **environmental events** can occur in an adolescent's life that may precipitate a depressive episode, such as the loss of a loved one or parental divorce. Other events such as physical or sexual abuse also can trigger depression in a susceptible teen. Major depressive disorder is diagnosed when symptoms last for at least 2 weeks and there is a change in usual function.

Differential Diagnosis

The differential diagnosis of depression includes any condition that may alter the patient's cognition or affect. For example, if a disease alters nutritional status and leads to malnourishment, this may alter affect and energy, which may resemble depression (D_x Box). Examples include cancer, tuberculosis, and eating disorders such as anorexia nervosa. Endocrine disorders such as hypothyroidism, hyperthyroidism, and Addison disease can mimic depression. Central nervous system (CNS) pathology, although rare, includes tumors, infections, postconcussion syndromes, and cerebrovascular accidents. Concomitant systemic illnesses such as systemic lupus erythematosus, diabetes mellitus, and AIDS can have CNS manifestations that may be mistaken for an isolated episode of depression. While these diseases can occur, they pale in comparison to the prevalence and significant contribution of substance and alcohol abuse. Comorbid conditions such as early-onset bipolar disorder can present initially with depressive symptoms. About 20% to 40% of children who have MDD eventually develop bipolar disorder. In contrast, longitudinal studies have found that very few of those diagnosed with bipolar disorder as children actually meet criteria as adults. For this reason, another diagnosis evolved with *DSM-5*. Disruptive mood dysregulation disorder was created to capture those children with irritability and persistent, prolonged tantrums; this diagnosis is an important differential. Another consideration is children with autism spectrum disorders who often develop comorbid depression during adolescence as a manifestation of their isolation and poor coping skills. Other psychiatric diagnoses to consider include adjustment disorders, uncomplicated bereavement, separation anxiety, and dysthymia, which is more chronic and sometimes less severe than major depression. Lastly, side effects of prescribed and over-the-counter medications may produce clinical symptoms consistent with depression and therefore should be considered in the differential diagnosis.

Evaluation

History

The assessment of an adolescent for depressive symptoms is an important part of any routine encounter, but the diagnosis of depression may be difficult to make after just one interview. At the initial visit, a complete psychosocial or **HEADDSSS** assessment (*h*ome, *e*mployment and education, *a*ctivities, *d*iet, *d*rugs, *s*afety, *s*exual activity/sexuality, *s*uicide/depression) should be performed on all adolescents (see Chapter 6). The parents or guardians should be included during the first part of the interview to review their observations and concerns regarding their adolescent's behavior and mood. The teenager then should be interviewed alone, and a thorough history of recent feelings, behaviors, and attitudes should be obtained (Questions Box: Adolescent Depression). Mood changes should be noted; a labile affect can be a symptom of ongoing

---

Adolescent Depression

SIG: E CAPS Mnemonic

S: Sleep changes
I: Interests—decreased interest in school or activities
G: Guilt, helpless, hopeless
E: Energy (decreased), fatigue
C: Concentration decreased
A: Appetite (increased or decreased)
P: Psychomotor agitation and retardation
S: Suicidal ideation

- Depressed or irritable mood
- Decreased interest in most daily activities, including school
- Significant weight changes
- Sleep problems
- Psychomotor agitation or retardation
- Low energy or fatigue
- Feelings of worthlessness or guilt
- Diminished ability to concentrate or think
- Preoccupation with death or suicide

Questions

Adolescent Depression

- Does the adolescent occasionally feel sad or "blue" and not understand why?
- Does the adolescent have unexplained crying spells?
- Does the adolescent feel "mad," "bored," or "grouchy"?
- Does the adolescent seem inappropriately jovial?
- Have there been any recent losses in the adolescent's life that may explain his or her feelings?
- Is the adolescent having trouble with concentration or memory?
- Does the adolescent have trouble falling asleep at night or have early morning awaking?
- Has the adolescent lost weight recently or shown any disinterest in food?
- Does the adolescent have feelings of hopelessness and have any desire to hurt himself or herself? Has the adolescent made any previous suicide attempts?
- Do the parents or siblings have a history of drug or alcohol use?
- Is there a family history of affective disorders? What has been their response to treatment?
- Is there a history of family violence?

depression. Physicians should keep in mind that patients who are malnourished for any reason can have a depressed or seemingly flat affect. A full psychiatric assessment also should be completed to obtain information about a possible comorbid condition, including features of psychosis, anxiety disorders, disruptive behaviors, and mania. However, severe depression can be accompanied by symptoms of psychosis. Information about a family history of psychiatric illness or substance abuse, including alcohol abuse, also should be reviewed with the teenager as well as the parents or guardians.

To identify youth at risk for suicide, practitioners must inquire about specific areas of adolescents' lives. This should include a history of sexual or physical abuse, violence, or neglect and current interpersonal conflicts such as fights, punishments, breakups, or traumas. An early history of sexual abuse has a strong association with the development of suicidal ideation by age 15 years. Feelings of hopelessness, agitation, and impulsivity should be identified, along with frequent thoughts of suicide or death. It has been reported that having frequent thoughts of suicide is the best predictor of suicide attempts. Use of any illicit substances also raises the risk of suicide attempts. Adolescents who are suspected of being at risk for suicide must be questioned directly about suicidal ideation, specifically whether they have a plan in mind and access to firearms, medications, or other means of suicide. Previous suicide attempts also need to be reviewed with the teenager because 35% to 45% of adolescents who complete suicide have a positive history of a previous attempt. Nonlethal suicide gestures or other methods of self-inflicted harm should never be taken lightly or minimized. As is recommended in other arenas, initial questions should be nonspecific and become more specific as the interview proceeds, especially if answers to previous questions are positive (Questions Box: Adolescent Suicide).

Promises to maintain confidentiality with depressed adolescents who are considered at risk for suicide are discouraged because parental involvement is strongly advised. Precipitating and motivating factors for any previous suicide attempts should be determined prior to the development of a treatment plan. More importantly, the lethality of previous attempts must be evaluated.

Physical Examination

A thorough physical examination and review of systems should be completed to rule out a chronic medical condition such as hypothyroidism, inflammatory bowel disease, lupus, or anemia, or an organic etiology for nonspecific complaints. If patients have a history of sexual abuse, assault, or sexual activity, a genital examination should be performed to evaluate for sexually transmitted infections. In most cases, the physical examination may be of little yield in the adolescent with a true affective disorder, but careful examination may reveal findings such as cut marks, track marks, skin picking, or loss of tooth enamel, any of which may be helpful in comorbid conditions such as substance abuse or eating disorders. A careful detailed neurologic examination, including a mental status examination looking at eye contact, rate of speech, spontaneity in conversation, thought content, affect, and processing, is essential in differentiating various psychiatric conditions such as bipolar disorder and schizophrenia.

Adolescent Suicide — Questions

- Is the adolescent on any prescribed medications (eg, phenobarbital)?
- Is the adolescent experiencing any psychiatric difficulties, social maladjustments, or family or environmental challenges (eg, recent parental divorce, school expulsion)?
- Does the adolescent have a history of symptoms of depression, conduct problems, or psychosis?
- How is the adolescent progressing in school?
- Does the adolescent have a history of substance abuse?
- Does the adolescent have any legal problems?
- Does the adolescent suffer any social isolation or have interpersonal conflicts with family or friends?
- Has the adolescent suffered any personal losses recently?
- Has there recently been a suicide in the school or community?
- Are there any family problems such as abuse or neglect?
- Has the adolescent ever thought that life was not worth living?
- Does the adolescent ever feel hopeless?
- Has the adolescent ever thought of hurting himself or herself?
- Does the adolescent have a previous history of suicide attempts?
- Does the adolescent presently have a plan for suicide?
- Does the adolescent have access to firearms, medications, or other means of suicide?

Laboratory Tests

While no routine laboratory studies are regularly recommended, there are a number of laboratory tests that one should consider in the evaluation for physiological contributions to depression. This would include a thyroid panel, fasting blood glucose, and complete blood cell count, electrolytes, and urine or serum toxicology screen. Laboratory studies are also important screening measures prior to pharmacotherapy, so that in addition to the aforementioned, one should also consider a blood urea nitrogen and creatinine test, liver panel, electrocardiogram, and, in females, pregnancy test. Psychometric testing may help rule out a concomitant learning disability or attention-deficit/hyperactivity disorder.

Imaging Studies

Radiographic imaging, such as computed tomography of the head or magnetic resonance imaging of the brain, would be indicated if the history of physical examination suggests a CNS process.

Management

Depression

Treatment for depression typically follows 1 of 3 paths: **psychotherapeutic, pharmacotherapy,** or a **combination.** The National Institute of Mental Health supports psychotherapeutic intervention for mild depression. The types of therapy shown to be most effective for adolescents with depression include cognitive behavioral therapy and interpersonal therapy for adolescents. For more severe depression or depression with suicidal ideation, the current first-line medical treatment in the primary care setting involves the use of SSRIs. Pharmacotherapy may be used with the aforementioned psychotherapies. It should be noted that not all therapists are trained in the delivery of these therapeutic methods and in many communities, these interventions are not readily available. Prescribing SSRIs earlier in these instances may be necessary.

If depressive symptoms are associated with a specific adjustment disorder such as divorce, a recent move, or death, and if family, peers, or school factors are affected, **supportive counseling** is indicated. The duration and depth of counseling depends, in part, on how comfortable the primary care practitioner feels performing this task and how receptive the youth and his or her family are to this intervention. Identification of the specific problem, exploration of the teen's response to the problem, and development of a reasonable solution with the adolescent and parents may be helpful to improve adherence to psychotherapy. Keep in mind, however, that regardless of a clear trigger for a depressive episode, medication may still be needed when the symptoms impair functioning.

If family difficulties or dysfunction is the major issue, family members and the physician or counselor should meet to assess the magnitude of the problem and the motivation required to address it. Physicians should use this opportunity to educate adolescents and families about the signs and symptoms of depression and the undeniable effect that depression has on school functioning, family and peer relationships, and social interactions. Cognitive behavioral therapy is a specific type of therapy that has been found to be particularly helpful in adolescents with depression. The need for individual cognitive-behavioral or family therapy should be discussed as well as the effectiveness of psychiatric medication in the appropriate setting. Attention to parental mental health and understanding the strategies necessary to manage the adolescent's irritability and isolation also are extremely important. Psychologic referral should be initiated if patients require more prolonged or intensive psychotherapeutic treatment, the degree of depression seems to increase, suicidal behavior becomes an issue and additional mental health consultation is needed, or a comorbid psychiatric condition is suspected.

Immediate **psychiatric consultation and referral** are indicated if adolescents have severe depressive features that interfere with daily functioning or if they are suicidal, homicidal, or psychotic. Ensuring the adolescent's safety is the priority. A mental health referral is also appropriate if supportive counseling by the primary care physician has been ineffective or when depression is recurrent or chronic.

Psychiatric intervention generally includes **pharmacotherapy** in conjunction with psychotherapy because most cases of depression include psychologic, social, and environmental components. Although much attention has been given to safety concerns about the use of antidepressant medications among children and adolescents, SSRIs are considered first-line medications for the treatment of moderate to severe depression in teenagers. While 2 SSRIs, fluoxetine (Prozac) and escitalopram (Lexapro), have been approved by the US Food and Drug Administration (FDA) for treating depression in adolescents, a number of other antidepressants are commonly prescribed in an off-label manner. Side effects of this class of

medication tend to be dose related, and most subside with time (1–2 weeks) or with a decrease in dosage. Common adverse effects include headache, abdominal pain, diarrhea, sleep changes, and jitteriness or agitation. Serious behavioral symptoms, such as aggression, hostility, and impulsivity, must be reviewed with a psychiatrist.

A black box warning for antidepressant medications was added by the FDA in 2004 stating that on rare occasions, children and adolescents treated with these drugs are more likely to display suicidal behavior, but no increase in the risk of completed suicides was noted. This was based on a meta-analysis conducted by the FDA. Subsequently, physicians decreased their use of antidepressants, which resulted in an increase in the rate of completed suicides. It now is generally accepted that although there may be a small risk of suicidal behavior, the benefits of prescribing antidepressants outweigh the risks if patients are monitored. This caution should be put in context with the risks of untreated depression and discussed openly with the parent or guardian and the adolescent. Prior to starting the medication, informed consent must be obtained from the parent or guardian as well as assent from the teenager. Patients should be observed closely for worsening of symptoms, suicidal behavior, or unusual changes in behavior. Families should be educated on the importance of close follow-up and immediate, open communication with the physician if these symptoms should occur. Initially, the adolescent should be seen or the family contacted frequently during the first 6 weeks. Improvements in vegetative functions such as sleep and appetite often can occur within the first 3 weeks. Family observations are initially more telling than self-observation. Often, the last feature to improve is the patient's self-report of mood elevation. An adequate trial of SSRIs is reported to be at least 4 to 6 weeks. Frequent medication adjustments are not advised, and abruptly stopping SSRIs is not recommended due to a possible withdrawal syndrome. Stopping medication after several weeks should include a slow taper.

Suicide and Suicidal Behavior

Adolescents who are considered at risk for suicide must be asked directly at every visit if they are, in fact, suicidal and if they have a plan (see Questions Box: Adolescent Suicide). Response to this inquiry determines whether adolescents will be treated on an inpatient or outpatient basis. In most cases, the adolescent with no previous suicide attempts, ambivalence toward suicidal thoughts, no real intent to die, and a good family support system may be managed as an **outpatient.** In patients who deny current suicidal ideation, a written or verbal "no suicide" contract can be made between the physician or psychologist and the adolescent, although research does not support the conclusion that such contracts actively prevent suicide. Unwillingness to sign such a contract should raise alarming concern. The patient is asked to agree to contact the clinician, parent, or another responsible adult if he or she feels a suicidal urge or experiences suicidal intent. The precipitants for possible suicidal behavior must be reviewed, and alternative methods for coping should be rehearsed with the teenager. In addition, all potential means of suicide, particularly firearms and toxic medications, must be removed from the home or place of residence. It is not enough to "secure" firearms; they must be removed. Referral to a therapist is recommended as soon as possible. Preferably, this should be arranged while adolescents are in the office, and they should be given a definite time and date for the appointment. Ideally, the therapist should meet with the family before the first appointment with the adolescent alone. Detoxification from drugs or alcohol, if necessary, also should be addressed.

Because all suicidal threats, gestures, or ideations by adolescents must be taken seriously, emergent psychiatric referral is required for most of these individuals. Adolescents judged to be at serious risk for suicide should be managed as **inpatients** and admitted to a pediatric or adolescent unit for 24 to 48 hours of observation. The purpose of this brief hospitalization is 3-fold: to stabilize patients medically, if necessary; to observe and evaluate patient-family dynamics; and to impress on patients and families that the attempt has been recognized and taken seriously. Intervention requires the involvement of mental health professionals and social services.

Prognosis

The risk of recurrence of major depression in adolescents who have recovered is substantial. One study reports that 5% of patients relapse within 6 months of recovery, 12% within 1 year, and an estimated 33% within 4 years. Higher rates of recurrence have been reported, however, with approximately 70% of teens with MDD experiencing another depressive episode within 5 years. In addition, youth who have a depressive disorder have a 4-fold risk of the same disorder as an adult. Prepubertal-onset depression is associated with an approximately 30% risk of developing future bipolar disorder or mania.

The risk of repeated suicidal behavior seems to be greatest within the first 3 months following the initial attempt. Reported reattempt rates are 6% to 15% in the first 1 to 3 years following the initial attempt.

CASE RESOLUTION

In the case study presented at the beginning of this chapter, the girl's symptoms may be indicative of depression because she has a flat affect and seems to be somewhat isolated (insufficient time for friends and just recently moved to the United States). She seems to be at low risk for suicide, however. The physician should nonetheless inquire about symptoms of depression and ask her directly about suicidal behaviors, then make arrangements to follow the girl's condition closely. If depression is confirmed at future visits or if she becomes suicidal, she and her family should be referred to a mental health professional for immediate consultation and intervention.

Selected References

Adler RS, Jellinek MS. After teen suicide: issues for pediatricians who are asked to consult to schools. *Pediatrics.* 1990;86(6):982–987

American Academy of Child and Adolescent Psychiatry. Practice parameter for the assessment and treatment of children and adolescents with suicidal behavior. *J Am Acad Child Adolesc Psychiatry.* 2001;40(7 Suppl):24S–51S

Birmaher B, Brent D; AACAP Work Group on Quality Issues, et al. Practice Parameter for the assessment and treatment of children and adolescents with depressive disorders. *J Am Acad Child Adolesc Psychiatry.* 2007;46(11):1503–1526

Bolfek A, Jankowski JJ, Waslick B, Summergrad P. Adolescent psychopharmacology: drugs for mood disorders. *Adolesc Med Clin.* 2006;17(3):789–808

Borowsky IW, Ireland M, Resnick MD. Adolescent suicide attempts: risks and protectors. *Pediatrics.* 2001;107(3):485–493

Bridge JA, Goldstein TR, Brent DA. Adolescent suicide and suicidal behavior. *J Child Psychol Psychiatry.* 2006;47(3-4):372–394

Brookman RR, Sood AA. Disorders of mood and anxiety in adolescents. *Adolesc Med Clin.* 2006;17(1):79–95

Campbell AT. Consent, competence, and confidentiality related to psychiatric conditions in adolescent medicine practice. *Adolesc Med Clin.* 2006;17(1):25–47

Copelan R. Assessing the potential for violent behavior in children and adolescents. *Pediatr Rev.* 2006;27(5):e36–e41

Eaton DK, Kann L, Kinchen S, et al. Youth risk behavior surveillance—United States, 2011. *MMWR Surveill Summ.* 2012;61(4):1–162

Emslie GJ, Mayes T, Porta G, et al. Treatment of Resistant Depression in Adolescents (TORDIA): week 24 outcomes. *Am J Psychiatry.* 2010;167(7):782–791

Gibbons RD, Brown CH, Hur K, et al. Early evidence on the effects of regulators' suicidality warnings on SSRI prescriptions and suicide in children and adolescents. *Am J Psychiatry.* 2007;164(9):1356–1363

Grossman DC, Mueller BA, Riedy C, et al. Gun storage practices and risk of youth suicide and unintentional firearm injuries. *JAMA.* 2005;293(6):707–714

Hammad TA, Laughren T, Racoosin J. Suicidality in pediatric patients treated with antidepressant drugs. *Arch Gen Psychiatry.* 2006;63(3):332–339

Hatcher-Kay C, King CA. Depression and suicide. *Pediatr Rev.* 2003;24(11):363–371

Jellinek MS, Snyder JB. Depression and suicide in children and adolescents. *Pediatr Rev.* 1998;19(8):255–264

Leslie LK, Newman TB, Chesney PJ, Perrin JM. The Food and Drug Administration's deliberation on antidepressant use in pediatric patients. *Pediatrics.* 2005;116(1):195–204

Lewinsohn PM, Clarke GN, Seeley JR, Rohde P. Major depression in community adolescents: age at onset, episode duration, and time to recurrence. *J Am Acad Child Adolesc Psychiatry.* 1994;33(6):809–818

March JS, Silva S, Petrycki S, et al. The Treatment for Adolescents With Depression Study (TADS): long-term effectiveness and safety outcomes. *Arch Gen Psychiatry.* 2007;64(10):1132–1143

Merikangas KR, He JP, Burstein M, et al. Lifetime prevalence of mental disorders in U.S. adolescents: results from the National Comorbidity Survey Replication—Adolescent Supplement (NCS-A). *J Am Acad Child Adolesc Psychiatry.* 2010;49(10):980–989

Prager LM. Depression and suicide in children and adolescents. *Pediatr Rev.* 2009;30(6):199–206

Shain BN; American Academy of Pediatrics Committee on Adolescence. Suicide and suicide attempts in adolescents. *Pediatrics.* 2007;120(3):669–676

Slap GB, Vorters DF, Khalid N, Margulies SR, Forke CM. Adolescent suicide attempters: do physicians recognize them? *J Adolesc Health.* 1992;13(4):286–292

Williams SB, O'Connor EA, Eder M, Whitlock EP. Screening for child and adolescent depression in primary care settings: a systematic evidence review for the US Preventive Services Task Force. *Pediatrics.* 2009;123(4):e716–e735

Woods ER, Lin YG, Middleman A, Beckford P, Chase L, DuRant RH. The associations of suicide attempts in adolescents. *Pediatrics.* 1997;99(6):791–796

Chronic Diseases of Childhood and Adolescence

CHAPTER 145

Cancer in Children

Eduard H. Panosyan, MD, and Joseph L. Lasky III, MD

CASE STUDY

A 10-year-old boy has a history of intermittent fevers of 102.2°F (39.0°C) for 1 month. For 2 days, he has experienced increasing shortness of breath with rapid respirations. His face is dusky and plethoric, and the veins in his neck are prominent. He has bilaterally enlarged cervical lymph nodes. The remainder of the examination is normal.

His blood cell count is normal, but the erythrocyte sedimentation rate is 110. A chest radiograph reveals a large mediastinal mass.

Questions

1. What signs and symptoms are associated with malignant conditions in children?
2. What oncologic emergencies require immediate attention?
3. What factors correlate with the development of cancer in children?

Epidemiology

Fortunately, childhood cancer is rare. Approximately 12,400 children and adolescents younger than 20 years are diagnosed with cancer each year in the United States. The likelihood of a child developing cancer before the age of 20 years is 1 in 300 for males and 1 in 333 for females. The overall incidence of childhood cancer has been slowly increasing since the mid-1970s, but death rates have declined dramatically for most childhood cancers and survival rates have improved markedly since the 1970s. However, cancer remains the leading disease-related cause of death in children younger than 15 years. The incidence is higher in children younger than 5 years and in children between the ages of 15 and 19 years. Acute hematologic malignancies, sarcomas, and embryonic neoplasms with fewer mutations are more typical in the pediatric age group compared with adults, who develop genetically more complex cancers and carcinomas of epithelial origin. Acute leukemia is the most common childhood cancer, followed by brain tumors, lymphomas, neuroblastoma, Wilms tumor (nephroblastoma), and other less common pediatric solid tumors (Figure 145-1).

Environmental factors, genetic predisposition, and developmental processes may all play a role in influencing the cancer risk of a child. Case-control epidemiology studies looking for the causes of pediatric cancer have evaluated foods, prenatal exposures of parents and affected offspring, electromagnetic fields, radon, and various other environmental factors with no conclusive evidence of causality to date. Although many environmental factors are known to induce carcinogenesis, current evidence does not support a major causative role for exogenous factors in childhood cancer. Most childhood cancers result from aberrations in early developmental processes. Some known risk factors for selected childhood cancers include *infectious agents* such as Epstein-Barr virus (B-cell lymphomas, Hodgkin lymphoma, nasopharyngeal carcinoma), HIV (B-cell lymphomas, Kaposi sarcoma, leiomyosarcoma), and hepatitis B and C (hepatocellular carcinoma); *ionizing radiation* (leukemia, osteosarcoma, brain tumors); *chemotherapeutic agents* (leukemia, osteosarcoma); *immunodeficiency* (non-Hodgkin lymphoma); and *genetic conditions*. Approximately 4% to 10% of childhood cancer results from known inherited genetic mutations that result in a cancer predisposition. Children with trisomy 21 (Down) syndrome have an increased risk of leukemia (lymphoid and myeloid). Beckwith-Wiedemann syndrome is associated with an increased risk for hepatoblastoma, Wilms tumor, rhabdomyosarcoma, and neuroblastoma and warrants appropriate surveillance screening. Inheritance of mutations in tumor suppressor genes such as the retinoblastoma gene or the p53 gene (Li-Fraumeni syndrome) predispose affected children in families with these mutations to particular malignancies at a greater frequency and an earlier age than in unaffected individuals. Some children with tuberous sclerosis (TS) or neurofibromatosis 1 (N1) will develop multiple types of brain tumors.

Clinical Presentation (Table 145-1)

Signs and symptoms of childhood cancer are varied, are often nonspecific at the start, and can mimic many common pediatric conditions. Acute lymphoblastic leukemia (ALL) is the most common childhood cancer, accounting for 80% of pediatric leukemia cases. Acute myeloid leukemia (AML) accounts for the remaining 15% to

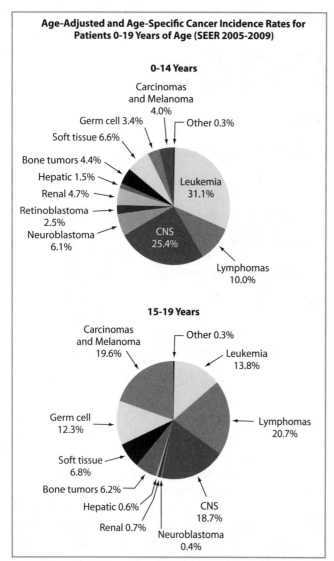

Age-Adjusted and Age-Specific Cancer Incidence Rates for Patients 0-19 Years of Age (SEER 2005-2009)

0-14 Years

- Carcinomas and Melanoma 4.0%
- Germ cell 3.4%
- Other 0.3%
- Soft tissue 6.6%
- Bone tumors 4.4%
- Hepatic 1.5%
- Renal 4.7%
- Retinoblastoma 2.5%
- Neuroblastoma 6.1%
- Leukemia 31.1%
- CNS 25.4%
- Lymphomas 10.0%

15-19 Years

- Carcinomas and Melanoma 19.6%
- Other 0.3%
- Leukemia 13.8%
- Germ cell 12.3%
- Lymphomas 20.7%
- Soft tissue 6.8%
- Bone tumors 6.2%
- Hepatic 0.6%
- Renal 0.7%
- Neuroblastoma 0.4%
- CNS 18.7%

Figure 145-1. Cancer incidence rates for patients aged 0 to 14 years and 15 to 19 years in the Surveillance Epidemiology and End Results (SEER) Program from 2005 to 2009. Incidence rates are age-adjusted and age-specific and are shown for leukemia, lymphoma, central nervous system (CNS) tumors, neuroblastoma, retinoblastoma, renal tumors, hepatic tumors, bone tumors, soft tissue tumors, germ cell tumors, carcinomas and melanomas, and other cancers. Retinoblastoma occurs infrequently in adolescents aged 15 to 19 years.

20% of cases. Children with **acute leukemia** present with signs and symptoms that reflect leukemic infiltration of the bone marrow and extramedullary locations. Children commonly present with generalized bone pain and signs and symptoms related to pancytopenia (fever, fatigue, pallor, bleeding, bruising, and infections). Disseminated intravascular coagulation is more characteristic of AML, especially acute promyelocytic leukemia. Leukemic infiltration of extramedullary sites can lead to hepatosplenomegaly, lymphadenopathy, chloromas, central nervous system (CNS), and sometimes testicular involvement. Children with high white blood cell counts at presentation (leukocytosis) can present with signs and symptoms of leukostasis typically involving the lung or brain. Tumor

lysis syndrome can occur spontaneously or with the initiation of intravenous (IV) hydration or chemotherapy. Tumor lysis syndrome occurs as a result of breakdown of leukemic blasts that results in the release of metabolic by-products. It is characterized by a metabolic triad of hyperuricemia, hyperkalemia, and hyperphosphatemia, which places a child at risk for renal dysfunction or failure secondary to precipitation of urate or calcium phosphate crystals within the renal tubules. Involvement of the CNS by leukemia can result in signs of increased intracranial pressure (ICP) (eg, headache, vomiting, hypertension, seizures, cranial neuropathies).

T-cell ALL or T-cell lymphoblastic lymphoma can present with a large anterior mediastinal mass and symptoms related to compression by the mediastinal mass on the trachea and blockage of venous return and lymphatic drainage (superior vena cava syndrome). Children with SVC syndrome can present with wheezing, dyspnea, dysphagia, plethora, and cyanosis. Pleural or pericardial effusions may also be present. Superior vena cava syndrome can rapidly progress and constitutes a true oncologic emergency that requires prompt intervention.

Lymphomas in children can be divided pathologically into Hodgkin or non-Hodgkin lymphoma. Children with **Hodgkin lymphoma** typically have a prolonged history (often at least 2–3 months) of painless enlarging cervical or supraclavicular lymphadenopathy. Affected lymph nodes can be firm, immobile, rubbery, and nontender. In two-thirds of cases, mediastinal adenopathy may be present, resulting in cough or wheeze. Constitutional symptoms such as fatigue, pruritus, and anorexia can occur, as well as the classic "B" symptoms (ie, fever, night sweats, and weight loss >10% of body weight). **Non-Hodgkin lymphoma** can be distinguished as lymphoblastic or non-lymphoblastic. Children with **lymphoblastic lymphoma** often present with supradiaphragmatic disease and may have cervical or supraclavicular lymphadenopathy, sometimes in association with a mediastinal mass or SVC syndrome (as previously described for T-cell lymphoblastic lymphoma). Central nervous system disease in such children is associated with signs of increased ICP. Patients with **non-lymphoblastic lymphoma** of the Burkitt or non-Burkitt type often present with intra-abdominal disease that can manifest as intussusception, abdominal obstruction, hepatosplenomegaly, or obstructive jaundice. Children with sporadic Burkitt lymphoma can present with a rapidly enlarging abdominal mass associated with tumor lysis syndrome. Endemic Burkitt lymphoma (African) presents with facial or isolated jaw tumors. In addition, patients with lymphoma can manifest a number of paraneoplastic syndromes. These include idiopathic thrombocytopenic purpura, autoimmune hemolytic anemia, nephrotic syndrome, and peripheral neuropathies, which may be mediated by abnormal and lymphoma-driven humoral or cell-mediated processes. Children with lymphomas are also at risk for tumor lysis syndrome as described for leukemia. In general, patients may have entirely normal blood cell counts or a mild anemia, but occasionally their bone marrow may be infiltrated, giving a clinical picture similar to leukemia with anemia, thrombocytopenia, or neutropenia.

Table 145-1. Signs and Symptoms of Childhood Cancer

Disease	Symptoms	Signs
Leukemia	Fatigue, pallor Bone pain Fever, infection Bruising, bleeding Disseminated intravascular coagulation SVC syndrome Headache Seizures Oliguria/anuria Abdominal pain, diarrhea	Anemia Neutropenia Thrombocytopenia Lymphadenopathy Hepatosplenomegaly Mediastinal mass Petechiae, purpura Papilledema Cranial neuropathies Renal failure
Brain tumors	Supratentorial tumors Seizures Visual dysfunction Unilateral motor dysfunction Infratentorial tumors Deficits of balance Difficulty breathing Increased intracranial pressure Headache Vomiting Diplopia Motor weakness Loss of developmental milestones	Upper motor neuron signs Marcus Gunn pupils Parinaud syndrome Diabetes insipidus Appendicular dysmetria Sixth nerve palsy Cranial neuropathies Horner syndrome Papilledema Systemic hypertension Setting sun sign Large head size
Lymphoma		
Non-Hodgkin	Supradiaphragmatic (lymphoblastic) Respiratory difficulty, cough SVC syndrome Enlarged/enlarging lymph nodes Infradiaphragmatic (small, non-cleaved) Abdominal obstruction Intussusception Abdominal distension	Mediastinal mass ±effusions Lymphadenopathy Abdominal mass Hepatosplenomegaly Obstructive jaundice
Hodgkin	Constitutional symptoms (fever, weight loss, pruritus)	Lymphadenopathy ± matted nodes
Neuroblastoma	Skin nodules Proptosis, raccoon eyes Nystagmus Diarrhea Spinal cord compression symptoms	Hypertension Abdominal mass Hepatosplenomegaly Horner syndrome
Rhabdomyosarcoma	Related to primary site (eg, urinary retention with GU tumors)	Head and neck mass Extremity swelling/mass
Wilms tumor	Rapid development of abdominal swelling Painless hematuria	Abdominal or flank mass Hypertension Associated congenital anomalies Aniridia Hemihypertrophy Urogenital anomalies
Ewing sarcoma	Painful swelling of bone or surrounding soft tissues Constitutional symptoms (fever, fatigue)	Pathologic fracture
Osteosarcoma	Painful swelling of bone	Pathologic fracture

Abbreviations: GU, genitourinary; SVC, superior vena cava.

Children with **brain tumors** can present with diverse signs and symptoms, depending on the anatomic location of the tumor (subtentorial, supratentorial, or brain stem), age of the child (eg, infants with open sutures), and presence and degree of increased ICP. Subtentorial tumors, which are more common in children, typically present with gaze palsies, cerebellar signs (especially truncal ataxia), dysmetria, or vomiting. Supratentorial tumors can cause seizures, upper motor neuron signs (ie, hemiparesis, asymmetrical hyperreflexia, and clonus), sensory changes, behavioral changes, decreased school performance, and disorders of the midbrain (Parinaud syndrome—paralysis of upward gaze). Signs and symptoms of ICP are often in the forefront of complaints. Recurrent morning headaches, headaches that awaken the child at night, intense headaches, vomiting (often followed by temporal relief of morning headaches), lethargy, sundowning (ie, eyes deviating downward like a sun setting on the horizon), increasing head circumference and loss of developmental milestones in infants, and change in school performance in older children all warrant close evaluation. Certain conditions, such as TS and N1, should increase the index of suspicion for brain tumors. Primary tumors intrinsic to brain (glial, neural, or choroid plexus origin) and extrinsic (craniopharyngioma and germ cell tumor) are encountered more often in the pediatric population. Neural/embryonic tumors such as medulloblastomas and primitive neuroectodermal tumors are more typical for childhood age group. Metastatic brain lesions are less common in children but may be encountered with neuroblastomas, lymphomas, or some renal tumors.

Children with spinal cord involvement from a primary spinal tumor or a paraspinal tumor (neuroblastoma, Ewing sarcoma, leukemic chloroma) may present with persistent back pain, intense radicular pain, local bony tenderness of the affected vertebrae, abnormal reflexes, abnormal dermatomal sensory examination, weakness/evolving paralysis, and subtle symptoms of bowel or bladder dysfunction (constipation, difficulty urinating). Suspicion of a spinal cord compression is an oncologic emergency for which timely, appropriate consultation must be sought.

Neuroblastoma is a malignancy of sympathetic ganglionic cell origin and can arise anywhere along the sympathetic nervous system. Most tumors arise in the abdomen (adrenal or paraspinal); additional sites include the neck, chest, pelvis, and, rarely, CNS. At presentation, tumors may be localized, with or without regional lymph node extension, or disseminated involving bone, bone marrow, liver, and CNS. Children with localized disease are often asymptomatic and the tumor is detected when radiographic imaging is performed for other medical purposes. Children with disseminated disease are ill-appearing and may present with fever, bone pain, and irritability. Paraneoplastic syndromes may also be present at diagnosis with a variety of features such as opsomyoclonus/myoclonus/ataxia (random dysconjugate eye movements, myoclonic jerking), cerebellar ataxia, and diarrhea. Proptosis and hemorrhage due to metastases involving the periorbital region can result in periorbital swelling and ecchymoses (raccoon eyes). A cervical tumor may be associated with unilateral Horner syndrome (unilateral ptosis, miosis, and anhidrosis). Central nervous system metastasis may present with signs and symptoms of increased ICP.

Nephroblastoma or **Wilms tumor,** an embryonic tumor of the kidney, usually presents as a painless abdominal mass, often detected by a parent while bathing the child. Associated symptoms may include fever, abdominal pain, or hematuria. If there is abdominal trauma, these bulky masses can rupture and hemorrhage and a child may present with acute abdominal pain and swelling. On examination, children may have hypertension, stigmata of associated genetic syndromes (eg, Beckwith-Wiedemann, Denys-Drash), or other isolated congenital anomalies such as aniridia, hemihypertrophy, or hypospadias.

Bone sarcomas that occur in children include Ewing sarcoma, osteosarcoma, and other rarer sarcomas. These tumors are most common in adolescents and rarely seen in young children. Bone tumors can present with pain at the site of tumor, with or without an associated soft tissue mass. Osteosarcomas classically involve the metaphyseal portions of the long bones, with the distal femur and proximal tibia being the most frequently involved sites. Metastatic disease, if present (15%–20% of cases), primarily involves the lung, although other sites of bone can be involved. Ewing sarcomas that occur in bone most commonly involve the flat bones of the axial skeleton. When affecting the long bones, they tend to arise in the diaphyseal region (unlike osteosarcoma). Twenty-five percent of cases will have metastatic disease at presentation involving lung, bone, or bone marrow. Children with Ewing sarcoma may also have associated constitutional symptoms such as low-grade fever, fatigue, and weight loss. Extraosseous soft tissue components are also more common with Ewing sarcomas than osteosarcomas.

Rhabdomyosarcomas, which account for about half of the soft tissue sarcomas in children, present with signs and symptoms dependent on the location of the primary tumor. Sites include the head, neck, chest, abdomen, genitourinary tract, or extremities. Fewer than 25% of children will present with metastatic disease, but when present it can involve lymph nodes, lungs, bone marrow, and bone. Head and neck sarcomas commonly arise in parameningeal and orbital sites and can present with recurrent headache, vomiting, visual problems, and proptosis. Abdominal and pelvic primary tumors can present with a palpable abdominal mass, pain, constipation, urinary obstruction, or dysuria. Genitourinary tract tumors most often involve the bladder or prostate and can present with pain, constipation, and urinary obstruction. One classic presentation occurs in girls who present with a grapelike mass at the introitus and vaginal bleeding. This is due to tumor involving the vagina or uterus and is known as sarcoma botryoides. Primary tumors involving an extremity present with swelling at the site of tumor that can be painful and tender on palpation.

Pathophysiology

Although the macroscopic causes of pediatric cancer are not well elucidated, significant research has been made in determining some of the cellular and molecular events that actively trigger or fail to prevent malignancy. Growth factors are responsible for stimulation of cellular proliferation, and growth factor receptors transduce this signal into the cell via cytoplasmic secondary messengers, which in turn transmit the signal to nuclear regulatory factors. These factors ultimately regulate transcription of new RNA and protein, resulting in the desired cellular response of stimulation or inhibition of growth. Malignant cells have a genetic makeup that differs from the constitutional karyotype of the host. A series of mutations occurs in genes that regulate cell growth and differentiation, resulting in dysregulation of cell growth, differentiation, and death. Oncogenes promote cell growth and tumor suppressor genes inhibit cell division. When there is inappropriate overexpression of an oncogene or underexpression of a tumor-suppressor gene, inappropriate cell growth and division may occur, resulting in a malignant transformation.

There are usually multiple genetic aberrations present that lead to malignant transformation of a cell. One of the most important tumor suppressor genes is p53. The p53 gene encodes for a nuclear protein that is expressed in all cells of the body and serves to induce cell cycle arrest or apoptosis in response to DNA damage. Inactivation of p53 has been identified in numerous cancers. An initial event can alter or knock out one allele of a p53 gene pair, and a second event results in loss of heterozygosity for that genetic locus. An inherited abnormality of p53 (Li-Fraumeni syndrome) or a serendipitous accident to p53 can cause heterozygosity for that gene. If a second event knocks out complete function of p53, a DNA-damaged cell can escape the signal to arrest its growth or undergo apoptosis. The result can be a malignant transformation that allows the abnormal cell to grow unchecked. Retinoblastoma gene is another classic and wellstudied tumor suppressor, loss of which results in malignant transformation of the cell.

Cancer's threat to a living organism lies in its uncontrolled growth. By growing unchecked and invading, compressing, and metastasizing to vital organs, malignant cells threaten normal life functions and cause symptoms specific to the affected area of the body.

Differential Diagnosis

Cancer is rare and often challenging to diagnose in children. Many of the presenting symptoms can be nonspecific and easily attributed to more common childhood complaints. To add to the difficulty, a pediatric practice will, on average, see a case every 5 to 7 years. Differential diagnoses for some common childhood complaints that may suggest an underlying malignancy are discussed herein.

Lymphadenopathy is a common pediatric complaint and is most frequently due to infections (see Chapter 88). Acute bacterial adenitis, usually involving the head and neck region, is typically associated with local signs of inflammation such as erythema, warmth, and tenderness. Cervical adenopathy due to viral illness is typically bilateral, and the lymph nodes are usually mobile, soft, and nontender. Generalized lymphadenopathy or regional lymphadenopathy characterized by firm, matted, rubbery lymph nodes should raise the suspicion for an underlying malignancy. Lymphadenopathy that is persistent or progressive, despite empiric antibiotic therapy or resolution of infectious symptoms, also merits further evaluation for malignancy. Leukemia often presents with generalized lymphadenopathy, usually in association with hepatosplenomegaly and abnormal laboratory findings. Lymphoma typically presents with regional lymphadenopathy, often in the cervical or mediastinal region, in conjunction with other signs of systemic illness. Metastatic disease (neuroblastoma, rhabdomyosarcoma) may also present with regional lymphadenopathy. Nonmalignant causes of neck masses that can be mistaken for cervical lymphadenopathy include structural anomalies such as branchial cleft cysts or cystic hygromas (see Chapter 82).

Bone and joint pain are common complaints in children with acute leukemia because of bone marrow involvement and may be generalized. This presentation can be confused with various rheumatologic conditions. Localized bone pain is a common presentation for children with primary bone cancers (osteosarcoma, Ewing sarcoma) and is often attributed by the child or parents to some trauma. It is not unusual for the diagnosis to be delayed several months. Differential diagnosis includes infection (osteomyelitis), trauma, musculoskeletal conditions, and benign bone lesions.

Headache is a common complaint facing the general pediatrician, and few of these headaches are caused by intracranial brain tumors. When evaluating a child with headaches, signs to raise the index of suspicion for a brain tumor include persistent vomiting, recurrent morning headaches or headaches that awaken the child, worsening headaches, associated neurologic abnormalities, and visual changes (papilledema on examination). In infants, increasing head size, sundowning, and loss of acquired developmental milestones are red flags. The differential diagnosis for headaches in children is broad and includes infections (meningitis, sinusitis), migraines, hydrocephalus, hemorrhage, and seizures.

An **abdominal mass** in an infant or child is always concerning and merits an evaluation. The most common malignant causes for an abdominal mass in this age range include neuroblastoma, nephroblastoma (Wilms tumor), hepatoblastoma, non-Hodgkin lymphoma (ie, Burkitt lymphoma), sarcomas, and germ cell tumors. Massive hepatosplenomegaly due to leukemic or lymphomatous infiltration can also be palpated as an abdominal mass. Nonmalignant etiologies of an abdominal mass may include hepatomegaly or splenomegaly, renal cysts, hemangiomas, or constipation.

Pancytopenia or **single cytopenias** are always worrisome for a malignancy involving bone marrow. Acute leukemia is the most common malignancy involving bone marrow and can present with leukopenia, anemia, thrombocytopenia, or in combination. Any malignancy that can metastasize to the bone marrow (neuroblastoma, lymphoma, Ewing sarcoma, rhabdomyosarcoma) can also produce pancytopenia or depression of one of the cell lines due to replacement of the bone marrow. Pancytopenia can also occur as a primary bone marrow failure syndrome, such as Fanconi anemia, or as an acquired aplastic anemia due to infections (post-hepatitis), drugs (chloramphenicol, anticonvulsants), radiation, or idiopathic causes. Transient mild depression of the cell lines (most often leukopenia or anemia) due to infectious causes is very common during childhood. Depression of more than one hematopoietic cell line merits a closer evaluation and pediatric hematologist consultation.

Evaluation

History

The history should focus on the duration and evolution of symptoms as well as the presence or absence of constitutional symptoms (eg, anorexia, fever, night sweats, weight loss). The effect of the symptoms on daily activities (eg, school attendance, sports) should be determined and will clue the physician to the scope of the illness. The presence of recent or persistent infections, medications (especially steroids), or unusual environmental exposures should also be ascertained (Questions Box). Relevant medical history should be considered. A previous cancer diagnosis would raise the index of suspicion for relapse or a secondary malignancy. Certain immunodeficiencies and genetic syndromes are associated with an increased risk for malignancy (eg, trisomy 21 syndrome and leukemia) and should also be considered. A family history of childhood cancers or genetic syndromes is also important.

Physical Examination

A thorough physical examination is essential, with particular attention to symptomatic areas (see Table 145-1). In general, the lymph nodes should be carefully assessed for enlargement or malignant characteristics (firm, fixed, rubbery nodes or nodular conglomerates) and the abdomen for organomegaly or masses. The skin should be evaluated for the presence of pallor, petechiae, or purpura that would suggest anemia or thrombocytopenia. A thorough search for signs of or persistent infection should be performed and, if present, may reflect bone marrow disease with neutropenia. Neurologic symptoms, including headache, vomiting, or focal complaints, warrant a full neurologic examination. Increased ICP may manifest as papilledema or sixth nerve palsy. In infants, increased ICP can manifest with a large head size, full fontanels, or sundowning. A complaint of back pain also merits a full neurologic examination with close attention to any signs of spinal cord compression, suggesting a possible spinal or paraspinal mass.

Questions

Cancer

- How long has the child had the symptoms?
- Does the child have a family history of cancer?
- Does the child have a history of constitutional symptoms (eg, fever, weight loss, night sweats)?
- Does the child have a history of recent onset of pallor, fever, bleeding/bruising, pain, swelling, hematuria, or malaise?
- Has the child been attending school or participating in routine activities?
- Has the child been exposed to any environmental toxins?
- Has the child been taking antipyretics/nonsteroidal anti-inflammatory drugs on a regular basis or any prescribed antibiotics or steroids?

Laboratory Tests (Table 145-2)

In a child with nonspecific or constitutional symptoms concerning for malignancy, it is reasonable to begin with a complete blood cell count (CBC), peripheral blood smear, and comprehensive chemistry panel (electrolytes, renal and liver function). If a malignancy is suspected, lactate dehydrogenase is useful as a nonspecific marker for increased cell turnover. If leukemia or lymphoma is suspected, evaluation for tumor lysis syndrome (by checking uric acid, potassium, phosphate, and calcium) should be performed. In addition, certain tumors secrete or synthesize characteristic markers and metabolites that are pathognomonic for their diagnosis. For example, elevated levels of the sympathetic neurotransmitter metabolites vanillylmandelic acid and homovanillic acid are found in the urine of individuals with neuroblastoma or pheochromocytoma. Tumor markers such as α-fetoprotein and β-human chorionic gonadotropin are characteristic of germ cell tumors. α-fetoprotein is a useful tumor marker for hepatoblastoma and, rarely, pancreatoblastoma as well. Monitoring of these levels is useful as an indicator of response to therapy or relapse. Other laboratory values, such as ferritin or erythrocyte sedimentation rate, can be elevated and reflect an underlying systemic illness (see Table 145-2).

Imaging Studies

Radiographic studies are a necessity in the initial evaluation and staging of most childhood cancers. Once the diagnosis of malignancy has been confirmed, appropriate imaging studies to assess the local and metastatic spread of the disease should be performed before the initiation of therapy. The type of studies performed depends on the specific malignancy and its associated pattern of metastatic spread. Common studies performed include plain radiographs, computed tomography (CT), magnetic resonance imaging, and gallium or positron emission tomography (PET) scans. For leukemias and lymphomas, an initial chest radiograph is necessary to evaluate for a mediastinal mass (most commonly seen in T-cell leukemia/lymphoma). Additional imaging is typically not necessary for leukemia; however, lymphomas warrant further diagnostic imaging for staging (CT, gallium, or PET scans). Required imaging for evaluation of specific childhood cancers is provided in Table 145-2.

Pathology

Children with suspected malignancies should be referred to a children's cancer center where there are specialized pediatric oncologists, radiologists, surgeons, and pathologists who can work together to establish the best approach for diagnosis (biopsy or removal of tumor) and handling of tissue. Collection of fresh tissue at biopsy for specialized genetic tests and tumor banking is important and can contribute significantly to a complete pathologic diagnosis.

There are certain clinical scenarios in which obtaining tissue for pathologic diagnosis is difficult. Children who present with a large mediastinal mass may be in respiratory distress (secondary to SVC syndrome) and at high risk during anesthesia. In this situation, coordinated efforts should be made to obtain pathology specimens in the least invasive manner, before the initiation of therapy. Diagnosis can

Table 145-2. Diagnostic Tests and Imaging Studies Used in the Evaluation of Common Childhood Cancers

Disease	Diagnostic Tests[a]	Imaging Studies
Leukemia	Bone marrow aspirate and biopsy Cytogenetic analysis of bone marrow CBC with platelet count, differential, reticulocytes Flow cytometry of peripheral blood PT, PTT, fibrinogen Serum electrolytes, Ca, PO_4 BUN, creatinine, uric acid, LDH CSF cell count, differential, cytology	Chest radiograph (look for mediastinal mass) Abdominal ultrasound for hepatosplenomegaly
Brain tumors	In case of suspected germ cell tumors: serum and CSF α-fetoprotein, β-human chorionic gonadotropin, carcinoembryonic antigen CSF cytology for medulloblastomas, primitive neuroectodermal tumors and ependymomas	MRI of brain with gadolinium MRI of spine for selected tumors
Lymphoma	CBC with platelet count, differential, reticulocytes Bilateral bone marrow aspirate and biopsy CSF cell count and cytology (EBV PCR for immunocompromised patients with suspected CNS lymphoma) Serum LDH, electrolytes, Ca, PO_4 ESR, ferritin	Gallium scan, PET scan CT of chest, abdomen, pelvis Brain MRI for CNS lymphomas
Neuroblastoma	CBC with platelet count, differential Serum electrolytes, liver and renal panel Serum ferritin Serum LDH, uric acid Urine HVA and VMA Bone marrow aspirate and biopsy	CT or MRI of primary tumor site CT of chest, abdomen, pelvis ($\pm$head) with contrast Bone scan Iobenguane scan
Rhabdomyosarcoma	CBC with platelet count, differential Electrolytes, liver and renal panel Bone marrow aspirate and biopsy CSF cell count and cytology (head and neck primary parameningeal tumors only)	CT or MRI of primary tumor site CT of chest, abdomen, pelvis Bone scan, PET scan
Nephroblastoma (Wilms tumor)	CBC with platelet count, differential Electrolytes, liver and renal panel Urinalysis PT, PTT, fibrinogen	Chest radiograph CT of primary tumor site Ultrasound of inferior vena cava CT of chest Bone scan
Ewing sarcoma	ESR CBC with platelet count Bone marrow aspirate and biopsy Serum LDH	Plain radiographs of primary site CT or MRI of primary tumor site CT of chest Bone scan
Osteosarcoma		Plain radiographs of primary site CT or MRI of primary tumor site CT of chest Bone scan
GCTs (extracranial)	Serum α-fetoprotein, β-human chorionic gonadotropin, carcinoembryonic antigen	Chest radiograph (for thoracic lesions) Abdominal (or testicular) ultrasound CT or MRI of primary tumor site CT of chest

Abbreviations: BUN, blood urea nitrogen; Ca, calcium; CBC, complete blood cell count; CNS, central nervous system; CSF, cerebrospinal fluid; CT, computed tomography; EBV, Epstein-Barr virus; ESR, erythrocyte sedimentation rate; GCT, germ cell tumor; HVA, homovanillic acid; LDH, lactate dehydrogenase; MRI, magnetic resonance imaging; PCR, polymerase chain reaction; PET, positron emission tomography; PO_4, phosphate; PT, prothrombin time; PTT, partial thromboplastin time; VMA, vanillylmandelic acid.

[a] Tumor biopsy (with few exceptions, eg, intracranial GCT secreting α-fetoprotein/β-human chorionic gonadotropin, inoperable brain stem gliomas) is required for diagnoses of most malignancies. Rarely, thoracic or abdominal hematologic lymphomas in an unstable patient may be diagnosed from cytology of pleural effusion or ascitic fluids.

often be made by less invasive procedures (eg, CBC, peripheral blood flow cytometry, bone marrow aspirate/biopsy, thoracentesis) that may require very minimal sedation. If therapy needs to be started, biopsy should be performed as soon as clinically tolerated.

Management

If a diagnosis of cancer is suspected or confirmed in a child, referral to a pediatric cancer center where appropriate diagnostic procedures, tissue handling, and treatment can be provided is important.

Diagnosing and treating childhood cancer requires a multidisciplinary team consisting of pediatric oncologists, surgeons, radiation oncologists, pathologists, and other pediatric subspecialists. In addition, supportive ancillary services such as social work, child life, child psychology, pain service, palliative care programs, and religious support are important. When making a referral for a child with a suspected cancer, the referring physician should prepare the family with his or her suspicions and the likely workup that will ensue at the accepting center. In addition, robust psychosocial support needs to be initiated.

Because the management of specific childhood cancers is beyond the scope of this chapter, the discussion will focus on the general principles of pediatric oncologic management. The primary therapeutic modalities for the treatment of childhood cancer include **chemotherapy** as a systemic treatment, **surgery** or **radiation** for local control, and myeloablative therapies followed by **hematopoietic stem cell transplantation. Neoadjuvant (preoperative) chemotherapy** sometimes is implemented for solid tumors to make surgery feasible with less morbidity and to treat undetectable micrometastases upfront. Increasingly, as the molecular aberrations of cancer are becoming understood, cancer-targeted therapies are becoming more prevalent. Conventional, cytotoxic anticancer therapy is likened to a "shotgun" approach in which cancer cells and normal cells are subject to toxicity. The effects of therapy on normal tissues and organs can manifest acutely (limiting dose) or in the long term (affecting quality of life). As more and more children are surviving childhood cancer, the late effects of therapy are increasingly evident, further emphasizing the need for risk-adapted therapy, cancer-targeted therapy, and a reduction of treatment-related toxicities.

Optimal outcome depends on several factors: correct pathologic diagnosis; careful medical management, including administration of chemotherapy and monitoring of side effects; precise customization of radiation fields if radiation therapy is necessary; optimal surgical resection for local control, if indicated; and therapeutic ability and experience with administration of treatment to children. Centers that specialize in the treatment of pediatric cancer are experienced in the diagnosis and treatment of rare malignancies and are thus best equipped to treat affected children. In addition, the standard of care for children with cancer is treatment according to research study protocols from national collaborative research groups (Children's Oncology Group), available at most specialized pediatric cancer centers. Posttreatment analysis of children treated on protocols at specialized pediatric cancer centers shows disease-free survival rates that are significantly better than those of children

treated outside this setting. Similarly, treatment of adolescents and young adults on protocols at specialized pediatric cancer centers yields better outcomes than those treated by oncologists who typically treat adults. These differences are perhaps due to more biological responsiveness of pediatric cancers, better tolerability of multi-agent chemotherapy regimens by younger patients, and, in part, compliance endorsed by parents.

The placement of indwelling central venous catheters is standard in cancer therapy in pediatrics, making frequent venous access for diagnostic and therapeutic purposes more easily tolerated by children. External catheters (eg, Broviac, Hickman) or internal subcutaneous catheters are selected depending on the underlying diagnosis and intensity of therapy. All indwelling catheters are at risk for infection from contamination of blood (line infections) or infections around the catheter site itself (tunnel infection). Most central line infections can be treated with IV antibiotic therapy; however, certain pathogens (fungi) are difficult to clear and require line removal. Central venous catheters may also be complicated, with thromboses requiring local thrombolytic therapy or long-term (3–6 months) anticoagulation therapy.

In the interest of cost containment and convenience as well as children's well-being, it is often more feasible for children to be closer to home between chemotherapy cycles. Primary care physicians should be familiar with the management of various infectious complications to which children undergoing cancer therapy are subject. Fever in children with neutropenia (especially with absolute neutrophil count <500 cells/μL) requires a different therapeutic approach than fever in otherwise normal children. Until proven otherwise, children with fever and neutropenia (usually induced by chemotherapy, sometimes in combination with radiation therapy) must be assumed to have a serious bacterial infection. They should be treated accordingly, with hospitalization, prompt initiation of IV antibiotics, thorough examination for site of infection, and careful hemodynamic monitoring. Initial treatment consists of wide spectrum antibiotic coverage for *Staphylococcus aureus,* gram-negative enteric organisms, and *Pseudomonas aeruginosa* (eg, cefepime with or without an aminoglycoside, vancomycin). Additional coverage for anaerobic infection (eg, mucositis), viral infection (eg, herpes stomatitis, varicella), and other pathogens (eg, fungi) depends on the child's treatment history and clinical findings. Additional proactive supportive care (including aggressive antiemetic, anti-constipation, and analgesic regimens, IV hydration, administration of granulocyte colony stimulating factors, and blood product transfusions) permits to minimize complications secondary to intensive chemotherapy. Standard of care for a child undergoing chemotherapy also includes *Pneumocystis jiroveci* prophylaxis. Live vaccines are omitted for these children, usually until near complete immune reconstitution takes place post-chemotherapy.

Prognosis

The prognosis for children with all forms of cancer has dramatically improved over the past 4 decades. Nearly 80% of children diagnosed with cancer can expect to be long-term survivors. Figure 145-2 shows

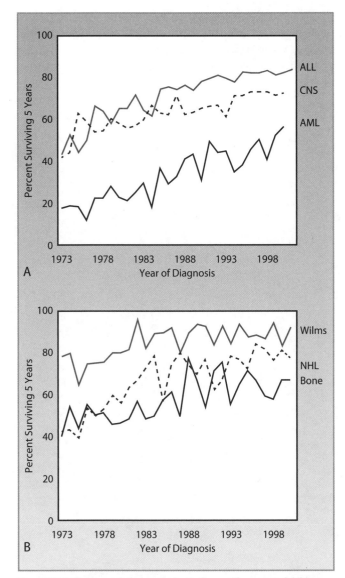

Figure 145-2. Five-year relative survival rates for specific cancers of children (0–19 years), 1973–2006. Data are from the Surveillance, Epidemiology, and End Results Program regions (9 areas). A, ALL, acute lymphoblastic leukemia; AML, acute myeloid leukemia; CNS, central nervous system. B, bone tumors; NHL, non-Hodgkin lymphoma; Wilms tumor.

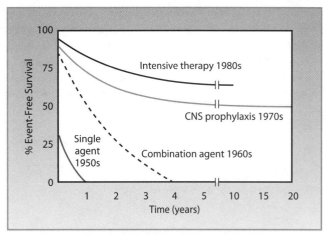

Figure 145-3. Historical perspective of the treatment of childhood acute lymphoblastic leukemia. The single-agent era resulted in few complete remissions and no cures. The combination-agent era without adequate central nervous system (CNS) treatment resulted in high complete remission rates but almost uniform mortality. Between the mid-1960s and 1970s, combination chemotherapy and CNS treatment resulted in prolonged, disease-free survival for approximately 50% of children. Intensive therapy in the 1980s and 1990s resulted in an event-free survival of 75% to 80% of children. (From Silverman LB. Acute lymphoblast leukemia. In Orkin SH, Fisher DE, Look AT, Lux SE, Ginsburg D, Nathan DG, eds. *Oncology of Infancy and Childhood*. Philadelphia, PA: Saunders Elsevier; 2009.)

CASE RESOLUTION

In the case study, the boy undergoes a mediastinoscopic biopsy of the mediastinal mass, which reveals lymphoblastic lymphoma. No evidence of disease in the bone marrow or spinal fluid is present, which would indicate a worse prognosis. Treatment involves chemotherapy, and the prognosis is quite good. Symptoms of superior vena cava syndrome due to obstruction from the tumor resolve with shrinkage of the tumor secondary to therapy.

Selected References

Golden CB, Feusner JH. Malignant abdominal masses in children: quick guide to evaluation and diagnosis. *Pediatr Clin North Am.* 2002;49(6):1369–1392

Meck MM, Leary M, Sills RH. Late effects in survivors of childhood cancer. *Pediatr Rev.* 2007;27(7):257–263

National Cancer Institute. SEER Cancer Statistics Review 1975-2009. http://seer.cancer.gov/csr/1975_2009_pops09/results_merged/sect_29_childhood_cancer_iccc.pdf. Accessed February 26, 2014

Oeffinger KC, Nathan PC, Kremer LC. Challenges after curative treatment for childhood cancer and long-term follow up of survivors. *Pediatr Clin North Am.* 2008;55(1):251–273

Park JR, Eggert A, Caron H. Neuroblastoma: biology, prognosis, and treatment. *Pediatr Clin North Am.* 2008;55(1):97–120

Poplack DG. Acute lymphoblastic leukemia. In: Pizzo PA, Poplack DG, eds. *Principles and Practice of Pediatric Oncology.* 5th ed. Philadelphia, PA: Lippincott Williams & Wilkins; 2006

the improvement in cure rates for the most common childhood cancers. This success is largely due to the efforts of national collaborative group science and treatment protocols and best can be exemplified by historical improvements of childhood ALL survival due to improved therapies (Figure 145-3). However, with increased survivorship, new concerns have arisen with respect to long-term effects of treatment, risks of secondary malignancies, and complex social and psychologic issues. In a large study of childhood cancer survivors, adults treated for a childhood cancer in the 1970s and 1980s were 3 times more likely than their siblings to have developed a chronic health condition. Risk-adopted therapies and continued multidisciplinary surveillance of childhood cancer survivors through adulthood will help to optimize more favorable outcomes.

Pui CH, Schrappe M, Ribeiro RC, Niemeyer CM. Childhood and adolescent lymphoid and myeloid leukemia. *Hematology Am Soc Hematol Educ Program.* 2004:118–145

Ries LAG, Smith MA, Gurney JG, et al, eds. *Cancer Incidence and Survival among Children and Adolescents: United States SEER Program 1975–1995, National Cancer Institute, SEER Program.* Bethesda, MD: National Institutes of Health; 1999. NIH Pub No 99-4649

Silverman LB. Acute lymphoblast leukemia. In Orkin SH, Fisher DE, Look AT, Lux SE, Ginsburg D, Nathan DG, eds. *Oncology of Infancy and Childhood.* Philadelphia, PA: Saunders Elsevier; 2009

Ullrich NJ, Pomeroy SL. Pediatric brain tumors. *Neurol Clin.* 2003;21(4): 897–913

CHAPTER 146

Chronic Kidney Disease

Mark Hanudel, MD; Justine Bacchetta, MD, PhD; Walter Jimenez, MD; and Isidro B. Salusky, MD

CASE STUDY

During a consultation for diarrhea and dehydration, the pediatrician notes that a 7-year-old boy has growth retardation. His parents report a decreased appetite, a decreased level of physical activity, and bed-wetting, despite having been previously potty trained. His medical history is significant for multiple episodes of fever due to presumed ear infections during his first years of life and one episode of urinary tract infection, without further studies. After hydration, the physical examination reveals a pale and short patient (height 101 cm [<fifth percentile]) with blood pressure above the 99th percentile for age, gender, and height. Routine laboratory studies reveal anemia, a serum creatinine of 1.4 mg/dL, and 3+ proteinuria.

Questions

1. How do you estimate renal function in children?
2. What are the relevant questions to ask about medical and family history in children who present with **chronic kidney disease (CKD)?**
3. What additional diagnostic tests should be performed to determine the etiology of the kidney disease?
4. What are the approaches to the management of children with CKD?

Although the kidney is mainly responsible for excretion or clearance of waste products, it also plays important roles in the regulation of acid-base status, electrolytes, and water and the synthesis of erythropoietin (EPO), renin, and 1,25-dihydroxycholecalciferol. When the kidney is affected, the regulation of multiple functions is disturbed. To differentiate chronic kidney disease (CKD) from acute kidney injury, CKD is defined as at least 3 months of abnormal renal function. Currently, **glomerular filtration rate (GFR)** is the best method to detect, evaluate, and manage CKD. The GFR varies according to gender, age, and body size and reflects the amount of plasma cleared by the kidney (Box 146-1). It can be challenging to evaluate

GFR in children; however, the 2009 Schwartz et al formula has been shown to be accurate for a range of GFRs, from 15 to 75 mL/min/1.73 m^2. Early recognition of children with CKD is important to prevent complications associated with progressive decline in renal function. Signs and symptoms of CKD in children are nonspecific; thus, it is vital that the primary medical professional, usually a pediatrician or family practitioner, recognizes the earliest signs and symptoms of CKD and institutes proper medical care. Prompt referral to a pediatric nephrologist must be made, and follow-up consultations by both physicians should be performed regularly to optimize management of these children.

The Kidney Disease: Improving Global Outcomes (KDIGO) "2012 Clinical Practice Guideline for the Evaluation and Management of Chronic Kidney Disease" states that pediatric CKD may be diagnosed by GFR less than 60 mL/min/1.73 m^2 for at least 3 months or GFR greater than 60 mL/min/1.73 m^2 accompanied by evidence of structural abnormalities or other markers of functional kidney abnormalities, including proteinuria, tubular disorders, or pathologic abnormalities detected by histology or inferred from imaging. In children at least 2 years old, depending on the GFR, the physician can classify kidney function into stages (Table 146-1). Stages 1 and 2 are defined by a GFR of more than 90 mL/min/1.73 m^2 and 60 to 89 mL/min/1.73 m^2, respectively. Chronic kidney disease staging is important because management guidelines are based on CKD stage, and CKD progression is associated with certain comorbidities. Ameliorating CKD-associated comorbidity may reduce long-term cardiovascular disease risk factors and improve clinical outcomes. Particular importance should be placed on managing **growth, proteinuria, acidosis, anemia, hypertension,** and **metabolic bone**

Box 146-1. How to Evaluate Glomerular Filtration Rate in Children

1. **Measuring the true glomerular filtration rate (GFR)**

   Reference standard: inulin clearance, iothalamate, iohexol

   Expensive, time-consuming

   Not for everyday practice

2. **Evaluating the GFR**

   A. **Measured from a 24-hour urine collection**

   $$GFR = \frac{\text{Urine creatinine (mg/dL)} \times \text{Volume of urine (mL)}}{\text{Time of urine sampling (min)} \times \text{Plasma creatinine (mg/dL)}}$$

   GFR (normalized for 1.73 m^2) = creatinine clearance × 1.73/body surface area

   B. **Estimated from a spot blood sample (2009 Schwartz et al formula)**

   GFR (mL/min/1.73 m^2) = 0.413 × Height (cm)/Plasma creatinine (mg/dL)

Table 146-1. Classification of Chronic Kidney Disease	
Stage	Glomerular Filtration Rate (mL/min/1.73 m²)
1	≥90
2	60–89
3a	45–59
3b	30–44
4	15–29
5	<15

disease. Once the GFR declines to 15 to 29 mL/min/1.73 m² (stage 4 CKD), patients and families should be prepared for **renal replacement therapy** and possible **renal transplantation. End-stage renal disease (ESRD)** (or stage 5 CKD) is defined as a GFR of less than 15 mL/min/1.73 m² or the need for **dialysis** or **transplant.** All children with CKD should be referred early to a pediatric nephrologist to facilitate management of the patient and education of the family. In adult patients with CKD, late referral is associated with increased rates of morbidity and mortality.

In newborns, normal GFR is less than 60 mL/min/1.73 m², and body surface area–adjusted GFR values do not reach adult levels until 2 years of age. As such, GFR threshold values used to stage CKD are not applicable to children younger than 2 years. There are many references for normal GFR in preterm and term newborns; one of the most comprehensive tables is included in a 2007 review by Schwartz and Furth (see Selected References). Glomerular filtration rate values between 1 and 2 standard deviations below the mean should be considered moderately reduced, and GFR values at least 2 standard deviations below the mean should be considered severely reduced.

As studies in adult CKD patients have found that morbidity and mortality associates not only with GFR level but also with degree of albuminuria, the 2012 KDIGO guidelines recommend classifying adult CKD by GFR and albuminuria category. Although similar large-scale trials assessing albuminuria severity and clinical outcomes in the pediatric CKD population are currently lacking, prospective studies are ongoing. As such, albuminuria is not currently used to classify pediatric CKD, although it may be employed in the near future, pending further clinical data accumulation.

Epidemiology

The incidence of CKD in children is unknown. Current estimates are based on the number of children accepted for dialysis and renal transplantation; however, some children do not require dialysis or transplantation until adulthood. In 2008, the North American Pediatric Renal Trials and Collaborative Studies (NAPRTCS) reported 7,037 patients with an estimated GFR of 75 mL/min/1.73 m² or less. The causes of CKD can be broadly categorized into 2 main groups: congenital and acquired. Congenital conditions such as **obstructive uropathy, aplasia/hypoplasia/dysplasia, reflux nephropathy,** and **prune-belly syndrome** accounted for the majority of diagnoses (53%) and are summarized as CAKUT (congenital *a*bnormalities of the *k*idney and *u*rinary *t*ract). Among the acquired conditions, **focal segmental glomerulosclerosis** is the most prevalent diagnosis at 9%. Overall, males are more often affected by CKD (64%). Age at registry entry varies, with 20% of children entered into the registry before 2 years of age, 16% between 2 and 5 years of age, 32% between 6 and 12 years of age, 28% between 13 and 17 years of age, and 4% after the age of 17 years; however, time at registry entry does not strictly correspond to age at time of CKD diagnosis.

Clinical and Biological Presentation

Children with CKD are often asymptomatic or present with nonspecific symptoms, and abnormal renal function is detected during routine health examinations or screening. For a small percentage of these patients, CKD is incidentally discovered when patients present with other illnesses, such as diarrhea and dehydration. Patients may be referred to the physician because of **growth retardation, hypertension,** or **anemia** (Box 146-2). Occasionally, a history of recurrent episodes of fever without a source or partially treated urinary tract infections (UTIs) secondary to undiagnosed vesicoureteral reflux is uncovered. Children may also complain of vague generalized symptoms, including malaise, anorexia, and vomiting, which may be associated with advanced renal failure.

Metabolic and Water/Electrolyte Abnormalities

Children with congenital abnormalities such as obstructive uropathy or renal dysplasia may develop polyuria due to an inability to concentrate urine. As such, salt wasting and polydipsia may become prominent features of the patients' diseases; in such cases, blood pressure is usually normal. A history of **bed-wetting** may therefore be a clue to CKD. In contrast, children with advanced CKD may have impaired sodium excretion leading to water retention and, consequently, fluid overload and secondary hypertension. **Hyperkalemia** is not an uncommon component of CKD, and it becomes evident when the GFR falls below 10 mL/min/1.73 m². **Hypokalemia** is a less common problem and may be secondary to excessive diuretic use or strict dietary restriction; it may also be the hallmark of tubulointerstitial disease (proximal tubulopathy) during the early stages of CKD.

Box 146-2. General Symptoms Associated With Chronic Kidney Disease
• Growth retardation/growth failure
• Anorexia
• Anemia
• Bone disease
• Metabolic acidosis
• Hypertension

Metabolic acidosis is mainly caused by the overall decrease in ammonia excretion from a reduced number of nephrons. Decreased excretion of titratable acid, as well as bicarbonate wasting in cases of proximal renal tubular acidosis, may also play a role.

Glucose intolerance may occur in some children with CKD despite elevated insulin levels, independent of genetic diseases such as hepatocyte nuclear factor 1β mutations, which induce renal cysts and atypical diabetes mellitus. The linear correlation between a decline in renal function and insulin resistance even at the early stages of CKD has been shown in adults. More than 50% of children develop **hyperlipidemia** by the time they reach ESRD. The characteristic plasma lipid abnormality is a moderate **hypertriglyceridemia.** There is also a high prevalence of **hypercholesterolemia** and low levels of high-density lipids and albumin. These derangements have a role in cardiovascular disease development.

Growth Failure

Failure to thrive is the hallmark of CKD in children, and the degree of growth retardation varies according to the age of presentation. Indeed, as maximal growth occurs during the first years of life, children with congenital renal problems are the most affected. In the NAPRTCS, height deficits were greatest for children younger than 5 years, with nearly 50% below the third percentile for age and gender. Growth failure develops early in the course of CKD and affects up to 35% of this population; by the time of renal transplantation, many children have severe short stature. Moreover, children with more severely impaired renal function tend to have greater height deficits. Sexual development is often delayed in affected patients as well as bone age. Uremia, anorexia, and frequent vomiting contribute to the **protein and calorie malnutrition** frequently observed in younger children with CKD. Early, intensive management is often required to maximize nutritional status and optimize growth.

Mineral and Bone Disorders Associated With Chronic Kidney Disease

The effect of CKD on mineral and bone disorders (MBD) may be immediate (eg, biological disequilibrium of calcium, phosphate, vitamin D, and parathyroid hormone [PTH]) or delayed (eg, growth retardation, bone pain, fractures, bone deformities, extraskeletal and vascular calcifications, increased morbidity and mortality). The development of CKD-MBD begins early in the course of CKD; clinical manifestations include growth retardation and skeletal deformities such as **genu valgum, ulnar deviation of the hands, pes varus,** and **slipped capital femoral epiphyses.** Whereas the term *renal osteodystrophy* refers specifically to different bone lesions as defined by bone histomorphometry, the term *CKD-MBD* is used to define clinical and biochemical abnormalities as well as the long-term consequences of alterations in bone and mineral metabolism associated with CKD. Thus, CKD-MBD is manifested by one or a combination of the following abnormalities: abnormalities of calcium, phosphorus, PTH, or vitamin D metabolism; abnormalities in bone histology, linear growth, or strength; and vascular or other soft tissue calcification.

Anemia

The anemia of CKD is normochromic and normocytic. Insufficient EPO production occurs when the GFR is less than 30 mL/min/1.73 m². Anemia is frequently accompanied by decreased serum iron levels, increased total iron-binding capacity, and low reticulocyte counts. Dialysis patients are predisposed to develop bleeding tendencies secondary to platelet dysfunction and mechanical hemolysis.

Hypertension

The incidence of **hypertension** in children with CKD varies from 38% to 78%. Prolonged hypertension may accelerate deterioration of renal function. An acute rise in blood pressure may cause seizures in children. Other manifestations include headache, epistaxis, congestive heart failure, nerve palsies, and cerebral hemorrhage. Hypertension is frequently seen in children with CKD secondary to polycystic kidney disease or chronic glomerulonephritis.

Cardiac Dysfunction

Patients are at increased risk of left ventricular hypertrophy (LVH), vascular calcification, and congestive heart failure. Left ventricular hypertrophy, as diagnosed by echocardiogram, is present in 75% of adults with CKD; hypertension and anemia are important contributing factors. Left ventricular hypertrophy is also seen in the pediatric CKD population, with a prevalence of 10% to 20% in CKD stages 3 and 4. Fluid overload, refractory hypertension, severe anemia, and uremic cardiomyopathy may contribute to **congestive heart failure**.

Neurologic Dysfunction

Children with CKD may have **impaired neurodevelopment** related to the age of presentation. Memory deficits, lack of concentration, depression, and weakness may occur. Children younger than 5 years are more affected because significant brain growth and maturation occur during the early years of life. Children who are severely uremic may suffer from global developmental delay and seizures. Unless neurodevelopmental delays are recognized promptly and early intervention is instituted, neurologic dysfunction is often progressive. Of note, some genetic diseases involving cerebral and renal development may play a role in developmental delay.

Pathophysiology

The Final Common Pathways in Nephron Loss

Regardless of the type of initial injury to the kidney, glomerular hyperfiltration and tubulointerstitial damage are the final common pathways of glomerular destruction. Hyperfiltration occurs as a response by the residual glomeruli to compensate for the loss of nephrons, as summarized in Figure 146-1. Reduced filtration results in increased production of **renin** and **angiotensin-converting enzyme (ACE)**. The consequent vasoconstriction of the efferent arteriole increases the hydrostatic pressure on the capillary wall, leading to a compensatory higher filtration rate per nephron but also to

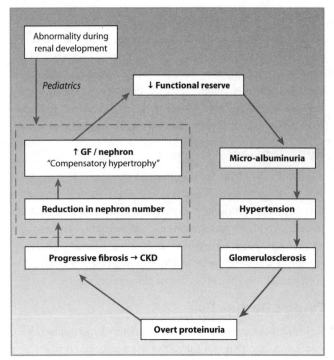

Figure 146-1. The consequences of reduction in nephron number. Abbreviations: CKD, chronic kidney disease; GF, glomerular filtration.

increased protein transit across the wall. Proteinuria recruits inflammatory cells and upregulates proinflammatory and profibrotic genes. Protein overload in tubular cells stimulates their differentiation into myofibroblasts, promoting fibrosis. Concurrently, the inflammatory cascade activates the complement system, leading to additional kidney damage. Interstitial fibrosis impairs oxygenation of the tubular cells; the chronic hypoxia then further activates the renin-angiotensin system. In addition to their antihypertensive properties, ACE inhibitors or angiotensin receptor blockers (ARBs) may reduce intra-glomerular pressure, proteinuria, and the consequent tubulointerstitial fibrosis, thus potentially slowing the rate of CKD progression.

Growth Failure

Multiple factors are involved in the pathogenesis of growth retardation in children with CKD, including deficient calorie and protein intake, decreased EPO production, metabolic acidosis, decreased serum levels of **insulinlike growth factor (IGF) 1**, peripheral resistance to growth hormone secondary to decreased levels of growth hormone binding proteins and growth hormone receptors, renal osteodystrophy, hypogonadism, and drug toxicity (corticosteroids). In children, renal osteodystrophy involves alteration of the growth plate cartilage architecture, contributing to growth failure. Adynamic bone lesions and severe hyperparathyroidism increase the severity of growth retardation. In teenagers with CKD, the loss of pulsatile secretion of gonadotropin-releasing hormone contributes to shortening of the pubertal growth spurt and reduced growth velocity.

Mineral and Bone Disorders Associated With Chronic Kidney Disease

The development of **renal osteodystrophy** is multifactorial. Reduced renal mass results in decreased synthesis of 1,25-**dihydroxycholecalciferol**; as such, the stimulus to absorb calcium from the gut decreases. The resultant hypocalcemia and lack of vitamin D feedback on the parathyroid glands stimulate the production of PTH, facilitating rapid mobilization of calcium from the skeleton, thus normalizing serum calcium at the bone's expense. As CKD advances, skeletal resistance to PTH occurs, and circulating levels of PTH increase.

Hyperparathyroidism and the resultant high bone remodeling produces fibrosis in bone, a condition termed **osteitis fibrosa.** Administration of exogenous vitamin D and its derivatives can suppress such bone remodeling but, if not adequately monitored, can result in low bone remodeling disease (adynamic bone). In this case, serum PTH and alkaline phosphatase levels usually are lower than in patients with secondary hyperparathyroidism and high bone remodeling disease.

Hyperphosphatemia develops when the few remaining nephrons lose the ability to excrete the daily load of phosphorus from the diet; it is a late phenomenon, usually occurring in CKD stages 4 and 5. In the past, aluminum-containing phosphate binders contributed to the pathogenesis of osteomalacia, characterized by poorly mineralized osteoid, and adynamic bone disease; currently, the use of large doses of calcium-based phosphate binders and active vitamin D sterols are implicated. Biochemical abnormalities present in CKD-MBD, including abnormal calcium-phosphate metabolism, hyperparathyroidism, and increased levels of fibroblast growth factor 23 (FGF23) (see following paragraph), in association with traditional cardiovascular disease risk factors, such as hypertension, hyperlipidemia, hyperhomocysteinemia, anemia, and oxidative stress, contribute significantly to the development of cardiovascular disease, the leading cause of death in ESRD. In young adults with childhood-onset CKD, the prevalence of coronary artery calcification can be as high as 92% when evaluated by sequential computed tomography (CT) scan with electrocardiogram gating.

In the early 2000s, FGF23 was identified as the pathogenic hormone in various forms of hypophosphatemic rickets and tumor-induced osteomalacia. Secreted by osteocytes, FGF23 functions as a phosphaturic hormone and as a suppressor of renal 1-α-hydroxylase. Circulating FGF23 levels have been observed to increase early in the CKD course. Contributing to these elevated levels may be decreased FGF23 clearance, increased synthesis by osteocytes, a compensatory mechanism attempting to maintain normal hypophosphatemia, or a response to treatment with active vitamin D analogs. In CKD populations, elevated FGF23 levels are associated with renal disease progression, cardiovascular morbidity, cardiovascular mortality, and all-cause mortality. In vitro and animal studies have shown that FGF23 may directly induce LVH.

Anemia

Chronic kidney disease anemia begins when the GFR falls below 30 mL/min/1.73 m² and is multifactorial, possibly also involving decreased EPO production, decreased red cell survival, bone marrow inhibition, iron deficiency, vitamin B_{12} and folate deficiency, inflammation, and osteitis fibrosa. In the past, aluminum toxicity was also implicated in CKD anemia. Blood loss during hemodialysis sessions may be contributory, as well. Recently, hepcidin, a hormone synthesized in the liver, was found to be central to the pathogenesis of CKD-associated anemia. Hepcidin causes the internalization of ferroportin, a protein that exports iron from the intracellular space to the extracellular compartment. Decreased hepcidin activity results in iron overload, whereas increased hepcidin activity is associated with anemia. Iron loading and inflammation increase hepcidin levels, and EPO treatment decreases hepcidin levels. As GFR declines, hepcidin levels increase, resulting in ferroportin internalization, intracellular iron sequestration, and functional iron deficiency, contributing to the anemia of CKD.

Differential Diagnosis

Instead of crafting a differential diagnosis, the main challenge for the physician initially will be to determine whether renal impairment is acute or chronic and, if chronic, its etiology. A variety of kidney problems, whether congenital, hereditary, acquired, or metabolic, may result in CKD. Although specific cures are not available for most of these renal conditions, it is essential to perform a complete diagnostic workup to determine the etiology of the renal disease. Such information may identify the presence of an inherited problem that may require genetic counseling and, in some cases, anticipation of problems associated with renal transplantation. Some renal diseases may recur after renal transplantation (eg, focal segmental glomerulosclerosis, atypical hemolytic uremic syndrome); parents and children must be informed early about this possibility in preparation for renal transplantation. The different etiologies of CKD, as well as their prevalence in the 2008 NAPRTCS registry, are summarized in Table 146-2.

At initial presentation, it is necessary to differentiate between acute and chronic renal failure because therapeutic strategies may differ and long-term renal prognoses can be quite different. Hereditary diseases commonly encountered include hereditary nephritis (Alport syndrome), branchio-oto-renal (BOR) syndrome, and juvenile nephronophthisis. Acquired diseases, such as chronic glomerulonephritis, membranoproliferative glomerulonephritis (MPGN), and focal and segmental glomerulosclerosis, affect a large percentage of older children who progress to CKD. Anemia, hypertension, and fluid and electrolyte abnormalities are often associated with chronic and acute renal failure. Suboptimal linear growth and signs and symptoms of renal osteodystrophy develop over time in patients with chronic renal impairment.

Evaluation

A complete evaluation of children presenting with renal failure must be performed.

History

A thorough history must be obtained, including a complete and detailed family history, as this may provide some clues to the patient's diagnosis (Questions Box). A prenatal history, including possible drug exposures and results of antenatal imaging, may also provide useful information.

Table 146-2. Etiologies of Pediatric Chronic Kidney Disease (2008 North American Pediatric Renal Trials and Collaborative Studies)

	Disease	Percentage
CAKUT	Obstructive uropathy	20.7
	Aplasia/hypoplasia/dysplasia	17.3
	Reflux nephropathy	8.4
	Prune-belly syndrome	2.7
Genetic diseases	Polycystic disease	4.0
	Cystinosis	1.5
	Oxalosis	0.1
	Denys-Drash syndrome	0.1
	Congenital nephrotic syndrome	1.1
	Medullary cystic disease	1.3
Glomerular diseases	FSGS	8.7
	Chronic GN	1.2
	MPGN type 1	1.1
	MPGN type 2	0.4
	IgA nephritis	0.9
	Henoch-Schönlein nephritis	0.6
	Idiopathic crescentic GN	0.7
	Membranous nephropathy	0.5
Systemic diseases	HUS	2.0
	SLE nephritis	1.6
	Wegener granulomatosis	0.4
	Other systemic immunologic diseases	0.4
	Diabetic nephropathy	0.2
	Sickle cell nephropathy	0.2
Miscellaneous	Familial nephritis	1.6
	Pyelonephritis/interstitial nephritis	1.4
	Renal infarct	2.2
	Wilms tumor	0.5
	Others	15.8
	Unknown	2.6

Abbreviations: CAKUT, congenital abnormalities of kidney and urinary tract; CKD, chronic kidney disease; FSGS, focal segmental glomerulosclerosis; GN, glomerulonephritis; HUS, hemolytic uremic syndrome; IgA, immunoglobulin A; MPGN, membranoproliferative glomerulonephritis; SLE, systemic lupus erythematosus.

Physical Examination

A complete physical examination is required. Height and weight must be measured accurately, and the results should be plotted on the same growth curves used for healthy children. Weight may be overestimated if fluid retention is present. Blood pressure, using an

Chronic Kidney Disease

Questions

- **Does the child have**
  — Abnormalities on prenatal ultrasound such as hydronephrosis or polyhydramnios/oligohydramnios?
  — A history of prolonged illness, pallor, weakness, vomiting, or loss of appetite?
  — Any history of headaches or visual or hearing problems?
  — Any history of hematuria, proteinuria (foamy or bubbling urine), urinary tract infections, or episodes of fever with unknown source?
  — Impaired growth or development compared with siblings and other children?
  — Any problems with micturition, such as dribbling or weak stream?
  — Polyuria or polydipsia?
  — Daytime or nighttime enuresis?

  If so, what was the age at presentation?

- **Does any family member have**
  — Any kidney diseases (including hematuria, proteinuria, kidney cysts, or urinary tract infections) or have they undergone any urologic surgery?
  — Need for dialysis or kidney transplantation?
  — History of ear/hearing problems or eye abnormalities?

Figure 146-2. Initial diagnostic workup of a pediatric patient with chronic renal failure. Abbreviations: ANA, antinuclear antibodies; ds, double-stranded; BUN, blood urea nitrogen; CBC, complete blood cell count; DMSA, dimercapto-succinic acid; GFR, glomerular filtration rate; HPF, high-power field; HSP, Henoch-Schönlein purpura; IgA, immunoglobulin A; MPGN, membranoproliferative glomerulonephritis; RBC, red blood cell; SLE, systemic lupus erythematosus; UTI, urinary tract infection; VCUG, voiding cystourethrogram.

appropriately sized cuff, must be taken. Blood pressure measurements should be compared to the 50th percentile for age, gender, and height (www.nhlbi.nih.gov). The presence of tachycardia, heart murmurs, or adventitious heart sounds that may indicate uncompensated anemia or cardiac or pericardial involvement must be noted. Gross eye examination should be performed, including fundal examination, to assess for evidence of chronic hypertension. Macular abnormalities or hearing problems may provide clues to heritable diseases, such as Alport syndrome. Ear abnormalities, such as preauricular pits or ear tags, accompanied by hearing deficits, may be associated with renal disease (eg, BOR syndrome). Undescended testes may be evident in some children with urogenital problems.

Laboratory Tests

For the initial laboratory workup, complete blood cell count, electrolytes, blood urea nitrogen, creatinine, calcium, phosphorus, and urinalysis should be obtained (Figure 146-2). Glomerulonephritis usually presents with numerous red blood cells, white blood cells, proteinuria, and a variety of casts in the urine. In cases of proteinuria, if a 24-hour collection is impossible, quantified excretion should be estimated by a protein-creatinine ratio in a spot urine sample. A ratio greater than 0.2 is abnormal and is well correlated with urinary protein excretion greater than 4 mg/m^2/hour in a 24-hour urine collection. In nephrotic syndrome, the proteinuria is usually greater than 40 mg/m^2/hour. Immunologic studies, including C_3, C_4, antinuclear antibody, and anti–double-stranded DNA, as well as a minimal infectious disease evaluation (hepatitis B and C), should be obtained if the renal disease suggests the presence of an immune

complex–mediated glomerulonephritis (eg, systemic lupus erythematosus, postinfectious glomerulonephritis, MPGN).

Imaging Studies

Ultrasound is by far one of the best radiographic tools in the assessment of patients with CKD. Renal ultrasound yields important information, such as kidney size, echogenicity, and the presence of hydronephrosis, cysts, or stones, that may help establish the diagnosis of the renal disease. The presence of small kidneys usually indicates chronic disease that may date back to fetal development. Increased echogenicity with normal kidney size indicates the presence of medical renal disease in most cases.

A **voiding cystourethrogram** is indicated in patients with hydronephrosis and recurrent UTIs to diagnose vesicoureteral reflux and evaluate the anatomy of the upper urinary tract. The use of the spiral CT scan in the evaluation of patients with renal failure has increased over the last few years. This procedure requires relatively less time than the standard CT scan and can be used to evaluate the kidney parenchyma as well as the upper and lower urinary tract.

Nuclear imaging of the kidneys has provided vital information in the workup of children with CKD. In general, nuclear studies are not routinely done unless specifically indicated. A technetium Tc 99m mertiatide scan may be used to assess renal plasma flow. A technetium Tc 99m dimercaptosuccinic acid scan may be used to assess renal parenchymal involvement in acute pyelonephritis and recurrent UTIs. This nuclear imaging study provides excellent images of the renal parenchyma and is frequently used to detect renal scarring in patients with recurrent UTIs. Significant renal parenchymal scarring portends the development of hypertension later in life.

Management

The management of children with CKD has markedly improved over the last 2 decades and is summarized in Figure 146-3. Newer treatment options and earlier intervention strategies have greatly improved the lives of affected children. These patients must be managed by multidisciplinary teams involving primary care physicians, nephrologists, nurses, social workers, nutritionists, and psychologists. Comprehensive management includes treatment of the primary disease and comorbid conditions, growth optimization, slowing disease progression, preserving residual renal function, preventing CKD-MBD and cardiovascular disease, and preparing for renal replacement therapy and renal transplantation as CKD progresses. To delay the progression toward ESRD and cardiovascular mortality, medical management of patients with CKD includes strict control of hypertension; prevention of obesity; control of proteinuria with ACE inhibitors or ARBs; management of serum calcium, phosphorus, and PTH levels; anemia treatment; and prompt treatment of infections.

Malnutrition; Metabolic and Water/Electrolyte Abnormalities

Dietary management remains an important and challenging aspect of the overall management of children with CKD. Frequently, these children are anorectic and require supplementation with fat, carbohydrates, and protein. Some patients, especially younger children, may require enteral feeding by nasogastric or gastrostomy tube to meet their daily nutritional requirements. Children with CKD should receive the recommended daily allowance for protein and calories according to age and gender; adjustments should be made depending on weight gain. Protein restriction is not advised; studies have shown that restriction of protein intake does not delay the progression of renal failure in these patients. Close monitoring of nutritional status should be performed at each visit, with serial measurements of height and body weight; in children younger than 3 years, head circumference should also be measured.

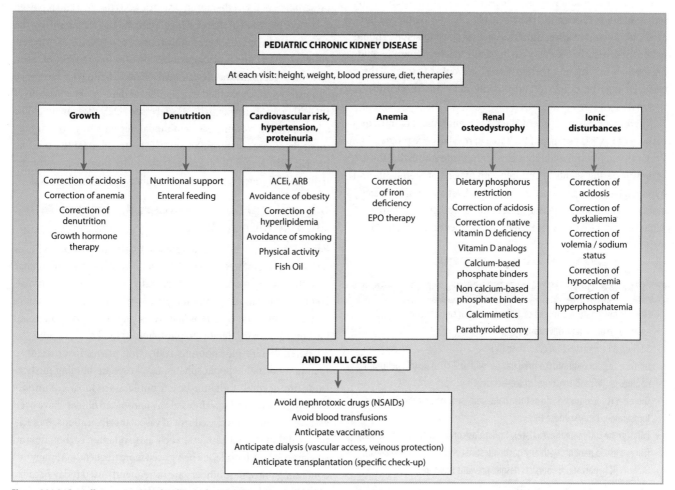

Figure 146-3. Overall management of pediatric chronic kidney disease. Abbreviations: ACEi, angiotensin-converting enzyme inhibitors; ARB: angiotensin receptor blockers; EPO: erythropoietin; NSAIDs: nonsteroidal anti-inflammatory drugs.

Daily salt and fluid intake among patients may vary. Patients with hypertension may require relative dietary salt restriction. Conversely, patients with congenitally obstructed, dysplastic kidneys or nephronophthisis often have polyuria and salt wasting, requiring increased fluid intake and sodium supplementation.

Oral base therapy should be used to maintain bicarbonate levels above 22 mEq/L, as recommended by the National Kidney Foundation Kidney Disease Outcomes Quality Initiative guidelines, as metabolic acidosis may have many deleterious effects, including worsening of bone disease, growth retardation, increased muscle wasting, decreased albumin synthesis, resistance to insulin, stimulation of inflammation, and increased overall mortality.

Most children with CKD do not become hyperkalemic unless their renal function falls below 10 mL/min/1.73 m^2. Initially, dietary intervention may be sufficient, but this is difficult in infants and small children whose diet is limited to formula and only a few solid foods. Pharmacologic interventions, such as diuretics and polystyrene sulfone, are used to manage **hyperkalemia** in these children. In situations in which there is an acute rise in the serum potassium level, emergent measures must be implemented (Box 146-3). Sodium bicarbonate, insulin/glucose, and β$_2$-agonists (eg, albuterol) acutely decrease the serum potassium level by facilitating intracellular potassium uptake. If the hyperkalemia is unresponsive to conservative medical measures, dialysis must be performed immediately. In the setting of fluid overload and hyperkalemia, diuretic use may be indicated; potassium-sparing diuretics such as spironolactone should not be used. Also, in patients with impaired concentrating and diluting mechanisms, diuretic therapy should be avoided, as some of these children may be polyuric and become dehydrated on diuretic therapy.

There is increasing concern about the management of **lipid disturbances** in CKD because of their role in renal disease progression. Presently, no recommendations have been made addressing the use of lipid-lowering agents in children with hypercholesterolemia and hypertriglyceridemia because of reported liver and muscle toxicity associated with some of these medications. Further studies are warranted to test the efficacy and safety of these medications in the pediatric population.

Box 146-3. Treatment of Hyperkalemia

- Calcium gluconate, 0.5 mL/kg of 10% solution, or calcium chloride, 0.2 mL/kg of 10% solution (intravenous)
- Sodium bicarbonate, 2 mEq/kg/dose (IV)
- Glucose-insulin solution, 0.5 g/kg glucose with 0.25 U of insulin per gram of glucose (IV; monitor serum glucose closely.)
- Diuretics (Loop diuretics; do not use potassium-sparing diuretics.): furosemide, 1 mg/kg/dose (IV)
- Polystyrene sulfonate (Kayexalate), 1 g/kg/dose orally (if awake) or rectally (Do not use in patients with any gastrointestinal problems or anomalies.)
- Dialysis (if hyperkalemia persists despite previous measures)

Growth Failure

Recombinant human growth hormone (rhGH) therapy has improved the management of growth retardation in children with CKD; it should be considered in children with height below the fifth percentile. The 2012 KDIGO international guidelines recommend that children and adolescents with CKD stages 2 through 5 with related height deficits should be treated with rhGH when further growth is desired, after first addressing malnutrition and the biochemical abnormalities of CKD-MBD. Several studies have demonstrated a positive effect of rhGH on linear growth but with variable results according to CKD stage at the initiation of rhGH. In the NAPRTCS database, catch-up growth after rhGH therapy was observed in 27% of children with chronic renal insufficiency, 25% of transplanted children, and only 11% of children undergoing renal replacement therapy, highlighting the need for early management of growth failure in pediatric CKD. Moreover, the response during the first year correlates with final height. Growth hormone administration is continued until the patient reaches the 50th percentile for mid-parental height or renal transplant is achieved. Of note, growth hormone therapy is contraindicated in patients with a history of malignancy, hyperglycemia, hyperinsulinemia, or significant scoliosis.

A recent retrospective multicenter US study noted the underprescription of rhGH therapy in pediatric CKD patients and reported that more than half of short CKD children did not receive rhGH. The most common reasons were family refusal, severe secondary hyperparathyroidism, and noncompliance; however, in up to 25% of cases, no evident rationale was determined. Of note, waiting for insurance company approval resulted in a significant delay in the initiation of rhGH therapy in 18% of patients. Access to rhGH therapy should be a high priority. Newer treatment modalities targeting growth hormone resistance (eg, recombinant IGF-1, recombinant IGF binding protein [BP] 3, IGF BP displacers) are under investigation for the treatment of growth retardation in pediatric patients with CKD.

Mineral and Bone Disorders Associated With Chronic Kidney Disease

For the management of renal osteodystrophy, dietary phosphorus restriction is reinforced in children with CKD; however, adherence with this dietary modification is generally poor secondary to unpalatability of the food. Additionally, many processed foods contain large amounts of phosphorous that are usually not taken into account but contribute considerably to phosphorous intake.

When dietary phosphorous restriction proves insufficient to maintain normal hypophosphatemia, phosphate-binding medications are needed. Calcium-based binders are most commonly employed; however, large doses of calcium-based binders have been associated with an increased risk of vascular calcifications. As such, non–calcium-based binders, such as sevelamer carbonate and sevelamer hydrochloride, are being used more frequently. Aluminum-containing phosphate binders are infrequently used today because of the risk of aluminum toxicity and should be avoided as first-line therapies. If used, precautions must be taken in children who are concomitantly treated with citrate-containing medications, as citrate enhances aluminum absorption, thus enhancing toxicity risk.

Secondary hyperparathyroidism often develops in children with CKD. The 2012 KDIGO guidelines recommend a serum PTH level within the normal range in CKD stages 1 and 2, and between 2 to 9 times the upper limit of normal in dialysis patients. Between 15 and 60 mL/min/1.73 m², the optimal level of PTH is unknown. Management of secondary hyperparathyroidism involves first correcting hyperphosphatemia, hypocalcemia, and vitamin D deficiency. If the patient is vitamin D sufficient with normal calcium and phosphorous and still has elevated PTH levels, treatment with activated vitamin D sterols, such as calcitriol or doxercalciferol, may be warranted. Patients receiving activated vitamin D sterols should be frequently monitored for the development of hypercalcemia or hyperphosphatemia; in such cases, dose modification or phosphate binder adjustment may be required.

Lastly, if present, 25-hydroxyvitamin D deficiency may require treatment. Optimal levels of 25-hydroxyvitamin D are greater than 30 ng/mL (75 nmol/L). Vitamin D deficiency is highly prevalent in pediatric patients across the spectrum of CKD (between 40% and 80% of children), resulting from several factors such as low dietary intake, chronic illness, skin changes, and sometimes urinary losses in proteinuric patients.

Anemia

The use of recombinant human EPO in the anemia associated with CKD has become a standard of treatment. The correction of anemia results in improved appetite, increased physical activity, and more importantly, avoidance of the risks associated with blood transfusion. Prior to the availability of EPO, most patients received frequent blood transfusions, increasing their risks of infection, transfusion reaction, and development of antibodies. The goal is to keep the hemoglobin between 11 to 12 g/dL. Iron stores are assessed by transferrin saturation and ferritin levels and should be maintained between 20% to 50% and 200 to 800 ng/mL, respectively. With the elucidation of the hepcidin pathway and a better understanding of the pathophysiology of anemia, new therapeutic modalities will probably be available in the future to improve the management of anemia during pediatric CKD, such as prolyl-hydroxylase inhibitors, EPO-receptor agonists (eg, Omontys), oxygen-carrier products, and *GATA* inhibitors.

Arterial Hypertension

For chronic management, antihypertensive medications should be started in children if blood pressure measurements are consistently above the 90th percentile for age, sex, and height. The 2012 KDIGO CKD guidelines suggest that the blood pressure goal should be should be less than or equal to the 50th percentile for age, sex, and height unless achievement of this target blood pressure is limited by signs or symptoms of hypotension. Drugs currently used to treat hypertension in children with CKD include ACE inhibitors, diuretics, adrenergic blockers, peripheral vasodilators, and calcium channel

blockers. Angiotensin-converting enzyme inhibitors are often used as first-line antihypertensive agents in children with CKD and, as mentioned, treatment with ACE inhibitors has been shown to be beneficial in reducing proteinuria, which may help to inhibit proteinuria-associated tubulointerstitial inflammation and fibrosis. Angiotensin-converting enzyme inhibitors must be used with caution in patients with a solitary kidney and those with renal artery stenosis, as these medications may acutely decrease kidney function and precipitate hyperkalemia in patients with renal failure. Sexually active adolescent females must be informed about the adverse effects of ACE inhibitors in pregnancy, including renal tubular dysgenesis in the fetus. Calcium channel blockers, especially nifedipine, have been used in cases of severe hypertension because of their rapid onset of action. For patients with poor adherence to daily oral medications, clonidine is currently available in the form of transdermal patches. However, patients should be warned of central nervous system side effects, as well as rebound hypertension if the patch is removed abruptly. If hypertension is secondary to fluid overload and salt retention, aggressive fluid removal with diuretic therapy should be initiated. Patients with long-standing hypertension must have regular echocardiograms to assess for LVH and serial ophthalmologic examinations to assess for pathologic eye changes. For uncontrollable hypertension, which is often secondary to fluid overload, dialysis may be indicated (Box 146-4).

General Measures

In all cases, anticipation of dialysis or transplantation should be performed early in the course of CKD, as many CKD patients may progress to ESRD and require renal replacement therapy. Protection of upper extremity veins, in anticipation of the need for possible future vascular access, is important. Additionally, blood transfusions should be avoided as much as possible to prevent the development of hyperimmunization, potentially compromising a future transplant.

Children with CKD, as well as their siblings and household contacts, should receive all standard vaccines, including varicella, influenza, and

---

Box 146-4. Indications for Initiation of Dialysis

Severe fluid overload
- Congestive heart failure
- Uncontrollable hypertension

Uremic neuropathy
- Paresthesia

Electrolyte abnormalities unresponsive to medical management
- Intractable metabolic acidosis
- Hyperkalemia

Pericarditis

Severe renal osteodystrophy
- Extraskeletal calcification
- Severe skeletal deformities

Progressive malnutrition and severe growth retardation, especially in the first year of life

Severe anemia or bleeding diathesis

Streptococcus pneumoniae. Patients on immunosuppressive treatment because of glomerulonephritis or after transplant should not receive live-virus vaccines. Every attempt to administer live-virus vaccines, such as measles, mumps, rubella, and varicella, should be done before transplantation. Because children with CKD have a decreased ability to mount an immunologic response, repeated vaccination to induce protective serum antibody titers may be needed.

A review of all medications should be performed at every visit to adjust dosages according to kidney function, detect possible adverse effects, and identify any potentially dangerous drug interactions. Monitoring drug levels may be desirable when using antibiotics, anticonvulsants, digoxin, theophylline, and anticoagulants. To prevent toxicity, dosages of all medications should be altered based on estimated GFR. Special care should be taken when using antibiotics such as aminoglycosides and vancomycin, as well as nonsteroidal anti-inflammatory drugs, because of possible detrimental effects on residual kidney function, even in the early stages of CKD.

For contrast-requiring imaging studies in patients with GFR less than 60 mL/min/1.73 m² undergoing elective investigation involving the intravascular administration of iodinated radiocontrast media, the 2012 KDIGO CKD guidelines recommend avoidance of high osmolar agents; use of lowest possible radiocontrast dose; withdrawal of potentially nephrotoxic agents before and after the procedure; adequate hydration with saline before, during, and after the procedure; and measurement of GFR 48 to 96 hours after the procedure.

As stated in the 2012 KDIGO CKD guidelines, indications for referral to a pediatric nephrologist include acute or chronic reduction in renal function, poorly treated or severe hypertension, severe electrolyte abnormalities, the finding of significant abnormalities in urinary tract structure, the presence of systemic diseases likely to produce renal effects, the need for education in progressive conditions, performance and interpretation of renal biopsies, or allaying parental or patient anxiety. Early referral may provide the opportunity to slow renal disease progression and may result in improved clinical outcomes.

Timing of Dialysis Initiation

For pediatric nephrologists, the conversation with the patient's family about renal replacement therapy is initiated early in the CKD course. When to start dialysis is determined not by a certain GFR threshold but rather by multiple factors, including patient signs and symptoms, laboratory values, possibility of transplantation, and family circumstance. As mentioned in the 2012 KDIGO CKD guidelines, a recent pediatric review by Greenbaum and Schaefer states that generally agreed-on absolute indications for dialysis initiation include neurologic consequences attributable to uremia, hypertension that fails to respond to antihypertensive therapy, pulmonary edema unresponsive to diuretics, pericarditis, bleeding tendency, and refractory nausea or vomiting. Relative indications may include less severe uremic symptoms, hyperkalemia, hyperphosphatemia, malnutrition, and growth failure. Such indications for dialysis often occur when the GFR declines to less than 15 mL/min/1.73 m²; however, some patients may remain asymptomatic despite a GFR less than 15 mL/min/1.73 m², and other patients may warrant dialysis consideration at higher GFRs.

Prognosis

The prognosis for children with CKD has changed in the last 2 decades. Options for dialysis (hemodialysis or peritoneal dialysis) and kidney transplantation (deceased or living-related donor) should be discussed prior to the occurrence of ESRD. Strategies such as preemptive transplantation (ie, transplantation before the need for dialysis) are probably preferred but may not be achievable because of the median time on the waiting list. Technical advances in dialysis allow pediatric nephrologists to offer dialysis options to children of any age and have made long-term survival possible while children await renal transplantation.

Kidney transplantation is the ultimate treatment for children with CKD. Improvements in immunosuppressive medications and availability of other therapeutic strategies have considerably increased patient and graft survival after kidney transplantation. Full rehabilitation should be achieved after these children have undergone successful renal transplantation.

CASE RESOLUTION

The patient at the beginning of this chapter presents with a glomerular filtration rate of 30 mL/min/1.73 m², estimated by the 2009 Schwartz et al formula. The initial evaluation reveals anemia (hematocrit 28%, normal 36–48), low serum bicarbonate (17 mEq/L, normal 22–26), hypocalcemia (8 mg/dL, normal 8.6–10), hyperphosphatemia (7 mg/dL, normal 2.7–4.5), and elevated PTH (700 pg/mL, normal 10–65). Ultrasonography reveals that both kidneys are small with increased echogenicity, and voiding cystourethrogram reveals bilateral vesicoureteral reflux. Management of the primary disease is started with antibiotic prophylaxis to prevent further urinary tract infections, and the patient is referred to pediatric urology. Measures to slow the progression to end-stage renal disease are initiated, involving dietary intervention and treatment of comorbid conditions. Bicarbonate is started for metabolic acidosis; iron and recombinant human erythropoietin are started for anemia; and calcium carbonate is started as a phosphate binder/calcium supplement. The hypertension associated with proteinuria is best treated with an angiotensin-converting enzyme inhibitor. Growth hormone will be considered once the acidosis, anemia, and hyperparathyroidism are corrected. Immunizations are up-to-date. An appointment with the pediatric nephrology team is scheduled.

Selected References

Boydstun II. Chronic kidney disease in adolescents. *Adolesc Med Clin.* 2005;16(1):185–199

Daschner M. Drug dosage in children with reduced renal function. *Pediatr Nephrol.* 2005;20(12):1675–1686

Geary DF, Hodson EM, Craig JC. Interventions for bone disease in children with chronic kidney disease. *Cochrane Database Syst Rev.* 2010;(1):CD008327

Greenbaum LA, Schaefer F. The decision to initiate dialysis in a pediatric patient. In: Warady BA, Schaefer F, Alexander SR, eds. *Pediatric Dialysis.* New York, NY: Springer; 2012:85–100

Hogg RJ, Furth S, Lemley KV, et al. National Kidney Foundation's Kidney Disease Outcomes Quality Initiative clinical practice guidelines for chronic kidney disease in children and adolescents: evaluation, classification, and stratification. *Pediatrics*. 2003;111(6 Pt 1):1416–1421

Jüppner H, Wolf M, Salusky IB. FGF-23: more than a regulator of renal phosphate handling? *J Bone Miner Res*. 2010;25(10):2091–2097

Kidney Disease: Improving Global Outcomes Chronic Kidney Disease Work Group. KDIGO 2012 clinical practice guideline for the evaluation and management of chronic kidney disease. *Kidney Int*. 2013:S1–S150

Kuizon BD, Salusky IB. Growth retardation in children with chronic renal failure. *J Bone Miner Res*. 1999;14(10):1680–1690

National Kidney Foundation. K/DOQI clinical practice guidelines for chronic kidney disease: evaluation, classification, and stratification. *Am J Kidney Dis*. 2002;39(2 Suppl 1):S1–S266

Neuhaus TJ. Immunization in children with chronic renal failure: a practical approach. *Pediatr Nephrol*. 2004;19(12):1334–1339

Schwartz GJ, Furth SL. Glomerular filtration rate measurement and estimation in chronic kidney disease. *Pediatr Nephrol*. 2007; 22(11):1839–1848

Schwartz GJ, Muñoz A, Schneider MF, et al. New equations to estimate GFR in children with CKD. *J Am Soc Nephrol*. 2009;20(3):629–637

Sedman A, Friedman A, Boineau F, Strife CF, Fine R. Nutritional management of the child with mild to moderate chronic renal failure. *J Pediatr*. 1996;129(2): S13–S18

Vimalachandra D, Hodson EM, Willis NS, Craig JC, Cowell C, Knight JF. Growth hormone for children with chronic kidney disease. *Cochrane Database Syst Rev*. 2006;(3):CD003264

CHAPTER 147

Diabetes Mellitus

Jennifer K. Yee, MD, and Catherine S. Mao, MD

CASE STUDY

A 10-year-old girl presents with a 3-week history of nocturnal polyuria. Her mother reports that her daughter, previously overweight, seems to have lost weight in the past 2 months after receiving nutrition education. Laboratory tests reveal that the girl's serum sodium level is 130 mEq/L; potassium, 3.2 mEq/L; glucose, 324 mg/dL; and 1+ ketones. Urinalysis reveals specific gravity of 1.025 and moderate glucose and ketones. Her height and weight are within normal ranges for her age, and the remainder of her physical examination is unremarkable.

Questions

1. What is the pathophysiology of type 1 and type 2 diabetes?
2. What are diagnostic criteria for differentiating type 1 and type 2 diabetes?
3. What are the objectives of therapeutic interventions in children with diabetes?
4. What diagnostic evaluations are used in ongoing management of diabetes?
5. What are the acute and chronic complications associated with diabetes?
6. What is the role of "tight glycemic control" in children and adolescents?

Diabetes mellitus is the second most common chronic illness after asthma among children in developed countries. Diabetes mellitus is a metabolic imbalance that results from insulin deficiency, impairment of insulin action, or both. Advancement in the knowledge of the pathophysiology supports the assessment that diabetes is a heterogeneous disease involving immunologic, environmental, and genetic factors. This has led to a categorization of diabetes based on its pathophysiology rather than the therapeutic intervention. Diabetes associated with absolute insulin deficiency and impaired beta cell function is called **type 1** (previously juvenile onset or insulin-dependent), and diabetes associated with insulin resistance as well as impaired beta cell function is called **type 2** (previously adult-onset or non–insulin-dependent).

Epidemiology

In the past, more than 97% of children with diabetes presented with type 1 diabetes mellitus (DM1), with an overall incidence of 18 in 100,000 cases per year. In the past decade, 2 population-based studies showed a dramatic increase in the number of older children and adolescents presenting with type 2 diabetes mellitus (DM2). One study reviewed newly diagnosed cases of diabetes over a 12-year period and found that DM2 made up 4% of such cases before 1992 and 16% in 1994 in one Midwestern metropolitan area. Among adolescents, the relative incidence of DM2 increased from 3% to 10% before 1992 to 33% in 1994. By 1999 the proportion of diabetes in children and adolescents attributed to DM2 ranged from 8% to 45% depending on geographic location. In addition, the populations affected by DM1 and DM2 seem to differ. Type 1 diabetes mellitus is seen equally among girls and boys, with the highest incidence among white youth. Type 2 diabetes mellitus is more prevalent among girls and has the highest incidence among African American, Mexican American, and Native American populations. The peak age of presentation for DM1 is between 5 and 15 years of age. Less is known about DM2 in children, but previous studies show a mean age of 13.8 years at presentation.

The SEARCH for Diabetes in Youth Study is a population-based, observational study of physician-diagnosed diabetes among youth younger than 20 years from 6 centers. The overall prevalence estimate for diabetes in children and adolescents was approximately 0.18%. Type 2 diabetes was found in all racial/ethnic groups but generally was less common than DM1, except in American Indian youth.

Clinical Presentation

Children can vary in their clinical presentation from being asymptomatic to having fulminant metabolic imbalance (D_x Box). Type 1 diabetes mellitus commonly presents with a classic triad of polydipsia,

---

 Diabetes Mellitus

- Symptoms (polydipsia, polyuria, and polyphagia) together with a random plasma glucose higher than 200 mg/dL
- Fasting blood glucose higher than 126 mg/dL (confirmed on a subsequent day)
- Oral glucose tolerance test with 2-hour peak plasma glucose higher than 200 mg/dL
- Hemoglobin A_{1c} 6.5% or greater

polyuria, and polyphagia. The most consistent presenting complaint is increased urinary frequency, manifested as nighttime polyuria or secondary enuresis. Alterations in appetite and thirst are most commonly recognized when disease onset occurs in the preschool years (probably because parents are most able to monitor eating and drinking behaviors during the first few years of life). Weight loss can be variable but is more common in DM1 than DM2. Diabetic ketoacidosis (DKA) occurs at the time of initial presentation in up to 45% in DM1 and 14% in DM2 and presents with vomiting, polyuria, dehydration, and Kussmaul respirations. Children and adolescents with DM2 also report having the classic triad of symptoms but are often identified through screening urinalysis. Type 2 diabetes mellitus is highly associated with obesity (body mass index ≥95th percentile [see Chapter 139]), acanthosis nigricans, and having a first-degree relative with DM2.

Pathophysiology

Patients with DM1 have an absolute insulin deficiency due to autoimmune destruction of the beta cells of the pancreas. The disease process is thought to be triggered by an environmental factor such as a virus or toxin in genetically susceptible individuals. Exposure occurs in early childhood, but disease progression can be variable. More than 90% of affected individuals carry HLA antigen DR3 or DR4. Discordance of disease among twins supports the theory that DM1 involves an environmental exposure in genetically susceptible individuals. Twin studies show evidence of a preclinical autoimmune process, which also has predictive value in identifying susceptible individuals at risk for developing DM1. Immune changes include an increase in activated T-cells expressing HLA-DR, islet cell antibodies (ICA), insulin autoantibodies (IAA), and glutamic acid decarboxylase antibodies (GAD Ab) (Table 147-1).

Disordered immune function, in which some antigenic components of pancreatic islet cells are not recognized as self, seems to be the pathogenic mechanism for the development of DM1. It is generally believed that at least 90% of beta cell mass must be destroyed before problems with glycemic regulation are manifest. Endogenous insulin deficiency, occurring as a natural consequence of islet cell destruction, results in the inappropriate use of carbohydrate. Cellular uptake of glucose by liver, muscle, and adipose tissue is blocked. Synthesis of glycogen, protein, and fat is reduced, and a catabolic state marked by lipolysis, proteolysis, and ketone body formation ensues. Increased serum glucose and ketones present an overwhelming osmotic load to the kidneys, resulting in urinary losses of volume and cations (Na^+, K^+, NH_4).

The autoimmune phenomena described previously are not evident in DM2 as demonstrated by the absence of ICAs, IAA, and GAD Ab. This disease, which is characterized by resistance to insulin, may assume different presentations in childhood. The more traditional form of DM2 presents in older children and adolescents and is highly associated with obesity and having a first-degree relative with DM2. Like adults with DM2, there is insulin resistance, but there must be a relative insulin deficiency to develop DM2.

Differential Diagnosis

Diagnosis is usually straightforward given the symptomatology, except in children who present at a very young age. Although the onset of diabetes is rare before 1 year of age, the disease does occur but with nonspecific symptoms (ie, irritability, vomiting, tachypnea, and poor weight gain). When diabetes presents before 1 year of age, monogenic causes of diabetes need to be considered. Chemotherapeutic agents (eg, L-asparaginase) and a variety of medications (eg, corticosteroids, diuretics, oral contraceptives, phenytoin, epinephrine) may induce glucose intolerance. Glycosuria without evidence of ketosis or elevated blood glucose occurs in certain renal conditions (eg, Fanconi syndrome, carbohydrate malabsorption syndromes, heavy metal intoxication). Transient hyperglycemia, with or without glycosuria, may occur in response to physiological stress (eg, burns, trauma, hyperosmolar dehydration). In most of these cases, glucose regulation returns to normal within several days.

Evaluation

Evaluation should focus on the diagnosis of diabetes (hyperglycemia) and the category because DM1 and DM2 can have different treatment modalities and disease courses.

History

The history should focus on classic symptomatology and whether there is a family history of diabetes. Up to 80% of youth with DM2 will report a positive family history of diabetes, compared with 20% of youth with DM1. In addition, exogenous causes of diabetes should be ruled out. Obtaining a history of viral infections or chemical exposures during early childhood may be useful (Questions Box).

Physical Examination

Growth parameters should be measured and plotted on standard growth curves. Obesity is present in 96% of youth with DM2, compared with 24% of youth with DM1. Even when obese, patients with

Table 147-1. Predictive Tests for Individuals Susceptible to Type 1 Diabetes Mellitus[a]

Immunologic Marker(s)	Risk of Developing DM1 (Within 5–8 y)
ICA	25%–70%
Anti-GAD antibodies	68% among siblings of DM1 proband and 50% in the general population
IA₂ antibodies	58% among siblings of DM1 proband and 43% in the general population
IAA	Variable (may not be specific to islet cell tissue)
Reduced first-phase insulin release	100%
ICA and IAA	90%
Human leukocyte antigen with index case	25%–30%

Abbreviations: DM1, type 1 diabetes mellitus; GAD, glutamic acid decarboxylase; IAA, insulin autoantibodies; ICA, islet cell antibodies.

[a]Individuals with first-degree relative with type 1 diabetes.

Type 1 Diabetes Mellitus

Questions

- Is the child having increased urination (eg, nighttime urination, unusual bed-wetting)?
- Is the child drinking or eating more than usual?
- Has the child experienced any weight loss?
- Has the child been taking or had access to any kind of medications (eg, corticosteroids, L-asparaginase, diuretics ["water pills"], birth control pills)?
- Are there any family members with diabetes (first- or second-degree relatives)?

diabetes may lose weight at the time of presentation. Youth with uncomplicated DM1 may have an unrevealing physical examination, while those with DM2 may have physical findings associated with obesity. One study demonstrated that 60% of adolescents with DM2 had acanthosis nigricans and 32% had hypertension at presentation. An intercurrent infection may trigger the symptomatology and should always be sought in cases of ketoacidosis. Children who present with ketoacidosis may have evidence of vomiting, dehydration, Kussmaul respirations, and in severe cases, altered mental status.

Laboratory Tests

Initial laboratory tests should include evaluation of the serum and urine for glucose and ketones. For patients presenting in DKA, evaluation should also include a full chemistry panel to assess for metabolic acidosis, hypokalemia, and serum osmolality. Once the diagnosis of diabetes is suspected, further testing can assist in categorizing the type of diabetes. Tests include anti-GAD and anti–islet cell antibodies whose presence support diagnosis of DM1 (see Table 147-1) and insulin and C peptide (a marker of insulin levels) levels. Insulin and C peptide levels are usually higher in patients with DM2 because they have insulin resistance rather than an absolute insulin deficiency. Insulin reserve can be measured by determining the basal and stimulated levels of C peptide ($>$0.6 ng/mL basal level, $>$1.5 ng/mL 90 minutes after nutritional supplement such as Sustacal). In categorizing diabetes, it is important to note that some with DM1 can have insulin reserves up to 2 years after diagnosis.

Oral glucose tolerance tests may be necessary to confirm the diagnosis of diabetes in cases in which the onset of symptoms is not obvious. Two-hour postprandial values in excess of 200 mg/dL or fasting glucose of 126 mg/dL or higher are evidence of diabetes. The introduction of the intravenous glucose tolerance test with measurement of first-phase insulin release has allowed early diagnosis of individuals at risk for the disease prior to development of symptoms.

Recently, the American Diabetes Association (ADA) added hemoglobin A_{1c} (HbA$_{1c}$) of 6.5% or greater as an additional criteria that may be used to diagnose diabetes. If such a value is found in a patient, a second test should be performed to confirm the result, and evaluation should proceed to assess for presence or absence of ketones and type of diabetes.

To assess children who are at risk for DM2, screening may be done every 2 years starting at age 10 years or at the onset of puberty (whichever comes first) using fasting plasma glucose (as recommended by the ADA), oral glucose tolerance test (as recommended by the World Health Organization), or HbA$_{1c}$ (ADA). Children who should be screened are those who meet criteria for obesity and have 2 or more of the following risk factors: family history of DM2 in first- or second-degree relatives, at-risk race/ethnicity (African American, Asian/Pacific Islander, Native American, Hispanic), or associated signs and symptoms of insulin resistance (acanthosis nigricans, dyslipidemia, hypertension, polycystic ovarian syndrome).

Management

Early diagnosis together with a comprehensive program of education and aggressive management are essential to prevent acute and long-term complications. Long-term objectives of therapeutic intervention in children with diabetes are to facilitate normal physical growth and psychologic and sexual maturation, promote euglycemia through regulation of glucose metabolism, prevent acute complications (ie, hypoglycemia, ketoacidosis), prevent or delay long-term sequelae, and accommodate physiological changes that alter therapeutic needs (eg, exercise, adolescence, intercurrent illness).

Effective management requires a multidisciplinary team of professionals skilled in handling the myriad issues that arise for families and children with diabetes. Most clinics specializing in the care of children with diabetes include a nurse educator, dietitian, social worker, psychologist or counselor, and pediatric endocrinologist. In settings where such special care centers are available, the primary care physician serves as a key adjunct, underscoring the importance of ongoing patient-family involvement in disease management and ensuring optimal growth, development, and nutrition. In the absence of special care centers, the primary care physician assumes responsibility for all aspects of management, including treatment of acute complications, monitoring compliance and control, and surveillance for long-term complications.

Effective therapeutic intervention is based on individual needs for energy, insulin, and exercise. A number of factors, including physical growth, insulin requirement, glycemic control, and activity level, influence those needs and must be assessed on a regular basis. For DM1, insulin therapy is the mainstay of management, whereas DM2 therapeutic options include weight control through diet and exercise (see Chapter 139), oral hypoglycemic agents, and insulin. Oral hypoglycemic agents can lower blood glucose by increasing insulin secretion, increasing insulin sensitivity, decreasing hepatic glucose output, or decreasing nutrient absorption. These agents include sulfonylureas and other insulin secretagogues, metformin, thiazolidinediones, and acarbose. While DM2 may initially be managed with exogenous insulin, metformin is the oral agent prescribed most often for DM2 in children and adolescents. A newer class of medication acts by an incretin effect and increases glucose-dependent insulin secretion. These medications include exenatide (administered by injection) and a drug that inhibits dipeptidyl-peptidase-4, thereby prolonging the effect of endogenous insulin release after a meal. Similar to most drugs for the treatment of DM2, these newer drugs do not have a pediatric indication.

Insulin

The purpose of insulin therapy is to enable children to approach euglycemia in response to adequate amounts of food, insulin, and exercise. The amount of daily insulin required is dependent on the child's age, weight, and development. On average for DM1, children younger than 5 years require 0.6 to 0.8 U/kg, children between 5 to 11 years of age require 0.75 to 0.9 U/kg, and 12- to 18-year-olds require 0.8 to 1.5 U/kg in a 24-hour period. Within 3 to 4 months of diagnosis, most individuals experience a partial remission, or honeymoon phase, during which time their insulin requirements decline dramatically. Conversely, illness, anxiety, and adolescence (ie, pubertal changes) may cause the insulin requirement to increase. Even under conditions of increased need, reported daily insulin dosages in excess of 2 U/kg of body weight should stimulate investigations into patient compliance.

A number of insulin regimens currently in use take advantage of the variable onset of action of different insulin preparations (Table 147-2). The new insulin analogs are monomers of insulin rather than insulin aggregates. They provide a rapid onset and a shorter duration of action. This allows for easier adjustment of insulin dose depending on the child's appetite because the injection can be given immediately before the meal. Children with newly diagnosed diabetes should use semisynthetic or recombinant human insulin preparations to minimize the possibility of allergic reactions. Any change in insulin preparation should be undertaken cautiously and only under medical supervision because brands vary in strength, purity, and glycemic response.

Morning hyperglycemia may result from 1 of 2 phenomena, which must be distinguished because the appropriate therapeutic responses are opposite. The **dawn phenomenon** probably involves

a nocturnal surge of growth hormone, resulting in hyperglycemia that is present during the night (2:00–4:00 am) and is sustained until morning. Treatment involves increasing the evening dose of intermediate-acting insulin or moving the evening insulin to bedtime. In the **Somogyi phenomenon,** morning glucose is high as a physiological response to nighttime hypoglycemia. Treatment of this condition requires decreasing the evening intermediate-acting insulin or increasing the carbohydrate content of a bedtime snack.

Adolescents require special consideration. The sexual maturation process occurs in the setting of relative insulin resistance, other hormonal alterations, and a burden of developmental tasks, which make glycemic control problematic at best. Daily insulin requirements may increase to 1.5 to 2 U/kg during adolescence but return to prepubertal levels at the end of the teenage years. Particular efforts must be made to ensure physical and psychologic growth in the context of these special tasks. Dietary manipulation and consideration of alternative (usually more intensive) insulin and monitoring regimens is critical for successful glycemic control during this challenging period.

External infusion pumps afford the advantages of programmed variable basal rates and insulin dosing during specific times of the day. In a long-term study on outcomes among children with DM1, children on pumps had fewer hypoglycemic events and hospitalizations for DKA and improved HbA$_{1c}$. While insulin pumps are not widely used in young children because of the potential risk of mechanical malfunction and catheter problems (leading to hypoglycemia or hyperglycemia), they may be considered in children with unstable diabetes or to provide very low doses of insulin.

Glucose Monitoring

Self-monitoring of glycemic response through the in-home assessment of blood glucose levels is critical to effective therapy. The introduction of reflectance meters (glucometers) has obviated the need for inaccurate, visually read strips of glucose-sensitive paper. Patients who are taking insulin should measure glucose 3 to 7 times daily. Most endocrinologists advocate testing before each meal and at bedtime during the first year after diagnosis. Testing may also be done at 2:00 am to test for hypoglycemia or hyperglycemia. Depending on the age of the child, an acceptable range for glycemic control is 80 to 150 mg/dL. Additional short-acting insulin may be given to correct for high blood glucose. Patients also need to monitor their urine for ketones whenever their blood glucose readings exceed 240 mg/dL.

Glycosylated hemoglobin (HbA$_{1c}$) measurements reflect glucose control over the preceding 2 to 3 months. The normal value is 4% to 6% of total hemoglobin. Glycosylated hemoglobin values less than 7% are excellent, between 7% to 8% are good, between 8% to 10% are average, and more than 10% are poor. The Diabetes Control and Complications Trial studied the effect of different levels of glycemic control on the complications of diabetes. Although the study only included pediatric patients 13 years or older, the study did show that patients with "tight glycemic control" had lower HbA$_{1c}$ levels and fewer long-term complications than patients not tightly controlled. Adolescents with tight glycemic control had a greater risk of

Table 147-2. Commonly Used Insulin Preparations[a]

Type	Onset of Action	Duration of Effect
Rapid-acting analogs Lispro, aspart, glulisine	Within 15 min	<5 h
Short-acting Regular	Within 30 min	5–8 h
Intermediate-acting (zinc or protamine) Neutral protamine Hagedorn	1.5–2.5 h	18–24 h
Long-acting Glargine Detemir	70 min 1.5–2.5 h	22–24 h 20–24 h

[a]Twice-daily injections: Two-thirds of the total daily dose before breakfast made up of intermediate- and short-acting insulin in 2:1 ratio. One-third before dinner made up of intermediate- and short-acting insulin in 1:1 ratio.

Basal/bolus: Intermediate-/long-acting insulin at bedtime with regular insulin or short-acting insulin analog before each meal.

hypoglycemic events than the control group, a fact that must be taken into consideration in determining ideal glycemic control for a child. In general, tight glycemic control is not recommended for children younger than 5 years; for older children, glycemic control should be individually tailored. Whenever children's routines undergo dramatic change, stepped-up home monitoring and medical consultation are advisable. Caution should be used in interpreting HbA_{1c} values in infants and others in whom fetal hemoglobin or other hemoglobin variants are present because these hemoglobin variants may falsely elevate or lower the value of HbA_{1c}. Although compliance with intensive regimens is an indisputable challenge (particularly as responsibility for management shifts from parent to child), increasing evidence underscores the importance of tight glycemic control.

Nutrition

The timing, amount, and types of foods eaten for meals and snacks should be relatively consistent from one day to the next to match the relative constancy of the exogenous insulin. Standard daily caloric requirements are distributed in the following way: carbohydrate, 50% to 55% (<10% in the form of sucrose); protein, 20% to 25%; and fat, 25% to 30% (6%–8% polyunsaturated, <7%–10% saturated). However, in DM2 with overweight/obesity, the patient may benefit from overall reduced calorie intake (carbohydrates minimum 130 g per day). The distribution of calories should be approximately 25% for breakfast, 25% for lunch, 30% for dinner, and 20% for snacks. Snacks are an important part of the nutrition regimen for children with diabetes. Most nutritionists recommend 3 snacks for young children (between meals and at bedtime) and 2 for older children. Dietary discipline is a tremendous challenge for many children. Introducing one change at a time may make such dietary manipulations more acceptable over the long run. In addition, establishing healthy eating habits requires availability of healthy choices in the child's environment. Cooperation from the school and home enhances the likelihood of a child developing healthy eating practices.

Carbohydrate counting is an important part of matching insulin requirements to nutritional intake. For patients on multiple daily insulin injection schedules, there is flexibility in tailoring each dose of insulin based on the carbohydrate content of each meal or snack. For patients on twice-daily insulin injection regimens, consistent carbohydrate content of meals and snacks is important in maintaining blood glucose levels. Learning carbohydrate counting takes time for patients and families, and they need ongoing nutrition support to become familiar and comfortable with how different foods affect their blood glucose levels.

Exercise

Exercise contributes to glucose control by facilitating the use of glucose without the assistance of insulin. If not carefully undertaken on a regular basis, exercise can precipitate acute hypoglycemia. Physical activity enhances the body's sensitivity to insulin and can even decrease the daily insulin requirement. Thoughtful planning of exercise involves compensatory changes in food intake and insulin doses. For example, extra energy intake at bedtime may offset the nighttime hypoglycemia that accompanies late afternoon exercise. Seasonal physical activities may necessitate an adjustment in the insulin regimen at certain times of the year.

Education

The role of education is pivotal to the successful management of diabetes in childhood and throughout life. During childhood, educational efforts must be focused on the entire family unit. Affected children must be involved as early as possible and in ways that are developmentally appropriate. The process should involve the early introduction of basic survival information, such as insulin therapy and management of complications. This can be followed by more detailed information, including strategies to reduce long-term sequelae.

Prognosis

Diabetic ketoacidosis is the major cause of morbidity and mortality in children and adolescents, followed by **hypoglycemia.** Clinical signs of hypoglycemia in older children include shakiness, blurred vision, and dysarthria. Concerns about the neurodevelopmental effect of hypoglycemia in young children have led to the recommendation of more liberal glycemic control in early onset disease. Diabetic ketoacidosis, precipitated by an intercurrent infection or poor compliance, is a metabolic derangement that always requires urgent medical attention and often necessitates hospitalization. Replacement of fluids, attention to electrolyte abnormalities, and insulin therapy are the mainstays of treatment in the face of this complication.

There has been an increase in the number of pediatric patients presenting with hyperglycemic hyperosmolar state (HHS). Because treatment of HHS is different from DKA, the clinician needs to be aware of this entity. In fact, treatment for children with HHS may be different than treatment of this disorder in adults.

Long-term complications include **proliferative retinopathy, nephropathy, peripheral and autonomic neurologic impairment,** and **early onset of cardiovascular disease.** Ophthalmologic evaluation, overnight urine protein measurement, and a detailed neurologic examination should occur once or twice each year depending on the duration of disease. Intensive therapeutic intervention results in significant reduction in retinopathy, nephropathy, and cardiac and peripheral vascular disease. Preliminary evidence warrants consideration of such therapy with the expectation of benefit in long-term outcomes.

CASE RESOLUTION

With the presence of ketones, the girl in the opening case study is admitted to the hospital to initiate insulin treatment and determine appropriate dosing. Anti–glutamic acid decarboxylase and anti–islet cell antibody levels are ordered to determine if she has autoimmunity, which would indicate type 1 diabetes mellitus. She and her family require ongoing education. Careful management is necessary to optimize normal growth and development as well as to delay or prevent long-term sequelae.

Selected References

American Diabetes Association. Diagnosis and classification of diabetes mellitus. *Diabetes Care*. 2010;33(Suppl 1):S62–S69

American Diabetes Association, Bantle JP, Wylie-Rosett J, et al. Nutrition recommendations and interventions for diabetes: a position statement of the American Diabetes Association. *Diabetes Care*. 2008;31(Suppl 1):S61–S78

Copeland KC, Silverstein J, Moore KR, et al. Management of newly diagnosed type 2 diabetes mellitus (T2DM) in children and adolescents. *Pediatrics*. 2013; 131(2):364–382

Gellar LA, Schrader K, Nansel TR. Healthy eating practices: perceptions, facilitators, and barriers among youth with diabetes. *Diabetes Educ*. 2007;33(4): 671–679

Hannon TS, Gungor N, Arslanian SA. Type 2 diabetes in children and adolescents: a review for the primary care provider. *Pediatr Ann*. 2006;35(12): 880–887

Johnson SR, Cooper MN, Jones TW, Davis EA. Long-term outcome of insulin pump therapy in children with type 1 diabetes assessed in a large population-based case-control study. *Diabetologia*. 2013;56(11):2392–2400

Kapadia C, Zeitler P; Drugs and Therapeutics Committee of the Pediatric Endocrine Society. Hemoglobin A1c measurement for the diagnosis of Type 2 diabetes in children. *Int J Pediatr Endocrinol*. 2012;2012(1):31

Leslie RD, Elliott RB. Early environmental events as a cause of IDDM. Evidence and implications. *Diabetes*. 1994;43(7):843–850

Mohamadi A, Clark LM, Lipkin PH, Mahone EM, Wodka EL, Plotnick LP. Medical and developmental impact of transition from subcutaneous insulin to oral glyburide in a 15-yr-old boy with neonatal diabetes mellitus and intermediate DEND syndrome: extending the age of KCNJ11 mutation testing in neonatal DM. *Pediatr Diabetes*. 2010;11(3):203–207

Pinhas-Hamiel O, Zeitler P. Acute and chronic complications of type 2 diabetes mellitus in children and adolescents. *Lancet*. 2007;369(9575):1823–1831

Pinhas-Hamiel O, Zeitler P. The global spread of type 2 diabetes mellitus in children and adolescents. *J Pediatr*. 2005;146(5):693–700

Scott CR, Smith JM, Cradock MM, Pihoker C. Characteristics of youth-onset noninsulin-dependent diabetes mellitus and insulin-dependent diabetes mellitus at diagnosis. *Pediatrics*. 1997;100(1):84–91

SEARCH for Diabetes in Youth Study Group, Liese AD, D'Agostino RB Jr, et al. The burden of diabetes mellitus among US youth: prevalence estimates from the SEARCH for Diabetes in Youth Study. *Pediatrics*. 2006;118(4):1510–1518

Siljander HT, Veijola R, Reunanen A, Virtanen SM, Akerblom HK, Knip M. Prediction of type 1 diabetes among siblings of affected children and in the general population. *Diabetologia*. 2007;50(11):2272–2275

Silverstein J, Klingensmith G, Copeland K, et al. Care of children and adolescents with type 1 diabetes: a statement of the American Diabetes Association. *Diabetes Care*. 2005;28(1):186–212

Springer SC, Silverstein J, Copeland K, et al. Management of type 2 diabetes mellitus in children and adolescents. *Pediatrics*. 2013;131(2):e648–e664

Tamborlane WV, Ahern J. Implications and results of the Diabetes Control and Complications Trial. *Pediatr Clin North Am*. 1997;44(2):285–300

Zeitler P, Haqq A, Rosenbloom A, Glaser N; Drugs and Therapeutics Committee of the Lawson Wilkins Pediatric Endocrine Society. Hyperglycemic hyperosmolar syndrome in children: pathophysiological considerations and suggested guidelines for treatment. *J Pediatr*. 2011;158(1):9–14

CHAPTER 148

Juvenile Idiopathic Arthritis and Benign Joint Pains of Childhood

Miriam F. Parsa, MD, MPH, and Deborah McCurdy, MD

CASE STUDY

A 4-year-old white girl is evaluated for limp. Parents are unclear about the duration of her symptoms, although they believe knee complaints started after she was playing with her brother 3 months ago. Parents have observed the patient to walk "like her grandmother" every morning, with marked improvement in her gait approximately 1 hour after moving around. Her activity level has remained about the same, although the morning limp does limit her ability to keep up with her siblings. She has no history of rash, fever, weight loss, severe pain complaints, or other joint involvement. On physical examination, vital signs are normal, her left knee is swollen with a 20-degree flexion contracture, and the left leg is 1.5-cm longer than the right leg.

Questions

1. What findings are indicative of juvenile idiopathic arthritis (JIA)?
2. What is the differential diagnosis for monarthric arthritis?
3. Which laboratory tests are important in the diagnostic workup of a child with suspected JIA?
4. What are the most common complications of uncontrolled JIA?
5. What are the long-term outcomes for patients with JIA?
6. What types of agents are used in the treatment of JIA?

Joint pain is a common complaint in the pediatric population, and etiologies include trauma, hypermobility, and chronic inflammatory arthritis, such as juvenile idiopathic arthritis (JIA). Differentiating between a benign, self-limited etiology and a potentially destructive, chronic process is critical to the preservation of growing bones and cartilage. The etiology of joint pain may be roughly divided into 2 categories: mechanical versus inflammatory. Mechanical or non-inflammatory causes include pes planus, hindfoot valgus, or hypermobility. Inflammatory causes can be infectious, postinfectious (immune complex mediated), or autoimmune mediated. Distinguishing between mechanical and inflammatory processes, and the subsequent need for a pediatric rheumatology consultation, may be straightforward after a detailed history, thorough physical examination, and focused laboratory investigation are performed.

Epidemiology

Juvenile idiopathic arthritis is the most common pediatric rheumatologic disease and one of the more common chronic diseases of childhood. The estimated US incidence is 14 per 100,000, and the estimated prevalence is 96 per 100,000 children. The disease can occur in all racial and ethnic profiles with variable frequencies. Juvenile idiopathic arthritis is most prevalent among whites and least prevalent in African Americans and Asian Americans. Consistent with most autoimmune diseases, females are affected more commonly than males.

The International League of Associations for Rheumatology system is most commonly used for classification of JIA. Juvenile idiopathic arthritis is an umbrella term for a set of diverse diseases with one common thread: chronic idiopathic inflammation of the joint space (Table 148-1). Juvenile idiopathic arthritis encompasses all of what was called juvenile rheumatoid arthritis and juvenile chronic arthritis. "Rheumatoid" was removed because rheumatoid factor (RF) antibodies are absent in the majority of children with JIA.

Clinical Presentation

Juvenile idiopathic arthritis presents with arthritis during the course of the disease. Arthritis is defined as joint edema on examination or joint(s) with pain on range of motion *and* limitation of range of motion. The onset may be insidious (ie, oligoarticular JIA), rapid (ie, RF+ polyarticular JIA), or delayed (ie, systemic JIA) (see Table

Table 148-1. International League of Associations for Rheumatology Classification of Juvenile Idiopathic Arthritis

JIA Subtype	Peak Age of Onset (y)	Number of Joints Involved	Type of Onset	Gender Predilection
Oligoarticular	4	≤4	Insidious	Girl > Boy
RF- polyarticular	2–5	≥5	Insidious	Girl > Boy
RF+ polyarticular	12	≥5	Rapid	Girl > Boy
Systemic	Any, <16	Variable	Variable	Girl = Boy
Enthesitis related	12	Variable	Insidious	Girl < Boy
Psoriatic	3	Initially ≤4	Insidious	Girl > Boy
	11	≤4		Girl = Boy

Abbreviations: JIA, juvenile idiopathic arthritis; RF, rheumatoid factor.

Data derived from Petty RE, Southwood TR, Manners P, et al. International League of Associations for Rheumatology classification of juvenile idiopathic arthritis: second revision, Edmonton, 2001. *J Rheumatol.* 2004;31(2):390–392; and Cassidy J, Laxler R, Petty R, Lindsley C. *Textbook of Pediatric Rheumatology.* 6th ed. Philadelphia, PA: Elsevier; 2011.

148-1). Adolescents 16 years and older with a new diagnosis of chronic idiopathic arthritis are considered to have adult rheumatoid arthritis, not JIA. Children may be observed to limp mostly in the mornings, have difficulties completing writing assignments, or regress with gross motor milestones. Complications of JIA, such as leg-length discrepancy and flexion contracture of the joint, may lead to difficulties in performing activities of daily living and may be a presenting symptom. Leg-length discrepancy is a product of persistent inflammation providing an abundance of blood flow to an open epiphysis (most obvious is the distal femoral epiphysis), causing premature growth with eventual premature epiphyseal closure.

Oligoarticular JIA (also known as pauciarticular JIA) is the most common form, making up approximately 50% of all JIA cases. It is defined by the presence of arthritis in fewer than 5 joints during the first 6 months of disease and most often involves the large joints (knees most common, hips rarely). Children may present with single joint involvement. Oligoarticular JIA is divided into persistent and extended forms, the latter associated with more severe disease course and mimicking adult polyarticular disease. Extended oligoarticular JIA can only be diagnosed after the first 6 months of symptoms in which patients extend the number of joints with arthritis to greater than 5 joints.

In addition to complications, such as leg-length discrepancy and joint flexion contracture, children with oligoarticular JIA are at an increased risk of developing anterior uveitis. Anterior uveitis is defined as inflammation of the anterior uveal tract and adjacent ciliary body, and it is not clear why the same types of inflammatory cells are targeting seemingly disparate parts of the body (eyes and joints). Anterior uveitis may be a clinically silent part of approximately 25% of all oligoarticular JIA patients' disease course and, in a minority of affected patients, may lead to blindness. Guidelines put forth by the American Academy of Pediatrics and American Academy of Ophthalmology define risk factors and ophthalmologic screening frequencies for the prevention of JIA-associated uveitis (Table 148-2).

Polyarticular JIA is defined as arthritis of 5 or more joints during the first 6 months of disease and represents approximately 30% of JIA cases. There are 2 peaks of the disease, suggesting 2 different genetic interplays. Rheumatoid factor–negative disease is the more common subtype, often with a positive antinuclear antibody (ANA) test and higher risk of anterior uveitis, and tends to present in early childhood. Rheumatoid factor–positive disease most commonly presents in early adolescent females with symmetric small joint disease. The arthritis is erosive and may result in boutonniere deformities (proximal interphalangeal joint flexion and distal interphalangeal

Table 148-2. Frequency of Ophthalmologic Examinations in Children With Juvenile Idiopathic Arthritis[a]

Disease Subtype	ANA	Age at Diagnosis (y)	Duration of Disease (y)	Risk Category	Frequency of Eye Examinations (mo)
Oligoarticular or polyarticular	+	≤6	≤4	High	3
	+	≤6	>4	Moderate	6
	+	≤6	>7	Low	12
	+	>6	≤4	Moderate	6
	+	>6	>4	Low	12
	-	≤6	≤4	Moderate	6
	-	≤6	>4	Low	12
	-	>6	N/A	Low	12
Systemic disease (eg, fever, rash)	N/A	N/A	N/A	Low	12

Abbreviations: ANA, antinuclear antibody test; N/A, not applicable.

[a]Recommendations for follow-up continue through childhood and adolescence.

From Cassidy J, Kivlin J, Lindsley C, Nocton J; American Academy of Pediatrics Section on Rheumatology and Section on Ophthalmology. Ophthalmologic examinations in children with juvenile rheumatoid arthritis. *Pediatrics.* 2006;117(5):1843–1845 joint hyperextension) and swan neck deformities (proximal interphalangeal joint hyperextension and distal interphalangeal joint flexion) if disease is uncontrolled.

Systemic JIA is present in 10% to 15% of patients with JIA and is associated with the greatest morbidity and mortality of all JIA subtypes. Systemic JIA lacks autoantibody, gender, age, or human leukocyte antigen (HLA) association seen among other JIA subtypes. It is characterized by fever, rash, lymphadenopathy, hepatosplenomegaly, and serositis. Classically, fevers are quotidian or daily in pattern and are accompanied by a migratory rash that consists of discrete salmon-colored macules seen predominantly on the trunk and proximal extremities (Figure 148-1). If arthritis is part of the presenting symptoms, pain complaints will be worst during the febrile period. The arthritis is typically polyarticular, affecting large and small joints, and is present within the first 6 months of symptoms. Patients are often initially categorized as "fever of unknown origin" because arthritis may be minimal or often absent at time of presentation.

A rare but life-threatening complication of systemic JIA is macrophage activation syndrome. Patients present with hepatosplenomegaly, lymphadenopathy, and purpura and may progress to multiorgan failure. A relative decrease in inflammatory laboratory tests (eg, erythrocyte sedimentation rate [ESR], platelets) is observed in macrophage activation syndrome, in contrast with an elevation during disease exacerbation, as liver and bone marrow function deteriorates. Treatment involves steroids and immunosuppressive therapy. Triggers to macrophage activation syndrome include viral infections and addition or change in medications such as nonsteroidal anti-inflammatory drugs (NSAIDs), sulfasalazine, and etanercept.

Enthesitis-related arthritis (ERA) is characterized by typically lower extremity arthritis and inflammation where tendons, ligaments, fascia, or joint capsule inserts at the bone (ie, enthesitis). Unlike pauciarticular and polyarticular JIA, in which autoantibodies are frequently present (eg, ANA, RF), ERA is generally seronegative with a strong association with HLA B27. Enthesitis-related arthritis most likely represents the earliest clinical stage of ankylosing spondylitis, which is defined by inflammatory axial disease.

Juvenile ankylosing spondylitis generally affects boys aged 8 years or older. Extra-articular symptoms include anterior uveitis, which is acute and painful, in contrast with uveitis seen in oligoarticular and polyarticular arthritis, which is more insidious in onset.

Psoriatic arthritis occurs in patients with chronic arthritis and psoriasis or those who meet 2 of the following criteria: dactylitis, nail pitting or onycholysis, and first-degree relative with psoriasis. The age at onset is biphasic, 3 years and 11 years of age. Clinical presentation of the younger cohort is similar to oligoarticular JIA, with the exception of higher frequencies of small joint involvement and dactylitis (sausage-like appearance of the digit). The older cohort resembles adult psoriatic arthritis and is characterized by axial skeletal involvement and enthesitis. The arthritis, which is asymmetric, may present before the psoriatic rash, making diagnosis difficult. Similar to polyarticular JIA, the biphasic nature suggests different genetic contributions. Up to 17% of patients will have asymptomatic uveitis, similar to ANA-positive oligoarticular JIA, and require routine slit-lamp examinations for diagnosis.

Differential Diagnosis

The differential diagnosis for joint pain in children is vast, including infectious, oncologic, immunologic, and autoimmune, and can be separated from a self-limited versus chronic etiology with a targeted history and thorough physical examination (Table 148-3 and D_x Box). Joint pains of childhood may be self-limited in nature and include growing pains, postinfectious arthralgia, and pain amplification as well as mechanical abnormalities such as hypermobility syndrome as causal.

Growing pains are a benign cause of pain in children and usually resolve within 1 to 2 years of onset. Growing pains are characterized by nocturnal pain without objective musculoskeletal manifestations. The pain complaints are generally localized to the bilateral lower extremities and are relieved by massage, heat, or NSAIDs. *Red flags necessitating further workup include* systemic symptoms (eg, fevers, weight loss), persistent pain during the day, objective musculoskeletal examination abnormalities, limping, and unilateral pain.

Mechanical or noninflammatory causes of joint pain in children may include joint hypermobility, hindfoot valgus or pronation, genu recurvatum, or pes planus. A typical presentation of a child with mechanical causes of joint pain contains a history of pain after activity, relief with rest, and typical physical examination findings. Further questioning may reveal a history of pain exacerbation of the

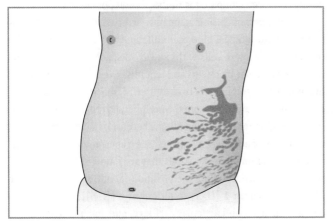

Figure 148-1. Salmon-colored rash seen in systemic juvenile idiopathic arthritis with Koebner phenomenon.

Dx · Juvenile Idiopathic Arthritis

- Systemic: arthritis with daily fevers, rash, and general malaise
- Oligoarthritis: arthritis affecting 1 to 4 joints in the first 6 months
- Polyarticular: arthritis affecting more than 5 joints in the first 6 months
- Enthesitis related: arthritis and enthesitis, ±human leukocyte antigen B27
- Psoriatic: arthritis and psoriasis or arthritis and dactylitis, nail abnormalities, and family history of psoriasis

Table 148-3. Differential Diagnosis of Joint Pain in Children			
Monarthric Arthritis	*Polyarticular Arthritis*	*Positive Systemic Features*	*Arthralgia*
Infectious			
Septic arthritis Osteomyelitis Lyme disease	Lyme disease	Bacterial infections (Lyme, TB, gonococcal, *Brucella*) Viral infections (parvovirus, EBV, hepatitis B) Parasitic infection (malaria)	
Autoimmune			
Oligoarticular JIA	Polyarticular JIA Connective tissue disease[a] Inflammatory bowel disease–associated arthritis	Systemic JIA Connective tissue disease[a] Inflammatory bowel disease–associated arthritis	
Oncology			
Malignancy (ALL)	Malignancy	Malignancy (neuroblastoma)	
Immunologic			
Reactive arthritis	Reactive arthritis Immunodeficiency-related arthritis Chronic recurrent multifocal osteomyelitis	Acute rheumatic fever	
Other			
Trauma Osteonecrosis Hemarthrosis (bleeding disorder)			Hypermobility Osteochondrosis Pain amplification Growing pains Legg-Calvé-Perthes disease Slipped capital femoral epiphysis

Abbreviations: ALL, acute lymphoblastic leukemia; EBV, Epstein-Barr virus; JIA, juvenile idiopathic arthritis; TB, tuberculosis.

[a]Systemic lupus erythematosus, mixed connective tissue disease, sarcoidosis, juvenile dermatomyositis, Henoch-Schönlein purpura.

knees, ankles, and feet when the child does not wear supportive shoes during physical activity. *Benign hypermobility syndrome* (BHS) is defined as generalized joint hypermobility in the absence of other connective tissue abnormality or congenital syndrome. Although approximately 8% to 20% of the white population meets BHS criteria, many more have hypermobility limited to a few joints. Patients with hypermobility syndrome commonly experience fibromyalgia (a pain amplification syndrome) and patellofemoral syndrome as comorbid conditions. Joint edema can occur but is not persistent, as in chronic inflammatory arthritis.

Generally, joint pain that is persistent, daily, worst in the morning, not severe in quality, and known to improve with activity is suggestive of a chronic inflammatory process, such as JIA. Joint pain that is acute in onset, monarthric, severe in quality, and accompanied by fever is suggestive of septic arthritis, an orthopedic emergency because of the rapid cartilage destruction if treatment is delayed. Monarthric joint pain that is localized to the *peri*articular region, severe in quality, and accompanied by weight loss and abnormal complete blood cell count suggests malignancy such as acute lymphoblastic leukemia.

Pathophysiology

The exact pathogenesis of JIA is unclear, and a monogenetic inheritance pattern has not been observed. Autoimmune diseases result from an alteration in the selection, regulation, or death of T cells or B cells, which results in an abnormal response to a particular antigen. Genetic factors increase an individual's vulnerability but are not sufficient for disease expression. It is the interplay of environmental triggers, immune mechanisms, and largely specific HLA predisposition that leads to clinical manifestations. Multiple HLA types have been associated with the development of JIA, with early-onset oligoarticular JIA having the most distinctive HLA associations. The level of risk to family members of a child with JIA seems to be only mildly increased compared with the general population.

The hallmark of chronic idiopathic arthritis is synovial cell proliferation with synovial fluid accumulation, also called pannus. The marked expansion of cells within a closed space results in stretching of periarticular ligaments and tendons. The cells responsible for inflammation (lymphocytes [mostly T cells], macrophages, and dendritic cells) are recruited from the peripheral circulation and able to penetrate into the synovial membrane because of factors that include proangiogenic and vasoactive proteins. An aberrant immune system produces inflammatory cytokines that are found in large numbers within the synovial membrane or fluid (eg, tumor necrosis factor [TNF], interleukin-1 [IL-1], interleukin-6 [IL-6]), enzymes that degrade collagen and articular cartilage, and signals that activate osteoclasts and result in bone erosions.

Evaluation

History

The history should clearly delineate the duration, severity, and extent of the symptoms (Questions Box). Which joints have been involved and for how long? Did the pain start acutely? Has the pain been persistent, intermittent, or migratory? Are there visible changes, such as swelling and erythema? Are the symptoms more pronounced at specific times of the day, such as in the morning on arising or only after activities? Does the pain wake the child up from sleep? Was there a precipitating event, such as trauma? What other symptoms are present, such as fever, rash, fatigue, gastrointestinal symptoms, and weight loss? Is there a history of other medical problems, such as inflammatory bowel disease and psoriasis? Is there a family history of autoimmune disease, growing pains, or hypermobility?

Physical Examination

Patients should undergo a complete physical examination that includes a full assessment of the skin, all joints, flexibility of the spine (particularly cervical and lumbosacral), and evaluation for leg-length discrepancy. Specific to the pediatric examination is the consideration of normal joint hypermobility when assessing for arthritis. Comparing bilateral joints is imperative in determining whether a subtle flexion contracture may be present, suggesting the presence of chronic arthritis. Patients suspected of having JIA should also undergo a slit-lamp examination of the eyes, performed by a pediatric ophthalmologist or uveitis specialist.

Laboratory Tests

A diagnosis of JIA is primarily based on physical examination and history. A targeted laboratory investigation helps to evaluate for other etiologies. For example, a young child presenting with monarthric arthritis and a marked elevation in acute phase reactants (ie, ESR >100) deserves an evaluation for malignancy and infection. Typically, children with oligoarticular JIA have normal acute phase reactants, with any persistent elevation considered a poor prognostic factor (Table 148-4). Evaluating for the presence of RF, anti–cyclic citrullinated peptide (CCP) antibody, ANA, and HLA B27 may help with diagnostic and

Table 148-4. Typical Laboratory Evidence of Systemic Inflammation in Juvenile Idiopathic Arthritis

Juvenile Idiopathic Arthritis Subtype	Acute Phase Reactants
Oligoarticular	Normal
Polyarticular	Elevated
Systemic	Elevated
Macrophage Activation	Relative Decrease
Enthesitis Related	Normal
Psoriatic	Normal

prognostic assessment. The most important laboratory test in the diagnostic evaluation of a young child with chronic arthritis is the ANA. A positive ANA test result helps in the risk stratification of the child for the development of JIA-associated uveitis (see Table 148-2).

Imaging Studies

Imaging is used to determine the extent and severity of joint damage as well as help exclude other diagnoses (eg, metaphyseal lines seen in leukemia on X-ray). Conventional radiography is used in the assessment of joint damage, such as bone erosions, joint space narrowing, joint subluxation, misalignment, or ankylosis. Advances in ultrasound technology have stimulated its increased use in the diagnosis and management of JIA. An ultrasound diagnosis of JIA is made when synovitis is detected, as measured by excess synovial fluid, synovial hypertrophy, and joint space hyperemia. Ultrasound provides multiple advantages over conventional radiology, including its lack of ionizing radiation, noninvasive nature, and cost. Magnetic resonance imaging (MRI) is the gold standard for detecting synovitis and is able to assess all structures for active inflammation and joint damage. Ultrasound and MRI are more sensitive than clinical examination in the assessment of arthritis.

Management

The objective of treatment for JIA is to control pain and inflammation while preserving function and normal growth, development, and well-being. Physical and occupational therapy are essential to maintain function but are limited in benefit when there is ongoing inflammation. In 2011, the American College of Rheumatology published guidelines for the management of JIA that describe initiation and monitoring of therapeutic agents including NSAIDs, disease-modifying antirheumatic drugs (DMARDs), and biologics. Nonsteroidal anti-inflammatory drugs are first-line therapy for JIA, including several available in liquid formulations (naproxen, meloxicam, ibuprofen). Biologics have greatly reduced the morbidity of disease and drug side effects once seen. Biologics include anti-TNF (etanercept, adalimumab), anti–IL-1 (canakinumab), and anti–IL-6 (tocilizumab); all have been US Food and Drug Administration (FDA) approved for subtypes of JIA. Medication side effects are generally well tolerated by the pediatric population; they include gastrointestinal complaints with NSAIDs and oral

---

Juvenile Idiopathic Arthritis

Questions

- Has the child ever had any swelling, warmth, or redness of joints?
- Does the child have difficulty walking or running?
- If so, does it occur at any particular time of the day?
- Has the child been experiencing fevers or weight loss?
- Has the family noticed any type of skin rash, like psoriasis?
- Has the child had any recent illnesses such as gastroenteritis?
- Has the child traveled recently or been bitten by a tick?
- Is there a family history of autoimmune disease, such as juvenile idiopathic arthritis?

methotrexate and increased number and duration of upper respiratory and skin infections with biologics. It is important to remember that all medications used to reduce the effects of a hyperactive immune system are inherently going to reduce the body's ability to fight infections. As always, carefully weigh the risks versus benefits of these medications. Live vaccines should not be administered to individuals receiving medications, such as methotrexate and chronic glucocorticoids.

Oligoarticular JIA is generally treated with NSAIDs, or intra-articular steroid injection is performed. Local therapy has been shown to induce remission in select patients and may avoid systemic medication exposure. Methotrexate, a DMARD, is used in those patients who have persistent disease despite joint injection and an adequate (2-month) NSAID trial. Rarely, anti-TNF therapy is used for this subtype.

Polyarticular JIA may be treated initially with NSAIDs; however, methotrexate and anti-TNF therapy is initiated more quickly given the worst prognosis of polyarticular versus oligoarticular JIA. Methotrexate is started if, after 1 month of NSAID use, there is persistent disease. Intra-articular steroid injections are also used when there are 1 or 2 joints with particularly large disease activity.

Systemic JIA treatment has progressed rapidly over the last several years. It is now possible to reduce the steroid burden with early initiation of biologic therapy, specifically IL-6 and IL-1 antagonists. Interleukin-6 is an inflammatory protein found to be one of the main drivers of systemic JIA inflammation. Tocilizumab and canakinumab have been FDA approved for the treatment of systemic JIA. Nonsteroidal anti-inflammatory drugs, methotrexate, intra-articular steroid injections, and glucocorticoids may also be part of disease management.

Anterior uveitis treatment is comanaged by a pediatric ophthalmologist or uveitis specialist and pediatric rheumatologist. First-line therapy includes topical glucocorticoids and dilating drops. However, if eye disease is refractory to treatment, antimetabolites, such as methotrexate, or anti-TNF therapy are considered.

Prognosis

Among individuals with persistent oligoarticular JIA, 75% report remission of disease, while only 12% of those with extended subtype report remission, with the remaining continuing to experience symptoms into adulthood. Children with polyarticular JIA experience the same remission rates as extended subtype, between 10% to 15%. Features of poor prognosis include arthritis of the hip or cervical spine, bone erosions on imaging, persistently elevated ESR with wrist or ankle arthritis in oligoarticular patients, and RF+ or anti-CCP antibodies in polyarticular patients.

In systemic JIA, systemic features such as fever and rash tend to subside during the initial months to years of the disease but may flare, as in most autoimmune diseases. About 40% of children with systemic JIA follow a *monocyclic* disease course and eventually recover. A small proportion of children have a *polycyclic* course characterized by recurrent episodes of active disease interrupted by periods of remission without medications, while more than half of children with systemic JIA have a *persistent* disease course.

The care of a child with chronic inflammatory arthritis also requires a multidisciplinary approach involving a primary care physician, rheumatologist, physical therapist, and subspecialists with expertise in affected target organs. The role of the primary care physician is to ensure optimal function of the patient as well as prevention of long-term disease and treatment sequelae. Because agents used to suppress chronic inflammation may have significant side effects, it is vital for the primary care physician to be well versed with a patient's medication regimen. Patients who require chronic steroid use to control systemic JIA often suffer from growth failure from the disease process or its treatment; therefore, ensuring appropriate diet and physical activity is vital. Supplementation with calcium and vitamin D is beneficial to prevent osteoporosis for all patients with chronic inflammation, but it is even more importantly for those on chronic steroids. Disease management for patients with chronic inflammatory arthritis is a balance of optimal function, minimal complications, and improved quality of life.

CASE RESOLUTION

The young girl in the case study has a presentation consistent with oligoarticular JIA based on the number of involved joints with arthritis, the chronicity of her complaints by history, and abnormal physical examination. She was found to be antinuclear antibody (ANA) positive, which puts her at high risk of developing anterior uveitis (age <6 years at diagnosis, new diagnosis, ANA positive). She is referred to a pediatric ophthalmologist for uveitis screening every 3 months for the first 4 years, every 6 months for the next 3 years, then yearly screening thereafter. She is also referred to a pediatric rheumatologist for assistance in managing her disease and a physical therapist to address her limitation of motion.

Selected References

Beukelman T, Patkar NM, Saag KG, et al. 2011 American College of Rheumatology recommendations for the treatment of juvenile idiopathic arthritis: initiation and safety monitoring of therapeutic agents for the treatment of arthritis and systemic features. *Arthritis Care Res (Hoboken)*. 2011;63(4):465–482

Cassidy J, Kivlin J, Lindsley C, Nocton J; American Academy of Pediatrics Section on Rheumatology and Section on Ophthalmology. Ophthalmologic examinations in children with juvenile rheumatoid arthritis. *Pediatrics*. 2006;117(5): 1843–1845

Cassidy J, Laxler R, Petty R, Lindsley C. *Textbook of Pediatric Rheumatology*. 6th ed. Philadelphia, PA: Elsevier; 2011

Petty RE, Southwood TR, Manners P, et al. International League of Associations for Rheumatology classification of juvenile idiopathic arthritis: second revision, Edmonton, 2001. *J Rheumatol*. 2004;31(2):390–392

Ravelli A, Varnier GC, Oliveira S, et al. Antinuclear antibody-positive patients should be grouped as a separate category in the classification of juvenile idiopathic arthritis. *Arthritis Rheum*. 2011;63(1):267–275

Remvig L, Jensen DV, Ward RC. Epidemiology of general joint hypermobility and basis for the proposed criteria for benign joint hypermobility syndrome: review of the literature. *J Rheumatol*. 2007;34(4):804–809

Riise ØR, Handeland KS, Cvancarova M, et al. Incidence and characteristics of arthritis in Norwegian children: a population-based study. *Pediatrics*. 2008; 121(2):e299–e306

Smith JA, Mackensen F, Sen HN, et al. Epidemiology and course of disease in childhood uveitis. *Ophthalmology.* 2009;116(8):1544–1551

Stoll ML, Lio P, Sundel RP, Nigrovic PA. Comparison of Vancouver and International League of Associations for rheumatology classification criteria for juvenile psoriatic arthritis. *Arthritis Rheum.* 2008;59(1):51–58

van Rossum MA, van Soesbergen RM, Boers M, et al. Long-term outcome of juvenile idiopathic arthritis following a placebo-controlled trial: sustained benefits of early sulfasalazine treatment. *Ann Rheum Dis.* 2007;66(11):1518–1524

Vastert SJ, Kuis W, Grom AA. Systemic JIA: new developments in the understanding of the pathophysiology and therapy. *Best Pract Res Clin Rheumatol.* 2009;23(5):655–664

Weiss JE, Ilowite NT. Juvenile idiopathic arthritis. *Pediatr Clin North Am.* 2005;52(2):413–442

CHAPTER 149

Autoimmune Connective Tissue Diseases

Deborah McCurdy, MD

CASE STUDY

A 14-year-old girl has a 1-month history of severe fatigue with difficulty sleeping and a non-restorative sleep, hand swelling, generalized aches, low-grade fever, weight loss, and facial and leg rashes. She has not felt well enough to go to school for several weeks and complains her fingers are stiff and she can't type. On examination, she appears fatigued and does not look well. Vital signs show a temperature of 100.5°F (38.1°C), blood pressure of 138/84 mm Hg, pulse of 98 beats/min, and respiratory rate of 22 breaths/min. Her eyes appear puffy and her ankles and feet are swollen. She has swelling over the joints of her fingers and is having difficulty with buttons.

Questions

1. What findings are indicative of systemic lupus erythematosus (SLE)?
2. How can the clinical history and laboratory evaluation assist in determining the diagnosis and treatment?
3. What are the long-term outcomes for patients with SLE?
4. What similar clinical findings are present in other autoimmune diseases?
5. What types of agents are used in the treatment of autoimmune diseases?

The diseases discussed in this chapter have been called *collagen vascular diseases* because of the collagen proteins in connective tissues and the involvement of the vascular system. However, these diseases are not caused by problems with connective tissues or blood vessels, but in fact are aberrant immune responses, with known anti–self-antibodies associated with each disease, that result in inflammation and damage to connective tissues, blood vessels, and other organs in the body. Significant progress has been made in classifying each disease with criteria for diagnosis, including clinical and laboratory findings.

Treatment algorithms have been proposed by the Childhood Arthritis and Rheumatology Research Alliance (made up of pediatric rheumatologists from Canada and the United States) and the Paediatric Rheumatology International Trials Organization (a similar European organization). In general, treatment for these diseases must be started early and often aggressively to prevent organ damage and usually includes steroids and immunosuppressive therapies. While there has been great progress in the treatment of juvenile idiopathic arthritis with new biological treatments, many other autoimmune diseases are still treated with medications used for the last several decades. One exception is belimumab (Benlysta), a B-lymphocyte stimulator (BLyS)–specific inhibitor approved in 2011 and used to treat systemic lupus erythematosus (SLE). This new medication increases the hope for better treatments of these diseases in the future.

Evaluation for Autoimmune Disease: General Considerations

History

As always, the history is important to determine if an autoimmune disease is likely and should clearly delineate the onset (eg, whether there was a prior illness or injury), duration (eg, continuous or intermittent symptoms), and extent of the symptoms (eg, systems involved, severity of pain, swelling) (Questions Box).

Questions

Autoimmune Disease

- Has there been fatigue that interferes with normal activities? Does this fatigue extend to the weekends?
- Has there been skin or joint involvement? If so, where is the rash? Is it photosensitive? Which joints are affected?
- Is there pain in the joints?
- Are there visible changes in the joints such as swelling, erythema, or tightening of the skin?
- Are the symptoms more pronounced at specific times of the day (ie, morning stiffness, morning periorbital edema, swelling of the ankles at night)?
- Has the patient experienced weakness?
- What other symptoms, such as headache, fever, and weight loss, are present?

Physical Examination

Patients should undergo a complete physical examination with vital signs that includes a full assessment of the skin, a complete musculoskeletal examination, flexibility of the spine, strength of the muscles, and a neurologic and neuropsychiatric assessment. Lymphadenopathy should be noted as well as the presence of organomegaly. The presence of edema may indicate renal disease.

Laboratory Tests

In general, laboratory tests should include a complete blood cell count, erythrocyte sedimentation rate (ESR), C-reactive protein (CRP), urinalysis, and other studies as determined by the differential diagnosis. Patients suspected of having SLE should have an evaluation of autoantibodies, including antinuclear antibody (ANA), anti-dsDNA, anti-ribonucleoprotein (RNP)/Sm, and anti–SS-A (Ro)/SS-B (La). Low complements (due to consumption) are important indicators of active disease. Electrocardiograms (ECGs) and echocardiograms are appropriate in patients with SLE suspected of having cardiac involvement. Patients suspected of inflammatory myopathies should have creatine phosphokinase, aldolase, and lactate dehydrogenase levels, and, in severe cases, myositis-specific antibodies. Electromyogram (EMG) and muscle biopsy may be indicated if the diagnosis is not clear.

Imaging Studies

Magnetic resonance imaging (MRI) and magnetic resonance angiography (MRA) are helpful in the evaluation of central nervous system (CNS) lupus, and an MRI of the muscle shows inflamed joints in juvenile dermatomyositis (JDM).

Management

The treatment of autoimmune diseases depends on the diagnosis and severity and is discussed in the following sections.

Systemic Lupus Erythematosus

Systemic lupus erythematosus is a classic autoimmune disease with most patients having 6 or more autoantibodies, although it is not always clear that the autoantibodies cause the pathogenesis. Systemic lupus erythematosus is characterized by multiorgan system involvement and a waxing and waning course. The clinical presentation is variable and may be mild, presenting primarily with rash and arthritis, but in the pediatric population, it is often more severe, with frequent renal and other organ system involvement. It can present in any organ and should be considered in any child with multiorgan system symptoms. Antinuclear antibodies are present in greater than 90% of patients with SLE but can also be seen in many other diseases or in normal populations. Other, more specific autoantibodies are usually present and may be associated with disease manifestations. Studies have shown that symptoms of SLE may be present well before the diagnosis is made and it may take time to see the full picture. The goal of treatment is to decrease the inflammation and bring the immune system into balance.

Epidemiology

In certain populations, SLE is not rare. Always more common in females, the incidence and prevalence of SLE is reported to be higher in those descended from Hispanic, African, Native American, or Asian background. It is difficult to determine the incidence and prevalence of SLE in the pediatric population because of a lack of extensive pediatric studies. Approximately 20% of the cases of SLE are diagnosed in the pediatric population (<19 years old). The incidence is approximately 6 to 18.9 per 100,000 among white females, 20 to 30 per 100,000 among African American females, and 16 to 36.7 per 100,000 among Puerto Rican females. The male-female ratio varies from 1:4 to 1:7 depending on the ethnicity of the cohort. Five- and 10-year survival rates have improved to greater than 95% and 92%, respectively, among pediatric patients. Survival is affected by socioeconomic status, access to health care, educational background, racial and ethnic background, endemic infection rates, disease activity, and renal or CNS involvement. In the first 2 years, mortality is often associated with severe disease, and death results from pancreatitis, pulmonary hemorrhage, infection, thromboembolic disease, and active neuropsychiatric disease. More than 5 years after diagnosis, causes of mortality include complications of end-stage renal disease, atherosclerosis, suicide, and, less commonly, active SLE or infection.

Etiology and Pathogenesis

Systemic lupus erythematosus is the prototype of autoimmune disease with multiple autoantibodies. The current hypothesis is that there is a genetic predisposition to SLE that is induced by environmental factors. The genome-wide association studies done in 2008 identified more than 40 robust susceptibility loci of genes associated with SLE. These candidate genes are mostly involved in a variety of pathways suspected of leading to lupus pathogenesis, including immune complex processing, toll-like receptor signaling, and type 1 interferon production. Environmental factors include ultraviolet radiation, primarily viral infections (there is a strong association of SLE with Epstein-Barr virus), and drugs and chemicals.

In addition, there is a well-studied immune dysregulation that involves the innate and adaptive immune systems. In SLE, there is a loss of tolerance that leads to recognition of a self-antigen as foreign with subsequent autoantibody production (antibodies to DNA, histones, and small RNA proteins), increase in proinflammatory cytokines, and immune complexes. Theories include the generation of self-antigens on cell surfaces following apoptosis; abnormalities of innate immunity, including toll-like receptors; abnormalities of all arms of the adaptive immune system (including antigen-presenting cells, T cells, and B cells); and abnormal regulation of interferon-α.

Clinical Presentation

In 1982, criteria for the diagnosis of SLE were established by the American College of Rheumatology and were modified in 1997 to include antiphospholipid antibodies. To fulfill the criteria for a diagnosis of SLE, 4 out of the 11 clinical and laboratory findings must be present at some point during the disease. The criteria are approximately 95% specific and sensitive for diagnosis (Box 149-1).

Usually, patients present with constitutional symptoms such as fever, fatigue, and weight loss. Often, there is a history of a photosensitive rash and swelling of the joints. There may also be systemic inflammation with lymphadenopathy and hepatosplenomegaly. In the pediatric population, more than 80% have renal involvement at onset or at some point in the disease.

Mucocutaneous Involvement

Although the butterfly rash is strongly associated with SLE, only 60% of patients have this type of rash at onset, though up to 85% will have the butterfly rash at some point in their disease. This rash is usually photosensitive and crosses the nose, is present on both cheeks, but spares the nasolabial folds. There are other photosensitive rashes, including palpable purpura. Less common in the pediatric population is the discoid rash, which involves the dermis and can leave scars. This rash most often occurs in those of African descent. Approximately 10% to 30% of patients will have painless oral and nasal ulcers. Raynaud phenomenon is seen in 15% to 20% of children but is not specific for SLE.

Musculoskeletal Involvement

Often at onset and throughout their course, most patients experience arthritis, arthralgia, or tenosynovitis. The arthritis is usually a symmetric polyarthritis affecting large and small joints, especially the membrane cofactor proteins (MCPs) and proximal interphalangeal joints of the fingers. The arthritis is nonerosive and usually responds to treatments given to control other aspects of the disease. Often, patients have myalgia and occasionally myositis, usually with good response to disease treatment. Of concern, however, is that up to 20% of patients with SLE may develop a secondary fibromyalgia-like picture, and some develop a myopathy related to steroid treatment.

Box 149-1. Systemic Lupus Erythematosus Criteria for Diagnosis

Four of the following 11 clinical and laboratory findings are required for diagnosis:

- Butterfly rash
- Discoid rash
- Photosensitivity
- Oral ulcers
- Nonerosive arthritis
- Pleurisy or pericarditis
- Renal disorder
- Seizures or psychosis
- Hematologic disorder
- Positive autoantibodies (anti-dsDNA, anti-Sm, or antiphospholipid antibody/lupus anticoagulant)
- Positive antinuclear antibody

From Hochberg MC. Updating the American College of Rheumatology revised criteria for the classification of systemic lupus erythematosus. *Arthritis Rheum.* 1997;40(9):1725, with permission.

Renal Involvement

Other than the skin and joints, the organ system most frequently involved in SLE in the pediatric population is the kidney. Approximately 50% of patients present with lupus nephritis and 80% to 90% develop renal involvement in the first year. Treatment and prognosis is based on the histologic classification of nephritis as established by the World Health Organization (WHO) using renal biopsy (class I–VI) (Box 149-2).

The clinical markers (proteinuria, hematuria, creatinine level) may not correspond to histologic classifications, but often WHO class III and IV are associated with hypertension and impaired renal function and are treated with high-dose steroids and immunosuppression. Patients with WHO class III, IV, and V may also present with peripheral edema requiring steroid therapy. With more aggressive and consistent treatment, overall survival for patients with renal involvement has improved, with markedly higher 5- and 10-year survival rates.

Neuropsychiatric Involvement

Often, neuropsychiatric manifestations are underappreciated because patients often present with headaches, poor school performance, and features of depression. There may be involvement of the CNS or peripheral nervous system (thus, the term *neuropsychiatric SLE*) in 20% to 95% of patients with SLE. Headaches are the most frequent presentation, with a *lupus headache* defined as a migraine-like, unremitting headache requiring narcotic analgesics. Those that are refractory to treatment can be indicative of active CNS vasculitis, increased intracranial pressure, or cerebral vein thrombosis. Thrombotic events in the CNS or elsewhere are often associated with antiphospholipid antibodies in patients with lupus, and a full workup with urgent imaging is indicated if thrombosis is suspected. In these cases, an MRA often shows vasculitis or evidence of bleeding or ischemia. Psychosis manifested by visual and tactile hallucinations may be present in 30% to 50% of patients. Hallucinations are usually visual but may also be auditory. Imaging studies in this case may be normal, but often autoantibodies are found in the blood or spinal fluid. When psychosis is in isolation, secondary effects of glucocorticoids need to be considered. More difficult to delineate is cognitive impairment, which may present as a broad range of symptoms from difficulty concentrating to confusion and coma. Other, less common neurologic symptoms include seizures, movement disorders including chorea, and cranial nerve abnormalities. Imaging studies are an important part of the workup and may show vasculitis, hemorrhage or clot, or demyelination, or can be normal in antibody-mediated CNS disease.

Box 149-2. Lupus Nephritis: World Health Organization Classification

I: Normal or minimal mesangial
II: Mesangial
III: Focal proliferative, <50% glomeruli
IV: Diffuse proliferative, >50% glomeruli
V: Membranous, subepithelial immune deposits
VI: Sclerosing

Hematologic Involvement

Anemia, thrombocytopenia, and leukopenia may be present in 50% to 75% of patients. During active disease, patients often have a normochromic, normocytic anemia typical of anemia of chronic disease. The Coombs test is positive in 30% to 40% of patients, but only 10% to 15% have significant hemolysis. Thrombocytopenia is present in 15% to 45% of patients. Patients with chronic autoimmune idiopathic thrombocytopenic purpura (AITP) and Evans syndrome (AITP and Coombs-positive anemia) with a positive ANA are more frequently diagnosed with SLE. Leukopenia is thought to represent a general marker of disease activity.

Cardiac Involvement

Pericarditis is not uncommon in SLE (15%–25% symptomatic, but ECG changes in up to 68%) and may be asymptomatic. The myocardium and pericardium may also be involved, as well as the valves (aortic, tricuspid, mitral) with sterile verrucous vegetations or Libman-Sacks endocarditis. Libman-Sacks endocarditis may be associated with antiphospholipid antibodies and increase the risk for subacute bacterial endocarditis. Patients may present with chest pain that is worse when lying down or taking a deep breath. With chronic inflammation, there is an increased risk of premature arthrosclerosis, and one of the highest mortalities in young adults with SLE is from myocardial infarction.

Pleuropulmonary Involvement

The lungs may be involved in 25% to 75% of patients with SLE, with higher numbers noted by abnormal pulmonary function tests (PFTs) in an otherwise asymptomatic patient. Pleurisy is the most common manifestation and may be associated with pericarditis. Symptoms include chest pain, orthopnea, and dyspnea, and a chest radiograph may show a pleural effusion (frequently unilateral). Patients may present with pleuritic chest pain and respiratory distress associated with acute lupus pneumonitis or pulmonary hemorrhage or have a more indolent course with interstitial lung disease and shrinking lung syndrome (ie, loss of lung volume resulting from diaphragmatic dysfunction or phrenic nerve dysfunction). Pulmonary hypertension may be insidious and is a life-threatening complication of pulmonary involvement in the lung. Because of the disease and medications, opportunistic infections are also problematic. Imaging studies, especially a high-resolution chest computed tomography (CT) scan, and PFTs are indicated if pulmonary disease is suspected.

Gastrointestinal Involvement

Gastrointestinal involvement may be difficult to diagnose and differentiate from adverse effects from medication. The gastrointestinal system is involved in approximately 20% of patients. During active inflammation, patients often have hepatosplenomegaly. If transaminases are high, lupoid hepatitis should be suspected. Symptoms may include abdominal pain and diarrhea. Underlying pathology may be lupus peritonitis, enteropathy, or, with copious diarrhea, protein-losing enteropathy. Severe abdominal pain is seen with mesenteric vasculitis. Celiac disease has been associated with SLE and should be considered with severe weight loss. Pancreatitis is seen associated with active lupus or with steroid use and often presents with abdominal pain, nausea, and vomiting.

Endocrine Involvement

Antithyroid antibodies are common in SLE (up to 35% with antithyroid antibodies), and 10% to 15% of patients develop hypothyroidism. Thyroid-stimulating hormone should be checked annually in patients with SLE. Diabetes can be associated with SLE, but more frequently, diabetes is induced by corticosteroid treatment. Growth failure is a consequence of active disease and corticosteroid therapy. There may be a delay in puberty and menstrual abnormalities and, rarely, a girl without a menstrual cycle may have autoimmune ovarian failure. Ovarian failure may occur as a result of immunosuppressive treatment with cyclophosphamide.

Ocular Involvement

Active disease with retinal vasculitis may cause cytoid bodies (cotton-wool spots) noted on the retinal examination. Antiphospholipid antibodies may cause retinal vein occlusion and vision loss. Episcleritis and scleritis may occur. Keratoconjunctivitis sicca is seen in patients with secondary Sjögren syndrome.

Autoantibodies in Systemic Lupus Erythematosus

Autoantibodies are the hallmark of SLE, and most patients have more than 6 autoantibodies (Box 149-3). A positive ANA is found in virtually all patients, but this is not specific for or associated with a certain disease manifestation. The antibodies of SLE are directed against histone, nonhistone, RNA-binding, cytoplasmic, and nuclear proteins. These include anti-DNA (65%–95%), anti–RNA-binding proteins, and anti-U1RNP (27%–34%) and anti-Sm antibodies (32%–34%). Anti–SS-A and anti–SS-B antibodies (27%–33%) are seen less frequently but are associated with skin disease and neonatal lupus. Anticardiolipin (19%–87%) and the lupus anticoagulant (10%–62%) are the most common antiphospholipid antibodies. The

---

Box 149-3. Autoantibodies Frequently Seen in Systemic Lupus Erythematosus

Autoantibodies (specific)

Antinuclear
- Positive in virtually every patient

Anti-dsDNA
- Fluctuate with disease activity
- Increased with active renal disease

Anti-Sm

Autoantibodies (seen in other disease but associated with a clinical sequelae)

Coombs—hemolytic anemia

Anticardiolipin or antiphospholipid—thrombosis, thrombocytopenia, hemolytic anemia

Anti-ribosomal P—psychiatric disease

greatest risk of thrombosis is associated with lupus anticoagulant rather than with the other antiphospholipid antibodies.

Treatment

Treatment of children and adolescents with SLE must be started early to prevent organ damage. Treatments must be tailored to the symptoms, but young patients are reported to have a more severe disease and often require aggressive treatments. Those having mild disease with primarily musculoskeletal or cutaneous symptoms can be treated with nonsteroidal anti-inflammatory drugs (NSAIDs) and antimalarial drugs (hydroxychloroquine). The patient must be monitored carefully for progression of disease. One adverse effect of NSAIDs that is of particular concern in SLE is the association of the use of ibuprofen with aseptic meningitis. Methotrexate is used in patients with arthritis as their primary manifestation. Most often, children with SLE present with renal or other organ system involvement, and more than 90% require the use of corticosteroids at some point. There is a great deal of variability in how corticosteroids are used, but they must be used judiciously because of the adverse effects of weight gain, poor skin healing, osteoporosis, and, in approximately 10% of patients with SLE on corticosteroids, avascular necrosis, usually of the femoral head of the hip. Immunosuppressive therapy is used routinely in severe renal disease (classes III and IV) and in neuropsychiatric manifestations of lupus, including seizures, psychosis, and coma. Cyclophosphamide (Cytoxan) may be indicated in the most severe cases. Often, azathioprine (Imuran) or mycophenolate mofetil (MMF) (CellCept) is used to induce or maintain a clinical response. Plasmapheresis is used in severe cases of thrombocytopenic, thrombotic purpura, catastrophic antiphospholipid syndrome, and pulmonary hemorrhage. In autoimmune cytopenias, intravenous immunoglobulin (IVIG) may be useful. Monoclonal antibodies, including rituximab (Rituxan, anti-CD20), may be useful in cytopenias, and in antiphospholipid syndrome, belimumab (Benlysta, anti-BLyS) may be useful in treating skin disease and musculoskeletal manifestations. In renal disease, angiotensin-converting enzyme inhibitors help to decrease proteinuria. In neuropsychiatric disease, antiepileptics and antidepressants are indicated. Aspirin or other anticoagulants are used in those with antiphospholipid syndrome to prevent a thrombotic event. The diet and physical activity of all patients should be reviewed to be sure they are getting a healthy diet with enough calcium, vitamin D, and exercise to maintain good bone health.

Inflammatory Myopathies

Although chronic inflammatory myopathies are not common in children, JDM is not rare; prevalence is approximately 3.2 per 1 million children in the United States. Juvenile dermatomyositis is a multisystem disease of uncertain etiology that is characterized by a vasculopathy and inflammation of muscles, primarily the striated muscles, and skin. Often, as healing occurs, there is calcinosis in the areas affected by chronic inflammation. Polymyositis rarely occurs in children but presents in a manner similar to JDM, except there are no skin manifestations, and it is associated with a cellular inflammatory response. Myositis may be associated with other connective tissue diseases, such as SLE, mixed connective tissue disease, and scleroderma, with other types of myositis occurring very rarely in children.

Epidemiology

Although JDM is not common, it is important to recognize the symptoms because early treatment can prevent sequelae. A bimodal peak of onset of dermatomyositis is noted with the age range of onset in children of 5 to 14 years, with a peak at 7.6 years, and the age range in adults of 45 to 64 years. Dermatomyositis in adults may be associated with malignancy, but in JDM, this is rare. Juvenile dermatomyositis is more frequent in females, with an overall female to male ration of 1.7:1. In children, this ratio may be as high as 2.7:1.

Etiology and Pathology

The etiology of JDM is unknown, but, as with most autoimmune diseases, it is thought to be an interplay between genetics and environmental stimuli. At the locus of the human lymphocyte antigen (HLA), there are known inheritance patterns that confer a risk of myositis. In these susceptible individuals, infectious agents may increase the risk of inflammation. Often, an upper respiratory infection or gastrointestinal illness precedes the onset of JDM. Infections, including coxsackievirus, influenza, group A streptococcus, toxoplasmosis, parvovirus, hepatitis B, *Borrelia,* and leishmania, have been reported in association with JDM. In addition, JDM has been reported after vaccinations. Several studies suggest that JDM may be a result of microchimerism, in which the mother's cells are present in the child's muscle tissue, leading to an immune response.

The pathogenesis is that of an autoimmune angiopathy with an immune attack on muscle capillaries and endothelium that leads to vascular damage and vessel occlusion. There may also be deposition of immune complexes that contribute to vascular injury. The skin and muscle, primarily the striated muscles but also muscles of the gastrointestinal tract, are involved. Muscle fibers demonstrate atrophy or necrosis.

Clinical Presentation

The criteria in Box 149-4 are useful in making a diagnosis of JDM; however, these criteria have not been validated.

Box 149-4. Criteria for the Diagnosis of Juvenile Dermatomyositis

- Symmetric proximal muscle weakness
- Characteristic cutaneous changes
  - Heliotrope rash: discoloration of the eyelids with periorbital edema
  - Gottron papules: erythematous, scaly rash over dorsal aspects of the metacarpal and proximal interphalangeal joints
- Elevated skeletal muscle enzymes: creatine kinase, aspartate aminotransferase, alanine aminotransferase, lactate dehydrogenase, aldolase
- Electromyogram: myopathy and denervation
- Muscle biopsy: necrosis and inflammation

Adapted from Bohan A, Peter JB. Polymyositis and dermatomyositis (first of two parts). *N Engl J Med.* 1975;292(7):344–347; and Bohan A, Peter JB. Polymyositis and dermatomyositis (second of two parts). *N Engl J Med.* 1975;292(8):403–407, with permission.

Muscle Involvement

Often, children with JDM have an insidious progression over 3 to 6 months of malaise, low-grade fevers, and fatigue. Muscle pain or tenderness occurs in 25% to 75%, and there may be edema over the affected muscles. The predominant feature is muscle weakness of the neck and abdominal muscles, limb girdle, and lower extremities. On examination, the child is unable to sit up from the supine position without rolling over and using the arms to push himself or herself into a sitting position, to rise from sitting to standing, or to squat or sit on the floor and get up without help. On getting up from the floor, the Gowers sign is often present, and on walking, there may be a truncal sway and a positive Trendelenburg gait indicating weakness of the hips.

Pharyngeal, hypopharyngeal, and palatal muscles can be affected, and such involvement must be recognized promptly to prevent aspiration or respiratory distress. It is important to evaluate this urgently with a barium swallow and PFTs.

Skin Involvement

More than 75% of children have cutaneous abnormalities that are pathognomonic of the disease at presentation. The heliotrope discoloration of the upper eyelids and edema of the eyelids is usually present at diagnosis, as are Gottron papules—shiny, erythematous, scaly plaques that are symmetric changes over the extensor surfaces of joints that occur from the vasculopathy and subsequent ischemia. They are especially common over the proximal interphalangeal and metacarpophalangeal joints of the hand, extensor surfaces of the elbows and knees, and, more rarely, malleoli of the ankles. Less frequently appreciated but usually present is the inflammation and erythema of periungual skin and capillary nail bed that often show the presence of dilatation of vessel loops, thrombosis and hemorrhage, and, ultimately, loss of the capillary nail bed vessels.

Related to ischemic changes, ulceration may occur. In the areas of chronic inflammation, calcification occurs in 12% to 43% of patients, sometimes within 6 months of onset. Calcification may occur in the skin or muscle belly or diffusely and is problematic because of recurrent skin ulcerations, limitation of motion, pain in the involved muscle, and increased risk of infection because of poor skin integrity. Treatment of calcinosis is difficult and may require surgical removal in some instances.

Lipodystrophy, loss of fat from the body and extremities or local fat loss, occurs in 7% to 50% of children and can be associated with other metabolic problems.

Gastrointestinal Involvement

The muscles of the gastrointestinal tract may also be involved with inflammation throughout the bowel and micro-perforations when the disease is active. The child presents with progressive abdominal pain, melena, and hematemesis, or an ileus. Imaging studies may show free intraperitoneal air, but because the perforations are multiple and small, they may be difficult to recognize. This is a medical emergency and children should be treated for sepsis and evaluated for possible surgical intervention.

Cardiovascular Involvement

Cardiac involvement is rare but may be life threatening. Myocarditis, conduction defects, or first-degree heart block may be delayed in presentation but can lead to death. Hypertension can occur in 25% to 50% of patients, especially with glucocorticoid therapy. Prior to surgery, children with JDM should have a careful cardiac evaluation.

Involvement of Other Systems

Arthritis and arthralgia are frequent complications seen in JDM and may occur in 10% to 65% of children. Lymphadenopathy occurs early in the disease course in 10% to 65% of cases and usually improves with treatment.

Laboratory Studies

Laboratory studies, including a CBC and inflammatory markers (ESR and CRP), may be normal, but if there is a lot of inflammation in the skin and muscle, the inflammatory markers may be elevated.

Leukocytosis and anemia are rare except in children with infection or gastrointestinal bleeding. Urinalysis is usually normal. Because of the vasculopathy, factor VIII-related antigen (von Willebrand factor) may be high in children with active disease. Flow cytometry studies show increased numbers of CD19+B cells.

Muscle Enzymes

Serum levels of the sarcoplasmic muscle enzymes—aspartate transaminase, creatine kinase, lactate dehydrogenase, and aldolase—contribute to making the diagnosis and monitoring the effectiveness of therapy. Aspartate transaminase and lactate dehydrogenase correlate the best with active disease. Usually, creatine kinase is elevated, but it may fluctuate and is the first to decrease with therapy. The other enzymes may remain high and decrease more slowly as the disease improves.

Autoantibodies

The ANA is positive in 10% to 85% of patients, and antibodies against small RNA antigens (RNP, SS-A/SS-B) may be present. Traditional myositis-specific autoantibodies are rare in JDM, although anti-Jo-1 is seen in 2% to 5% of children with JDM, especially those with severe Raynaud disease and interstitial lung disease, and anti-Mi-2 is seen in 1% to 7% of those with more mild disease. Of note, several myositis-associated autoantibodies, including anti-p155 (associated with more severe cutaneous involvement and lipodystrophy) and anti-p140 (MJ) (associated with calcinosis, contractures), have recently been identified in 13% to 29% of children with JDM. These tests may not be available in all laboratories and are most helpful if the child has a specific disease manifestation but are not necessary for the diagnosis or treatment. The titers of these autoantibodies fluctuate with the level of disease activity and may become negative when disease enters remission.

Imaging Studies

Radiographs may show muscle edema and osteoporosis, but to determine the extent of muscle edema, MRI, especially the fat-suppressed T2 weighted or short T1 inversion recovery sequences, is required.

Short T1 inversion recovery is optimal to show hyper-intensity indicating muscle edema.

Electromyogram and Muscle Biopsy

An EMG showing a myopathic pattern and muscle biopsy with inflammation and loss of muscle fibers are rarely needed for the diagnosis. Usually, these are used in cases that are unclear and for which another criteria for diagnosis is needed.

Treatment

The use of corticosteroids has changed the prognosis for children with JDM. Corticosteroids decrease inflammation, improve skin manifestations and muscle strength, and prevent the chronic inflammation that leads to calcinosis. Almost all children require corticosteroid therapy; generally, a methylprednisolone sodium succinate pulse (30 mg/kg each day for 3 days) or a daily oral prednisone dose of 2 mg/kg is the first line of treatment. As strength improves and muscle enzymes return to normal, steroids are tapered. An adverse event of note with the use of corticosteroids is the onset of steroid-induced myopathy. However, in this case, muscle enzymes are not elevated. If there is an inadequate response to steroids, methotrexate is generally the second line of therapy, and if this is not sufficiently effective, IVIG is used. Hydroxychloroquine is useful for skin manifestations and may decrease the risk of calcinosis. Immunosuppressants may be necessary to treat vasculopathy of the bowel or other organs. For severe involvement, cyclophosphamide is indicated, but in less severe cases, azathioprine or cyclosporine is used. More recently, rituximab has been found to reverse severe muscle disease. Most children with JDM benefit from physical therapy. It is important to protect the skin from ultraviolet light and prevent tissue injury. The diet and physical activity are important to promote optimal intake of calcium and vitamin D and prevent osteopenia, muscle atrophy, and contractures.

Systemic Sclerosis (Scleroderma)

Scleroderma means "hard skin," but the term is not currently used to define this pleomorphic disease process. Instead, it is classified into systemic sclerosis, which is subdivided by the extent of the skin disease into diffuse cutaneous systemic sclerosis (dSSc) and limited cutaneous systemic sclerosis (lSSc). (Scleroderma was previously designated as CREST syndrome [*c*alcinosis cutis, *R*aynaud phenomenon, *e*sophageal dysfunction, *s*clerodactyly, *t*elangiectasia], localized scleroderma [LS], and morphea or linear scleroderma.) Fortunately, the systemic form of the disease is rare in children.

Epidemiology

There are worldwide reports of dSSc with an incidence of 0.45 to 1.9 per 100,000 and a prevalence of 24 per 100,000. The disease is more frequent in African Americans and Choctaw Native Americans. Children younger than 20 years comprise only about 1.2% to 9% of cases. In younger children, boys and girls are affected equally, but in older children, girls are affected more frequently.

Etiology and Pathogenesis

There is still much to be learned about the scleroderma spectrum. The skin thickening is believed to be caused by a dysfunction of the immune system that activates the endothelium and fibroblasts that promotes fibrosis. The genetic influence is not clear, but there is association with certain HLA markers. This is felt to be an autoimmune process because there are disease-specific autoantibodies and multiple abnormalities of T cell function (cellular immunity) with increased cytokines, adhesion molecules, and growth factors resulting in endothelial injury and fibroblast proliferation. Some studies suggest microchimerism may play a role in the pathogenesis of the sclerodermas, as well as dermatomyositis.

Clinical Manifestations

The Pediatric Rheumatology European Society, American College of Rheumatology, and European League Against Rheumatism developed criteria useful in diagnosis and research. Juvenile systemic sclerosis involves children younger than 16 years with one major criterion (presence of skin sclerosis, induration proximal to MCP or microsomal triglyceride transfer protein) and at least 2 of the 20 minor criteria (Box 149-5).

Because early on the course and progression of dSSc and lSSc may be insidious, the diagnosis may not be made for several years. The course is waxing and waning, and children and their parents may not notice subtle changes until there is significant effect on function or mobility. The characteristic presentation is a child with Raynaud phenomenon; tightening, thinning, and atrophy of the skin of the hands and face; or the appearance of cutaneous telangiectasias about the face, upper trunk, and hands. At the onset, there may be edema of the skin for a few weeks or months, and this may offer a window of opportunity for treatment to decrease the inflammation and decrease the resulting fibrosis. Following this, there is the sclerotic phase, noticeable especially over the digits (acrosclerosis, sclerodactyly) and face (circumoral furrowing). Finally, there is atrophy of the skin. Telangiectasia and calcinosis may be seen during this process.

Arthritis may be a symptom in approximately 36% of children with morning stiffness and pain of the small joints of the hands, knees, and ankles. Joint contractures progress slowly and most often involve the proximal interphalangeal joints and elbows.

The greatest morbidity and mortality is related to involvement of the cardiovascular, pulmonary, renal, and gastrointestinal systems. Cardiac involvement usually presents later in the course. Pericardial effusions may be the initial presentation, but morbidity is from cardiac ischemia of the coronary arteries and cardiac fibrosis. Systemic hypertension may be a complication and must be monitored carefully, especially because it may indicate a renal crisis. Pulmonary parenchymal disease is often asymptomatic early, but there may be symptoms of a dry cough or dyspnea on exertion. Patients may eventually develop interstitial pneumonitis or pulmonary hypertension with significant morbidity and mortality. Complications of this sort can be monitored by high-resolution chest CT scans and pulmonary PFTs. Renal disease is also an ominous complication of dSSc. A

Box 149-5. Criteria for Juvenile Systemic Sclerosis

Major Criterion

Sclerosis/induration of the skin proximal to the metacarpophalangeal or metatarsophalangeal joints

Minor Criteria

Skin

Sclerodactyly

Vasculopathy

Raynaud phenomenon

Nail fold capillary abnormalities

Digital tip ulcers

Gastrointestinal

Dysphagia

Gastroesophageal reflux

Renal

Renal crisis

New-onset arterial hypertension

Cardiac

Arrhythmias

Heart failure

Respiratory

Pulmonary fibrosis (high-resolution computer tomography/radiograph)

Decreased diffusion lung capacity for carbon monoxide

Pulmonary hypertension

Musculoskeletal

Tendon friction rubs

Arthritis

Myositis

Neurologic

Neuropathy

Carpal tunnel syndrome

Serology

Antinuclear antibodies

Systemic sclerosis selective autoantibodies (anti-centromere, anti-topoisomerase 1, anti-fibrillarin, anti-PM-Scl, anti-fibrillin, or anti-RNA polymerase 1 or 3)

From Zulian F, Woo P, Athreya BH, et al. The Pediatric Rheumatology European Society/American College of Rheumatology/European League Against Rheumatism provisional classification criteria for juvenile systemic sclerosis. *Arthritis Rheum.* 2007;57(2):203–212, with permission.

---

database in children noted that 5% had renal involvement and one developed renal crisis. The presence of anti-topoisomerase 1 antibody and rapidly progressing skin involvement are thought to be predictors of renal and cardiac involvement. Concern among rheumatologists caring for adults is the relationship between the use of high-dose steroids and the development of scleroderma renal crisis; thus, corticosteroids to reverse skin involvement must be used with caution and close monitoring. Gastrointestinal involvement is fairly common, affecting one-third of patients during the course of the disease. The oral cavity may have telangiectasia, and often patients complain of dry mouth or the sicca syndrome. Esophageal involvement may present early in the disease with heartburn and delayed gastric emptying that can lead to aspiration. The small bowel is often involved with decreased motility and malabsorption and the large bowel with constipation.

Laboratory Studies

The CBC shows anemia in about 25% of patients and may reflect anemia of chronic disease or caused by vitamin B_{12} or folate deficiency resulting from chronic malabsorption. Leukocytosis is rare, but eosinophilia occurs in approximately 15% of patients.

Autoantibodies

High titers of ANAs in the speckled pattern are frequently seen in approximately 80% of patients. Anti-topoisomerase 1 (anti–Scl-70) autoantibodies are present in 28% to 34% of patients and are usually seen in patients with dSSc with peripheral vascular disease, digital pitting, pulmonary interstitial fibrosis, renal involvement, and higher rate of mortality. Anti-centromere antibodies occur almost exclusively in patients with lSSc in association with calcinosis and telangiectasias; they are seen less frequently in children.

Cardiopulmonary Function

If the heart is involved, there may be ECG abnormalities such as first-degree heart block, right and left bundle branch block, premature atrial and ventricular contractions, nonspecific T wave changes, and evidence of ventricular hypertrophy, but most concerning is cardiac arrhythmia, which in children is of supraventricular origin. Pulmonary function tests show a decrease in vital capacity and forced expiratory flow, an early decrease in diffusion, and an increase in functional residual volume. Restrictive lung disease occurs in up to 23% of patients. Electrocardiograms and PFTs should be done every 6 to 12 months to monitor for heart and lung involvement in patients with dSSc and lSSc.

Radiologic Examination

Radiographs may show resorption of the distal tufts of the digits. Chest radiographs and high-resolution chest CT scans are indicated to detect interstitial lung disease or signs of pulmonary hypertension.

Treatment

The optimal treatment is not yet worked out for dSSc and lSSc, and often, patients do not seem to respond to therapies. Raynaud phenomenon and digital ulcers are treated with calcium channel blockers and sildenafil. More recently, iloprost (synthetic analogue of prostacyclin PGI_2) and bosentan (competitive antagonist of endothelin-1) are used for severe digital ulcers. Iloprost and bosentan are useful in pulmonary hypertension to increase vascular dilatation and decrease pulmonary vascular resistance. To decrease inflammation in the lung, cyclophosphamide may be used in severe cases and other immunosuppression drugs (MMF or azathioprine) and hydroxychloroquine in more mild cases. Angiotensin-converting enzyme inhibitors play an important role in preventing renal crisis. The skin disease is treated cautiously with low-dose steroids early in the disease during the edematous phase and with methotrexate during the sclerotic phase. Gastroesophageal reflux disease is treated with proton pump inhibitors. Supportive care is of great importance with attention to skin integrity, joint range of motion, and gastrointestinal issues with weight loss. The family and child need to be educated on the disease and its complications, and information for the school and community should be available. Despite all treatment efforts, the prognosis is guarded.

Localized Scleroderma

Despite the fact that systemic sclerosis and LS are associated with accumulation of collagen and fibrosis, the diseases are distinct in that LS is limited to the skin and almost never involves internal organs. Often, the lesions are called morphea.

Epidemiology

Linear scleroderma is seen predominantly in the pediatric population, with 67% of cases diagnosed before 18 years of age. The prevalence of morphea in children younger than 17 years is estimated to be 50 per 100,000. The incidence of LS is approximately is 2.7 cases per 100,000.

Etiology and Pathogenesis

Often, the picture of LS is like graft-versus-host disease, with abnormalities of regulation of fibroblasts, production of collagen, and immunologic abnormalities. Immune activation and autoantibody production are consistent with an autoimmune disease. The pathology is similar to that seen with systemic sclerosis.

Clinical Manifestations

Recently, the Pediatric Rheumatology European Society proposed a new classification for LS with 5 subtypes: circumscribed morphea, linear scleroderma, generalized morphea, pansclerotic morphea, and the new mixed subtype, in which a combination of 2 or more of the previous subtypes is present (Box 149-6).

Linear scleroderma is the most common subtype in children and adolescents, characterized by one or more linear streaks that typically involve an upper or lower extremity. With time, the streaks become progressively more indurated and can extend through the dermis, subcutaneous tissue, and muscle to the underlying bone.

Box 149-6. Classification of Juvenile Localized Scleroderma

1. Circumscribed morphea: round circumscribed areas
2. Linear scleroderma: affecting the trunk or limb, the head (en coup de sabre ["blow of a saber"]); Parry-Romberg syndrome or progressive facial hemiatrophy
3. Generalized morphea: induration of the skin that becomes confluent, eventually involving a large area
4. Pansclerotic morphea: circumferential involvement of limb(s) affecting the skin, subcutaneous tissue, muscle, and bone
5. Mixed morphea: combination of 2 or more of the previous subtypes

From Laxer RM, Zulian F. Localized scleroderma. *Curr Opin Rheumatol.* 2006;18(6):606–613, with permission.

En coup de sabre involves the scalp and head (at once thought to look like the depression caused by the strike from a sword); progressive facial hemiatrophy may occur. Parry-Romberg syndrome is characterized by progressive facial hemiatrophy of the skin and tissue below the forehead. Patients with facial hemiatrophy may experience associated seizures and dental and ocular abnormalities.

Morphea—areas of indurated, waxy skin with an ivory center and violaceous halo—are most commonly found on the trunk. The lesions may be small (<1 cm) and called guttate or larger and may become confluent or generalized morphea. Deep morphea, in which the entire skin is thickened and feels bound down, involves subcutaneous morphea and eosinophilic fasciitis. This form is the least common and considered the most disabling. Although LS involves primarily the skin, some patients will develop musculoskeletal complaints.

Laboratory Studies

Antinuclear antibodies are present in 23% to 73% of patients but do not predict the disease course. Anti-histone antibodies are detected in 47%, are associated with more extensive localized disease, and may be useful in assessing disease activity.

Treatment

Topical imiquimod, an immunomodulator that inhibits the collagen production by fibroblasts, is used with reports of success. Ultraviolet phototherapy is sometimes used for superficial lesions. Treatment with methotrexate in combination with corticosteroids should be considered for linear scleroderma because of the progressive process. If lesions do not improve or expand, MMF is useful to inhibit further fibrosis. Unfortunately, the difficulty in measuring lesion size makes it difficult to fully assess response to treatment.

Prognosis

Prognosis is improving for most autoimmune diseases because there is increased understanding of the pathogenesis. Criteria are being established and validated to aid in the diagnosis of each disease and to optimize treatment. Consultation with rheumatologists, neurologists, nephrologists, and infectious disease specialists may be required to assist in the final diagnosis.

The care of a child with an autoimmune disease requires a multidisciplinary approach involving a primary care physician, rheumatologist, and subspecialists with expertise in affected target organs. The role for the primary care physician is to ensure routine care of the patient as well as prevent long-term disease and treatment sequelae. Because many of the agents used to manage autoimmune disease have significant side effects, it is vital for the primary care physician to be well versed with a patient's medication regimen. Patients with autoimmune disease often experience growth failure from the disease process or its treatment. Ensuring appropriate diet and physical activity is vital. Supplementation with calcium and vitamin D is beneficial to prevent osteoporosis. Periodic ophthalmologic screening, essential to assess for disease activity or adverse effects from medication, should be done at least annually. In the long term, patients with autoimmune disease are at a higher risk for cardiovascular disease secondary to chronic inflammation. They may require annual cardiovascular risk assessments that include a review of the diet and lipid profiles. Individuals who have suffered thrombolytic events or are at high risk for thrombosis may benefit from low-dose aspirin prophylaxis. As with any patient with a chronic disease, maintaining a feasible quality of life is essential. Disease management for patients with autoimmune disease is a balance of optimal function, minimal complications, and improved quality of life.

CASE RESOLUTION

The adolescent in the case study has findings consistent with systemic lupus erythematosus and mild hypertension consistent with lupus nephritis. She undergoes a number of laboratory studies, including a complete blood cell count, erythrocyte sedimentation rate, antinuclear antibody (ANA), and anti-dsDNA and complements. Her ANA and anti-dsDNA results are positive. The complements are low. She is referred to a pediatric rheumatologist and nephrologist and a renal biopsy confirms lupus nephritis (class III). She is started on treatment with steroids and immunosuppression and improves over the next 6 months.

References

Benseler SM, Silverman ED. Systemic lupus erythematosus. *Pediatr Clin North Am.* 2005;52(2):443–467

Christen-Zaech S, Hakim MD, Afsar FS, Paller AS. Pediatric morphea (localized scleroderma): review of 136 patients. *J Am Acad Dermatol.* 2008;59(3): 385–396

Cunninghame Graham DS. Genome-wide association studies in systemic lupus erythematosus: a perspective. *Arthritis Res Ther.* 2009;11(4):119

Feldman BM, Rider LG, Reed AM, Pachman LM. Juvenile dermatomyositis and other idiopathic inflammatory myopathies of childhood. *Lancet.* 2008;371(9631): 2201–2212

Hochberg MC. Updating the American College of Rheumatology revised criteria for the classification of systemic lupus erythematosus. *Arthritis Rheum.* 1997;40(9):1725

Horowitz DL, Furie R. Belimumab is approved by the FDA: what more do we need to know to optimize decision making? *Curr Rheumatol Rep.* 2012;14(4): 318–323

Laxer RM, Zulian F. Localized scleroderma. *Curr Opin Rheumatol.* 2006;18(6): 606–613

Reed AM, McNallan K, Wettstein P, Vehe R, Ober C. Does HLA-dependent chimerism underlie the pathogenesis of juvenile dermatomyositis? *J Immunol.* 2004;172(8):5041–5046

Rider LG, Lindsley CB, Cassidy JT. Juvenile dermatomyositis. In: Cassidy JT, Laxer RM, Petty RE, Lindsley CB, eds. *Textbook of Pediatric Rheumatology.* Sanders; 2013

Silverman E, Eddy A. Systemic lupus erythematosus. In: Cassidy JT, Laxer RM, Petty RE, Lindsley CB, eds. *Textbook of Pediatric Rheumatology.* Sanders; 2013

Tan EM, Cohen AS, Fries JF, et al. The 1982 revised criteria for the classification of systemic lupus erythematosus. *Arthritis Rheum.* 1982;25(11):1271–1277

Wedderburn LR, Rider LG. Juvenile dermatomyositis: new developments in pathogenesis, assessment and treatment. *Best Pract Res Clin Rheumatol.* 2009; 23(5):665–678

Zulian F. Systemic sclerosis and localized scleroderma in childhood. *Rheum Dis Clin North Am.* 2008;34(1):239–255

Zulian F, Cassidy JT. The systemic sclerodermas and related disorders. In: Cassidy JT, Laxer RM, Petty RE, Lindsley CB, eds. *Textbook of Pediatric Rheumatology.* Sanders; 2013

Zulian F, Laxer RM. Localized scleroderma. In: Cassidy JT, Laxer RM, Petty RE, Lindsley CB, eds. *Textbook of Pediatric Rheumatology.* Sanders; 2013

Zulian F, Woo P, Athreya BH, et al. The Pediatric Rheumatology European Society/American College of Rheumatology/European League Against Rheumatism provisional classification criteria for juvenile systemic sclerosis. *Arthritis Rheum.* 2007;57(2):203–212

CHAPTER 150

Nephrotic Syndrome

Elaine S. Kamil, MD

CASE STUDY

A 2-year-old boy is brought to the office because of abdominal distention. He has just recovered from a runny nose that lasted a week, with no fever or change in activity. His mother complains that his eyelids were very swollen that morning, and she says that his thighs look "fat." She has noticed that he has fewer wet diapers. He has always been a healthy child, and his immunizations are up-to-date. The family has a history of asthma and allergic rhinitis. Physical examination shows an active 2-year-old boy. Head and neck examination is clear, except for a few shotty anterior cervical lymph nodes and some minimal periorbital edema. Chest examination reveals some decreased breath sounds at the bases. The abdomen is moderately distended; bowel sounds are active and a fluid wave is detectable. There is 2+ pitting edema of the lower legs, extending up to the knees. The urine has a specific gravity of 1.030; pH 6; 4+ protein; and trace, non-hemolyzed blood. Microscopic examination shows 4 to 6 red blood cells per high-power field and 10 to 20 hyaline and fine granular casts per low-power field.

Questions

1. What is the differential diagnosis of edema and ascites in previously healthy young children?
2. What criteria are used to determine if children with nephrotic syndrome require hospitalization or can be managed as outpatients?
3. What laboratory evaluation and therapy are instituted initially?
4. What are the important issues to address in parent education?
5. What is the prognosis of young children with nephrotic syndrome?

Although nephrotic syndrome is not a common childhood disease, every pediatrician can expect to care for 1 to 3 nephrotic children at some time. Nephrotic syndrome may have serious or even fatal complications, and the disease tends to follow a chronic, relapsing course. Thus, it is important for the pediatrician to become familiar with the signs and symptoms of the disease and with the most current treatment modalities aimed at keeping affected children healthy and active.

Nephrotic syndrome occurs when an individual excretes a sufficient quantity of plasma proteins, primarily albumin, in the urine to cause hypoalbuminemia. Substantial urinary protein losses, hypercholesterolemia, and hypoalbuminemia characterize nephrotic syndrome. The condition is usually accompanied by obvious edema, but occasionally edema is not clinically detectable (D_x Box).

In children, proteinuria of more than 40 mg/m²/hour (>50 mg/kg/24 hours) is considered nephrotic range proteinuria. (In adult-sized patients, proteinuria of more than 3.5 g in 24 hours is associated with nephrotic syndrome.) Collection of a 24-hour urine sample is cumbersome in children, and the urinary total protein-creatinine (TP-Cr) ratio done on a random urine sample, preferably a first morning urine, is a useful alternative. Whereas a ratio greater than 3.5 is considered nephrotic range proteinuria in adults with normal renal function, a ratio greater than 1.0 may occur in nephrotic children (see Chapter 98). Twenty-four–hour urine protein losses (g/m²/day) in children can be estimated by multiplying the urinary TP-Cr by 0.63.

Epidemiology

Minimal change disease (MCD) is the most common form of nephrotic syndrome in childhood. The annual prevalence of new cases of nephrotic syndrome is 2 to 3 in 100,000 children in the population younger than 16 years. The cumulative prevalence of this chronic disease is 16 in 100,000. Ninety percent of childhood cases are not associated with any systemic disease, and two-thirds of cases of childhood nephrotic syndrome present before age 5 years. The ratio of boys to girls in young children with nephrotic syndrome is 2:1. By late adolescence, both sexes are equally affected, and diseases other than MCD are much more prevalent in adolescents.

Clinical Presentation

The typical child presenting with nephrotic syndrome is a preschool-aged boy who is brought to the physician because he appears swollen

Nephrotic Syndrome

- Heavy proteinuria (>40 mg/m²/hour or 50 mg/kg/24 hours in children)
- Hypoalbuminemia
- Hypercholesterolemia
- Edema

to the parents. Some children are active and relatively asymptomatic despite the edema, whereas others may be very uncomfortable, with markedly swollen eyelids, abdominal discomfort, scrotal or labial edema, and even respiratory compromise. Usually children have a history of preceding infection, most typically an upper respiratory infection (URI). Occasionally, children develop diarrhea secondary to edema of the bowel wall.

Occasionally, children with nephrosis are critically ill because of peritonitis, bacteremia, or, rarely, a major thrombotic episode. Because their immune state is compromised, rapid evaluation and treatment of children with these complications of nephrotic syndrome are essential for survival. The primary peritonitis associated with nephrotic syndrome may be confused with an acute abdomen, such as may be seen with appendicitis. Some children who are experiencing a severe relapse have hypotensive symptoms secondary to intravascular volume depletion.

Pathophysiology

The exact cause of MCD and focal segmental glomerulosclerosis (FSGS) is not known. Recent genetic and biomarker studies suggest that MCD and FSGS are different diseases, although they both exhibit intrinsic structural defects in the glomerular podocyte. For MCD, the best current theory postulates that some stimulus (usually infectious) causes a clone of cells to proliferate and produce one or more soluble factors that are toxic to the glomerular epithelial cells (podocytes), cells that maintain the glomerular basement membranes. Active MCD shows a reduction in the net negative charge across the glomerular basement membrane and causes a diffuse abnormality in capillaries throughout the body, leading to leakage of albumin in the peripheral capillaries and increases in interstitial fluid. The constituents of the glomerular basement membrane and chemicals coating the glomerular epithelial and endothelial cells normally bear a net negative charge. The presence of these negatively charged chemicals creates a charge-selective barrier to filtration. This barrier plays a significant role in the ultrafiltration of macromolecules present in the plasma, enhancing the filtration of molecules bearing a positive electrical charge and retarding the filtration of molecules bearing a negative electrical charge. During episodes of relapse, patients with MCD show a breakdown in the normal charge-selective barrier to filtration, often resulting in massive proteinuria. Kidney biopsies from patients with nephrotic syndrome demonstrate a net reduction in anionic sites during periods of relapse. In addition, some children have mutations in podocyte proteins such as nephrin and podocin that lead to nephrotic syndrome. Children presenting with nephrosis before 1 year of age have a high likelihood of having a genetic mutation causing nephrotic syndrome, and any child with steroid-resistant nephrotic syndrome should also be screened for such genetic mutations.

Recent studies have shown evidence that the soluble factors in FSGS and MCD are probably different. For example, 70% of patients with FSGS have been shown to have elevated plasma levels of soluble urokinase plasminogen activator receptor, but patients with MCD have undetectable levels. Evidence indicating that the proteinuria in the patient with MCD or FSGS may be caused by soluble factors is manyfold. Some patients who develop end-stage renal disease from idiopathic nephrotic syndrome (particularly FSGS) have experienced a relapse of the nephrotic syndrome with massive proteinuria immediately after transplantation of a normal kidney. Infusion of peripheral blood mononuclear cell products from nephrotic children induces albuminuria in rats. Removal of serum proteins by adsorption to a protein A Sepharose column or by plasmapheresis has led to remission of proteinuria in some patients who have experienced a recurrence of nephrotic syndrome after transplantation. Mixing plasma from a patient in relapse with FSGS with glomeruli in vitro can lead to swelling of the glomeruli. The remission of the proteinuria after treatment with immunosuppressive medication provides further evidence that nephrotic syndrome is mediated in some way by the immune system. Children with MCD have been shown to have higher helper T–regulatory T cell ratios.

Normal adults are able to synthesize 12 g of albumin per day in the liver, and adults with nephrotic syndrome may synthesize 14 g of albumin per day. Therefore, the **hypoproteinemia** characteristic of nephrotic syndrome cannot be explained completely by measured amounts of urinary protein losses (about 3.5 g/day). The difference between the hepatic synthetic capacity for albumin and measured urinary losses can be explained by protein catabolism in the kidney. Renal tubular epithelial cells reabsorb filtered plasma proteins and catabolize them to amino acids, which then reenter the amino acid pool of the body. Thus, the magnitude of losses of plasma proteins at the glomerular level is far greater than the amount measured in a 24-hour urine sample.

The **hypoalbuminemia** seen in nephrotic syndrome is a result of the massive proteinuria, and the **hypercholesterolemia** occurs as a consequence of the hypoalbuminemia. The hyperlipidemia is partially the result of a generalized increase in hepatic protein synthesis that also involves overproduction of lipoproteins. In addition, less lipid is transported into the adipose tissue because the activity of lipoprotein lipase is reduced in adipose tissue during active nephrotic syndrome. Hyperlipidemia is most pronounced in children with MCD. Serum albumin and serum cholesterol are generally inversely correlated. The hyperlipidemia is the last biochemical abnormality to clear after the child achieves remission from an episode of nephrotic syndrome.

Differential Diagnosis

Nephrotic syndrome is considered primary or secondary. Primary nephrotic syndrome is not associated with a systemic disease, while secondary nephrotic syndrome is a feature of a systemic disease such as anaphylactoid purpura, immunoglobulin (Ig) A nephropathy, or systemic lupus erythematosus (SLE). Most young children with nephrotic syndrome have the primary form of the disease, although secondary causes become more prevalent during adolescence.

Children with primary nephrotic syndrome are also classified according to their response to steroid therapy. Affected individuals may be categorized as steroid-sensitive, steroid-dependent, or steroid-resistant. Typically, children who are steroid-sensitive and remain so have MCD, although, strictly speaking, a renal biopsy must be performed before the diagnosis of MCD is made. Sensitivity to or dependence on corticosteroids is a critical factor in determining a child's prognosis.

Nephrotic syndrome is also classified by the appearance of the glomeruli on renal biopsy. A summary of the histologic lesions causing nephrotic syndrome appears in Table 150-1. About 95% of young children with nephrotic syndrome have MCD. In these children, light microscopy shows normal-appearing glomeruli. Immunofluorescent microscopy is generally negative but may show some mesangial IgM deposits, and electron microscopy simply shows foot process effacement of the podocytes. In individuals with FSGS, light microscopy may show enlarged glomeruli and glomeruli with segments of sclerosis. Immunofluorescence may reveal some IgM and complement in the sclerotic segments, and electron microscopy shows areas of foot process effacement of podocytes. Biopsies performed later in the disease course show some totally sclerotic glomeruli, areas of interstitial fibrosis, and atrophy. Several recent series have noted an apparent increase in the incidence of FSGS among nephrotic children.

Other primary renal diseases that can cause nephrotic syndrome in children include membranous nephropathy, membranoproliferative glomerulonephritis (MPGN), IgA nephropathy and other forms of chronic glomerulonephritis, congenital nephrotic syndrome, and diffuse mesangial proliferative glomerulonephritis. Chronic hepatitis B infection may cause membranous nephropathy or MPGN. In endemic areas, the incidence of hepatitis B–associated membranous nephropathy has been reduced since the implementation of universal hepatitis B vaccination programs. Rarely, poststreptococcal acute glomerulonephritis and other forms of postinfectious acute glomerulonephritis may also cause nephrotic syndrome. With the exception of congenital nephrotic syndrome, all of these diseases show the presence of immune deposits in the glomerular mesangial regions or along the glomerular basement membrane as well as some element of cellular proliferation, which may be severe. In these disease states, the presence of nephrotic syndrome is indicative of marked injury to the glomerular capillary wall. Neonates with congenital nephrotic syndrome, Finnish type, have a mutation of the gene encoding the nephrin molecule, a podocyte protein with a large extracellular domain that is an integral part of the glomerular slit diaphragm. These neonates have massive proteinuria beginning in utero and have severe nephrotic syndrome presenting in the first month of life.

Because of the varying distribution of edema fluid at presentation, nephrotic syndrome may be confused with sinusitis or an allergic reaction (periorbital edema), obesity (ascites), or an abdominal mass (ascites). Other causes of generalized edema, such as congestive heart failure, hypoproteinemia from inflammatory bowel disease, or liver disease, can be easily excluded.

Evaluation

History

The clinical evaluation should include a careful history (Questions Box).

Physical Examination

A complete physical examination is necessary. Blood pressure should be monitored because hypertension or hypotension may occur. The extent of peripheral and central edema, including swelling of the eyelids, should be assessed. The physician should obtain a reliable, overall impression of the child's level of comfort and activity. Examination should also include a careful search for infection, particularly life-threatening infections such as pneumonia or peritonitis. Examination of the head and neck should focus on signs of recent infection, such as otitis media. The presence of dullness to percussion at the bases of the thorax is consistent with large pleural effusions. Ascites may be minimal or massive. With severe ascites, scrotal or labial edema may occur. If the child has a history of abdominal pain, a careful check for signs of peritoneal irritation should be made. The skin should be inspected for infection and rashes.

Table 150-1. Distribution of Histologic Type by Age of Onset in Children With Nephrotic Syndrome					
Age (y)	MCD[a]	FSGS	MN	MPGN	Other GN
1–4	95%	3%	2%	—	—
4–8	75%	15%	1%	7%	2%
8–16	52%	15%	2%	25%	6%

Abbreviations: FSGS, focal segmental glomerulosclerosis; GN, glomerulonephritis; MCD, minimal change disease; MN, membranous nephropathy; MPGN, membranoproliferative glomerulonephritis.
[a]MCD remains the dominant histologic type through mid-adolescence but becomes relatively less important in later childhood and adolescence.

Questions

Nephrotic Syndrome

- Has the child recently had any infections, such as pharyngitis or an upper respiratory infection? Is he from a group at high risk for hepatitis B or C infection?
- Are the child's eyelids swollen? Do they look more or less puffy at certain times during the day, especially on awaking or after crying?
- Does the child have a history of rashes characteristic of diseases that are associated with nephrotic syndrome?
- Is there a history of fever, oliguria, or abdominal pain?
- Is there a family history of nephrotic syndrome or kidney disease?
- Is the child playful and active, or is the edema so significant that movement is uncomfortable?
- Are the ascites and pleural effusions so severe that some respiratory compromise is evident?

Laboratory Tests

The laboratory evaluation of children with nephrotic syndrome begins with a urinalysis. The dipstick shows 3+ or 4+ protein, although a dilute urine may be only 2+. Microscopic hematuria may be present in up to 25% of children with MCD. The presence of associated glycosuria in a nephrotic child who is not on steroid therapy raises a concern for FSGS. Careful microscopic examination of the urine is necessary. Casts are seen frequently because urinary proteins precipitate in the tubules. The casts are hyaline, fine, and coarse granular. White blood cell (WBC) casts are sometimes seen because some children with nephrotic syndrome may also have increased amounts of leukocytes in their urine. Large amounts of red blood cells (RBCs) and RBC casts are not seen in uncomplicated MCD and, if present, indicate another cause for the nephrotic syndrome. If RBC casts are seen together with substantial hematuria, an antistreptolysin-O titer should be added to the preliminary evaluation outlined as follows. A random urinary TP-Cr should be done to determine whether children have nephrotic range proteinuria.

If the urine shows only proteinuria, with perhaps some microscopic hematuria, blood tests should include a complete blood cell count (CBC), serum creatinine and blood urea nitrogen (BUN), electrolytes, serum calcium, serum albumin, cholesterol, complement component 3 (C3), and antinuclear antibody (ANA). The CBC may show a high hematocrit from hemoconcentration because many children experience volume contraction as a complication of hypoproteinemia. Children may also have very high platelet counts (sometimes >1 million/µL). The BUN and creatinine help assess renal function. A hyperchloremic metabolic acidosis is sometimes seen. The serum albumin and cholesterol are required to differentiate nephrotic syndrome from other edematous states. A low level of C3 is associated with other renal diseases such as MPGN, acute postinfectious glomerulonephritis, and SLE. The ANA is useful in screening for SLE and other collagen vascular diseases. Hepatitis B serology is helpful in children who come from a population at risk for hepatitis B infection, such as recent immigrants from Southeast Asia or children of intravenous (IV) drug abusers. Although not part of the routine laboratory evaluation, measurement of quantitative Ig often shows low IgG levels and elevated IgM levels. The febrile child should also have blood and urine cultures and, if there are signs of peritoneal irritation, a culture of peritoneal fluid. Though not part of the routine evaluation, if there is a family history of thrombotic events, a thrombophilia evaluation should be considered because of the association between renal vein thrombosis and nephrotic syndrome, particularly in adults.

Imaging Studies

Chest radiographs help assess the severity of pleural effusions in children with marked ascites and respiratory compromise.

Management

Hospitalization

The decision to admit a child with nephrotic syndrome to the hospital is determined by the child's functional status. All children with severe edema compromising ambulation or respiration should be admitted. Other indications for admission include unstable vital signs, fever, marked oliguria, and hemoconcentration (hematocrit >48%–50%).

Most children with nephrotic syndrome are hospitalized for control of edema or treatment of a complication such as infection. The management of children in relapse is aimed at minimizing edema and preventing complications until the disease can be controlled with immunosuppressive therapy. Intake, output, and weight need to be closely monitored. Blood pressure should be followed, although hypertension is not common. If children have a fever (temperature >100.7°F [38.2°C]), blood and urine cultures should be obtained and antibiotics started pending culture results. If signs of peritoneal inflammation are evident, paracentesis should also be performed to obtain samples of the ascites fluid for Gram stain, cell count, and culture. Broad-spectrum antibiotics should be given to cover respiratory pathogens, especially pneumococcus, and enteric pathogens. All children who are newly diagnosed with nephrotic syndrome should have a purified protein derivative (PPD) test because immunosuppression associated with steroid therapy may facilitate reactivation of tuberculosis infection. Treatment with corticosteroids should be delayed until there is confirmation of a negative PPD.

Intravenous albumin (25%) should be used selectively because albumin infusions are expensive, and the infused albumin is excreted very rapidly in the urine. Infusions are indicated in children with marked ascites, scrotal or labial edema, or significant pleural effusions. They are also helpful in maintaining blood pressure and renal perfusion in septic children with nephrotic syndrome. The usual dose is 1 g/kg, up to 25 g, infused over 2 to 4 hours, with close monitoring of blood pressure. Furosemide (1 mg/kg IV) is usually administered post-infusion. Albumin infusions may be repeated every 12 to 24 hours as necessary. If children with oliguria fail to increase their urine output after the first or second albumin infusion, they need to be evaluated immediately for the presence of acute kidney injury (see Chapter 70). The albumin-induced mobilization of edema fluid in nephrotic children with acute kidney injury can precipitate pulmonary edema.

Children with nephrotic syndrome have an increased tendency to thromboembolic phenomenon. Increased risk factors for this complication include loss of antithrombin 3 in the urine, age 12 years or older, the existence of a central line, and secondary causes of nephrotic syndrome such as SLE.

Supportive Therapy

Diet

Because sodium plays a key role in edema formation, children with nephrotic syndrome should be placed on a no-added-salt diet that limits dietary sodium to 2 or 3 g/day. Technically, sodium restriction is indicated only during times of relapse, but a consistent no-added-salt diet helps entire families maintain a healthy diet. Even though the children have hyperlipidemia, it is not advantageous to implement a low-fat diet because hyperlipidemia is not caused by fat intake and should resolve after the child goes into remission. In general, fluid restriction is not necessary except in unusual circumstances (eg, a steroid-resistant patient with persistent edema). Although earlier teachings recommended the use of high-protein diets, newer research has shown that high-protein diets may actually increase urinary protein losses.

Activity

In the past, children with nephrotic syndrome were treated with bed rest because the supine position somewhat reduces urinary protein losses. No evidence shows that bed rest has a significant effect on children's clinical state, however. Therefore, most pediatric nephrologists recommend that children be allowed full activity. Boys with marked scrotal edema may be more comfortable resting in bed while diuresis is being initiated. Children with nephrotic syndrome should not be isolated from other children and should be allowed to attend school.

Diuretics

Diuretics are often helpful in children in relapse, particularly in children with steroid-resistant disease. Serum potassium levels, as well as clinical signs of intravascular volume, should be monitored. If children have moderate intravascular volume contraction, the injudicious use of diuretics could precipitate hypotension and increase the risk of thrombosis and acute kidney injury. The most commonly used diuretic is furosemide (1–2 mg/kg per dose given orally or via IV). Spironolactone is sometimes added to the diuretic regimen for its potassium-sparing effect.

Long-term Management

The goal of long-term management is induction and maintenance of remission from active nephrotic syndrome. At the same time, the side effects of medications should be minimized. Spontaneous remission may eventually occur in children with MCD, but the 70% historical mortality rate makes waiting for a spontaneous remission unacceptable. Remissions are induced and maintained with the use of immunosuppressive medications. Figure 150-1 summarizes an approach to the overall management of nephrotic syndrome with these agents. A list of commonly used medications and dosages appears in Table 150-2.

Corticosteroids

More than 90% of younger children with primary nephrotic syndrome respond to corticosteroid therapy. Steroids are, therefore, diagnostic and therapeutic because failure to respond to steroids can be a marker for disease other than MCD or for a genetic cause of nephrotic syndrome. Even so, some children with MCD are steroid-resistant at some time in their disease. Steroids can be started promptly in children who are newly diagnosed with nephrotic syndrome if they have no signs of systemic disease, no more than microscopic hematuria, a normal C3 (or results pending), a negative PPD, and normal renal function. Acute infection should be managed with specific antimicrobial therapy to avoid infection-related steroid resistance.

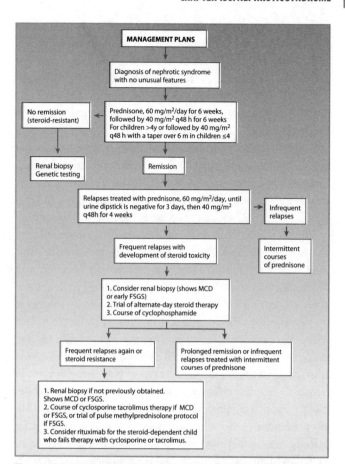

Figure 150-1. Management of nephrotic syndrome in children. Abbreviations: FSGS, focal segmental glomerulosclerosis; MCD, minimal change disease; q, every.

Table 150-2. Treatment Options in Childhood Nephrotic Syndrome

Medication	Dose	Length of Therapy
Prednisone	Initial course: 60 mg/m²/d for 6 wk, then 40 mg/m2 every 48 h for 6 wk	Varies
Cyclophosphamide	2–2.5 mg/kg/d (cumulative dose <168 mg/kg)	12 wk
Chlorambucil	0.15 mg/kg/d (cumulative dose ≤8.2 mg/kg)	8 wk
Cyclosporine	2–3 mg/kg every 12 h, monitor levels, target trough 100–200 ng/mL	Varies
Levamisole[a]	2.5 mg/kg every other d	Varies
Mycophenolate mofetil	12-18 mg/kg every 12 h; adults 1–1.5 g every 12 h	Varies
Tacrolimus	0.05–0.3 mg/d in divided doses, monitor levels, target trough 4–8 ng/mL	Varies
Rituximab	375–1,000 mg/m²/dose, 2 doses, 2 wk apart	

[a]Levamisole is no longer available in the United States.

Prednisone is usually started at 60 mg/m^2/day. It can be given once a day in the morning or divided into 2 daily doses. If first episodes of nephrotic syndrome are treated with a prolonged course of corticosteroids (60 mg/m^2/day for 6 weeks followed by 40 mg/m^2/48 hours for 2 to 5 months), children are subsequently less likely to follow a frequently relapsing course. Proteinuria resolves within 2 weeks in many children with MCD and by 4 weeks in more than 90%. Serum albumin normalizes soon after proteinuria clears, but hypercholesterolemia may take many weeks to return to normal. Children who fail to respond to 4 weeks of daily prednisone may be treated with a course of IV methylprednisolone at a dose of 15 mg/kg/day for 3 to 5 doses prior to declaring them steroid-resistant.

The pediatrician can easily manage steroid-sensitive children, but children with more difficult nephrotic syndrome should be managed in conjunction with a pediatric nephrologist. Children with relapses are treated with daily prednisone (60 mg/m^2) until the urine is protein-free for 3 days. This regimen is followed by 4 weeks of 40 mg/m^2 every other morning. An increased incidence of side effects (eg, cushingoid appearance, hypertension, obesity, glucose intolerance, cataracts, osteopenia, decreased growth rate) occurs when children require frequent courses of prednisone therapy. In frequently relapsing children, a chronic course of alternate-day steroid therapy may eliminate relapses and reduce steroid toxicity. Usually prednisone 40 mg/m^2 is given every other morning initially for at least 3 months with tapering over the subsequent several months to the lowest dose that keeps the child in remission. A recent study has found that children on chronic low-dose alternate-day therapy are less likely to experience a relapse following a URI if they receive daily prednisone at their stable prednisone dose for 7 days during the illness.

Other Agents for Difficult Nephrotic Syndrome

If alternate-day steroid therapy fails to maintain remission or when children develop signs of steroid toxicity, cyclophosphamide or chlorambucil may be administered. Either of these alkylating agents may induce a long-lasting remission that persists for years in children with steroid-dependent or frequently relapsing nephrotic syndrome. Either agent is started while children are in remission on steroid therapy, and the steroids are gradually tapered during the course of treatment with the alkylating agent. In the past, a diagnostic renal biopsy was routine prior to starting an alkylating agent. Many pediatric nephrologists now consider such therapy in steroid-sensitive or steroid-dependent children without a biopsy, however, provided that renal function is normal. Initially a daily dose of cyclophosphamide (2 mg/kg) was recommended for 8 weeks. However, a 12-week course is more likely to induce a prolonged remission and still be safe. The maximum cumulative dose of cyclophosphamide should not exceed 168 mg/kg. Chlorambucil at 0.1 to 0.2 mg/kg/day may be given as an alternative to cyclophosphamide, but it may be more toxic.

Potential toxicities of cyclophosphamide include bone marrow suppression with increased risk of infection, alopecia, hemorrhagic cystitis, gonadal toxicity, and possibly a small but indeterminately increased risk of developing a malignancy at some time. Some nephrologists advocate the use of oral mesna along with the oral cyclophosphamide to reduce the development of hemorrhagic cystitis. Mesna is always used when individuals receive IV cyclophosphamide. Complete blood cell counts should be monitored weekly, and parents should be cautioned about the increased risk of overwhelming varicella infections in children who have not yet had a varicella infection or immunization. The cyclophosphamide dose should be withheld if the WBC count falls below 4,000/μL and restarted when the WBC returns to or exceeds 4,000/μL. Alopecia and hemorrhagic cystitis are rare when the recommended dose is used and when children are asked to drink extra fluids while on cyclophosphamide. A 12-week course of cyclophosphamide (2 mg/kg/day) does not seem to increase the risk of infertility, but longer courses are associated with oligospermia, aspermatogenesis, and ovarian dysfunction. Postpubertal individuals may be at greater risk for gonadal toxicity than prepubertal children.

When steroid-sensitive or steroid-dependent children have failed to achieve prolonged remission after cyclophosphamide therapy, a diagnostic renal biopsy should be performed. Renal biopsy is indicated early, however, in the course of illness for steroid-resistant children. If FSGS is identified on biopsy, treatment may involve a prolonged course of IV methylprednisolone therapy, cyclosporine, or tacrolimus. Therapeutic options for children with MCD who continue to be steroid-dependent after a course of cyclophosphamide include treatment with mycophenolate mofetil, cyclosporine, tacrolimus, or levamisole. Although cyclosporine and tacrolimus are more likely to induce prolonged remission, they only maintain remission while being administered. Children trade steroid dependence for cyclosporine or tacrolimus dependence. Nevertheless, for children with steroid toxicity, a 12-month course of cyclosporine or tacrolimus allows resolution of the adverse effects of steroids and is generally well tolerated when administered by an experienced physician. Side effects such as hirsutism and gingival hyperplasia are frequent at the onset of therapy with cyclosporine. These effects regress as the dose is decreased or the drug is discontinued, however. Hypertension is not uncommon. The most common metabolic abnormality seen with cyclosporine use is hypomagnesemia. Long-term therapy may lead to significant nephrotoxicity and, rarely, patients experience liver toxicity. Tacrolimus, like cyclosporine, is a calcineurin inhibitor. It has a similar toxicity profile to cyclosporine, but it does not cause gingival hyperplasia or hirsutism and is now being used more frequently.

Because of potential toxicity, cyclosporine and tacrolimus should only be prescribed by a physician familiar with the drug. Dosing requirements may change with remission and relapse, and the family and physician should be aware of several drug interactions. Any medication interfering with the cytochrome P 450 enzyme system in the liver, such as erythromycin, greatly increases cyclosporine and tacrolimus levels and should be used only under extraordinary circumstances. Diarrhea may increase tacrolimus blood levels to a toxic range. Children who require prolonged treatment with cyclosporine or tacrolimus should have follow-up kidney biopsies performed after a year or two of therapy to assess for any nephrotoxicity.

Mycophenolate mofetil has been shown to be useful as a corticosteroid-sparing agent in the steroid-dependent, frequent relapsing child. It is typically used for at least 12 months because most children will relapse if it is withdrawn sooner. Some children have been on this medication for years without apparent adverse events. Levamisole, which is an immune modulating agent, has also been shown to be useful in the frequently relapsing child. However, it is not available in the United States. Rituximab, an anti-CD20 monoclonal antibody, is also promising for use in the steroid-dependent child. The use of rituximab should be reserved at this point for children who have continued relapses despite optimal use of prednisone and corticosteroid-sparing agents.

Nephrotic children who fail to achieve good remission with immunosuppressive therapy are given supportive therapy with angiotensin-converting enzyme inhibitors or angiotensin blockers, which reduce proteinuria and have been shown to reduce the progression of glomerulosclerosis. These medications are also first-line therapy for nephrotic children who develop hypertension. Other supportive measures for children with persistent edema include sodium restriction and the chronic use of diuretics. Genetic testing should be performed early in steroid-resistant children, and further immunosuppressive therapy should be withheld until the results of the genetic testing are available.

Immunization Issues

Because of the unusual susceptibility to pneumococcal infections, children older than 2 years with nephrotic syndrome should receive the 23-valent pneumococcal vaccine, even if they have previously received the 13-valent conjugated pneumococcal vaccine. The vaccine is best administered while children are in remission, but it produces protective titers even in children who are on alternate-day steroid therapy at the time of immunization. Patients on multiple immunosuppressive medications should have their pneumococcal antibody titers measured, and a second dose of vaccine should be administered if they fail to seroconvert. Influenza vaccine should be administered each autumn to children with nephrotic syndrome using the age-appropriate schedule and dosage.

Some of the routine childhood immunizations (eg, diphtheria-tetanus-pertussis, *Haemophilus influenzae* type b, hepatitis B, inactivated poliovirus vaccine) should be administered by the usual schedule but while children are in remission, if possible (see Chapter 34). Some controversy exists concerning the use of live-virus vaccines in children who require long-term immunosuppressive therapy. No vaccines should be administered if children are currently being treated with an alkylating agent. The measles-mumps-rubella vaccine could potentially cause a relapse. Based on limited data on the use of varicella vaccine in nephrotic children, it is probably safe to administer varicella vaccine while children are in remission and not on immunosuppressive medications.

Parent Education

Because nephrotic syndrome follows a chronic, relapsing course, parent education is essential for effective long-term management.

Parents need to be instructed about using urinary dipsticks to monitor protein excretion. Generally, urine dipsticks should be used daily during periods of active relapse and when medication is being tapered. Otherwise, the dipstick should be checked whenever children have infections, including URIs; whenever they look "puffy"; and weekly when asymptomatic.

Weight should also be monitored, especially during relapse. Children should be weighed each morning when they awake. Urine output should be measured in more difficult cases. As parents become more familiar with nephrotic syndrome, they may become partners with the physician about medication changes. Parents should also contact the physician about "danger signs" such as fever (temperature >100.7°F [38.2°C]), significant abdominal pain, or exposure to varicella. If children do not have protective antibodies against varicella and are taking any immunosuppressive medication (including prednisone), the varicella-zoster Ig should be administered within 72 hours of exposure to varicella. If varicella infection develops, IV acyclovir should be instituted.

Prognosis

In the pre-antibiotic era, nephrotic syndrome was frequently fatal, usually because of overwhelming infection. After the introduction of antibiotics, the mortality rate fell significantly. The use of corticosteroids has led to a further reduction in mortality. Currently, the mortality rate is about 5%, almost exclusively caused by infections from encapsulated organisms or thrombosis. The greatest risk of death in children with nephrotic syndrome (approaching 50% over 20 years in some series) is among children with resistance to corticosteroid therapy.

The long-term outlook for most children with nephrotic syndrome is favorable, particularly for steroid-sensitive patients. Relapses often disappear by the completion of puberty. Occasionally, individuals continue to have relapses into adulthood. Approximately 20% of children with steroid-sensitive MCD still experience relapses 15 years after the onset of their disease. Disease recurrence is highly unlikely if 8 years pass without a relapse. Fewer than 10% of initially steroid-sensitive children with nephrotic syndrome develop end-stage renal disease. This occurs almost exclusively in children with FSGS. Focal segmental glomerulosclerosis may recur after kidney transplants, particularly in young children with aggressive FSGS.

> ### *CASE RESOLUTION*
>
> In the case study, the child most likely has minimal change disease. He appears stable enough to be managed as an outpatient and should be placed on a salt-restricted diet and prednisone. The overall prognosis depends on a close interaction among the parents, pediatrician, and consulting pediatric nephrologist.

Selected References

Benoit G, Machuca E, Antignac C. Hereditary nephrotic syndrome: a systematic approach for genetic testing and a review of the associated podocyte gene mutations. *Pediatr Nephrol.* 2010;25(9):1621–1632

Bernard DB. Extrarenal complications of the nephrotic syndrome. *Kidney Int.* 1988;33(6):1184–1202

Filler G. Treatment of nephrotic syndrome in children and controlled trials. *Nephrol Dial Transplant.* 2003;18(Suppl 6):vi75–vi78

Guan N, Ding J, Zhang J, Yang J. Expression of nephrin, podocin, alpha-actinin, and WT1 in children with nephrotic syndrome. *Pediatr Nephrol.* 2003;18(11): 1122–1127

Gulati S, Sharma AP, Sharma RK, Gupta A. Changing trends of histopathology in childhood nephrotic syndrome. *Am J Kidney Dis.* 1999;34(4):646–650

Hladunewich MA, Avila-Casado C, Gipson DS. Focal segmental glomerulosclerosis. In: Gilbert SJ, Weiner DE, Gipson DS, et al, eds. *Primer on Kidney Diseases.* Philadelphia, PA: Elsevier Saunders; 2014:170–175

Hodson EM, Willis NS, Craig JC. Interventions for idiopathic steroid-resistant nephrotic syndrome in children. *Cochrane Database Syst Rev.* 2010;(11):CD003594

Kemper MJ, Gellermann J, Habbig S, et al. Long-term follow-up after rituximab for steroid-dependent idiopathic nephrotic syndrome. *Nephrol Dial Transplant.* 2012;27(5):1910–1915

Kerlin BA, Blatt NB, Fuh B, et al. Epidemiology and risk factors for thromboembolic complications of childhood nephrotic syndrome: a Midwest Pediatric Nephrology Consortium (MWPNC) Study. *J Pediatr.* 2009;155(1):105–110

Lewis MA, Baildom EM, Davis N, Houston IB, Postlethwaite RJ. Nephrotic syndrome: from toddlers to twenties. *Lancet.* 1989;1(8632):255–259

Lombel RM, Gipson DS, Hodson EM; Kidney Disease: Improving Global Outcomes. Treatment of steroid-sensitive nephrotic syndrome: new guidelines from KDIGO. *Pediatr Nephrol.* 2013;28(3):415–426

Lombel RM, Hodson EM, Gipson DS; Kidney Disease: Improving Global Outcomes. Treatment of steroid-resistant nephrotic syndrome in children: new guidelines from KDIGO. *Pediatr Nephrol.* 2013;28(3):409–414

Minimal change nephrotic syndrome in children: deaths during the first 5 to 15 years' observation. Report of the International Study of Kidney Disease in Children. *Pediatrics.* 1984;73(4):497–501

Mubarak M, Kazi JI, Lanewala A, Hashmi S, Akhter F. Pathology of idiopathic nephrotic syndrome in children: are the adolescents different from young children? *Nephrol Dial Transplant.* 2012;27(2):722–726

Munyentwali H, Bouachi K, Audard V, et al. Rituximab is an efficient and safe treatment in adults with steroid-dependent minimal change disease. *Kidney Int.* 2013;83(3):511–516

Quien RM, Kaiser BA, Deforest A, Polinsky MS, Fisher M, Baluarte HJ. Response to the varicella vaccine in children with nephrotic syndrome. *J Pediatr.* 1997; 131(5):688–690

Roberti I, Vyas S. Long-term outcome of children with steroid-resistant nephrotic syndrome treated with tacrolimus. *Pediatr Nephrol.* 2010;25(6):1117–1124

Shenoy M, Plant ND, Lewis MA, Bradbury MG, Lennon R, Webb NJ. Intravenous methylprednisolone in idiopathic childhood nephrotic syndrome. *Pediatr Nephrol.* 2010;25(5):899–903

Trachtman H, Hogan J, Radhakrishnan J. Minimal change disease. In: Gilbert SJ, Weiner DE, Gipson DS, et al, eds. *Primer on Kidney Diseases.* Philadelphia, PA: Elsevier Saunders; 2014:164–169

Vester U, Kranz B, Zimmermann S, Hoyer PF. Cyclophosphamide in steroid-sensitive nephrotic syndrome: outcome and outlook. *Pediatr Nephrol.* 2003;18(7): 661–664

CHAPTER 151

Seizures and Epilepsy

Kenneth R. Huff, MD

CASE STUDY

A 6-year-old boy is evaluated for unusual episodic behaviors. The previous week his mother was awakened by the boy's brother and found her son lying in bed unresponsive and drooling, with his head and eyes averted to the right, his right arm slightly raised, and his body stiff. His face was jerking intermittently. When the paramedics arrived, the boy's posturing and movements had stopped. After the event, he could speak but was somewhat incoherent. He was taken to the local emergency department, where his examination and mental status were normal. Screening blood and urine tests were normal, and he was discharged with instructions to see his pediatrician for further recommendations.

His father remembers 2 or 3 other episodes of a somewhat different nature in the past month. These occurred as the boy was being put to bed. They involved some body stiffening and facial grimacing, with the mouth slightly open and the tongue twisted and deviated to one side. The child could not speak but appeared to be trying to talk. The episodes lasted 20 to 30 seconds. Afterward the boy was his usual self and could tell his father what had been said to him.

The child has had no intercurrent illnesses or abnormal behavior apart from these "spells," and he has lost no abilities. A paternal cousin and grandfather had seizures during childhood but "grew out of them." The examination is completely normal.

Questions

1. How likely is it that the episodic behavior represents a seizure?
2. What historical data about an event support the diagnosis of a seizure disorder?
3. How does an electroencephalogram help in classifying the type of seizure disorder?
4. What rationale should be used to formulate short-term and long-term treatment plans?

Seizures are a common medical problem in children. Diagnosing an episode that does not contain generalized convulsing movements as a seizure is sometimes problematic, however. Seizures are defined as episodic, stereotypical behavior syndromes of abrupt onset with loss of voluntary control by the patient, resulting in loss of responsiveness and rarely provoked by external stimuli. Frequently, the occurrence of this behavior correlates with interictal brain electrical discharges on electroencephalogram (EEG), and the behavioral ictus (seizures) should match temporally with a period of electrical hyper-synchrony if it occurs during the EEG recording.

A detailed history of the nature of the episodic behavior from an eyewitness is paramount in making the diagnosis of a seizure disorder and elucidating the type of seizure problem. The EEG is most often an adjunct to diagnosis. It is abnormal in many individuals who do not have clinical seizures and it may be normal interictally in many patients with clinical seizures because of its sampling limitations. Special techniques can sometimes help alleviate these limitations.

The type of seizure problem is important information in devising the management plan. Seizures can simply be classified as primary generalized seizures (involving the whole cerebrum from the outset) or partial seizures. However, some partial seizures can secondarily generalize, thereby clinically mimicking primary generalized seizures after their onset. Distinguishing these entities illustrates the importance of eyewitness information. Many treatment options are available, but the therapeutic plan must be individualized to the child's seizure type or clinical syndrome to optimize seizure control and minimize side effects. With appropriate treatment, most children with seizure disorders are not handicapped scholastically or socially and can enjoy normal lives.

Epidemiology

About 0.5% to 1.0% of all children experience at least one afebrile seizure. The new onset epilepsy incidence rate per year is about 0.05% in children younger than 18 years. Recurrent seizures can occur as a component of a static encephalopathy after brain malformation or dysgenesis, encephalitis or meningitis, metabolic disorder, hypoxic-ischemic injury, or severe head trauma. Such secondary or symptomatic seizures make up approximately one-third of childhood epilepsies. The remaining two-thirds of epileptic seizures occur presumably as part of a genetic epileptic syndrome. As genetic knowledge increases, eventually it may no longer be true that most often seizures occur in children without any known cause or association.

Clinical Presentation

Children present with a history given by observers of an episode of abrupt onset characterized by a loss of ability to respond to external stimuli (D_x Box). The child may experience various difficult-to-describe sensory, emotional, or psychic phenomena (aura) before

Seizures

- Abrupt loss of responsiveness
- Rhythmic clonic movements
- Sustained changes in posture or tone
- Simple automatic movements
- Completely unresponsive
- Staring without change in tone or posture
- Simultaneous change in cerebral electrical activity (repetitive discharges)

losing consciousness. Observers then see convulsive muscle activity, following which the patient may be sleepy. With some seizures, observers may note only an akinetic or staring spell, but with others, there are dramatic, rhythmic spasms of the face, extremities, or torso. Major motor seizures are frequently also associated with systemic autonomic changes, including changes in skin vascular supply causing color change, sweating, saliva production, and loss of sphincter control. About 10% of children have a headache before or after their seizure. Most seizure episodes are neither provoked nor attenuated by environmental factors (except for the common provocative factors of fever, intercurrent illness, and sleep deprivation and the much rarer provocative factors of the reflex epilepsies). Between episodes, children's general physical and neurologic examination may be entirely normal.

Pathophysiology

A seizure represents a sudden, synchronous depolarizing change in the electrical activity of a network of neurons that becomes widely propagated over the cortex, affecting awareness, responsiveness to external stimuli, and motor control. The propagation may be enhanced by defects in cell ion channels. Partial seizure disorders may result from a focal cortical lesion, such as a glial scar or dysplasia caused by a remote insult (eg, an infarct), or dysgenesis or primary cortical dysplasia that disrupts the electrical circuitry. The focal abnormality could also contain hamartomatous immature cells and abnormal synaptic properties and allow for periodic, abnormal transmission of impulses.

Exactly what initiates the synchronous depolarization of the neurons and the widespread network propagation is not well understood, and a rigorous analysis of abnormal neuronal and cerebral neurophysiology is not within the scope of this chapter. Several physiological mechanisms, including disrupted neuronal circuitry; voltage- and ligand-gated membrane ion channel abnormalities; abnormal excitatory or inhibitory neurotransmitter or receptor production, degradation, or uptake; and perhaps glial support mechanisms, are probably involved. It is known, for example, that familial childhood absence epilepsy results from abnormal thalamocortical circuitry. A further understanding of the mechanism involved in familial epilepsy syndromes awaits the definition of relevant genes, their expression and product functions, and the effects of variability in base pair sequence, transcription, and splicing on membrane

polarization, synaptic function, and circuitry physiology. Another example is cryptogenic West syndrome (infantile spasms), an "interneuronopathy" that has been associated with several genes, including *LIS1*, *DCX*, and *ARX* (sometimes resulting in agyria), which are important in GABAergic inhibitory interneuron development. A third example is the neuronal voltage-gated sodium channel subunit gene, SCN1A, which is mutated in the mild phenotype of "generalized epilepsy with febrile convulsions plus" and also mutated but in different regions of the gene sequence in the much worse phenotype of severe myoclonic epilepsy of infancy (Dravet syndrome).

Seizure Types

Seizures can be simply classified as **primary generalized seizures,** which include grand mal seizures, generalized tonic-clonic convulsions, and petit mal (absence) seizures (so named because of the child's complete loss of awareness at the outset of the episode), or **partial (localization-related) seizures,** which include focal motor, psychomotor, and other partial disorders (Box 151-1). The examples presented here should not be considered an exhaustive list of seizure syndromes but some of the more important types encountered in practice.

Two-thirds of nonfebrile seizures in children result from a partial seizure disorder. **Psychomotor seizures** are partial seizures that are usually preceded by a sensory aura or sometimes emotional behavioral manifestations and have a wide range of ictal behaviors, including focal clonic jerking, aversive or asymmetric hypertonic posturing, and more complex stereotypic fumbling or fingering behaviors. Seizures may be followed by postictal confusion or drowsiness. In some instances, children have partial sensory awareness but are unable to respond during seizures. In other cases, however, they are completely unconscious. The initial partial motor manifestations may not be seen by the observer before the movements rapidly generalize. Partial seizures are more often associated with focal brain pathologic processes, including traumatic lesions, infarcts, malformations, infections (eg, viral encephalitis, cerebral cysticercosis), and hippocampal sclerosis. The latter is rare in children but may be associated after many years with a history of a prolonged

---

Box 151-1. Classification of Epileptic Seizures

Partial Seizures (Seizures Beginning Locally)
- Elementary symptoms: focal seizures
- Complex symptoms: psychomotor seizures
- Partial seizures evolving secondarily to generalized seizures

Generalized Seizures (Bilaterally Symmetric; Onset Not Local)
- Absence seizures (petit mal): typical and atypical
- Tonic-clonic seizures
- Tonic seizures
- Myoclonic seizures (minor motor)
- Atonic seizures (drop attacks)
- Infantile spasms

Unclassified Seizures (Includes Neonatal "Subtle" Seizures)

febrile seizure. These etiologies each may have a characteristic appearance on magnetic resonance imaging (MRI), although, in many cases, the etiology is not apparent on MRI.

Benign epilepsy syndromes occur in children with normal developmental history, respond well to therapy, and remit without sequelae. **Rolandic seizures, or benign epilepsy with central temporal spikes,** is a relatively common partial seizure syndrome that sometimes is familial and has a good prognosis for resolving by adolescence. These episodes commonly occur when children are falling asleep, during sleep, or on awaking. Motor manifestations involve the tongue, mouth, or face but can sometimes generalize to the rest of the body. The clinical syndrome is accompanied by a characteristic focal EEG discharge over the central temporal region of the scalp. Other benign syndromes include **benign familial infantile seizures, benign infantile seizures with mild gastroenteritis, childhood occipital epilepsy** characterized by visual symptoms and EEG occipital spike-wave discharges, and **Panayiotopoulos syndrome,** which is characterized by paroxysmal autonomic dysfunctions such as vomiting and other gastrointestinal (GI) motility problems, pallor, mydriasis, and cardiorespiratory and thermoregulatory abnormalities (lasting up to 30 minutes), ending often in generalized convulsing and largely occurring in sleep.

An **absence seizure** may sometimes be difficult to distinguish from a partial seizure (Table 151-1). The absence spell is a brief (2–15 seconds) loss of consciousness without loss of tone. Staring into space and minor movements such as lip smacking or semi–purposeful-appearing movements of the hands are often the only observed behaviors. There is no postictal period. Because absence seizures occur multiple times a day and children are often unaware of them, parents may dismiss the subtle behavior change as selective attention or daydreaming; however, these seizures may adversely affect learning and carry a risk of injury. Hyperventilation, a useful diagnostic test that can be performed in the office, may provoke absence

seizures. The EEG is generally confirmatory and may also distinguish classic petit mal seizures with 3-per-second spike-wave discharges from variant syndromes. The classic petit mal is more often familial with dominant inheritance, age-specific occurrence between 4 and 16 years as childhood or juvenile absence, and sensitivity to ethosuximide treatment, whereas the atypical variant has a poorer prognosis for early resolution and is more resistant to anticonvulsant therapy. **Juvenile myoclonic epilepsy** begins in teen years but extends into adulthood and is characterized by upper extremity myoclonus and convulsive seizures in the mornings.

Neonatal seizures may be tonic, focal clonic, or multifocal clonic. The seizure problem is less often primary, and a vigorous search for an etiology of the seizure is more often successful than with older children. Problems commonly leading to neonatal seizures include hemorrhage (germinal matrix in the premature neonate or subarachnoid or subdural from birth trauma in older neonates); hypoxic-ischemic damage from asphyxia; infections producing postnatal sepsis or meningitis or prenatal encephalitis; drug withdrawal in the newborn of a substance-abusing mother; metabolic problems including hypoglycemia, hypocalcemia, or hypomagnesemia in the neonate of a diabetic mother; amino or organic acidopathies occurring a few days after feedings have begun; and congenital brain malformations.

A number of age-related seizure syndromes exist, perhaps related to maturational events in brain circuitry or ion channels. Although the appearance of the seizures within each of these syndromes is stereotypical and ultimately cognition is usually affected, resulting in an epileptic encephalopathy, there may be a wide variety of etiologic diagnoses.

Infantile spasms are an age-related seizure syndrome with typical movements of flexion contraction of the trunk with the head bowed or sudden raising of the arms, sometimes accompanied by a cry. These behaviors occur stereotypically several times in succession in a series. This syndrome occurs in infants and children between 3 months and 2 years of age. Another, perhaps related, but rarer syndrome of frequent tonic spasms, **Ohtahara syndrome,** occurs at a younger neonatal age and is associated with an abnormal neurologic examination and structural brain abnormalities. It is characterized by a different burst-suppression EEG pattern but carries a similar ominous prognosis for impaired intellectual development. **Dravet syndrome** arises out of typical febrile seizures which then occur without fever and subsequently manifest as staring spells and myoclonic seizures accompanied by delayed cognition. **Landau-Kleffner syndrome** involves loss of language abilities at age 3 to 5 years in the context of epileptic seizures and a very abnormal EEG pattern. A fifth syndrome in older children that is also associated with a different but characteristic EEG pattern, **Lennox-Gastaut syndrome,** has the same poor prognosis for seizure control and cognitive development but produces several different behavioral seizure types, including tonic, absence, and drop attacks. Different types of brain lesions in these age groups (including focal lesions) can result in the same generalized seizure syndromes. Examples include tuberous sclerosis; neonatal ischemia, hemorrhage, or meningitis; and major central nervous system (CNS) malformations.

Table 151-1. Partial Complex Versus Absence Seizures

Characteristic	Partial Complex	Absence
Aura	Frequent	None
Loss of consciousness	Sometimes partial	Complete
Motor movements	Sometimes complex	Blinking or none
Postictal state	Frequent	None
Duration	>30 sec	<15 sec
Frequency	Few per month to few per day	Many per hour or day
Hyperventilation provoked	No	Yes
Electroencephalogram findings	Variably localized discharge or normal	3/sec spike-wave generalized
Prognosis past adolescence	Frequently persists	Rarely occurs

Differential Diagnosis

Seizures are distinguished from nonepileptic paroxysmal disorders on the basis of history. The circumstances of place and time as well as details about the symptoms and nature of the behavior are important pieces of data. A diagnosis often confused is **syncope.** The syncopal episode is frequently situational, unlike a seizure. It occurs when children are in hot or stuffy environments; when they have been standing in one place for a long time, such as during a ceremony or physical education class; or when they see or experience a painful event, such as an injection or phlebotomy. Boys may experience micturition syncope standing in the bathroom shortly after arising in early morning. **Syncope** is often preceded by symptoms of light-headedness, nausea, tinnitus, and eventually a gradual darkening of vision, sometimes without total loss of auditory perception. Observers may note pale color and cool damp skin.

Breath-holding spells are characterized by apnea and loss of responsiveness accompanied by cyanosis or pallid skin color. Breath-holding spells are also situational. Infants or children are often upset or crying just before such spells. They may be frightened by a seemingly minor injury or angry after a toy is taken away or they are disciplined. Children may then throw themselves backward and stiffen while closing their glottis in expiration, and they may even have a few clonic jerks after losing consciousness (see Chapter 51).

Selective attention is frequently mistaken for absence seizures. This behavior often occurs when children are involved in relative passive activities (eg, watching television, playing a video game, daydreaming) and do not respond to verbal stimuli such as hearing their own name called. Generally, the attention lapses do not occur during talking or eating; seizures will occur, however, even during these activities.

Epileptic seizures must also be differentiated from **pseudoseizures (psychogenic nonepileptic seizures),** which actually occur most often in patients who have true seizures. Such episodes may include ictal eye closure and pelvic thrusting but also may resemble true seizures accurately, the psychodynamics of secondary gain or other motivation for the behavior may not be readily apparent, and the "need" for attention may be legitimate. The finding that the standard EEG is normal does not exclude a true seizure and thus is not helpful. Pseudoseizures should be suspected in children who may have witnessed seizures in relatives or close friends, who have seizures that consistently recur in the same situations, whose seizure frequency is not decreased with therapeutic levels of anticonvulsants, and whose seizures appear suggestible. Diagnosis can often be supported in complicated cases by simultaneous video EEG monitoring, which will show a lack of correlation of electrical abnormalities with the behavior in question. Immediate postictal serum prolactin level also may be normal, and psychologic assessment may detect underlying emotional problems related to prior trauma (eg, sexual abuse, other major psychologic trauma). The prognosis of pseudoseizures in children generally is better than in adults and relates to the more acute psychosocial genesis of the problem in most children.

Infants and older children have several behaviors that mimic seizures. Infantile gastroesophageal reflux (Sandifer syndrome) may look like brief epileptic tonic spasms but should have a consistent temporal relationship to feeding. Benign paroxysmal vertigo occurs in the infant or toddler and presages migraine later in childhood. Infantile shuddering is brief, rapid side-to-side shaking of the head and trunk. Older children can experience a paroxysmal dystonia, which is provoked externally and produces a change in truncal tone and posture and a brief cessation of movement. Tics are sudden, brief stereotypical movements preceded by an urge and partially suppressible. None of these disorders produces a loss of responsiveness of the child.

Paroxysmal events in sleep may also be a challenge for accurate diagnosis because the motor behaviors of non–rapid eye movement sleep or other **parasomnias** may mimic nocturnal frontal lobe epileptic seizures. Video EEG polysomnography will also help distinguish these, as the former will not be associated with ictal discharges.

Evaluation (Box 151-2)

History

The history should determine the exact events surrounding the seizure episode. A detailed history of the nature of the behavior from an eyewitness is extremely important (Questions Box). The physician must determine whether children experienced any loss of their normal level of responsiveness. Most often, this change in mental status is abrupt, although a warning behavior or aura that lasts for a few seconds may precede complete loss of responsiveness. The warning behavior or aura may be a cry, an expression of fear or anxiety, or nonspecific irritability. If children are articulate, they may be able to describe a discrete sensory phenomenon or relate a less distinct or even indescribable sensation.

A change in muscle tone and activity is frequently associated with the abrupt change in mental status unless the spell is an absence seizure. Most often, the tone is increased with general extensor posturing, more focal hypertonicity, or more complex torsion or aversive upper-body posturing. The patient may fall if not supported. Rhythmic jerking or clonic movements (focal or general), including the

---

Box 151-2. Initial Evaluation of Seizure Patients

- Eyewitness account of the episode
- Description of children's own experiences before, during, and after the episode if they are articulate enough
- History from caregiver concerning remote injuries to the nervous system, progressive neurologic symptoms, or intercurrent illness
- Careful neurologic examination looking for signs of cerebral hemisphere lateralization
- Brain imaging study when a partial seizure is observed, a crescendo history of neurologic symptoms is obtained, focal neurologic signs are found on interictal examination, or postictal encephalopathy persists too long
- Waking and sleep electroencephalogram with hyperventilation

Seizures

- Where was the child and what was he or she doing when the episode began?
- Did the child experience a loss of responsiveness?
- Did the child show any warning behavior or aura (eg, a cry, a facial expression of fear, irritability)?
- Did any part of the child's body become stiff? Was any shaking or jerking apparent?
- What did the child's eyes do, and was saliva produced at the mouth?
- Did the child's skin change color?
- Did the child experience a loss of sphincter control?
- How long did the episode last?
- Has the child been well recently?
- Did the child have a complicated birth, head trauma, meningitis, or other previous brain damage?
- Have episodes of a similar nature occurred previously? If so, when did they begin and how frequently do they occur?
- Has the child's development and school experience progressed normally?
- Does the child have any relatives who have had seizures?

trunk, limbs, face, and eyes, may occur concomitantly. Respirations may involve gagging sounds, rhythmic grunting, or silent, nearly imperceptible movements. Swallowing may not occur, so that saliva pools or forms bubbles at the lips. Autonomic changes, including skin color change (circumoral cyanosis), increased pulse, and loss of sphincter control, frequently occur with major motor spells. The ictal period generally lasts 30 seconds to 2 minutes, although observers frequently overestimate this time. Postictal periods of sleepiness or lethargy may occur. Their length is often correlated with the length or intensity of the seizure.

Children and those around them are often unaware of the occurrence of absence seizures. Often, an observant teacher brings the child's problem to a physician's attention. During a spell, a child has no change in tone or clonic movements and may have only subtle facial or hand movements. The episode lasts only a few seconds, and there are no preictal or postictal behaviors.

Historical information can also help determine potential etiologies of the seizure problem. A known distant brain insult or a hereditary disposition or consanguinity may be related to the cause. A progressive loss of skills indicates a need for a degenerative disease investigation.

Physical Examination

Children should be examined carefully for focal neurologic signs, particularly cerebral hemisphere-related asymmetries in strength, tone, or tendon reflexes. The examination should include a developmental assessment and mental status examination. The physician should look for signs of potential genetic problems, such as dysmorphic features, microcephaly, or organ malformations, which often correlate with cerebral dysgenesis; abnormal skin pigmentation or vessels, suggesting a neurocutaneous disorder; and organomegaly or bony abnormalities, indicating the possibility of a storage disorder. A careful eye examination or ophthalmologic consultation might also reveal evidence of a neurocutaneous, neurodegenerative, or dysgenic disorder. Children who are old enough to cooperate should be asked to hyperventilate, which might provoke an absence spell if the history is suggestive of this type of seizure.

Laboratory Tests

An EEG should be requested to help with the diagnosis of the type of seizure disorder, although the diagnosis should not rest on the EEG alone. In children with partial seizure disorders, the interictal discharge is helpful in localizing the initial site of abnormal electrical activity. A sleep record is often essential for observing the most useful abnormalities; 40% of children with epilepsy have a normal EEG. If a normal waking EEG is obtained and seizures continue to recur, it is sometimes useful to help ensure sleep during the record by prior sleep deprivation carried out by the parents or caregivers. Special techniques (eg, prolonged monitoring with telemetry, special anatomic electrode placements) can sometimes help overcome the standard EEG limitations of sample time and inaccessible areas of cerebral cortex. It should be noted, however, that even the standard EEG is rarely normal in petit mal disorders.

Historical information can frequently guide the need for metabolic tests. A blood sugar determination should be done acutely, but electrolytes are rarely abnormal in older children who have been well prior to the seizure. Urine toxicology should be done in a teenager with possible illicit drug use. Neonates and infants with recurrent unexplained seizures should have metabolic screening, including urine organic acid and amino acid levels, ammonia level, and acyl and free carnitine levels. If seizures persist with mental status changes, cerebrospinal fluid glucose, lactate, and amino acids; lysosomal and peroxisomal screens; and a diagnostic or therapeutic trial of pyridoxine should be considered. Tissue biopsy histologic analysis and specific assays may be indicated when physical signs suggest possible storage or other metabolic etiologies. Dysmorphic features may suggest chromosome analysis, a gene copy number variant screening array, or exome sequencing unless together they suggest a specific diagnostic gene test.

Imaging Studies

Magnetic resonance imaging scans are particularly helpful if a progression in neurologic symptoms or signs has occurred, there is a history of prior neurologic insult, an asymmetry of strength or tone is noted on examination, or signs of dysgenesis are present in other parts of the body. Even in the absence of these factors, partial or focal seizures have a higher yield of abnormal imaging results than do febrile seizures or petit mal disorders, which have a low yield. Finding a structural abnormality can obviate the need for expensive metabolic testing. Acutely, intravenous contrast should generally be given because loss of focal blood-brain barrier with an inflammatory or neoplastic lesion can help with diagnosing the cause of the seizure. Children with recurrent or resistant seizures should have an MRI scan, particularly when surgical treatment is under consideration. Coronal MRI scans can detect mesial temporal sclerosis, a lesion in the hippocampus seen in chronic temporal lobe epilepsy, and 20% of these will have had febrile seizures. Helpful additional modalities in studying surgical candidates include ictal positron emission tomography (PET) using fludeoxyglucose F18, interictal PET using α-methyl-L-tryptophan, single photon emission computerized tomography, functional MRI, and magnetoencephalography. These studies help define the nature of damaged or epileptic cortex and differentiate it from normal cortex.

Management

When there has been an episode of abrupt loss of consciousness or tone with a potential for recurrence, families need to be cautioned about the risks of drowning, falls from high places, and accidents with operating machinery, including vehicles. Anticonvulsants are the mainstay of management of seizure disorders (Table 151-2). At the same time, the clinician must realize that seizures and antiepileptic drugs affect brain development and could have long-term consequences, such as altered cognition and even subsequent epilepsy susceptibility. (This observation may be especially true in the case of neonatal seizures in which the seizures themselves may contribute to adverse outcomes and the standard treatment of phenobarbital has been shown in some long-term treatment models to be inhibitory of learning.) Half of first-time seizures in an otherwise neurologically normal child do not recur. Anticonvulsants are prescribed if the risk of recurrence of seizures, particularly prolonged seizures; the physical danger of a recurrence; or the social stigma is

Table 151-2. Drugs Useful for Treating Seizures		
Seizure Type	**Dose**	**Toxic Symptoms/Side Effects**
Partial Seizures		
Carbamazepine	Approximately 15 mg/kg/d	Gastrointestinal distress, headache
Phenytoin	4–8 mg/kg/d	Ataxia, nystagmus, bone changes
Primidone	12–25 mg/kg/d	Drowsiness, ataxia
Oxcarbazepine	30 mg/kg/d	Drowsiness, rare sodium depletion
Lamotrigine	4–7 mg/kg/d	Dizziness, sedation, rash (Stevens-Johnson syndrome)
Gabapentin	4–8 mg/kg/d	Somnolence, ataxia
Vigabatrin	15–50 mg/kg/d	Drowsiness, visual field defects
Topiramate	6–10 mg/kg/d	Weight loss, sedation, speech disturbance, metabolic acidosis
Zonisamide	4–6 mg/kg/d	Sedation, metabolic acidosis
Levetiracetam	10–60 mg/kg/d	Behavior or personality change
Rufinamide	10–45 mg/kg/d	Sedation, headache
Lacosamide	1.5–6 mg/kg/d	Dizziness, ataxia, caution with cardiac disease
Neonatal Seizures		
Phenobarbital	5–6 mg/kg/d	Lethargy, irritability, osteopenia
Topiramate	6–10 mg/kg/d	Sedation
Levetiracetam	10-60 mg/kg/d	Sedation
Generalized Seizures		
Valproic acid	20–60 mg/kg/d	Tremors, hair loss, thrombocytopenia, weight gain, pancreatitis
Felbamate	45 mg/kg/d	Insomnia, anorexia, bone marrow aplasia
Topiramate	6–10 mg/kg/d	Weight loss, sedation, speech disturbance, metabolic acidosis
Clorazepate	0.3–1.5 mg/kg/d	Drowsiness
Clonazepam	0.01-0.2 mg/kg/d	Drowsiness, ataxia
Clobazam	0.15-0.5 mg/kg/d	Drowsiness
Absence Seizures		
Ethosuximide	30 mg/kg/d	Nausea, hiccups
Valproic acid	20–60 mg/kg/d	Tremors, hair loss, thrombocytopenia, weight gain
Infantile Spasms		
Adrenocorticotropic hormone	40 U/m²	Increased appetite, irritability, acne, immunosuppression
Valproic acid	20–60 mg/kg/d	Tremors, hair loss, thrombocytopenia, weight gain
Vigabatrin	15–50 mg/kg/d	Drowsiness, visual field defects

significant based on seizure classification and individual factors. A known structural or physiological lesion demonstrated by the EEG may also suggest a higher recurrence risk. The choice of anticonvulsant depends on age, gender, neurologic diagnosis, seizure type or epilepsy syndrome, other conditions or medications, and social factors. The doses and combination of anticonvulsants prescribed for children depend on a balance of seizure resistance, risk of recurrence, and potential toxicity of medication. The initial goal is complete control with a single medication and as little toxicity as possible. When this goal is not achieved, doses are advanced to an individualized optimal balance of seizure control and tolerated toxicity.

Oxcarbazepine and carbamazepine are often recommended for partial seizures. Toxicity is generally mild or nonexistent, but adverse effects can include GI upset, dizziness, and headache. Carbamazepine has been known to aggravate idiopathic generalized and myoclonic epilepsies, including Lennox-Gastaut syndrome, however. Phenytoin is also effective for partial types of seizures and can be given intravenously for status epilepticus, but it can worsen absence seizures. Phenobarbital is effective in neonatal seizures but may have deleterious effects on behavior and learning in older children. Ethosuximide is used for petit mal seizures. Valproic acid is used for more common atypical petit mal and other seizure disorders resistant to other anticonvulsants. It should not be used in female adolescents who might conceive because of an increased risk of fetal neural tube defects and offspring learning disabilities and used with caution in infants younger than 2 years at higher risk of metabolic disorders. Felbamate is also effective in many difficult-to-treat epilepsy syndromes, although a very small but nevertheless frightening incidence of irreversible severe bone marrow suppression and liver toxicity has limited its use. Other anticonvulsants, including gabapentin, lamotrigine, vigabatrin, topiramate, zonisamide, levetiracetam, clonazepam, clorazepate, and clobazam, have proven effective. Gabapentin and levetiracetam are useful as adjunctive agents because of their lack of interaction with other anticonvulsants. Lamotrigine is useful in partial and primary generalized seizure disorders but may worsen seizures in Dravet syndrome. Vigabatrin is useful in infantile spasms when caused by tuberous sclerosis. Topiramate is effective in partial seizures, generalized seizures, and Lennox-Gastaut syndrome. Rufinamide and clobazam are also effective in the latter syndrome, particularly. Zonisamide and levetiracetam are effective in partial and generalized seizure disorders, and lacosamide is effective in partial disorders. The latter 2 medications can also be used intravenously. Clonazepam, clorazepate, and clobazam are adjunctive benzodiazepines effective in several seizure types. Rectal diazepam empowers the family to begin treatment at home before paramedic arrival for a long seizure or cluster of seizures.

Periodic monitoring of efficacy and side effects is essential in children who take medication daily on a long-term basis. A log of seizure frequency helps assess medication efficacy. Gastrointestinal and neurologic symptoms (sedation and ataxia) are the most common side effects. The perception of symptoms being related to the medication as well as the actual presence of side effects or toxicity contribute to the complex issue of compliance. Serum drug levels are useful in monitoring compliance, dosage, and the likelihood that symptoms are the result of drug side effects. Compliance is improved if a medication formulation with less frequent dosing can be chosen. Organ toxicity (bone marrow, liver, and pancreas) must be considered and monitored with many medications, although routine laboratory tests after a few months on stable doses are rarely necessary. Hypersensitivity reactions and Stevens-Johnson syndrome usually, but do not always, occur within 2 months of beginning the medication. Ethnic variability in drug metabolism and drug interactions can be important and involve the liver cytochrome P450-inducing potential of barbiturates and the potential of other medications, such as erythromycin, to inhibit other liver detoxification systems, such as that involved with carbamazepine metabolism, which produce acutely high levels and clinical toxicity. New educational problems in a child with epilepsy deserve aggressive evaluation to determine a common etiology to the underlying seizure condition and alternatively for assessing medication toxicity or long-term detrimental effects.

Non-medication therapeutic options are also available for refractory cases. The ketogenic diet has success in about 50% of cases but requires considerable knowledge and commitment. The vagal nerve stimulator delivers a regular electrical stimulus afferently to the CNS and also allows for an abortive intervention by the caregiver with an external magnet. It is effective in about 50% of cases, and when this occurs, less medication may be used, allowing a better overall quality of life. Intracranial resection surgery for epilepsy in childhood must sometimes be considered. Children with hemispheric seizure-associated syndromes, including Sturge-Weber syndrome, Rasmussen encephalitis, hemimegalencephaly, perinatal hemispheric infarction, catastrophic seizure disorders of early childhood such as infantile spasms related to a localized zone of epileptogenic cerebral tissue, and hamartomatous cortex–producing seizures, have benefitted the most often, but patients with refractory partial seizure disorders, including temporal lobe epilepsy, may also be candidates for surgical resection. Extensive staged presurgical imaging and physiological monitoring are necessary for these surgery candidates.

Attention-deficit/hyperactivity disorder is quite common in children with epilepsy, and concomitant therapy should be considered when it is diagnosed. Because of frequent behavioral and learning disability comorbidities, as well as social stigmatization, patients and their families often benefit from psychologic and social therapy and support groups.

Prognosis

In general, approximately two-thirds of children who have experienced a tendency for seizure recurrence have a good prognosis for prevention of further recurrence and little or no problem with side effects of medication. They can lead normal lives without handicap. The etiologic diagnosis is the most important prognostic factor. The type of epilepsy, EEG findings, child's age, difficulty of initial seizure control, and time since the last seizure are also important. Partial complex disorders sometimes have a poorer prognosis for early resolution and may be more resistant to treatment with anticonvulsants. Some seizure types have intrinsically poor prognoses. For example, infantile spasms are prognostically ominous because even in the absence of a metabolic diagnosis, children frequently suffer temporary brain growth and developmental arrest unless the seizures are controlled with medication. About 10% to 25% of children, most often those with generalized symptomatic epilepsies, frequent seizures, high anticonvulsant use, and early onset of epilepsy, show some intellectual decline. A small percentage develop an epileptic encephalopathy and are significantly handicapped. Children with seizures resistant to 2 concomitant medications have a much lower chance of responding to a third medication or other combinations. These children also have a higher risk of sudden unexplained death, particularly if they have symptomatic epilepsy. However, some of the seizure syndromes with a familial tendency, such as rolandic seizures and typical petit mal seizures, have a good prognosis for control by medication and ultimate complete resolution by the teenage years.

The individualized decision to discontinue medication is often complex. As a general rule, withdrawal of medications should be considered in most children after 2 years of seizure freedom. The prognosis for recurrence of seizures, the parents' and children's reactions to seizures and to the prospect of their recurrence, and social factors such as school participation may all contribute to the decision. Children and parents must be aware that none of the prognostic factors, whether considered individually or in combination, is an absolute predictor of seizure recurrence or non-recurrence in a given child.

CASE RESOLUTION

The boy described in the case study at the beginning of the chapter had a generalized seizure when he was taken to the emergency department. The previous episodes recalled by the father have characteristics of partial seizures. The tonic-clonic seizure was probably a secondary generalized rather than a primary generalized seizure. The possibility of rolandic seizures is suggested by the circumstances of the prior episodes, drowsiness, facial or oral symptomatology, and family history. This diagnosis was confirmed by electroencephalogram. Oxcarbazepine was prescribed. The boy experienced no side effects or seizure recurrences and was successfully able to discontinue the medication 3 years later.

Selected References

Camfield P, Camfield C. Pediatric epilepsy: an overview. In: Swaiman K, Ashwal S, Ferriero D, eds. *Pediatric Neurology: Principals and Practice.* 4th ed. Philadelphia, PA: Elsevier; 2006

Clancy RR; Neurology Group on Neonatal Seizures. The newborn drug development initiative workshop: summary proceedings from the Neurology Group on Neonatal Seizures. *Clin Ther.* 2006;28(9):1342–1352

Faught E. Epilepsy case studies. *Neurol Clin.* 2006;24(2):291–307

Glauser T, Ben-Menachem E, Bourgeois B, et al. Updated ILAE evidence review of antiepileptic drug efficacy and effectiveness as initial monotherapy for epileptic seizures and syndromes. *Epilepsia.* 2013;54(3):551–563

Kato M. A new paradigm for West syndrome based on molecular and cell biology. *Epilepsy Res.* 2006;70(Suppl 1):S87–S95

Koh S, Menkes J, Sankar R, Wu J. Paroxysmal disorders. In: Menkes J, Sarnat H, Maria B, eds. *Child Neurology.* 7th ed. Philadelphia, PA: Lippincott, Williams & Wilkins; 2006

Marsh ED, Brooks-Kayal AR, Porter BE. Seizures and antiepileptic drugs: does exposure alter normal brain development? *Epilepsia.* 2006;47(12):1999–2010

Werz MA, Pita IL. *Epilepsy Syndromes.* Philadelphia, PA: Elsevier Saunders; 2010

CHAPTER 152

Pediatric Palliative Care: Principles and Practice

Kevin Madden, MD, and Rick Goldstein, MD

CASE STUDY

Jason is a 17-year-old boy with spastic quadriplegia, severe global developmental delays, a seizure disorder, cortical blindness, and dystonia. Since leaving the neonatal intensive care unit (NICU) at 3 months of age, he has lived in a skilled nursing facility and spends weekends at home with his family. He was born after 24 weeks' gestation and had a turbulent NICU course. During that hospitalization, in accord with his neonatologists, he was treated for comfort and extubated due to his severe respiratory failure but managed to survive and breathe independently. Once beyond the newborn period, his medical course was fairly stable, notable for episodic respiratory decompensations requiring hospitalization and numerous orthopedic procedures. In the past 2 years, however, he has spent substantially more time in the intensive care unit due to increasing respiratory fragility. With so much time spent in the hospital and so little time when he is comfortable "at home," his parents have begun questioning whether the intensive medical care he has been receiving translates into quality of life and whether they should begin to limit efforts at resuscitation. They do not know what it would mean to place limitations on his care and, whatever their choices, they do not want Jason to suffer.

Questions
1. What is palliative care?
2. What is involved in the practice of palliative care?
3. How do children understand death? How does their understanding vary with their age?
4. What role does a primary care pediatrician play in the palliative care of her patients?

During the typical career of primary care pediatricians, only a few of their patients will die. Many more patients will suffer from complex medical conditions, sometimes life-threatening, generally requiring high levels of management. Caring for these patients can be among the most challenging yet rewarding experiences a pediatrician may have. Close, long-standing relationships with a family make it apparent how the effect of the illness on the child and family goes beyond biomedical issues, and many pediatricians make important contributions to addressing the suffering that occurs. These children especially benefit from a medical home providing care that is accessible, continuous, comprehensive, family centered, coordinated, and compassionate, led by an invested primary care pediatrician empathetic of their experience.

Even with the best of intentions, the care of these patients can accentuate changes in modern medical care. There can be a divide between the goals of subspecialty-based care provided in hospitals and those of generalist care in the community. The increasing use of new medical technologies in the home setting can leave primary care pediatricians uncertain even as they are asked to sign the orders for home care. There can be uncertainty about whether unexpected symptoms can be managed quickly, effectively, and authoritatively in the community setting. Continuity of care can be challenging with prolonged hospitalizations. And lastly, there is the matter of case ownership: Who is "in charge" and who will help the family and patient not simply with disease management but in accord with their hopes and wishes for their child?

Pediatric palliative care addresses many of the central concerns in the care of these children. It builds on an important cornerstone from hospice care, namely, acceptance of the fact that some children do die, and the circumstances of their death can be improved with specialized expertise directed toward improving the process and relieving pain and suffering. In all cases, it exists to help children and their families live as well as possible in the face of complex, life-threatening illness. The developing expertise of this subspecialty supports and augments the important work that emanates from the patient's medical home. Palliative care also deals with more complex cases that require enhanced care and coordination and can assist primary pediatricians when they need help or when most patient care is hospital-based. Far from signaling an abandonment of hope, palliative care practitioners work with families to redefine hope in a realistic way and clarify what the family may need to align treatment decisions with the child and family's vision of what is best.

Scope of Pediatric Palliative Care

Each year, more than 50,000 children in the United States will die and 10 times that number will cope with life-threatening conditions. In 2011, 54% of deaths of children younger than 19 years occurred in children younger than 1 year, with 20.8% of those infant deaths attributed to congenital malformations, deformations, and chromosomal abnormalities; 17.2% to short gestation and low birth weight; 7.2% to sudden infant death syndrome; 6.6% to newborns affected by maternal complications of pregnancy; and 4.6% to unintentional injuries. For older children, aged 1 to 19 years, the leading causes of death were unintentional injuries (35.6%), homicide (11.4%), suicide (10.1%), malignant neoplasms (9.2%), and congenital malformations, deformations, and chromosomal abnormalities (5.2%). Approximately 47% of US children die outside of a hospital.

Research by Feudtner et al and others has increased our understanding of children with complex chronic conditions (CCCs) in the United States. These children are estimated to make up one-fifth of all pediatric deaths. *Complex chronic conditions* have been defined as medical conditions that can be reasonably expected to last at least 12 months (unless death intervenes) and that involve several different organ systems or one organ system severely enough to require specialty pediatric care and probably some period of hospitalization in a tertiary center. The major categories of CCCs leading to death are cardiovascular (22.2%), malignancy (21.4%), congenital/genetic (19.4%), neuromuscular (18.1%), and respiratory (9.3%). Increasingly, these children are dying at home, perhaps due to longer survival, the migration of advanced medical technology into the home, and shifting attitudes about what is better care, with a greater focus on quality of life among children with life-threatening conditions. Many studies indicate that, overall, home is the preferred site of ongoing care for children with life-threatening illnesses, regardless of their condition.

The American Academy of Pediatrics (AAP) endorses an integrated model of palliative and curative treatment in which components of palliative care are offered at diagnosis and continued throughout the course of illness, whether the outcome is cure or death. The prevailing view is that the palliative care "approach should be instituted when diagnosis, intervention, and treatment are not limited to a disease process, but rather become instrumental for improving the quality of life, maintaining the dignity, and ameliorating the suffering of seriously ill or dying children in ways that are appropriate to their upbringing, culture, and community" (Himelstein et al). Palliative care is often incorrectly equated with end-of-life and hospice care. Hospice is a program of coordinated services offering comfort-centered care at the end of life in the home or community setting. While there is a shared philosophy and an overlap of many of the priorities of care, palliative care should not be considered only at the end of life, nor is it exclusive of curative care. Although death may be imminent in some cases and end-of-life care is a part of palliative care, the true scope of palliative care is much broader. The misperception of this limited focus of palliative care can impede the timely referral to a palliative care specialist with unintended and important consequences not only to the death of a child and the bereavement that parents experience afterward but also on the child's life during illness.

Palliative care should be considered in 4 categories of illness: conditions for which curative treatment is possible but may fail (eg, cancer with a poor prognosis), conditions requiring intensive long-term treatment aimed at maintaining quality of life (eg, cystic fibrosis, advanced muscular dystrophy), progressive conditions in which treatment is exclusively palliative after diagnosis (eg, progressive metabolic disorders), and conditions involving severe, nonprogressive disability causing extreme vulnerability to health complications (eg, holoprosencephaly, other severe brain malformations) (Box 152-1).

In addition, there is an emerging role for palliative care in the neonatal intensive care unit (NICU). At this point, it is unclear whether, from a palliative care perspective, the needs of newborns and their families in NICUs are fully addressed. Neonatologists certainly have expertise dealing with the medical needs of critically ill neonates and the care-related concerns of their families. The pace of

---

Box 152-1. Conditions Appropriate for Pediatric Palliative Care[a]

Conditions for which curative treatment is possible but may fail
- Advanced or progressive cancer or cancer with a poor prognosis
- Complex and severe congenital or acquired heart disease

Conditions requiring intensive long-term treatment aimed at maintaining quality of life
- HIV infection
- Cystic fibrosis
- Severe gastrointestinal disorders or malformations, such as gastroschisis
- Severe epidermolysis bullosa
- Severe immunodeficiencies
- Renal failure in cases in which dialysis, transplantation, or both are not available or indicated
- Chronic or severe respiratory failure
- Muscular dystrophy

Progressive conditions in which treatment is exclusively palliative after diagnosis
- Progressive metabolic disorders
- Certain chromosomal abnormalities, such as trisomy 13 or trisomy 18
- Severe forms of osteogenesis imperfecta

Conditions involving severe, nonprogressive disability causing extreme vulnerability to health complications
- Severe cerebral palsy with recurrent infection or difficult-to-control symptoms
- Extreme prematurity
- Severe neurologic sequelae of infectious disease
- Hypoxic or anoxic brain injury
- Holoprosencephaly or other severe brain malformations

[a]Premature death is likely or expected with many of these conditions.

Reprinted with permission from Himelstein BP, Hilden JM, Boldt AM, Weissman D. Pediatric palliative care. *N Engl J Med.* 2004;350(17):1752–1762.

the NICU and the absence of a primary care practitioner no doubt have some effect on the priorities of care. A palliative care approach emphasizes critical communication, symptom management, and assistance with shared decision-making and articulating goals. Alternatively, pediatric deaths that are sudden and unexplained or due to traumatic injuries, intentional and unintentional, occur largely outside of medical settings. First responders and emergency medicine clinicians would benefit from palliative care guidance about symptom management in the face of imminent death and decision-making related to resuscitation.

Not every dying child requires the involvement of pediatric palliative care specialists. Most children with life-threatening illnesses lead lives and receive at least some of their care in the community setting. For example, among children with complex chronic illnesses, only half will spend more than 2 weeks of their last year hospitalized, and more than one-third spend less than a week in the hospital at all. These children receive their care in the community setting. There may be differences in the willingness of primary care practitioners to become involved or in the ability of practices to manage complexities of care, but the primary care pediatrician can be the central coordinating figure in the medical care offered to these children. At the very least, primary care pediatricians will provide essential contributions to the care of these children. The literature describes a role for general pediatricians in the care of these children, although research suggests that parental expectations and physician involvement do not reflect vigorous involvement. Primary care physicians play a supportive and appreciated, albeit limited, role in end-of-life care and decision-making in children with complex medical issues. Collaboration with pediatric palliative care specialists offers a promise of enhancing that involvement.

Efforts to improve the quality of life for these children require a willingness to address biomedical, psychologic, sociocultural, and spiritual matters. Families need guidance in navigating the administrative, financial, and coping challenges placed on them. Importantly, there is a fundamental need to promote the sense of a lived life of value and identity, in contrast with a life determined by the course of illness alone. These needs are best served when an interdisciplinary team attends to the unique needs of each child. Such a team may have a pediatrician leader but benefits from involvement by nurses, social workers, psychosocial clinicians, and pastoral care. Subspecialists are often involved, with varying relationships with the family. There may be a hospice or community-based palliative care program. The care of children additionally may involve representatives from the school, child life, and practitioners of functional therapies, whether occupational therapy, physical therapy, and speech therapy or massage, hippotherapy, and Feldenkrais, a method used to increase a patient's kinesthetic and proprioceptive self-awareness. Strong communication and reliable continuity within the team are essential to success.

Pain and symptom management for chronically ill or dying children is a foundation of quality of life and a core concern of pediatric palliative care. When parents of children dying from cancer were asked about symptoms, 89% reported that their children suffered "a

lot" or "a great deal" from at least one symptom as they were dying. Other research has found that parents list emotional distress, fatigue, nutritional concerns, and pain as troubling areas at the end of life. While the medical focus is on pain, there also is concern about symptoms such as dyspnea, nausea and vomiting, constipation, secretions, fatigue, anorexia, pruritus, sleep issues, anxiety, and anorexia. A full discussion of pain and symptom management can be found in Chapter 12.

Prognosis, Disclosure, Decision-making

The care of these children is marked by periods of intense uncertainty and fearful realities. Helping families determine the goals of care, appropriate treatment choices, and all aspects of planning for the child's life is facilitated when they understand their child's prognosis. To accomplish this, careful and thoughtful communication is of paramount importance. Yet research has found that many parents feel they receive confusing, inadequate, or uncaring communication related to prognosis and treatment. They are expected to reach decisions with a different understanding of medical details than their children's health care professionals. Such decisions are especially difficult in a setting of misunderstanding, disagreement, or, worse, lack of trust. Recent research documents that the frequency with which parents use positive words to describe their child's illness was inversely related to how positive they felt emotionally about their child's illness, potentially setting the stage for tremendous miscommunication between the physician and family.

Most illness has prognostic uncertainty. Despite this, parents benefit from direct communication about the disease severity and the timeline for progression and potentially death. This is a difficult task, not only because imparting bad news is an uncomfortable and complex task but also the exact prognosis is truly uncertain. Studies of prognosis have found that physicians are accurate only 20% of the time and tend to be overly optimistic. While more experienced clinicians tend to err less, there is also a correlation between the length of a relationship with a patient and a lowered likelihood that the prognosis will be correct. Parents nonetheless seek a clear disclosure. They interpret hidden or minimal information as their doctor withholding frightening information. Alternatively, parents who receive more elements of prognostic disclosure are more likely to report communication-related hope, even when the likelihood of cure is low. The benefits of honest communication about the prognosis exceed the hazards.

When parents and some children ask about prognosis, they are asking about the time remaining and the pace of expected decline. Three typical trajectories for progressive chronic illness have been described in adults and are informative for pediatric patients as well (Figure 152-1). The first is a pattern of illness with a modest effect on function during most of its course followed by a precipitous decline near the time of death. Cancer death classically fits this pattern, and cancer research has led to models in which timelines can be discussed with some accuracy. An implication for care with this trajectory is that there is life to live even in the face of imminent

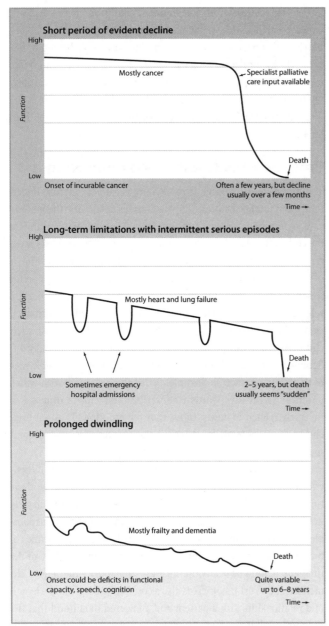

Figure 152-1. Typical illness trajectories for people with progressive chronic illness. (Modified with permission from Lynn J, Adamson DM. *Living Well at the End of Life. Adapting Health Care to Serious Chronic Illness in Old Age.* **Washington, DC: Rand Health; 2003.)**

death and also that when decline comes, there has been time to review the priorities of care before circumstances at the end of life.

The second trajectory is one of long-term limitations with intermittent serious episodes. Cystic fibrosis and severe disability following prematurity are 2 examples of this trajectory. Although there is slow, steady decline that can generally be discussed with some clarity, there are unpredictable decompensations that often bring the child close to death and which will affect the overall rate of decline. A predicted timeline to death can only be described in general terms. These patients sometimes survive their decompensations after seeming, to all appearances, beyond recovery. This can make it very difficult for parents to feel confident about placing limitations on

resuscitation, even when quality of life is extremely compromised. The third trajectory, described as prolonged dwindling, can apply to children with severe metabolic abnormalities, trisomy 13 or 18, or severe brain abnormalities. It is a life of ever-diminishing function. Families tend to become quite medicalized and organize their lives around the child's care. A key challenge in these cases is to help the family articulate what it sees as giving the child's life meaning and helping the family evaluate interventions in terms of its goals, not simply whether interventions are possible.

Uncomfortable as it is, anticipating death and addressing it clearly and frankly allows families, and some patients, to make choices about the time remaining. The early recognition of a poor prognosis predicts an earlier do-not-resuscitate (DNR) order, less use of disease-directed therapies in the last months of life, and a greater chance of incorporating the child's comfort as a goal. It allows a narrative to evolve of who this child was and the terms under which he or she lived. It allows for some sense of control and expression of values in overwhelming circumstances. Mack and Wolfe have nicely outlined an approach to communicating with children and families once prognosis has been shared and palliative care is under consideration (Table 152-1).

The Burden of Suffering and the Power of Hope

It is indeed surprising that the topics of suffering and hope can seem, at first glance, to be nontechnical and not properly "medical." It is hard to imagine how concepts so central to the call to heal can seem peripheral. This may be rooted in a bias that matters of the body are appropriate areas of treatment whereas matters of the mind and soul are left to other subspecialties or areas outside of medicine.

Disease and its treatment can cause physical distress, but suffering is much larger and more complex. Cassel defines *suffering* as "the state of severe distress associated with events that threaten the intactness of a person." When a child or parent worries "what will happen, . . ." or their complaints seem greater than their physical basis, they may be reflecting the suffering that comes from a threat to any of the multiple aspects of personhood—"the lived past, the family's lived past, culture and society, roles, the instrumental dimension, associations and relationships, the body, the unconscious mind, the political being, the secret life, the perceived future, and the transcendent dimension." In caring for patients with life-threatening illness, understanding all aspects of suffering is critical to effective care, and reflection and understanding are prerequisite to a healing presence. Pain and symptom management are foundational, but the relief of suffering requires helping a child and family struggle with issues of meaning and transcendence.

Hope involves expectations or belief in a worthy future. It carries a sense of trust and reliance. Life-threatening illness makes it complicated to know what to hope for, trust in, or rely on. Medical particulars aside, as Cassell has written, "The imperative to tell the truth seems an insufficient guide to what you should tell patients." It is not that truth or the best understanding should be withheld, but rather

Table 152-1. Communicating With Children and Families About Integrating Palliative Care	
Beginning the conversation	• What is your understanding of what is ahead for your child? • Would it be helpful to talk about how your child's disease may affect him or her in the months and years ahead? • As you think about what is ahead for your child, what would you like to talk about with me? • What information can I give you that would be helpful to you?
Introducing the possibility of death	• I am hoping that we will be able to control the disease, but I am worried that this time we may not be successful. • Although we do not know for certain what will happen for your child, I do not expect that your child will live a long and healthy life; most children with this disease eventually die because of the disease. • I have been noticing that your child seems to be sick more and more often. I have been hoping that we would be able to make him or her better, but I am worried that his or her illness has become more difficult to control and that soon we will not be able to help him or her to get over these illnesses. If that is the case, he or she could die of his or her disease.
Eliciting goals of care	• As you think about your child's illness, what are your hopes? • As you think about your child's illness, what are your worries? • As you think about your child's illness, what is most important to you right now? • You mentioned that what is most important to you is that your child be cured of his or her disease. I am hoping for that too. But I would also like to know more about your hopes and goals for your child's care if the time comes when a cure is not possible.
Introducing palliation	• Although I hope that we can control your child's disease for as long as possible, at the same time I am hoping that he or she feels as good as possible each day. • Although it is unlikely that this treatment will cure your child's disease, it may help him or her to feel better and possibly to live longer.
Talking about what to expect	• Would it be helpful to talk about what to expect as your child's illness gets worse? • Although we cannot predict exactly what will happen to your child, most children with this disease eventually have [eg, difficulty breathing]. If that happens to your child, our goal will be to help him or her feel as comfortable as possible. We can use medications to help control his or her discomfort.
Talking to children	• What are you looking forward to most of all? • Is there anything that is worrying you or making you feel afraid? • Is there anything about how you are feeling that is making you feel worried or afraid?

From Mack JW, Wolfe J. Early integration of pediatric palliative care: for some children, palliative care starts at diagnosis. *Curr Opin Pediatr.* 2006;18(1):10–14, with permission from Wolters Kluwer Health.

it should be communicated with the goal of reducing uncertainty and providing a basis for action. Hope can be sustained when a meaningful way forward is elucidated even in the face of dismal diagnosis.

Barriers to Palliative Care

Parenting a child with chronic and potentially terminal illnesses can be frightening, confusing, frustrating, and exhausting. While a decision to involve palliative care practitioners is in no sense a decision by parents to stop working strenuously for their child's life, it is crucial that palliative care is introduced with sensitivity to this misinterpretation. If palliative care is viewed by the parents or child as an act of abandonment or disloyalty, the benefits of the consultation may not be forthcoming. Primary care physicians identify a family's reluctance to accept palliative care and a family's perception that palliative care is akin to "giving up" as the primary obstacles preventing a referral to a palliative care specialist. With that in mind, it is crucial that parents be advised of the growing body of research demonstrating that involvement of palliative care strategies leads not only to an improved quality of life for extremely ill patients, even as their illness progresses, but also longer survival. The involvement of a palliative care specialist can also empower families to be more

thoughtful and proactive in determining the location of their child's death. Recent research shows that increased availability of pediatric palliative care had led to a significant change in the number of patients receiving palliative home care. Additionally, children who receive palliative care receive fewer medications, are less likely to undergo invasive interventions, and are less likely to die in an intensive care unit. Palliative care offers much more than "doing nothing and letting the disease take its toll."

One of the greatest obstacles to palliative care and hospice has been a payment model based on Medicare hospice benefits, which required patients in hospice to forego curative care and gear care toward survival of 6 months or less. Parents, understandably, find it very hard to give up curative efforts for their children. They appreciate quality of life in a developing though ill child that is different than in a dying geriatric patient. Because hospice was associated with the elderly, parents felt a disincentive against selection of hospice insurance as a benefit. While certain states offer palliative care programs to remedy this, the Patient Protection and Affordable Care Act of 2010 removed the prohibition against curative treatment as a hospice benefit by or on behalf of a Medicaid or Children's Health Insurance Program–eligible child. States are not required to provide hospice services, although this is increasingly the norm, but where hospice services are provided, concurrent curative treatment must be offered. Despite these changes, eligibility still requires a physician to certify the child as likely to die in the next 6 months.

A Child's Understanding of Death

Ultimately, death is a singular transcendent experience, likely beyond the understanding of the living. But parents want to know what their children can understand as they go through the process. Caregivers, too, wonder what a child knows as they try to anticipate needs or reckon with enigmatic statements from them. Most would agree that a child's suffering due to avoidance of discussions of their fears about their condition and death is especially tragic and counterproductive.

The pediatrician should, when possible, communicate with children about what is happening to them, while respecting the cultural and personal preferences of the family. A developmental understanding of children's concepts of health and illness can help frame the discussion with children or serve to advise parents in their discussions. The understanding of a child's concept of death has changed very little from that extrapolated from Piaget's work in cognitive development and is based on the stages of sensorimotor, preoperational, concrete operations, and formal operations.

Up to 2 years of age (sensorimotor), there is probably no concept of death per se. Death in others is understood and responded to as a separation. Grief relates to the loss of an attachment figure and is expressed through protest and difficulty attaching to other adults. The degree of difficulty dealing with the loss depends on the availability of other nurturing adults who have cared for the child and with whom the child has had a good previous attachment.

Once they are 3 years of age, children can recognize death as a changed state. In the preoperational stage (ages 3–5 years), however, they cannot understand the meaning of a severe illness nor the finality and universality of death. Limited language abilities can give the appearance of little insight, and moods or behavior can be the means of expression. Bad things happen for an immediately identifiable reason, and death may be viewed as punishment. For instance, if a child's newborn sibling suddenly dies and the child had previously wished them to have died or gone back to where he or she came from, they may feel their wish was the cause of the death. Children this age can feel overwhelmed when confronted with the strong emotional reactions of their parents at the time of loss. They may talk about dying in a way that does not grasp its finality, worrying about where they are going, who will be there, what it will be like, or how their parents will manage.

Ages 6 to 11 years (school age) are considered the late preoperational to concrete operational stages of cognitive development. In this age range, the finality of death comes to be understood. Eight-year-olds are aware of personal mortality, and work by Hinds et al has found that children as young as 10 years are able to speak about their experiences and decisions at the end of life. Magical thinking gives way to a need for detailed information to gain a sense of control. Older children in this range will often feel a need to control their emotions by compartmentalizing and intellectualizing.

The developmental stage of adolescents ($\geq$12 years old) is considered formal operations. The concept of death includes universality and finality, and adolescents can understand personal mortality. Adolescents handle death issues at an abstract or philosophical level and can be realistic. They may seem closed off to information and resist frank discussions with undercurrents of deep emotion, relying on anger or disdain. Communication with peers, perhaps involving social networking technologies, can be more open, although critically ill children are sensitive about not burdening their friends, just as they often feel their friends are unable to fully comprehend their situation. Adolescents can discuss withholding of treatments. Their personal goals should be understood, respected, and discussed on their own terms.

A child's cognitive limitations will obviously have an effect on his or her understanding. Another matter is how illness has affected development—it is observed that chronically ill children may possess a precocious and advanced understanding of certain things, such as the details of their illness or the way to address their symptoms, while simultaneously being less mature in other developmental areas.

Parents can struggle with whether they should talk with their child about the child's imminent death. While research supports a bias toward speaking frankly to dying children, each individual case presents its own complexities based on the child's age, cognitive development, disease, timeline of disease, and parental psychologic state. In a study by Kreicsberg et al of parental disclosure to children with impending cancer death, no parent who talked with their child about his or her death regretted doing so, and of those who did not speak frankly about imminent death, 27% regretted not having done so. Among those who did not talk with their child about death, parents who sensed their child was aware of imminent death, parents of older children, and mothers more than fathers were more likely to feel regretful.

Primary Care at the End of Life: Normal and Extraordinary

There is no disputing the important role that primary care pediatricians can play in the care of children with life-threatening illness. The medical home is especially beneficial to these children. A constant, continuous physician who understands the child and family holistically can contribute profoundly to their care. Because caring for these children is a rare experience in general practice, the complexities of care can be daunting. There is a need to understand an appropriate role and develop a supportive structure for primary care pediatricians in a way that supports best practice.

Primary care is provided outside of the hospital and "at home." Families and children may develop strong feelings about returning to the hospital, having spent difficult times there. They may feel relief in not having to deal with the logistic, seemingly less personal, hurdles of hospital-based care. Care provided in the normal setting of primary care tends to be more tolerable.

General pediatric care under the guidance of the primary care physician also can be an important affirmation of the normal and can contribute to quality of life. For the patient, routine health care visits, vaccinations, and developmental assessments are important because the rationale for this care is not the patient's disease but the positive and ordinary characteristics of childhood. The focus on development, education and learning, social engagement, play, and involvement with family and community affirms the whole child and the importance of his or her life. The primary care pediatrician is often seen as a trusted advisor who understands the family and child in the normal context and thus "knows" them best. The pediatrician is the child's doctor without qualification.

A trusted primary care pediatrician also has a role in complex disease management. The primary care pediatrician is in the best position to assess the family's level of understanding and address any gaps. Importantly, the pediatrician can help families understand complex medical information, terminology (medical jargon), or other specific medical details. An involved primary care pediatrician also can help the medical team better understand the patient and family perspective. He or she can ease the adjustment between home and hospital and help ensure a more seamless transition in either direction. For the pediatrician to have relevant involvement in crucial developments, there must be a timely sharing of information among all members of the team, the generalist, and the specialist. Ideally, the primary care pediatrician should participate in hospital rounds on the patient and in team meetings. This is especially important for meetings with the family at which goals of care and medical decision-making are the focus. Fostering collaboration between the primary care pediatrician and the palliative care specialist is essential (Box 152-2).

When a child is facing the end of life at home, the primary care pediatrician has additional opportunities to facilitate things for the child and family. The primary care pediatrician works with the hospice team to continuously fine-tune approaches to pain and symptoms. The pediatrician's greater availability and sense of the family are important assets. Primary care pediatricians can also play a central role in delineating resuscitation orders.

Research finds that parents consider end-of-life decisions to be the most difficult treatment decisions they face. It is not unusual for them to operate in a way that continues to seek a cure even as they accept the inevitability of death, and these decisions reveal the tensions of holding both views. It is not surprising that DNR orders are frequently instituted near the time of death. Paradoxically, the child may spend less time at home as the parents still expect efforts toward an impossible cure. The proper timing to introduce these issues is early in the course of the child's illness, not in the midst of crisis or very late in the patient's course. Thoughtful conversation with a trusted primary care pediatrician who has a broad perspective on the medical details as well as the family identity and values is invaluable.

Most important is to help the family determine realistic goals for the child. This is facilitated by a frank discussion of whether resuscitation efforts support the goals or not. A powerful guide for these discussions is the document *Voicing My Choices* for adolescents and young adults, or for younger children up to approximately age 11 years, *My Wishes*, distributed by Aging With Dignity. These are guided conversations that approach advance directives derived from the *Five Wishes* document that was originally designed for adults and is legally recognized in 42 states (Box 152-3). Simply addressing "DNR orders" is inadequate. Another important contribution that differs in each state are comfort care forms and physician orders for life-sustaining treatment. These are DNR orders that are not particular to the inpatient setting. For instance, emergency medical technicians in the field must resuscitate a child found in cardiac or respiratory failure unless orders exist to refrain. Once a family has come to the difficult decision to limit interventions, it is important to advocate for these wishes in all potential settings.

Case coordination should explicitly address outpatient management and clarify the responsibilities of the primary care team as well as each subspecialist. The potential for this collaboration to improve the care offered by all members of the child's medical team is enormous.

Loss and After

The loss of a child or sibling changes life forever. It begins a process of bereavement, the psychologic and spiritual accommodation to death on the part of the child and the child's family, and grief, the

---

Box 152-2. Fundamental Elements of Successful Collaboration Between Primary Care and Palliative Care

- Timely sharing of information
- Mutual inclusion in clarifying goals of care and medical decision-making
- Coordinated designation of responsibilities
- Explicit review of case management and social work needs
- Technical backstopping for pain and symptom management
- Trusted, timely collaboration and assistance with urgent symptom management issues

Adapted from Steinhorn D, Goldstein R, Orloff S. Relationships with the community: palliative care and beyond. In: Wolfe J, Hinds P, Sourkes B. *Textbook of Interdisciplinary Pediatric Palliative Care*. Philadelphia, PA: Saunders; 2011.

Box 152-3. My Wishes and Five Wishes

My Wishes (for children up to approximately 11 years)
- How I want people to treat me
- How comfortable I want to be
- What I want my loved ones to know
- What I want my doctors and nurses to know

Five Wishes
- The person I want to make care decisions for me when I can't
- The kind of medical treatment I want or don't want
- How comfortable I want to be
- How I want people to treat me
- What I want my loved ones to know

Reprinted with permission from Aging with Dignity. Available at www.agingwithdignity.org.

emotional response caused by the loss. Grief can cause pain, distress, and physical and emotional suffering, but, except in cases of prolongation, it is a normal adaptive human response, not a disease. Anticipatory grief begins with the awareness of impending loss or death in parents and children with sufficient awareness and cognitive development. Palliative care attends to the grief reaction before and following death. Assessing the coping resources and vulnerabilities of the affected family system before death takes place is central to the palliative care approach.

Parental grief is more intense and sustained than other types of grief. Parents may never completely accept the loss of the child. Most parents work through their grief, though studies have found that more than one-fourth had not worked through their grief in 4 to 9 years after the loss of the child. Research suggests that parents who share their problems with others during the child's illness, who have had access to psychologic support during the last month of their child's life, and who have had closure sessions with the attending staff are more likely to resolve their grief.

Surviving siblings are also burdened. The AAP recommends that primary care pediatricians reach out to children and families at the time of loss, evaluate their bereavement to understand the personal meaning of their loss and their process of mourning, and monitor their process, especially in the year following a death. There is a further role of explaining to parents how surviving children are managing their loss and that children often reexamine the meaning of loss in their lives during each developmental period. When necessary, referrals to skilled mental health professionals should be offered.

Those involved in the care of children and families should appreciate how meaningful simple things like condolence letters and attendance at funerals or memorial services are to families. Notes remembering the anniversary of the deceased child's birthday or helping the family think about developing the child's legacy or a remembrance also contribute to an improved bereavement. Helping bereaved children safely remember their deceased siblings and appreciating their success as they integrate the loss can be a powerful part of a health care visit.

CASE RESOLUTION

The hospital-based palliative care team arranges to meet with the parents. During their conversations, they help the parents articulate what gives Jason's life meaning, what happiness and unhappiness are for him, and what is a hopeful versus a hopeless existence. The parents decide they would still opt for intubation and respiratory interventions should he become compromised by an acute, likely reversible issue but could not imagine that a further deterioration of his condition after the need for cardiac resuscitation would prove consistent with their goals. Therefore, a limitation is placed on cardiac resuscitation. With their permission, the palliative care team speaks with personnel at the skilled nursing facility, their primary care pediatrician, and the palliative care team at the community hospital where Jason would be taken if ill. Documents are prepared and shared for use in all of the settings. The palliative care team continues to meet with Jason and his family for each hospital admission and has made visits to his nursing facility to help the staff.

Selected References

Aging With Dignity. *Five Wishes.* http://www.agingwithdignity.org/five-wishes.php. Accessed February 26, 2014

American Academy of Pediatrics Committee on Bioethics and Committee on Hospital Care. Palliative care for children. *Pediatrics.* 2000;106(2):351–357

American Academy of Pediatrics Committee on Psychosocial Aspects of Child and Family Health. The pediatrician and childhood bereavement. *Pediatrics.* 2000;105(2):445–447

Cassel EJ. The nature of suffering and the goals of medicine. *N Engl J Med.* 1982;306(11):639–645

Feudtner C, Feinstein JA, Satchell M, Zhao H, Kang TI. Shifting place of death among children with complex chronic conditions in the United States, 1989-2003. *JAMA.* 2007;297(24):2725–2732

Goldstein R, Rimer KP. Parents' views of their child's end-of-life care: subanalysis of primary care involvement. *J Palliat Med.* 2013;16(2):198–202

Hamilton BE, Hoyert DL, Martin JA, Strobino DM, Guyer B. Annual summary of vital statistics: 2010-2011. *Pediatrics.* 2013;131(3):548–558

Hexem KR, Miller VA, Carroll KW, Faerber JA, Feudtner C. Putting on a happy face: emotional expression in parents of children with serious illness. *J Pain Symptom Manage.* 2013;45(3):542–551

Himelstein BP, Hilden JM, Boldt AM, Weissman D. Pediatric palliative care. *N Engl J Med.* 2004;350(17):1752–1762

Hinds PS, Drew D, Oakes LL, et al. End-of-life preferences of pediatric patients with cancer. *J Clin Oncol.* 2005;23(36):9146–9154

Keele L, Keenan HT, Sheetz J, Bratton SL. Differences in characteristics of dying children who receive and do not receive palliative care. *Pediatrics.* 2013;132(1):72–78

Knapp C, Thompson L. Factors associated with perceived barriers to pediatric palliative care: a survey of pediatricians in Florida and California. *Palliat Med.* 2012;26(3):268–274

Kreicbergs UC, Lannen P, Onelov E, Wolfe J. Parental grief after losing a child to cancer: impact of professional and social support on long-term outcomes. *J Clin Oncol.* 2007;25(22):3307–3312

Mack JW, Wolfe J. Early integration of pediatric palliative care: for some children, palliative care starts at diagnosis. *Curr Opin Pediatr.* 2006;18(1):10–14

Mack JW, Wolfe J, Cook EF, Grier HE, Cleary PD, Weeks JC. Hope and prognostic disclosure. *J Clin Oncol.* 2007;25(35):5636–5642

Murray SA, Kendall M, Boyd K, Sheikh A. Illness trajectories and palliative care. *BMJ.* 2005;330(7498):1007–1011

Schmidt P, Otto M, Hechler T, Metzing S, Wolfe J, Zernikow B. Did increased availability of pediatric palliative care lead to improved palliative care outcomes in children with cancer? *J Palliat Med.* 2013;16(9):1034–1039

Wolfe J, Grier HE, Klar N, et al. Symptoms and suffering at the end of life in children with cancer. *N Engl J Med.* 2000;342(5):326–333

Index